PSYCHIATRIC
MENTAL HEALTH NURSING

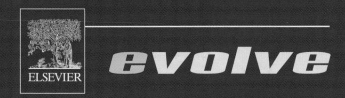

PSYCHIATRIC
MENTAL HEALTH NURSING

THIRD EDITION

Katherine M. Fortinash, MSN, RNCS, CNS

Certified Clinical Specialist
Adult Psychiatric-Mental Health Nursing;
Associate Faculty
Mt. San Jacinto College
Menifee, California;
Clinical Nurse Specialist and Educator
Sharp HealthCare, Mesa Vista Hospital
San Diego, California;
Consultant
San Diego, California

Patricia A. Holoday Worret, MSN, RNCS, CNS

Certified Clinical Specialist
Adult Psychiatric-Mental Health Nursing;
Professor, Psychiatric Mental Health Nursing
Palomar College
San Marcos, California;
Consultant
San Diego, California

M Mosby

An Affiliate of Elsevier

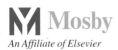
An Affiliate of Elsevier

11830 Westline Industrial Drive
St. Louis, Missouri 63146

PSYCHIATRIC MENTAL HEALTH NURSING, THIRD EDITION   0-323-02011-9

NOTICE

Nursing is an ever-changing field. Standard safety precautions must be followed, but as new research and clinical experience broaden our knowledge, changes in treatment and drug therapy may become necessary or appropriate. Readers are advised to check the most current product information provided by the manufacturer of each drug to be administered to verify the recommended dose, the method and duration of administration, and contraindications. It is the responsibility of the licensed prescriber, relying on experience and knowledge of the patient, to determine dosages and the best treatment for each individual patient. Neither the publisher nor the author assumes any liability for any injury and/or damage to persons or property arising from this publication.

Previous editions copyrighted 1996, 2000

Library of Congress Cataloging-in-Publication Data

Psychiatric mental health nursing / [edited by] Katherine M. Fortinash, Patricia A.
    Holoday Worret.—3rd ed.
        p. ; cm.
    Includes bibliographical references and index.
    ISBN 0-323-02011-9
    1. Psychiatric nursing. I. Fortinash, Katherine M.   II. Holoday-Worret, Patricia A.
    [DNLM: 1. Mental disorders—nursing. 2. Psychiatric Nursing—methods. WY 160
P972035 2003]
    RC440.P7338 2003
    616.89′0231—dc22

                                                    2003049347

Acquisitions Editor: Tom Wilhelm
Associate Developmental Editor: Jill Ferguson
Publishing Services Manager: Deborah Vogel
Senior Project Manager: Mary Drone
Senior Designer: Kathi Gosche
Cover Art: Jennifer Brockett

Printed in the United States of America

Last digit is the print number: 9   8   7   6   5   4   3   2

We dedicate this book to all clients

who struggle to overcome their mental disorders

and strive to maintain dignity in a complex world;

to the families and friends who support them;

and

to the students, nurses, and caregivers

who are involved in their lives.

Contributors

Merry A. Armstrong, DNSc, CS, ARNP
Associate Professor
Intercollegiate College of Nursing
Washington State University College of Nursing
Spokane, Washington

Donna Oradei Berger, MSN, RNCS, CNAA
Director, Inpatient Behavioral Health Services
Sharp HealthCare, Mesa Vista Hospital
San Diego, California

Pauline Chan, RPh, MBA, BCPP, FCSHP, FASHP
Pharmacy Manager
Mesa Vista Hospital and
Mary Birch Hospital for Women
Sharp HealthCare
San Diego, California

Anne Clarkin-Watts, MSW, LCSW
Private Practice
San Diego, California

Phillip R. Deming, MA, MS, MDiv
Doctoral Student
University of San Diego
San Diego, California;
Chaplin and MFT Intern
Grossmont Partial Hospital Program
La Mesa, California

Robert L. Erb, Jr., MA, RNCS, CLNC
Advanced Clinician
Sharp HealthCare
San Diego, California

Chantal M. Flanagan, RN, MS
Carlsbad, California

Sandra S. Goldsmith, MSN, RN, APRN, BC CS (ANCC), CNS
Clinical Nurse Specialist
Clinical Care Coordinator
Department of Mental Health Services
San Diego County Psychiatric Hospital
San Diego, California

Ruth N. Grendell, DNSc
Professor Emerita
Point Loma Nazarene University
San Diego, California

Bonnie Hagerty, PhD, RN, CS
Associate Professor
School of Nursing
University of Michigan
Ann Arbor, Michigan

Linda Hollinger-Smith, PhD, RN
Director of Research
Mather Institute on Aging
Mather LifeWays
Evanston, Illinois

Charles Kemp, FNP, FAAN
Senior Lecturer
The Louise Herrington School of Nursing
Baylor University
Dallas, Texas

Richard C. Lucas, MD, JD
Adolescent Unit Director
Aurora Hospital
San Diego, California;
Assistant Clinical Professor of Psychiatry
University of California, San Diego
La Jolla, California

Shelly F. Lurie, MS, RN, CS-P
Director of Specialized Treatment Services
Clifton T. Perkins Hospital Center
Jessup, Maryland

Pamela E. Marcus, RN, MS, CS-P
Advance Practice, Nurse Psychotherapist
Private Practice
Upper Marlboro, Maryland

Susan Fertig McDonald, MSN, RNCS
Clinical Nurse Specialist
Inpatient Psychiatric and Chemical Dependency Units
San Diego VA Medical Center
San Diego, California

Kathleen Pace Murphy, PhD, RN-CS, GNP
Therapeutic Team Director
Gastrointestinal/Arthritis/Bon Metabolism for Western
    United States
Novartis Pharmaceuticals Corporation
United States Medical Affairs/Scientific Operation
Houston, Texas

Kathleen L. Patusky, PhD, RN, CS
Assistant Professor
College of Health and Human Sciences, School of Nursing
Georgia State University
Atlanta, Georgia

Susan Selverston, MA, PHN, APRN, BC
Program Manager
North Coastal Mental Health Clinic
San Diego Health and Human Services Agency
Oceanside, California

Alwilda Scholler-Jaquish, PhD, ANCC, APRN, BC
Assistant Professor and Interim Director
Orvis School of Nursing
University of Nevada, Reno
Reno, Nevada

Kathryn Thomas, PhD, CS-P, FAACS
Associate Professor
Baccalaureate Nursing Program
Villa Julie College
Stevenson, Maryland;
Founder and Director
The Baltimore Institute of Sexology
Baltimore, Maryland;
Clinical Sexologist
The Human Ecology Center
Baltimore, Maryland

James M. Turnbull, MD
Medical Director
Frontier Health
Gray, Tennessee

Joan C. Urbancic, PhD, APRN, ANCC, CS
Professor
University of Detroit Mercy
Detroit, Michigan

Gwen van Servellen, RN, PhD, FAAN
Professor and Chair, Acute Care Section
School of Nursing
University of California, Los Angeles
Los Angeles, California

Kathleen M. Walker, RN, PhD, CS
Frontier Health
Kingsport, Tennessee

Mary Magenheimer Webster, RN, MS, CS
Clinical Instructor in Psychiatric Mental Health Practice
Intercollegiate College of Nursing
Washington State University College of Nursing
Spokane, Washington

Reviewers

Lois Angelo, MSN, RN, CS
Massachusetts General Hospital
Boston, Massachusetts

Vicki Britt, ARNP
Process Improvement/Staff Development
Fairfax Hospital
Kirkland, Washington

Jacqueline Rosenjack Burchum, DNSc, APRN, BC
Family Nurse Practitioner;
Assistant Professor
Loewenberg School of Nursing
The University of Memphis
Memphis, Tennessee

Amy Coenen, PhD, RN, CS
Associate Professor
College of Nursing
Marquette University
Milwaukee, Wisconsin

Janine Graf-Kirk, RN, BC, MA
Faculty/Course Coordinator
Trinitas School of Nursing
Elizabeth, New Jersey

Rebecca Crews Gruener, RN, MSN
Associate Professor of Nursing
Louisiana State University at Alexandria
Alexandria, Louisiana

Benita W. Harris, PhD, MSN, RN
Delaware Technical & Community College
Georgetown, Delaware

Coleen L. Heckner, MS, APRN, BC
Acadia Hospital
Bangor, Maine

Connie S. Heflin, MSN, RN
Professor
Paducah Community College
Paducah, Kentucky

Kay Jansen, MSN, RN, CS
Clinical Assistant Professor
College of Nursing
Marquette University
Milwaukee, Wisconsin

Ellen Kirking, RN, MSN
Chippewa Valley Technical College
Eau Claire, Wisconsin

Deborah Klaas-Kindy, RN, PhD
Associate Professor
Sonoma State University
Rohnert Park, California

Nancy Kostin, RN, MSN
Assistant Professor of Nursing
Madonna University
Livonia, Michigan

Charlotte M. Lorentson, MSN, RN, CS, BC
Clinical Specialist in Psychiatric Mental Health Nursing
Certified Gerontological Nurse
Eastern State Hospital
Williamsburg, Virginia

Anne W. Ryan, MSN, RN, C, MPH
Associate Professor
Chesapeake College/MGW Nursing Program
Wye Mills, Maryland

Barbara Jones Warren, PhD, APRN, BC
Associate Clinical Professor
College of Nursing
The Ohio State University
Columbus, Ohio

Harriet Wichowski, PhD, RN
Associate Professor of Nursing
University of Tennessee at Chattanooga
Chattanooga, Tennessee

Judith A. Wilson, MS, RN, CS
Clinical Nurse Specialist
University of Alabama at Birmingham Hospital
Birmingham, Alabama

Preface

As we move through the changes evolving from the 1990s "Decade of the Brain," psychiatric nurses are required to blend their broad base of scientific knowledge and interpersonal skills to meet the challenges of biologic and technologic advances in treating clients with mental disorders and their families. Even as the impetus continues to move toward biology and technology, the combination of psychopharmacology and psychotherapy remains the treatment of choice in the psychiatric setting.

Another challenge for psychiatric nurses is the managed care organizations that continue to influence the health care delivery system, resulting in the shift of client care from inpatient facilities to less costly alternatives for treatment. These include partial hospital programs, outpatient clinics, and community agencies. Ongoing advances in biology and technology and the changing health care environment strongly encourage psychiatric nurses to continue to deliver quality client care in the midst of emerging treatment complexities.

APPROACH AND INTENDED USE

The third edition of *Psychiatric Mental Health Nursing* is designed to help nurses successfully meet today's health care challenges by presenting the newest information from psychiatric mental health nursing, psychiatry, and the sciences. The balanced nursing and medical approach, with strong emphasis on DSM-IV-TR guidelines and related treatments, remains a distinguishing feature of this textbook. Although psychiatric nursing is thoroughly discussed as it relates to various well-regarded theorists, the text does not advocate any one specific nursing framework. This timely, state-of-the-art text is primarily intended to help students and practicing psychiatric nurses deliver professional nursing care for clients and their families, regardless of time, place, or circumstances.

The nursing process, a time-proven, six-step problem-solving method, is featured as a distinct section in relevant chapters. A discussion of each nursing process step is accompanied by many features that provide additional relevant information. Interesting case studies depicting "real-life" situations followed by a series of questions are interspersed throughout the various stages of the nursing process section to stimulate student learning and critical thinking. This section also includes comprehensive nursing care plans that begin with a case study, followed by DSM-IV-TR multiaxial diagnoses and relevant NANDA nursing diagnoses. Client outcomes are identified based on the nursing diagnosis statement, interventions with rationales are presented, and an evaluative statement is noted.

The major organizing structure for the disorders chapters includes both the diagnoses of the North American Nursing Diagnosis Association from *NANDA Nursing Diagnoses and Classification 2003-2004* and the American Psychiatric Association from the *Diagnostic and Statistical Manual of Mental Disorders,* Fourth Edition, Text Revision. We strongly believe in the practicality and effectiveness of the collaborative efforts of nursing and medicine whenever possible. We contend that the use of current NANDA terminology most accurately describes the therapeutic services and contributions of nurses and also reflects contemporary nursing actions and responses. Application and use of refined diagnostic labels are essential to the evolution of the language and discipline of nursing.

STRUCTURE AND ORGANIZATION

This book is organized into five sections. **Part I, Introduction to Psychiatric Mental Health Nursing,** presents concepts that not only define nursing as an art and a science but also reveal the substantive changes and trends that currently shape and challenge the traditional professional nursing roles in the area of mental health. **Part II, Psychiatric Disorders,** focuses on ten major disorders generated by DSM-IV-TR criteria. Each chapter follows a consistent, standardized format including a separate nursing process section to facilitate learning. **Part III, Therapeutic Modalities,** emphasizes the major therapeutic modalities used to treat clients in the psychiatric setting. **Part IV, Aggressive Behaviors,** addresses the critical issues of violence and suicide. **Part V, Care in the Community,** describes a variety of timely issues and concerns experienced by clients in different settings and treated by psychiatric nurses.

DESIGN AND KEY FEATURES

Bright and vivid full-color design permeates this text to promote visual appeal, emphasize and distinguish key pedagogic features, and graphically portray illustrations of critical psychiatric nursing concepts for students. Numerous full-color brain scans and drawings of psychobiologic concepts are presented in relevant chapters throughout the text. Many boxes, tables, and other figures summarize and highlight important information.

Each chapter has several standard features that make critical information more accessible for learning:

- **Objectives,** placed at the beginning of the chapter, emphasize the most important concepts.
- **Key Terms** are presented at the beginning of the chapter with page number references and are highlighted in bold in the chapter.
- A **Chapter Summary** concludes each chapter, summarizing the most significant ideas to be remembered.
- Multiple-choice **Review Questions** can be found at the end of each chapter for immediate reinforcement of chapter content. Answers to the review questions are provided in Appendix D.

Other important key features are highlighted by a unique design and included in relevant chapters:

- **DSM-IV-TR Criteria** boxes present the DSM-IV-TR criteria for specific mental disorders.
- **Nursing Assessment Questions** boxes present questions that are included in a client assessment.
- **Clinical Symptoms** boxes summarize the symptoms that indicate a certain disorder.
- **Collaborative Diagnoses** tables present DSM-IV-TR and NANDA diagnoses relevant for the disorders.
- **Clinical Alert** boxes throughout the text highlight critical information relevant to clinical practice.
- **Case Study** boxes offer realistic depictions of psychiatric disorders and integrate critical thinking questions or statements to foster students' problem-solving skills and application of the concepts presented.
- A detailed **Nursing Care Plan** is presented as part of the nursing process section. It begins with a case study, followed by DSM-IV-TR multiaxial diagnoses and relevant nursing diagnoses. Client outcomes based on the nursing diagnoses statements are identified, interventions with rationales are presented, and an evaluative statement is noted.
- **Additional Treatment Modalities** boxes summarize various modalities and interventions that are used in conjunction with nursing interventions in the treatment of a particular disorder.
- **Client and Family Teaching Guidelines** provide valuable education for both the client and the family to facilitate insight and skills concerning the client disorders.
- **Understanding and Applying Research** boxes summarize a research study related to a disorder and its application to nursing interventions.
- **Nursing Care in the Community** boxes discuss community perspectives on particular disorders and issues.
- **Clinical pathways,** for various disorders and from different institutions, are presented to demonstrate the importance and usefulness of this interdisciplinary tool in the treatment of psychiatric disorders.

A **Glossary** at the end of the book provides concise, updated definitions for key terms found throughout the text. **Appendixes** include the complete DSM-IV-TR Classification, American Nurses Association Standards of Psychiatric-Mental Health Nursing Practice, a discussion of the NIC and NOC classification systems, as well as the answers to the chapter review questions.

TEACHING AND LEARNING PACKAGE

A complete ancillary package to enhance teaching and learning is provided for this text.

The **Instructor's Resource (CD-ROM)** is available free to adopters of the textbook and includes: (1) an **Instructor's Manual** with critical thinking exercises, enrichment activities, and multimedia resources for each chapter of the book; strategies for teaching psychiatric nursing; and suggested course outlines for courses of varying lengths; (2) **Computerized Test Bank** with more than 800 NCLEX-style questions organized by chapter and including objective, stage of the nursing process, cognitive level, correct answer, rationale, and text page reference; (3) **PowerPoint** slide presentations, including relevant text and illustration slides for each chapter of the book.

The **Evolve Learning Resources** to accompany the third edition of *Psychiatric Mental Health Nursing* are available for both students and instructors. Students will find valuable resources in learning exercises, drug monographs, and WebLinks. In addition to the information available to students, instructors are able to access all of the components of the Instructor's Resource (CD-ROM), rationales for the critical thinking questions that accompany the case studies throughout the textbook, and expanded answers to the chapter review questions (including topic, stage of the nursing process, type of question, correct answer, and rationale).

TERMINOLOGY AND LANGUAGE

We recognize the contribution of both men and women to the nursing profession. Whenever possible, we have attempted to use plural nouns and pronouns in place of the singular *his* or *her.* However, clarity sometimes has dictated the use of *she* for nurse and *he* for client.

We have chosen to use the term *client* instead of *patient* because we view individuals receiving treatment as significant participants in the reciprocal process of treatment. We also recognize that *family* can refer not only to blood relatives but friends and significant others. However, the term *family* is generally used for simplicity.

We are proud to launch this new edition of our textbook and invite psychiatric nursing students and nurses at all levels to meet the challenges presented and to apply the concepts in clinical practice. We wish you well in your professional journey and feel confident that you will successfully meet these challenges while experiencing the satisfaction and wonder of psychiatric nursing.

Kathi Fortinash and Pat Holoday Worret

Acknowledgments

We thank the entire staff at Elsevier for their dedication and support in helping us complete this textbook. Special thanks to those who worked directly with us throughout this project: Tom Wilhelm, Acquisitions Editor; Jill Ferguson, Associate Developmental Editor; and Mary Drone, Senior Project Manager.

We also thank our family and friends who tolerated long hours spent away from them. We love you.

A special acknowledgement goes to our contributors, past and present, who helped make this textbook a success, and to their families.

Contents

PART I
INTRODUCTION TO PSYCHIATRIC MENTAL HEALTH NURSING

1

Foundations of Psychiatric Mental Health Nursing

Patricia A. Holoday Worret

KEY TERMS

adaptive (p. 8)
autodiagnosis (p. 14)
defensive functioning (p. 10)
eclectic approach (p. 17)
evidence-based practice
  (p. 11)
judgment (p. 4)
label (p. 4)
maladaptive (p. 10)
neuropsychiatric (p. 2)
protective factors (p. 8)
risk factors (p. 8)
severe and persistent (p. 16)
stereotypes (p. 14)
stigma (p. 4)
therapeutic alliance (p. 11)

OBJECTIVES

- Discuss the projected statistical increase for psychiatric disorders by 2020.
- Discuss mental and emotional effects of terrorism on the general population after September 11, 2001.
- Describe the ongoing threat of mental disorders to individuals, families, and the community.
- Identify factors that contribute to stigmatization of mental illness and ways to decrease stigma, judgment, and stereotyping of this population.
- Describe four specific reasons for diagnoses of mental disorders.
- Identify levels of prevention of mental illness.
- Identify similarities and differences of risk factors and protective factors associated with mental illness.
- Discuss the role of the nurse in psychiatric mental health nursing.
- Discuss the art and science of nursing as related to psychiatric mental health.
- Describe six possible reasons for entering a helping profession.

It was clear by the end of the last century that mental health, a basic human right, is fundamental and essential for the overall health, well-being, and productivity of every man, woman, and child. The first major *Report on Mental Health* in the United States by the Surgeon General presents multiple entries throughout the document in support of that statement (Department of Health and Human Services, 1999). However, this report also reveals that in the United States and other developed countries, mental disorders are among the leading causes of disability, with a leading mental disorder being major depression.

Several recent world health documents reiterate the importance of ensuring mental health for all people. The following salient reports illuminate the existing and pending problem of mental disorders in the United States and other nations. The *World Health Report 1999: Making a Difference* offers statistics demonstrating that **neuropsychiatric** disorders are the world's leading cause of disability from noncommunicable diseases (World Health Organization, 1999) (Figure 1-1). The 1999 *Global Burden of Disease* and current reports in World Health Organization (WHO) bulletins continue to state that mental disorders are projected to be a leading worldwide cause of disability for developed countries by the year 2020 (World Health Organization, 1999, website: www3.who.int/whosis/menu.cfm).

Researchers from Harvard School of Public Health and WHO collaborated to complete the series entitled the *Global Burden of Disease and Injury,* which reports current worldwide patterns of mortality and disability from diseases and injuries and predictions for the year 2020. Using traditional approaches of assessment that examined death, but not disability, the burdens of mental illnesses such as depression, schizophrenia, and alcoholism have been seriously underestimated in the past. Although psychiatric disorders account for only 1% of deaths, they account for 11% of the world's entire disease burden. That number is significant when considering all worldwide causes of death and disability, which also include communicable diseases, maternal and perinatal conditions, nutritional deficiencies, and the tobacco epidemic. Deaths from noncommunicable diseases that include mental disorders are expected to rise 77% by 2020.

These statistics are obvious evidence of the need for educated and clinically prepared, licensed professionals. These include psychiatric nurses, psychiatrists, psychologists, psychiatric social workers, and therapists from other disciplines, who focus on all aspects of mental health in individuals, their families, and the community (National Council on Disability, 2002). The number of professionals necessary to fill today's need falls short. What will the need be in 2020?

Psychiatric mental health nurses interact with clients in the *promotion* of mental health, the *prevention* and *treatment* of mental disorders, and *restoration* of health in the aftermath of dysfunction. At this time in history there is a remarkable shortage of nurses from all specialty areas, and, from the statistics previously presented, the need for educated, clinically prepared psychiatric mental health nurses is great.

THREATS TO SECURITY
Violence and Terrorism

Currently the specters of violence and terrorism are also threatening the basic human right of mental health. The United States is focused to deal with the threats. Since the turn of the century the entire world has changed because of increased violence. In an executive summary of world violence and health, violence was ranked the twelfth leading cause of disability throughout the world. In addition, injuries due to accidents and violence may rival infectious diseases by the year 2020 (see Figure 1-1).

Inhabitants of the United States of America, although never naïve about world strife and violence, were empathic but generally insulated by a relative sense of safety and security that existed within our shores for hundreds of years. America experienced some internal violence and terrorism but was seemingly removed from major violent threats and upheavals that were often experienced in other parts of the world.

That era ended in New York City, in Washington, DC, and in a Pennsylvania field on September 11, 2001 (911), a date that is burned into the history of the United States. That date made visible a major threat, but, more important, it ushered in a change in the way many Americans perceive the world, their country, their homes, the safety and security of their families, their well-being, and their lives in general. Beyond the tangible evidence that manifested in multiple

Increasing Burden of Noncommunicable Diseases and Injuries

Change in rank order of DALYs for the 15 leading causes (baseline scenario)

1999 Disease or Injury	2020 Disease or Injury
1. Acute lower respiratory infections	1. Ischaemic heart disease
2. HIV/AIDS	2. Unipolar major depression
3. Perinatal conditions	3. Road traffic injuries
4. Diarrhoeal diseases	4. Cerebrovascular disease
5. Unipolar major depression	5. Chronic obstructive pulmonary disease
6. Ischaemic heart disease	6. Lower respiratory infections
7. Cerebrovascular disease	7. Tuberculosis
8. Malaria	8. War
9. Road traffic injuries	9. Diarrhoeal diseases
10. Chronic obstructive pulmonary disease	10. HIV
11. Congenital abnormalities	11. Perinatal conditions
12. Tuberculosis	12. Violence
13. Falls	13. Congenital abnormalities
14. Measles	14. Self-inflicted injuries
15. Anaemias	15. Trachea, bronchus and lung cancers

FIGURE 1-1. Rank order of disease burden for 15 leading causes. From World Health Organization: *The global burden of disease: a comprehensive assessment of mortality and disability from diseases, injuries, and risk factors in 1990 and projected to 2020,* vol 1, 2000. (*DALY,* Disability-adjusted life year.)

deaths and injuries, as well as disruptions in the government, businesses, the economy, and travel, and eventual war (Iraqi freedom), other factors emerged that were of utmost importance to psychiatric nurses. Nurses are among those who are concerned with and are treating the grief of thousands of survivors, the sorrow of the nation, the terror and anxiety that gripped people of all ages, and the emotional upheaval that is still being measured.

Within the first 6 months after 911 and thereafter, numerous reports of increased mental disorders in both adults and children appeared in the literature. Statistics are being gathered with the intention of identifying numbers and types of mental disorders and symptoms of stress that resulted from this national trauma (Silver et al, 2002). The World Health Organization is investigating violence and its outcomes (World Health Organization, 1996).

On a positive note, in the aftermath of this tragedy there were also numerous reports of affiliation, with families and strangers coming and working together, helping and valuing each other and the time they spent together. There is hope that positive studies of resiliency and affiliation will result from this North American tragedy. In addition, educational facilities (Pfefferbaum, 2003; Lensch, 2003), government agencies (Federal Emergency Management Agency, 2003) and businesses across the United States are educating, training, and serving communities with safety and security as a primary focus. Nurses who are prepared can be a major part of this activity in *primary prevention* (educating and instructing about safety in the face of violence or terrorism); in *secondary prevention* (treating depression, grief, anxiety that occurs from any trauma); and *tertiary prevention* (reha-

bilitating clients and families). Additional discussion about primary, secondary, and tertiary prevention appears later in this chapter.

Incidental vs. Ongoing Threats to Security

The 911 tragedy was notably dramatic and copiously reported in the media. The number of people affected from that traumatic event and the continued threats of bioterrorism and physical and chemical aggression are rivaled by the less advertised, yet very real, ongoing, daily threats to security and well-being of millions of people because of the existence of mental disorders in their lives.

Mental disorders disrupt life for the individual, the family, the employer, the community, the nation, and the world. The cost in personal and economic losses resulting from mental disorders is substantial, which is validated in the reports cited previously. A looming threat is the risk for increasing numbers of people with mental disorders and the current and projected lack of resources and personnel to meet the needs (Figures 1-2 and 1-3).

The recent reports cited here provide information and education about advances made in research within the last two decades. These include the explosion of information that occurred during the "Decade of the Brain," the 1990s, and other notable advances in neuroscience and technology that occurred at the end of the last century. However, there was little mention in the reports about actual treatment proposals or specific expected outcomes to be met in the near future. Although laws for parity for the mentally ill were passed early in the 1990s, mental illness is still not receiving its

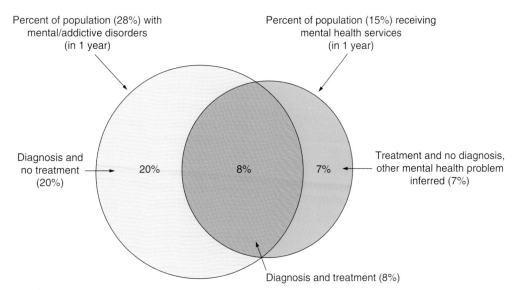

Percent of population (28%) with mental/addictive disorders (in 1 year)

Percent of population (15%) receiving mental health services (in 1 year)

Diagnosis and no treatment (20%)   20%   8%   7%   Treatment and no diagnosis, other mental health problem inferred (7%)

Diagnosis and treatment (8%)

FIGURE 1-2. Annual prevalence of mental/addictive disorders and services for adults. (From Regier D et al: The de facto US mental and addictive disorders service system: epidemiologic catchment area prevalence rates of disorders and services, *Arch Gen Psychiatry* 50:85, 1993; and Kessler RC et al: The 12 month prevalence and correlates of serious mental illness. In Manderscheid R, Sonnenschein M, editors: *Mental health, United States 1996*, Department of Health and Human Services Publication No. (SMA) 96-3098, Washington, DC, 1996, US Government Printing Office.)

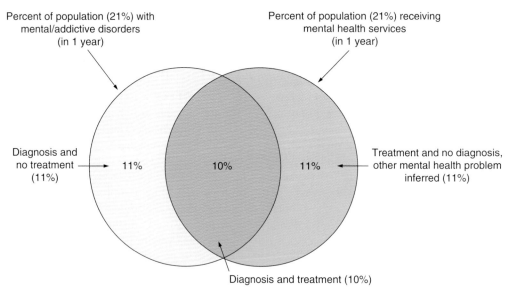

Percent of population (21%) with mental/addictive disorders (in 1 year)

Percent of population (21%) receiving mental health services (in 1 year)

Diagnosis and no treatment (11%) → 11%

10%

11% ← Treatment and no diagnosis, other mental health problem inferred (11%)

Diagnosis and treatment (10%)

FIGURE 1-3. Annual prevalence of mental/addictive disorders and services for children.(From Schaffer D et al: The NIMH diagnostic interview schedule for children: methods for the epidemiology of child and adolescent mental disorders study, *J Am Acad Child Adolescent Psychiatry* vol 35, 1996.)

share of federal or state budgets to care for mental disorders. However, the reports do provide impetus for changes toward what the surgeon general calls "a healthy era of mind and body for the nation" (Department of Health and Human Services, 1999).

Stigma

Political and economic rationale are offered for the lack of adequate attention toward mental disorders, but a major cause for inadequate care and services is continued stigmatization of the mentally ill (A Report of the Surgeon General, 1999). The **stigma** placed on mental illness is a primary reason why millions fail to have their needs met. Increased progress is being made in the direction of reducing stigma and responding with action to the needs of this population. Although the general public is improving, they still lack understanding about mental illness, and uninformed people fear those who demonstrate symptoms of mental illness. Their main fear centers on violence, although only a small percentage of individuals with mental disorders are violent (Link et al, 1999).

In most instances the diagnosis of a mental disorder brings two burdens. The primary burden comes from having to suffer and bear the symptoms of the mental illness. A second burden results from having to carry the **label** that accompanies a mental disorder, which usually has a negative connotation and results in the **judgment** cast on the already burdened individual and the family.

All forms of the media are a primary source of stigmatization of the mentally ill and their families and must take responsibility for the burden borne by this population. Each week new films, magazine articles, television programs, and novels emerge, portraying the mentally ill in a negative

light. Only rarely does a character from one of these money-making media forms receive empathy from a voyeuristic public. Instead, portrayals are directed at highlighting sinister, frightening, offensive characters that cause the public to make false conclusions based on inadequate information and become less accepting of this population.

Resources for Reduction of Stigma

Many disciplines are working tirelessly to decrease stigmatization. Nurses particularly act as advocates for clients with mental disorders in helping to increase respect and reduce **stereotypes**, stigma, judgments, and labels that unfortunately accompany mental disorders. Each national psychiatric nursing organization is continually engaged in reduction of the stigma attached to mental disorders.

Several other national organizations such as the National Association for Mental Illness (NAMI) strongly support and legislate for respect and acceptance of the mentally ill. Some methods include providing family and public education and personally involving the clients and families in their care and helping them take responsibility for their futures. NAMI lobbies in the legislation for changes in treatment and care of this population.

In addition, the American Psychiatric Association, in an effort to decrease stigma, plainly states in the Diagnostic and Statistical Manual of Mental Disorders (DSM-IV-TR) that their diagnostic manual categorizes and classifies disorders and does not classify or stigmatize people (APA, 2000).

Many religious organizations have taken on the cause of caring for the mentally ill. Exact statistics are not available, but the probability is high that a significant amount of daily basic care is provided by these beneficent organizations.

A major force in the effort to eradicate stigmatization lies within the nursing profession in the everyday encounters with clients and in the interdisciplinary communication between nurses and other health care professionals. An end to stereotyping and the beginning of acceptance for mental illness begin with nurses and their colleagues. Examples of nurses demonstrating respect/disrespect for clients in direct clinical care appear below:

Respectful remark:

"Charles has a diagnosis of Paranoid Schizophrenia and is experiencing an acute episode of psychosis. We'll admit him to Room 23B."

Disrespectful remark:

"Charles is back again and acting crazy as ever. Put him in Room 23B this time."

Respectful remark:

"Sonia is from a family that has experienced several traumatic events and losses in the past 2 years. Her father died, her brother was killed in a gang fight, and her best friend moved out of town. Sonia is depressed and acting out by taking drugs, and her mother is unable to manage her behavior."

Disrespectful remark:

"We are admitting another adolescent addict. Her mother brought her in . . . who knows where the father is."

Note the attitudinal shift that occurs when clients with mental illness are thought of, spoken about, and treated with disdain.

Nurses have every opportunity to help change the general public opinion about people with mental disorders. Those opportunities exist in acute care facilities; outpatient settings; local, national, and international nursing and psychiatric organizations; the legislature; and governmental bodies that can make the ultimate necessary monetary changes. Before clients can be dignified, accepted, respected, and treated fairly in the health care system, stigma against this population must be eradicated. There is still much to be done in this direction.

MENTAL HEALTH AND MENTAL DISORDER

It is widely agreed that defining mental health and mental disorder is difficult and furthermore that no one definition of either mental health or mental disorder is universally accepted. There are many reasons why it is difficult to simplify a definition. One reason is the problem that arises when an attempt is made to separate mind and body of individuals, because the mind and body are inextricably interrelated (APA, 2000; Department of Health and Human Services, 1999). Another reason is the unique ways that human beings express themselves, their wellness, and their disorders. Those with clinical experience agree that clients with the same psychiatric diagnosis express their symptoms differently. Among other factors that make defining mental health/disorder difficult are the variances

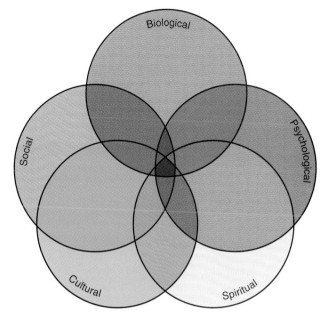

FIGURE 1-4 Biopsychosocial-cultural-spiritual model.

in culturally accepted and rejected norms that dictate health and illness.

Nursing Perspective

Nursing has traditionally viewed wellness and illness holistically and taught that human well-being depends on intrinsic components and extrinsic factors of a person's working in relative harmony (Figure 1-4). That is not an abstract concept. When internal and external factors harmoniously coexist, the person is healthy.

What Is Mental Health?

Mental health is not merely the absence of mental disorder. It consists of many factors. Healthy human function depends on a structurally whole and intact human biologic organism with well-orchestrated interactive physiology of multiple biologic systems. It also depends on an external environment that provides resources, encourages healthy living, and reinforces and fosters healthy function. Boxes 1-1 and 1-2 depict major components and influencing factors for mental health. When these components and factors are present, mental health is an expectation.

What Is Mental Disorder?

Current national reports and research on the causes of mental disorders favor the stress diathesis model that focuses predominantly on the convergence of (1) human constitutional and biologic predisposition or vulnerablity (i.e., genetics, structural defects, neurotransmitter dysfunction) with (2) environmental and psychosocial stressors (i.e., diseases, viruses, parenting deficiencies, poverty, lack of social sup-

Box 1-1   Components of Mental Health

Presence of anatomic and physiologic components necessary to function in the world

Absence of signs and symptoms of mental disorder

Freedom from excessive mental and emotional disability and pain

Ability to:

  Demonstrate mental and physical competence and skills

  Perceive self, others, and events correctly

  Recognize own strengths, weaknesses, capabilities, and limitations

  Separate fantasy from reality

Think clearly

  Problem solve

  Use good judgment

  Reason logically

  Reach insightful conclusions

Negotiate each developmental stage

Attain and maintain positive self-system

  Self-concept

  Self-image

  Self-esteem

Accept self and others as uniquely different but humanly similar

Appreciate life

Find beauty, joy, and goodness in self, others, and environment

Be creative

Be optimistic but realistic

Be resilient

Use talents to fullest

Involve self in purposeful, meaningful life work

Engage in play

Develop and demonstrate appropriate sense of humor

Express emotions

Exhibit congruent thoughts, feelings, and behaviors

Accept responsibility for actions

Control impulses and behavior

Be accountable for own behaviors

Respect societal rules and sanctions

Learn from experiences

Maintain wholesome values and belief system

Cope with internal and external stressors in constructive and adaptive ways

Return to usual or higher function after crises

Delay gratification

Function independently

Maintain reasonable expectations concerning self and others

Adapt to social environment

Relate to others

  Form relationships

  Maintain close, meaningful, loving, adaptive relationships

  Work and play well with others

  Be intimate, appropriately and selectively

  Respond to others in need

  Feel and exhibit compassion and empathy toward others

  Demonstrate culturally and socially acceptable interpersonal interactions

  Manage interpersonal conflict constructively

  Give and receive gracefully

  Learn from and teach others

  Function interdependently

Seek self-actualization

Attain self-defined spirituality

Box 1-2   Influencing Factors for Mental Health or Disorder

Inherited factors

  Predisposition

  Capacities

  Limitations

Pregnancy environment and experience (from conception to birth)

Psychoneuroimmunologic factors

Biochemical influences

Hormonal influences

Family

  Composition

  Birth position

  Bonding

  Members' mental health

Developmental events

  Completion of clearly defined stages

  Resolution of developmental crises

Cultures

Subcultures

Values

Belief systems

Perception of self

Cognitive abilities

  Capacity

  Volition

Personality traits and states

  Competence

  Resilience

Goals, aspirations

World view

Internal stressors

External stressors

Support system

  Choice

  Availability

Negative influences

  Internal/external

  Mental disorders

  Crime

  Drugs

  Psychosocial stressors

  Poverty

Demographic factors

Geographic location

Health practices and beliefs

Spirituality/religion

ports) that exceed the individual's ability to adapt and cope (Department of Health and Human Services, 1999).

When internal and external components as described in Boxes 1-1 and 1-2 are absent or become dysfunctional, disorder may occur. Chapters 9 through 18 of this textbook describe multiple etiologies in detail to increase understanding of mental disorders. Another factor to consider when attempting to understand mental disorders is that the mind and body are inextricably associated and the outcome of dysfunction in one may result in dysfunction of the other. This concept is represented in the following examples:

> Stephen was a high-functioning executive who had everything to live for. He had a close and caring family, a satisfying, well-paying position with a company he joined 15 years ago, community ties with several organizations, an ample complement of good friends, and close connections with his church. During an annual routine medical examination, Stephen was diagnosed with cancer of the pancreas with metastasis and an unfavorable prognosis. Stephen, a self-made man who had taken good care of himself and valued his physical health, was devastated by this diagnosis and, despite the reassuring words of his physician, family, and friends, became deeply depressed and soon was diagnosed with major depression.

This example illustrates that psychiatric disorders may develop from medical illnesses.

Conversely, because mind and body are inseparable, a disturbed mind often manifests in disturbances of body function, as illustrated in the following example:

> Promise was 18 years old when she experienced her first episode of schizophrenia. She had graduated from high school, moved away from her family into a shared apartment, and worked during the summer, intending to enter college in the fall semester. She met new "friends" at work and started to casually experiment with drugs and sex during rave parties. Promise started to hear voices while sober and at work, telling her she was "a no-good slut, was worthless," and "would fail at anything she tried." Promise soon stopped working because she was afraid co-workers could hear the voices and believed them. The voices also told her that the water and any food in the apartment were poisoned. She stayed in the apartment; stopped going out of the building; stopped eating, drinking, or bathing; and stayed in bed most of the day with the covers over her head. She lost several pounds and became dehydrated and incoherent. She refused any contact with friends or family. Her worried roommates called the police, who brought her to the hospital where she was admitted to the psychiatric unit with symptoms of psychosis.

This is a clear example of dysfunctional behavioral and body responses to a mental disorder, and the inseparable mind body connection.

Mental disorders are not easily defined but are formally described in the *Diagnostic and Statistical Manual of Mental Disorders* (APA, 2000) and in the *International Classification of Diseases* (World Health Organization, ICD-9-CM, 1992). These texts specifically describe symptoms of mental disorders in classifications that are widely recognized and accepted. Authors of the DSM-IV-TR also write that it is counterproductive to separate mind and body in determining mental health and disorder (APA, 2000). In addition, the first report of the surgeon general of the United States repeatedly states that the relationship between mental and physical health is inseparable (Department of Health and Human Services, 1999). For the purposes of this text, each chapter on specific mental disorders describes and discusses the diagnoses in a particular category of mental disorders. Although the diagnosis of a mental disorder often carries negative connotation and stereotyping in the general public, psychiatric professionals know that diagnoses are essential.

DIAGNOSES: PROS AND CONS
Importance of Diagnoses

It is clear after reading the section about stigma that mental disorders and their diagnostic labels may result in problems for clients and their families. Diagnoses of mental disorders have both positive and negative aspects and purposes, but they are necessary. Diagnoses are precise classifications and descriptions of mental disorders and have several useful purposes that include *communication, treatment, prognosis, funding,* and *research.*

Communication

Each psychiatric diagnosis represents a specific set of symptoms or a syndrome. The criteria for each disorder enable mental health care providers to communicate with each other without having to explain symptoms when discussing the diagnoses. Staff should bear in mind that each client presents a unique expression of his or her disorder.

Educating individuals about psychiatric disorders is effective because the psychiatric classification of disorders is clearly defined and therefore can be communicated to learners in an organized way.

Treatment

Staff members are prepared to begin symptom-specific treatment based on a client's diagnosis. They know that the approaches (biologic and interpersonal) vary, depending on the diagnosis. For example, preparation of the staff and the psychiatric setting is different for a client with a diagnosis of paranoid schizophrenia with acutely psychotic symptoms and aggressive behavior toward others than is preparation for a client with a diagnosis of major depression and severely withdrawn behavior.

Prognosis

Some psychiatric diagnoses have more favorable prognoses than do others. Mental health care providers remain hopeful and convey that hope to clients. However, they are aware that a goal of treatment may be to return a client to a level of function that existed before an acute exacerbation of a chronic disorder, without expecting a cure of the disorder. For example, the prognosis for some adjustment disorders is more favorable than the prognosis for one of the schizophrenias that has a chronic course, with *severe and persistent* symptoms.

Funding

It is a well-established fact that money is required to pay for services delivered during the care of clients, regardless of the psychiatric setting. Whether the source is private or public, certain criteria must be met to receive payment, and the client's diagnosis is a major factor.

On a larger scale, research money is targeted for investigation of designated diagnoses. Research may be carried out in the private sector (e.g., pharmaceutical companies) or public sector (e.g., government mental health agencies).

Research

Diagnostic labels are instrumental in guiding and governing research directed toward mental illness. Private and public universities, medical centers, biologic and psychosocial research facilities, and pharmaceutical companies rely on acceptance of accurate diagnostic criteria to operate their projects. Each organization uses exact diagnostic criteria to reach reliable and valid conclusions, regardless of the focus. Government funding of mental health/illness research projects is also based on accurate diagnoses.

PREVENTION OF MENTAL DISORDERS

Prevention of mental illness is more than an ideal. It is a right of every human being as stated in the introduction of this chapter. A classic definition of prevention of illness was proposed for public health in the 1950s and, although modified several times, remains widely accepted today. Gerald Caplan used the concept to define prevention of mental disorders in his text, *Principles of Preventive Psychiatry* (1964), naming *primary, secondary,* and *tertiary* levels of prevention.

The early prevention principles were modified again in the 1990s during the Decade of the Brain by the Institute of Medicine, in their report on prevention (IOM, 1994). The modification identified three primary activities as *prevention, treatment,* and *maintenance;* and, although the new definition shifted some components to other areas, the newly adapted definition remains conceptually similar. The concept works well for psychiatric nurses when levels of prevention are considered and used in practice. Caplan's concept is still widely used.

Levels of Prevention
Primary Prevention

Focus is on reduction of incidence of mental disorders in the community. Emphasis is on health promotion and prevention of disorders. Screening plays a vital role in early identification of any disorder. Examples follow.

- Teach pregnant couples about normal child development and help them learn and practice parenting skills.
- Teach stress reduction/management skills to any population.
- Present a seminar for elementary and middle school children and their families on the topic of preventing use of illegal drugs.
- Assist a group of neighbors to clear a vacant lot in an inner city neighborhood and plant and maintain a neighbor-operated garden, sharing the fruits of their labor.

Secondary Prevention

Focus is on reducing the prevalence of mental disorders through early identification of symptoms and early treatment of symptoms that occur. Examples follow.

- Treat clients after diagnoses of mental disorders is made. Treatment may take place in any psychiatric

setting (inpatient, clinic, day treatment). Treatment may be any approved biologic or interactive type of therapy.
- Refer clients to other therapists for additional treatment (family therapy, couples therapy).

Tertiary Prevention

Focus has a dual purpose of (1) reducing residual effects of the disorder, and (2) providing rehabilitation and restoration. Examples follow.

- Lead ongoing outpatient therapy group of clients with the same diagnosis to offer support, monitor, and evaluate members' progress.
- Continue to meet with family who has a member with a mental disorder. Assist and reinforce willingness to care for member and help identify symptoms that recur.
- Conduct seminars and workshops to teach clients job skills and match potential employers with potential client employees.

Risk Factors and Protective Factors

Risk factors and protective factors are inherent in prevention of mental disorders.

When certain internal characteristics and external influences (**risk factors**) are present before a disorder occurs, the individual is considered more vulnerable to develop a disorder. Risk factors can be biologic (genetics, gender) or psychosocial (lack of family supports, school problems). Some risk factors may be altered over time and may in turn influence the outcome of the disorder.

Other factors in prevention include those that help the individual guard against the risks (**protective factors).** Protective factors may be either *internal* (capacity for tolerating stress; learned skills and techniques; competence) or *external* (caring, facilitative teacher; planned after-school programs). Protective factors may also be modified and help improve a client's response to potential or actual risk factors.

Defense Modes

Healthy people desire, work toward, and function best when they think positively and feel good about themselves and their accomplishments, goals, and relationships. They want to be content within their environment, accepting of self, and accepted and loved by others. At the same time, they also desire and work toward avoidance of anxiety, discomfort, distress, and mental or physical pain. All of these at one time or another are an inevitable part of the human condition.

People use numerous ways to avoid anxiety and contend with stress. Some of these are conscious methods or techniques that may be learned and may be adaptive or maladaptive, whereas others are unconscious and operate automatically (Box 1-3). The unconscious mechanisms are sometimes referred to as protective ego defenses.

Box 1-3   Defense Mechanisms and Strategies

Repression: The active unconscious process of keeping out or ejecting from the consciousness ideas or impulses that are unacceptable to the person.
Example: An adult male who was sexually abused as a child has no recollection of the events.

Denial: Refusal to perceive or face unpleasant reality as it actually exists.
Example: Nonacceptance of a fatal diagnosis such as AIDS.

Rationalization: Use of a contrived, socially acceptable and logical explanation to justify unpleasant material and to keep it out of consciousness.
Example: A high-school graduate who does not get accepted to a prestigious military academy says he could never tolerate the regimentation anyway.

Projection: Attributing one's own unacceptable motives or characteristics to another person or group.
Example: A paranoid person uses projection frequently in always seeing "the others" as hostile, threatening, or dangerous.

Displacement: The discharge of pent-up feelings (frequently hostility) onto something or someone else in the environment that is less threatening than the original source of the feelings.
Example: After her boss berates her publicly, a woman comes home and starts an argument with her neighbor over parking rights.

Reaction formation: Prevention of awareness or expression of unacceptable desires by adoption of opposite behaviors in an exaggerated way.
Example: A woman who does not want her child before it is born becomes overly protective after the birth, refusing to leave the child's side.

Intellectualization: The overuse of abstract thinking or generalizations to control or minimize painful feelings.
Example: A man who faces a pending divorce engages in lengthy and lofty discourse about divorce statistics and process during a support group but never talks about his own fears and feelings.

Undoing: Atonement for or attempt to dissipate unacceptable acts or wishes.
Examples: (1) A man has an affair with another woman and then buys his wife a new car. (2) A professional berates her colleague and causes her to lose her job and then invites her out for dinner and the theater.

Compensation: Counterbalance for deficiencies in one area by excelling in another area.
Example: A young man who fails at sports studies hard and becomes valedictorian of his graduating class.

Identification: Incorporation of the image of an emulated person, then acting, thinking, and feeling like that person (unconscious mental mimicry).
Example: Gang members dress exactly like their leader and steal from neighbors as the leader does.

Introjection: Treating something outside the self as if it is actually inside the self.
Example: A child who fears dragons "becomes" a dragon in serious play, thus assimilating the fearful experience.

Sublimation: Modification of an instinctual but socially unacceptable impulse into a constructive acceptable behavior.
Examples: (1) An aggressive young man becomes a star hockey player. (2) A woman with strong sexual urges becomes a sculptor.

Regression: Returning to an earlier level of adaptation.
Examples: (1) An adolescent who is under stress curls up on his bed with a stuffed teddy bear, sucks his thumb, and does not speak. (2) An adult client admitted to the psychiatric unit with a diagnosis of psychosis is found smearing feces on the wall.

Suppression: The conscious inhibition of an impulse, idea, or affect. The person has full awareness of the behavior.
Example: A man on his way to give a major speech is told by his wife that she is divorcing him. He decides not to think about it until his speech is over, and puts it out of his mind so he can complete his task.

Humor: Emphasis on ironic or amusing components of a crisis, conflict, or stressor.
Example: Two people leave a room after being strongly disciplined by their boss and burst into laughter, which they had restrained. They jokingly discuss the only thing each focused on—a large piece of spaghetti and sauce from lunch on his white tie.

Splitting: Compartmentalization of opposite-affect states and failure to integrate positive and negative aspects of self or others, resulting in polarized images of self and others as all good or all bad.
Example: A client on a psychiatric unit tells Nurse A that she is "the kindest, smartest, most well-prepared nurse on the unit." She tells Nurse B, who sets limits on the client's behavior, that she is "stupid and insensitive, and it's a miracle she ever got an RN license."

Self-Observation: Reflection on one's own behavior, thoughts, and feelings, followed by appropriate response.
Example: A man leaves the store after joking with the clerk and discovers he received too much change. He returns the excess money.

Self-Assertion: Expression of thoughts and feelings in direct ways that are not manipulative or intimidating.
Examples: A young attorney asks the senior attorney in the firm to include her in a major case and then proceeds to outline her reasons and ideas for winning the case.

Altruism: Devotion of self to serving others as a way to manage conflict and stress; differs from reaction formation in that it is gratifying but not self-sacrificing.
Example: Some nuns, priests, rabbis, ministers, nurses, physicians, firefighters, and paramedics, to name a few, often serve people for unselfish reasons and gain satisfaction through giving.

Affiliation: Turning to others for support and help when stressed or conflicted, without attempting to make others responsible for taking care of the person.
Example: A woman is widowed and moves across the country to be near her family of origin and friends from her past.

Anticipation: Anticipating consequences of events yet to come and thinking of options, solutions, and alternatives; also can include experiencing the feelings associated with these thoughts (a "mental rehearsal" of future events).
Example: A hard-working engineer, called to interview for partnership in a firm, spends the rest of the day rehearsing and experiencing the event.

Continued

Box 1-3   Defense Mechanisms and Strategies —cont'd

Help-Rejecting Complaining: Repeated requests for help, suggestions, or advice that is then rejected; request disguises covert feelings of reproach or hostility for others; complaints may be about problems of life or physical or psychologic symptoms.

Example: A woman constantly calls her grown and married children to complain about her physical pains and loneliness but constantly refuses to take any helpful steps they suggest to alleviate her situation.

Passive Aggression: Expression of aggression toward others in indirect and nonassertive ways; covert hostility and resentment masked by overt compliance.

Example: A girl who is jealous because her best friend dated a boy she wanted to date agrees to meet her friend for lunch and then arrives an hour late, apologizing profusely and begging forgiveness.

Omnipotence: Feeling or acting superior to others or as if one has special abilities or power.

Example: An inept and underachieving son of a dynamic business tycoon struts around his own plush but token office and treats others condescendingly.

Isolation of Affect: Separation of feelings from thoughts and ideas that are originally associated with them.

Example: A woman describes in full detail the traumatic event of watching her friend get hit by a truck and killed but displays no emotion.

Fantasy: Gratification of frustrated desires, achievements, and relationships by substituting them with daydreams and imagery.

Example: An unpopular high school senior is left out of social events but spends her spare time imagining herself dressing for and going to the senior prom with the class football hero.

Acting Out: The use of actions versus reflection or true experiencing of feelings to deal with stress and conflict.

Example: A student learns he or she has failed a course, then smashes a window in the classroom, leaves, and drinks six beers.

Box 1-4   Conscious Techniques to Manage Anxiety

Examples of Adaptive Methods
Exercising
Calling a friend
Talking to a parent or significant other
Going to a movie
Crying
Eating
Dancing
Reading
Volunteering time
Writing in a journal
Sleeping
Practicing relaxation techniques
Going to the theater
Attending church or community meetings
Writing letters to friends, family, or others
Getting involved in purposeful work

Examples of Maladaptive Methods
Drinking alcohol excessively
Taking mind- and mood-altering illegal drugs
Isolating self
Getting involved in destructive confrontations or altercations
Excessive involvement on computer (pornography, buying)
Compulsive gambling
Excessive spending or sexual activity
Exercising excessively to exclusion of other activities
Calling others continually on the phone
Watching television all day long
Overeating

Each individual develops a pattern of mechanisms and techniques that are either adaptive or maladaptive, with **adaptive** signifying preservation or enhancement of health and **maladaptive** the opposite. Unconscious mental mechanisms serve to protect the individual from anxiety, but they may also prevent realistic appraisal of self, other people, situations, or events. Some mechanisms are considered high-level **defensive functioning** (affiliation, humor, sublimation), whereas others are considered dysfunctional methods of adaptation. Conscious adaptive and maladaptive defenses are presented in Box 1-4.

ROLE OF THE NURSE

The role of the nurse is crucial in all levels of care. Psychiatric nurses specialize in the care of clients (individuals, families, community) when life crises and mental disorders exist or are risk factors in clients' lives. Nurses who specialize in psychiatric mental health nursing work with clients in the multileveled prevention of dysfunction and disorders, as well as in the treatment of mental disorders when they occur. Nurses in this field are prepared to use keen assessment skills and specific psychiatric nursing interventions with their clients, while incorporating both biologic modalities and therapeutic interpersonal communication techniques during interactions.

Preparation of the Nurse
Theoretic Background

Knowledge is the core of the nursing profession, and it is essential that nurses are educated in many areas. Among these are basic physical, natural, and behavioral sciences; the humanities; and languages. After successful completion of basic courses, nurses learn the art and science of nursing. Skilled clinical practice is based on knowledge, research, and actual interventions that use learned evidence-based techniques to ensure client safety and well-being.

Knowledge and understanding of theory relating to psychiatric mental health nursing, plus safe, effective practice is necessary and expected by client consumers and by those who govern nursing practice. Psychiatric nursing is a specialty within registered nursing in which nurses use their knowledge and skills to therapeutically interact with clients who are experiencing emotional distress, life crises, and mental disorders. Each level of education and practice is governed by standards.

Practice Standards

Principles and standards of nursing practice ensure that the public experiences consistent and safe measures of care. Principles and standards are clearly delineated by several governing organizations, including:

- *Individual accredited nursing education programs* that provide psychiatric mental health curriculum and guide students through theory and practice levels until graduation.
- *State boards of nursing* that issue licenses to registered nurses to practice only after completion of comprehensive testing that ensures a standard of excellence. In addition, the boards of nursing monitor nursing practice and continued education, and provide disciplinary measures when necessary. Some state boards also certify psychiatric nurse clinical specialists and psychiatric nurse practitioners in advanced practice.
- *National and state nursing organizations* provide direction (ANA Standards of Practice, NLN Core Components and Competencies [2000]), affiliation (psychiatric nursing associations and organizations), support, and continued education opportunities for specific disciplines; some provide certification for advanced levels of practice in nursing.
- *Place of employment* ideally provides specific guidelines in policies and procedures for interventions with clients while maintaining state and national standards of practice.

Psychiatric nursing standards and organizations appear in Appendix B.

Nurses prepare for practice by learning and using standards and principles and adhere to them to maintain their licenses but, more important, to give safe and effective care to their clients. Nurses welcome and embrace guidelines, knowing that their use paves the way to client health. However, knowledge without **evidence-based practice** is ineffective. It is through experience and research in the psychiatric clinical setting that nurses hone skills and procedures they have learned. With experience nurses can then adapt skills in safe yet creative ways while still adhering to the principles that assist clients on their journey to wellness.

It is important for nurses to understand their roles and the roles of other health team members. Box 1-5 explains member roles.

The Art and the Science of Nursing

During actual practice, the art and the science of nursing are inextricable. The art of caring is professionally embodied in a **therapeutic alliance** that develops between the nurse and the client, and is referred to as the *nurse-client relationship*. The alliance is a vehicle for the client to learn and practice skills for the purposes of gaining insight, effecting change, healing mental and emotional wounds, and promoting growth. A strong and healthy alliance between client and nurse is one of the most crucial aspects of the therapeutic process. Its purpose is to collaboratively bring the client to an optimal state of health within the client's capacity for change or acceptance. Comprehensive therapy for the client includes many other modalities, but the individual, one-on-one nurse-client relationship or alliance is a key factor in any client's successful participation in therapy.

The science of nursing includes understanding and use of principles of nursing on all levels. In addition, there is required commitment to remain current in knowledge and to practice all learned skills and procedures that ensure client safety and well-being. The science of nursing also includes the operationalization of the principles of the nurse-client relationship. The therapeutic alliance or the nurse-client relationship is also discussed in Chapter 7.

Principles of the Nurse-Client Relationship

The therapeutic interpersonal relationship that develops between the nurse and client is an important factor for effecting client change and growth. The following are principles and guidelines for developing and maintaining the relationship:

- The relationship is therapeutic rather than social.
- The focus remains on the client's needs and problems rather than on the nurse or other issues.
- The relationship is purposeful and goal directed.
- The relationship is objective versus subjective in quality.
- The relationship is time limited versus open ended.

Therapeutic vs. Social. A therapeutic relationship is formed to help clients solve problems, make decisions, achieve growth, learn coping strategies, let go of unwanted behaviors, reinforce self-worth, and examine relationships. The meetings between nurse and client are not for mutual satisfaction. Although the nurse can be friendly with the client, the nurse is not there to be the client's friend. Because boundaries define nurses and their roles and are important in any relationship, especially in a therapeutic relationship, trying to be a client's friend blurs boundaries and confuses roles. The nurse helps the client increase awareness of

Box 1-5   Roles of the Mental Health Team

Psychiatric Nurse

Nurses have the most widely focused position description of any of the member roles. This depends on their license and certification mandates, the policies of the psychiatric facility or care setting, and their experience. They interact with clients in individual and group settings; manage client care; administer and monitor medications; assist with numerous psychiatric and physical treatments; participate in interdisciplinary team meetings; teach clients and families; take responsibility for client records; act as a client advocate; interact with clients' significant others; and assess and intervene with clients' psychiatric, biologic, psychosocial, cultural, and spiritual problems.

Licensed vocational nurses provide direct client support. Registered nurses have expanded roles of unit management and decision making in addition to client interaction. Master's- and doctoral-prepared nurses act as clinical specialists in individual, group, and family therapy, with expanded roles within psychiatric settings, or they act autonomously in private practice.

In some states clinical nurse specialists prescribe medications and manage client caseloads. A master's or doctoral degree is required to teach nursing education. Graduate nurses frequently conduct psychiatric research or act as administrators of psychiatric settings.

Psychiatric Social Worker

This graduate-level position allows members to work with clients on an individual basis, conduct group therapy sessions, work with clients' families, and act as liaisons with the community to place clients after discharge. They emphasize intervention with the client in the social environment in which he or she will live.

Psychiatric Technician

The licensed psychiatric technician has direct client contact in a psychiatric setting and usually reports to the registered nurse. Technicians are trained to observe and record symptoms and intervene under supervision. In some states they can administer medications under the supervision of a registered nurse.

Mental Health Worker

Some facilities call this position mental health counselor. It is an unlicensed position in which the member acts only under the supervision of an RN in assisting clients with activities of daily living, maintaining the schedule, and providing general support. Some mental health workers have minimal education in psychiatry; others may work in this position while accruing hours toward master's or doctoral degrees. They do not administer medications.

Psychiatrist

A psychiatrist is a licensed medical physician who specializes in psychiatry. Responsibilities include admitting clients into acute care settings, prescribing and monitoring psychopharmacologic agents, administering electroshock therapy, conducting individual and family therapy, and participating in interdisciplinary team meetings that focus on his or her clients.

Psychologist

A psychologist is a licensed individual with a doctoral degree in psychology. There are several different psychology tracks. Preparation is for assessment and treatment of psychologic and psychosocial problems of individuals, families, or groups (including industrial, educational, environmental). Psychologists do not prescribe or administer medications. Many psychologists administer psychometric tests that aid in the diagnosis of disorders.

Marriage, Family, Child Counselor

These are licensed individuals who frequently work in private practice. They are prepared to work with individuals, couples, families, and groups, and emphasize the interpersonal aspects of achieving and maintaining relationships.

Case Managers

This position is continuously redefined. Nurses are qualified for this position because of their diverse education. Case managers facilitate delivery of individualized, coordinated care in cost-effective ways. Managed care and case management are not interchangeable concepts. *Managed care* refers to a system of cost-containment programs that are utilized to direct, control, and approve access to services and costs within the health care delivery system. *Case management* is a process in the managed care strategy (Mullahy, 1995). Case managers need to know the various types of hospitalization and outpatient care settings, the coverage offered by different payers (insurance companies, health maintenance organizations, preferred provider organizations), and the impact of federal and state legislation. Case managers serve as a connection between agencies to provide the most favorable outcomes for the client.

---

boundaries and practice boundary setting. Box 1-6 gives some examples the nurse may use to assist clients to recognize boundary violations.

Some social conversation is usual at the beginning of meetings and may help to establish or maintain rapport. Occasionally during meetings, superficial or social conversation may briefly reappear, but the majority of conversation is focused and therapeutic. Table 1-1 compares therapeutic and social interactions.

Client Focus. Frequently during a session, a client redirects the focus away from self by changing the subject, talking about the weather, focusing on the nurse (nurse's appearance, personal problems, problems in the milieu), or other issues. The nurse recognizes this as a divergent tactic that is probably a form of resistance. The nurse then confronts the behavior in a matter-of-fact way and refocuses the client. Clients do this for one or more of several reasons: resistance to discussing anxiety-producing material, boredom, repetition of material previously discussed with other therapists, or inability to stay cognitively focused because of a mental disorder.

Goal Direction. The primary purpose of a therapeutic relationship is helping clients to meet adaptive goals. Together the client and nurse determine problematic issues and collaboratively decide what the client needs and is able to achieve. Once goals are established, the nurse and client

Box 1-6   Signs of Unhealthy Boundaries

Going against personal values or rights to please another
Not noticing when someone displays inappropriate boundaries
Not noticing when someone invades your boundaries
Talking at an intimate level on the first meeting
Falling in love with a new acquaintance
Falling in love with anyone who reaches out
Being overwhelmed by (preoccupied with) a person
Acting on first sexual impulse
Being sexual for your partner, not yourself
Accepting food, gifts, touch, or sex that you do not want
Touching a person without asking
Taking as much as you can for the sake of getting
Giving as much as you can for the sake of giving
Allowing someone to take as much as they can from you
Letting others direct your life
Letting others describe your reality
Letting others define you
Believing others can anticipate your needs
Expecting others to fill your needs automatically
Falling apart so someone will take care of you
Self-abuse
Sexual and physical abuse
Food abuse
Loaning money you do not have
Flirting; sending mixed messages
Telling all

Table 1-1   Therapeutic vs. Social Interactions

Therapeutic	Social
Offer client therapeutic assistance	Give and receive friendship equally
Focus on client's needs	Meet both person's needs
Discuss client's perceptions, thoughts, feelings, and behaviors	Share mutual ideas and experiences
Actively listen and use therapeutic communication, skills, and techniques	Give opinions and advice
Encourage client to choose subject for discussion	Randomly discuss topics at will or whim
Encourage client to problem solve toward independence	Insist on helping as a friend; tolerate dependence
Keep no secrets that may harm client	Promise to keep secrets at any cost
Set goals with client	Goals of relationship are not important
Remain objective	Become subjectively involved
Maintain healthy boundaries	Accept blurred boundaries
Evaluate interactions with client	Avoid relational evaluations

agree to work toward those goals and put intentions into action and modify strategies when necessary until the identified goals are achieved. The activities involved are usually many and varied, but each activity is purposefully planned with the client's goals in mind.

Objective vs. Subjective. Nurses can be therapeutic only if they remain objective. Objective refers to remaining free from bias, prejudice, and personal identification in interaction with the client and being able to process information based on facts. On the other hand, subjective refers to emphasis on one's own feelings, attitudes, and opinions when interacting with the client. When nurses act subjectively in relation to the client's problems or situations, they lose effectiveness in the relationship. With conscious intent to remain objective, the nurse will see things realistically rather than identifying with the client or becoming overly and personally involved with the client's issues. Of course, this approach does not imply that the nurse withdraws from feeling or constructs barriers to protect himself or herself by intellectualizing or avoiding responses. With knowledge, awareness, and practice, the nurse can be both objective and fully attentive to clients' situations and needs.

An example of objectivity versus subjectivity is the nurse's ability to remain empathic instead of becoming sympathetic when interacting with a client, even though the nurse may have experienced a similar, painful situation. For example, consider a nurse who has lost a child in an accident and then encounters a client who is depressed and grieving the recent death of his or her own child. The nurse demonstrates objectivity by allowing and facilitating the client's full expression of thoughts and feelings and then responding in a warm, empathic way that remains client centered. This approach helps the client relieve pent-up feelings in a normal grieving process, allows the client to feel understood, and helps the client to process and organize thoughts directed toward solving problems.

An example of nontherapeutic subjectivity is a nurse in the same situation who hears the client's expression of feelings and responds with excessive self-disclosure about his or her own similar experience. This approach represents a loss of therapeutic boundaries by identifying with the client's problem—becoming enmeshed in the situation by personalizing it. The client's response will most likely be negative. The client will probably stop sharing information because he or she feels unimportant and negated, or because he or she worries that the nurse is fragile or inept and cannot even manage his or her own problems. Clients compromised by their own conditions and situations cannot be burdened by the nurse's problems. Healthy nurses seek supervision or private therapy when personal problems arise.

Time-Limited Interactions. Before the relationship is established, the nurse sets necessary parameters of the relationship by agreeing with the client on the days and times when they will meet and on the numbers of times meetings will take place. Such structure helps the client realize that this relationship has limits and is not open ended (e.g., the client cannot see the nurse whenever he or she wants and for as long as he or she wants).

The principle of time-limited interaction is important for several reasons. Sometimes clients have not learned during formative relationships that limits are important for all relationships and that without limits problems are inevitable. When participants define the amount of time they are willing and able to give, then anxiety-provoking guesswork is eliminated and individuals can decide how to make appropriate use of the time they have together. Also, all relationships have inevitable endings. Much grief is avoided if both the nurse and client are certain of the parameters of their relationship and enforce them together. The relationship is a microcosm of the client's relationships outside of their meetings and serves as a model for the client to successfully begin and appropriately let go of subsequent relationships.

Stages of the Nurse-Client Relationship

Every relationship between the nurse and client is unique because of the qualities each participant brings to the interaction process and because of the human chemistry that develops between them. However, relationships undergo definitive stages. The astute nurse identifies these stages as they occur to more effectively facilitate the client's progress.

Preorientation Stage. During this initial phase before the nurse and client ever meet, the nurse must accomplish several tasks. The first is to gather data about the client, his or her condition, and the present situation. Information is taken from all available sources (client's chart, staff report, physician's report, input from family or other reliable sources such as police and ambulance attendants).

From the information gathered, the nurse engages in a period of **autodiagnosis** regarding his or her thoughts, feelings, perceptions, and attitudes about this particular client. Judgmentalism, biases, or stereotyping may arise that may influence the pending contact in a nontherapeutic way. For example, if the nurse learns information that reminds him or her of a personal loved one or of a despised or feared person, the nurse's response to the client could be subjective, nontherapeutic, and ineffective if the facts are not recognized and closely examined by the nurse. The following example can be used as critical thinking tool.

> Consider Nurse A, whose father was dependent on alcohol and verbally abused her mother when he drank. What are some possible responses Nurse A may demonstrate in the following situations if she does not engage in autodiagnosis?
>
> A male client is admitted to the unit because of inebriation and wife abuse.
>
> A matronly female is admitted to the unit with major depression. Her husband drinks and abuses her.

Nurse A's conscious efforts to examine each situation and put it in an objective perspective are important so that identification, judgmentalism, and stereotyping can be avoided.

Orientation Stage. After the nurse-client introduction, the relationship begins to grow. During this stage, participants become acquainted, build trust and rapport, and demonstrate acceptance of the process that will take place when the client begins to work on important issues.

The Contract. A contract is established in the orientation phase of the relationship. The contract may be formal or informal, written or verbal. Nurses most frequently use verbal, informal contracts with clients in acute care settings in which the client and nurse are more continually together. It may be necessary for the nurse to write a more specific, formalized contract for clients who are seen outside of an acute care setting or when there is an expectation for a client behavior to continue (e.g., no self-harm contract).

The contract may be succinct and still be effective and efficient. For example, the nurse on an inpatient unit may say to the client: "I will be your contact person while you are in the (facility). I work Monday through Friday from 8 AM to 4 PM. Because of your schedule on this unit, it seems that the best time for us to meet is 9 AM. Is that a good time for you?" If the client agrees, the contract is established.

In a community setting (e.g., home care, partial-day treatment program, halfway house), the nurse would probably write a contract for the client, specifying dates, days, and times of meetings, and phone numbers where the nurse can be reached if the client has questions between appointments. Some contracts specifically identify client behaviors (expected outcomes) that the client may practice between meetings, as well as goals that may be achieved.

Regardless of the type of contract, the nurse explains the purpose of the meetings, what may be expected during the meetings, and roles of both nurse and client. Together, they determine long-term goals and short-term objectives for reaching those goals.

Dependability is imperative, and nurses must keep all appointments with clients. When circumstances prevent this, the nurse contacts the client to explain and sets a new meeting time. Client dependability is also expected and conveyed.

During the orientation stage client strengths, limitations, and problem areas are identified by both the client and the nurse. Outcome criteria are established, and a plan of care is formulated. Client's responses to this phase vary widely.

Working Stage. The orientation stage ends and the working stage begins when the client takes responsibility for his or her own behavior change. This means committing to working on problems and concerns that caused disruptions in the client's life.

Prioritizing clients' needs helps to determine those problems that will require immediate attention and promotes an organized way to manage the problems. A general principle is that safety and health problems supersede any others. For example, it is always determined first that clients are free from danger to self or others and that physical needs are met before traditional therapy begins. Then, within the established relationships, behaviors that are socially unacceptable are modified (e.g., hostile remarks, swearing, isolation, poor hygiene). The nurse assists the client to change problematic behaviors in a safe environment in which the client can practice new skills and behaviors and reinforces positive outcomes achieved by the client.

As nurses gain experience, they are better able to recognize when their clients are in the working phase. Sometimes clients tell their "story" but do not do the work to change. Seasoned nurses are able to separate the provocative content from actual process and growth.

Termination Stage. In this stage the relationship comes to a close. Termination actually begins in the orientation phase when the nurse states meeting times with the client. This lets the client know that the relationship is about to begin, but that it also has parameters and will end. It avoids confusion on the part of the client, who occasionally is unable or unwilling to recognize the boundaries of the relationship and wants to contact the nurse outside of the facility or after the client has been discharged. The nurse does not continue relationships after the client leaves treatment.

Termination generally occurs when the client has improved and has been discharged, but it may also occur if the client or nurse is transferred. When termination is anticipated, the nurse uses strategies to prepare for the event. Ending treatment may sometimes be traumatic for clients who have come to value the relationship and the nurse's attention and assistance. Some methods that the nurse may use when preparing for termination include:

- Reduce the amount of time spent with the client in each session and increase the amount of time between sessions as the client's condition improves.
- Begin to work on preparation for the client's postdischarge situation (plans for future) rather than focus on new or past problems.
- Have the client identify changes he or she has made toward growth; share perceptions of the client's growth.
- Help the client express feelings about ending the relationship; tell the client if the relationship has been pleasant.

When nurses recognize relationship stages and are aware of the strategies and responses during each stage, the course of the therapeutic process runs more smoothly. The nurse is not caught off guard or shocked when responses are other than anticipated. When nurses are unaware of potential client responses, they may take responsibility for what seems like failure or may even abandon the relationship because it is unrewarding or unfulfilling. When the nurse is aware of responses that may occur, however, he or she is prepared to use strategies that facilitate client growth.

Motives for Helping

Nursing in the psychiatric setting also includes a thorough understanding of the concept of helping. A predominant motivator for nurses to enter the nursing profession is usually that they enjoy being with others and they also like to help others. The process of helping is complex, and several motives may generate helping behaviors. Nurses work with vulnerable clients in the psychiatric setting, so they must approach the helping process in a healthy way. Brammer (1993) described some of the reasons why nurses and others enter the helping professions. Here are some helpful examples that will raise consciousness about this concept and assist nurses to choose healthy reasons for helping others.

- *Desire to contribute to society.* A feeling of wanting to give back to the world describes this altruistic urge to make things better than they are. By contributing to society, the person feels more worthwhile. Beginning to help in tangible, concrete ways versus grandiose ways is recommended.
- *Need to protect others.* Helping may take the form of protecting the individual. Sometimes rescuing others from consequences of their own decisions and behaviors is counterproductive (e.g., a family member's co-dependent protective behavior toward a person with alcoholism). Objective assessment of the client's condition and situation is necessary to know when protection for health and safety's sake is legitimate and when it fosters dependence or encourages, rather than eliminates, maladaptive behavior.
- *Need for love.* If when helping others the focus is on the helper's own need for love and attention, the result becomes counterproductive. Awareness of the need to be needed is important, because a consequence of serving others to the exclusion of getting one's own needs met leads inevitably to disappointment and burnout, resulting in decreased capacity and ability to help others. Nurses must not look to clients as a source of this love but must find healthy sources outside of their jobs.
- *Need for control or power.* Clients often see helpers as more powerful because of their presumed knowledge, coupled with the client's sense of vulnerability during both acute and chronic dysfunction or disorder. When helpers are aware of this need to influence others or to gain prestige and praise, they can act to correct their motive for helping and focus on the client's needs. Gratitude and praise are then received appropriately.
- *Need for personal satisfaction.* Balanced, healthy individuals who work in helping professions often describe personal satisfaction from working with and watching individuals overcome adversity, achieve goals, and experience growth. To know that the helper facilitated these changes is rewarding and often brings great satisfaction to the helper.
- *Need for personal insight.* While working with clients who have personal problems, helpers may use the relationship to solve their own problems. Awareness of this vicarious learning is important as a constant re-

minder that the nurses focus on clients and their issues rather than their own problems. However, many helpers who have worked through their own similar problems become effective therapists and are able to offer empathy and insight to their clients who move toward change and growth.

Above are some reasons why helpers enter the psychotherapeutic arena. Many motives are unconscious and can be brought to awareness through a process of autodiagnosis: examination of one's own thoughts, feelings, perceptions, and attitudes about a particular client. Motives can also be discovered through continual education and supervision by effective instructors, mentors, or professional peers, who will assist the helper to confront areas that may be problematic.

Outcomes of Helping. Helping is a process that aims to assist another person as follows:
- Help himself or herself
- Choose a direction in life
- Find purpose for existing
- Solve problem
- Survive crises
- Share life with others in work, play, and love

Helping is not about doing "to" or "for" another when the person can function autonomously or with guidance and assistance. Only when the client takes responsibility for life through independence (within his or her own ability, age, stage of development, life situation) can that person experience the freedom to grow. The helper's task is awareness of self, awareness of client needs, and use of skills to set the client free, with tools to forge his or her own life.

TREATMENT

When mental disorders occur, treatment is required. Symptoms may be mild and treated on an outpatient basis or be very severe and require hospitalization.

Historical Overview

Treatment of clients with mental disorders has varied widely throughout history. Although currently in some cases treatment is inadequate in scope as discussed in the beginning of this chapter, it is generally humane and governed by standards of practice at many levels. However, review of the history of mental disorders reveals that in the distant past there were only a few periods when humane treatment of this population existed. More often, individuals who had mental illness were misunderstood and feared as they sometimes are today; but, unlike today, they were often openly mistreated by being shunned, alienated, imprisoned, beaten, or worse.

Treatment Systems

Today clients enter treatment systems voluntarily or involuntarily. If a client or family determines that intervention for disruptive symptoms is desirable or necessary, they may voluntarily seek help through any one of many sources discovered by word of mouth, referral, or even by looking in a telephone book. Some ways clients are initially helped are by family physician, nurse practitioner, clergy, school nurse, community clinic, inpatient psychiatric facility, psychiatrist, psychologist, or other licensed mental health counselors.

If clients have disruptive mental disorders, are not in touch with reality and are unaware of their condition by reason of psychosis, or otherwise resist necessary treatment, they may be brought into treatment involuntarily under laws that govern treatment of mental disorders. Chapter 4 has detailed descriptions of this topic.

Reasons for Treatment

There are many reasons for a person or family to seek help for mental disorder. These are some reasons why intervention and treatment are initiated:
- *Symptoms are intolerably painful for the individual.* Example: A father is so depressed that he can't go to work or meet his family's needs, so he calls his family doctor.
- *Symptoms are unmanageable.* Example: A 20-year-old client with a diagnosis of **severe and persistent** schizophrenia decides to stop taking his medications and becomes floridly psychotic and disruptive in the neighborhood. The family calls the psychiatrist.
- *Symptoms interrupt daily function.* Example: A woman compulsively cleans her house continuously and is unable to interrupt her cleaning to get her children to school or to make meals.
- *Symptoms cause life crises.* Example: An adolescent tries to commit suicide by cutting her wrists in the school restroom when she finds out she has failed to pass her final exam and go on to high school with her friends.
- *Symptoms result in a crime.* Example: A mother who is dependent on illegal drugs is discovered selling drugs to care for her children and support her habit.

Therapeutic Modalities

A virtual revolution in mental health care has occurred in the past few years in which traditional inpatient hospitalization has been replaced with an entire range of care options. These optional care modalities may offer cost-effective, creative, client-focused alternatives to traditional treatment. Nurses' awareness of the shift in treatment methods ensures optimum client care.

Multiple methods may be used during intervention with clients in any psychiatric setting that include, but are not limited to, inpatient hospital or treatment center, outpatient day treatment program, clinic, home, community center, crisis center, place of employment, and school. The choice of methods for intervening with clients' needs and problems is influenced by several factors, including:
- The client's presenting problems
- The client's knowledge about treatment methods
- The client's ability to make treatment choices

- The client's ability to engage in treatment modality
- The therapist's theoretic background, training, and philosophy
- Type of setting
- Available resources

Approaches vary widely among the scores of available therapies, and it is not an uncommon practice to incorporate several methods (**eclectic approach**) during treatment. Generally clients admitted to an acute care psychiatric setting receive both interactive and biologic types of therapy. Any range of methods may be used in community settings.

Interactive therapies include those in which the client has interpersonal contact with one or more therapists and interaction with other clients. Biologic therapies include use of medications, electroshock therapy, and, more rarely, psychosurgery. Interactive therapies most often used regardless of the theoretic framework, or conceptual model on which they are based, take the form of individual therapy, group therapy, and adjunctive therapies. Box 1-7 lists therapeutic treatment modalities that may be offered in traditional and nontraditional settings. A description of therapies is presented in Part III.

SIGNIFICANCE FOR NURSING

Nurses in the psychiatric setting use many techniques that are derived from nursing theories, as well as theories from other disciplines. It is important for nurses to continue to seek interventions for their clients that are safe and effective, regardless of their origin. Nurses also remain current in their own discipline, learning and using new evidence-based interventions that are continually evaluated for having met expected outcomes. Nurses in the psychiatric setting are adaptable and ready for inevitable change that is the hallmark of the psychiatric arena. This includes learning and practicing new skills to manage threats of violence and terrorism.

Psychiatric nurses must also remain active in their professional organizations and have a voice for increased attention, legislation, and resource allocation for their clients. Individuals with mental disorders, their families, and the community are all affected directly and indirectly by involvement of nurses and other health team members in the care and disposition of their clients.

NURSE ADVOCATES

In psychiatric mental nursing, never has it been more important than now for nurses to consciously take on the role as advocates for clients living with mental disorders. Laws have been passed to provide the mentally ill with equal opportunity for treatment of their disorders, but to date this has not come to full fruition. The general public has great empathy for and volunteers to support treatment for many medical disorders, yet it continues to perceive mental illness as something to be feared, denied, and at worst, ignored. Nurses at the front line of treatment have every opportunity to make changes in the way treatment is delivered to this population and their families.

Box 1-7	Therapeutic Modalities

Medical/biologic treatments
  Medications
  Electroconvulsive therapy (ECT)
Psychotherapy
Crisis intervention
Milieu therapy
Support, psychosocial
  Caregiver support
Therapeutic processes
  Transference (psychology)
  Countertransference (psychology)
Transactional analysis
Reality therapy
Validation therapy
Symbolism (psychology)
  Metaphor
Socioenvironmental therapy
  Client passes
  Group psychotherapy
Psychodrama
Role playing
Support groups
Residential care
Family therapy
Marital therapy
Behavior modification
  Assertiveness training
  Behavior contracting
  Behavior therapy
  Cognitive therapy
  Biofeedback
  Relaxation techniques
    Distraction
    Guided imagery
    Meditation
Biofeedback
Hypnosis
Art therapy
Play therapy
Pet therapy
Music therapy
Dance therapy
Bibliotherapy
Guided imagery
Substance dependence program
Rehabilitation, psychosocial

Nurses begin by demonstrating respect for their clients with mental illness, by continuing to collaborate with other members of the health care team, by supporting organizations that openly and publicly advocate for the mentally ill, by becoming active in legislative decision making, and by voting for individuals who advocate for these clients. Nurses have a large voice that is not being heard in this regard. How might you help in this important cause?

CHAPTER SUMMARY

- Statistics support the worldwide problem of mental disorders and the lack of trained, skilled professionals to meet the challenge.
- Violence and terrorism are real, but the numbers of people affected by either of these is small compared to the number of people with mental disorders.
- Stigma is an obstacle to adequate treatment of those with mental disorders.
- Judgment, stereotypes, and labels emerge from stigma and are detrimental to the population with mental disorders and their families.
- Nurses and other health team members play a major role in reducing stigma for clients.
- Mental health and mental disorder are thoroughly discussed.
- The practical necessity for diagnoses of psychiatric disorders remains even in the face of stigma.
- Primary, secondary, and tertiary levels of prevention of mental disorders are presented, with rationale and practical applications for nurses.
- Humans use conscious and unconscious defensive modes of coping that may be adaptive or maladaptive. Some are healthy modes that lead to productivity, whereas others are unhealthy and inhibit growth.
- The role of the nurse in the psychiatric setting remains a major force in mental health.
- Theoretic background and practice standards are an integral part of preparation for the nurse in the psychiatric setting.
- The art and science of nursing is the basis of effective, evidence-based care of clients in psychiatric mental health nursing. The therapeutic alliance in nursing, the nurse-client relationship, is an essential component of care.
- Nurses need a full understanding of reasons for seeking positions in helping professions. Guidelines describe positive and negative influences for helping relationships.
- The involvement of nurses and other health team members is the cornerstone of client care.

REVIEW QUESTIONS

1. To increase community awareness and decrease the incidence of youth violence the nurse should plan to:
   a. Present seminars for parents at elementary schools.
   b. Provide support groups for juvenile offenders.
   c. Develop an anger management program on the adolescent unit.
   d. Teach anger management classes to youth offenders.

2. A child who pushes over a desk, throws a pencil, and bangs his chair against the wall because his parents did not come to visit him for visiting hours is an example of which defense mechanism:
   a. Reaction formation
   b. Displacement
   c. Acting out
   d. Regression

3. Only a certified clinical nurse specialist in psychiatric mental health nursing may use which of the following?
   a. Counseling
   b. Family therapy
   c. Health teaching
   d. Milieu therapy

4. A client is hospitalized for depression and suicidal ideation after her husband asked her for a divorce. The best nursing response would be:
   a. "I understand that you've been depressed because your husband asked you for a divorce. I know that when I got divorced I was devastated."
   b. "Tell me why you are here."
   c. "Attempting suicide is not the answer to your problems."
   d. "I think that you should forget your husband and move on with your life."

5. A mother of a 10-year-old boy asks the nurse if she could explain the results of her son's psychologic testing. The nurse's response would be to:
   a. Direct her to the treating psychiatrist.
   b. Read the psychologic report and explain the results to the mother.
   c. Explain to the mother that psychologic reports are too difficult to understand and are only meant to be discussed among the treatment team.
   d. Give the phone number of the psychologist's office and explain that the psychologist who conducted the testing will explain the results to her.

REFERENCES

American Nurses Association: *Standards of clinical nursing practice,* Washington, DC, 1998, ANA Publishing.

American Psychiatric Association: *Diagnostic and Statistical Manual of Mental Disorders,* Fourth Edition, Text Revision. Washington, DC, American Psychiatric Association, 2000.

American Nurses Association, American Psychiatric Nurses Association, and International Society of Psychiatric Mental Health Nurses: *Scope and standards of psychiatric mental health nursing practice.* Washington DC, 2000, American Nurses Publishing.

Federal Emergency Management Agency: website: www.fema.gov/areyouready/, March, 2003.

Lensch E: The fight against terrorism, *Commun Coll J* Feb/Mar, 2003

Link B et al: Public conceptions of mental illness: the labels, causes, dangerousness, and social distance, *Am J Public Health* 89:1328-1333, 1999.

Meier D: Skeletal aging. In Kent B, Butler R, editors: *Human aging research: concepts and techniques,* New York, 1988, Raven Press.

Pfefferbaum R: Homeland security: a role for community colleges, *Commun Coll J* Feb/Mar, 2003.

Silver R et al: Nationwide longitudinal study of psychological responses to September 11, *JAMA* 288:10, 2002.

US Department of Health and Human Services: *Health data on older Americans,* Public Health Services, Centers for Disease Control and Prevention, National Center for Health Statistics, No. PHS93-1411, Hyattsville, Md, 1993, USDHHS.

US Department of Health and Human Services: *Mental health: a report of the Surgeon General,* Washington, DC, 1999, USDHHS, Substance Abuses and Mental Health Services Administration, Center for Mental Health Services, National Institutes of Health.

World Health Organization: *International statistical classification of disease and related health problems,* revision 10, ICD-10, Geneva, 1992, WHO.

World Health Organization: *Global burden of disease and injury,* Geneva, 1999, WHO, website: www3.who.int/whosis/menu.cfm.

World Health Organization: *World health report, 1999: making a difference,* Geneva, 1999, WHO, website: www.who.int/whr/1999/.

WHO, website: www.whoint/mipfiles/2008/NCDDiseaseBurden.pdf, p. 11

SUGGESTED READINGS

Andreason NC: *Brave new brain: conquering mental illness in the era of the genome,* London, 2001, Oxford Press.

Brammer L: *The helping relationship: process and skills,* Boston, 1993, Allyn and Bacon.

Caplan G: *Principles of preventive psychiatry,* New York, 1964, Basic Books.

Catalano JT: *Nursing NOW: today's issues, tomorrow's trends,* Philadelphia, ed 3, 2003, FA Davis.

Center for Mental Health Services: *Cultural competence standards in managed care mental health services for underserved/underrepresented racial/ethnic groups,* Rockville, Md, 1998, The Center.

Gazzaniga M et al: *Cognitive neuroscience: the biology of the mind,* New York, 1998, WW Norton.

Institute of Medicine: *Reducing risks for mental disorders: committee on prevention of mental disorders,* Washington, DC, 1994, National Academy Press.

Institute of Medicine Violence in Families: *Assessing, prevention, and treatment programs,* Washington, DC, 1998, National Academy Press.

Kandel ER: A new intellectual framework for psychiatry, *Am J Psychiatry* 155:457-469, 1994.

Lamb HR: A century and a half of psychiatric rehabilitation in USA, *Hosp Commun Psychiatry* 45:1015-1020, 1994.

Marjoribanks D: Ethnicity, birth order and family environment, *Psych Rep* vol 84, 1999.

Martin C: The theory of critical thinking of nursing, *Nurs Educ Perspective* 23:5, 2002.

Montgomery S: Understanding depression and its treatment, *J Clin Psychiatry* 61:6, 2000.

National Council on Disability Report: *The well-being of our nation: an intergenerational vision of effective mental health services and supports,* website: www.ncd.gov.

National League for Nursing: *Educational competencies for graduates of associate degree nursing programs,* Boston, 2000, Jones and Bartlett.

National League for Nursing: *Educational competencies for graduates of baccalaureate degree nursing programs,* Boston, 2000, Jones and Bartlett.

NANDA International (2003). NANDA Nursing Diagnoses: Definitions and Classification 2003-2004. Philadelphia: NANDA.

NIH News Release: NIMH awards new grants in response to terrorist attacks of September 11, 2001, website: www.nih.gov/news/pr/apr2002/nimh-18.htm.

Peplau H: *Interpersonal relations in nursing,* New York, 1952, Putnam.

Peplau H: Interpersonal relations: a theoretical framework of application in nursing practice, *Nurs Sci Q* vol 5, no 1, 1992.

Regier D, Burke J: Epidemiology. In Sadock B, Sadock V (editors): *Comprehensive textbook of psychiatry,* vol 7, Philadelphia, 2000, Lippincott Williams & Wilkins.

Sadock B, Sadock V: *Comprehensive textbook of psychiatry,* vol VII, Philadelphia, 2000, Lippincott, Williams & Wilkins.

Silver RC: Nationwide longitudinal study of psychological responses to September 11, *JAMA* 288:10, 2002.

US Department of Health and Human Services: *Healthy people 2010: understanding and improving health and objectives for improving health,* ed 2, Washington, DC, 2000, US Government Printing Office.

Veenema T: Chemical and biological terrorism, *Nurs Educ Perspectives* 23:2, 2002.

Veenema T: Shortage of nurses: looking for a few good men, *Minority Nurse* Spring, 2002.

World Health Organization: *Global consultation on violence and health. Violence: a public health priority,* Geneva, 1996, WHO.

ONLINE RESOURCES

American Nurses Association: www.nursingworld.org

American Psychiatric Nurses Association: www.apna.org

FAQ's educational requirements and schools: www.allnursingschools.com

Harvard Medical School/Beth Israel Deaconess Medical Center—Mind/Body Medical Institute: www.mbmi.nih.gov

Health Resources and Services Administration, Bureau of Health Professionals: http://bhpr.hrsa.gov/nursing/

Healthy People 2010 report: www.health.gov/healthypeople

International Society of Psychiatric–Mental Health Nurses: www.ISPN-Psych.org

Initiative on depression in public health: www.who.int/ncd

National Council on Disability; features full reports on public mental health system in United States: www.ncd.gov

National Institute for Mental Health: www.nln.org

National League for Nursing: www.nimh.nih.gov

National Library of Medicine, with nursing and mental health information and articles through PUBMED: www.nlm.nih.gov

National Mental Health Association: www.nmha.org

Nothing to Hide: Mental Illness in the Family: information about the book and exhibit by the same name: www.familydiv.org

Rehabilitative services for people with schizophrenia: www.reintegration.com

Stem cell research: www.stemcellresearch.org

Substance Abuse and Mental Health Statistics Bureau national statistics on alcohol, tobacco, illegal drug use, treatment programs: www.samhsa.gov/oas/oasftp.htm

2

Clinical Experiences: Rewards, Challenges, and Solutions

Patricia A. Holoday Worret

OBJECTIVES

- Identify rewards and challenges that occur when working with clients in the psychiatric mental health setting.

- List solutions for challenges that arise in the psychiatric mental health setting.

- Discuss the necessity for synthesizing versus compartmentalizing knowledge and skills in the psychiatric mental health area.

- State the importance for the nurse to prioritize all aspects of activity when working with clients who have mental disorders.

- Describe how the characteristics of adaptability and flexibility serve the nurse when working in any psychiatric setting.

- Describe the necessity for overcoming fears of the psychiatric mental health area.

- Describe the outcome of keeping secrets with or making promises to psychiatric clients.

- State ways to reinforce strengths of clients and families.

- State benefits to individuals, families, and the community from reinforcing strengths and offering support.

The nurse who engages with clients in the psychiatric setting receives many rewards and also meets many challenges. **Rewards** come in several forms. Some are obvious and easily identified; others are not obvious, but rather are subtle, and are recognized and enjoyed only by nurses who are aware and open to receiving the rewards. Nurses who can reframe most situations into becoming rewards are particularly fortunate.

Challenges also exist in this field and are the reason why many nurses choose to work in a psychiatric setting. **Solutions** are available for the challenges that may arise and are found in both the theoretic principles of psychiatric nursing and actual experiences within the clinical practice setting. This chapter discusses some of the rewards, challenges, and solutions that nurses encounter in their psychiatric experiences. Many additional rewards, challenges, and solutions will be a part of the reader's own clinical experience in psychiatric nursing. It is suggested that nurses maintain a written personal journal (a reward in itself), that will measure and record their evolving growth in nurse-client interactions, as well as identify many gifts that emerge in this specialty.

REWARDS

Some of the many rewards nurses experience become evident in their direct statements. The following examples were offered in interviews with several nurses who spoke of their rewards for working in the psychiatric setting:

"When a client is being discharged after having been suicidal, looks me in the eye, and sincerely says thank you for helping him or her choose life again, that is the ultimate reward for any work."

"In all my nursing experience, I have come to think there is no greater pain than the kind these clients endure, some of them for a lifetime. I consider that helping them to meet their needs is a profound privilege."

"One thing about the acute care psychiatric setting is that it is never the same two days in a row, and is never boring."

"When a client suddenly gains insight into a situation or problem that they have defended against for a long time….when their own light bulb turns on and they understand, I find that rewarding."

"After working with a family whose members have been estranged due to one member's disruptive disorder, and seeing them heal their relationships, I feel rewarded, and fortunate to have helped and observed the growth."

"At the end of some days I feel exhausted; then a client with Alzheimer's who has not spoken all day will have a glimmer of recognition for me and I feel the day's work was worthwhile."

"No other discipline of nursing calls for the use of so many different skills. In psychiatric nursing the nurse has to be prepared for anything. It is so much more than caring for just the mind. In that way it is stimulating and rewarding."

"It was a reward when I finally understood that what I thought were only minor changes in some clients were actually giant steps for the client who was compromised by a severe and persistent mental disorder. When clients were trying hard to make a difference in their own lives, I subsequently saw them as minor heroes. I was thankful for the insight and felt rewarded to have assisted in any way."

It is a fortunate nurse who can find the rewards in this challenging discipline. These rewards are the reason nurses remain in psychiatric nursing.

CHALLENGES AND SOLUTIONS

As stated in the first chapter, knowledge and practice are inseparable components of successful nursing care. The core of the nursing profession is *knowledge* that is derived from a variety of sources, namely the basic sciences, as well as the art and science of nursing. Adequate research-based theoretic background forms a foundation for the next level in the complex matrix of interacting with humans, and that next level is *practice*. Knowledge and practice together are necessary to meet client's needs and problems in any psychiatric setting.

The following section consists of challenges that may exist in the psychiatric setting with some suggested solutions. Readers are provided with practical principles and examples for focusing on specific client-centered problems and needs that the nurse may encounter, as well as solutions for solving the problems. It is by no means a complete list, but is meant to assist nurses to recognize what may occur in the psychiatric arena. Readers are encouraged to add their own experiences to this list of suggestions. The following challenges and solutions offer a compass for navigating on the journey through psychiatric nursing.

Challenge: Synthesize Knowledge and Skills

General principles of nursing provide a basis on which the nurse continues to build when the nurse reaches the specialty discipline of Psychiatric Mental Health Nursing. General nursing principles are never forsaken, but are incorporated to provide comprehensive care for clients, individuals, families, and the community. The nurse synthesizes all principles and skills learned in early levels of nursing education with skills that are specific for psychiatric nursing. Basic medical nursing knowledge and skills often save many psychiatric clients from undue pain and suffering when the psychiatric nurse can critically integrate nursing principles, as revealed in the following example:

Jason was admitted to the adult psychiatric intensive care unit over the weekend because of an acute episode of severe and persistent schizophrenia, a disorder he had had for several years. Jason's condition was exacerbated by his recent refusal to take his prescribed antipsychotic medications and his symptoms returned soon after that point. He had been a patient on the unit many times and staff thought they were prepared to help him manage his symptoms by using techniques and methods that had proven successful in the past.

However, the treatment team became frustrated because Jason did not respond as expected. They continued to discuss and report his symptoms, and chart about his persistent delusions and his lack of progress. Jason kept talking about the "fire in his stomach that was put there by the devil." His delusional system was elaborate and included a theme that staff had not encountered with him before. Regardless of the interventions tried by the staff, he could not be distracted from his obvious fear and suffering from what staff called his "delusion."

On Monday, Sue, the RN unit manager, returned from vacation. She was in the habit of making rounds on all clients on her unit each day after report. She did a basic mental status assessment on each client and physical assessments on those clients about whom she had questions. She actively listened and talked with Jason, did a mental status assessment and a physical assessment, and concluded that Jason seemed to have a genuine physical problem in his abdomen that was not entirely delusional. She called both the psychiatrist and the medical physician, suggested an order for diagnostic tests, explained procedures to Jason, and assured him that the staff was trying everything they could to help him. Laboratory tests revealed that Jason had a stomach ulcer and treatment was begun.

Alleviation of Jason's stomach symptoms cleared the way for him to engage in his therapeutic medical regimen and psychosocial treatment plan.

Sue used communication plus several other nursing skills to help Jason describe the pain he was having. She was not stuck solely in psychiatric interpretations. She gathered data and then critically analyzed and synthesized information. Sue correctly determined that perhaps Jason's symptoms included an overriding medical condition that interfered with the psychosocial interventions and that his current condition was due to a combination of psychiatric and medical problems, manifesting as psychiatric symptoms.

Solutions

- The nurse considers all possible sources of each problem. A good question to ask self while assessing a client is, "*What else* can this be?" Even after coming to a conclusion, avoid becoming complacent. It is human nature to want closure, so nurses reach an answer, feel satisfied, and may conclude prematurely when a feasible answer is found. That first answer reached may be only part of the whole. Always ask the question, "What else can this be?" at that time. Identifying the client problem is like detective work. Curiosity rather than complacency is a desirable component of the nurse's role.
- Draw from all nursing knowledge each day. Avoid compartmentalizing information. A good psychiatric nurse is also a good medical nurse. Conversely, nurses who choose to work in other nursing areas frequently "forget" skills of psychiatric nursing that may be a client's priority regardless of the admitting diagnosis. The body, mind, and spirit are one—wise nurses avoid dismembering it.

Challenge: Determine Priorities

Prioritization of nursing diagnoses, expected client outcomes, and nursing interventions are the most essential actions that psychiatric nurses learn and practice. Often there

is time to carefully consider priorities, but frequently emergencies in the acute care psychiatric setting demand that the nurse prioritize diagnoses and interventions immediately.

Carmine, a 25-year-old woman, was admitted to the psychiatric facility after medical clearance for a serious suicide attempt. She had moved to town a year ago because of a job opportunity and was currently living alone. According to a friend who brought her to the facility, Carmine recently had abused multiple street drugs, was depressed for several weeks, and had lost 20 pounds during the last few months.

After assessment by a psychiatric intake nurse who determined that Carmine was definitely a potential risk but not an imminent risk for harming herself, Carmine was assigned a room near the nurse's station on the Psychiatric Intensive Care Unit for close observation. She was put on suicide precautions using a 15-minute-close-watch protocol. Because the nurse observed that Carmine was dehydrated, her fluid and food intake was closely monitored and managed by the staff. Carmine was able to sign a contract for safety while in the facility but explained that she couldn't stop thinking of jumping off a particular bridge.

Carmine displayed no withdrawal symptoms from the drugs she apparently took in the recent past, so the nurse determined that this problem would be addressed in the near future.

Next the client was assigned a contact nurse on each shift who set aside specific time to meet with and encourage Carmine to verbalize her thoughts and feelings about her situation and condition and her continued ability to adhere to the contract she signed for maintaining safety.

Carmine's parents were called. They revealed her past history of hospitalization as an adolescent for severe anorexia nervosa. They explained that she did respond favorably to that treatment and remained out of the hospital until this time. The parents described Carmine's present inability to adjust to separation from the family and a recent breakup with a boyfriend.

Carmine remained free from self-harm on the unit and soon began attending groups that focused on cognitive therapy, substance abuse, and relationship topics. A social worker was then assigned to follow through with discussions about her plans for family contact and job decisions.

The nurse in this scenario first addressed Carmine's most salient problem, which was to help her avoid self-harm, and then followed through in order of priority to assist her toward wellness.

Solutions

Prioritization means following these steps:
- Obtain all necessary data
- Sort and organize information
- Identify most immediate problems/needs
- Intervene with the client in order of importance using the following sequence:
  - Safety
  - Health
  - Intrapersonal problems and needs
  - Interpersonal problems and needs

The preceding steps were carefully followed in the former example to ensure the client's well-being. It is also important to know that priorities sometimes must be modified on the basis of each unique situation, and nurses are called on to be flexible and to carefully discern when priorities seem equally important. This is explained in the next example.

Challenge: Practice Dynamic vs. Static Prioritization

Prioritization is a necessary nursing action, but understanding, assimilating, and adhering to the dynamic nature of prioritizing are also essential for nurses in the psychiatric setting. This implies that (1) the nurse is continually rearranging the priorities list; (2) what was most important 5 minutes ago may quickly move to a less important position, being replaced by another priority; and (3) the nurse is alert and always ready for changes on the unit. Psychiatric nurses with experience have little difficulty changing their own action direction; they can also delegate to appropriate staff when necessary.

Nurses who need absolute sameness in schedules, activities, and tasks every day when they come to work may not be comfortable or effective in a psychiatric setting. A psychiatric nurse is able to see the plan for the day as potentially fluid and unpredictable while continually maintaining a safe unit.

Some nurses meet this challenge and are comfortable and effective in psychiatric nursing; other nurses find it difficult to work in an unpredictable setting. When it is established that the nurse is effective in a changing environment, priorities are carefully arranged according to clients' problems and needs; but change is expected, welcomed, and met throughout each day.

Richard, the unit nurse manager on an acute care unit, made it a habit to be out on the unit several times a day to assess and interact with clients. Monique was admitted with a diagnosis of severe, recurrent major depression. She had been admitted to the facility several times in the past for suicide ideation, and this time because she made a serious attempt on her life. She reluctantly signed a "no-suicide" contract.

Monique's physician asked Richard to use his communication skills and meet with her each day. Richard and Monique agreed to meet and talk after lunch each day, which they did on the first day after admission. On the second day, at the start of their scheduled meeting time, Jose, a client admitted that morning for treatment of acute psychosis, began shouting and pacing up and down the hall, screaming that he had to get out of this "prison" to take care of his children. He claimed that the end of the world was coming today, and he needed to be with his children or they would not go to heaven.

Richard realized how important the meeting time was to Monique, whose condition was fragile, but he explained that he had to leave because of Jose's acute need at this time, and Richard's position as unit manager made his presence on the unit a priority. He left Monique and told her he would return as soon as he could. Richard assigned a mental health counselor to stay with Monique, and then he gathered the rest of the staff to assist Jose.

Richard returned to his meeting with Monique as soon as the crisis was over.

This example demonstrates the necessity for determining priorities and acting on them when they change. Both client situations were important and each client was in an acute need state. These were probably two equally important priorities, but the nurse determined that Jose's situation needed his attention first. Frequently the events necessitating prioritization are less acute, but nevertheless are important enough to demand continual scrutiny, action, and flexibility by the nurse.

Solution

- Carefully follow the steps for prioritizing diagnoses, client expected outcomes, and nursing interventions as outlined in an earlier example, but be prepared to change order of priorities when an immediate crisis demands it.

Challenge: Overcome Fear of the Psychiatric Setting

As described in Chapter 1, clients with severe psychiatric disorders are sometimes treated unfairly by the public. They are frequently feared, avoided, alienated, or treated with disgust; they often fail to find sustained compassion. The beginning nurse's preconceived ideas about the psychiatric environment are largely influenced by negative stereotypes portrayed in films, television, books, magazines, and video or Internet games. In addition to stereotyping, other sources of avoidance and worry are fear of the unknown, fear of being injured or rejected by the client, doubt about nurse's own skills and ability, and fear of being exposed or embarrassed. A student or a nurse who is new to the experience in this setting may have difficulty entering a psychiatric unit for the first time. Of course, nurses are constantly aware of clients' behaviors and take necessary precautions to ensure safety for clients and staff. This section focuses on the nurse who wishes to modify his or her own responses to fear.

Nurses who can avoid general stereotyping find that their fear diminishes once they gain experience interacting with these clients. Nurses about to enter a psychiatric setting for the first time who are anxious, however, may miss many opportunities for meaningful therapeutic interaction with clients. Because avoidance is a companion of anxiety, the new nurse who is anxious avoids interacting with clients who are in need of contact and, as a result, misses both valuable moments to learn from the interaction and opportunities to provide therapeutic interventions for the client.

Learning in this setting happens through doing. By practicing new skills, the nurse learns about clients and about self in relation to the clients. All that is lost when the nurse fails to take the first steps into what initially appears to be a risk by approaching the client. Success comes from setting aside personal fears and taking client-focused action.

Chuck was about to enter his first day on the unit in the nursing program's psychiatric rotation. He and his family lived in the same neighborhood with Mr. Tanner, a man who had had what his parents and neighbors described as a "nervous breakdown," and had been in the psychiatric hospital. After discharge Mr. Tanner was unpredictable. Sometimes he seemed lucid and polite, but at other times he had episodes of loud shouting and cursing in his house and on the street in front of his house. His family always apologized for him, and sometimes he had to go back into the hospital.

Chuck's parents told the children to stay away from Mr. Tanner and not to play with the Tanner children anymore. Mrs. Tanner dropped out of the neighborhood women's bridge club. The Tanner children were alienated in the neighborhood. Families were sometimes afraid for their own and their children's safety. Everyone talked about the Tanners and some people called them names.

Three days before Chuck was to enter the psychiatric clinical rotation he saw Mr. Tanner taken to the hospital again. He would be there when Chuck arrived. Chuck was scared but did not tell anyone. Without knowing this situation, his instructor assigned Chuck and two other students to the psychiatric intensive care unit where Mr. Tanner was a patient. Chuck told the instructor when he saw the printed schedule, but the instructor did not change his schedule. Instead the instructor assured Chuck he could do this, reviewed with Chuck what he had learned in class and in the textbook about beginning interactions, and reviewed the confidentiality policy with him.

Chuck heard the unit report and then went to the unit where he met with Mr. Tanner who was recovering from a recurrent episode of bipolar mania. Mr. Tanner still had some of the symptoms Chuck read about, but was beginning to gain control of his behavior. Mr. Tanner recognized Chuck and agreed to talk with him each day after Chuck told him about the confidentiality policy. They established a contract. Chuck's fears quickly were dispelled as he began to see Mr. Tanner as a man, a husband, and a father with a mood disorder problem rather as the problem itself. When Mr. Tanner was able, he told Chuck how remorseful he was about his family having to suffer this disorder with him. Chuck felt privileged to have this learning opportunity and growth experience. He was professional with Mr. Tanner and kept his interactions confidential.

When Mr. Tanner was discharged, Chuck made it a point to greet him and his family each time he saw them. Chuck was able to slowly assist his own family and the other neighbors to see Mr. Tanner and his family as human beings who deserved respect. Confidentiality was never breached, but the Tanner's slowly began to feel welcome in the neighborhood.

Solutions

- Begin interactions! Talking with clients, even if the nurse does not want to, breaks the avoidance pattern. Each client reserves the right to refuse interactions (e.g., may need to finish a project, timing is off), and the nurse must not take this personally.
- Approach each client on the unit using therapeutic communication techniques and open-ended questions and statements whenever possible.
- Make a conscious effort to avoid stereotyping. If this is a planned objective, it is easier to accomplish.
- Focus on the client versus self and performance. When thinking about what the client has to say and showing genuine concern, it is less probable that the nurse will worry about own appearance or performance. The connection with a client and the result is usually rewarding to both client and nurse. The client becomes less threatening when the nurse interacts with him and sees the client as a human being instead of a psychiatric label to be feared.
- Learn basic communication techniques and skills and practice at every opportunity.
- Challenge self to work with clients with varied diagnoses. Learn about the symptoms associated with each psychiatric diagnosis and learn specific interventions intended for these symptoms. The outcome is effective nursing care. Perfecting skills brings a sense of control in each situation that further reduces fear.
- Keep expectations about performance realistic. Nurses are not expected to be therapists by the end of the first few clinical experiences, so relax about performance.
- Nurses become more skilled and feel better each day as they practice and continue to learn about this specialty. Increased skill will be its own reward.
- Use positive affirmations such as, "I am doing well and am exactly where I should be in the level of my performance."
- Review theory and policies about safety, confidentiality, and boundaries.
- Write actual objectives before each clinical day. These objectives will become the nursing plan and function as rehearsal tools for the actual clinical experience. An increase in confidence follows. Some examples of objectives are:
  - Interact with a client who has major depression and use the following interventions:
    - Ensure client safety by following the unit procedures (suicide assessment and precautions)
    - Interact with the client, allowing time for answers
    - Create a safe environment for client to interact
    - Encourage client to express thoughts and feelings
    - When client is able, assist client to join milieu groups and activities
    - Remembering that the client with depression may defy an alliance; continue to initiate contacts
  - Use the following therapeutic communication techniques with a depressed client:
    - Silence
    - Reflection
    - Giving recognition
    - Offering self
    - Encouraging comparisons

Safety is always the most important nursing intervention and should be the primary objective of the unit manager, instructor, and student or new nurse. It is assumed that either the unit will be safe for new nurses to practice their skills, or the inexperienced nurses will be reassigned to other units. Learning the agency policies and procedures is necessary, and selected policy and procedures are part of the orientation process for students and employees.

Challenge: Keep No Secrets and Avoid Making Promises

When clients are admitted to an acute psychiatric setting, they may have important information concerning their lives that they are withholding or have withheld for a long time. Content of the "secret" can be anything, but if it is significant, the secret is a burden that the client is bearing alone, and it may reach a point when it becomes unbearable. When the client begins to trust staff in a clinical situation or setting, the client realizes how difficult it is to hold onto the closely held secret and that help is as close as the next trustworthy nurse.

When the client feels safe and able to trust, the client frequently chooses a staff member who has been helping to process the client's problems. In some cases the client resists telling the physician or the staff about the secret, but feels compelled to share the secret and chooses a student who seems the least likely to tell anyone else. In some cases the student has been interacting with a client for several clinical days and may be in the working phase of the nurse-client relationship when the student becomes the recipient of the client's "secret." The student or staff nurse knows about this principle and acts according to guidelines. The following example clarifies this principle.

Cheryl was in her fifth week of the psychiatric rotation in a registered nursing program. She felt comfortable on the psychiatric unit, having diligently studied the theory and practiced all the skills she could each day that she was assigned to the clinical setting. Cheryl established a contract with Ophelia, a 15-year-old female client on the adolescent locked unit, and met with her each clinical day. The client had been admitted by her parents for out of control behaviors that included polysubstance abuse, running away from home for weeks at a time, not attending school, and hanging out with "friends" who were many years older and who had past drug histories that worried her parents. Ophelia said they were good friends because they gave her what she needed. She said she didn't get what she needed at home.

One day Cheryl was preparing to leave the unit to attend a scheduled adjunctive therapy session. Ophelia stopped her and quietly said she had a secret. Cheryl told Ophelia that she was scheduled to attend a meeting and had 20 minutes to talk. The client continued to say that she wanted to tell Cheryl but that Cheryl had to promise not to tell anyone else. Cheryl was surprised by the disclosure but maintained her composure because she remembered from class discussion and her reading what she had to do. She told Ophelia that she couldn't keep a secret that may affect her care, and that the physician and the staff work as a team who together would be able to help her. Then Cheryl continued with the next step. Instead of stopping there, Cheryl told the client that her secret probably was very important or she wouldn't have brought it up and then offered to talk with her about it for the next 15 minutes.

Ophelia cried as she told Cheryl that she had been sexually abused for 3 years by an uncle who came to her home often and frequently offered to stay with her and her younger sister when her parents went out for the evening. She said the uncle threatened to abuse her sister if she told, and that her parents would not believe her, but would blame Ophelia if they found out.

Cheryl listened and responded therapeutically, using many of the recently learned communication skills to facilitate the client's disclosure. The student empathized with what Ophelia had been through. Ophelia said that her recent "craziness" and acting out made her scared for her life, and she was worried about her sister. Cheryl commented on Ophelia's bravery in telling what had to be told. Ophelia said she felt relieved.

Cheryl reminded Ophelia that she had to leave for the meeting but that she would be back the next clinical day, and would get another nurse to be with her now. Cheryl reported the incident to RN unit manager who assigned an RN to respond to the client's needs. Cheryl discussed this incident with her instructor, and the class processed this important learning experience in postconference, learning vicariously and gaining insight from Cheryl's experience.

This example amplifies the importance of the nurse telling the client that the information will have to be shared when the client asks the nurse to keep a secret. Clients usually choose to tell the information anyway because of the need for relief from their burden, and also to get some help. If the inexperienced nurse or student makes the mistake of promising to keep the secret and then tells significant material that must be told to the treatment team, the result is almost without exception traumatic for client, nurse, or both. The client feels betrayed "again" by someone she trusted and usually refuses to talk with that nurse thereafter. This perceived betrayal may also hinder trust in other members of the treatment team. All the actual and potential good work that was and could be done through the nurse-client relationship is disrupted or ended for the time being.

Solutions

- Learn the theory for avoiding making promises and keeping client "secrets."
- Practice and role play telling a client that you cannot keep secrets and why, so that, when the actual situation occurs, the nurse is ready for appropriate therapeutic intervention.
- Resolve to keep the communication open after the nurse says she cannot keep a secret, by offering to discuss the client's information because it is important to the client.
- List several topics that may fit the category of a client secret, and use the list as a rehearsal and preparation tool.

Challenge: Emphasizing Client and Family Strengths

When nurses begin a psychiatric specialty they have a great deal to learn about mental disorders and life crises. As a result much energy and interest are channeled in that direction, namely gathering information and remembering all the details about client's disorders and the crisis situation that may surround a disruptive psychiatric episode. In addition mental disorders are often fascinating and sometimes dramatic to read about, so it is understandable that the focus quickly shifts away from the healthy aspects and strengths of every client and toward the disorders. However, client

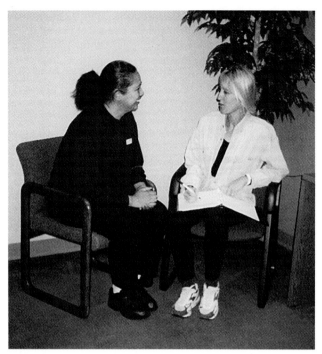

FIGURE 2-1. An interaction between a psychiatric nurse and client. The nurse and client are discussing the client's strengths while she makes a list to keep for personal reference and reflection.

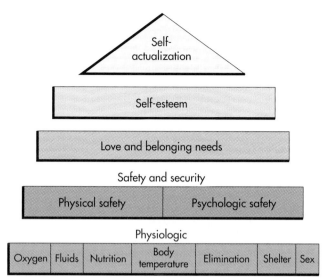

FIGURE 2-2. Maslow's hierarchy of needs. (Redrawn from Maslow AH: *Motivation and personality,* Upper Saddle River, NJ, 1970, Prentice Hall.)

strengths are the key to wellness, and nurses keep that in mind as they assist clients to help themselves through their own crisis.

Nurses and all other members of the health care team must assist the client, family, and staff to identify client strengths and work with the clients to build strengths, increase competence, and reinforce reasons for seeking health and for living (Figure 2-1). Unless the client and family become invested in this pattern, the client is at risk for failing to succeed in overcoming life crises, or to learn to live with a recurrent disorder.

For many reasons clients and their families are not always able to identify strengths at the beginning of an acute psychiatric episode. For example, one or more members may be in shock or denial, or may be angry about the episode or the client's behavior. When clients are psychotic, severely depressed, under the influence of substances, or have low self-esteem, they are frequently unable to identify strengths. The family may be able to focus on only one thing at a time, and it may not be client strengths at that time. The nurse is able to assess client/family readiness for moving toward positive aspects of the current disruptive event and gives them time to understand and accept what has occurred.

At a time like this, nurses can recall Maslow's hierarchy of needs. Clients are usually not ready to self-actualize when their basic needs are unmet as a result of a disruptive episode of a severe mental disorder (Figure 2-2). When the time is right, however, ideally the nurse assists client and

family to identify and reinforce the client and family's strengths. When strengths are discussed, negative aspects of the situation are minimized, whereas courage, self-esteem, and motivation increase.

Nurses are continually reminded and aware that the allotted time for helping clients has been greatly diminished because of managed care and premature discharges. Thus clients are often discharged well before the staff has time to intervene in all areas they know are important for clients to maintain wellness. Nurses must act much sooner in the treatment plan to discuss strengths, or miss the opportunity to help in this regard.

Solutions
- Assess client and family readiness for identifying strengths. Nurse may have objective input but does not make a list of strengths for the client(s) but encourages client.
- Assist client to name specific reasons and benefits for client getting and staying well.
- If client is unable to verbalize strengths, modify the plan, or use other methods: (1) the client may be able to make a list after the meeting with the nurse; assign it as homework before next meeting; (2) the nurse may need to allow more time for clients to process the information; (3) the client may be able to draw the "reasons" in art therapy, or express strengths in recreational therapy or in other types of alternative therapy.
- Ask the client what another member of the family, clergy, or friend would say about him or her concerning his or her strengths.
- Have client attend multidisciplinary team meeting and hear what the physician and other staff members say are his or her strengths.
- Assign a task to a client process group where client's strengths are discussed.

Challenge: Expect Variations of Change vs. Dramatic Change

Unlike most physical sciences that are predictable and exact, psychiatry and psychology will sometimes seem elusive and ambiguous to the nurse. The definition, description, and categorization of psychiatric diagnoses in the *Diagnostic and Statistical Manual of Mental Disorders*, fourth edition, text revision (DSM-IV-TR), appear exact. Because of the complex nature of human beings, however, symptoms of the same name are manifested and expressed in unique ways by each client.

The nurse may initially think in absolutes, seeing symptoms as being totally present or totally absent (i.e., *all or none*). In reality, the client's symptoms may change slightly or dramatically over hours or days (i.e., *more or less*). Because psychiatric symptoms cannot always be measured by laboratory values, charts, and graphs, they are sometimes overlooked or missed completely by beginning nurses. Subtle changes may be clues that more dramatic changes are coming, so increases or decreases in symptoms need to be carefully noted, as in the following clinical situation.

Angela was admitted to the psychiatric acute care unit because she was jogging down the center of a busy two-way traffic boulevard and taunting motorists. She was wearing multiple layers of brightly colored clothes, high heels, and excessive jewelry. On admission she shouted out about the indignity of having to be in this facility against her will, which she termed a violation of her "personal, important rights." She was diagnosed with bipolar disorder, mania type.

After several days of quiet surroundings, consistent unit routines, staff interventions, and medication (which she had stopped taking before admission), she calmed down. Staff reports and charting stated that she seemed ready to return home.

However, just before discharge, her contact staff person noted that she began to change her clothes every few hours and that the content of her conversation centered on "very important" things she was planning to accomplish when she got home. The staff member asked her if she had been taking her medication. Angela admitted she had been putting it in the toilet because she was getting too "normal" to get her plans accomplished. Discharge was postponed.

Solutions

Solutions to this challenge include:
- Keep clients' expected outcomes hopeful but realistic.
- Avoid predicting client progress.
- Be prepared for and accept an unpredictable course toward wellness.
- Avoid absolute "black and white" thinking.

Symptoms are **dynamic** and are more like shades of gray than black and white. The nurse should observe for fluctuation of symptoms rather than **static**, set patterns of behaviors and responses.

For example, a client who is paranoid may demonstrate mistrust by being loud and accusatory on admission. He may then quiet down but remain guarded, suspicious, and controlled on subsequent days. The symptom of paranoia is the same, but the manifestations change depending on the client's internal stimuli, the unit environment, the present situation or events, and the client's personality style.

Another point is to write care plans reflecting realistic appraisal of the client's symptoms, as seen in the following partial nursing care plan. Note that the correct realistic expectations indicate symptom reduction (more or less) rather than total absence (all or none).

Nursing Diagnosis. Disturbed thought processes related to inability to process internal and external stimuli, secondary to Bipolar disorder; psychosocial stressors that exceed ability to cope; noncompliance with medication regimen.

Expected Outcomes

REALISTIC	UNREALISTIC
Client will verbalize that her thinking was disturbed and put her in danger (within 1 week).	Grandiose delusions will be absent in 1 week.

In some cases it is unrealistic to expect complete absence of symptoms. Interdisciplinary treatment plans aim at symptom reduction within reasonable time limits, with concurrent expectations that clients will achieve these objectives with assistance. Symptom "cure" is an unreasonable expectation for some clients.

Challenge: Avoid Evaluative Responses

A general principle in psychiatric nursing states that when communicating with clients the nurse should avoid using **evaluative responses** and statements that indicate approval or disapproval (e.g., good or bad, right or wrong) about the client's appearance, progress, or behavior. A more effective response from the nurse is neutral recognition. Consider the following clinical situation.

Mrs. Ravella, a 72-year-old woman, was hospitalized after the death of her spouse of 53 years. Although she had been suffering from major depression and chronic low self-esteem for several decades, she had remained loyal and loving. After admission, Mrs. Ravella wore dark, drab clothing every day and cared for her hygiene only after constant encouragement from staff. After several days, she showered and came to breakfast wearing a brightly flowered dress. Jane, a nurse with little experience, was assigned to the unit. She said, "Oh, Mrs. Ravella, you look so pretty in that dress. It's so much better than all those dark clothes you've been wearing." Mrs. Ravella lowered her head and returned to her room. She refused breakfast, lunch, and activities, saying she didn't feel well. She came to dinner in her dark, drab clothing.

Withdrawn or depressed people reject praise because it is the opposite of their own present negative self-image. Praise conflicts with the client's mind-set of, "I'm ugly," "I'm worthless," "I deserve nothing." The client either fails to hear the praise, or the praise is discredited. Disapproval only serves to reinforce pathology, so it also needs to be avoided. Both strong approval or disapproval also signify an authorative or judgmental position.

On the other hand, nurses sometimes learn to avoid direct approval or disapproval but mistakenly substitute indifference. Neutrality and indifference are not the same. **Indifference** manifests as disconnected, unconcerned, aloof separation from the client's needs and situation; it is the antithesis of psychiatric nursing. Nurses can still provide a necessary warm human experience and environment by maintaining **neutrality**—interaction with the client that shows respect and acceptance but not excessive approval or disapproval. Showing indifference toward a client who is mentally or emotionally compromised is like having the person take an ice cold shower in the dead of winter. It is certain to snuff out any spark of remaining spirit or hope.

Solutions

Solutions to showing appropriate evaluative responses include:

- Focus on behaviors, not on the person.
- Be neutral but not indifferent.
- Avoid evaluative statements.
- Use statements of recognition.

Of course, limits may need to be set appropriately on self-defeating behaviors. When doing the latter, the nurse comments on behaviors while avoiding statements about the person's worth. Compare the nurse's comments to the client in the following two examples:

Correct: "During group yesterday, it was agreed that each client would be ready to go on the field trip by 8 AM. Because you are refusing to dress, the trip is behind schedule. The bus will leave in 15 minutes." (Comment on behavior)

Incorrect: "You are so slow and undependable. Everyone is on the bus and thinks you're terrible for holding up the field trip." (Comment on the person's worth)

Neutral statements recognize the person's behavior. Recall Mrs. Ravella and the brightly flowered dress. Appropriate neutral statements to her would be, "I see you showered before breakfast, Mrs. Ravella," and "You're wearing a brightly flowered dress today." These statements, which imply neither approval nor disapproval, offer recognition and may elicit responses from the client that promote further insight into her problems. On the other hand, evaluative statements close communication, and the client either withdraws from the interaction or becomes defensive.

Two more examples of neutral statements follow.

"You decided to join the group today, Tom. Seats are not assigned, so sit anywhere you wish."

"I notice you received all your points yesterday for attending school and the scheduled activities, Amber."

Evaluative statements are discouraged for other reasons as well. If staff praises the client too soon, he or she may

fear support will be withdrawn. Even though he or she is rehearsing new behaviors, the client may still feel vulnerable and revert to old behaviors to regain imagined loss of support. Or, a client may believe he or she is acceptable only if he or she looks or behaves in the specified evaluative way. If the client cannot comply with the evaluation, he or she may feel even more unworthy.

Some psychiatric nurses may disagree with this practice and freely offer praise for positive behavior. This practice has merit when it is clear that the client is ready to receive praise. Each case is unique, but the nurse has a responsibility to understand the client and the situation before choosing responses. False praise is nontherapeutic.

Challenge: Make Observations vs. Inferences

It is sometimes difficult for the nurse who is new to the psychiatric setting to avoid inferences about a client's behavior. An **inference** is an interpretation of behavior that is made by finding motive and forming conclusions without having all of the information. When inferences are made, the nurse interprets the client's behavior, decides on a reason, assigns a motive, and forms a conclusion. There is great potential for error and unfairness in this process.

Some dangers in drawing inferences are that the nurse is operating from his or her own experience and frame of reference that may have little or no connection to the client's actual behavior. In addition, when the nurse makes an inference and forms a conclusion, the client is robbed of the opportunity to problem solve and share thoughts and ideas about important issues. A false conclusion may also misdirect treatment objectives.

Experienced nurses often interpret client behaviors and make inferences that do not lead to negative conclusions. The difference is that experienced nurses take additional steps before final conclusions are reached, as stated in the following paragraphs.

Solutions

Solutions to this challenge include:

- Respond through observation instead of inference.
- Validate interpretations with the client to reach mutual conclusions.
- Explore conclusions with the client.

To avoid making inferences, the nurse operates from an understanding of the importance of obtaining a client's viewpoint about situations and events that affect his or her own life instead of forming a personal opinion. Also, the nurse draws conclusions by responding to client behaviors without interpreting them. This means that the nurse simply observes behaviors. For example:

"I saw your wife leave, Joe, and now you're crying."

"Yesterday you sat alone, Mike, but today the other children joined you."

"Janet, what you just said got a major reaction from the group."

Notice that the nurse does not offer any conclusions to these obviously significant situations. It may be difficult for the nurse to relinquish giving his or her concluding opinion, but it is a necessary, rewarding tactic.

The client usually responds to the nurse's statement, and then communication, reasoning, and problem solving can begin. The more experienced nurse continues beyond observation to interpretation. The critical difference is that the nurse immediately validates the interpretation with the client, and a mutual conclusion is formed or at least brought to awareness for future discussion. Here is an example of the entire four-step process.

1. "I saw your wife leave, Joe, and now you're crying." *(Observation)*
2. "You said earlier that she was coming in today to discuss a divorce." *(Interpretation)*
3. "Is that the reason you're feeling sad now?" *(Validation)*
4. "This might be a good time for us to discuss your relationship." *(Offer to explore the issue)*

Notice that the nurse is not guessing but rather is reasoning based on past information. Also, the client now has an opportunity to validate. The last important step is the nurse's willingness to be available to the client for processing this event through therapeutic communication.

Challenge: Offer Alternatives vs. Resolutions

Nurses may feel inadequate before beginning to work in the psychiatric setting because they worry that they do not have answers for clients' problems. However, clients, not nurses, are responsible for their choices.

Solutions

Solutions to this challenge include:
- Help the client express concerns and problems.
- Allow expression of feelings.
- Help the client problem solve toward solutions.
- Avoid giving advice.
- Offer multiple alternatives or options only when the client is unable to do so.
- Facilitate choices.

The nurse engages in therapeutic communication with the client, facilitating expression of thoughts and feelings. When the client is able to hear his or her own words, the problem-solving process has begun and the client starts to reach his or her own solutions.

Often the client will ask the nurse what he or she would do in the situation. The client probably does not want the nurse's opinion as much as he or she wants the nurse to stay engaged while the client talks; there is a relief in expressing problems openly to a willing listener. If the client asks, "What would you do?" or "What do you think I should do?" the nurse can reply, "I think it is more important for you to decide what works best for you. Let's talk about your ideas."

Telling the client what to do or how to do it negates the client's experience. He or she feels less worthwhile and maybe even infantilized, as if a parent were dictating how the client should conduct his or her life. Also, the nurse's solutions may not fit the client's lifestyle or self-image.

If the client for any reason (depression, cognitive impairment or deficit, state of crisis) is unable to come up with answers, the nurse can then offer alternatives or options. This means offering assistance and giving some prompting without providing answers or advising. For example:
"Some things that have worked for other people in similar situations are . . . [*name several options*]. Do any of these seem reasonable for you?"
"Have you considered . . . [*give several choices*]?"
"What are some of the options you have for placement when you're discharged? Some that come to mind are . . . [*give several realistic and appropriate choices*]."

The nurse may need to be more definitive in helping the client when the client sees no solutions. For example: "You said you are a workaholic and can't relax since you got your own business. What leisure activities have you enjoyed in the past? Which of those would you enjoy now if you had the time? What did you like most about [golfing, fishing]? Who do you trust to run the business while you take vacations? Since the business is open Monday through Friday, when could you find time to [golf, fish]?"

Most clients know the solutions they need and only require assistance to bring these solutions to their awareness.

Challenge: Address the Nurse's Frustration

To frustrate means to nullify, defeat, make worthless, or negate plans or directions of another person. **Frustration** is a difficult state to experience, tolerate, or, sometimes, let go. It arises when efforts or plans fail to materialize according to expectations. Frustration may prevail in health care, especially when the caregiver is new at his or her field, and nurses in the psychiatric setting are no exception in this matter.

Prepared with carefully studied and learned theory and ready to apply the theory through utilization of skills based on principles, the nurse enters the arena of psychiatric mental health to care for clients with mental disorders who are probably also undergoing life crises as a result. Plans are carefully made to interact with the client and intervene in current problems and client needs. Assessment is made of the client and the events and situations surrounding the client. Problems and needs are identified with the client, and a plan directed at solutions is formulated, with the intent of carrying out the plan and evaluating the progress.

The nurse may use one or more of the planned interventions with success. It is not uncommon, however, in this setting for clients not to cooperate with the best-made plans. Frustration can occur when the client has different plans or refuses to engage in the plan they both formulated because of one or more reasons. In addition to frustration, the nurse may experience loss of confidence, embarrassment, rejection, anger, and/or thoughts of failure. These can be exaggerated responses toward the noncompliant client and with time should be modified or eliminated, as they are usually unproductive.

Solutions

When frustration occurs in an exaggerated way, the nurse must step back, put the situation into realistic perspective, and review some basic principles of psychiatric mental health nursing. This may involve validating and discussing the situation with appropriate staff, the instructor, and peers.

The nurse may have lost contact with the fact that client plans and interventions must be:

- Client focused versus nurse focused and require client input.
- Goal directed (client's goals versus nurse's goals). If the nurse ignores the client's needs or objectives when making the plan, the goals usually fail to materialize.
- Objective versus subjective in approach. The nurse must keep appropriate perspective and boundaries regarding the client and the problems.

A reaction to frustration for some beginning nurses is to abandon the plan and, in extreme cases, the client. When the nurse has insight into the need of all individuals to have some control over their lives (even though limited in many cases because of symptoms), the nurse begins to come closer to working *with* the client, rather than *on* the client. When clients believe they have had sufficient input into their plan of care, cooperation usually increases relative to the client's capacity to engage. The nurse needs to collaborate with the client on a mutually formulated plan of care.

Some specific client-focused objectives for the nurse to follow are:

- Maintain awareness of the client's capability and capacity to engage in his or her own care.
- Include the client in the plan of care.
- Assist the client toward understanding positive aspects of self-help.
- Encourage the client to engage in behaviors directed toward eliminating problems and maintaining health and well-being.
- Teach client skills that will assist in making change possible.
- Praise attempts to improve.
- Continually evaluate progress and reassess changes.

The nurse benefits from incorporating personal goals toward meeting the client's needs. These include:

- Remain acceptant of the client's need to maintain some control over his or her own life.
- Refrain from the need to complete your own agenda.
- Refrain from abandoning the client if frustration arises (look for alternatives).
- Remain objectively involved with problems.
- Lighten up. Use appropriate humor and relaxation techniques when needed to diffuse tension.
- Review principles frequently.
- Get supervision (staff, instructor) to validate your own and the client's progress.

ADDITIONAL CLINICAL PRINCIPLES

Many principles of nursing practice are incorporated by the nurse as clinical experience continues. In addition to the detailed principles described previously, the following principles are briefly described for nurses' interventions with clients.

1. *Accept client's feelings, but it is not necessary to accept all client's behaviors.* Assist by setting limits on client behaviors that are self-defeating or that threaten self or others in any way. Limits do not imply punishment but rather provide external controls when client is unaware or unable to use own internal controls. Clients need to learn that their actions result in consequences. Allowing them to do anything that is socially unacceptable not only hinders their progress and insight while under treatment, but also interferes with acceptance by society when they are discharged. The nurse sets limits and then follows through by processing the incident with the client for the purpose of assessing client's understanding, reinforcing any positive attempts, and encouraging and assisting the client to continue the effective behavior.

2. *Avoid false reassurances, clichés, and global statements.* Give hope but not false reassurances. New nurses sometimes are uncomfortable with the client's strong emotions and want to fix the situation or see the client cured. They may say things like, "Don't worry, I bet your wife will come back to help you," or "You'll be better in just a few weeks as soon as the medications take effect," or "Everyone gets sick some time, and you'll get through this," or "There is a light at the end of every tunnel!" Statements with superficial content only serve to negate the client and the severe problems he or she is facing. The nurse must learn to tolerate the fact that all clients in the psychiatric setting are not cured of their mental disorders.

3. *Avoid giving advice.* A nurse's advice may seem to her to be the perfect solution, but may not fit the client's situation as he perceives it or his way of addressing a problem. Unless clients can think through their own situation, they will not be equipped to make changes. Instead, assist a client to identify and formulate alternatives and options and to select what the client believes will work in his or her unique situation. If the client is completely blocked and cannot think of any solutions, the nurse may offer several options from which the client may choose. When it is evident that a client is stuck for any answers, some helpful statements may be, "Have you ever tried…" (then offer two or three choices), or "In the past I knew some people with similar situations and they were successful by doing. . ." (here, name two or three solutions from which the client may choose).

4. *Avoid "rescue fantasy."* When a nurse thinks he or she is the only one who can help a specific client, it is time to talk with a supervisor. Members of the health team collectively assist clients to make changes toward wellness. No one staff member does this alone. Nurses who form the idea that they are special in a client's life may act outside or even against the treatment plan, or may do the client favors that are actually nontherapeutic. Stay with the collective treatment plan of the client, or discuss ideas with the entire health care team before acting unilaterally.

5. *Use simple, concrete, direct language with clients.* Avoid psychiatric jargon. Clients in the acute care setting in particular respond better to plainly spoken conversation versus using language that they do not understand or that they may misperceive. Clients with low self-esteem are embarrassed or ashamed in their belief that they are not smart enough to understand what the nurse or physician is telling them when medical terminology is used. The client who is cognitively impaired cannot track long or complex sentences, particularly when they contain psychiatric terms or are abstract in content. Clients who have delusions may misperceive content. Speaking plainly is most therapeutic.

6. *Avoid heroics!* When a staff member notices a client beginning to escalate in behavior, get help. Failing to act soon enough often leads to a client's loss of control over own behavior, and the client or others may be unnecessarily injured. The nurse or other staff needs to use good discernment and judgment and err on the side of safety in all cases, alerting and getting help from other staff members versus trying to change the behavior by themselves.

7. *Consider the clinical setting the client's "laboratory."* Create a physically and emotionally safe, supportive environment for clients to practice newly learned skills. Encourage clients to discuss and role play situations and events with the nurse in individual therapy, or in supportive group therapy sessions. Often clients are able to solve many of their own problems when nurses make themselves available to discuss clients' ideas and let them practice new behaviors with the nurse's guidance.

8. *Encourage clients to take responsibility* for their own actions, decisions, choices, and lives whenever they are capable. Avoid fostering dependence. This may have to happen in stages, with a healthy mixture of nurturing, encouragement, limit setting, teaching, coaching, releasing control, and role modeling. There is no one absolute recipe, and the ingredients vary with each client. With genuine support from staff, most clients can learn to structure their own lives within the parameters of their abilities and support groups.

CHAPTER SUMMARY

- Psychiatric mental health nursing is often very rewarding.
- Multiple practice challenges are presented in this chapter to assist the nurse in gaining awareness about the clinical setting.
- Solutions are offered for solving some of the problems that arise when interacting with clients.
- Multiple techniques are offered for working with clients in the psychiatric setting.
- Nurses are assisted in recognizing that each client's success depends on avoiding judgment on the quantity or quality as measured against any other capability but the client's.

REVIEW QUESTIONS

1. A psychiatric nurse may decide to seek supervision or counseling after:
   a. Feeling angry after a client tried to hit her.
   b. Avoiding talking to a client because the client's depressive statements remind her of her own depression.
   c. Making a medication error.
   d. A client refused to talk to her and insisted on another staff person.

2. The best time to identify the adolescent client's strengths is:
   a. On admission while the client's parents are present.
   b. After the client has become acquainted with the adolescent program, approximately 7 days.
   c. On admission with the adolescent.
   d. During a group therapy session.

3. An adult client is admitted to the hospital after attempting suicide. His wife died 3 months earlier. He has lost 15 pounds and has been unable to sleep more than 3 hours a night since her death. The first nursing intervention would be to:
   a. Discuss with the attending physician the need for a medication to help the client sleep.
   b. Arrange for the client to attend grief-counseling groups.
   c. Place the client on continuous staff observation.
   d. Obtain a dietary consult.

4. The following is an example of an observation:
   a. "I see by the way your wife left that you must have had an argument."
   b. "I noticed that you were crying after your mom left."
   c. "You need to take a shower now because not bathing is unhealthy and your peers are starting to complain."
   d. "Why don't you just focus on the positive things you have in your life?"

5. A client has been hospitalized after becoming addicted to Xanax. He verbalizes his addiction as resulting from work-related stress because he works long hours and has a very demanding boss. He asks you what he should do about his job after he leaves the program. Your best response would be:
   a. "I think that you need to find another job if this job leaves you feeling stressed and unable to cope."
   b. "You need to have some income so maybe you need to work on some stress-reduction techniques."
   c. "Let's review your options."
   d. "Why don't you stay with your sister for awhile until you feel more able to cope with the demands of life."

SUGGESTED READING

Peplau H: Interpersonal relations in nursing, New York, 1982, Putnam.

3

Psychobiology

Kathleen M. Walker, James M. Turnbull,
and Chantal M. Flanagan

KEY TERMS

action potential (p. 39)
allele (p. 42)
amygdala (p. 37)
association cortex (p. 36)
axon (p. 39)
basal ganglia (p. 37)
central nervous system
  (CNS) (p. 35)
cerebral cortex (p. 35)
cerebrum (p. 35)
corpus callosum (p. 35)
dendrites (p. 39)
extrapyramidal motor
  system (p. 37)
fissures (p. 36)
frontal lobe (p. 36)
gray matter (p. 35)
gyri (p. 36)
hippocampus (p. 38)
human genome (p. 42)
hypothalamus (p. 38)
limbic system (p. 37)
motor cortex (p. 36)
neuron (p. 39)
neurotransmitter (p. 39)
neuroplasticity (p. 44)
occipital lobe (p. 37)
parietal lobe (p. 37)
peripheral nervous system
  (PNS) (p. 35)
premotor area (p. 36)
sulci (p. 36)
temporal lobe (p. 37)
thalamus (p. 38)
white matter (p. 35)

OBJECTIVES

- Identify the basic anatomic structures of the central nervous system.
- Describe the physiologic functions of the central nervous system.
- Describe normal functioning of neurons.
- Discuss the role of common neurotransmitters in the functioning of the central nervous system.
- Describe the electrochemical mechanism of the central nervous system.
- Identify common client care concerns for clients having neuroimaging testing.
- Identify the common behavioral symptoms demonstrated by clients with brain-based abnormalities who are diagnosed with psychiatric disorders.
- Understand uses for new neurobiologic knowledge in planning care for clients with a psychiatric disorder.
- Review potential areas for further nursing research related to neurobiology.

The explosion of new knowledge about the brain that occurred in the past two decades has greatly influenced the care of individuals and families experiencing psychiatric disorders. Psychiatric disorders are being discussed more openly, and much more attention is being paid to psychiatric illnesses as common and debilitating disorders. Many articles have appeared in general publications about the genetics, brain changes, and treatments of psychiatric disorders, and the increased knowledge has altered the way in which these disorders are conceptualized. Psychiatric disorders are becoming increasingly recognized as "brain-based" illnesses and, although stigma still persists, the accelerated learning about the biology of the brain has helped to reshape perceptions of mental illness. Today's psychiatric mental health nurse is faced with significantly different client care issues from those of nurses even 10 years ago. The shift to thinking about psychiatric disorders from a brain-based perspective requires the psychiatric mental health nurse to be familiar not only with the anatomy and physiology of the brain but also with approaches to client care that are based in psychobiology.

UNDERSTANDING NEUROBIOLOGIC FUNCTIONS

The biologic model of psychiatric illness is not a new phenomenon, but the availability of new tools has made it more sophisticated. We can now move beyond making educated guesses about how the brain works and develop scientific models that allow for testing brain-based interventions and developing new effective treatments (Gur, 2002). Models of nursing care using neurobiology incorporate information from many recently developed neuropharmacology and neuroimaging tools. The mapping of human genes and research on psychoimmunology are exciting new fields that will contribute even more to current understanding of brain-based disorders.

The best psychiatric mental health care begins with an understanding that the symptoms associated with psychiatric disorders are usually manifested behaviorally. Clients with psychiatric disorders frequently do not behave in ways society considers normal. They may express their disorders through behavior such as hearing voices, considering suicide, or wearing a winter coat on a hot summer day. These abnormal behaviors all have a neurobiologic basis. Understanding the structural or neurochemical defect experienced by clients with psychiatric disorders allows psychiatric mental health nurses to assess these clients' behaviors and plan interventions to improve health. Effective psychiatric mental health nursing care requires an understanding of normal brain functioning and how it has been altered by illness. Whether a client has bipolar disorder, schizophrenia, panic disorder, major depression, or dementia, the basis for all aspects of nursing care in clients with these brain-based illnesses starts with understanding the normal brain and how it operates (see Nursing Care in the Community).

NEUROANATOMY AND NEUROPHYSIOLOGY OF THE HUMAN NERVOUS SYSTEM

Human thoughts, feelings, and actions begin in the nervous system. The brain is the basis, the control center for our interaction with the world. The complex interplay of environment, brain function, emotions, and actions that leads to human thought and behavior is the result of the underlying neuroanatomy, neurophysiology, and of the genetic factors that influence those systems. This chapter reviews basic structures and functions of the brain and briefly discusses the growing field of molecular genetics that will influence psychiatric nursing in the coming decade.

NURSING CARE IN THE COMMUNITY — Psychobiology

Tremendous advances have been made in the field of neurobiologic research related to mental disorders. Discoveries about the mechanisms and role of the neurotransmitters, their functions, and their pathways have revolutionized the treatment of a variety of psychiatric illnesses from schizophrenia to eating disorders. These discoveries have brought about a whole new market of antipsychotic, antidepressant, and related drugs for the treatment of mental disorders and other behavioral problems.

Because of the rapid advances in neurobiology and/or diseases of the brain, newer psychiatric nursing paradigms are emerging. These paradigms stress the integration of this neurobiologic perspective into community-based treatment and clinical practice approaches. The integration of neurobiologic concepts with psychosocial and spiritual dimensions of care will truly move nursing toward holistic models of working more intimately with our clients in the community.

In addition to medication education related to brain malfunction, social skills training must have a greater impact. Supportive nursing interventions for meeting these defects of neurobiologic functioning must be very basic (e.g., how to introduce oneself, how to stay focused and make small talk, when to join in a conversation and when to stay quiet and just listen—all important survival skills for living and fitting into the community).

Also, in working with clients using these newer paradigms, nurses must be able to deal with disease/symptom management and, more important, the ever-present economic realities of managed care and capitation. Mental health experts are already pointing out that behavioral care systems are becoming multidisciplinary, integrated systems for the delivery of care. This will require that all disciplines involved in the care of clients and families with psychiatric disorders be more resourceful in allocating and coordinating services to client groups. No longer will one discipline have a monopoly on providing all services to this group.

The significant opening of the scientific frontier of "diseases of the brain" means that nurses will have to deal with our clients' behavioral limitations, their cognitive deficits, and their emotional responses in new and more meaningful ways.

Neuroanatomy

The brain is one of the most complex structures in the human body. Although it weighs only 3 to 5 pounds, the brain contains approximately 140 billion neurons, making it the most complex and vital of human organs (Gribbin, 2002). The nervous system of human beings is composed of two separate but interconnected divisions. The first division, the **central nervous system (CNS)**, is composed of the spinal cord and brain and is commonly thought of as any nervous system tissue that is protected by the bones of either the skull or vertebrae. The second division, the **peripheral nervous system (PNS)**, contains peripheral nerves and includes the cranial nerves starting from just outside of the brainstem.

Although the PNS is of critical importance to human functioning, understanding of psychiatric disorders most often involves in-depth understanding of the structure and function of the CNS. For that reason, the rest of this chapter focuses on understanding the CNS and how that knowledge can be used to provide nursing care to individuals who have disorders.

Understanding the normal structures of the brain and their functions in directing human behavior is one of the best ways to comprehend the complexity of the brain. Brain tissue is categorized as either white or gray matter. **White matter** is composed of the myelinated axons of neurons, and **gray matter** is composed of nerve cell bodies and dendrites. The gray matter is the working area of the brain, and because the gray matter contains the cell bodies, it also contains the synapses between the cell bodies.

Cerebrum

The **cerebrum**, the largest part of the brain, is divided into two halves called cerebral hemispheres. The cerebral hemispheres compose the bulk of the CNS and include the cerebral cortex, limbic system, and basal ganglia. These structures are described in more detail within this chapter.

The cerebral hemispheres account for more than 70% of the neurons in the CNS and are responsible for functions such as hearing and vision. In most people one hemisphere is dominant and is responsible for language expression. The left hemisphere, dominant in almost 95% of people, controls functions mainly on the right side of the body. The right hemisphere, dominant in only about 5% of people, controls functions on the left side of the body. Most right-handed people, as well as about half of left-handed people, have a dominant left hemisphere. In rare cases people may have mixed dominance, with one side dominant for language expression and the other for motor functions such as handwriting.

Although differences between the hemispheres have been of interest to researchers, effective coordinated human activity requires a complex interrelationship and communication between the two hemispheres. The hemispheres are connected by a large bundle of white matter referred to as the **corpus callosum**. Sensorimotor information constantly flows between the two hemispheres via nerve pathways that are contained in the corpus callosum. Because information from one hemisphere is continuously transmitted to the other hemisphere via this connection, the corpus callosum must be intact for full, smooth, and coordinated bilateral behavior.

The **cerebral cortex** is the thin layer of gray matter that makes up the surface of the two hemispheres (Figure 3-1). The cerebral cortex is responsible for much of the behavior that makes us human. Control for brain functions such as sensations, speech, thinking, voluntary motor function, and perceptions merge in this area of the CNS. The sheer size of the cortex speaks to its importance in the behaviors that make us uniquely human. In humans, approximately three fourths of total brain volume is cortex. The human cortex, if

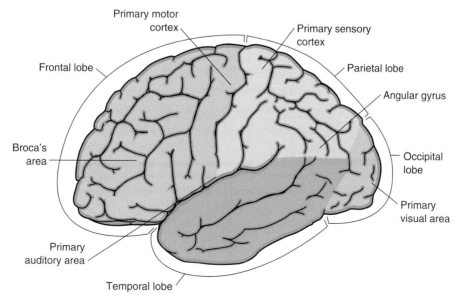

FIGURE 3-1. Map of the cortex. (From Hamdy R et al: *Alzheimer's disease: a handbook for caregivers*, ed 3, St Louis, 1998, Mosby.)

spread flat, would cover a surface area of four regular sheets of paper, $8\frac{1}{2} \times 11$ inches. In contrast, the cortex of a chimpanzee would cover only a single sheet of paper, and a rat's cortex would occupy an area roughly equal to the size of a postage stamp (Gribbin, 2002).

The outermost surface of the brain cortex contains corrugated wrinkles with many grooves and indentations. Shallow grooves are called **sulci**, and the deeper grooves extending deep into the brain are called **fissures**. The raised areas are called **gyri**. These fissures, sulci, and gyri give the brain its characteristic look and provide identifiable landmarks indicating specific areas of the brain. The wrinkles and grooves also dramatically increase the overall surface area of the cerebral cortex. Because the brain has wrinkles and grooves, the cerebral cortex contains almost 70% of the total neurons in the CNS, with more than 70 miles of axons and dendrites; the surface area, if spread out, equals almost 2.5 square feet.

The cerebrum can be further divided into four distinct regions referred to as lobes. Although these lobes work in an interrelated manner, each has a distinct function. These lobes are the frontal lobe, temporal lobe, occipital lobe, and parietal lobe. Each lobe is covered by a layer of cortical tissue that performs, based on its location, one of four functions: primary sensory function, primary motor function, secondary sensory function, or association function. Many of the symptoms exhibited by clients with psychiatric illness can be understood as a disturbance in the normal functioning of one or more these lobes. The normal functions of each lobe, along with typical symptoms of disturbances in each cerebral region of the brain, are shown in Table 3-1.

The **frontal lobe** is the largest lobe, and human beings as a species have the best-developed frontal lobes of all mammals. Much of what makes human behavior unique can be explained by the functioning of the frontal lobe. The frontal lobe contains several important structures that give it its important function. The motor strip, or **motor cortex**, lies in front of a large sulci and is also called the *precentral gyrus*. The motor cortex of the frontal lobe is responsible for controlling voluntary motor activity of specific muscles. Nerves from the frontal lobe can be directly traced to the peripheral nerves that innervate the muscle of the body; they form a pyramid-shaped bulge called the *corticospinal nerve tract*. Because of its unique shape, this system of nerves is also referred to as the *pyramidal tract*. The pyramidal tract passes through the intersection of the medulla and spinal cord. It is at this point that the nerve tract crosses over, or decussates. This helps to explain why the right motor cortex actually controls voluntary motor activity on the left side of the body and the left motor cortex controls motor activity on the right side of the body.

The frontal lobe also contains two other important structures, the **premotor area**, which is responsible for coordinated movement of multiple muscle, and the **association cortex**. The association cortex performs many of the processes and functions of daily living. The association cortex

Table 3-1	Normal Functions and Symptoms of Dysfunction of the Cerebrum		
Lobe	Location	Normal Function	Symptoms of Alterations in Brain Functioning
Frontal	Anterior, or front area, of brain	Programming and execution of motor functions Higher thought processes such as planning, ability to abstract, trial-and-error learning, and decision making Intellectual insight, judgment Expression of emotion	Changes in affect such as flattening Alteration in language production Alteration in motor functioning Impulsive behavior Impaired decision making Concrete thinking
Parietal	Lies beneath skull, posterior to central sulcus	Sensory perception: taking in information from environment, organizing it, and communicating this information to rest of brain Association areas that allow for such things as accurately following directions on a map, reading a clock, building a birdhouse, or dressing oneself	Altered sensory perceptions such as decreased consciousness of pain sensation Difficulty with time concepts such as inability to keep appointment times Alteration in personal hygiene Alteration in ability to calculate numbers Inability to adequately perform common motor actions of writing Mixing up right and left Poor attention span
Temporal	Lies beneath skull on both sides; commonly called the temple	Primarily responsible for hearing and receiving information via ears	Auditory hallucinations Increased sexual focus Decreased motivation Alterations in memory Altered emotional responses Sensory aphasia
Occipital	Most posterior of brain lobes—back of head	Primarily responsible for seeing and receiving information via eyes	Visual hallucinations

is the area of the brain most responsible for personality, and damage to this area of the frontal lobe has been demonstrated to cause changes in personality. Other functions of the association cortex, commonly labeled *executive functions*, include reasoning, planning, prioritizing, sequencing behavior, insight, flexibility, and judgment (Young and Pigott, 1999). Executive functions help suppress and modulate more primitive impulses and actions and allow a person to focus on tasks, respond to social cues, and attend in appropriate ways to incoming sensory stimuli. Difficulty in performing these executive function activities often manifests as symptoms of psychiatric disorders. Two key executive functions, working memory and behavioral inhibition, have increasingly become targets of research interest as the neurobiology of psychiatric disorders is explored (Dubin, 2002). Another important area in the left frontal lobe is Broca's area, which controls motor speech. Damage to Broca's area results in the inability to speak (motor aphasia).

The **temporal lobe** is most involved with language, memory, and emotion. Wernicke's area is a specialized area of the temporal lobe responsible for speech capacity. Written speech, verbal speech, and the visual recognition that is critical to communication are all functions of the temporal lobe. Sensory aphasia occurs when there is damage to the temporal lobe resulting in inability to comprehend written or spoken words. Other structures of the temporal lobe are involved with memory, especially those connected to visual and auditory cues.

The **occipital lobe** is most responsible for visual functioning. Color recognition, the ability to recognize and name objects, and the ability to track moving objects are functions of the occipital lobe. The occipital lobe is sensitive to hypoxia, and trauma to this region of the brain can result in blindness, even if the optic nerves remain intact. Lesions of the occipital lobe can cause visual hallucinations and other abnormalities of visual functioning, such as alexia (the inability to read).

The **parietal lobe** of the brain functions as a processing center. Sensory information such as visual, tactile, and auditory information is interpreted in the sensory strip area of the parietal lobe.

Basal Ganglia

The **basal ganglia** are made up of cell bodies closely involved with motor functions and association. The basal ganglia interpret movements such as walking while it is happening, and modulate and correct muscle functioning to allow movements to occur. The basal ganglia lie beneath the frontal cortex and have many connections to both the cortex above and the midbrain structures below. The basal ganglia are involved in the learning and programming of behavior. Activities that are well learned and rehearsed over the course of one's life often become automatic. Complex motor skills involved in walking, eating, or driving become so ingrained that one does not have to think consciously to perform them. Much of these complex activities are functions of the basal ganglia. This helps to explain why some of these complex behaviors are retained in people with dementia long after the severe loss of memory or language has occurred as a result of damaged frontal lobes. Alterations in this area also help explain odd associations or loose and illogical associations often seen as a symptom of severe psychiatric disorders such as schizophrenia (Mujica-Parodi et al., 2002).

The **extrapyramidal motor system**, a collection of nerve fibers responsible for much of the involuntary motor functioning of the CNS, is a nerve pathway starting in and connecting the basal ganglia with the thalamus and the cerebral cortex. Muscle tone, common reflexes, and automatic motor functioning of walking (posture) are controlled by this nerve track. The extrapyramidal tract works by maintaining balance between excitatory and inhibitory neurons. Conditions such as Huntington's disease and Parkinson's disease cause dysfunction of this motor track and produce symptoms of abnormal muscle movements.

Alteration in functioning of the basal ganglia is also seen as a consequence of medications used to treat psychiatric disorders. Hypertonicity, for example, is seen as a common side effect of the older neuroleptic antipsychotic medications such as chlorpromazine (Thorazine) and haloperidol (Haldol).

Limbic System

Instincts, drives, needs, and emotions are considered part of the functions of the deeper structures of the brain called the **limbic system** or limbic lobe. It is often called a "system" because its functions are thought to be a result of the interrelated, closely coordinated actions of its various structures. Table 3-2 and Figure 3-2 identify the structural components of the limbic system.

Part of the limbic system, the **amygdala**, is instrumental in emotional functioning and in regulating affective responses to events. The amygdala modulates common emotional states such as feelings of anger and aggression, love, and comfort in social settings. The amygdala has direct connection to areas of the brain involved with smell. The limbic system's function of emotional regulation is inte-

Table 3-2	Structures of the Limbic System
Structure	**Function**
Amygdala	Modulate emotional states
	Regulate affective responses to events
Thalamus	Relay all sensory information, except smell
	Filter incoming information regarding emotions, mood, and memory to prevent cortex from becoming overloaded
Hypothalamus	Regulate basic human functions such as sleep-rest patterns, body temperature, and physical drives of hunger and sex
Hippocampus	Control learning and recall of an event with its associated memory

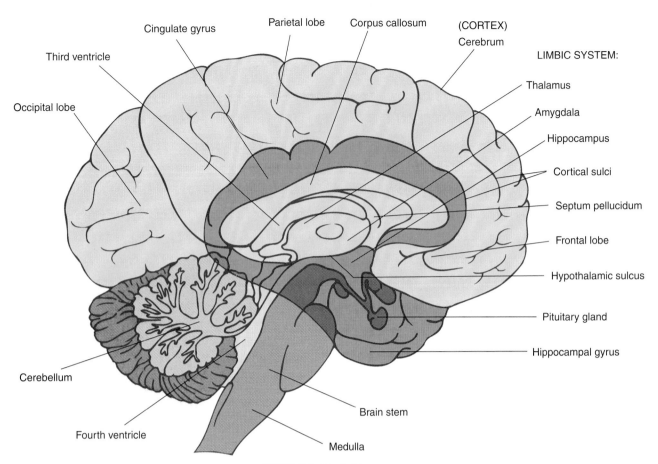

FIGURE 3-2. The limbic system.

grally linked with the olfactory pathways that connect to the amygdala. Primitive drives such as sexual arousal, fear, and aggressions are also functions of the amygdala. This area of the limbic system has been of increasing interest to researchers trying to identify the biologic etiology of bipolar disorder. Some researchers have hypothesized that rapid misfiring of neurons in the amygdala are instrumental in the development of the typical symptoms of bipolar disorder. The amygdala is also being studied in an attempt to better understand abnormal fear reactions such as panic and violent-rage behaviors (Carlson, 1998).

The **thalamus** is another part of the limbic system and is primarily a regulatory structure that acts as the gateway to the cerebral cortex. The thalamus functions to relay all sensory information, except smell, from the PNS to the cortex of the CNS. This critical structure helps to filter incoming information to prevent the cortex from becoming overloaded. Most incoming information regarding emotions, mood, and memory passes through and is regulated by the thalamus.

The **hypothalamus** is another part of the limbic system that rests deep within the brain and helps regulate some of the most basic human functions such as sleep-rest patterns, body temperature, and physical drives of hunger and sex. Dysfunction of this structure is common in many psychiatric disorders. Appetite and sleep problems seen in the depressed

client, the seasonal mood changes of seasonal affective disorder, and temperature regulation problems often manifested in clients with schizophrenia (e.g., wearing winter coats in the summer) can be understood in part as hypothalamic dysregulation.

The **hippocampus** is located in the inside fold of each temporal lobe below the thalamus. It has direct connections with the hypothalamus and the amygdala. The hypothalamus is the site of the intersection between the storage of memories and their reproduction with emotional coloring. The hippocampus allows us to recall even a remote event with its associated memory, allowing a memory to make us cry or cause us to laugh. It plays a major role in the encoding, consolidation, and retrieval of memories. Alzheimer's disease causes damage to the hippocampus, resulting in defects and difficulties with short-term memory and learning ability.

Neurophysiology

The brain is made up of approximately 140 billion nerve cells. Twenty billion of these cells are directly involved in information processing. Each of these cells has up to 15,000 direct physical connections to other brain cells. This massive network of brain cell connections is what allows the many different areas of the brain to communicate with one another. Nerve stimuli are constantly being sent and received within these cells, and those stimuli or messages turn on and off the various structures of the brain. This constant brain nerve cell activity accounts for the intricate perceptions and behaviors that make us human. The vast numbers of synaptic interconnections also help us to understand why the brain is far more complex and sophisticated than any computer that has been constructed at this time.

Each nerve cell (**neuron**) has a cell body, a stem (axon), and connecting dendrite branches. The **dendrites** collect incoming signals from other neurons and send the signal to the neuron's cell body. The **axon** transmits signals from the neuron's cell body to connect with other neurons and cells. Figure 3-3 shows the complex nature of neuron connections.

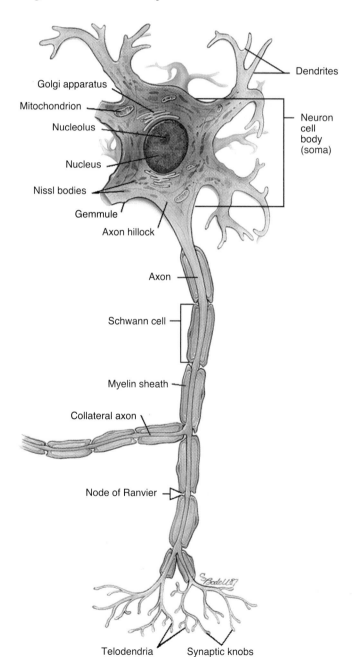

FIGURE 3-3. Structural features of neurons: dendrites, cell body, and axon. (From Lewis SM et al: *Medical-surgical nursing: assessment and management of clinical problems*, ed 5, St Louis, 2000, Mosby.)

Nerve Cell Electrical Functioning

Neurons within the brain are interconnected and operate both via electrical impulses and chemical activity. When a neuron is stimulated, by chemical or physical stimuli, it sends an **action potential** wave of electrical depolarization down the neuron. These electrical impulses move along the nerve cell, and when an impulse reaches the end of the neuron, it stimulates the production and release of chemical compounds called **neurotransmitters**. These neurotransmitters move across the synaptic gap, or cleft, between neurons, and cause the adjacent neuron to be stimulated to produce an action potential. This space, less than 20 mm in size, separates one neuron from another. This process is shown in Figure 3-4.

When a neurotransmitter moves across the synapse and reaches the dendrite of an adjacent neuron, that cell is stimulated. This newly stimulated neuron then transmits an impulse via depolarization waves down the axon to the synaptic space, or cleft. The stimuli, now in the form of a chemical messenger, goes across the synapse and in this way stimulates neighboring cells. This process is repeated billions of times a day and allows for the complex working of the structures of the CNS.

Many of the medications used to treat psychiatric disorders operate at the cellular level by affecting the ability of the neurons to initiate impulses through cell membrane depolarization. The neuron's cell membrane action potential, or ability to depolarize, can be increased or decreased by medication. When a medication decreases the membrane potential of neurons, it is said to have an *excitatory* action that makes the neuron more easily stimulated. Conversely,

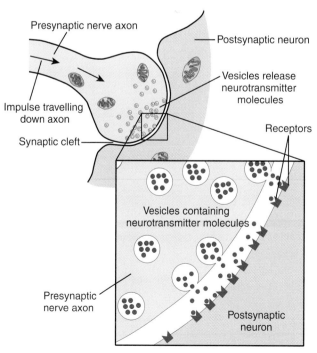

FIGURE 3-4. A synapse. (From Lewis SM et al: *Medical-surgical nursing: assessment and management of clinical problems*, ed 4, St Louis, 1996, Mosby.)

medications that increase the membrane potential, making it harder to stimulate the neuron, are *inhibitory* in nature.

Neurotransmitters: Nerve Cell Chemical Functioning

Many new advances in the understanding and treatment of psychiatric disorders are related to increased understanding of neurotransmitters. As the depolarization of neurons reaches the synapse, the stimuli transfer from an intracellular electrical signal to an extracellular chemical signal. Therefore medications that are used to treat psychiatric disorders operate in and around the synaptic cleft and have action at the neurotransmitter level. The discovery of new drugs has been concerned mainly with the study of neurotransmitters that make up the chemical messenger system of the brain.

Once a neurotransmitter has done its job by transferring a stimulus to an adjacent neuron, the chemical messenger is removed from the synaptic area by one of three naturally occurring processes:

1. The neurotransmitter leaves the area through natural diffusion of a substance from an area of high concentration to one of low concentration.
2. The neurotransmitter can be broken down by enzymatic degradation.
3. The neurotransmitter can undergo reuptake and be transported back into storage in the presynaptic neuron.

Many medications used to treat psychiatric disorders involve these three mechanisms. The selective serotonin reuptake inhibitor (SSRI) class of antidepressants works by influencing the reuptake mechanism, whereas monamine oxidase inhibitors affect the degree of enzyme degradation that occurs in the synaptic cleft.

Neurotransmitters carry two different types of messages. Some neurotransmitters carry excitatory messages, whereas others carry inhibitory messages. Nerve cells stimulated by an excitatory neurotransmitter will be "turned on" or stimulated to start some action. Glutamate, one of the most abundant neurotransmitters in the brain, is the brain's principal excitatory chemical. Glutamate makes it possible for nerves to fire and to carry out the action of exciting other cells to action. Excessive glutamate activity has been theorized to be part of the neurodegenerative process seen in such illnesses as schizophrenia and Alzheimer's disorder (Alexander et al., 2002; Goff and Coyle, 2001; Stahl, 2000). γ-Aminobutyric acid (GABA) is the brain's principal inhibitory neurotransmitter. Nerve cells stimulated by inhibitory neurotransmitters such as GABA will be "turned off," causing slowing or stopping of actions. Many antianxiety medications such as diazepam (Valium) or alprazolam (Xanax) act on the GABA system, producing a calming action in clients experiencing anxiety.

The intricate interaction of nerve cells in different areas of the brain is the basis for all complex activities of the CNS. Different neurotransmitters are found in different regions and areas of the brain, allowing for highly differentiated functions of brain tissue. Interruptions in the normal functioning of the brain can be caused by dysfunction in either the structure or chemistry of the brain. Problems with either structure or chemistry interrupt the normal flow of impulses and stimuli and result in symptoms of psychiatric disorders that manifest as unusual behaviors.

More than 100 substances have been identified as actual or potential chemical messengers in the CNS. Not all of these can be considered neurotransmitters. Sir Henry Dale formulated a fundamental rule about synaptic transmission: Any given neuron produces the same transmitter substance at all of its synapses. This rule has led to the identification of four criteria that must be met before a chemical substance can be considered a neurotransmitter. Box 3-1 outlines these criteria.

Neurotransmitters can be classified into one of three groups: the biogenic amines, the amino acids, and the peptides. Five common neurotransmitters are important to the understanding of psychiatric disorders. Table 3-3 describes these common neurotransmitters.

Acetylcholine was the first substance discovered to be a neurotransmitter. It can be found almost everywhere in the

Box 3-1   Criteria for a Substance to be Labeled a Neurotransmitter

The chemical must be synthesized in the neuron.
The chemical must be present in the presynaptic terminal and released in amounts sufficient to exert a particular effect on a receptor neuron.
When applied exogenously (as a drug) in a reasonable concentration, the drug mimics exactly the action of the endogenously released neurotransmitter.
A specific mechanism exists for removing it from its site of action, the synaptic cleft.

Table 3-3   Neurotransmitters

Neurotransmitter	Type	Action	Synthesis Substrate	Synthesis Location
Acetylcholine	Monoamine	Excitatory	Acetyl coenzyme + choline	Nucleus basalis in cortex
Dopamine	Monoamine	Excitatory	Tyrosine	Substantia nigra
Norepinephrine	Monoamine	Excitatory	Tyrosine	Locus ceruleus
Serotonin	Monoamine	Excitatory	Tryptophan	Raphe nuclei in brainstem
γ-Aminobutyric acid (GABA)	Amino acid	Inhibitory	Glutamate	No localized cell bodies

brain, but particularly high concentrations occur in the basal ganglia and motor cortex of the brain. Acetylcholine is the neurotransmitter primarily involved in Alzheimer's disease. Decreased levels of the neurotransmitter are thought to produce many of the behavioral manifestations of the disease. This helps to explain why drugs such as donepezil (Aricept) are useful in the treatment of Alzheimer's disease. Aricept and other similar drugs inhibit cholinesterase (the enzyme that degrades or breaks down acetylcholine), thus increasing the amount of available acetylcholine to improve symptoms of Alzheimer's disease (Stahl, 2000).

Acetylcholine receptors can be divided into two types: muscarinic and nicotinic. Many drugs, such the older neuroleptic antipsychotics, interact with acetylcholine and its receptor sites to produce anticholinergic side effects. These occur when muscarinic acetylcholine receptors are blocked, and the client experiences dry mouth, blurred vision, constipation, and urinary retention. These side effects can be troubling to clients and are a common reason for noncompliance with treatment. In severe cases muscarinic receptor blockade can produce confusion and delirium in clients, especially in older clients. Good client teaching and nursing care designed to manage the side effects are a significant aspect of psychiatric mental health nursing.

The neurotransmitter dopamine is well localized in the CNS. Dopaminergic pathways include the substantia nigra, midbrain, and hypothalamus. Dopamine-containing cells in the midbrain project to the limbic cortex, which is thought to be the part of the brain that is disturbed in schizophrenia. Dopamine levels are thought to be excessively elevated in some clients suffering from schizophrenia, and most of the drugs used to treat schizophrenia act in part by decreasing dopamine levels or transmission.

Norepinephrine or noradrenaline is concentrated in a small area of the brain known as the *locus ceruleus*. It has some modulating effect, and many studies now indicate that clients suffering from mood disorders, particularly major depression, may suffer from a deficit of norepinephrine. Norepinephrine is found in heavy concentrations in sympathetic nerves, which helps to explain its role in the "fight or flight" response.

Serotonin has a pattern of action similar to norepinephrine. Serotonin production begins in the brainstem and is primarily concentrated in the raphe nuclei, but it is also widely dispersed throughout the cerebral cortex. Serotonin is involved with many functions that we all take for granted. Maintaining a normal body temperature, having a normal sleep-rest pattern, eating well, and having normal moods are all dependent in large measure on adequate levels of serotonin. Clinically significant problems occur when clients have too little serotonin, and many behavioral symptoms common to such disorders as depression occur when available serotonin levels are low. The illness of depression is helpful in demonstrating the role that neurotransmitters play in the development of psychiatric illness. It is widely believed that there are two subtypes of major depression: one

---

caused by abnormal norepinephrine balance and the other by abnormal serotonin balance. These are discussed in greater length in Chapter 10. The two major classes of antidepressants—tricyclic and SSRI agents—differ primarily in their effect on either norepinephrine or serotonin levels. This explains why certain drugs that specifically target serotonin, such as fluoxetine or paroxetine, do not work for some clients but work well for others (see Case Study).

Nitric oxide is a somewhat surprising, newly discovered, and somewhat improbable neurotransmitter. Nitric oxide does not share many of the characteristics of other neurotransmitters. It is not stored in synaptic vesicles, does not get released through typical pathways, and has no known specific receptor sites. It is a poisonous unstable gas that is a component of automobile emissions. Yet it also seems to function as a chemical messenger in the brain and in peripheral blood vessels. It is involved in blood vessel contraction in the clitoris and penis during sexual arousal, and recent research has suggested that nitric oxide may play a role in the brain's memory function and may be part of the complex illness of major depression (McLeod, Lopez-Figueroa, and Lopez-Figueroa, 2001). Other chemicals, such as adenosine and adenosine triphosphate, whose functions are less well known, but that are found at multiple sites in the brain, are increasingly seen as playing a role in the complex functioning of the brain.

EMERGING CONCEPTS IN PSYCHOBIOLOGY
The Role of Genetics

Genetics is the study of genes and the role they play in the functioning of living organisms. Genes are found inside the cells of every organism from the smallest of viruses to humans and can be thought of as a set of instructions that tell the cell what to do and how to function. The genetic instructions used by a cell are encoded and transmitted in deoxyribonucleic acid (DNA). DNA is double helix-shaped molecule that is organized into structures called chromosomes. Genes are simply segments of a DNA molecule that direct the production of specific proteins, which are the building blocks for all other cellular functions. As cells duplicate themselves, the information encoded in genes is transmitted from that cell to all future offspring cells made by the original cell. If the genes of a cell are healthy and normal, the newly replicated cells function normally. If the genes are abnormal or become abnormal, however, they may instruct the cell incompletely or incorrectly, causing abnormal protein production, which in turn can lead to abnormal cell structure and/or function. Researchers are increasingly interested in understanding how small variations in genes can disrupt the function of a cell and how these disruptions may contribute to the development of a disease. As knowledge grows regarding the role genes play in the development of illness, researchers are looking to genetic engineering techniques to provide new diagnostic and treatment strategies for many common illnesses.

The **human genome** is a term used to refer collectively to all of the genes carried on human chromosomes. Recent research in understanding and mapping the human genome has increased understanding of the affect of gene variation on health. Small defects or variations in genes, called **alleles**, are common and account for much of the rich diversity seen in humans. Differences in hair color or blood type, for example, are the result of inheritance of different alleles of a gene. Although some alleles may simply produce diversity such as different blood types, some allele forms can produce illness. The defective gene, or allele, may cause disturbances in the cell's ability to function, leading to such problems as inhibiting the action of a critical enzyme or stimulating overproduction of an enzyme to toxic levels. Increasingly, psychiatric disorders are being identified as being caused, in part, by mutation or alleles of specific genes. Understanding this process helps to explain why certain psychiatric disorders run in families and why first-degree relatives of individuals with psychiatric disorders have increased risk for developing the same or similar disorders. Research has led to identification of genes that are linked to schizophrenia, bipolar illness, and substance addiction, leaving little doubt that these conditions do have a genetic component (Schindler et al, 2001). Other psychiatric disorders such as attention deficit hyperactivity disorder, antisocial personality disorder, and violent behaviors are areas of current research (Doyle, Roe, and Faraone, 2001; Raine et al., 2000).

Although few researchers believe that a single gene causes psychiatric illness, genetics clearly plays a significant role in influencing complex human behavior. The work of identifying the genetic basis of psychiatric disorders is slow and difficult. The interplay of genes is highly complex, and the link of genes to behavior remains controversial. It appears that psychiatric illness and the dysfunctional behaviors that are symptomatic of those illnesses are influenced by many genes, as well as by personal experiences.

INTERRELATED SYSTEMS

Evidence is now clear that the CNS operates in delicate union with other body systems. Research demonstrates that the CNS both affects and is affected by the immune system, the endocrine system, and the body's natural biologic rhythms, to name a few. Following are some examples of the interplay between body systems that may ultimately result in mental, emotional, and behavioral dysfunction and disorder.

Psychoneuroimmunology

Psychoneuroimmunology studies the relationship between the neurologic, endocrine, and immune systems and behaviors associated with these systems. Cytokines, chemical messengers between immune cells, are associated with signaling the brain to produce changes in behavior and the endocrine system as well as the immune system. Research studies have focused on the relationship of cytokines and the pathophysiology of medical diseases such as cancer, allergies, and autoimmune diseases but more recently in psychiatric disorders such as major depression, schizophrenia, and Alzheimer's disease (Kronfol and Remick, 2000).

Receptor sites for neuropeptides of the immune system are associated with emotions, feelings, and behaviors. Stress causes the release of corticotrophin-releasing factors that suppresses the immune system. Studies have found that emotions such as anger, fear, grief, loneliness, and anxiety and psychiatric disorders such as schizophrenia and mood disorders are associated with a decreased functioning of the immune system. Posttraumatic stress syndrome is associated with long-term immunosuppression (Kawamura et al, 2001).

Neuroendocrinology

Neuroendocrinology studies the relationship between the nervous system and the endocrine system and how it manifests behaviorally. Chemical messages are communicated between hormones within the endocrine system and neurons within the nervous system. An imbalance of the endocrine system results in medical disorders as well as psychiatric symptoms. Research studies have correlated hypothyroidsim with depressive symptoms and Addison's disease with depression and fatigue. Other endocrine disorders have been linked to autoimmune conditions such as Graves' disease, which often follows acute infection or emotional stress exhibited as nervousness, fatigue, weight loss, heat intolerance, and gastrointestinal symptoms. Clients with Alzheimer's disease had a lower glucose metabolism in the parietal, temporal, occipital, frontal, and posterior cortices (Alexander et al., 2002). Schizophrenia has been found to occur during the reproductive period. Negative symptoms of schizophrenia have been associated with prefrontal cortical pathology.

Chronobiology

Chronobiology studies the biologic rhythms such as circadian rhythms and normal sleeping patterns. Psychiatric and medical disorders occur when the biologic rhythm has been disrupted. Dreams are thought to be brain circuits activating recent memories and reinforcing long-term memories. It has been postulated that mental disorders are conditions where the brain circuits are not activating competently because of decay producing abnormal brain waves. When incompetent brain circuits are activated while the client is awake, the client experiences hallucinations and illusions. While the client is asleep these incompetent brain circuits produce bizarre or illusory dreams (Kavanau, 2000).

Psychoactive drugs are thought to modify these abnormal brain waves for psychotic clients, which temporarily restores the brain circuits. Antidepressants increase the brain waves and suppress or reduce rapid eye movement (REM) sleep. Electroconvulsive therapy suppresses abnormal brain waves, allowing more normal slow-waves to dominate.

Studies have correlated *sundowning* with the disturbance of circadian rhythms. Sundowning is the exacerbation of psychotic or depressive symptoms during the afternoon or evening resulting in confusion and disorientation. Circadian rhythms regulate body function such as body temperature, heart rate, secretion of hormones, and red blood cell production. Psychiatric and medical conditions such as Alzheimer's disease disrupt the client's circadian rhythm (Volicer et al, 2001). Decreased light during the winter months has also shown to produce depressive symptoms in clients suffering from seasonal affective disorder.

DIAGNOSTIC AND EVALUATION PROCEDURES
Neuroimaging

Within the last 20 years the development of imaging techniques has dramatically altered our understanding of brain functioning. Brain anatomy can now be mapped in exquisite detail, providing valuable information. Techniques that permit observation of the brain can be divided into two groups: those that measure structure (*anatomic imaging*) and those that measure function (*functional imaging*). Anatomic imaging techniques include computed tomography (CT) and magnetic resonance imaging (MRI). Functional imaging techniques include single photon emission computed tomography (SPECT) and position emission tomography (PET), which measure metabolic and neurotransmitter functions.

Anatomic Imaging

Computer Tomography. The first of these new neuroimaging techniques was discovered by scientists at Electronic Music Industry, a branch of Capitol Records, who were funded in part by money from the sale of records of the Beatles. A CT scan of the brain provides a three-dimensional view of brain structures that can differentiate fine densities, unlike a normal x-ray film. Abnormalities in CT scans are not specific to any type of psychiatric disorder and do not serve as a specific test for disorders. How-

CLINICAL ALERT

Causes of Chronic Insomnia
MEDICAL
Hyperthyroidism
Chronic renal failure
Restless leg syndrome
Chronic lung disease
Neurologic disorders
Heart failure
Arthritis

PSYCHIATRIC
Depression
Substance dependence/abuse
Anxiety
Bipolar
Delirium

DRUGS
Alcohol
Bronchodilators
Decongestants
Nicotine
Central nervous system stimulants
Calcium channel blockers
Stimulating antidepressants
Beta blockers
Corticosteroids
Thyroid hormones

CIRCADIAN RHYTHM DISORDERS
Delayed sleep phase syndrome
Advanced sleep phase syndrome

SPECIFIC SLEEP DISORDERS
Insomnia/hypersomnia
Breathing-related sleep disorder
Narcolepsy
Dyssomnia

BEHAVIORAL
Irregular sleep schedule
Caffeine, alcohol, nicotine intake
Exercise or mental stimulation near bedtime
Negative sleep associations (reading, TV)
Excessive napping

Beneficial Sleep Practices
Cut down on time in bed
Avoid trying to sleep
Avoid naps
Exercise about 6 hours before bedtime
Establish a regular schedule
Avoid caffeine, alcohol
Eat light bedtime snack
Deal with worries before bedtime

Presented by Sonia Ancoli-Israel, PhD, at the Second Annual Psychopharmacology Conference for Primary Care Physicians & Allied Mental Health Professionals, 2002.

ever, they do provide suggestive evidence of brain-based problems. Nonspecific abnormalities in CT scans have been found in clients with schizophrenia, bipolar disorder, other mood disorders, alcoholism, multiinfarct dementia, and Alzheimer's disease. The CT scan is widely used because it is available and costs relatively little. Its disadvantages include lack of sensitivity, underestimation of brain atrophy, and inability to image in the sagittal and coronal views.

Magnetic Resonance Imaging.

MRI is unaffected by bone and, unlike CT, can view brain structures close to the skull and can separate white matter from gray matter tissue. MRI is now readily available in most hospitals. It cannot be performed with all clients, however, because of several contraindications to its use that have been identified. Box 3-2 indicates the client groups who must avoid MRIs.

Clients with claustrophobia are often unable to complete the study because of the design of the machinery for the MRI. The MRI machine is an enclosed tubelike structure in which clients are required to lie still. Because of the confining environment of the machine, focused client teaching is necessary before testing, and close monitoring of anxiety levels occurs during testing. MRIs have shown neuroanatomic changes in clients with schizophrenia. Changes include increased size of ventricles, temporal lobe reductions, hippocampal reductions, and cortical atrophy.

Functional Imaging

The basis of PET and SPECT scanning is resultant information about blood flow to the brain. Both PET scans and SPECT scan use radiopharmaceuticals that readily cross the intact blood-brain barrier. PET scanning remains at the forefront in neuroimaging procedures because of the resultant information it provides. PET scans, however, are extremely expensive because they require use of a cyclotron machine.

Positron Emission Tomography.

PET relies on "coincidence scanning." Images of the brain are produced when a positron-emitting radionuclei interact with an electron. Both particles cease to exist and are converted into two photons that travel in opposite directions. A cyclotron can only produce positron-emitting radionuclei. The machine and procedure require a support team of physicists, chemists, and computer experts.

Box 3-2	**Client Group Contraindications for MRI**

Individuals with pacemakers
Individuals with metallic objects such as screws, prostheses, and orthopedic devices
Clients on life-support systems

Single Photon Emission Computed Tomography and Other Advances in Neuroimaging.

SPECT is more widely available and less expensive than PET. SPECT scans have detected abnormalities in the frontal cortex, occipital and temporal lobes, and parahippocampal gyrus in clients with panic disorders. Other neuroimaging techniques that are showing promise are the three-dimensional event-related functional MRI, dopamine receptor binding, and fluorine magnetic spectroscopy used to examine brain biochemistry (Raemaekers, 1999). As an example, Table 3-4 identifies the common nursing considerations for clients having a neuroimaging test.

NEUROBIOLOGY AND PSYCHIATRIC NURSING

Psychiatric mental health nursing provides nursing care to clients with brain-based illnesses. All steps of the nursing process need to occur within the context of the nurse's understanding of the client's biochemical problem. By putting together the findings of the nursing assessment discussed in Chapter 6 and the nurse's understanding of normal psychobiology, effective nursing care can assist clients in achieving wellness.

Each structure and each chemical produced and used by the brain have a specific function. Increasingly, the complexities of the brain are being revealed, and the brain is being understood as a dynamic, highly changing environment. Concepts such as **neuroplasticity** (Mohr and Mohr, 2001), or the ability of the brain to alter its structure and function, are providing insights into the role of certain brain areas in the development of illness. As illness affects different areas of the brain, certain abnormalities in normal brain activity are produced and frequently manifest in clients as alterations in behavior. Table 3-5 shows, in an abbreviated way, the link between neurotransmitter dysfunction and the expression of symptoms of psychiatric disorders.

New understanding and application of concepts such as the neuroplastic nature of brain tissue are also leading to new approaches to treating disorders. The ability of the brain to grow, proliferate, and migrate cells is just beginning to be understood. The capacity of the brain to repair itself after injury or to replace degenerative cells appears to be less flexible than in other parts of the body. Stem cell research is opening the door to potential treatments for these problems. Stem cells are a population of cells that are capable of extended self-renewal and the ability to generate both neurons and glia cell types. Stem cell research holds promise for establishing new ways to study CNS cell development and degeneration, as well as for new ways to treat degenerative illnesses such as Parkinson's and Alzheimer's disorders (Shihabuddin et al., 1999).

Psychiatric mental health nurses are increasingly required to apply principles of psychobiology to their care of clients with mental disorders. Increasingly a strong background in neurobiology is considered part of the standards of practice for psychiatric mental health nursing (American

Table 3-4 Nursing Considerations With Neuroimaging Procedures

Test	General Considerations	Common Nursing Care	Common Contraindications
Anatomic Imaging			
Computed tomography (CT)	Three-dimensional view of structures of brain Differentiate fine-density structures, unlike normal x-ray film Examination time: 15-30 min Clear fluids meal before test	Explain purpose of test and all procedures. Reassure client that test is safe and that radiation exposure is not a concern. Assess client's anxiety level and monitor for symptoms of claustrophobia. Reassure client that monotonous noise is commonly heard. Instruct client on need to lie very still to ensure good imaging. If contrast iodine is used, monitor for gastrointestinal upset, flushing, and perceptions of excess warmth.	Allergy to iodine (not all CT requires iodine) Inability to lie completely still Claustrophobia
Magnetic resonance imaging (MRI)	Separates view of white matter from gray matter tissue Examination time: 15-60 min	Explain purpose of test and all procedures. Reassure client that test uses magnets, not radiation. Radiation exposure is not a concern. Assess client's anxiety level and monitor for symptoms of claustrophobia. Instruct client on need to lie very still to ensure good imaging. Instruct client that a clear plastic helmet with antenna will be put over head. Reassure client that monotonous noise is commonly heard.	Inability to lie completely still Claustrophobia Pacemakers Metallic implants, plates, or screws Life support equipment needed for client Infusion pumps Generally not used when client is pregnant
Functional Imaging			
Positron emission tomography (PET)	Two-dimensional image Measures physiologic and chemical functioning such as glucose uptake by cells in brain, as well as information on anatomic structures Long half-life isotopes used No on-site cyclotron required	Explain purpose of test and all procedures. Reassure client that test uses magnets. Radiation exposure is not a concern. Assess client's anxiety level and monitor for symptoms of claustrophobia. Explain that there will be time interval of about 45 min between injection of isotope and scanning procedure. Explain that client may be blindfolded and have earplugs to decrease environmental stimulus during testing. Instruct client on need to lie very still to ensure good imaging. Client should not fall asleep during procedure—test results will be affected.	Inability to lie completely still Claustrophobia Severe anxiety level Recent use of sedating/tranquilizing medication because these medications alter cellular glucose use patterns Breast-feeding Requires expensive cyclotron machine
Single photon emission computed tomography (SPECT)			Breast-feeding Inability to lie completely still Claustrophobia

Nurses Association, 2000). Much of the stigma that has been attached to psychiatric illness has come from a lack of understanding regarding the biologic basis of these disorders. Therefore client teaching is an important function of the role of the psychiatric mental health nurse as new information is discovered regarding the structures and functioning of the CNS. The Client and Family Teaching Guidelines box on p. 46 displays the highlights of effective client teaching regarding the biologic basis of psychiatric disorders.

Table 3-5 Relationship of Neurotransmitter Dysfunction to Mental Disorders

Neurotransmitter	Dysfunction	Mental Disorder
Dopamine	Increase	Schizophrenia
Serotonin	Decrease	Depression
Norepinephrine	Decrease	Depression
γ-Aminobutyric acid (GABA)	Decrease	Anxiety disorders
Acetylcholine	Decrease	Alzheimer's disease

CLIENT AND FAMILY TEACHING GUIDELINES

Determine a mutually acceptable time and location for the teaching session.

Identify the client's readiness for learning.

Identify the client's motivation for learning.

Identify what the client already knows about the topic and accuracy of that knowledge.

Mutually identify with the client what content learning is requested.

Mutually define a measurable outcome that will be used to determine that learning has occurred.

Define the evaluation method used to determine the efficacy of teaching.

Use multiple teaching-learning approaches such as visual and auditory.

Monitor the client's anxiety level during the teaching session, as increased anxiety will decrease information processing.

Identify alternative resources available to the client to increase learning potential.

Identify the process for the client to access support persons if the client is having difficulty with learned content.

UNDERSTANDING and APPLYING RESEARCH

It has been reported that the brains of individuals who commit suicide are different from the brains of individuals who have died of natural causes. Postmortem examination of the receptor/transport binding sites of the brain tissue of suicide victims and of individuals who have died of natural causes show that the brains of suicide victims have unique, specific neurochemical characteristics that make "suicide brains" different from brains of individuals who have died of natural causes. Such studies are being used to formulate a hypothesis of molecular markers that could help define and identify individuals at risk for suicidal behavior. Tests to measure such identified markers are expected in the near future. Once these markers are identified and prove to be reliable in their ability to predict suicidal behavior, the test is expected to become a routine aspect of mental health evaluation.

Gross-Isseroff R et al: The suicide brain: a review of postmortem receptor transporter binding studies, *Neurosci Biobehav Rev* 22(5):653, 1998.

New research findings continue to alter the care of the psychiatric disordered. The Understanding and Applying Research box highlights the critical thinking needed by psychiatric mental health nurses as they encounter these alterations in care based on new research findings.

The explosion of information regarding the structure and functioning of the brain will continue. Because of this, the role and function of the psychiatric mental health nurse will continue to evolve. Knowledge of the psychobiologic basis of psychiatric disorders is now essential in effective psychiatric mental health nursing practice. All aspects of nursing care, from assessment to evaluation, need to incorporate biologic principles for comprehensive and quality nursing care to occur.

CHAPTER SUMMARY

- More has been learned about brain function in the last 10 years than was learned in all preceding time.
- The brain is the most complex organ in the human body and one of the most important because of its many functions.
- Psychiatric disorders are beginning to be understood as brain-based illnesses that have anatomic and/or physiologic components.
- It is imperative that nurses understand the anatomy and physiology of the brain and other systems that interact with the nervous system and become familiar with psychobiologic approaches to treat psychiatric disorders.
- This chapter begins to explain human brain structure and function and names some of the disorders that may occur when these systems are disrupted.
- Modern neuroimaging techniques have greatly expanded the capacity to understand psychiatric illnesses and are presented in this text.
- Continued study of emerging fields of psychobiology will bring new concepts and techniques to nursing.

REVIEW QUESTIONS

1. A client walks into the doctor's office 30 minutes late with disheveled clothes saying that she got lost on the way. She complains that she can't hold the pen to sign in. When the nurse calls her name and directs her to enter the second room on the left, she enters the first room on the right. The client is experiencing symptoms of dysfunction of what part of the cerebrum:
   a. Temporal lobe
   b. Occipital lobe
   c. Parietal lobe
   d. Frontal lobe

2. A nursing goal for the client to sleep 6 to 8 hours/night and eat a minimum of 75% of his meals would be a goal for a dysfunction of what part of the limbic system:
   a. Thalamus
   b. Amygdala
   c. Hippocampus
   d. Hypothalamus

3. The nurse must assess the client for which contraindication if the client is undergoing a magnetic resonance imaging (MRI) test?
   a. Allergy to iodine
   b. Pregnancy
   c. Angina
   d. Full stomach

4. The medication donepezil (Aricept) is used for the treatment of Alzheimer's disease because it:
   a. Inhibits the amount of acetylcholine
   b. Inhibits the amount of cholinesterase
   c. Decreases dopamine levels
   d. Inhibits the GABA neurotransmitter

5. The nurse will need to educate the client for the following side effects while taking antipsychotic medications such as haloperidol (Haldol) and chlorpromazine (Thorazine):
   a. Dry mouth, blurred vision, constipation
   b. Diarrhea, increased blood pressure, palpitations
   c. Agitation, insomnia, decreased appetite
   d. Sensitivity to temperature, muscle tremors, confusion

REFERENCES

Alexander et al: Longitudinal PET evaluation of cerebral metabolic decline in dementia: a potential outcome measure in Alzheimer's disease treatment studies, *Am J Psychiatry* 159(5):238-245, 2002.

Amen DG: Brain SPECT imaging in psychiatry, *Primary Psychiatry* 5:83-87, 1998.

American Nurses Association: *Scope and standards of psychiatric mental health practice*, Washington DC, 2000, American Nurses Publishing.

Carlson NR: *Physiology of behavior*, ed 6, Boston, 1998, Allyn and Bacon.

Doyle AE, Roe CM, Faraone SV: The genetics of attention deficit hyperactivity disorder, *Primary Psychiatry* 8(9):65-71, 2001.

Dubin MW: *How the brain works*, Williston, Vt, 2002, Blackwell Science.

Goff D, Coyle J: The emerging role of glutamate in the pathophysiology and treatment of schizophrenia, *Am J Psychiatry* 158(9):1367-1377, 2001.

Gribbin J: *How the brain works: a beginner's guide to the mind and consciousness*, New York, 2002, Doring Kindersley.

Gross-Isseroff R et al: The suicide brain: a review of postmortem receptor transporter binding studies, *Neurosci Biobehav Rev* 22(5):653, 1998.

Gur R: Functional imaging is fulfilling some promises, *Am J Psychiatry* 159(9):693-694, 2002.

Kavanau J: Sleep, memory, maintenance and mental disorders, *J Neuropsychiatry* 12:199-208, 2000.

Kawamura N, Kim Y, Asukai N: Suppression of cellular immunity in men with a past history of posttraumatic stress disorder, *Am J Psychiatry* 158:484-486, 2001.

Keltner NL et al: *Psychobiological foundations of psychiatric care*, St Louis, 1998, Mosby.

Kronfol Z, Remick, D: Cytokines and the brain implications for clinical psychiatry, *Am J Psychiatry* 157:683-694, 2000.

McLeod TM, Lopez-Figueroa A, Lopez-Figueroa MO: Nitric oxide, stress and depression, *Psychopharmacol Bull* 35(1):24-41, 2001.

Mohr WK, Mohr B: Brain, behavior, connections, and implications: psychodynamics no more, *Arch Psychiatr Nurs* 15(4):171-181, 2001.

Mujica-Parodi LR et al: Are cognitive symptoms of schizophrenia mediated by abnormalities in emotional arousal? *CNS Spectrums* 7(1):58-69, 2002.

Raemaekers M et al: Neuronal substrate of the saccadic inhibition deficit in schizophrenia investigated with 3-dimensional event-related functional MRI, *Arch Gen Psychiatry* 59:313-320, 1999.

Raine A et al: Reduced gray matter volume and reduced autonomic activity in antisocial personality disorder, *Arch Gen Psychiatry* 57:119-129, 2000.

Schindler KM et al: Candidate genes for schizophrenia: further evaluation of KCNN3, *Primary Psychiatry* 8(9):51-53, 2001.

Shihabuddin LS et al: Stem cell technology for basic science and clinical applications, *Arch Neurol* 6:29-32, 1999.

Stahl SM: *Essential psychopharmacology: neuroscientific basis and practical applications*, ed 2, New York, 2000, Cambridge University Press.

Thibodeau G, Patton K: *Anatomy and physiology*, ed 4, St Louis, 1998, Mosby.

Volicer L et al: Sundowning and circadian rhythyms in Alzheimer's disease, *Am J Psychiatry* 158:704-711, 2001.

Young GB, Pigott SE: Neurobiologic basis of consciousness, *Arch Neurol* 56:153-157, 1999.

ONLINE RESOURCES

National Sleep Foundation: www.sleepfoundation.org
Society of Light Treatment and Biological Rhythms: www.sltbr.org

4

Legal and Ethical Implications in Clinical Practice

Donna Oradei Berger and Robert L. Erb, Jr.

OBJECTIVES

- Review key events in the history of mental illness and its legal treatment.

- Describe and discuss the various forms of admissions to mental health facilities.

- Explain the difference between confidentiality and privileged communication.

- Relate the impact of federal legislation on patient privacy.

- Identify situations in which the duty to warn should be invoked.

- List the rights of mental health clients and identify how these rights apply in practice.

- Distinguish between the concepts of competency to stand trial and insanity defense.

- Apply the elements of malpractice to a current practice situation.

HISTORICAL REVIEW

According to Sales and Shuman (1994), law and mental health have been intertwined for many years. Even in ancient Rome the law was concerned about the legal status of the mentally disabled. Should the individual have a guardian? Could the individual enter into a contract? According to Roman law, the person with a mental disability could not form a marriage contract and, if made a ward, could not have any legal capacity (Brakel, Parry, and Weiner, 1985).

During the Middle Ages people with mental illnesses were considered to be possessed by demons. The king could hold custody of property of these people. Profits were applied to the maintenance of the individuals and their households. When a person was thought to be incompetent because of mental illness, a jury of 12 men would decide whether to commit the individual to the care of a friend, who would receive an allowance for maintenance (Brakel, Parry, and Weiner, 1985).

In the American colonies of the seventeenth century, the lack of facilities meant that families were expected to care for people with mental illnesses. If a person had no family or friends, the individual might wander from town to town—in some instances in the company of transient groups. There was no distinguishing between a vagrant and a person with a mental illness; therefore all were treated as itinerant, poor persons. As early as 1676, a law was passed in the state of Massachusetts to manage people who were considered to have mental illnesses and be dangerous. The individual could be detained, but generally no procedures for commitment of a person with a mental illness were instigated at this time (Brakel, Parry, and Weiner, 1985).

It was not until 1752 that Pennsylvania Hospital in Philadelphia opened to treat people with mental illnesses (Laben and MacLean, 1989). In Williamsburg, Va., in 1773, a facility was opened by the state, specifically for treatment of people with mental illnesses. The next state institution erected was in Lexington, Ky., in 1824 (Brakel, Parry, and Weiner, 1985).

In 1841 Dorothea Dix began her crusade for placing individuals with mental illnesses in specially built hospitals rather than placing them in almshouses and jails. During the following years, Dix traveled throughout the United States, pressing for moral and humane treatment of people with mental illnesses (Laben and MacLean, 1989).

During the late nineteenth and early twentieth centuries, laws were passed by various states enacting civil commitment procedures for people with mental illnesses. From 1900 to 1955, the population in mental institutions grew from 150,000 to 819,000 inpatients in state and county mental hospitals (LaFond, 1994). Passage of the Community Mental Health Centers Act of 1963 authorized funds to build community treatment centers. Shortly thereafter, civil rights lawyers began to challenge the treatment of people with mental illnesses. During the Vietnam War era, a distrust of government emerged. Judicial activism began with concern about the treatment of people with mental illnesses and maintenance of their rights. More consideration was given to individual rights; especially questioned was the long-standing practice of hospitalizing individuals for many years, in some instances without much treatment (LaFond, 1994).

Large numbers of individuals were released into the community, raising concerns that there were not appropriate facilities and services to adequately care for them within the community. Because of the increasing number of people with mental illnesses in the community and the appointment of more conservative judges who were reluctant to become involved in the administration of hospitals, recommendations for expanding the mental health commitment laws emerged. In California, legislation (Lanterman-Petris-Short Act of 1969) was passed that allowed psychiatrists and other designated professionals to hold for an evaluation period of 72 hours, individuals who *on the basis of a mental disorder* are judged to be a danger to self, danger to others, or "gravely disabled" (i.e., unable to provide or use food, clothing, or shelter for themselves).

In an extensive review of the literature Lamb and Weinberger (1998) describe a variety of factors limiting adequate access to mental health services: closure of long-term treatment facilities (state hospitals), lack of developed treatment resources in the community, lack of understanding by police officers and the general population, and the creation of rigid civil commitment standards. As a result, a large number of mentally ill individuals can now be found in jails and prisons; it is estimated that up to 15% of inmates have severe mental illness.

Most recently the impact of managed behavioral health organizations on hospitals, clinics, and clients themselves is a growing concern with ethical and legal ramifications. In an effort to control the escalating costs associated with psychiatric treatment, many insurance plans "carve out" the management of mental health benefits to managed behavioral health organizations. Authorization for access to treatment and ongoing use of mental health benefits can be a complicated maze for clients and clinicians alike. Insurance mental health benefits (if they are offered at all) have historically had many more restrictions on their use and/or are paid at significantly lower rates than health benefits for other chronic medical illnesses such as diabetes and heart disease. The stigma still associated with mental illness is thought to be a relevant factor in that discrepancy.

Nurses and physicians must consider their legal and ethical responsibilities when managed care organizations pressure to limit or deny client access to treatment or payment for services. Pressure to prematurely discharge clients from inpatient facilities is mounting (Simon, 1998). The advocacy role of nurses to assist clients to obtain, maintain, and fully utilize mental health benefits is critical. Although managed care organizations can deny authorization or terminate payment for mental health services, the potential liability for denying services remains with the physician, nurse, and hospital (Simon, 2001).

COMMITMENT

Commitment is a term referring to the various ways that an individual may enter mental health treatment. States have varying terms and mechanisms associated with commitment, but in general there are three common types: voluntary commitment, emergency commitment, and longer term judicial or civil commitment.

An important concept related to the location and nature of mental health treatment is the concept of **least restrictive alternative.** Least restrictive alternative means providing mental health treatment in the least restrictive environment, using the least restrictive treatment. About 35 years ago an elderly woman who was hospitalized at St. Elizabeth's in Washington, DC, filed a writ of habeas corpus so that she could be released into the community. At that time, there were few alternatives to hospitals for treatment. The court ruled that there should be alternatives to inpatient facilities, including halfway houses, nursing homes, and day treatment programs (*Lake v. Cameron*, 1966).

Developing a treatment plan involves consideration of all alternatives, including such options as inpatient treatment, partial hospitalization or intensive outpatient treatment, home health services, and foster and respite care. An individual residing in a community that has developed many care options is the least likely to be hospitalized. The cost of health care services is also an important factor. The least restrictive, most clinically appropriate, and most cost-effective intervention to assist the client should be selected.

Voluntary Commitment

Nurses are the most familiar with clients who access treatment voluntarily by consenting to be admitted and treated. Clients whose clinical conditions vary widely in their psychiatric severity may be treated on a voluntary basis. However, voluntary clients who are seeking a discharge from the hospital but who are assessed to be an immediate danger to themselves or others may be placed on an emergency commitment status pending further evaluation and treatment.

Emergency Commitment

Severe mental illness may affect a client's cognitive functions so that he or she refuses treatment for a variety of reasons. Individuals with psychosis, paranoia, delusions, and/or hallucinations may reject psychiatric treatment for fear of being harmed or on the basis of some idiosyncratic rationale that only they can understand. Persons suffering from severe mood disturbances who are depressed and suicidal may refuse to enter treatment on the basis of a sense of hopelessness and a wish to die. When the effects of the client's mental illness result in an immediate risk of self-harm or harm to others, an emergency commitment may be appropriate. In some states, if the effect of the mental illness is such that the client is unable to provide food, clothing, or shelter for himself or herself (i.e., "gravely disabled"), an emergency commitment may also be instituted.

Emergency commitment differs from a judicial or indefinite commitment in that it is for a shorter period and generally has more restrictive criteria for admission. Usually a state requires that the individual be seen initially by a mental health official, such as a physician, psychologist, social worker, or advanced practice nurse. Some states require a licensed physician. Once the individual is brought to the inpatient unit, examination by a second mental health professional, usually a physician, must take place. This procedure protects the rights of the individuals. Usually within a short period (5 days or less, excluding weekends and holidays) a probable cause hearing must take place to continue the person's hospitalization.

Depriving an individual of liberty through a commitment procedure is a serious matter. The U.S. Supreme Court has established the standard of **clear and convincing evidence** as the standard of proof that must be met to uphold the commitment. The criminal standard of "beyond a reasonable doubt" is not used.

Civil or Judicial Commitment

A judicial or civil commitment is for a longer time than an emergency commitment. The legal basis for extended detention of an individual for treatment lies in the *parens patriae* power of the state to protect and care for individuals with disabilities and the police power of the state to protect the community from persons who pose a threat. For a judicial commitment the individual must be given time to prepare a defense to state why hospitalization is not necessary. The client has the right to have his or her attorney cross-examine the mental health professionals regarding the necessity for continued inpatient treatment.

Although judicial or civil commitment is generally used for longer term inpatient or residential treatment, legislation for **mandatory outpatient treatment** has been enacted in at least 35 states (Torrey and Kaplan, 1995). In California, A.B. 1421 Court-Ordered Outpatient Treatment was effective January 1, 2003, but was applicable only in those counties adopting a resolution authorizing its application. The purpose of mandating outpatient mental health treatment is to break the cyclical pattern of clients who, on discharge from an inpatient treatment facility, discontinue medication, deteriorate, exhibit dangerous behavior, and subsequently require rehospitalization. Nurses must acknowledge their advocate role and yet balance clients need for progressive mental health treatment, including mandating participation in outpatient treatment programs that address the recidivism nature of chronic mental illness.

CONFIDENTIALITY

The protection and privacy of health information are now regulated at the federal level through the Health Insurance Portability and Accountability Act (HIPAA) of 1996. This law guarantees the security and privacy of health information and outlines standards for enforcement. The final

Legal Case Report: Clinical Case Implications

Sexually Violent Predator: Commitment Standard Kansas v. Hendricks (1997)

In a controversial 5 to 4 decision the U.S. Supreme Court upheld a statute enacted by the state of Kansas. Leroy Hendricks had been convicted of sexual offenses against children. He had a 40-year history of sexual involvement with children, for which he had been convicted on several occasions. Before his release, the state of Kansas petitioned to have Hendricks civilly committed under the state's Sexually Violent Predator Act. When he was stressed or pressured, he was unable to control his impulses. A jury in a lower state court found him to be a sexually violent predator, and the court civilly committed him. The court defined his pedophilia as a mental abnormality, but on appeal to the Kansas State Supreme Court, the commitment was invalidated on the basis of an assessment that a mental abnormality did not meet the commitment standard, which was predicated on mental illness.

On appeal to the U.S. Supreme Court, the justices commented that "states have, over the years, developed numerous specialized terms to define mental health concepts. Often these definitions do not fit precisely with the definitions employed by the medical community." The court maintained that the person must have an inability to control behavior and can be held until he or she is no longer dangerous to others. Hendricks had admitted at the jury trial that he could not control his behavior. "This admitted lack of volitional control, coupled with a prediction of future dangerousness, adequately distinguishes Hendricks from other dangerous persons who are perhaps more properly dealt with exclusively through criminal proceedings. Hendricks' diagnosis as a pedophile, which qualifies as a 'mental abnormality' under the Act, thus plainly suffices for due process purposes."

Because no effective treatment was being offered at this point, treatment was "nonexistent." The court asserted, "We have never held that the constitution prevents a state from civilly detaining those for whom no treatment is available, but nevertheless pose a danger to others." Treatment is not required for those who are dangerously mentally ill. There are built-in safeguards to ensure against an indefinite duration. The commitment is reviewed annually, and if the person can demonstrate in the future that there is no longer dangerous behavior, release can be granted.

The dissenting opinion focused on several issues; the Act was meant to segregate violent sexual offenders and be a meaningful attempt to provide treatment. This had not been accomplished. "As of the time of Hendricks' commitment, the state had not funded treatment, it had not entered into treatment contracts, and it had little, if any, qualified staff." Offenders were not committed until sentences were near completion, there were no less restrictive alternatives, and any treatment available was not offered until the sentence had been completed.

Since this ruling, some states have moved toward enacting laws that would place sexual offenders who have completed their sentences in mental health facilities. This action places a responsibility on mental health professionals to develop programs of intervention that will lead to diminution of symptoms of these sexual offenders.

HIPAA Privacy Rule mandated compliance effective April 14, 2003 for all health care providers (individuals or organizations who furnish bills or are paid for health care). The Privacy Rule defines Protected Health Information (PHI) as any individually identifiable health information that is kept, filed, used, or shared in an oral, electronic, or written form (Sharp HealthCare publication, 2002). Both civil and criminal penalties of fines or prison sentences were established under HIPAA for the knowing violation of patient privacy. Mental health records, including psychotherapy and drug and alcohol treatment, have special additional privacy protection under the regulation.

Nursing Implications

Nurses need to be knowledgeable about federal and state privacy regulations, and understand their relevance to information management in the nurse's practice area. The American Nurses Association Code of Ethics (ANA, 1982) also defines the importance of confidentiality of client information. At the time of admission to a mental health facility, clients are often requested to sign a Release of Information document specifying what information may be released, for what purpose, to whom it may be released, and over what period of time. The release of confidential client information even for the best intended purposes is fraught with risk. Even when presented with a subpoena for the release of PHI, consulting with an attorney from the nurse's place of employment before releasing any information may be advised.

The confidentiality of the client's information and the necessity for having a signed release from the client before releasing information, even to family members who are closely involved with the client's daily care, can pose challenges for the nurse. For instance, a paranoid client who refuses to sign a release of information for his parents who are the caregivers can result in the nurse having to tell the parents when they telephone, "I'm sorry, but I'm not able to give you any information at this time." However, it may be possible to also say, "but if you have information that you think would be important for me to know, I can listen to you." In this way, important medical or behavioral history may be conveyed from the family to the treatment facility without releasing any information about the client without his or her permission.

Privileged Communication

Privileged communication is different from confidentiality. It is enacted by statute to designated professionals such as the clergy, attorneys, psychologists, or physicians. Reflecting a major change in direction, several states are now including nurses and other health care professionals under these conditions. The provisions of these statutes allow certain information given to the professionals by clients to remain secret during any litigation. The privilege belongs to

Legal Case Report: Clinical Case Implications

Privileged Communication   Jaffee v. Redmond (1996)

In a U.S. Supreme Court decision the justices ruled that a social worker, according to Illinois law and the Federal Rule of Evidence 501, did have privileged communication and that her client could invoke privilege in keeping communications between them confidential. The client, Mary Lu Redmond, a police officer, had in the process of her duties shot and killed Ricky Allen. In a wrongful death lawsuit filed by Allen's estate after his death, the social worker and Redmond declined to answer questions concerning what transpired in the therapeutic sessions. The judge directed the jury that it could deduce that notes concerning the sessions must be negative in relation to the defendant. The jury sent back a verdict of $545,000 against the defendant, Redmond, on state and federal claims. Even though the therapist was not an advanced practice nurse, if a state has a nurse therapist–client privilege, it seems likely that federal courts, on the basis of this decision, would recognize the privilege. Nurses should be cognizant of the privileged communication in the state where practicing.

the client and can be asserted or waived only by the client. These statutes exclude the mandatory reporting of child, elder, impaired adult and (in some instances) domestic violence, some communicable diseases relating to public safety, and information that could prevent the commission of a felony such as murder.

Duty to Warn and Protection: Tarasoff

Nearly 30 years ago a landmark case changed the manner in which mental health professionals dealt with warning their clients' intended victims. That case, *Tarasoff v. Regents of the University of California* (1976), concerned a young University of California student from India, Prosenjit Poddar. He had formed a relationship with Tatiana Tarasoff and had misinterpreted a New Year's Eve kiss as a serious romantic gesture. After several months had passed, she conveyed to him that she wished to date other men and that she did not view their relationship as serious. He subsequently became depressed and sought mental health counseling. He communicated to his therapist that he might harm Tarasoff, who at that time was in South America. One day he ran out of the therapist's office and was detained by the campus police and released. After Tarasoff's return, he went to her home and fatally wounded her with a knife. The family of the victim brought suit against the University of California, and after the case reached the Supreme Court of California, the justices ruled "protective privilege ends where the public peril begins." This ruling, **Duty to Warn,** established the responsibility of a treating mental health professional to notify an intended, identifiable victim.

Additional statutes have been enacted in some states since that time that further delineate the duty to warn potential identifiable victims.

Nursing Implications

Nurses should be aware of any case law related to Duty to Warn/Tarasoff within their jurisdiction. Nurses, especially advanced practice nurses, should know when to refer a client for commitment and when to warn their client's potential intended victims. In mental health treatment facilities there may be Duty to Warn/Tarasoff Policies and Procedures in place that can help guide nurses and other clinicians in the notification and documentation process.

RIGHTS OF CLIENTS

Up until the last quarter of the twentieth century, there was little attention paid to the rights of individuals in mental health facilities. Mental health laws protecting client rights are little more than 25 years old (Wexler and Winick, 1992). These days, when individuals enter a mental health facility their civil rights usually remain intact. These individual rights are defined and understood unless clearly restricted using due process by certification as lacking capacity or competency. These individuals retain the right to vote, to manage financial matters, to enter into contractual relationships, and to assert the constitutional right to seek the advice of an attorney. Other basic rights usually include the right to send and to receive unopened mail, to wear one's own clothes, to receive visitors, to keep and use personal possessions, and to have access to a telephone.

Clients also have a right to be informed regarding potential risks, benefits, and reasonable alternatives before giving consent for any specific therapy, surgery, or treatments, including medication. Serious side effects that may be uncomfortable or irreversible should be disclosed. Clients are considered to be able to give informed consent unless there has been a judicial ruling to the contrary. In documented emergency or endangering situations, however, medications and treatment can be administered without the client's consent.

Many states require that all clients receive a written summary of their rights in their own language on admission to an inpatient facility. In California a list of patient rights (including the name and telephone number of the Office of Patient Advocacy) is required to be publicly posted in every mental health treatment facility. For non-English-speaking clients it is important that the patient rights be presented in their own language or via a qualified interpreting service. Treatment facilities are expected to know the dominant languages of the clients that they serve and to make provisions to have client rights available in those languages. See Nursing Care in the Community box for a discussion of legal issues and community psychiatric nursing.

Nursing Implications

The education of clients regarding their rights is an ongoing advocacy process and a major focus for nurses. Clients' diminished mental status and cognitive function at the time of admission when client rights are reviewed may necessitate a variety of educational methods and repetition of the material by nurses as a part of the treatment plan.

NURSING CARE IN THE COMMUNITY Legal and Ethical Issues

The expansion of nursing mental health care into the community presents unique legal and ethical concerns. The community psychiatric mental health nurse's role is greatly limited by laws that were originally intended to promote and protect the rights of the individual client. Often, the right of the individual to receive treatment seems to conflict with the right of the individual to refuse treatment. The right to refuse treatment usually takes precedence unless the client is deemed by law to be a danger to self or others or to be in some way gravely disabled. The nurse often makes decisions balancing the expressed desire of the client against what would be in the client's best interest mentally, emotionally, and physically.

These decisions may challenge the trust implicit in the nurse-client therapeutic relationship. A broader impact may be felt in the community, as other individuals might respond defensively regarding the involuntary hospitalization of a friend. A nurse's commitment to advocacy may be called into question, jeopardizing her position in the mental health community. Alternative solutions should be thoroughly explored to ensure that the principle of least restrictive environment for the individual is upheld while maintaining the integrity of the environment for the surrounding community.

Nurses may also experience an internal conflict between the expectations of meeting legal requirements, containing costs, and satisfying personal ethical values. Psychiatric mental health nurses practicing in the community have expanded independence, which demands increased responsibility. Their documentation must be rigorous, thorough, and accurate, leaving no opportunity for challenge, especially in the current managed care environment.

Treatment plans are required to be clear and concise, including rationales and anticipated outcomes. The standards of care and outcomes should be measurable in concrete ways and treated as if they were part of a research study. The nurse's ethical ideals will be mollified by painstaking attention to the details of patient care in accordance with the requirements of the law. An adequate support system should be in place for addressing these issues, including a consultant to explore legal ramifications of specific interventions and a working collegial network in which to discuss and explore treatment options.

Seclusion and Restraints

Since the Middle Ages seclusion and restraints (S/R) have been used to control the behavior of persons with mental disorders. In October 1998 the *Hartford Courant* published a five-part investigative series of articles on "Deadly Restraints." It included a national survey that documented 142 deaths over the most recent decade that were directly related to the use of S/R. Congressional hearings followed, and federal reforms were proposed and implemented shortly thereafter (see Understanding and Applying Research box).

Effective August 2, 1999, the Health Care Financing Administration (HCFA), now called the U.S. Centers for Medicare and Medicaid Services (CMS), introduced new standards for the use of S/R for all Medicare and Medicaid participating hospitals. CMS declared that, "the patient's right to be free of restraints is paramount" (Pennsylvania, 2000). The new rules stated that S/R could be used only when less restrictive alternatives to ensure patient safety had failed. Coercion, discipline, punishment, or staff convenience were identified as unacceptable reasons for placing a person in seclusion or restraints. However, the most notable change was the implementation of the "1-hour rule," which requires a face-to-face evaluation by a licensed independent practitioner (LIP) within 1 hour of the initiation of restraints used for behavioral management. The face-to-face assessment is required even if the client has been released from restraints before the arrival of the LIP. The definition of the LIP varies by state. In addition to physicians, psychologists and advanced practice nurses may be able to order restraints, depending on the scope of his or her license.

The second major wave of reform came from the Joint Commission on Accreditation of Healthcare Organizations (JCAHO). JCAHO issued new Restraint and Seclusion Standards for Behavioral Health effective January 1, 2001 (JCAHO website, November 2000). The new JCAHO stan-

UNDERSTANDING and APPLYING RESEARCH

A phenomenologic study was conducted with 10 adult participants—5 men and 5 women—relating to their experiences of being restrained. Interviews were transcribed in their entirety. All participants had been controlled with leather restraints on a psychiatric unit. Generally, the attitude of psychiatric nurses had been that assisting clients with external limits helped them to feel safe and protected. Usually the restraint resulted from failure to conform to unit rules or from a feeling on the part of the staff that the behavior of these clients was escalating and out of control. Results of the study indicated that the participants felt coerced, vulnerable, helpless, and dehumanized. Johnson comments that "We need to use restraints as a last resort."

This study aptly supports the need to use least restrictive interventions before physical restraint whenever possible.

Johnson ME: Being restrained: a study of power and powerlessness, *Issues Ment Health Nurs* 19(3):191, 1998.

dards concurred with CMS's "1-hour rule" and, in addition, added a new requirement that the client's family be notified when restraints are used. Staff is also now required to perform continuous in-person observation of any client in restraints for the duration of the restraint procedure. Clients who are in seclusion only are to be monitored in person for the first hour and thereafter the simultaneous use of audio and video equipment is permitted.

The third set of reforms were included in the Children's Health Act of 2000 that included national standards restricting the use of seclusion and restraints in psychiatric facilities and in nonmedical community children's programs that were previously not covered by CMS and JCAHO standards.

The use of S/R has been dramatically reduced in recent years, partly as a result of the stringent new standards, but also because of a new commitment on the part of mental health professionals to change S/R practice.

From 1997 to 2000, Pennsylvania successfully reduced the incidence of restraint and seclusion in its nine state hospitals by 74%, with no increase in staff injuries and without any additional funds. Key concepts that were implemented included identifying the use of seclusion/restraints as a treatment failure, restriction of the use of S/R to emergency situations only, having adequate numbers of staff, and providing staff training in crisis prevention and intervention.

Nursing Implications

In inpatient settings nurses play a primary role in maintaining or changing unit culture with regard to the use of S/R. The leadership role of nurses in staff training, treatment planning, and performance improvement activities related to decreasing S/R is critical. "Never underestimate the difference one person can make." (Studer, Quint, Sharp Experience, November 2002).

Right to Treatment

More than 20 years ago a movement began in Alabama that was directed at the right to treatment for people with mental illnesses. With financial constraints within the mental health system, employees at Bryce Hospital were laid off because of a budget shortfall. As a result of this situation, a class action suit on behalf of the employees and clients was filed, alleging that with fewer employees the clients could not receive the proper treatment. The case was settled by consent decree in 1986. Many jurisdictions continue to follow some of the standards and guidelines specified including the right to privacy and dignity, the right to the least restrictive treatment, and individual treatment plans that include a statement of problems and intermediate and long-range treatment goals (with a timetable for attainment with rationale for the specified treatment) (Laben and MacLean, 1989; *Wyatt v. Stickney*, 1972).

In a U.S. Supreme Court decision it was ruled that an individual cannot be kept in a mental hospital without treatment if he or she is nondangerous and capable of defining and carrying out a plan of self-care in the community. Mr. Donaldson had been hospitalized in Florida for more than 14 years and desired to be released. Because of his religion, he declined to take medication or other treatment. He was denied the privilege of going out on the grounds. He had a friend who was willing to assist him on discharge from the hospital. The ruling was limited, but it did set forth the premise that the state cannot detain individuals who are nondangerous without providing some mode of treatment (*O'Connor v. Donaldson*, 1975).

In the later decision *Youngberg v. Romeo* (1982), the U.S. Supreme Court ruled that a young man with profound retardation was entitled to "minimally adequate training" to provide him with safe conditions. The court stated that a qualified professional's judgment about this matter is considered "presumptively valid." There was great concern at the time that the right-to-treatment movement was over, but that has not proved to be true: courts have upheld the concept of pro-

viding adequate treatment (*Woe v. Cuomo*, 1986; Appelbaum, 1987). However, Stefan (1993) reports that "conditions and treatment in many state institutions are still so appalling that plaintiffs still can establish a departure from professional judgment in a well-litigated case." Therefore the new generation of mental health nurses has a professional obligation to assist patients seek out and engage treatment for mental illness at the least restrictive level, thereby providing greatly needed protective vigilance regarding health care discrimination for this underserved health care population (Mental Health Equitable Treatment Act of 2001).

Right To Refuse Treatment

In the late 1970s and early 1980s two well-known cases were litigated in the states of Massachusetts and New Jersey, based on the right to refuse psychotropic medication. In the New Jersey case, Mr. Rennie was diagnosed with a psychotic disorder (schizophrenia) at one point and manic depression (bipolar disorder) at another time. There was no unanimous conclusion about the appropriate medication to

Legal Case Report: Clinical Case Implications

Involuntary Commitment In the Interest of R.A.J. (1996)

In a recent case a son petitioned for involuntary commitment of his 62-year-old father, R.A.J. The court found probable cause at a preliminary hearing to commit R.A.J. for no more than 14 days to the state hospital. At the hospital he was diagnosed with bipolar disorder and alcohol abuse. At a later hearing it was not concluded that he had a chemical dependency, but a judgment was issued that he was mentally ill, had impairment, and could be hospitalized for up to an additional 90 days. Because he was refusing to take medication, the court ordered that this intervention was the least restrictive and that he could be involuntarily medicated with haloperidol (Haldol) and carbamazepine (Tegretol), or with risperidone (Risperdal) and carbamazepine, for 90 days. R.A.J. then appealed the decision related to the forced medication order. R.A.J. contended that he had agreed to take the risperidone but not the other medication. The hospital argued that if one medication was refused, the client had "effectively refused necessary treatment." The court noted that it must find by clear and convincing evidence that the treatment was necessary, that the client refused it, that medication was the least restrictive alternative, and that the benefits outweighed the risks. The following items also had to be taken into consideration:

- The danger that the client represented to himself or others
- The client's current condition
- The client's past treatment history
- The results of previous medication trials
- The efficacy of current or past treatment modalities concerning the client
- The client's prognosis
- The effect of the client's mental condition on his capacity to consent

The court ruled that refusal to take one medication instead of the two prescribed amounted to refusal of treatment for the "purposes of the forced medication statute." The medication haloperidol could be given in injectable form if R.A.J. refused the oral risperidone. The benefits outweighed the risks, and medication was the least restrictive form of treatment.

be administered. He was given the antipsychotics fluphenazine (Prolixin) and chlorpromazine (Thorazine) at different times. He suffered from documented side effects such as akathisia (a restlessness manifested by the inability to lie down or sit still) and wormlike movements of the tongue (symptoms indicative of tardive dyskinesia, a serious side effect). He refused to take his medication. Rennie filed suit to prevent the involuntary administration of medications. After the suit was heard on four different occasions, it was decided that voluntary and involuntary clients had the right to refuse medication.

During emergency situations, if potential danger is involved, clients can be forcibly medicated. In the case of an involuntary client, as long as due process guidelines are followed as established and the administration complies with accepted professional judgment, medication can be given (*Rennie v. Klein*, 1979, 1981). The administrative procedure includes the physician communicating with the client about his or her mental health condition and outlining the plan of care with the client when possible. If the client refuses, the medical director of the facility reviews the treatment recommendations and is authorized to call in an outside psychiatrist for consultation (Weiner and Wettstein, 1993).

Rogers v. Okin was originally filed in 1975 (Rogers, 1979, 1980) as a class action suit to enjoin a state hospital from certain seclusion practices and forcibly medicating clients. In this case, the courts reached a different conclusion. Instead of deferring to administrative procedures that rely on professional judgment, the right to refuse treatment is upheld if the client is involuntary and competent. If the person is ruled incompetent, the judge uses the substituted judgment standard to determine administration of medication. The judge looks at whether the client, if competent, would have chosen medication administration. In this decision the court ruled that only a judicial authority, and not the decision of the physician or the guardian, was paramount (Weiner and Wettstein, 1993).

Nursing Implications

Nurses practicing in mental health facilities should be aware of the state and case laws and policies and procedures for that jurisdiction relative to administration of medication to voluntary and involuntary competent clients. Frequent nursing assessment for side effects and careful documentation of clients' complaints related to side effects are imperative for adjustment or discontinuance of medication. The reason for the refusal of medication should be carefully analyzed and questioned by nurses: Is it because of the clients' denial of the illness or symptomatology of the pathologic condition, or is it because of side effects or displeasure with the treatment staff? Client and family medication education by nurses, in collaboration with physicians and pharmacists, and a reassuring therapeutic relationship, can greatly assist in medication adherence, and minimizing refusal (Laben and MacLean, 1989; Sharp HealthCare Medication Guidelines, 2002).

Electroconvulsive Therapy

The administration of electroconvulsive therapy (ECT) continues to be controversial, resulting in part from its portrayal in movies as a punitive and traumatic procedure. However, in many instances it can be an effective treatment for life-threatening depression. Informed consent for the procedure, including the risks and benefits, should be carefully obtained from the client. A potential side effect continues to be some varying degree of memory loss that can be temporary but that sometimes is irreversible.

The question of who can give informed consent is an issue. Previously, the American Psychiatric Association (1978) advised that if an incompetent client could not give informed consent, then a relative of the client should be sufficient. Later, Parry (1985) stated that if there is a question of competency, legal consultation or court guidance should take place. California recognizes that both voluntary and involuntary clients may be capable of giving informed consent and that both voluntary and involuntary clients may be incapable of giving informed consent. A court hearing is held for incapable clients to determine whether the ECT treatment will be administered.

In the state of Washington a client has the right to refuse ECT unless there is clear and convincing evidence that it is needed. The state must have compelling evidence that ECT is necessary and would be effective, and that other forms of treatment have not been beneficial or are not available (Washington; Antipsychotic Medication; ECT, 1993). Some states, such as Tennessee, have regulations related to administration of ECT to minors (Tenn. Code Ann. §33-3-105). Other states limit the number of treatments that can be given to an individual within a certain time frame (Weiner and Wettstein, 1993). California limits the duration of the validity of the client's informed consent to 30 days during which a maximum of 15 treatments may be administered. In addition, an oversight ECT Committee consisting of three ECT qualified psychiatrists must review each series of ECT treatments that is administered to a client to determine the appropriateness and efficacy of that treatment (Title 9, Calif. Welfare & Institutions Code). Data regarding the number of ECT treatments administered by age group, including any serious medical complications, is required to be reported quarterly to the state Department of Health (see Chapter 19 for more information on ECT including Nursing Implications).

Research

Guidelines have been established by the federal government that apply to research on human subjects. The major objective is to provide informed consent to the person who has agreed to participate in research projects. Some of the guidelines include a clear statement of the following: the purpose of the research, the risks and possible discomforts to the subject, the possible benefits to the individual or to others, alternative treatment procedures, confidentiality of records, sources for further information, and availability of compensation if injury occurs. Perhaps the most important fact to convey is that the

Box 4-1 Experimental Subject's Bill of Rights

1. A statement that the procedure or treatment involves research, an explanation of the purposes of the research, the expected duration of the subject's participation, an estimate of the subject's expected recovery time after the experiment, and identification of any procedures that are experimental.
2. An explanation of the procedures to be followed and any drug or device to be used, including the purposes of such procedures, drugs, or devices. If a placebo will be given to a portion of the subjects involved in a medical experiment, all subjects must be informed of this fact; however, they need not be informed as to whether they will actually receive a placebo.
3. A description of any reasonably foreseeable or expected risks or discomforts to the subjects.
4. A description of any benefits to the subject or to others that may reasonably be expected from the research.
5. A disclosure of appropriate alternative procedures or courses of treatment, if any, that may be advantageous to the subject and their relative risks and benefits.
6. A statement describing the extent, if any, to which confidentiality of records that identify the subject will be maintained. For research subject to the Food and Drug Administration (FDA) regulations, this statement must also specify that the FDA may inspect the records of subjects participating in studies involving a drug or device subject to FDA regulation.
7. For research involving more than minimal risk, an explanation as to whether any compensation and/or medical treatments are available if injury occurs and, if so, what they consist of, or where further information may be obtained.
8. A statement that participation is voluntary, refusal to participate will involve no penalty or loss of benefits to which the subject is otherwise entitled, and the subject may discontinue participation at any time without penalty or loss of benefits to which the subject may otherwise be entitled.
9. The name, institutional affiliation, if any, and address of the person or persons actually performing and primarily responsible for conducting the experiment.
10. The name of the sponsor or funding source, if any, or manufacturer if the experiment involves a drug or device, and the organization, if any, under whose general authority the experiment is being conducted.
11. The name, address, and telephone number of an impartial third party not associated with the experiment to who the subject may address complaints about the experiment.
12. An offer to answer any inquiries concerning the experiment or procedures involved, an explanation of who to contact for answers to pertinent questions about the research and the research subject's rights, and who to contact in the event of a research-related injury.

From California Health and Safety Code Section 24172.

research is voluntary and clearly reflects autonomy on the participants part (45 CFR §46.116) (Box 4-1).

Alzheimer's disease and other dementias will increase in numbers as the population ages. Because there are no animal models of this degenerative process, human experimentation is necessary (Dukoff and Sunderland, 1997). The National Institutes of Health has discovered that clients in the early stages of dementia can select health care proxies despite some "minimal memory problems and word-finding difficulties"; in the early stages they continue to "possess the capacity to make independent decisions." As a safeguard to this process, all clients are assessed by a bioethicist. In this manner, as the disease progresses and informed consent can no longer be given by the participant in the research, the client will have a health care proxy to speak for him or her.

Nursing Implications

Nurses should be aware of research guidelines in their particular area of practice, especially when they are involved with research projects to fulfill educational or clinical requirements. Many health care facilities are encouraging staff nurses to participate in research, and a thorough awareness of guidelines, including legal and regulatory implications, is imperative.

THE AMERICANS WITH DISABILITIES ACT

The Americans With Disabilities Act (42 USC §12101) is a substantial breakthrough in discrimination against people with mental illnesses; however, there are specific exclusions. The definition includes mental impediments that limit the ability of the individual in one or more major activities. Enforcement of the statute depends on the person's limitations. It has been ruled that if a person's mental condition is stabilized, there is no disability (*Mackie v. Runyon*, 1992). However, such people are protected if the fact that they once had a mental disability (such as depression) is used against them in the employment situation. Some exclusions include persons who use controlled substances for unlawful purposes and individuals who take prescribed drugs without the supervision of a health care professional (Parry, 1985). In addition, people who pose a direct threat to others are excluded. However, it is important to recognize that this must be based on actual behavior of the individual and not on the mental disability itself.

A person cannot be asked about a prior history of mental health treatment as part of an application process for employment. The individual can be evaluated as to the ability to perform the job functions. Questions about prior use of health care insurance coverage are also not permissible (Weiner and Wettstein, 1993).

Advocacy

The term *advocacy* refers to speaking in favor of or arguing for a cause. As a result of the mental health movement begun in the 1970s, states developed advocacy programs for clients. Internal grievance procedures allowing clients to express views on their treatment have been initiated in many states. Under the Protection and Advocacy for Mentally Ill Individuals Act of 1986, all states were required to designate an agency that is responsible for maintaining the rights of people with mental illnesses. The names vary from state to state. For example, in Tennessee, Tennessee Protection and Advocacy, Inc. (TPA) is the organization responsible for implementation of this Act. There has been some controversy in regard to this movement; some mental health professionals say that advocacy sets up adversarial relationships. Advocates should have some understanding of the nature of mental illness and how the mental health system works (Laben and MacLean, 1989).

Nursing Implications

With the increasing prevalence of managed care, patient or client advocacy has become a major part of the nurse's responsibility, especially in the case of nurse psychotherapists and psychiatric case managers who are seeking appropriate care for their clients from third-party payers. Simon (1998) writes that psychiatrists must advocate with managed care organizations for the care they consider necessary. This strategy incorporates nurses calling for authorization from managed care companies. Nurses need to be well informed about the client's right to appeal denial of services that a mental health provider believes is a "medical necessity." Appeals should be pursued with zeal, particularly in a case where the client is living in the community and the mental health provider believes there is a potential for dangerousness to self and others. Documentation that the client has been clearly informed of these rights is also advisable. In addition to the responsibility to pursue appeals, the nurse may be responsible for providing adequate data on which a utilization reviewer can base an informed decision.

It is critical that nurses have a keen understanding of each client's rights and report to the health care provider and administration when those rights are observed to be violated. Nurses have a long history of being in the best position to serve as outspoken advocates for the client; to continue in this role, they need to be aware of the changing laws and guidelines relative to mental health treatment.

FORENSIC EVALUATIONS

Individuals who have mental health problems and who are charged with or convicted of crimes fall within the category of forensic mental health services. In the 1960s and 1970s, exposés of treatment of these individuals were prevalent in the professional journals and newspapers. In many instances persons were sent to institutions for evaluation and remained there for many years without resolution of criminal charges. Procedural due process for many was nonexistent. Many forensic units were isolated and provided inadequate treatment. These conditions began to change in 1972 with the landmark decision *Jackson v. Indiana.* Jackson was mentally challenged and hearing and speech impaired. He was found incompetent to stand trial. Because of his disabilities, he probably would never become competent to stand trial. At that time Indiana required hospitalization in a mental hospi-

tal until return to competency. Jackson was not going to become competent, so hospitalization would literally sentence him to a form of detention for life. His criminal charge was robbery for a total of $9.

The U.S. Supreme Court ruled that an individual could be hospitalized only for a reasonable length of time (not defined) and that the 3½ years that Jackson had been detained was too long. If the state wanted to hospitalize him longer, he had to be civilly committed, meeting commitment standards. Otherwise he had to be released. Because of this ruling, in the state of Tennessee, the population of the forensic unit went from 185 to 50 within 2 years (Laben and Spencer, 1976).

Competency To Stand Trial

Competency to stand trial is a very narrow concept. Criteria include the following: Does the individual charged with the crime understand the criminal charges? Is there an understanding of the legal process and the consequences of the charges? Can the individual advise an attorney and defend the charges? Essentially it is the person's awareness of the legal process that must be evaluated by the mental health professional (see Understanding and Applying Research box).

If the judge, prosecuting attorney, or defense attorney believes that competency is an issue, a request by the attorney results in a *court ordered evaluation (COE)* asking for the evaluation of the person's competency to stand trial. Many states recognize not only the psychiatrist as the competent evaluator on this issue but also psychologists, social workers, and advanced practice psychiatric nurses who have been educated and trained in this evaluation process. Many evaluations are now performed on an outpatient basis, resulting in return to the courts and a more timely resolution of the charges (Laben and MacLean, 1989).

UNDERSTANDING and APPLYING RESEARCH

A survey was completed of Massachusetts district court judges related to forensic evaluations; 58 of 160 responded. The question presented to the judges was, when civil commitment was available and the charge was a minor offense, why were individuals committed for a 20-day forensic evaluation for competency to stand trial? An overwhelming majority (93.1%) admitted concerns about the treatment of individuals in a civil commitment to a mental health facility. Some of the reasons for this strategy included that the defendant did not meet commitment standards and that on some occasions psychiatric hospitals deny admission to offenders who meet commitment criteria unless the court orders the admission. A forensic commitment does not allow for early discharge; the defendant must remain for 20 days and must appear in court before discharge. "This study confirms suspicions that judges order pretrial evaluations to fill perceived gaps in the civil system."

Applebaum KL, Fisher WH: Judges' assumptions about the appropriateness of civil and forensic commitment, *Psychiatr Serv* 48(5):710, 1997.

Criminal Responsibility (Insanity Defense)

Competency to stand trial relates to the present mental condition of the defendants and their current ability to make a defense in court. The insanity defense relates to the state of mind at the time of the offense. This concept stems from the legal doctrine of *mens rea.* For a person to be found guilty, the individual must be able to form intent. If, because of mental illness, intent cannot be formed and the person is possibly responding to hallucinatory voices, there is no guilt involved (Shah, 1986).

The first well-known case came from England where the M'Naghten Rule was promulgated. The set of circumstances involved Daniel M'Naghten, who shot and mistakenly murdered the secretary to the prime minister instead of his intended victim, Sir Robert Peel. M'Naghten was found not guilty by reason of insanity, which caused great consternation in that country. Subsequently, a panel of 15 judges met and defined what has become known as the M'Naghten Rule. An accused will not be held responsible if at the time of the commission of the act, he was "laboring under such a defect of reason, from disease of the mind, as to not know the nature and quality of the act he was doing, or if he did know it, that he did not know he was doing what was wrong" (Shah, 1986).

Much criticism of this doctrine emerged in the 1960s and 1970s, and some states subsequently adopted a modern interpretation of the insanity defense, which states that a person is not responsible for criminal conduct if at the time of such conduct, as a result of mental disease or defect, the person lacks substantial capacity either to appreciate the criminality (wrongfulness) of the conduct or to conform his or her conduct to the requirements of the law (*Graham v. State of Tennessee,* 1977). This definition is derived from the Model Penal Code.

After a person is found not guilty by reason of insanity, he or she is usually hospitalized and sent to a psychiatric unit for evaluation of commitability. Many states have stricter release standards for individuals found not guilty by reason of insanity because, although they have been found not guilty, they have committed a criminal act (Laben and MacLean, 1989).

Guilty but Mentally Ill

Recently several states have adopted a new plea of guilty but mentally ill (GBMI). The individual is found guilty, but, because of the plea that mental illness caused commission of the crime, is sent to prison and treated for the mental illness. It was thought that fewer people would adopt an insanity defense with the GBMI plea. This has not always proved to be the case; in Michigan the numbers of those pleading this form of the insanity defense increased, although in Georgia the numbers have decreased (Callahan et al, 1992).

Nursing Responsibilities in the Criminal Justice System

In at least one state advanced practice nurses can testify to the issue of competency to stand trial. This should not be undertaken lightly, and special education should be sought out before testifying on this issue. In most states psycholo-gists with doctoral degrees and psychiatrists testify concerning the insanity defense.

MALPRACTICE

Because of the irreversible side effects of some medications given to individuals with mental health problems and the trend of short-term hospitalizations, nurses working in psychiatric settings must be aware of situations that might later lead to a malpractice lawsuit. *Negligence,* the primary basis for malpractice lawsuits, is a civil dispute between two or more citizens or a health care facility. A person alleges that a professional omitted or committed an act that a reasonably prudent professional would not do. The action of the professional causes injury resulting in measurable damages.

Elements of a Malpractice Suit Based on Negligence

To bring a suit, the plaintiff must establish that a nurse had a **legal duty** or relationship to that person to provide a certain standard of care. The second aspect that must be defined in that relationship is a **breach of duty.** The care is then measured by the reasonably prudent nurse standard: What would another nurse working in a mental health facility have done in the same situation? Usually **expert witnesses** are brought in to testify regarding adherence or departure from the standard of care. Some jurisdictions look to a reasonably prudent nurse standard; however, with the development of standards of care by the American Nurses Association and American Psychiatric Nurses Association in relationship to psychiatric nursing practice, these guidelines could be adopted in a lawsuit (Statement on Psychiatric Mental Health Nursing Practice, 1994). An act of negligence is never imputed simply because of a poor outcome. The next element that is explored is whether the injury (*damages*) was foreseeable based on the nurse's actions and the set of circumstances that followed. The court explores whether the nurse was the causal link in the injury that ensued. This is defined by establishing the connection between the nurses acts of negligence and the alleged damages using two tests that are accepted throughout the United States: (1) *But for Test*—the alleged damages would not have occurred but for the act of negligence, and (2) *Substantial Factor Test*—the negligence was a substantial factor in causing the alleged damages. For example, did the nurse give the wrong medication, or did the nurse not know about drug interactions with certain medications that led to the injury? The last element that must be determined is whether there is a proven injury because of the nurse's behavior. The most damaging and reckless behavior a nurse could be associated with would involve *gross negligence,* defined as acting with willful and conscious disregard of the rights and safety of others.

Documentation

The information that must be kept in a mental health record is often regulated by the state or the mental health facility where the nurse is practicing. Although many mental health professionals view comprehensive charting as a challenge,

Legal Case Report: Clinical Case Implications
Nurse's Responsibility Hatley v. Kassen (1992)

Pennie Johnson had been mentally ill for 10 years. She had been an outpatient in a forensic unit, because long-term inpatient treatment was considered nontherapeutic. Because of her long-term history, a difficult client file had been established to assist treating physicians. In February 1988, she was picked up by a state trooper on a tollway road, at which time she threatened suicide. She was taken to a county hospital. In the nursing assessment Johnson stated that she was feeling increasingly depressed and had ingested medication that exceeded the prescribed dosage. She continued to take this medication in front of the hospital staff, at which time it was removed from her.

She was examined by Dr. Kalra, who decided to discharge her because he thought her condition had not changed. Johnson asked both the nurse who assessed her and the nursing supervisor, Ms. Kassen, RN, to return her medication. She announced that, if the medication was not returned, she would throw herself in front of a car. Kassen told Johnson that, if she would return home in a taxicab paid for by the hospital, Kassen would return the medication. Johnson declined the offer. A security officer was instructed to escort her out of the hospital. There was disputed testimony as to whether the physician knew of her threats. Thirty minutes after leaving the hospital, Johnson stepped in front of a truck and was killed.

An action for damages was brought by Johnson's parents. In the lower court decision, a summary judgment (granted when no genuine issue of material fact is presented) was awarded to the physician and the hospital, and a directed verdict was entered in favor of Kassen (a decision that is directed to the jury by the judge because the opposing party has not sufficiently presented its case) (Weiner and Wettstein, 1993). The Court of Appeals of Texas reversed the decision and remanded the case back to the lower court for further litigation, stating that the doctor and the nurse were not entitled to official immunity because of employment at a government hospital.

The court, in its decision, did note the testimony of three expert witnesses regarding Kassen's nursing care. Two nurse experts testified that Kassen's actions were substandard once she knew that Johnson had communicated suicidal intentions with a specific plan. A psychiatric expert in the field of suicidology testified that Kassen should have sought the advice of the physician or supervisor before releasing Johnson after the suicidal threats.

One judge wrote a dissenting opinion. This justice believed that Johnson had threatened for 10 years to commit suicide and had never done so; therefore it was not foreseeable that Johnson would follow through with her threat, and therefore it was not negligence on Kassen's part. "I would hold that threats of suicide cannot enslave the intended victim to either submission or damages—especially threats that have been 'empty' for years."

This case was remanded for retrial, so the final results are unknown. However, elements of the case can be analyzed. The nurses and doctor had a duty to a client who was brought to the Emergency Department. Several experts testified that, once a client has a suicide plan, some form of hospitalization should be instituted, or—at the least—a supervisor notified or another discussion held with the physician. On the basis of this testimony, it might be concluded that the nurse fell below the standard of care. Because the nurse permitted the client to leave the hospital, she could be targeted as a causal agent in the resulting death. Damages could be awarded for the incident (Weiner and Wettstein, 1993).

---

reflected clinical information is not just a record of the care of the client; it is also a legal document that might be valuable in any litigation that might take place.

Adequate legible documentation is the best means of defense against a lawsuit and the best way to validate that the nurse and other health care professionals adhered to their scope of practice and a safe standard of care. It is important to be specific and to document symptoms by writing in quotes what the client expresses to you, such as, "I am hearing voices that say I am a bad person." Recording the actual words of the client is more definitive than simply noting, "The client is hallucinating," especially if the words are destructive to the client or others. Charting should be done in a timely and legible manner. Recording at the time something happens is considered more adequate than block charting, which is usually more brief and not as definitive (*Nurse's Handbook of Law and Ethics*, 1992). A client's record is a sequential document; thus space should not be "saved" for late entries. Late entries should be labeled as such and initialed.

In a mental health record it is especially important to document when the person has achieved the goals outlined in the treatment plan. If the individual has an exacerbation of the illness, the treatment plan should reflect the change. Informed consent concerning the giving of psychiatric medications is an important aspect of the chart, especially medications such as some neuroleptics, which can cause irreversible side effects or provide chemical restraint.

Records are an excellent source for communicating with other mental health professionals on the staff of a facility, as well as other agencies where the client is being treated. It is also validation for reimbursement that care was given for particular symptoms. Because managed care is becoming prevalent, a clear outline of all of the client's symptoms should be carefully recorded to document a necessity for continued, decreased/increased level of care (e.g., controlled structured environment, increased observation, medication stabilization, and continued hospitalization). For example, if routine hospitalization is for 5 days, but the client continues daily to verbalize suicidal thoughts, recording this information is critical for extended permission to continue the hospitalization.

Improper abbreviations not authorized by the agency should not be used. Records from other facilities or other treating professionals should be obtained to provide an accurate long-term picture of how the client was treated on prior occasions.

All client education, aftercare plans, participation in treatment team, or referral to other agencies for care should be written. Accurate recording of vital signs is essential, especially in relation to the taking of psychotropic medications. The observed efficacy of prescribed medication needs to be defined and communicated in the chart and to the physician. All notifications and order clarifications need to be clearly documented. Any nursing assessments that are re-

Legal Case Report: Clinical Case Implications

Responsibilities of Treating Therapists   Estates of Morgan v. Fairfield Family Counseling Center (1997)

Matt Morgan was playing a card game with his parents and sister when he left the room, returned with a gun, and shot and killed his parents. His sister was injured but survived. Matt had problems in his senior year in high school and after graduation had difficulty retaining employment. He was "verbally abusive" to his parents, and they had become afraid of him. In January 1990 he was removed from his home by police as he was attempting to fight with his father.

After a period of wandering, Matt eventually presented to the Emergency Department at a hospital in Philadelphia. He was diagnosed with schizophreniform disorder and transferred to a mental health facility. He had delusions that the government was affecting his body and the air waves so that he was unable to watch television or listen to tapes or radio, and he had delusions of persecution, ideas of reference, and thought broadcasting. He was given thiothixene (Navane) and was admitted to a respite unit.

During the 12-week stay at the respite unit, Matt continued to receive thiothixene and intensive therapy. He had paranoia concerning his family, but this decreased, and he was able to admit that the medication helped him to manage his symptoms. He acknowledged that his conflicts with his family, especially his relationship with his father, could be attributed to his mental illness. The treating physician thought it would be in Matt's best interest to return to his home and be followed at the Fairfield Family Counseling Center (FFCC). His parents came to get him at the end of June 1990, and he was first seen in the FFCC on July 16, 1990.

He was initially seen by a psychotherapist and was then referred to Dr. Brown, a contract psychiatrist for medication evaluation, on July 19, 1990. Dr. Brown reported that Matt had been in a mental health unit "of some sort" in Philadelphia and that he was out of medication. He wrote, "He comes to the mental health clinic for his medication, continued care, and help in completing a Social Security Disability form." Dr. Brown concluded that Matt had some form of atypical psychosis and did not appear to have a thought disorder or schizophrenia. Dr. Brown also noted that he thought Matt might be malingering in an attempt to obtain disability. Dr. Brown wrote that it was "wise to defer diagnosis, continue the medication, obtain Matt's records from Philadelphia, and schedule another appointment for a month later." When Matt returned for his appointment, the records from the mental health unit in Philadelphia were available, but the court reported that it was clear from Dr. Brown's testimony that he never read them or attempted to contact the treating physician.

Dr. Brown reduced the dosage of thiothixene and wrote again about the possibility of malingering. Dr. Brown saw Matt on October 11, 1990 for the last time; he prescribed a tapering and discontinuation of the thiothixene. He stated that Matt would continue in psychotherapy. Matt was referred to a vocational counselor to assist him in finding employment. Between October and January 1991, Matt remained in psychotherapy and vocational counseling. However, his mother reported that Matt's condition was deteriorating, as evidenced by his pacing, quiet demeanor, withdrawal, and irritability. She asked that he be placed back on medication and shared that Matt had given a deposit toward the purchase of a gun. The vocational counselor thought that the mother was overprotective. When Matt failed to keep his appointment with the psychotherapist in January of 1991, it was decided that the only person who should see him was the vocational counselor. Matt continued to decompensate, his parents

became afraid of him, and he once again developed symptoms of paranoia. During the month of May 1991, Matt's mother continued to report Matt's deterioration. An appointment was scheduled with Dr. Brown, but Matt did not keep it. Matt's employer also reported that he was "too weak to push a lawnmower, was on the verge of passing out, and did not seem to be totally in touch with reality." On June 14, 1991, Matt's mother wrote a letter to FFCC seeking help for her son. She explained her concerns about his potential violence. An assessment was conducted by the vocational counselor and a licensed social worker. FFCC had an unwritten policy that no involuntary commitment would be initiated without family involvement; but when the family attempted such course of action, the probate court informed them that it would need the vocational counselor's approval.

On July 20, 1991, Matt's parents sent a letter to a psychologist employed at FFCC who reviewed the record, talked with the vocational counselor and social worker, and determined that Matt could not be given medication against his will and could not be hospitalized. Another social worker commented on July 25, 1991, that Matt was losing weight and deteriorating. That evening Matt shot his family.

In an action for negligence brought by the parents' estate, expert witnesses for the plaintiffs, the Morgan estates, testified that Dr. Brown's treatment of Matt was negligent for failure to read the prior treatment reports, for failure to diagnose, for discontinuing needed medication, and for failure to closely monitor Matt after discontinuation of the medication. The fact that a vocational therapist was making commitment decisions was of particular concern. One expert testified that it was foreseeable that without medication, a potential for violent behavior was created. "The only reason Matt killed his parents is because he was taken off medication and didn't receive good care."

The expert witnesses testified that, at the point Matt refused medication because of his deteriorating condition, the action should have included "strong family involvement, making Matt's participation in vocational therapy contingent upon continued treatment, and telling Matt that he faced involuntary hospitalization unless he resumed taking his medication."

The court in its ruling stated that "a relationship between the psychotherapist and the patient in the outpatient setting constitutes a special relationship justifying the imposition of a duty upon the psychotherapist to protect against the patient's violent propensities. The outpatient setting embodies sufficient elements of control to warrant the imposition of such a duty, and such a duty would serve the public's interest in protection from the violently inclined mental patient in a manner that is consistent with Ohio law."

The trial court had dismissed this action, and the Court of Appeals affirmed in part and reversed in part. The Supreme Court held that the psychotherapist had a duty to protect against the client's potentially violent behavior. The case was returned to the trial court to settle the issues of whether the defendants were negligent and whether a summary judgment in the defendant's favor was warranted.

What can be learned from this case is that any treating therapist must be aware of the duty to hospitalize and protect families and the public when appropriate. Consultation by nurse clinicians with mental health professionals who have legal authority to commit is essential.

quired by the organization should be completed. Words should be spelled correctly and sentences should be grammatically correct. Errors in documentation should be noted by placing a single line through the words without obliterating them and then initialing each instance.

Sexual Misconduct

In studies that have been conducted with social workers, psychiatrists, and psychologists, it is estimated that up to 14% of these professionals have had a sexual relationship with a client (Weiner and Wettstein, 1993). There has been no known study of nurses; however, cases for removal of a nursing license for such activity are recorded (*Heinecke v. Department of Commerce,* 1991). All mental health professions consider such behavior unethical, and in many states this behavior is considered criminal, especially if it is within a few months of the therapeutic relationship. Some states have mandatory reporting laws for a second therapist who becomes knowledgeable about such behavior (Strasburger, Jorgenson, and Randles, 1991).

Many of the cases are settled out of court (*Hall v. Schulte,* 1992). When information about the relationship is presented to a jury, members tend to be sympathetic to the client, except when a client appears to have encouraged the relationship. Because the client comes to a therapist with a problem, the issue of the transference phenomenon becomes pronounced, resulting in true lack of consent to become involved with the therapist (Weiner and Wettstein, 1993).

Suicide and Homicide

Malpractice suits and wrongful death actions for homicidal clients' injury to a third party and death from suicide have become prevalent. Some states have ruled that individuals working in government agencies have sovereign immunity and can be protected from liability in malpractice situations (*Poss v. Department of Human Resources,* 1992; *Smith v. King,* 1993). When conducting nursing assessments that include a suicidal component, extreme caution is suggested. For example, when an individual threatens *intent* of suicide with a defined plan and demonstrates *lethality* and access to the *means* to commit suicide, timely communication of this information to a mental health provider, followed by appropriate steps to provide client safety, including involuntary commitment, must be taken to escape liability. If there is a question, legal consultation should be sought. However, "clinicians are not liable for errors of clinical judgment; they are liable only for departures from the relevant standard of care, given the clinical situation" (Weiner and Wettstein, 1993).

Because of the previously described decision regarding *Tarasoff v. Regents of the University of California,* it is important to communicate with the mental health treatment team when a client threatens to harm someone. Many states require that a potential victim and/or police be notified of this occurrence. Some states have limited the warning to include only identifiable victims (*Leonard v. Iowa,* 1992; Rudegair

and Appelbaum, 1992). Failure to comply with the required notification could lead to exposure and major liability.

ETHICAL ISSUES

Ethical issues are closely tied to legal implications for nursing care. *Ethics* is that body of knowledge that explores the moral problems that are raised about specific issues. In nursing practice one should look at the rules, principles, and ethical guidelines that have been developed by the nursing profession to guide conduct (Davis and Aroskar, 1991). Laws reflect the moral fiber of a society and are developed (it is hoped) with an ethical basis; therefore ethical principles should be considered when evaluating a dilemma. Many ethical problems are raised in the arena of mental health law when statutes conflict with a nurse's personal beliefs.

Autonomy

The term *autonomy* refers to having respect for an individual's decision or self-determination about health care issues. This point is especially important with problems such as the right to die and, in mental health, treatment in the least restrictive alternative. When involuntary commitment is necessary, it is difficult for mental health providers to have to follow the law rather than what the client currently desires. The caregiver may want to allow the client to make decisions, but if the individual is demonstrating intent by threatening suicide with an active plan of a lethal nature, proceeding against the wishes of the person may be necessary for safety and compliance with the law. This kind of decision in ethical terms is called a *paternalistic decision,* or *parentalism* (Purtilo, 1993). This can cause a great deal of inner turmoil for the health care professional who is just beginning to participate in this kind of decision making.

In addition, it is sometimes difficult for families when the member who is mentally ill and refusing treatment has to be involuntarily hospitalized. Educating the family about the illness, being supportive, and allowing all of the family to ventilate their frustration, anxieties, and (perhaps) anger can be helpful in this time of crisis for the family.

Olsen (1998) has raised an interesting question about autonomy and privacy in relation to video monitoring of psychiatric clients who are placed in seclusion. One loses autonomy when secluded or restrained, and compounding this situation with video monitoring can be threatening to a client. To justify the use of such strategies, Olsen recommends that there should be a record that a monitor is being used and the therapeutic reason for such use. The client should be informed of the monitoring, perhaps by placing a sign in the seclusion room. Olsen contends that only staff with clinical responsibility for care of the client should have access to the monitor, that only clinically competent staff should be monitoring clients, and that personal visualization and assessment of the client should be carried out by the nurse. "Ethical treatment means balancing the good of a safer environment with the potential of harm from a loss of privacy."

Beneficence

Individuals who work in the health care field have a special duty and responsibility to act in a manner that is going to benefit and not harm clients. The term *beneficence* refers to bringing about good (Purtilo, 1993). The goal in mental health treatment is to assist individuals in returning to a mentally healthy way of life.

Fidelity

The moral imperative of *primum no nocere* ("first do no harm") should be paramount in clinical interventions with persons with mental illnesses. Situations in which this issue might arise include giving neuroleptic medications when it is known that certain side effects may be irreversible. Another instance is the consideration of giving ECT to a client who has failed to respond to antidepressive medication and continues to be suicidal. It is known that memory loss can be a side effect. Do the beneficial aspects of the treatment outweigh the possible side effects? This dilemma can cause anxiety for the client, family, and mental health professional in the decision-making process.

Certainly, when a mental health professional considers a sexual relationship with a client, preventing harm should be the major consideration. According to the literature, the professional who becomes involved with a client uses denial and rationalization that the client desires the relationship, that the therapeutic relationship has been discontinued, or that it took place outside of the therapeutic time (Russell, 1993). Russell writes that it is important for students to become aware of their own sexual feelings and possible attraction to a client, and that this be an important part of the mental health curriculum, especially for students who later hope to specialize in this area.

Distributive Justice

According to Purtilo (1993), *distributive justice* refers to the "comparative treatment of individuals in the allotment of benefits and burdens."

"The principle of justice holds that a person should be treated according to what is fair, given what is due or owed" (Chally and Loriz, 1998). During times of health care cost constraints, who is going to get treatment and for how much are frequently asked questions. In managed care, provisions for mental health care are not always treated equally with provisions for physical health; the mental health needs of clients can be compromised. Nurses working in a mental health setting may find that it is necessary to become an active advocate for the client with the primary care provider to access mental health care. When there is an annual cap on the amount of money that a managed care organization is allowing for each individual in a health care plan, resistance to treating a person with a serious and persistent mental illness can arise, especially when this person needs a variety of services over a long time.

A major question is the treatment site for individuals with medical and mental health problems. It is not uncommon for a mental health unit to not want to admit a person with serious physical health problems, and a medical unit may not want to admit someone with severe mental health problems who also has a physical problem. These issues are going to become more prevalent as the nation moves more toward managed care to control health care costs. How is the health care dollar going to be divided, and where will individuals with mental illnesses fit into the picture when it comes to the division of resources (Lazarus, 1994)?

In a recent editorial in the *American Journal of Psychiatry*, it was reported that "under managed care, the actual dollar amounts spent on all mental illness treatment have gone down." There is growing concern that because people with the diagnosis of major depression have high rates of health care utilization, they will be "dumped" by the managed care organizations or not provided with adequate care, resulting in longer incapacity.

Mental health parity bills have been introduced and passed in some states. In addition, some states have passed their own statutes giving clients a bill of rights in relation to reimbursement for mental health care. Maryland has a law that requires coverage for mental health and substance abuse care (Goldstein, 1998).

CHAPTER SUMMARY

- Balancing the rights of the mentally ill versus the community has been and continues to be a struggle.
- Alternatives to inpatient mental health treatment should consider the least restrictive environment using the least restrictive treatment.
- There are three types of commitments for a client with a mental illness: an emergency commitment, a voluntary commitment, and an involuntary indefinite commitment.
- Clients should be informed about treatment, including risks and alternatives, on admission.
- A civil or judicial commitment of a client is legally based in *parens patriae*, the power of the state to protect and care for disabled individuals, and the police power of the state to protect the community from persons who pose a threat.
- Half of the states in the United States have enacted preventive or mandatory outpatient treatment, in which clients can be returned to the hospital if they discontinue treatment medication, deteriorate, and/or exhibit dangerous behavior after discharge.
- Clients with mental illnesses retain their civil rights on entering a mental hospital or other inpatient treatment center. Clients should receive a summary of their rights on admission.
- Clients should be restrained only to prevent physical injury to themselves or others, and only a psychiatrist or licensed physician can order nonemergency seclusion or restraint.
- Clients who are ruled competent and are voluntarily or involuntarily committed have a right to refuse treatment and medication.

- The U.S. Supreme Court ruled that individuals charged with or convicted of a crime could only be hospitalized for a reasonable length of time. To be committed longer requires a person to be civilly committed or released.
- Competency to stand trial is based on a person's current awareness of the legal process as evaluated by a mental health professional.
- The insanity defense stems from the concept that for a person to be found guilty, the person must be able to form intent and relate to his or her state of mind at the time of the offense.
- A new plea, guilty but mentally ill (GBMI), has recently been adopted by several states. Because of the plea that states mental illness caused the commission of the crime, the person is sent to prison and treated for mental illness.
- Nurses working in psychiatric settings must be aware of situations that may lead to potential malpractice lawsuits.

REVIEW QUESTIONS

1. A client enters the Emergency Department, stating that he is going to kill his boss because his boss is trying to poison him. After further assessment the nurse discovers that the client stopped taking his Zyprexa 2 months ago. The nurse determines that:
   a. The client needs to agree to sign himself into the hospital voluntarily because he needs treatment.
   b. The client needs to be admitted to the psychiatric hospital involuntarily because he is a danger to others.
   c. The client needs to be given Prolixin Decoanoate because of his medication noncompliance.
   d. The client needs a conservatorship because he cannot manage his mental illness on his own.

2. The nurse's supervisor evaluates that the nurse in training understands the legal issues of admitting a psychiatric patient after the nurse explains to the client:
   a. The hospital staff cannot acknowledge that the client was admitted into the hospital unless the client gives permission.
   b. The client has to be admitted because he failed outpatient therapy.
   c. The client must participate in this new research study because prior medications have failed.
   d. The client's employer may view the hospital records on request.

3. After a client verbally threatened to harm his father, the therapist notifying the father is an act of:
   a. Breaking confidentiality
   b. Releasing critical information
   c. Demonstrating his duty to warn
   d. Collaborating his client's care with the client's family

4. A client storms out of a group session and proceeds to destroy furniture in his room. When the hospital staff attempts to intervene, the client assaults a staff member. He is then placed in seclusion and restraints to protect himself and others. During a 15-minute check the nurse concludes that the restraints are no longer necessary after:
   a. The client is found sleeping.
   b. The client is struggling against the restraints and yelling.
   c. The client verbally threatens her when he notices her.
   d. The client spits at her as she enters the room.

5. When documenting a client's behavior, which chart entry adequately documents the client's actions and responses?
   a. The client is calmer today and is attending groups.
   b. The client appears to be hallucinating.
   c. The client is isolative and withdrawn.
   d. The client is wearing a short skirt and short-sleeved shirt, despite it being January with heavy make-up on her face. She stated, "The devil is in me. I need an exorcism."

REFERENCES

American Nurses Association: *Code for nurses,* Kansas City, Mo, 1982, The Association.
American Psychiatric Association: *Electroconvulsive therapy: task force report 14,* Washington, DC, 1978, The Association.
Americans With Disabilities Act (42 USC §12101).
Appelbaum P: Resurrecting the right to treatment, *Hosp Community Psychiatry* 38(7):703, 1987.
Brakel SJ, Parry J, Weiner BA: *The mentally disabled and the law,* ed 3, Chicago, 1985, American Bar Foundation.
California Health & Safety Code 24172 "Experimental Subject's Bill of Rights." California Welfare & Institutions Code, Title 9.
Callahan LA et al: Measuring the effects of the guilty but mentally ill (GBMI) verdict, *Law Hum Behav* 16(4):441, 1992.
Chally PS, Loriz L: Ethics in the trenches: decision making in practice, *Am J Nurs* 98(6):17, 1998.
45 CFR §46.116.
Davis AJ, Aroskar MA: *Ethical dilemmas and nursing practice,* ed 3, Norwalk, Conn, 1991, Appleton & Lange.
Dukoff R, Sunderland T: Durable power of attorney and informed consent with Alzheimer's disease patients: a clinical study, *Am J Psychiatry* 154(8), 1070, 1997.
Goldstein A: Ahead of the fed: how some states are already regulating managed care, *Time,* p 30, July 13, 1998.
Graham v. State of Tennessee, 541 SW2d 531 (Tenn 1977).
Hall v. Schulte, 836kP2d 989 (Ariz Or of App 1992).
Heinecke v. Department of Commerce, 810 P2d 459 (Utah App 1991).
Health Insurance Portability and Accountability Act of 1996.
Jackson v. Indiana, 406 US 715 (1972).
Laben JK, MacLean CP: *Legal issues and guidelines for nurses who care for the mentally ill,* Owings Mills, Md, 1989, National Health Publishing.
Laben JK, Spencer LD: Decentralization of forensic services, *Community Ment Health J* 12(4):405, 1976.
LaFond JQ: Law and the delivery of involuntary mental health services, *Am J Orthopsychiatry* 64(2):409, 1994.
Lake v. Cameron, 364 F2d 657 (DC Cir 1966 *en banc*).
Lamb HR, Weinberger LE: Persons with severe mental illness in jails and prisons: a review, *Psychiatr Serv* 49(4):483, 1998.
Lanterman-Petris-Short Act of 1969.
Lazarus A: Disputes over payment for hospitalization under mental health "carve-out" programs, *Hosp Community Psychiatry* 45(2):115, 1994.

Leonard v. Iowa, 491 NW2d 508 (Iowa Sup Ct 1992).

Mackie v. Runyon, 804 F Supp 1508 (1992).

Mental Health Equitable Treatment Act of 2001.

Nurse's handbook of law and ethics, Springhouse, Penn, 1992, Springhouse.

O'Connor v. Donaldson, 422 U5 563 (1975).

Olsen DP: Ethical consideration of video monitoring psychiatric patients in seclusion and restraint, *Arch Psychiatr Nurs* 12(2):90, 1998.

Parry J: Mental disabilities under the APA: a difficult path to follow, *Ment Phys Disabil Law Rep* 17(1):100, 1985.

Pennsylvania Department of Public Welfare, Office of Mental Health and Substance Abuse Services: *Leading the way toward a seclusion and restraint-free environment—Pennsylvania's Seclusion and Restraint Reduction Initiative,* Harrisburg, 2000, Office of Mental Health and Substance Abuse Services.

Poss v. Department of Human Resources, 426 SE2d 635 (Go Or App 1992).

Purtilo R: *Ethical dimensions in the health professions,* ed 2, Philadelphia, 1993, WB Saunders.

Rennie v. Klein 416 F Supp 1294 (1979); 653 F2d 836 (3rd Cir 1981); 454 US 1978 (1982).

Restraint and Seclusion Standards for Behavioral Health effective January 1, 2001, Joint Commission for the Accreditation of HealthCare Organizations website, November 2000.

Rudegair TS, Applebaum PS: On the duty to protect: an evolutionary perspective, *Bull Am Acad Psychiatry Law* 20(4):419, 1992.

Russell J: *Out of bounds sexual exploitation in counseling and therapy,* London, 1993, Sage Publications.

Sales BD, Shuman DW: Mental health law and mental health care: introduction, *Am J Orthopsychiatry* 64(2):172, 1994.

Shah S: *Criminal responsibility in forensic psychiatry and psychology,* Philadelphia, 1986, FA Davis.

Sharp HealthCare publication, San Diego, California, 2002.

Simon RI: *Psychiatry and law for clinicians,* ed 3, 2001, American Psychiatric Publishing.

Simon RI: Psychiatrists' duties in discharging sicker and potentially violent inpatients in the managed care era, *Psychiatr Serv* 49(1):62, 1998.

Smith v. King, 615 So2s 69 (Ala Sup Ct 1993).

Statement on psychiatric mental health nursing practice and standards of psychiatric mental health clinical nursing practice, Washington, DC, 1994, American Nurses Publishing.

Stefan S: What constitutes departure from professional judgment? *Ment Phys Disabil Law Rep* 17(2):207, 1993.

Strasburger L, Jorgenson L, Randles R: Criminalization of psychotherapist-patient sex, *Am J Psychiatry* 148:859, 1991.

Studer, Quint, Sharp HealthCare Leadership Development session, November 2002.

Tarasoff v. Regents of the University of California, 529 P2d 553 (Cal 1974) and 551 P2d 334 (Cal 1976).

Tenn Code Ann §33-6-201, 33-10-103, 33-3-105.

Torrey EF, Kaplan RS: A national survey of the use of outpatient commitment, *Psychiatr Serv* 46(8):778, 1995.

Washington Antipsychotic Medication: ECT: legislative and regulatory developments, *Ment Phys Disabil Law Rep* 17(2):206, 1993.

Weiner BA, Wettstein RM: *Legal issues in mental health care,* New York, 1993, Plenum Press.

Wexler DB, Winick BJ: Therapeutic jurisprudence and criminal justice mental health issues, *Ment Phys Disabil Law Rep* 16(2):225, 1992.

Woe v. Cuomo 638 F Supp 1506 (ED NY 1986).

Wyatt v. Stickney 344 F Supp 373 (1972).

Youngberg v. Romeo 461 US 308 (1982).

SUGGESTED READINGS

American Psychiatric Nurses Association: *Seclusion and restraint: position statement & standards of practice,* Arlington, Virginia, 2001.

California Senate Office of Research, *Seclusion and restraints: a failure, not a treatment,* March 2002.

Dee V, van Servellen G, Brecht ML: Managed behavioral health care patients and their nursing care problems, level of functioning and impairment on discharge, *J Am Psychiatr Nurses Assoc* 4(2):57, 1998.

Treatment for major depression in managed care and fee-for-service systems, *Am J Psychiatry* 155:859, 1998.

5 Cultural and Spiritual Issues

Merry A. Armstrong and Phillip R. Deming

KEY TERMS

acculturation (p. 66)
assimilation (p. 66)
cultural competence (p. 69)
culture (p. 67)
ethnicity (p. 67)
ethnocentrism (p. 66)
faith (p. 82)
heritage consistency (p. 70)
religion (p. 82)
socialization (p. 68)
spirituality (p. 82)
xenophobia (p. 68)

OBJECTIVES

- Discuss the need for a nurse's self-evaluation when providing care to patients from other sociocultural backgrounds.

- Analyze socialization issues—acculturation, assimilation, ethnocentrism, and xenophobia—as they interrelate with heritage and mental health.

- Compare and contrast cultural issues that define mental health perspectives.

- Differentiate general examples of both health and illness and mental health beliefs and practices of various ethnic and cultural groups.

- Identify selected social issues that interface with mental health beliefs and practices.

- Perform a cultural assessment using the Heritage Assessment Tool.

- Discuss the concept of spirituality in mental health nursing.

- Formulate potential nursing diagnoses related to a client's cultural or ethnic orientation.

- Discuss ways in which planning and implementation of nursing interventions can be adapted to a client's cultural or ethnic orientation.

- Compare and contrast the meanings of spirituality, religion, and faith.

- Develop a spiritual assessment that can be conducted by nurses when pastoral care is not available.

Cultural and spiritual aspects play a significant role in each person's life. Whether or not an individual openly chooses to identify with a specific ethnic, racial, or religious group, inextricable and inherent ties to cultural and spiritual issues remain an influence. Therefore it is necessary for any member of the health care team not only to consider the psychiatric focus on a person's mental health or disorder, but also to include all remaining aspects.

Nursing traditionally has taken a holistic view when caring for clients and their families and has incorporated cultural and spiritual content in academic text and in all levels of actual client care, including assessment, diagnosis, plan of care, intervention, and discharge planning. Psychiatry also now recognizes the necessity for inclusion of cultural and spiritual content. The *Diagnostic and Statistical Manual of Mental Disorders* (DSM-IV-TR) includes several problems that may cause noncompliance with treatment. Among those are ". . . decisions based on personal values, judgments, or religious or cultural beliefs about the advantages or disadvantages of the proposed treatment . . ." (APA, 2000). In the first report on mental health by the United States Surgeon General, multiple entries appear that emphasize influence of culture and spirituality in the role of mental wellness and illness (Department of Health and Human Services, 1999).

This chapter discusses the importance of culture and spirituality in mental health. It describes theoretic content pertaining to the topics and provides suggestions for practical applications when working with clients in the mental health care arena.

CULTURAL ISSUES

Becoming familiar with concepts of psychiatric mental health nursing within a cultural and social context is a professional responsibility (American Nurses Association, 1993, 1994, 1997, 2000), and supports an enriched professional nursing practice that evolves and deepens through appreciation and understanding of one's own culture and the culture of others. The provision of health care is a social exchange, and all health care takes place within a social structure. Represented within the social structure of the United States and most other countries are multiplicities of cultures, traditions, and ethnicities.

This chapter presents ideas about culture and describes several predominant types of cultural organizations as a beginning point of inquiry in this area. Becoming familiar with cultural issues in psychiatric mental health nursing provides the reader with cultural awareness and becomes another tool to use when conducting a cultural assessment within a mental health context. The professional nurse strives to become acquainted with cultural and ethnic criteria that identify clients in his or her geographic area and the predominant thinking and perception of mental health and illness in that area. Likewise, the nurse must be able to think critically

about his or her own ideas, values, and assumptions regarding mental health and illness. This sensitivity to personal worldviews helps the nurse to avoid **ethnocentrism,** a universal human characteristic of judging others by one's own standards of believing, acting, thinking, and valuing. Without inclusion of the cultural perspective of self and others, it is impossible to provide adequate psychiatric nursing care. Actualizing social and cultural theory is evidenced in a caring clinical practice and can be defined as cultural competence, which is discussed at a later point in the chapter.

UNDERSTANDING CULTURE

The need for cultural understanding is evident in everyday life, and although it may be a cliché to refer to the United States as a land of immigrants, except for native peoples, this is true. Ten percent of U.S. residents were born elsewhere (www.census.gov/), an increase of 44% from 1990 and the highest rate since 1930. Figure 5-1 demonstrates the countries of origin and state of residence for these immigrants, and Figure 5-2 represents the education of these groups. Some geographic areas in the country are more diverse than others, but wherever nursing care occurs, cultural differences among and between persons exist. This is not to say that the majority of cultural variations occur with clients who are foreign born, because cultural variations among people in the United States also occur as a result of regional differences and the influences of individual heritage. In particular dimensions of culture, differences between people sharing the same culture may be greater than differences across the culture in general (Hofstede, 1991). For example, Kevin and Nadia live in the same city, belong to the same political party, and share the same American culture, but each possesses characteristics that make each of them unique individuals. It is clearly an erroneous belief that one can generalize about individuals according to culture or ethnicity. As people live in and adjust to new environments, several processes occur and are important to understand.

The voluntary and/or involuntary process described as **acculturation** occurs when a member of a cultural group adapts to the new dominant culture in order to survive. This involuntary process evolves, but the person usually can be identified, through language or some other characteristic, as a member of a nondominant culture. The model of second-culture acquisition is what an individual experiences when he or she lives within or between cultures (LaFromboise, Coleman, and Gerton, 1993).

The development of a new cultural identity is known as **assimilation.** This term means becoming, in all ways, like the members of the dominant culture. The process comprises several stages, such as cultural or behavioral assimilation, marital assimilation, identification assimilation, and civic assimilation. The underlying assumption is that the person loses his or her original cultural identity to acquire the new one. However, this is not always possible, and the process of assimilation may cause stress and anxiety (LaFromboise, Coleman, and Gerton, 1993). Stress and anx-

Foreign-Born Population by Region
of Birth: 1970 to 2000
(Percent distribution)

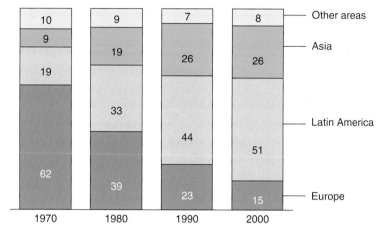

Source: U.S. Census Bureau, P23-206, Figure 2-2.

Foreign-Born Population by State: 2000

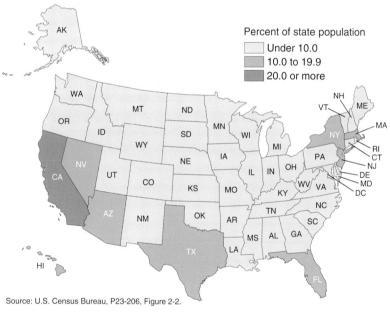

Source: U.S. Census Bureau, P23-206, Figure 2-2.

FIGURE 5-1. United States foreign-born population 2000 (www.census.gov/).

iety may bring this individual into the mental health system for care. How are nurses prepared to serve this diverse population? One effective way to begin the study of culture is to become familiar with one's own culture. Understanding the differences between culture and ethnicity is a beginning point for exploration.

ETHNICITY VS. CULTURE

Useful distinctions are made between the terms *ethnicity* and *culture* and understanding the differences becomes important in psychiatric mental health nursing. **Ethnicity** refers to people from common geographic origins who share language and religion, among other characteristics. Ethnic identification may be considered an internal and personal identification or distinctiveness (Mensah, 1993). **Culture** is a broad term that is related to but is not the same as, or as specific as, ethnicity. For example, one may be culturally American and also share an ethnic relatedness, through traditions, language, and customs, to others who have, for example, Hispanic ancestry. Knowing that someone is from Louisiana does not indicate his or her ethnicity, which may be Cajun, Indian, Middle Eastern, Native American, Germanic, Scandinavian, Hmong, or that of any other group.

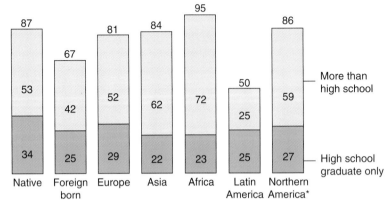

High School Completion or Higher by Nativity and
Region of Birth of the Foreign-Born Population: 2000
(Percent of the population 25 years and older)

*Northern America includes Canada, Bermuda, Greenland and St. Pierre and Miquelon.
Source: U.S. Census Bureau, P23-206, Figure 14-1 and 14-2.

FIGURE 5-2. United States foreign-born population education 2000 (www.census.gov/).

Culture is the whole collective process of acquiring shared beliefs, dominant patterns of behavior, values, and attitudes learned through **socialization**. Culture is acquired, transmitted from generation to generation, and shared. Culture determines appropriate dress, language, values, norms for behavior, economics, politics, law and social control, technology, and health care (Germain, 1992). Although people from individual cultures share many aspects of that culture, every person has a unique response to and relation to that culture. A culture does not indicate a "king-sized personality" (Hofstede, 1994) but rather refers to a social group that encompasses many different and interdependent people. Culture is influenced by the environment of the area in which people live and has been likened to a biotype in biology, or the population that belongs to a particular ecosystem (Hofstede, 1994).

For example, the culture of a particular high school may contain subsets of persons involved and identified with sports, computers, drama, music, or academics. Thus, an entire society or subgroups within that society, including lifestyles and habits, can be described in terms of culture. Members of those subsets may have their own special ways of talking about areas of interest, probably select friends among those interested in similar activities, and value certain activities above others. Considering society in greater depth, Geuss (1981) further considers aspects of culture to be areas of beliefs, concepts, attitudes and psychologic dispositions, desires, works of art, and religions and religious rituals. Included in this view of culture are values, principles, and standards that guide a person's actions in the world. For example, one's culture provides rules for touching; styles of communication, including appropriate eye contact; and relationships with others. The values set forth in a culture connect us to (and/or set us apart from) our families, communities, and social groups. In addition to positive values, negative values are manifested in "isms" or phobias:

| Box 5-1 | Common Prejudices or Biases |

Racism
The belief that members of one race are superior to those of other races.

Sexism
The belief that members of one sex are superior to the other sex.

Heterosexism
The belief that everyone is or should be heterosexual and that heterosexuality is best, normal, and superior.

Ageism
The belief that members of one age group are superior to those of other ages.

Ethnocentrism
The belief that one's own cultural, ethnic, or professional group is superior to that of others. One judges others by his or her own "yardstick" and is unable or unwilling to see what the other group is really about.

Xenophobia
The morbid fear of strangers and those who are not of one's own ethnic group.

From American Nurses Association: *Multicultural issues in the nursing workforce*, Washington, DC, 1993, The Association.

racism, sexism, ageism, classism, **xenophobia**, homophobia, anti-Semitism, and others. "Isms" are often reflected as stereotypes that we have about others that can manifest as prejudicial thinking and behavior (Box 5-1).

CULTURE AND MENTAL HEALTH

The influence of a culture is so pervasive that people can fail to recognize cultural aspects of life. Cultural differences deem what behavior is normal and what behavior is aber-

Box 5-2   Ensuring Cultural Competence in Health Care: Recommendations for National Standards and an Outcomes-Focused Research Agenda

Preamble: Culture and language have considerable impact on how patients access and respond to health care services. To ensure equal access to quality health care by diverse populations, health care organizations and providers should:

1. Promote and support the attitudes, behaviors, knowledge, and skills necessary for staff to work respectfully and effectively with patients and each other in a culturally diverse work environment.

2. Have a comprehensive management strategy to address culturally and linguistically appropriate services, including strategic goals, plans, policies, procedures, and designated staff responsible for implementation.

3. Use formal mechanisms for community and consumer involvement in the design and execution of service delivery, including planning, policy making, operations, evaluation, training, and, as appropriate, treatment planning.

4. Develop and implement a strategy to recruit, retain, and promote qualified, diverse, and culturally competent administrative, clinical, and support staff who are trained and qualified to address the needs of the racial and ethnic communities being served.

5. Require and arrange for ongoing education and training for administrative, clinical, and support staff in culturally and linguistically competent service delivery.

6. Provide all clients with limited English proficiency (LEP) access to bilingual staff or interpretation services.

7. Provide oral and written notices, including translated signage at key points of contact, to clients in their primary language informing them of their right to receive no-cost interpreter services.

8. Translate and make available signage and commonly used written patient educational material and other materials for members of the predominant language groups in service areas.

9. Ensure that interpreters and bilingual staff can demonstrate bilingual proficiency and receive training that includes the skills and ethics of interpreting, and knowledge in both languages of the terms and concepts relevant to clinical or nonclinical encounters. Family or friends are not considered adequate substitutes because they usually lack these abilities.

10. Ensure that the client's primary spoken language and self-identified race/ethnicity are included in the health care organization's management information system, as well as any patient records used by provider staff.

11. Use a variety of methods to collect and use accurate demographic, cultural, epidemiologic, and clinical outcome data for racial and ethnic groups in the service area, and become informed about the ethnic/cultural needs, resources, and assets of the surrounding community.

12. Undertake ongoing organizational self-assessments of cultural and linguistic competence, and integrate measures of access, satisfaction, quality, and outcomes for CLAS into other organizational internal audits and performance improvement programs.

13. Develop structures and procedures to address cross-cultural ethical and legal conflicts in health care delivery and complaints or grievances by patients and staff about unfair, culturally insensitive or discriminatory treatment, or difficulty in accessing services, or denial of services.

14. Prepare an annual progress report documenting the organizations' progress with implementing CLAS standards, including information on programs, staffing, and resources.

rant, what beliefs are tolerable and acceptable, and what beliefs are not acceptable. These collective beliefs change over time and are influenced by many factors. Cultural assumptions become the basis for decisions and actions, are part of one's fundamental psychologic realities, are deeply ingrained, are difficult to identify, and are difficult to change (Fielo and Degazon, 1997). Definitions of mental health and illness, as well as entire concepts of mental health and illness, may be different in different societal structures. To illustrate this point, note that Appendix I of DSM-IV-TR (APA, 2000), provides information about syndromes that are predominantly found in particular cultures (culture-bound syndromes) that may be of interest to nursing students. This appendix also notes that certain psychiatric syndromes are found in the *Chinese Classification of Mental Disorders,* illustrating that different cultures regard normal and abnormal behaviors in different ways. Because of differences in pharmacokinetics and pharmacodynamics, culture may be a variable when considering drug therapy (Keltner and Folks, 1992).

Mental health team members contribute different skills to the care of the client and how that person's particular worldview influences mental health care. Definitions of mental

health and illness can be examined from the perspective of the individual, the perspective of the family or immediate social group, and the perspective of the trained professional. Kleinman (1980), a medical sociologist, proposes that perceptions of normal and abnormal behavior are influenced and shaped by culture. It is clear that many social systems are involved in the care of the mentally ill and that social systems are culturally based. The nurse must identify those social systems and their foundational cultural principles in order to function most effectively to advocate for appropriate patient care. A necessary collection of skills and knowledge the nurse uses in these circumstances is culturally competent practice.

CULTURAL COMPETENCE

One set of national practice standards developed and instituted by health care professionals addresses **cultural competence.** Various versions of competency standards are required components of care by specific managed care and other health care payers who monitor quality of care. Recent federal standards (Office of Minority Health, 2000) for cultural competency include 14 statements found in Box 5-2. These important standards, reviewed by numer-

UNDERSTANDING and APPLYING RESEARCH

This case study illustrates the conflicts that arose when a 90-year-old Orthodox Jewish South African woman was referred to a nursing center in the United States. Placement in a nursing home was not acceptable to the client because she could not choose who would care for her. The client had been raised in Pretoria, South Africa, while apartheid was prevalent. She was accustomed to thinking of Africans as being in service positions and largely uneducated. Although caregivers visited her home, the client ignored those who were Hispanic or Afro-Carribean, or otherwise made them feel uncomfortable. These conflicts were addressed by the nursing director. The Jamaican nurse felt rejected but at the same time honored the client's right to choose who would care for her. The nurse appreciated opportunities in the United States and was learning to cope with expressions of discrimination. Her verbalizations that this situation was not troublesome was doubted by some other team members. Team conferences were held that included the client and her son. The conferences centered on open discussions on thinking processes and were not intended to influence the client to accept care from someone she found problematic. A compromise was reached when a British-born nursing student offered to help with this client's care. This was acceptable to all, and the plan of care continued until the client had further health problems.

This case study presents a difficult situation and a plan to address that difficulty. The author encourages clear commitment to fostering a climate that recognizes cultural needs and to establishing clear policies to encourage problem solving and decision making.

Fielo S: When cultures collide: decision making in a multicultural environment: an elder-care case study illustrates the concept of culturally competent nursing care and its implications for nurse-client relationships, *Nurs Health Care Perspect* 18(5):238, 1997.

Box 5-3   Health Care Practices

Health-Seeking Beliefs and Behaviors
Identify predominant beliefs that influence health care practices.
Describe the influences of health promotion and prevention practices.

Responsibility for Health Care
Describe the focus of acute care practice (curative or fatalistic).
Explore who assumes responsibility for health care in this culture.
Describe the role of health insurance in this culture.
Explore behaviors associated with the use of over-the-counter medications.

Folklore Practices
Explore combinations of magicoreligious beliefs, folklore, and traditional beliefs that influence health care behaviors.

Barriers to Health Care
Identify barriers to health care such as language, economics, and geography for this group.

Cultural Responses to Health and Illness
Explore cultural beliefs and responses to pain that influence interventions. Does pain have a special meaning?
Describe beliefs and views about mental illness in this culture.
Differentiate between the perceptions of mentally and physically handicapped in this culture.
Describe cultural beliefs and practices related to chronicity and rehabilitation.
Identify cultural perceptions of the sick role in this group.

Modified from Purnell L, Paulanka B: *Transcultural health care: a culturally competent approach,* Philadelphia, 1998, FA Davis.

---

ous groups interested in the provision of culturally competent care to all individuals, are being integrated into professional and institutional standard statements. Some national standards address health care systems and require time to implement, such as the provision of signage and institutional self-assessment processes. Other standards address the cultural competence of individuals providing care to patients.

The purpose of cultural competence is to ensure that patients of all cultures are given every opportunity to receive information about treatment in ways that they understand, considering their education, acculturation, and language (see Understanding and Applying Research box). One definition of cultural competency is the following: "Cultural and linguistic competence is a set of congruent behaviors, attitudes, and policies that come together in a system, agency, or among professionals that enables effective work in cross cultural situations" (Meadows, 2000).

How do nurses approach thinking about culture and mental illness, sickness, and disease? Why is a working knowledge of cultural influences in mental health important? The experience of illness from the individual and family point of view can be ascertained in various ways. Health care practices, including health-seeking behaviors, responsibility for

health care, folklore practices, barriers to health care, and cultural responses to health and illness including mental illness, are summarized in Box 5-3.

Spector's Heritage Assessment Tool (Box 5-4) may be used when assessing persons who identify with a traditional culture within the modern American culture. As the nurse begins to develop skills in this form of assessment, it is suggested that the initial assessment of an individual be a personal one, followed by assessments of the individual's parents, family members, and friends. Because most clients (especially those in mental health settings) often do not react well to pencil-and-paper questionnaires, it is helpful to memorize the scope and nature of these questions and then piece together the information needed to determine a client's level of **heritage consistency.**

Considering Self in Cultural Competence

Nurses may think of themselves as being continually in the process of becoming culturally competent, rather than being culturally competent (Camphina-Bacote, 2002). This suggestion implies that we are lifelong learners about culture and constantly work to understand individuals, and ourselves, as part of a culture and within that culture. Purnell

Box 5-4   Heritage Assessment Tool

1. Where was your mother born?
2. Where was your father born?
3. Where were your grandparents born?
   a. Your mother's mother?
   b. Your mother's father?
   c. Your father's mother?
   d. Your father's father?
4. How many brothers and sisters do you have?
5. What setting did you grow up in?
   a. Urban
   b. Rural
   c. Suburban
6. What country did your parents grow up in?
   a. Father
   b. Mother
7. How old were you when you came to the United States?
8. How old were your parents when they came to the United States?
   a. Mother
   b. Father
9. When you were growing up, who lived with you? (ask this way)
   a. Nuclear family
   b. Extended family
   c. Single-parent family
   d. Other
10. Have you maintained contact with:
    a. Aunts, uncles, cousins?   (1) Yes   (2) No
    b. Brothers and sisters?   (1) Yes   (2) No
    c. Parents?   (1) Yes   (2) No
    d. Your own children?   (1) Yes   (2) No
11. Did most of your aunts, uncles, and cousins live near to your home when you were growing up?
    a. Yes
    b. No
12. Approximately how often did you visit your family members who lived outside of your home when you were young?
    a. Daily
    b. Weekly
    c. Monthly
    d. Once a year or less
    e. Never
13. Was your original family name changed?
    a. Yes
    b. No
14. Do you have a religious preference?
    a. Yes (if yes, please specify)
    b. No (1 point for yes, but 0 for no)
15. Is your spouse the same religion as you?
    a. Yes
    b. No
16. Is your spouse the same ethnic background as you?
    a. Yes
    b. No
17. What kind of school did you go to?
    a. Public (0)
    b. Private
    c. Parochial

18. As an adult, do you live in a neighborhood where the neighbors are the same religion and/or ethnic background as yourself?
    a. Religion   (1) Yes   (2) No
    b. Ethnicity   (1) Yes   (2) No
19. Do you belong to a religious institution?
    a. Yes
    b. No
20. Would you describe yourself as an active member?
    a. Yes
    b. No
21. How often do you attend your religious institution?
    a. More than once a week
    b. Weekly
    c. Monthly (0)
    d. Special holidays only (0)
    e. Never
22. Do you practice your religion in your home?
    a. Yes (please specify, 1 point for each example)
    b. Praying
    c. Bible reading
    d. Diet
    e. Celebrating religious holidays
    f. No
23. Do you prepare foods of your ethnic background?
    a. Yes
    b. No
24. Do you participate in ethnic activities?
    a. Yes (if yes, please specify, 1 point for each)
    b. Singing
    c. Holiday celebrations
    d. Dancing
    e. Festivals
    f. Costumes
    g. Other
    h. No
25. Are your friends from the same religious background as you?
    a. Yes
    b. No
26. Are your friends from the same ethnic background as you?
    a. Yes
    b. No
27. What is your native language (the language your parents may have spoken other than English)?
28. Do you speak this language?
    a. Prefer
    b. Occasionally (0)
    c. Rarely (0)
29. Do you read this language?
    a. Yes
    b. No

The greater the number of "yes" answers, the more likely the client is to strongly identify with a traditional heritage. (The one "no" answer that indicates heritage identity is "Was your name changed?") This assessment may be scored 1 point for each yes from question 10, except where noted (0), and 2 points for no if the person's family name was not Americanized. Again, a high score, usually greater than 15 points, is indicative of identification with a traditional background.

From Spector RE: *Cultural diversity in health and illness,* ed 4, Norwalk, Conn, 1996, Appleton & Lange.

Box 5-5	Cultural Self-Assessment for Nurses

- Who am I with respect to my cultural identity?
- What is my personal heritage, and how deeply do I adhere to it?
- What is my nursing heritage, and how deeply do I adhere to it?
- What biases and assumptions do I have, and how do these affect my ability to interact with clients?
- What do I know about mental health and illness from my formative years?
- What have I learned about mental health and illness in nursing?

and Paulanka (1998) define a person who is culturally competent as one who:

- Develops an awareness of his or her own existence, sensations, thoughts, and other environment without letting it have an undue influence on those from other backgrounds
- Demonstrates knowledge and understanding of the client's culture
- Accepts and respects cultural differences
- Adapts care to be congruent with the client's culture

One proposition of this model is that one progresses from unconscious incompetence (not being aware at all of lacking information about other cultures) to conscious incompetence (being aware that one lacks information about other cultures), to conscious competence (actively learning about other cultures and verifying this information), and finally to unconscious competence, when one automatically provides culturally competent care. These authors believe that most caregivers achieve conscious competence but must always be on the alert for ethnocentrism and the effect of deeply held values on attitudes and behaviors toward others. Being culturally competent is an expectation of professionals working in the United States and is a requirement of accrediting bodies that examine the quality of care in health care institutions. Having a culturally competent practice means that one is able to render care in a cultural environment different from one's own and that one can relate, communicate, and sensitively provide care in a manner appropriate for clients and their families. Pertinent questions that nurses may ask themselves about their own cultural perspective are found in Box 5-5.

The nurse and other health care providers are important advocates in helping clients and families understand various treatment components in our multilingual and ethnically diverse environments. This is particularly critical in the area of mental health, given the complex terminology and myriad behaviors and symptoms that require accurate interpretation by a culturally aware staff. Interpreters must be able to attach accurate meaning and purpose to a client's language so that nursing implications for effective treatment are clearly understood. Cultural diversity helps nurses and professionals in other health care disciplines recognize that people are more alike than different and that everyone deserves the best possible physical and psychologic treatment regardless of language, culture, and ethnicity. A summary of cultural competence standards in clinical practice is located in Box 5-6.

Box 5-6	Summary of Cultural Competence Standards in Clinical Practice

- Availability of professional interpreters who are capable of effectively communicating with the population they serve
- A multicultural, multilingual staff who effectively represent the community they serve
- Psychologic testing that is culturally sound and appropriate for the ethnically diverse population
- Cultural components as part of the patient admission interview, treatment plan, education plan, interventions, and discharge plan
- Use of resources, including family and community, in helping patients meet cultural needs
- Physician recognition that cultural factors play a role in treatment compliance
- Involvement in culturally competent community research and training
- Provider involvement in ongoing cultural competence self-assessment
- Agency/facility involvement in ongoing cultural competence self-assessment

Each cultural competence standard is accompanied by a series of objectives and outcomes for that standard. Methods of outcome measurement include:

- Submission of written protocols such as documentation in the medical record of how the language needs of the client were met
- Quarterly and annual reports, including an annual program review of the bilingual proficiency of staff and other agency support positions
- Periodic site reviews by designated county reviewers
- Client satisfaction survey reports in culturally sensitive areas
- Documentation in the medical record of client orientation, education, treatment goals, legal issues, program expectations of the client and provider, and confidentiality that meet cultural needs
- Availability of a clinic/hospital brochure describing treatment services in the preferred language of the client
- Minimum of 4 hours required for staff training per year, with submission of a report listing staff names and hours of cultural competence training (Staff training log must be kept on site.)
- Procedure/protocol for psychologists to access consultation when needed for assessment of ethnically diverse clients (This is to be documented in the client's medical record.)

COMMUNICATION

As health care professionals, we communicate through words, gestures, and our dress and deportment. Written, spoken, and nonverbal forms of language are equally important aspects in communicating with clients. More information is transmitted nonverbally than verbally. Nonverbal communication provides the process and context through which messages are communicated and is used extensively for much of the world's population. *Although generalizing about individuals solely on the basis of their culture is impossible, understanding low- and high-context cultures helps the nurse understand barriers to dynamic communication and expression.*

Low-Context and High-Context Cultures

Many approaches to understanding culture can be found in various disciplines such as anthropology, sociology, and psychology. Examination of those disciplines yields a sociologic model that is helpful in psychiatric mental health nursing. This model addresses behavioral and communication aspects of culture and considers societies whose foundations are low context (individualistic) or high context (collectivistic). This sociologic framework suggests that one universal characteristic of culture is the way that individuals relate to one another. Hofstede (1991) suggests that an individualistic, or low-context, society is one in which people are expected to care for themselves and their immediate family. Low-context societies emphasize thinking and values that are centered on the individual: autonomy, individual initiative, the right to privacy, emotional independence, and universalism (arriving at rules of conduct that are applied to everyone). Although there are wide variations among persons in any culture, these qualities are generally characteristic of persons who function in a democratic environment in which most members of the society have a legal voice and are expected to advocate for themselves. These cultures emphasize individual thinking and an analytic style of approaching a situation without considering the context or social situation in which the individual is acting. In general, this kind of thinking is typically American and is found in other Western cultures. Successful communication in this type of culture includes being assertive (including making direct eye contact), advocating for oneself, thinking through problems independently, and arguing for a point of view. It is typical for Americans to use this type of interactional style as a standard; however, many of the world's peoples do not function with these understandings.

In contrast, a high-context society is one in which people are included in strong, cohesive groups throughout their lifetime. These persons stress a "we" consciousness, collective identity, group solidarity, sharing, group decision making, collective duties and obligations, emotional dependence, and particularism (arriving at rules of conduct that are applied to persons depending on their particular role in society) (Hofstede, 1980; Kim, 1994). These cultures are referred to as high context because the emphasis is on the individual as part of a societal structure and within relationships whose rules may be inferred by those who are part of that culture.

Several high-context cultural cues are present and noticeable to the observer. For example, those from a high-context culture orientation tend to use communication that is more global and based on standards external to the person, such as social position. Successful communication in this culture may depend on the physical context and the cultural information internalized in the communicators. More of the message is developed from nonverbal symbolization and cultural roles in the society.

Many Asian, some South American, Hispanic, African-American, and some Native American cultures may share high-context culture characteristics. This cultural environment supports the development of persons who base their decisions on group input, may not want to argue in public, may use indirect language to communicate, and may also be hesitant to make direct eye contact. Roles of women and men in some cultures may dictate appropriate interaction with professional persons or those outside the family. (It must be remembered, however, that wide individual variations exist within any culture, and knowing that a client is from a particular culture is just a starting point.)

The reader is encouraged to remember that any description of culture is not to be confused with stereotyping cultures, and examples of high-context culture responses may provide perspective. A client from a high-context culture stated that he could not offer an opinion about treatment because he did not know what to say. This stance was not due to lack of information or intellectual ability but was based on his lack of training in making arguments and inability to refute or question another's opinion. His culture had taught him that important statements were based on authority, which as a client he did not possess. Thus he believed that his own observations and feelings were not appropriate to verbalize. Another client thought that she could not speak in public because she might be wrong and would embarrass her family by this action. It is important to ascertain clients' levels of comfort in speaking for themselves. Some questions suggested by Swanson (1993) are:

- When is it appropriate to express yourself publicly?
- What subjects are appropriate to express publicly?
- When is it appropriate to disagree?
- When do you think it is appropriate to express disagreement?
- To whom is it appropriate to express disagreement?

These two styles of communication and relationship to society are important to include in one's assessment of culture because clients may come from a high-context culture and find themselves as clients in a low-context culture. For the nurse to appreciate the patient's experience of illness, investigation of the client's comfort level in a high- or low-context culture must occur, because the American system of health care requires individuals to speak for themselves, articulate a dissenting opinion, and function apart from their families. Those from cultures who function with different assumptions can present perplexing situations (Lester, 1998). The nurse's role as a client advocate may be of the utmost importance in this situation, as clients with chronic mental illness often have low self-esteem, have difficulty processing information, and may thus have a great deal of difficulty speaking for themselves. If the caregivers are from a low-context culture (analytic and objective) and the client is from a high-context culture (identification with a group and symbolic meanings), these problems may be intensified.

Obtaining Translation Services

Guidelines for obtaining translation services are important. The reader can imagine that trying to communicate about an important and often complex health care matter is difficult without specific language. Nurses are often in the position of using translation services, and a good interview question before accepting a position in a particular health care facility is the provision of translation services. It is important to acquire accurate translation, using a trained, credentialed, or certified translator if possible. Using a family member or ancillary hospital staff is often convenient but not recommended, because the client may wish to avoid embarrassing the translator or reveal information that would be culturally inappropriate. Accuracy of translation may be affected by many factors, and care must be taken to avoid bias on the part of the translator. It is a good idea to use standard communication techniques when asking questions through an interpreter, beginning with general information and asking sensitive questions after communication has been established. Communication patterns in low-context cultures may be characterized by fewer words and more nonverbal communication. Therefore the translator may seem not to be asking the questions posed by the interviewer. It is important to consider the communication context and preference of the client and translator. The care team needs to incorporate a plan of adequate translator involvement for adequate ongoing assessment of the client's status. Box 5-7 provides suggestions for communicating with and obtaining translation for clients who speak other languages.

Important cultural needs may include dietary needs. In addition, reading materials, especially client education materials, need to be provided in the client's language. Some hospitals with large populations have specific units for clients with specific cultural needs (Foster, 1990).

Meeting Spiritual Needs

Akin to obtaining translation services is the provision of spiritual support or pastoral counseling to psychiatric clients. It is helpful for clients when the nurse obtains a representative of traditional faith to offer them support, and access and provision of these services are a standard of credentialing organizations. A person's spirituality includes the core beliefs about people, the divine, and the relationship between them (Deming, 2000). Expressions of spirituality can take many forms through music, art, poetry, and stories, among others. Religion, as differentiated from spirituality, is one way that a person expresses his or her spirituality, either through an organized faith community or personal expression, and may also include music, art, and beliefs and practices.

In general, one of the pastoral services offered by institutions or within communities is to contact appropriate representatives of the patient's faith tradition. Having these services available is often of great comfort to the mentally ill. Certified Pastoral Counselors (CPCs) are skilled in communicating with mentally ill patients. The nurse's role is to ascertain if the patient wishes to make use of these persons by visitation, prayer, or other faith tradition. Part of the typical

Box 5-7   Communicating with Patients Who Speak a Foreign Language

- Use interpreters rather than translators. Translators just restate the words from one language to another. An interpreter decodes the words and provides the meaning behind the message.
- Use dialect-specific interpreters whenever possible.
- Use interpreters trained in the health care field.
- Give the interpreter time alone with the client.
- Provide time for translation and interpretation.
- Be aware that interpreters may affect the reporting of symptoms, insert their own ideas, or omit information.
- Avoid the use of relatives who may distort information or not be objective.
- Avoid using children as interpreters, especially with sensitive topics.
- Use same-age and same-gender interpreters whenever possible.
- Maintain eye contact with both the client and the interpreter to elicit feedback and read nonverbal cues. (NOTE: Some cultures interpret constant eye contact as disrespectful or aggressive, so nurses will vary eye contact.)
- Remember that clients can usually understand more than they can express; thus they need time to think in their own language. They are alert to the health care provider's body language, and they may forget some or all of their English in times of stress.
- Speak slowly without exaggerated mouthing, allow time for translation, use the active rather than the passive tense, wait for feedback, and restate the message. Do not rush; do not speak loudly. Use a reference book with common phrases, such as *Roget's International Thesaurus* or *Taber's Cyclopedic Medical Dictionary*.
- Use as many words as possible in the client's language, and use nonverbal communication when you and the client are unable to understand each other's language.
- If an interpreter is unavailable, the use of a translator may be acceptable. The difficulty with translation is omission of parts of the message, distortion of the message, transmission of information not given by the speaker, and messages not being fully understood.

NOTE: Social class differences between the interpreter and the client may result in the interpreter's not reporting information that he or she perceives as superstitious or unimportant.

psychiatric intake assessment includes concerns about spirituality or religion. Patient concerns are usually addressed by contacting a representative of the patient's faith tradition to meet with the patient and/or the health care team to share issues and make plans to meet the patient's needs.

Patients with depression or crisis are often comforted by having a religious practitioner visit them (Andrews and Hanson, 1999). Frequently, representatives of faith traditions such as elders, rabbis, or ministers may visit psychiatric units to visit people from their communities. Occasionally, patients with serious mental disorders experience delusions that are spiritual or religious. As explained in Chapter 11, challenging or debating the veracity of a patient's delusions is not therapeutic, and spiritual delusions are no exception. The nurse is advised to avoid arguing or debating the specifics of a delusion and to focus on decreasing the patient's anxiety or agitation.

Nurses must be consciously aware of their own personal beliefs about spirituality and religion to avoid sending confusing messages to the patient. For example, advising the patient that mental illness can be cured with a particular spiritual practice is inappropriate, even if the nurse believes this is true. Engaging in spiritual or religious practice with patients on a psychiatric unit is inappropriate. The nurse must gain skill in eliciting information about what is causing the patient distress without delving into specific spiritual or religious material. CPCs are skilled in counseling patients and consulting with staff about these problems and can assist the health care team in ways to address particular concerns of individual patients.

CROSS-CULTURAL PERSPECTIVES OF MENTAL HEALTH

Vast differences occur between and among individuals. Beliefs, values, and behaviors of persons of various cultures and ethnic groups can be discussed only with conscious awareness of the differences between each and every individual. The nurse provides sensitive, culturally competent care by first completing a thorough assessment that identifies these individual differences. Table 5-1 provides a beginning point for approaching persons from different cultural groups, but making the assumption that every person in a particular group shares these characteristics is cultural stereotyping (Foster, 1990) and must be avoided. The degree to which people are influenced by other people and cultures may influence their beliefs about mental illness. Although persons with mental illness are still negatively viewed in much of the world (Purnell and Paulanka, 1998), advances in neuroscience that promote the biochemical model of mental illness are helping to alleviate this social response.

An overview of mental health beliefs and practices from different selected cultures follows, and is preceded by the statement that this information is not intended to stereotype any group but merely to describe the known traditional means by which an individual member or family of a given group may cope with a mental health problem. The nurse cannot begin to understand a client with only previously held views of that client's cultural group. Sincere dialog and genuine interest in the client and his or her culture are necessary elements for beginning the process.

African-Americans

Members of the African-American communities in the United States have their origins in Africa and a cultural heritage that is a mixture of the Caribbean cultures, Native American cultures, and northern European cultures (Baker, 1994). In 2000 there were 34,659,190 African-Americans in the United States, or 12.3% of the total population (www.census.gov/).

The family often has a matriarchal structure and there are strong, large, extended family networks. There is a continuation of tradition and a strong religious affiliation within the community. Many African-Americans tend to use traditional medicines and healers when they are knowledgeable in this area and have access to this resource.

Traditional African-Americans may choose to be treated by a traditional healer, and herbs are frequently used to treat

mental symptoms. Several diagnostic techniques include the use of Biblical phrases and material from folk medicine books, observation, and entering the spirit of the client (see Understanding and Applying Research box).

Asian Americans

Members of the Asian–Pacific Island communities in the United States have their origins in China, Hawaii, the Philippines, Korea, Japan, and Southeast Asia (Cambodia, Laos, and Vietnam). In 2000 there were 10,242,998 Asian Americans in the United States, or 3.6% of the total population (www.census.gov/).

The family has a hierarchical structure, and loyalty among members is valued. There is a devotion to tradition; many religions, including Taoism, Buddhism, Islam, and Christianity, are practiced. Many people tend to use traditional medicines and healers and herbs are frequently used to treat mental symptoms.

Knowledge regarding mental health therapy is often scant in the Asian communities, especially among recent emigrants. Two points that must be noted: the importance placed on the family in caring for the mentally ill and that Asian peoples may tend to describe mental illness in somatic terms. A tremendous amount of stigma is attached to mental illness. Asian clients tend to come to the attention of mental health workers late in the course of their illness, and they come with a feeling of hopelessness (Lin, 1982).

European Origin

Members of this community have origins throughout Europe and constitute 15% of the foreign-born population of the United States (www.census.gov/). The 2000 census counted 211,460,626 people who indicated their heritage as European, or 75.1% of the population. Those noting two races (Caucasian was one) constituted 77.1 of the population. Many languages comprise the communication, and in general, this population

Table 5-1 Cross-Cultural Examples of Selected Communication Phenomena That Affect Nursing Care

Nations of Origin	Language	Space	Time Orientation	Mental Illness*
Asian Origin				
China	National language	Noncontact people	Present	Metabolic imbalance and organic problem
Hawaii	preference			Evaluate (many other beliefs)
Philippines	Dialects, written			
Korea	characters			
Japan	Use of silence			
Southeast Asia	Nonverbal and contextual			
Laos	cueing			
Cambodia				
Vietnam				
African Origin				
West Coast (as slaves)	National languages	Close personal space	Present over future	Spiritual distress
Many African countries	Dialect			Evaluate for religious beliefs
West Indian islands	Pidgin			Evaluate (many other beliefs)
Dominican Republic	Creole			
Haiti	Spanish			
Jamaica	French			
European Origin				
Germany	National languages	Noncontact people	Future over present	Evaluate (many beliefs)
England	Many learn English	Aloof		
Italy	immediately	Distant		
Ireland		Southern countries: closer		
Other European countries		contact and touch		
Native American				
170 Native American tribes	Tribal languages	Space is very important	Future over present	Placing of a curse (Navajo)
Aleuts	Many learn English	and has no boundaries		Evaluate (many other beliefs)
Eskimos	immediately			
Hispanic Origin				
Spain	Spanish or Portuguese	Tactile relationships	Present	Spells or bad spirits
Cuba	primary languages	Touch		Evaluate (many other beliefs)
Mexico		Handshakes		
Central and South America		Embracing		
		Values physical presence		
Arab Origin				
Yeman	Arabic	Variable; many customs,	Assess for religion	Consequence of physical or
Lebanon-occupied Palestine	Colloquial Arabic and di-	formal manners		emotional trauma
Oman	alects in many areas			Attributed to supernatural
Saudi Arabia				beings
Morocco				Evaluate (many other beliefs)
Tunisia				
Algeria				
Sudan				
Libya				
Egypt				
Syria				
Jordan				
Iraq				
Kuwait				
Bahrain				
Qatar				
United Arab Emirates				

Data from Spector RE: *Cultural diversity in health and illness,* ed 4 Norwalk, Conn, 1996, Appleton & Lange; Giger JN, Dividhizar RE: *Transcultural nursing,* ed 3, St. Louis, 1999, Mosby; and Purnell L, Paulanka B: *Transcultural health care,* Philadelphia, 1998, FA Davis.
*See DSM-IV-TR for culture-bound syndromes.

expresses a low-context cultural heritage. Individual strengths and independence are valued and community identification is less emphasized than in some of the other groups mentioned here. Traditional religious practice is common and many nationalities are represented in this group. Careful assessment, as in all the other groups, is key to understanding the individual. Individuals in this population may seek traditional medical care; many use alternative health care before seeking allopathic treatment. Mental illness is becoming more understood but is still often viewed as a moral failing.

Hispanics

Members of the Hispanic community have their origins in Spain, Cuba, Central and South America, Mexico, Puerto Rico, and other Spanish-speaking countries. In 2000 there were 35,305,818 Hispanics in the United States, or 12.5% of the total population. One half of the foreign-born population of the United States are from Latin American countries, primarily Mexico, Cuba, the Dominican Republic, and El Salvador (www.census.gov/).

The family often has a nuclear structure, with strong, large, extended family networks and *compadrazzo* (godparents). There is continuation of tradition and a strong church affiliation within the community. Many use traditional medicines and healers and are knowledgeable about these resources. People may be treated by a traditional healer such as a *curandero*, *santero*, or *señora*; herbs are frequently used to treat mental symptoms (see Case Study, top right).

Native American Indians

The ancestors of Native American Indians living in the United States today immigrated to this land long before the Europeans and other immigrants. Today there are approximately 170 Native American nations, or tribes, located mostly in the western states. Many Native Americans have remained on reservations, whereas others live in urban and rural areas off the reservations on the East Coast. In 2000 there were 2,475,958 Native Americans and Native Alaskans in the United States, or 0.9% of the total population, the smallest ethnic group in the American population. Although each group has many differences, in general the family often has a nuclear structure, with strong, large, extended family networks, and children are taught to respect traditions and community organizations. Some Native Americans and Native Alaskans use traditional medicines and healers (see Case Study at right).

OUTCOMES OF HEALTH CARE FOR MINORITY POPULATIONS

In two recent documents, Culture, Race, and Ethnicity (USDHHS, 2001) and A Report of the Surgeon General (USDHHS, 1999), it is clearly stated that ethnic and racial minorities are underserved by the mental health system. Both reports cite problems accessing and utilizing services, and effectiveness of treatment when they are accessed. Culturally competent professionals are needed who respect and understand the values, beliefs, histories, and traditions of racial and ethnic groups (CMHS, 1998).

CASE STUDY

Maria, a 20-year-old Hispanic woman, is seen in the psychiatric unit to rule out schizophrenia. She was admitted after she was found screaming in her front yard and acting irrationally. She sat in her room and was well groomed and quiet. She isolated herself from other clients and appeared suspicious of staff. She had poor eye contact and spoke softly when questioned by the nurse. She remarked that her mother, who has been deceased 3 years, appears to her and speaks to her. The nature of these "appearances" is comforting; no commands are given.

Critical Thinking

1. What culture-specific issues may be influencing Maria?
2. How might the assessment process be improved with an understanding of Maria's cultural heritage?
3. It is known that Hispanic people often report hearing the voice of deceased relatives in times of stress. How could the nurse differentiate between this cultural phenomenon and a psychotic thought process?
4. What communication barriers may be operating between Maria and the nurse?

CASE STUDY

Mr. Looie is a 40-year-old Native American Indian who has been diagnosed and treated for paranoid schizophrenia for about 20 years. During an acute phase of his illness, he is hospitalized. While hospitalized, he wishes to have his fan of eagle feathers to control his auditory hallucinations. He waves the fan in front of himself and talks to himself in his native language when he is distressed. This activity frightens some of the other clients. Some of the staff think that the fan should be taken away because it disturbs other clients, but other staff think Mr. Looie has a right to keep the fan if it helps him cope with his symptoms.

Critical Thinking

1. How can the nurse balance the needs of Mr. Looie and the needs of the other clients?
2. Should the nurse support Mr. Looie in the use of this device?
3. What should the nurse's intervention be, if any, when Mr. Looie is seen using his fan?
4. What is the meaning of the fan to Mr. Looie?
5. What other cultural supports might be available to Mr. Looie during his hospitalization?

High degrees of poverty and stress result in an increased incidence of physical and mental illness (ANA, 1997). The cultural expression and personal experience of illness (Kleinman, 1980) may be misinterpreted by the health care practitioner who diagnoses disease using a Western medical model. Diagnosticians may be limited or biased in their application of cross-cultural differences (Davis, 1995) as evidenced by the disproportionate number of diagnoses of schizophrenia given to African-Americans and Hispanics (Davis, 1995; Mandersheid and Sonnenachein, 1996). Persons in poverty are apt to experience more stress and are diagnosed with more severe disorders than those not in poverty situations. Patients from some cultural groups believe that medicine should be taken until the symptoms abate (Andrews and Herberg, 1999). Further, recent developments in identifying unique patterns of pharmacokinetics in various ethic groups are discussed in Chapter 20.

Because employment is tied to most health care plans, many persons from minority cultures either lack access to health care or have access only to very limited health care that often excludes or severely limits mental health care, and persons from minority groups are often handicapped when seeking employment. In addition, among adults considered poor according to defined federal guidelines for poverty, there was a 1.92 greater probability for the development of new (Axis I) psychiatric disorders than among the nonpoor population (Bruce, Takeuchi, and Leaf, 1991). Different cultural and ethnic presentations of symptoms contribute to this disparity, and persons who are less acculturated are not adept at gaining entry into a caregiving system (Ruiz, Venegas-Samuels, and Alarcon, 1995). Therapeutic and treatment issues are also affected if the client is treated by someone not culturally competent (Fielo, 1997). It is estimated that one third to two thirds of clients discharged from psychiatric hospitals return to their families (Cook, 1988; Goldman, 1982; Lefley, 1987). How are these clients managed if their family members are not able to negotiate the often-complicated mental health system or do not agree with the diagnosis? The cycle of poverty depicted in Figure 5-3 perpetuates a closed social and economic system that includes an increased incidence of mental illness, physical illness, and substance abuse.

THE NURSING PROCESS

The principal nursing tool in mental health is the therapeutic use of self. It is in the relationship between the nurse and client that the sensitive and usually embedded cultural issues manifest themselves and impact client care. Therefore understanding the significance of culture and its impact on clients' mental and physical health is of foundational importance for nurses in all settings of health care delivery. This understanding and awareness are integral to the nursing process; they affect assessment, diagnosis, outcome identification, planning, intervention, and evaluation of clients. As the nurse applies the nursing process in the mental health setting, understanding the meanings of the health care problem from both the client's and nurse's cultural perspective is important. Each step of the nursing process is impacted by an understanding of the complex cultural issues that affect clients and their interpretation of life events.

ASSESSMENT

The assessment process is the foundation for all other steps of the nursing process. It is during assessment that the nurse formulates a perspective of the client's needs and issues. Far from being objective, this process is greatly influenced by the nurse's personal biases, assumptions, cultural meanings, and nursing experience.

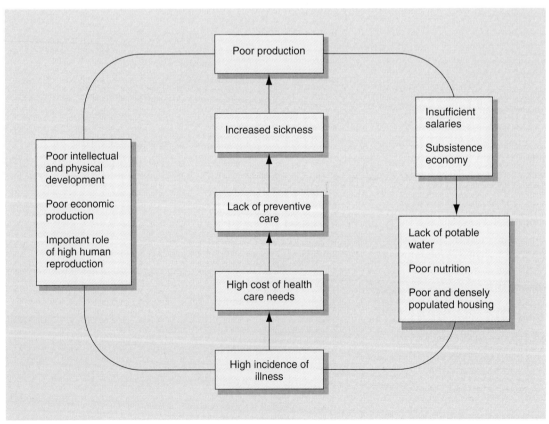

FIGURE 5-3. The cycle of poverty. (From Spector RE: *Cultural diversity in health and illness,* ed 4, Norwalk, Conn, 1996, Appleton & Lange.)

Numerous researchers describe race as a factor that can alter the assessment of symptoms and level of functioning. Lawson et al (1994) describe how racial differences between client and clinician can lead to a failure to appreciate cultural differences in the presentation of symptoms and thus lead to misdiagnosis. In addition, clients from minority groups may delay seeking treatment because of mistrust of the system, which can lead to the application of more serious diagnostic labels. Warren and Lutz (2000) offer a consumer-oriented model of nursing care for recovery and monitoring of mental illness that includes cultural factors. They suggest that cultural patterns and influence contribute significantly to patients' recovery processes.

The client must be truly "heard" to allow for accurate diagnosis. The nurse must be informed and sensitive to advocate for the patient to prevent stereotyping and labeling, major problems in mental health care. The nurse needs to be aware of his or her own personal and professional cultural heritage, as well as the client's cultural heritage and what mental health means in its context. The use of the Heritage Assessment Tool (see Box 5-4) in assessing the client is an entry point for gathering culture-specific data. In addition, the following questions may be asked to gather cultural data:

- *Cultural background.* What is the client's ethnic, religious, spiritual, and racial heritage? If unfamiliar with the client's culture, the nurse should seek information about the specific cultural group by interviewing the client's family and members of the group. Although the nurse might feel uncomfortable initially, most people are happy to be asked and to help inform caregivers about particular issues.
- *Values orientation.* What are the attitudes of the given client, family, or community, based on their cultural heritage, in regard to this mental health problem?
- *Cultural sanction and restrictions.* What are the "rules" in this client's cultural background with respect to this mental health problem? Does the client identify with a high-context or low-context culture?
- *Communication.* What primary language does this client speak? If necessary, the nurse should obtain an interpreter.
- *Health/illness beliefs and practices.* What cultural factors do the client and family associate with the identified problem? What types of traditional healers are available to the family?
- *Nutrition.* What are the specific dietary restrictions to consider, if any?
- *Economic considerations.* What economic resources are available to the family?
- *Educational background.* What is the level of education of both the client and family? Are they able to read, understand, and follow instructions in English or in their native language? Where have they attended schools and for how long? Have they attended schools in the United States? What role does informal education play in their lives?

CLINICAL ALERT

Mrs. Williams is a 50-year-old woman whose husband died about 14 months ago of a myocardial infarction. She has come to the family practice clinic because she has begun to have chest pain and wonders if she might also have cardiac problems. While obtaining a history, the practitioner notices that Mrs. Williams is still dressed in black and adds the diagnosis of delayed bereavement to the history. The practitioner failed to assess Mrs. Williams in terms of her cultural expression of grief. Mrs. Williams is Hispanic, and it is customary for people of many Hispanic cultures to wear black for a year or longer. It would be socially unacceptable for Mrs. Williams to do otherwise.

- *Spiritual or religious affiliation.* What role does spirituality or religion play in the life of the client and family? Is a spiritual advisor or a member of the clergy readily available? What are the religious views of this client and family? Do they have special prayers?

NURSING DIAGNOSIS

The nurse should be as specific as possible in conducting an assessment to determine that an identified problem is individualized for client needs. The nursing diagnoses are much the same for clients from diverse cultural backgrounds, with a few exceptions. Actual culture-related nursing diagnoses include those related to communication barriers, sociocultural dissonance, language barriers, and differences in health and illness beliefs and practices.

The process of deriving a nursing diagnosis is an important one because these diagnostic categories often enable other staff to "frame" a client's health concerns. They must be as accurate as possible and reflect the unique cultural perspective of the client. In other words, they must be culturally congruent.

A nursing diagnosis cannot be correct if made on the basis of an inaccurate assessment. The nurse, viewing client behavior through an ethnocentric lens, interprets the client's behavior as dysfunctional. Box 5-8 describes common nursing diagnoses that are often misapplied to clients as a result of culture-related misunderstandings.

OUTCOME IDENTIFICATION

An understanding of cultural issues is crucial to ensure that the determination of outcomes of nursing care uses client input and is congruent with the clients' needs and wishes. Often clients fail to achieve desired outcomes because such outcomes are inconsistent with their cultural worldview. Many clients will defer to the nurse, whom they see as the "expert." In reality, however, the clients do not plan to follow through with the client educational and discharge planning because it does not make sense to them and is not relevant to their problems from their perspective. This may lead to further misdiagnosis, especially the diagnosis of noncompliance. This happens most often when a client

| Box 5-8 | Commonly Misapplied Nursing Diagnoses |

Common NANDA nursing diagnoses frequently misapplied because of a lack of understanding of cultural issues:

Defensive Coping and Noncompliance
Clients from minority cultures that have experienced discrimination, bias, and stereotyping may be resistant to appropriate nursing interventions, especially in the area of teaching and discharge planning. Suspicion and mistrust may cause the nurse to misunderstand a client's behaviors and mislabel them.

Ineffective Role Performance and Impaired Parenting
Use of these diagnoses requires an understanding of the client's culture-specific roles and parenting activities. They may be different from those of the nurse and the majority culture.

Impaired Social Interaction and Impaired Verbal Communication
Misunderstanding occurs when the nurse fails to take into account culture-specific interaction patterns. Silence, infrequent eye contact, shame, fear, and language barriers all affect clients' ability to interact. The gender of the nurse and the gender of the client may also influence communication because many cultures have specific gender-role behavioral codes.

Disturbed Thought Processes
Thought patterns and processes that may appear to be distorted can be related to culture-specific expressions of anxiety and fear. Careful assessment will enable the nurse to accurately diagnose anxiety or fear in many clients, rather than assume that underlying thought processes are altered.

wants to use a traditional healing method or other culture-specific approach and sees the allopathic-oriented nursing intervention as conflicting with the traditional ways of achieving health.

PLANNING
A client's beliefs are more likely included in a client's mental health care plan when the nurse is aware of the meaning of the client's behavior and verbalizations in the context of his or her culture and traditions. When establishing goals of care and planning nursing interventions, the nurse considers each client's particular situation and challenges. The family is generally included in the client's treatment plan and, as often as possible, the client's community as well.

IMPLEMENTATION
Holistic and culturally sensitive care plans congruent with the patient's culture and needs evolve over time. The care plan is a living document, adjusted as goals are met and other goals are identified. For example, if the client is using ethnomedications, determine what type and how they react with conventional medications. Maintain effective verbal and nonverbal communication between the client and caregivers and obtain an interpreter if necessary. Promote the client's understanding of the allopathic system and the rationale behind the care that is being delivered.

Clients who are members of cultural communities may have a deep-seated mistrust of the system in general and the nurse in particular, especially if the nurse comes from a different cultural background. The nurse must be aware that trust issues are important in mental health nursing care and because of their professional role, they own the responsibility for the therapeutic relationship. For example, researchers have noted that race is a powerful issue in treatment. In particular, it can affect how medication is administered, the level and frequency of interventions, and the outcome of intervention.

In a study of the psychiatric treatment of older African-American clients, Baker (1994) noted that the use of social support mechanisms in the intervention process was crucial in effectively caring for these older clients. This study is typical of many suggesting that mental health intervention must be done within the framework of culture if it is to be effective (Friedman, Paradis, and Hatch, 1994; Hickling and Griffith, 1994; Morris and Silove, 1992; Nelson et al, 1992; Kim et al, 2002). Use of family members and other members of the client's cultural group in the assessment, planning, and intervention process can facilitate nursing care and ensure more effective client outcomes.

EVALUATION
The nurse must evaluate whether the client has been able to maintain his or her cultural beliefs regarding mental health and illness. By so doing, the nurse evaluates mental health care from a multicultural nursing perspective by determining if the client outcomes have been achieved. The client's needs and beliefs should be respected with open lines of communication. The discharge plan should be realistic and culturally congruent. If the client does not feel invested in the treatment choices, he or she is less likely to be effective after discharge. Thus evaluation of nursing interventions is based on the attainment of client outcomes that have been determined to be culturally sensitive and realistic.

SPIRITUALITY
Culture can be a strong influence and significantly affect a person's spirituality. Some cultures place great emphasis on spirituality and religious practices that become traditional and are incorporated into worship and important celebrations that take place in stages from birth to death.

A person's spirituality addresses core beliefs and images about humanity and the divine, as interpreted by the individual, and the relationship between them. These beliefs and images can be healing and sustaining, or punitive and crippling. In the treatment of any illness, including mental illness, it is necessary to attend to the spiritual dimensions of the person.

Serious or persistent and severe mental illness often is associated with increased feelings of loss and powerlessness. Mental illness, especially chronic mental illness, can lead to a cycle of loss: feelings of powerlessness, leading to hopelessness, leading to a sense of despair, which in turn feeds back into a deeper sense of loss. When quality spiritual care is provided in a consistent and effective manner as a key part of a multidisciplinary approach to treatment, both research (Dossey, 1999) and anecdotal evidence indicate that there are significant benefits. These benefits can have both an impact on the client and an impact on other members of the health care team. One benefit is in the reduced length of inpatient stay for those clients who have had their spiritual concerns and questions addressed in an effective and helpful manner. Addressing client spiritual issues may also contribute to a decreased use of total system resources, in that client anxiety may be lessened, symptom control may be more effective, and there may be a reduced number of client complaints, all of which result in an increased level of client satisfaction (Perrin and McDermott, 1997).

RESEARCH

The science/spirituality/health connection has become mainstream knowledge, and research on the power of spirituality and healing has proliferated in the past two decades. Larry Dossey, MD (Dossey, 1997, 1999, 2001), author of several books on that and related subjects, has spent more than 20 years researching and describing the synergy of health and spiritual awareness and practice. For well over a decade, Herbert Benson, MD, and associates from the Mind Body Medical Institute for Spirituality and Health have offered seminars each year that highlight research and modalities of intervention incorporating spirituality and prayer in healing. Emphasis is on diminishing the dichotomy between science and spirituality by presenting hard scientific evidence that spiritual and religious means are effective in facilitating healing and fostering wellness. Great progress has been made in the research, but more focus can be placed on mental illness/wellness aspects.

SPIRITUALITY IN MENTAL HEALTH

Spirituality is an essential and integral part of who we are as individuals. Our spirituality is the thread that connects us with other people, with the world in which we live, and with the divine nature as we experience it. Through our spirituality we can make sense of powerful life experiences that would otherwise be confusing or devastating, and use them in ways that become life sustaining. Our spirituality allows us to make sense of the cycle of life and death. Spirituality gives us the hope and strength to laugh and celebrate life while consciously acknowledging the reality of illness and tragedy. Spirituality also connects us with our human potential and creativity, which are important elements of mental health.

Spirituality plays an important role in mental health (see Nursing Care in the Community box). For many afflicted individuals, their spirituality gives them a powerful sense of hope in the face of an often devastating and chronic illness. For those who experience rejection by family and friends because of the illness's impact on their relationships, spiri-

---

NURSING CARE IN THE COMMUNITY   Spirituality and Well-Being

Spiritual well-being among our mentally ill clients is a relatively unexplored area. It is the one aspect of care that we often neglect and/or overlook during our assessment. As an integral part of our assessment, do we even give any thought to the spiritual needs of our clients? Most likely we have a tendency to be caught up in the all-consuming task of trying to assist our clients in dealing with their multiple problems: behavioral, medication taking, money management, living arrangements, and possibly alcohol/drug usage. Unfortunately, we let these tasks of everyday living take precedence. Perhaps we ourselves are unable to deal with or be comfortable addressing our clients' religious needs. Or we just assume that spirituality is not important in their lives.

Assessment of the spiritual needs of our clients should include their religious and nonreligious beliefs and values. Their religious beliefs and values are going to be complex, personal, and private. For example, one client shared that her religious beliefs gave her a sense of space from a chaotic board-and-care environment, a sense of peace, and, more important for her, time for herself. Although a client's religious beliefs and values may not fit into what we consider accepted religious practices, they do serve a purpose by providing a tangible idea to hold onto. This client believed that the presence of a Higher Power outside herself could be guiding and supporting. Even for those clients who profess nonreligious beliefs in a mystical way—not delusional—these inner experiences of beliefs give them a sense of worth and promote self-esteem and self-confidence.

The available literature on spirituality and the mentally ill is sparse. However, the literature does point out that attending to our client's spiritual needs can serve as a buffer against the increased anxiety they confront in their daily lives. Despite this anxiety, affirmation of self is made easier through a spiritual presence. For many of our clients, their spiritual beliefs may be all they have, as family support, caring friends, and social networks may be nonexistent. Painfully aware of their losses, spirituality can serve to allay the angst associated with being mentally ill or perceived as different. Religion can help to improve the quality of life for our clients, who are often isolated, afraid, lonely, and frequently ignored.

The use of prayer can serve as a source of strength in helping to overcome the uncertainty of living, managing, and surviving in what to them is a hostile, unfriendly world. We need to be able to facilitate and share in prayer with our clients as part of our therapeutic interventions.

In providing spiritual nursing interventions, we need to be comfortable in discussing religious beliefs and values, including our belief in God or a Higher Power, and be able to participate with our clients in their experiences. It is important for us to take the lead from our clients to determine from their perspective what it is that is needed at a particular moment. By bridging onto our client's expressed spiritual interests, we, as nurses, can foster a sense of hope and self-worth for giving meaning and purpose to their lives.

tuality can help maintain a sense of connection and belonging. For those who may feel abandoned, a healthy spirituality can provide a sense of being loved and accepted for who they are as unique individuals, in spite of having a mental illness. Spirituality can also be a solid anchor for those individuals whose illnesses may create feelings of internal chaos. Left unattended, the same spiritual beliefs that help an individual feel accepted and that provides hope can also become punitive or crippling in nature, rather than be a source of healing.

Defining the Terms

Spirituality is a search for the sacred, a need to have a conscious experience of the divine, or a transcendence of self, a meaning of life, however one conceives of it. Spirituality is that part of the person that deals with the transcendent and the universal. Spirituality recognizes one's relationship to the divine and sees how that relationship affects one's experience with people and all of creation. One's spirituality encompasses an understanding of the sacred, of the holy, of faith, and of all those things that are not physical. Spirituality may take expression in religion and ritual, but it is not limited to those things. Music, art, poetry, dance, and stories can all be spiritual expressions. Spirituality is the recognition that some connecting thread weaves through all creation; it is the search to more fully experience that connecting thread. Some spiritual belief goals are listed in Box 5-9.

Religion is a manner of expressing one's spirituality. It may be experienced through membership in a particular community that accepts a formal and organized system of beliefs, or it may be a less formal and more individual set of beliefs and practices. Religious expression may include ritual, ceremonies, music, art, and one's intentional participation in a community that has a specific understanding of history and the future. Christianity, Judaism, Buddhism, Hinduism, Taoism, and Islam are all formal systems of religious beliefs through which individual members are able to experience their spirituality. New Age spirituality is a collection of individual practices that are largely unconnected to formal communities.

Faith is the ability to draw on spiritual resources without having physical and empiric proof. It is an internal certainty that comes from one's own experience with the divine. Faith, although only a part of spirituality, is an essential component. It is through one's experience of faith that a deep individual spirituality can be mobilized to assist one in the challenges and celebrations of life.

MAJOR SPIRITUAL ISSUES

Some major spiritual issues include the fear of death and loss, both of self and others. Spirituality allows one to cope with these feelings by providing a sense of hope and meaning to experiences that would otherwise be crippling. Having a spiritual understanding that one's connection with creation is more than merely physical helps to ease the fear and pain of loss. Feeling connected to the divine eases feelings of abandonment, grief, and alienation, as well as promoting a sense of self-acceptance. Spirituality is thought to be a key component in the healing process and an integral part of the client's treatment plan.

The significant spiritual questions tend to remain constant, regardless of the health care need. Such issues as loss, fear, death, abandonment, and feelings of alienation may be present in clients with both physical and psychiatric illnesses. Responses to these feelings can range from finding new meanings and strength, to acceptance, to grief, to a sense of hopelessness. It is often a spiritual intervention to first acknowledge and validate these feelings, and then help the client to look at ways to rewrite their life story in such a manner as to encompass these experiences. One's spirituality can be a significant help during these times.

Before one can provide effective spiritual interventions, it is critical to identify people who are at significant spiritual risk. Individuals at spiritual risk are defined by Fitchett (1997) as those who have a high spiritual need, coupled with low spiritual resources to meet that need. These individuals have more risk for poor outcomes and should be the primary focus for outcome-based spiritual care.

Intervention Tools

There are a variety of spiritual interventions for use and they range from formal rituals and practices to informal types. Formal Christian rituals, for example, include sacraments, such as baptism, communion, and anointing. Additional formal practices include worship or memorial services, as well as formal confession and absolution. On many of these occasions a chaplain involves members of a local faith community, either in a leadership or a support role. Often a chaplain is in contact with local worship communities to provide appropriate information for formal prayer services at a local church or synagogue when requested by a client.

Informal rituals and practices include pastoral counseling, use of individual or group prayer at the hospital, reading of scripture, and the distribution of devotional books, cards, and

---

Box 5-9   Goals of Spirituality Beliefs

- Providing an image of the divine
- Providing an image of humanity
- Providing an understanding of the relationship between the divine and humanity
- Helping to examine thoughts of divine punishment, reward, or neutrality
- Helping to give belief and meaning to life
- Helping to find a sense of duty, vocation, calling, or moral obligation
- Helping to examine one's experience of the divine and sacred
- Helping to cope with situations and conflict with spiritual understanding
- Providing a format for spiritual rituals and practices
- Providing a faith community
- Providing authority and guidance for one's system of belief, meaning, and ritual

other related materials. The use of rosaries or prayer beads, the playing of music, and the use of icons or pictures often allow the more experiential, noncognitive side of a patient's spirituality to be expressed. Verbal imagery is present in the telling of sacred stories from various traditions. Other forms of visual imagery are also used. Audiotapes and videotapes may be especially helpful. If the client has access to tapes of his or her own community worshipping, that can augment any mass media material that is available.

The nurse is aware that religious practices often are beneficial for clients, but for those who do not pursue formal religion, other spiritual interventions are useful. Group therapies that encourage clients to extend themselves and to find meaning in life are helpful. In addition, several other creative forms of expression such as art, music, and dance therapy often address clients' spiritual needs.

Spiritual Assessment

Assessing an individual's spiritual need and determining interventions that will be helpful and appropriate in addressing that need is an essential component of a chaplain's role in a health care system. Approaching the client where he or she "is" in terms of spirituality requires the ability to acknowledge one's own biases and a willingness to put them aside during the interaction.

Spirituality may be most commonly addressed by a pastor or chaplain. If there is no pastoral care department in the facility, and if the client has no specific faith community, these spiritual issues may never be addressed. Even in cases where one has a faith community, a client may be reluctant to delve too deeply into areas of spirituality that deal with mental illness. Therefore interventions by the nurse addressing these issues may be crucial. Box 5-10 provides a spiritual assessment tool.

Other helpful assessments may focus on the following seven items.

Belief and Meaning

Belief and meaning form the central and foundational principle underlying this model. An individual views life in terms of what he or she perceives is life's meaning. In other words, whatever the individual believes in is important and gives meaning to life. This axis examines how a person makes sense of the world that he or she lives in, and what meanings are ascribed to people, relationships, events, thoughts, actions, and consequences. Some questions that may be included as one examines this axis include:

- What are the beliefs a person has that give meaning and purpose to life, and what are the important symbols that reflect these?
- How does a person's life story reflect or demonstrate these underlying themes?
- Do any areas of the person's life story come into conflict with these underlying, foundational beliefs?
- Do any current situations or problems come into direct conflict with these beliefs?

- In what ways is the person able to consciously articulate these beliefs?
- In what ways do these beliefs seem to be an unconscious part of the person's worldview?

Vocation and Obligation

Out of one's perception of belief and meaning flows a sense of what one needs to do with, and in, life. This axis is very closely linked to the first, in that one usually does what one considers important to do. If a task, action, or thought has no meaning, one is much less likely to do that action or to follow through on thoughts regarding that task. When life circumstances place one in a position in which actions come into conflict with core belief and meaning systems, crisis and significant stress may result. Questions that may be included in this axis are:

- What sense of duty, vocation, calling, or moral obligation does this person have?
- How actively has this client been able to express these in the past?
- What impact does the client's current situation/illness have on these?

Experience and Emotion

In this axis, one examines questions that surround the emotional experience, both helpful and punitive, that one has encountered in experiencing one's own faith. Questions that may be examined in this axis include:

- What experience of the divine or sacred has this person had?
- What emotions or moods are associated with these contacts?
- How does the client's current situation relate to these experiences?

Courage and Growth

This axis examines how one adapts to situations that may confront and conflict with the core beliefs and meanings that one holds. Questions in this axis examine how a client may deal with extremely stressful and challenging issues and include:

- How spiritually adaptable is the client?
- How has the client coped in the past with situations that were in conflict with his or her current spiritual understanding?
- Must new experiences fit into existing belief systems, or can the person's beliefs adapt with new experiences?
- How concrete is the person's spirituality?
- How adaptable is the person currently?

Ritual and Practice

- What are the spiritual rituals and practices of this individual?
- Are they formal or informal?
- Does the individual experience them on a regular basis?
- How do they support the individual?
- How does the client's current circumstances affect these rituals?

Box 5-10   Spiritual Assessment Tool

The following reflective questions may assist you in assessing, evaluating, and increasing awareness of spirituality in yourself and others.

Meaning and Purpose

These questions assess a person's ability to seek meaning and fulfillment in life, manifest hope, and accept ambiguity and uncertainty:
What gives your life meaning?
Do you have a sense of purpose in life?
Does your illness interfere with your life goals?
Why do you want to get well?
How hopeful are you about obtaining a better degree of health?
Do you feel that you have a responsibility in maintaining your health?
Will you be able to make changes in your life to maintain your health?
Are you motivated to get well?
What is the most important or powerful thing in your life?

Inner Strengths

These questions assess a person's ability to manifest joy and recognize strengths, choices, goals, and faith:
What brings you joy and peace in your life?
What can you do to feel alive and full of spirit?
What traits do you like about yourself?
What are your personal strengths?
What choices are available to you to enhance your healing?
What life goals have you set for yourself?
Do you think that stress in any way caused your illness?
How aware were you of your body before you became sick?
What do you believe in?
Is faith important in your life?
How has your illness influenced your faith?
Does faith play a role in recognizing your health?

Interconnections

These questions assess a person's positive self-concept, self-esteem, and sense of self; sense of belonging in the world with others; capacity to pursue personal interests; and ability to demonstrate love of self and self-forgiveness:
How do you feel about yourself right now?
How do you feel when you have a true sense of yourself?
Do you pursue things of personal interest?
What do you do to show love for yourself?
Can you forgive yourself?
What do you do to heal your spirit?

These questions assess a person's ability to connect in life-giving ways with family, friends, and social groups and to engage in the forgiveness of others:
Who are the significant people in your life?
Do you have friends or family in town who are available to help you?
Who are the people to whom you are closest?
Do you belong to any groups?
Can you ask people for help when you need it?
Can you share your feelings with others?
What are some of the most loving things that others have done for you?
What are the loving things that you do for other people?
Are you able to forgive others?

These questions assess a person's capacity for finding meaning in worship or religious activities, and a connectedness with a divinity:
Is worship important to you?
What do you consider the most significant act of worship in your life?
Do you participate in any religious activities?
Do you believe in God or a higher power?
Do you think that prayer is powerful?
Have you ever tried to empty your mind of all thoughts to see what the experience might be?
Do you use relaxation or imagery skills?
Do you meditate?
Do you pray?
What is your prayer?
How are your prayers answered?
Do you have a sense of belonging in this world?

These questions assess a person's ability to experience a sense of connection with life and nature, an awareness of the effects of the environment on life and well-being, and a capacity for concern for the health of the environment:
Do you ever feel a connection with the world or universe?
How does your environment have an impact on your state of well-being?
What are your environmental stressors at work and at home?
What strategies reduce your environmental stressors?
Do you have any concerns for the state of your immediate environment?
Are you involved with environmental issues such as recycling environmental resources at home, work, or in your community?
Are you concerned about the survival of the planet?

From Dossey BM: Holistic modalities and healing moments, *Am J Nurs* 6:44, 1998.
Sources: Burkhardt MA: Spirituality: an analysis of the concept, *Holist Nurs Pract* 3(3):69, 1989; and Dossey BM et al, editors: *Holistic nursing: a handbook for practice,* ed 2, Gaithersburg, Md, 1995, Aspen.

Community

- Family of origin: How did the client's family of origin share spiritual experiences?
- Current family structure: How does the client's current family share spiritual experiences?
- How does the client view participation in a faith community?
- Faith community of origin:
  How formal was the client's faith community of origin?
  How informal?

How active or inactive was the client?
- Current faith community:
  How formal is the client's current faith community?
  How informal?
  How active or inactive is the client?

Authority and Guidance

- What is the source of this client's system of belief, meaning, and ritual?
- When faced with problems, tragedy, or doubt, where does the client look for guidance?

- Does the client look for answers from internal or external sources?
- Is this source fixed, or is it flexible? (Fitchett, 1997)

The Case Study on p. 86 illustrates assessment of a client's spiritual needs and the use of appropriate interventions.

STAGES OF FAITH

A key concept in understanding spiritual development is that one's faith tends to become internalized as one develops. As one develops, one's sense of faith, meaning, moral values, and judgment moves from an external locus of control to an internal locus of control (Santrock, 1997). In assessing how best to assist a client in using his or her spirituality to address mental illness, it is essential to determine where the client is in his or her spiritual development. This is important to determine what interventions, if any, are appropriate. Several significant models of both faith development and moral/spiritual development can help inform a chaplain of the relative foundations in which a patient is grounded.

The first model is James Fowler's stages of religious development theory (Box 5-11). In this theory, Fowler posits that an individual passes through various stages in a linear

---

Box 5-11   Fowler's Stages of Religious Development

Stage 1: Intuitive-Projective Faith
A developmental stage that begins in early childhood
Intuitive images of good and evil
Fantasy and reality are the same

Stage 2: Mythical-Lyrical Faith
A developmental stage that can begin in middle to late childhood
More logical, concrete thought
Literal interpretation of religious stories
God is like a parent figure

Stage 3: Synthetic-Conventional Faith
A developmental stage that can begin in early adolescence
More abstract thought
Conformity to the religious beliefs of others

Stage 4: Individuating-Reflexive Faith
A developmental stage that can begin in late adolescence to early adulthood
Individuals begin to take full responsibility for their religious beliefs
In-depth exploration of one's values and religious beliefs

Stage 5: Conjunctive Faith
A developmental stage that can begin in middle adulthood
Becoming more open to paradox and opposing viewpoints
Stems from awareness of one's finiteness and limitations

Stage 6: Universalizing Faith
A developmental stage that can begin in late adulthood
Transcending belief systems to achieve a sense of oneness with all beings
Conflictual events are no longer viewed as paradoxes

---

fashion, based on age. As such, this theory is much like many of the other individual development theories (Santrock, 1997).

STAGES OF MORAL DEVELOPMENT

A second important model that can help assess a client's spirituality and how illness or the current situation has challenged the client's spirituality is Kohlberg's six stages of moral development theory, in which Kohlberg posits that individuals move, in a linear fashion with age, through key areas of faith and spiritual reasoning. The theory indicates that individuals all move through one or more of the following stages:

Preconventional	I. Avoid breaking rules to avoid punishment
	II. Moral action based on satisfying needs
Conventional	I. Pleasing others and doing what is expected
	II. Maintaining order and following the law
Postconventional	I. Moral actions determined by individual rights and community standards
	II. Belief in universal ethical principles that can guide actions

Based on the work of Kohlberg and Fowler, the following model looks at four areas of spirituality, each having implications for effective pastoral interventions.

Impartial Spirituality
- Individuals are considered to be "amoral."
- They tend to do things in their own interest. ("What's in it for me?")
- They are generally individuals who are not involved in faith communities or are only nominally involved.
- They may have a casual, cultural acquaintance with a formal faith community.
- They are a significant minority of the population.

Institutional Spirituality
- Individuals are regular church attendees.
- They adhere to outside, institutional rules.
- They do things because they are told to do them.
- They follow a good person/bad person concept.
- They probably make up the largest percentage of the population.

Individual Spirituality
- Individuals are seekers who have left a formal religious community.
- They often challenge the tenants of formal religious communities.
- They seek new answers or personal answers to questions, problems, or crises.
- They can appear on the surface to be in the impartial stage of faith.
- They are a smaller minority of the population.

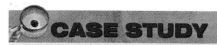
CASE STUDY

This case illustrates the use of the assessment and intervention tools referred to in this chapter. It also reflects some of the significant aspects of spiritual care as they apply to both clients and nurses. The value of spiritual care as perceived by a client and physician is also demonstrated.

Holistic Assessment

The client is a 66-year-old woman who has been hospitalized for an extensive period (approximately 6 weeks). The initial problems were major depression, anxiety, and a degenerative spinal condition that required several surgeries. The spinal condition is treatable, but the process will leave her with some permanent restrictions in movement and some possible residual pain. The client currently has significant chronic leg and lower back spasms and states that medication gives her little relief. Both the pain and the restrictions resulting from surgery have exacerbated her depression and anxiety.

The client has been divorced for almost 40 years. Immediately after her divorce she and her four children moved 1500 miles away from her family and friends to seek employment in a manufacturing environment. Although two of her children live close by, only one child is in regular contact with the client. Although the client has a nominally Lutheran background, she has no local connection to a congregation and has not attended church regularly since leaving her home town. Both the client and her physician are extremely interested in her having regular visits for spiritual care, and both have stated that the visits provide the client with significant help and support.

The Client's Belief and Meaning

Being independent, stoic, and self-sufficient are important goals in life, which are to be valued and pursued.

The Client's Vocations and Obligations

The client's goal was to support, raise, and care for herself and her children without being dependent on others. She still seeks to care for her adult daughter—asking the spiritual caregiver to meet with her daughter to talk about performing a marriage ceremony.

The Client's Experience and Emotion

The client has had a life of struggle, which has been balanced against the rewards of accomplishing her goal to be independent and her pride in being self-sufficient.

The Client's Courage and Growth

The client is now struggling to find some meaning in her pain and suffering.

The Client's Ritual and Practice

The client has a strong, dependent need to have the poem "Footprints," the Twenty-Third Psalm, and the Lord's Prayer read to her; she requests few other institutional rituals.

The Client's Community

The client's community is small, consisting of her children, their spouses, and several grandchildren, mostly living some distance from the client.

The Client's Source of Authority and Guidance

The client's source of authority and guidance is largely external and is derived from her early Midwestern social norms and experiences with institutional religion. She grants pastors a great deal of power, authority, and control; the client also believes that common religious articles such as the Bible and prayer cards have an almost magical authority and power.

The Client's Stage of Faith Development

The client is basically in stage 1, the impartial stage of faith, and is now possibly seeking to move into the early phase of stage 2, the institutional religion stage.

Level of Spiritual Risk

This client is considered to be at significant spiritual risk. She has an extremely high need for spiritual care and has very limited to nonexistent resources with which to meet this need. In making a triage assessment of how to allocate scarce pastoral care resources, this client's particular situation would dictate that a significant amount of qualified pastoral care be provided.

Spiritual Care Plan

Using the assessment tools as previously described, the spiritual pastoral care plan was to see the patient often—daily if possible. During these visits the spiritual intervention tools of prayer, presence, and short scripture readings were used to help bolster the client's sense of God's care for her and to support her in the healing process. Another intervention strategy was to help the patient explore her stated desire to be connected to a local Lutheran church and to help identify ways in which she might do this. In addition, the spiritual caregiver helped the client explore, to the extent of her desire and capability, what meaning there might be for her in this illness and in her future physical limitations. The intent of this goal was to help the client find possible new meanings in her life as a result of this illness.

The benefit to the client in pursuing these spiritual care plan goals was the provision of help, support, and comfort. This spiritual support helped ease her sense of torment and pain, resulting in a reduced experience of suffering. The benefit to the hospital in pursuing these spiritual care plan goals was greater client satisfaction. As the client experienced significant relief in the periods after her spiritual care, her requests for nursing interventions decreased. The client was also more satisfied with her overall care and was less anxious about her prognosis. The client's physician reported that she was quite satisfied with the hospital's ability to address the client's spiritual needs and that in doing so the hospital helped the client to experience less pain and discomfort.

Critical Thinking

1. Assess and prioritize the client's psychiatric, physical, and spiritual areas of concern, ensuring that all areas are addressed.
2. Describe the benefits of collaborating with the hospital chaplain in addressing the client's spiritual needs as part of a holistic assessment.
3. Given your knowledge of the stages of faith and the client's spiritual and religious background, which stage of faith best fits this client? What is the rationale for your choice?
4. How can your assessment of this client's family history of struggle, pride, and pain be used to guide you in your spiritual assessment? Consider the stages of the spiritual dimension as a guide.

Integrated Spirituality

- Individuals have internalized their faith.
- These people obey "rules" because they fully accept them and feel that they are just and right.
- They may or may not belong to formal faith communities.
- They can be seen as teachers or mystics.
- They make up a very small percentage of the population.

• • •

An accurate assessment of the client's stage of faith is extremely important in that it helps determine the nature of interventions that may be used. As in all models, these also have their limitations, and individuals tend to move along a continuum of spirituality and faith, rather than being locked into a particular stage. In some instances a crisis may in fact be the initiator of a person's movement, in either direction, along the continuum. An individual in the first stage might likely be operating out of a "bargaining" position when dealing with a spiritual crisis that questions a core meaning held by the individual. An intervention that helped that individual become connected with a faith group, perhaps a return to a youthful experience of faith, may provide some additional spiritual tools that were not otherwise available to the person. It would probably be less effective to attempt to use interventions that encouraged and supported challenges to existing spiritual norms for a person in either the first or second stage, but it might be a very effective intervention to use when dealing with an individual in the third stage. For individuals who are in the fourth stage, often older adults, the best possible pastoral intervention may be in learning from them, in being a student, and accepting their unique spiritual legacy.

SELECTED CASES OF CLINICAL SPIRITUAL INTERVENTIONS
Pain

Kathleen, a patient with depression and anxiety, also had an extremely difficult case of pancreatitis, which required an inpatient stay of about 30 days. A few weeks after her discharge, she returned to talk. As she talked, she confessed that the experience had made a significant impact on her faith and spiritual viewpoint. When faced with agonizing pain for the first time in her life, this middle-age woman confided that the physical agony she felt connected her emotionally for the first time with the concept of "torment and damnation." Although her existing spiritual beliefs helped her to cope with the symptoms of her illnesses, the experience of excruciating pain caused her to question some of the fundamental spiritual principles that had guided her up to that point. Especially challenged during this illness was her understanding of the relationship between the divine and humanity, and her concept of ultimate punishment and reward.

Spiritual Torment

Steven, a devout Mormon in his mid-fifties, was in spiritual torment. His permanent developmental delay, coupled with his bipolar illness, had prevented him from marrying. His own understanding of his religious principles, whether or not they were completely accurate according to that faith tradition, led him to believe that he would never "be able to enter heaven." This statement was always made as part of a tearful, tormented lament. His own strong faith was "punishing" him. An appropriate intervention in this case was to listen to and acknowledge Steven's pain and help connect him with responsible members of his faith community, where he could address his concerns.

Punishment

Mary, a woman in her mid-fifties, was a devout Catholic. She believed that her lifelong bouts of major depression were an appropriate "punishment" for the sexual abuse she had experienced as a child. She clung to the belief that she was responsible for the abuse and that the enjoyment and attention she felt at the time only confirmed her worthlessness and lack of capacity to be loved as an adult. In this case, where Mary was deeply entrenched in her denominational faith system, religious authority figures were seen to speak with much more authority than either physicians or other health care team members. Mary was introduced to a sympathetic priest who was also a trained psychotherapist. The interventions all centered around Mary's own belief system and included helping Mary to see herself as a survivor of abuse rather than as the responsible party. A sacramental ritual particular to her denomination was also included to eliminate Mary's deeply held "need" to be punished.

Voices

Fred, a patient with schizophrenia and a member of a charismatic Protestant group, stated that he had the "gift of wisdom"; Fred's schizophrenic symptoms included auditory hallucinations. On further discussion with Fred, it was revealed that during worship services it was quite common for him and others to rise and to "speak in tongues," a regular occurrence within his denomination. He also revealed that the voices he heard were quite malevolent and frequently urged him to harm himself. In Fred's case the hospital chaplain provided the interventions. Without challenging the faith experience that Fred described having in worship services, the chaplain was able to help Fred see a distinction between the malevolent voices that urged him to harm himself and any prophetic experience that Fred might have within the understanding of his own religious concepts. Out of this distinction, Fred's reluctance to maintain his antipsychotic medication regimen diminished. This improved medication maintenance resulted in a better quality of life for Fred and fewer hospitalizations.

Guilt

Terry, a woman with bipolar disorder in her mid-forties, was riddled with guilt because of behaviors that she had demonstrated during previous manic phases of her illness. These actions had included both risky sexual acting out and behaving in ways that were financially irresponsible. Terry came from a mainstream, liturgical Protestant tradition whose culture had emphasized both "personal responsibility" and "spiritual consequences" for one's own actions. Terry believed that she was "condemned" and that there was nothing she could do to change that. In ongoing discussions Terry was provided with education about her illness and instructed on how her symptoms could be more effectively contained by correctly using and monitoring her medications. Terry was eventually able to view her illness in the same way she viewed a chronic physical illness, such as diabetes. This diminished her feelings of guilt. To help maintain her medication compliance, Terry also began to incorporate part of her faith tradition in her ongoing care by using the daily prayer rituals of her faith to help her take her medication.

Hyperreligiosity

Hank, a religiously preoccupied individual with schizoaffective disorder, would often respond in a tangential fashion when anyone engaged him in conversation. Any attempt to relate to Hank using the more traditional religious language of his own faith background would propel him into long, rambling, confused, and pressured ranting about his "special connection" to God "as a prophet." To engage Hank in spiritual discussions for either assessment or intervention purposes, it was necessary to use language that he did not identify as "religious." When Hank was engaged by staff in discussions about meaningful areas of spirituality that were couched in ordinary language rather than "spiritual language," the words that would usually trigger Hank's tangential responses were avoided, and he would enter into more meaningful dialog with staff.

• • •

The role of spiritual caregiver, even in today's increasingly diverse and secular environment, still plays a significant part in the lives of individuals and health care organization. Chaplains, who most commonly hold these positions and who provide spiritual care on a variety of levels, have made an effective impact on the overall quality of client care. The various disciplines within the multidisciplinary health care team are usually seen by clients as having different levels of authority and expertise regarding spirituality and mental illness. For some clients, the physician is the "ultimate authority" when dealing with a health crisis and the subsequent challenges and interpretations of meaning that the crisis may hold. For others the "ultimate expertise" may be vested in a nurse, social worker, or therapist. For some individuals a chaplain may reflect an important image of "ultimate authority." To help clients with mental illness attempt to undertake a healing journey without addressing their spirituality and its authority in their lives may significantly impede the healing process.

CHAPTER SUMMARY

- The best way to understand any culture is to be deeply knowledgeable about one's own culture.
- Psychiatric mental health nurses must assess and evaluate clients and implement care plans with a holistic and culturally sensitive perspective toward care.
- Multicultural nursing in mental health involves an understanding of many issues, including demographic change, heritage consistency, socialization, acculturation, and assimilation.

- To effectively assist someone from another culture, nurses need to have an awareness of their own cultural heritage.
- Heritage consistency is the concept that describes the degree to which a person identifies with his or her cultural background.
- The Heritage Assessment Tool can assist nurses in assessing a client's heritage consistency.
- Health can be viewed as three-dimensional, encompassing the body, mind, and spirit.
- The communication aspects of language, space, and time orientation have various practices among different cultures.
- A person's spirituality can be influenced by culture, as well as life experiences.
- Belief and meaning make up the central, foundational principle underlying an individual's spiritual dimension.
- Spirituality is an essential human dimension that helps connect people to each other, the community, and the world.
- Spirituality, religion, and faith may be experienced and expressed in a variety of ways.
- There is a growing belief that quality spiritual assessment can be significantly beneficial in reducing a client's feelings of powerlessness and despair.
- For some individuals a chaplain may represent the "ultimate authority" for one's spiritual health, much as the nurse or physician is the authority for one's physical or mental health.
- Research on spirituality and healing has proliferated but more focus needs to be on mental health and spirituality.

REVIEW QUESTIONS

1. Which nursing intervention is appropriate for a hearing-impaired African-American client?
   a. Arrange for the client's 14-year-old daughter to be present 2 hours a day to interpret during individual and group sessions.
   b. Arrange for a sign-language interpreter to assist with the assessment process and for individual and family sessions.
   c. Arrange for a sign-language interpreter for the client during waking hours.
   d. Train the staff to learn basic sign language.

2. Which nursing intervention demonstrates the nurse's understanding of the Asian geriatric client's cultural needs?
   a. Encourage the client's family to assist with activities of daily living.
   b. Provide educational pamphlets to explain the client's mental illness.
   c. Restrict the home-made herbal remedies the family brought to the hospital.
   d. Encourage the family to attend support groups.

3. It is critical for the psychiatric nurse to be culturally competent so that:
   a. The client will not feel prejudice from the nurse.
   b. The psychiatric nurse will understand her own cultural identity.
   c. Clients may receive information about their illness and treatment in terms that they will understand.
   d. The psychiatric nurse will be able to serve in other countries.

4. A 50-year-old American Indian woman is admitted after experiencing auditory and visual hallucinations. She stated that her deceased father told her to kill herself to save herself from the bad spirits. What would be an appropriate nursing intervention for the nursing care plan?
   a. Consult with the client's family once the client has given consent for a spiritual healer from the client's tribe.
   b. Request that the hospital chaplain see the client.
   c. Request that the physician order a vegetarian diet.
   d. Allow her time alone to meditate and pray.

5. A 50-year-old Hispanic woman was seen by her family practitioner after the urging of her children. Her husband had died 4 months before, and since then she has lost 25 pounds and has not been able to sleep. She reports that her husband has come to visit her several times with a message she does not understand. An appropriate nursing diagnosis would be:
   a. Ineffective coping
   b. Disturbed thought processes
   c. Grieving
   d. Ineffective denial

REFERENCES

American Nurses Association: *Multicultural issues in the nursing workforce,* Washington, DC, 1993, The Association.

American Nurses Association: Addressing cultural diversity in the profession, *Am Nurse* 30(1):25, 1994.

American Nurses Association: Improving minority health outcomes through culturally specific care, *Nurs Trends Issues* 2(3):1, 1997.

American Nurses Association: Scope and standards of psychiatric mental health nursing practice. Washington, DC, 2000, American Nurses Publishing.

American Psychiatric Association: *Diagnostic and Statistical Manual of Mental Disorders,* Fourth Edition, Text Revised. Washington, DC, American Psychiatric Association, 2000.

Andrews M, Hanson P: Religion, culture and nursing. In Andrews M, Boyle S, editors: *Transcultural concepts in nursing care,* Philadelphia, 1999, Lippincott Williams & Wilkins.

Andrews M, Herberg D: Transcultural nursing care. In Andrews M, Boyle S, editors: *Transcultural concepts in nursing care,* Philadelphia, 1999, Lippincott Williams & Wilkins.

Baker F: Psychiatric treatment of older African-Americans, *Hosp Community Psychiatry* vol 45, no 32, 1994.

Bruce M, Takeuchi E, Leaf P: Poverty and psychiatric status: longitudinal evidence from the New Haven Epidemiologic Catchment Area Study, *Arch Gen Psychiatry* 48:470, 1991.

Camphina-Bacote J: Cultural competence in psychiatric mental health nursing: a conceptual model, *Nurs Clin North Am* vol 29, no 1, 1994.

Camphina-Bacote J: Cultural competence in psychiatric nursing: have you asked the right questions? *J Am Psychiatric Nurses Assoc* 8:183-187, 2002.

Center for Mental Health Services: *Cultural competence standards in managed care: mental health services for four underserved/underrepresented racial/ethnic groups,* Rockville, Md, 1998, Author.

Cook J: Who "mothers" the chronically mentally ill: *Fam Relations* 37:42, 1988.

Davis K: *Mental health training and black colleges: identifying the need,* Keynote speaker at the September African-American Behavioral Health Conference in Atlanta, 1995.

Dossey L: *The power of meditation and prayer,* Carlsbad, Calif, 1997, Hay House.

Dossey L: *Healing words: the power of prayer and the practice of medicine,* San Francisco, 1997, Harper.

Dossey L: *Healing: beyond the body,* Boston, 2001, Shambhala Publications.

Dossey L: *Reinventing medicine: beyond mind-body to a new era of healing,* Pittsburgh, 1999. Harper Collins.

Dossey L: *Medicine, meaning, and prayer,* Carlsbad, Calif, 1997, Hay House.

Fielo S, Degazon C: When cultures collide: decision making in a multicultural environment, *Nurs Health Care Perspect* 18(5):238, 1997.

Fitchett G: *Developing outcome-focused spiritual care: facing the challenge of filling a new wineskin.* Unpublished monograph presented to the national meeting of the College of Chaplains, 1997.

Foster S: The pragmatics of culture: the rhetoric of difference in psychiatric nursing, *Arch Psychiatr Nurs* 4(5):292, 1990.

Fowler JW: *Stages of faith,* San Francisco, 1981, Harper San Francisco.

Friedman S, Paradis C, Hatch M: Characteristics of African-American and white patients with panic disorder and agoraphobia, *Hosp Commun Psychiatry,* vol 45, 1994.

Germain C: Cultural care: a bridge between sickness, illness, and disease, *Holistic Nurs Pract* 6(3):1-9, 1992.

Geuss R: *The idea of a critical theory,* New York, 1981, Cambridge University Press.

Goldman H: Mental illness and family burden: a public health perspective, *Hosp Community Psychiatry* 33:557, 1982.

Hickling F, Griffith E: Clinical perspectives on the Rastafari movement, *Hosp Community Psychiatry,* vol 45, 1994.

Hofstede G: *Culture's consequences: international differences in work-related values,* Thousand Oaks, Calif, 1980, Sage Publications.

Hofstede G: *Cultures and organizations: software of the mind,* New York, 1991, McGraw-Hill.

Hofstede G: In Kim U et al, editors: *Individualism and collectivism: theory, method, and applications,* Thousand Oaks, Calif, 1994, Sage Publications.

Keltner N, Folks D: Psychopharmacology update, *Perspect Psychiatr Care* 28(1):33, 1992.

Kim M et al: Primary health care for Korean immigrants: sustaining a culturally sensitive model, *Public Health Nurs* 19(3), 2002.

Kim U: Individualism and collectivism: conceptual clarification and elaboration. In Kim U et al, editors: *Individualism and collectivism: theory, method and applications,* Thousand Oaks, Calif, 1994, Sage Publications.

Kleinman A: *Patients and healers in the context of culture,* Berkeley, Calif, 1980, University of California Press.

Kohlberg L: The development of children's orientations toward a moral order. In Damon W, editor: *Social and personality development,* New York, 1983, WW Norton.

LaFromboise T, Coleman H, Gerton J: Psychological impact of biculturalism: evidence and theory, *Psychol Bull* 14:395, 1993.

Lawson W et al: Race as a factor in inpatient and outpatient admissions and diagnoses, *Hosp Community Psychiatry* vol 45, no 72, 1994.

Lefley H: The family's response to mental illness in a relative. In Hatfield A, editor: *Families of the mentally ill,* New York, 1987, Guilford Press.

Lester N: Cultural competence: a nursing dialogue, *Am J Nurs* 98(8):26, 1998.

Lin K: Cultural aspects of mental health for Asian Americans. In Gaw A, editor: *Cross-cultural psychiatry,* Boston, 1982, John Wright.

Mandersheid R, Sonnenachein M: Percentage of clinically trained mental health personnel. In *Mental health, United States,* Washington, DC, 1996, U.S. Department of Health and Human Services.

Meadows M: Moving toward consensus on cultural competency in health care, Closing the Gap, Office of Minority Health, January 2000.

Mensah L: Transcultural, cross-cultural, and multicultural health perspectives in focus. In Masi R, Mensah L, McLeod K, editors: *Health and cultures: exploring the relationships,* vol 1, New York, 1993, Mosaic Press.

Morris P, Silove D: Cultural influences in psychotherapy with refugee survivors of torture and trauma, *Hosp Community Psychiatry* vol 43, no 3, 1992.

Nelson S et al: An overview of mental health services for American Indians and Alaska natives in the 1990s, *Hosp Community Psychiatry* vol 43, no 3, 1992.

Office of Minority Health, Assuring cultural competence in health care: recommendations for national standards and an outcomes-focused research agenda, website: http/www.omhrc.gov/clas/ds/htm.

Perrin KM, McDermott RJ: The spiritual dimension of health: a review, *Am J Health Stud* 13(2):90, 1997.

Purnell L, Paulanka B: *Transcultural health care: a culturally competent approach,* Philadelphia, 1998, FA Davis.

Ruiz P, Venegas-Samuels K, Alarcon R: The economics of pain: mental health care costs among minorities, *Psychiatr Clin North Am* 18(3):659, 1995.

Santrock JW: *Life-span development,* Chicago, 1997, Brown & Benchmark.

Spector RE: *Cultural diversity in health and illness,* ed 4, Norwalk, Conn, 1996, Appleton & Lange.

Swanson D: *Considering the communication traits of expressiveness, advocacy, and argumentativeness in the multicultural student population at the University of Guam,* 1993, Unpublished manuscript.

US Department of Health and Human Services: *Mental health: a report of the Surgeon General,* Rockville, Md, 1999, DHHS.

Warren J, Lutz, W: A consumer-oriented practice model for psychiatric mental health nursing. *Arch Psychiatr Nurs* vol 14, no 3, 2000.

SUGGESTED READINGS

Anderson H, Foley E: Experiences in need of ritual, *Christian Century* 114(31):1002, 1997.

Appleby C: Integrated delivery: organized chaos, *Hosp Health Netw,* 71(14):50, 1997.

Barber E: Racism and mental health, *J Am Psychiatr Nurses Assoc* 8:6, 194-199, 2002.

Bartol G, Richardson L: Using literature to create cultural competence, *Image J Nurs Sch* 30(1):75, 1998.

Becker V, editor: *Recovery devotional Bible, new international version,* Grand Rapids, Mich, 1993, Zondervan.

Culligan K: Spirituality and healing in medicine, *America* 175(5):17, 1996.

Episcopal Church: *The book of common prayer,* Philadelphia, 1979, Seabury Press.

Evans F: *New St. Joseph's people's prayer book,* New York, 1993, Catholic Book Publishing.

Ford-Grabowsky M: *Prayers for all people,* New York, 1995, Doubleday.

Go H: Changing populations and health. In Edelman CL, Mandle CL, editors: *Health promotion throughout the lifespan,* ed 3, St Louis, 1994, Mosby.

Hall BA: Spirituality in terminal illness: an alternative view of theory, *J Holist Nurs* 15(1):82, 1997.

Hines-Martin V: American consumers: what should we know to meet their mental health needs? *J Am Psychiatric Nurses Assoc* 8:188-193, 2002.

Holst L: *Hospital ministry,* New York, 1992, Crossroads.

Hunter RJ, editor: *Dictionary of pastoral care and counseling,* Nashville, 1996, Abingdon Press.

Job R, Shawchuck N: *A guide to prayer,* Nashville, Tenn, 1983, The Upper Room.

Kelly EW: *Spirituality and religion in counseling and psychotherapy,* 1995, American Counseling Association.

Kessler R, MicKelson K, Willliams D (1999): The prevalence, distribution, and mental health correlates of perceived discrimination in the United States. *J Health Soc Behav* 40, 208-230.

Kleinman A: *The illness narratives: suffering, healing, and the human condition,* New York, 1988, Basic Books.

Leininger M: *Culture, care, diversity, and universality: a theory of nursing,* New York, 1991, National League of Nursing.

Moore T: *Care of the soul,* New York, 1992, HarperCollins.

Morrison, E, Thornton K: Influences of southern spiritual beliefs on perception of mental illness, *Issues Mental Health Nurs* 20:443-458, 1999.

National Alliance for the Mentally Ill: Families on the brink: the impact of ignoring children with serious mental illness, 1999, Retrieved September 24, 2001 from http://www.nami.org/youthbrink3.html.

Nichols JE: *The relationship between meaning in life and chronic illness,* master"s thesis, San Diego, 1998, San Diego State University.

Nouwen H: *The wounded healer,* New York, 1990, Doubleday.

Oman M: *Prayers for healing,* Berkeley, Calif, 1997, Conari Press.

Richards PS, Bergin AE: *A spiritual strategy for counseling and psychotherapy,* Washington, DC, 1997, American Psychological Association.

Roukema RW: *The soul in distress,* New York, 1997, Haworth Pastoral Press.

Schlooser S: Social, cultural, and spiritual aspects of health care. In Berger K, Williams M: *Fundamentals of nursing,* Stamford, Conn, 1999, Appleton & Lange.

Smith J: *The HarperCollins dictionary of religion,* New York, 1995, Harper Collins.

Spector R: *Cultural diversity in health and illness,* ed 5, Norwalk, Conn, 2000, Appleton & Lange.

Spurlock J: Black Americans. In Comas-Diaz L, Griffith E, editors: *Cross-cultural mental health,* New York, 1988, John Wiley & Sons.

Tripp-Remier T: *Cultural assessment: a multidimensional approach,* Monterey, Calif, 1995, Wadsworth.

Warter C: *Recovery of the sacred,* Deerfield Beach, Fla, 1994, Health Communications, website:www.census/gov/www.socdemo/foreign/cps.200.html.

Yamamoto J: Japanese Americans. In Gaw A, editor: *Cross-cultural psychiatry,* Boston, 1982, John Wright.

6

The Nursing Process

Katherine M. Fortinash

OBJECTIVES

- Define the nursing process and describe its cyclic nature.

- Identify the six steps of the nursing process and explain the nursing actions for each step.

- Discuss the roles of intuition, expertise, and critical thinking and how they apply to the nursing process.

- Describe the North American Nursing Diagnosis Association (NANDA) taxonomy and explain its effect on nursing and other disciplines.

- Compare and contrast nursing and medical assessment frameworks, with specific focus on the NANDA taxonomy.

- Explain the meaning of actual, risk, and health promotion/wellness diagnoses; and give an example of each one using current NANDA labels, etiologies, risk factors, and defining characteristics.

- Develop outcomes that accurately measure clients' achievable behaviors based on their nursing diagnoses.

- Describe nursing-sensitive outcomes and the Nursing Outcomes Classification (NOC) and their influence on NANDA diagnoses and the nursing process.

- Formulate nursing interventions that are prescriptive and directive, for both actual and risk diagnoses.

- Define the Nursing Interventions Classification (NIC) and explain its relationship to NANDA diagnoses and the nursing process.

- Construct rationale statements for each proposed nursing intervention.

- Develop evaluations for outcomes that effectively measure client progress within an appropriate time frame.

The nursing process is a time-tested, organized, scientific method consisting of six distinctive steps and actions designed to help nurses treat and evaluate clients' responses to actual or potential health problems. This chapter examines the six steps of the nursing process, according to the American Nurses Association (ANA) in the *Standards of Clinical Nursing Practice* (ANA, 2000) (see Appendix B). Standards of care refer to the professional activities of the nurse as she or he goes through the six steps of the nursing process:

Standard I—Assessment
Standard II—Nursing Diagnosis
Standard III—Outcome Identification
Standard IV—Planning
Standard V—Implementation
Standard VI—Evaluation

HISTORY AND PERSPECTIVES OF THE NURSING PROCESS

The nursing process is a long-standing, systematic, problem-solving method that encompasses all of the components necessary to care for clients. It also addresses the needs of the family, significant others, and the community. Many nursing theorists agree that the nursing process is not like most linear or episodic problem-solving methods in which a problem is identified, diagnosed, treated, and resolved. They believe that the nursing process is an ongoing, multidimensional, cyclic approach in which data are continually collected, critically analyzed, and incorporated into the treatment plan according to the client's fluctuating responses to health and illness. Figure 6-1 shows the cyclic nature of the nursing process. There-fore the steps of the nursing process are not necessarily taken in strict sequence (beginning with assessment and ending with evaluation). They may be taken concurrently because nurses may be evaluating their assessment or even their plan of action at any given time. The dynamic nature of the nursing process continues to guide and challenge both the seasoned nurse and the new graduate in making sound clinical judgments and decisions.

Kritek (1978) states that the phases or steps of the nursing process are interactive as well as continual; therefore the phases influence each other and the client at the same time. There are points throughout the process in which the phases converge (come together). The nurse can attend the client at any point throughout this interactive, fluctuating process. For example, the nurse can continue to assess the client as necessary while also planning interventions.

Mental Status Examination

Components of the mental status examination include mood, affect, thoughts, and perceptions; they are the nurse's primary focus for assessing and treating mental and emotional disorders. The nurse conducts a client interview based on this time-tested, holistic assessment that reflects the individual's mental and emotional functioning at the time of the interview. The mental status examination is the basis for both the psychiatrist's and nurse's diagnoses, as well as management of care by all disciplines that collaborate with psychiatric mental health nursing. Psychosocial criteria such as stressors, coping skills, and relationships are also included in the overall examination of the client (see Box 6-1).

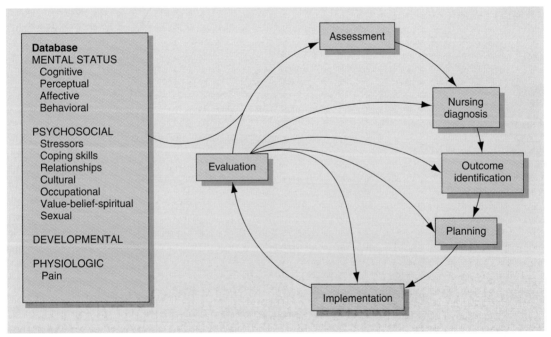

FIGURE 6-1. Cyclic nature of the nursing process. (From Fortinash KM, Holoday Worret PA: *Psychiatric nursing care plans,* ed 4, St Louis, 2003, Mosby.)

Multisystem Assessment

Psychiatric nurses must be equally prepared to conduct a multisystem assessment similar to that used in a medical-surgical setting because clients may have medical illnesses, dual diagnoses (concomitant substance abuse), or problems resulting from medication effects, self-neglect, or self-harm. Some clients require placement in special medical units within the psychiatric facility. These are generally older adults with multiple physical problems or clients experiencing symptoms related to alcohol- or other substance-related disorders. Although the majority of clients treated in a psychiatric facility are not attached to intravenous tubing, oxygen, or a cardiac monitor, the wounds resulting from mental illness are equally painful and debilitating. Therefore psychiatric nurses are keenly aware that clients are biopsychosocial beings and that all symptoms may affect both the mind and the body.

Intuition and the Nursing Process

Intuition, also known as intuitive reasoning, is an individual's insight into a situation without critical analysis. A strong "hunch" or a "gut feeling" is an example of intuition. Westcott (1968) said that a person operating on intuition needs little data to support his or her insights. Many experienced nurses have credited intuition with their ability to make the right decisions in client care. As technology grew, nursing focused more toward scientific reasoning and away from the intuitive approach (Munhall and Oiler, 1993). During this scientific revolution, nurses resisted using intuitive terms and opted for more researched-based problem-solving methods.

More recently, intuition has appeared in nursing journals as a valid part of the complex nature of clinical reasoning. Although intuition has not replaced nursing science as the primary basis for clinical judgment and problem solving, some clinicians consider intuition as a component of critical thinking. Fidaleo (2002) believes that a "gut feeling" does not emerge out of nowhere. He notes that it generally comes from a client who transfers his or her pain to a nurse who approaches the client in a "neutral state," meaning that the nurse is open and accessible to the client's feelings and emotions. This type of intuitiveness is especially critical when assessing clients who are suicidal (see the following example).

> A client tells a nurse that staff told him he is no longer suicidal and does not need to be watched so closely. He says he is looking forward to some privacy and proceeds to enter his room.

Although the client appears calm and self-assured, the nurse decides to follow the client into the room. As the nurse quietly stands there, the client sits on his bed and begins to cry. The nurse sits down next to the client and the client confesses that he was thinking about taking a whole bottle of medication that he had been saving. When the nurse was later questioned about his actions, he stated that he had a "gut feeling" that prompted him to remain with the client at this particular time. The client admitted that it was the nurse's caring and concern that made him express his suicidal feelings and intentions.

Benner's significant work, *From Novice to Expert: Excellence and Power in Clinical Nursing Practice* (2001), described the role of intuition in critical care nurses and concluded that many of them were not consciously aware of the higher level reasoning processes they used to assess and deliver client care. Yet the nursing interventions based on these intuitive forces often reflected superior insights and sound judgment. Smith (1988) noted that these nurses somehow had the ability to sense impending deterioration in their clients before such crises actually occurred.

Whiteside (1997) said that "intuition is rapid critical thinking." An example is: A nurse recognizes a pattern of behavior, applies common sense and skilled know-how, sorts out important from unimportant problems, and views situation from different perspectives.

Although the precise mechanism by which intuition works is elusive, it continues to play a major role in the psychiatric setting, where assessment is focused primarily on the client's behavior and its meaning beyond the spoken word. Combined with scientific reasoning and the unique skills and experience of the nurse, intuitive reasoning definitely has a place in the future of nursing research and practice.

Expertise and the Nursing Process

Both expertise and intuition are necessary for making sound clinical judgments. Only through clinical experience can nurses develop expertise in selected areas of practice (Benner, 2001). Expertise, like intuition, influences the phases of the nursing process. Although it is said that intuition cannot be taught, it can be learned through clinical practice. However, the exact process by which this learning occurs remains vague and complex. Both expertise and intuition are worthwhile goals that nurses should continue to pursue and develop throughout their professional lives. Many nurses agree that expertise can incorporate intuition in clinical practice.

The Nurse's Role in the Nursing Process

The nursing process, like other decision-making methods, does not guarantee instant improvement of symptoms. Psychiatric clients seldom leave the hospital completely symptom free, given the complex nature of mental illness. However, it is anticipated that clients will achieve a higher level of functioning because of nurses who are willing to try a variety of acceptable, time-tested approaches with patience, understanding, and hope. In the final analysis, it is the nurse and his or her unique spirit who adds a critical dimension to the nursing process and brings it to life.

Critical Thinking and the Nursing Process

Critical thinking is an important component in the nursing process and includes judgment, intuition, and expertise. Critical thinking skills develop over time, and enhance and become a part of the nurse's expanding knowledge base. It is the nurse's critical thinking ability that determines which data are meaningful and which take priority in the client's care. When using the nursing process, the nurse incorporates experience and knowledge from nursing and other courses to apply theories and principles in practice. Knowledge of basic human needs; anatomy and physiology; disease processes; growth and development; sociologic trends and patterns; and various cultures, religions, and philosophies are all crucial elements of the critical thinking framework. The following critical thinking skills are used in all phases of the nursing process (Wilkinson, 1992):

- *Observing* (observations are planned and ongoing versus casual and singular)
- *Distinguishing* (sorting relevant from irrelevant data)
- *Validating* selected data through observations and communication
- *Organizing* data into meaningful parts via a time-tested data collecting system
- *Categorizing* data for easy retrieval and communication with nursing and other disciplines

Critical thinking is similar to the nursing process in that it is a diffuse rather than a linear method. The nurse generally selects a course of action based on knowledge and past experiences. This requires hypothesizing many possible reasons for a problem; therefore diagnoses should not be hastily made. Productive memory, which requires a blending of diagnostic reasoning and experience, is the basis for critical thinking and generally increases as one's knowledge and experience increase (Whiteside, 1997).

ASSESSMENT (STANDARD I)

The nurse collects data relevant to the client's overall health status.

Assessment is perhaps the most critical phase of the nursing process because it is where nurses collect enormous amounts of data about clients' holistic health status. *Holistic assessment provides nurses with relevant data from which to accurately formulate and prioritize nursing diagnoses, the crux of treatment planning, according to clients' needs or immediate conditions.* Throughout the assessment phase, nurses collect data through learned, time-tested, interactive and interviewing skills, and observations of verbal and nonverbal behaviors based on a broad biopsychosociocultural background and knowledge of functional and dysfunctional behaviors.

In psychiatric nursing, assessment takes place in a number of settings (e.g., inpatient, outpatient, or community and home environments). This gives the nurse many opportunities to observe the client and modify assessment data according to the client's continued adjustment to the milieu and progress made throughout hospitalization. Ideally the client is the primary source of information during the assessment phase. Occasionally, however, the client may be unable to offer a complete or accurate health history, given the acuity of his or her illness. In such cases a reliable source may be interviewed on the client's behalf, with the understanding that such information will be evaluated in terms of that person's relationship with the client (Fortinash, 1990).

Assessment of the individual includes the following criteria: physical, psychiatric, psychosocial, mental status, developmental, cultural, spiritual, and sexual. The method of assessment includes the client's subjective report of symptoms and problems and the nurse's objective findings (Fortinash, 1990). Box 6-1 details mental status and psychosocial criteria that should be covered during assessment.

A major focus of a client's mental status is identification of his or her strengths and capabilities for interaction with and within the environment. This includes the ability to initiate interactions, sustain meaningful communication and relationships, and attain satisfaction consistent with his or her developmental and sociocultural lifestyle. Knowledge and appreciation of the psychodynamics and psychopathology of human behavior are essential for effective assessment of the individual's adjustment or maladjustment to internal and external life stressors.

The Nurse-Client Interview

The nurse as a primary communicator

The interview is the most critical method of collecting information about the overall health status of clients with psychiatric disorders. It is a more meaningful, flexible way of gathering important data than are questionnaires or computers, and it allows the nurse to use all of the senses to explore specific topics and key themes or concerns expressed by the client through verbal and nonverbal responses. Box 6-2 lists samples of some general questions that can be asked during the nurse-client interview.

In assessing a client's mental status, the primary instrument, or "tool," of evaluation is the nurse interviewer. The success of the interview depends largely on the development of trust, rapport, and respect between the nurse and the client and between the nurse and the family. Keen therapeutic communication skills such as active listening and reflective questioning are used throughout the interview in an effort to determine the client's immediate needs and actively engage him or her in treatment (Fortinash, 1990). Throughout the communication process, the nurse is aware of each client's unique qualities, including age, culture, and ethnicity, and how these qualities may influence the client's response to illness and treatment. Care must be taken, however, not to assume that all clients who share these same qualities will think or behave the same way. Each client is treated as an individual, avoiding *stereotyping* or *biases* that may compromise quality care (see Chapter 7 for more information on therapeutic communication).

Assessment Frameworks

Data collecting systems

Assessment frameworks are organizational systems by which to store and collect data for easier access to in-

Box 6-1   Components of Assessment: Mental Status and Psychosocial Criteria

Mental Status Examination

APPEARANCE
Dress, grooming, hygiene, cosmetics, apparent age, posture, facial expression

BEHAVIOR/ACTIVITY
Hypoactivity or hyperactivity, rigid, relaxed, restless or agitated motor movements, gait and coordination, facial grimacing, gestures, mannerisms, passive, combative, bizarre

ATTITUDE
Interactions with the interviewer: cooperative, resistive, friendly, hostile, ingratiating

SPEECH
Quantity: Poverty of speech, poverty of content, voluminous
Quality: Articulate, congruent, monotonous, talkative, repetitious, spontaneous, circumlocutory, confabulations, tangential, pressured, stereotypic
Rate: Slowed, rapid

MOOD AND AFFECT
Mood (intensity, depth, duration): Sad, fearful, depressed, angry, anxious, ambivalent, happy, ecstatic, grandiose
Affect (intensity, depth, duration): Appropriate, apathetic, constricted, blunted, flat labile, euphoric, bizarre

PERCEPTIONS
Hallucinations, illusions, depersonalization, derealization, distortions

THOUGHTS
Form and content: Logical vs. illogical, loose associations, flight of ideas, autistic, blocking, broadcasting, neologisms, word salad, obsessions, ruminations, delusions, abstract vs. concrete

SENSORIUM/COGNITION
Levels of consciousness, orientation, attention span, recent and remote memory, concentration; ability to comprehend and process information; intelligence

JUDGMENT
Ability to assess and evaluate situations, make rational decisions, understand consequences of behavior, and take responsibility for actions

INSIGHT
Ability to perceive and understand the cause and nature of own and others' situations

RELIABILITY
Interviewer's impression that individual reported information accurately and completely

Psychosocial Criteria

STRESSORS
Internal: Psychiatric or medical illness, including pain, perceived loss, such as loss of self-concept/self-esteem
External: Actual loss (e.g., death of a loved one, divorce, lack of support systems, job or financial loss, retirement, dysfunctional family system)

COPING SKILLS
Adaptation to internal and external stressors; use of functional, adaptive coping mechanisms and techniques; management of activities of daily living

RELATIONSHIPS
Attainment and maintenance of satisfying, interpersonal relationships congruent with developmental stage; includes sexual relationship as appropriate for age and status

CULTURAL
Ability to adapt and conform to prescribed norms, rules, ethics, and mores of an identified group

SPIRITUAL (VALUE-BELIEF)
Presence of a self-satisfying value-belief system that the individual regards as right, desirable, worthwhile, and comforting

OCCUPATIONAL
Engagement in useful, rewarding activity, congruent with developmental stage and societal standards (work, school, recreation)

From Fortinash KM, Holoday Worret PA: *Psychiatric nursing care plans,* ed 4, St Louis, 2003, Mosby.

formation. Because nurses gather large amounts of complex, holistic, client data, these frameworks are valuable assessment guides that contain categories corresponding to qualities accepted by nursing, such as the nature of humans, health, illness, and nursing. Table 6-1 depicts three separate assessment frameworks. The traditional medical framework (body systems) model listed in the first column is considered insufficient for the holistic assessment required in psychiatric nursing, and most likely in other nursing specialty areas. The other two columns describe the two frameworks most commonly used in today's nursing practice and are discussed in the following paragraphs.

Functional Health Pattern Framework

Functional health patterns were developed in 1984 by Dr. Marjory Gordon, nurse theorist and a chair of NANDA's Board of Directors from 2000 to 2003 (NANDA, 2003). These patterns are categories of human, biologic, physiologic, psychologic, developmental, cultural, social, and spiritual assessments. Health patterns related to these categories are assessed over time, as either functional or dysfunctional. Functional patterns reflect the client's strengths and adaptive coping strategies, whereas dysfunctional patterns form the basis for client problems and nursing diagnoses. Functional health patterns are accepted framework methods currently used in educational and practice settings (Gordon, 1987).

Box 6-2   The Nurse-Client Interview: Sample General Questions

Presenting Problem
Tell me the reason you are here (in treatment).

Present Illness
When did you first notice the problem?
What changes have you noticed in yourself?
What do you think is causing the problem?
Have you had any troubling feelings or thoughts?

Family History
How would you describe your relationship with your parents?
Did either of your parents have emotional or mental problems?
Were either of your parents treated by a psychiatrist or therapist?
Did their treatment include medication or electroconvulsive therapy (ECT)?
Were they helped by their treatment?

Childhood/Premorbid History
How did you get along with your family and friends?
How would you describe yourself as a child?

Medical History
Do you have any serious medical problems?
How have they affected your current problem?
Are you experiencing pain? If yes, complete a pain history and assessment.

Psychosocial/Psychiatric History
Have you ever been treated for an emotional or psychiatric problem? Have you been diagnosed with a mental illness?
Have you ever been a patient in a psychiatric hospital?
Have you ever been in counseling/therapy for an emotional or psychiatric problem?
Have you ever taken prescribed medications for an emotional problem or mental illness? Did you ever have ECT?
If so, did the medication or ECT help your symptoms/problem?
How frequently do your symptoms occur? (About every 6 months? Once a year? Every 5 years? First episode?)
How long are you generally able to function well in between onset of symptoms? (Weeks? Months? Years?)
What do you feel, if anything, may have contributed to your symptoms? (Nothing? Stopped taking medications? Began using alcohol? Street drugs?)

Recent Stressors/Losses
Have you had any recent stressors or losses in your life?
What are your relationships like?
How do you get along with people at work?

Education
How did you do in school?
How did you feel about school?

Legal
Have you ever been in trouble with the law?

Marital History
How do you feel about your marriage? (If client is married)
How would you describe your relationship with your children? (If client has children)
What kinds of things do you do as a family?

Social History
Tell me about your friends, your social activities.
How would you describe your relationship with your friends?

Support Systems
Who would you turn to if you were in trouble?
Do you feel you need someone to turn to now?

Insight
Do you consider yourself different now from the way you were before your problem began? In what way?
Do you think you have an emotional problem or mental illness?
Do you think you need help for your problem?
What are your goals for yourself?

Value-Belief System (Including Spiritual)
What kinds of things give you comfort and peace of mind?
Will those things be helpful to you now?

Special Needs (Including Cultural)
How can staff help you during your treatment?
What kinds of things will be most helpful to you now?

Discharge Goals
How do you want to feel by the time you're ready for discharge?
What do you think you can do to help yourself reach that goal?
What things will you do differently from the way you did them before?
What things can you do to help prevent your symptoms from recurring and stay out of the hospital?
What are your goals for daily medication compliance?
How will you manage your leisure time?

Modified from Fortinash KM, Holoday Worret PA: *Psychiatric nursing care plans*, ed 4, St Louis, 2003, Mosby; Fortinash KM: Assessment of mental states. In Malasanos L, Garkauskas V, Stoltenberg-Aller K, editors: *Health assessment*, ed 4, St Louis, 1990, Mosby.

NANDA Taxonomy II—Human Response Patterns

NANDA developed human response patterns, a framework that categorizes nursing diagnoses, in 1986 at their seventh conference. It continues to be a part of Taxonomy II. After going through many changes, Taxonomy II was presented at the fourteenth biennial conference in April, 2000, and remains intact as the taxonomic structure for the nursing diagnoses framework. See Table 6-1 for a list of NANDA's nine human response patterns (Taxonomy II). However, NANDA continues to evolve. See Nursing Diagnosis Standard II for further information on NANDA's development in 2003-2004.

Both the NANDA **taxonomy** (a hierarchic framework) and the nursing diagnoses help guide nurses toward building a solid, scientific foundation for the profession. They also

Table 6-1	Comparison of Medical and Nursing Assessment Frameworks	
Medical	**Nursing Models**	
Body Systems	**NANDA Taxonomy II Human Response Patterns**	**Functional Health Patterns**
Cardiovascular	Exchanging	Health perception/ health management
Respiratory	Communicating	Nutritional/metabolic
Neurologic	Relating	Elimination
Endocrine	Valuing	Activity/exercise
Metabolic	Choosing	Sleep/rest
Hematopoietic	Moving	Cognitive/perceptual
Integumentary	Perceiving	Self-perception/ self-concept
Gastrointestinal	Feeling	Role/relationship
Genitourinary	Knowing	Sexuality/reproductive
Reproductive		Coping/stress tolerance
Psychiatric		Value-belief

Modified from Davie JK: The nursing process. In Thelan LA et al, editors: *Critical care nursing: diagnosis and management*, ed 3, St Louis, 1998, Mosby; Gordon M: *Nursing diagnosis: process and application*, ed 3, St Louis, 1994, Mosby.

provide nursing with a standardized, more efficient method of communication, so that nurses everywhere speak the same professional language (NANDA 2003).

Frameworks are necessary tools with which to process the large amount of data collected by nurses in assessing clients. Frameworks form a basis for diagnostic reasoning (discussed later) by gathering assessment information and organizing it into manageable pieces. An organized collection system ensures easier access to critical client information and shows important relationships among the data. The selection of one framework over another is an individual choice.

NURSING DIAGNOSIS (STANDARD II)

The nurse diagnoses the client from data analyzed in the assessment phase.

Nursing diagnoses are statements that describe an individual's health state or an actual or potential alteration (known as a risk diagnosis) in a person's life process. The nursing diagnosis statement may reflect one's biologic, psychologic, sociocultural, developmental, spiritual, or sexual process (Table 6-2). At NANDA's ninth conference, nursing diagnosis was defined as ". . . a clinical judgment about individual, family, or community responses to actual or potential health problems/life processes. Nursing diagnoses provide the basis for selection of nursing interventions to achieve outcomes for which the nurse is accountable" (American Nurses Association, 1990).

The continual development and refinement of nursing diagnoses is a challenging task. Taxonomy II (NANDA, 2001-2002) resulted in the changing of many of the diagnostic names and approved seven new diagnoses and six revised diagnoses. Taxonomy II remains intact. NANDA's international work on the development of nursing diagnosis (NANDA,

Table 6-2	Nursing Diagnosis Statements in Relationship to Life Processes	
Nursing Diagnoses		**Life Processes**
Readiness for enhanced nutrition		Biologic
Readiness for enhanced self-concept		Psychologic
Impaired social interaction		Sociocultural
Delayed growth and development		Developmental
Readiness for enhanced spiritual well-being		Spiritual
Ineffective sexual pattern		Sexual

2003-2004) produced 12 new diagnoses, including 11 health promotion/wellness diagnoses and 3 revisions. A complete list of the current NANDA diagnoses is found on the inside back cover of this text. Table 6-2 contains three health promotion/ wellness diagnoses (i.e., "readiness for..."). A complete account of the diagnostic changes can be found in *NANDA Nursing Diagnoses: Definitions & Classificaton 2003-2004.*

Nursing diagnoses provide nurses with a vocabulary that is distinctive to nursing. This unique language enhances communication among nurses and clarifies nursing's purpose and role in assessing and treating clients. By using its own vocabulary, nursing grows as a profession and gains respectability. Carpenito (1996) stated that "NANDA's attempt to upgrade nursing's status as a profession by its unifying vocabulary..." is as much for purposes of a social policy as it is for "clarifying nursing for nurses."

Diagnostic Reasoning
Interpreting the data

After the data have been collected and recorded, the next step is interpretation of what the data actually mean in terms of the client's health-illness status. Critical thinking in diagnostic reasoning consists of the following two major cognitive processes (Wilkinson, 1992):

1. **Analysis:** Taking apart the collected data to examine and interpret each piece and identify variations from typical behaviors or responses. Analysis also includes discovering patterns or relationships in the data that may be cues that require further investigation.
2. **Synthesis:** Combining several parts of relevant data into a single piece of information. Synthesis also involves comparing behavioral patterns with learned theories or typical patterns of behavior to identify strengths and seek explanations for symptoms.

The term *inference* has been defined as "the process of arriving at a conclusion by reasoning from evidence." Inherent in the use of inference, however, is a tendency to assume that the evidence is slight or has not been fully examined. Therefore to avoid (as much as possible) a rush to judgment or an "inferential leap," the nurse reaches conclusions and formulates diagnoses based on logical and factual data. This goal can be achieved by limiting the amount of bias that can influence the diagnostic process and by remaining as objective as possible (Benner, 2001; Carnevali and Thomas, 1993; Tanner et al., 1987).

Definition of Health Problems

Explaining the health problem

Nearly all approved diagnoses are accompanied by definitions that more clearly describe or explain the health problem, which is a useful feature for students and practicing nurses as well. The following are NANDA definitions for two sets of similar diagnoses that are often confused with one another, currently published in NANDA *Nursing Diagnoses: Definitions & Classification 2003-2004*:

Fear: "Response to perceived threat that is consciously recognized as a danger"

Anxiety: "Vague uneasy feeling of discomfort or dread, accompanied by an automatic response (the source often nonspecific or unknown to the individual); a feeling of apprehension caused by anticipation of danger. It is an alerting signal that warns of impending danger and enables the individual to take measures to deal with the threat"

Powerlessness: "Perception that one's actions will not significantly affect an outcome; a perceived lack of control over a current situation or immediate happening"

Hopelessness: "Subjective state in which an individual sees limited or no alternatives or personal choices available and is unable to mobilize energy on own behalf"

Qualifying Statements

Clarifying the root or etiology of the problem for each individual client

For additional clarity, some nursing diagnoses require qualifying statements based on the nature of the health problem as it is manifested in each particular client response or situation.

It is not advisable to use medical diagnoses as etiologies for nursing problems. It is more difficult for nurses to treat an etiology that is stated as a medical diagnosis, such as schizophrenia, as that type of label suggests a whole array of treatment strategies that are not uniquely nursing (for example, nurses don't treat schizophrenia as a whole disorder, but they do treat client symptoms, behaviors, and responses related to the disorder).

However, many symptoms and behaviors resulting from mental disorders and medical conditions are of great concern to nurses and require management and treatment by nurses. Some examples of *medically based etiologies* are:

- Imbalanced nutrition: less than body requirements, *as a result of anorexia nervosa*
- Disturbed thought processes, *as a result of schizophrenia*
- Impaired verbal communication, *as a result of bipolar disorder*

In such situations the nurse isolates those aspects that contribute to the symptoms that can be treated by nursing interventions and cites them as etiologies. Some examples of *nursing etiologies* are:

- Imbalanced nutrition: less than body requirements, related to:
  Inadequate intake and hypermetabolic need
  Loss of appetite secondary to constipation

- Disturbed thought processes, related to:
  Internal and external stressors
  Impaired ability to process internal and external stimuli
- Impaired verbal communication, related to:
  Rapid thought processes secondary to manic state

The previously cited etiologic factors that accompany the nursing diagnoses more clearly specify the focus of care for nursing interventions.

Guidelines for Defining Characteristics

Signs and symptoms or client responses to the diagnosis

Defining characteristics, also known as signs and symptoms and labeled "as evidenced by" (AEB) in many nursing care plans, are the observable, measurable manifestations of clients' responses to the identified health problems (nursing diagnoses). As with diagnoses and etiologies, defining characteristics are generally in nonspecific terms and often need to be modified to reflect the particular situation or response presented by the client. For example, the diagnosis of ineffective coping has as one of its defining characteristics "inadequate problem solving" (NANDA, 2003). The nurse can clarify the defining characteristic statements by quoting the client. Examples of inadequate problem solving:

"I can't decide if I should stay with my family or move to a board-and-care home."

"I can't decide what to do first—get a job or begin day treatment."

Therefore defining characteristics, when applicable, should be present in the nurse's assessment criteria to help validate the health problem that is being diagnosed. Some examples of defining characteristics used to define the diagnosis of chronic low self-esteem are:

- Self-negating verbalization
- Expression of shame or guilt
- Evaluation of self as unable to deal with events
- Hesitancy to try new things or situations

Risk Diagnoses

Problems at risk for becoming actual

A risk diagnosis refers to an individual's vulnerable health status. It means that the person is exposed to factors that increase chances for injury or illness. If the risk is not addressed by the preventable efforts of the nurse, the potential problems may become actual, and an actual diagnosis will replace the risk diagnosis. There are no defining characteristics in a risk diagnosis, as the actual problem has not been manifested. Also, there are no etiologies in a risk problem, as etiologies mean there is a cause, and cause cannot exist without effect. Thus, a risk diagnosis has a two-part statement (*risk diagnosis* and *risk factors*), and an actual nursing diagnosis consists of a three-part statement (*diagnosis, etiology,* and *defining characteristics*). Box 6-3 presents the two types of nursing diagnosis formats, with two examples of each type (NANDA, 2003).

Risk problems can be assigned to any individual in a compromised health state. For example, a client taking a tricyclic antidepressant medication may be at risk for several potential problems as a result of the actions of these drugs on many of the body systems, such as risk for injury (hypotension, dizziness, blurred vision), risk for constipation, risk for urinary retention, or risk for altered mucous membranes (dry mouth).

Examples of a risk diagnosis:

Part 1 Nursing diagnosis:	Risk for constipation
Part 2 Risk factors:	Tricyclic antidepressant medications
	Refusal to drink water, juice, etc.
	Noncompliance to high-fiber foods

Several of the approved diagnoses address potential dysfunctional states and cite risk factors. The following are examples of such diagnoses:

- Risk for impaired parenting
- Risk for trauma
- Risk for other-directed violence

In addition to those diagnoses formally listed as risk diagnoses, any actual diagnosis can be stated as a risk diagnosis if it meets the criteria for an "at risk" problem. For example, situational self-esteem can be written as "risk for situational low self-esteem" if risk factors exist that could make the risk problem actual (NANDA, 2003).

Guidelines for Health Promotion/Wellness Diagnoses

Readiness for enhanced level of functioning

A wellness nursing diagnosis is a clinical judgment about an individual, family, or community in transition from one level of wellness to a higher level of wellness or functioning. NANDA (2003) is now using the prefix "readiness for enhanced" to describe wellness diagnoses. Most wellness diagnoses are one-part statements. Here are two examples: readiness for enhanced communication, and readiness for enhanced community coping. Wellness diagnoses may have either defining characteristics, or both defining characteristics and etiologies (NANDA, 2003).

OUTCOME IDENTIFICATION (STANDARD III)

The nurse projects client behaviors as a result of nursing interventions.

Outcome statements consist of specific, measurable indicators that are used by nurses to evaluate the results of their interventions. Outcome criteria illustrate:

- The actual nursing diagnosis has been resolved or reduced.
- The risk diagnosis has not occurred (or become actual).

Outcomes derive from nursing diagnosis statements and are projections of the expected influence that nursing interventions will have on the client. Figure 6-2 shows the nurs-

---

Box 6-3   Format of Nursing Diagnosis

Two-Part Statements

RISK PROBLEM

Part 1: Nursing diagnosis
Risk for other-directed violence
Part 2: Risk factors (predictors of risk problem)
History of violence
Hyperactivity secondary to manic state
Low impulse control
Aggressive verbal remarks

RISK PROBLEM

Part 1: Nursing diagnosis
Risk for loneliness
Part 2: Risk factors (predictors of risk problem)
Social isolation
Deprivation of love/affection
Physical isolation
Long-term institutionalization

Three-Part Statements

ACTUAL PROBLEM

Part 1: Nursing diagnosis
Post-trauma syndrome
Part 2: Etiologic factors (related to)
Overwhelming anxiety secondary to:
    Rape or other assault
    Catastrophic illness
    Disasters
    War
Part 3: Defining characteristics
Reexperience of traumatic event (flashbacks)
Repetitive dreams or nightmares
Intrusive thoughts about traumatic event
Excess verbalization about traumatic event

ACTUAL PROBLEM

Part 1: Nursing diagnosis
Chronic confusion
Part 2: Etiologic factors (related to)
Disorientation secondary to Alzheimer's disease
Psychosis secondary to Korsakoff's syndrome
Trauma secondary to recent head injury
Memory loss secondary to dementia
Part 3: Defining characteristics
Altered interpretation/response to stimuli
Progressive long-standing cognitive impairment
No change in level of consciousness
Impaired socialization
Impaired short-term memory

---

ing process depicting the actual and risk diagnosis format of the six-step process. Outcomes are often confused with client goals or nursing goals, but they are more specific, descriptive, and measurable. Outcomes also do not describe nursing interventions. Box 6-4 lists examples of outcome statements.

Outcome criteria for an actual diagnosis are generally considered the opposite of the defining characteristics. In

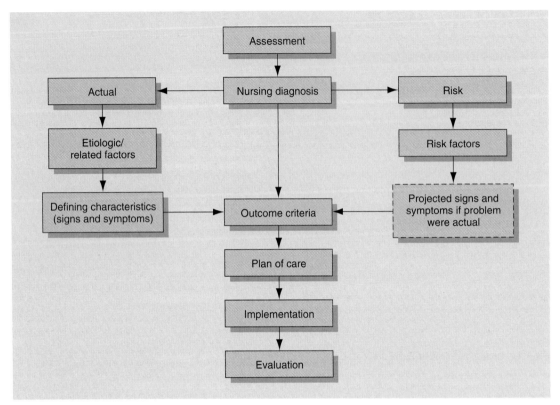

FIGURE 6-2. Nursing process depicting actual and risk diagnosis format of the six-step process. (Modified from Fortinash KM, Holoday Worret PA: *Psychiatric nursing care plans,* ed 4, St Louis, 2003, Mosby.)

Box 6-4   Examples of Outcome Statements

Client will:
Verbalize absence of suicidal thoughts and plans.
Demonstrate absence of self-mutilation and other self-destructive be-
    haviors.
Interpret environmental stimuli accurately.
Interact socially with clients and staff.
Participate actively in group discussions.
Seek staff when experiencing troubling thoughts and feelings.
Comply with treatment and medication regimen.

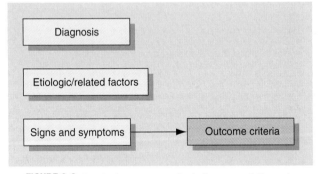

FIGURE 6-3 Developing outcome criteria for an actual diagnosis.

---

other words, the signs and symptoms discovered in the assessment phase to help establish the nursing diagnosis are also used to identify outcomes for improvement or resolution (Figure 6-3). For example:

NURSING DIAGNOSIS

Self-care deficit, bathing/
    hygiene; dressing/
    grooming
Related to: Psychotic state
As evidenced by: Disheveled
    appearance; poor hygiene/
    grooming

OUTCOMES

Neat, clean appearance
Cleans and grooms self

Outcome criteria for a risk diagnosis are developed from the risk factors that replace the defining characteristics found in an actual diagnosis. Clinical symptoms are absent

in a risk diagnosis, as it is a two-part statement (Figure 6-4). For example:

NURSING DIAGNOSIS

Risk for self-directed
    violence

OUTCOMES

Verbalizes absence of
    suicidal intent
Absent demonstration of
    suicidal gestures/acts

RISK FACTORS

History of suicide attempts
Verbalizes suicidal intent

Measurable outcomes should include client statements, behaviors, and/or psychosocial or physical conditions that are observable. This presents a challenge to psychiatric nurses, however, as concepts such as anxiety, hopelessness, powerlessness, or ineffective coping require the client's subjective perceptions

Table 6-3 Correct and Incorrect Outcome Statements

Nursing Diagnosis	Incorrect Outcome	Correct Outcome
Anxiety	Exhibits decreased anxiety; engages in stress reduction	Verbalizes feeling calm, relaxed, with absence of muscle tension and diaphoresis; practices deep breathing
Ineffective coping	Demonstrates effective coping abilities	Makes own decisions to attend groups; seeks staff for interactions vs. remaining isolated in room
Hopelessness	Expresses increased feelings of hope	Makes plans for the future (e.g., to continue therapy after discharge); states, "My kids need me to be well."

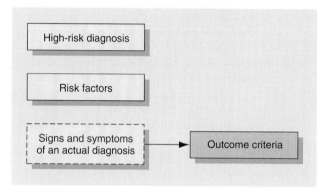

FIGURE 6-4 Developing outcome criteria for a risk diagnosis.

Table 6-4 Comparison of NANDA Diagnoses and NOC Outcomes

NANDA Diagnosis	NOC Outcome
Impaired physical mobility	Mobility level
Hopelessness	Hope
Deficient knowledge	Knowledge: disease process
	Knowledge: medication
	Knowledge: health behaviors
	Knowledge: treatment regimen
Constipation	Bowel continence
Diarrhea	Bowel elimination
Stress urinary incontinence	Urinary elimination
Reflex urinary incontinence	Urinary continence
	Tissue integrity: skin and mucous membranes
	Well-being
Interrupted family processes	Family functioning
	Family environment: internal
	Family coping

Modified from Johnson M, Maas M, Moorhead S: *Nursing outcomes classification (NOC),* St Louis, 2000, Mosby.

and often resist measurability. Outcome statements such as "reduced anxiety," "more hopeful," or "copes effectively" offer minimal criteria for measuring client outcome achievements. Therefore, when measuring client behaviors, the nurse should:

- Phrase the outcomes so that they clearly describe client behaviors
- Use the client's own words to describe feelings and thoughts whenever relevant
- Incorporate some type of measurement tool or parameters by which to quantify client progress or resolution of problem/symptoms

Table 6-3 provides examples of correct and incorrect outcome statements.

In some instances nurses place a specific target date for each outcome criterion to predict the evaluation time for each outcome attainment. Designated dates ensure that certain problems do not exceed specified, acceptable time periods. The outcome criteria throughout this text do not include projected target dates or time lines, as this practice is better applied to actual situations, not hypothetical client symptoms and behaviors. Developing clear, measurable outcomes assists the nurse in managing, resolving, preventing, and improving clients' multiple health and illness states. Effective client outcomes also justify reimbursement for nurses and ensure quality client care (Olsen, Rickles, and Travlik, 1995).

Wheeler (1999) indicates that clinical nurse specialists are in key positions to influence the care of clients that leads to positive client outcomes, as a result of their involvement in outcome studies currently being conducted in many health care systems. This type of research forces clinical nurse specialists and other advanced practice nurses to be accountable and responsible for the results of their care and to act as role models for nursing and other disciplines.

Nursing Outcomes Classification

The **Nursing Outcomes Classification (NOC)** was developed by the Iowa Outcomes Project and published in 1997 and 2000 to help nurses identify outcomes that are most influenced by the actions of nurses. NOC developed the first standardized language describing client outcomes that are responsive to nursing interventions. NOC defined nursing-sensitive outcomes as "neutral" concepts that can be measured on a continuum. Neutral concepts are such things as mobility and hydration (physical states) or coping and grieving (psychologic states). These concepts differ from discrete goals that are either met or unmet. The project members report that the precise impact that nursing care has on client outcomes and satisfaction helps distinguish nurses as major contributors to quality client care. NOC is continually developing precise client satisfaction outcomes with concomitant nursing care (see Nursing Interventions Classification [NIC], described in Interventions). For nurses to work effectively with managed care companies to improve quality and reduce costs, they must be able to measure and document the client outcomes that are most sensitive to nursing interventions (Johnson, Maas, and Moorhead, 2000). Table 6-4 compares NANDA diagnoses and NOC outcomes. See Appendix C for expanded description of NIC and NOC.

PLANNING (STANDARD IV)

The nurse plans client care with client, physician, and interdisciplinary team.

The planning phase consists of the total planning of the client's overall treatment to achieve quality outcomes in a safe, effective, timely manner. Nursing interventions with rationales are selected in the planning phase based on the client's identified risk factors and defining characteristics. The process of planning includes:

- Collaboration by the nurse with clients, significant others, and treatment team members
- Identification of priorities of care
- Critical decisions regarding the use of psychotherapeutic principles and practices
- Coordination and delegation of responsibilities according to the treatment team's expertise as it relates to client needs

Planning client care builds on the prior phases of the nursing process and is vital for the ultimate selection of relevant nursing interventions by which to achieve successful client outcomes.

Interdisciplinary Treatment Team Planning

Interdisciplinary treatment team planning is a typical method used to plan and monitor a client's treatment. The treatment plan is generally constructed on a standard form and consists of various sections in which to document diverse information relevant to client care, such as strengths, legal status, discharge plans, medical and nursing diagnoses, therapies, and social work data.

The treatment plan is implemented the first time the treatment team meets to discuss the client (ideally, no later than 3 days after the client's admission). The team is generally represented by nursing, social work, occupational and recreational therapy, and the client's physician. The client may also be present during a portion of the meeting unless contraindicated. Each team member is given an opportunity to discuss the client from the perspective of his or her own discipline and expertise. The treatment plan may be updated after the initial treatment team meeting as each discipline has more opportunity to spend time with the client and elaborate on its specific criteria.

The interdisciplinary treatment plan for a client with bipolar disorder in Figure 6-5 was developed in conjunction with the sample standard care plan in Figure 6-6. The information on each form should be reflected on the other. For example, the nursing diagnoses identified during the treatment team meeting should be the same diagnoses initiated on the client's standard care plan. Thus client assessment and treatment flow from one document to the other, illustrating consistency and reliability. Treatment plans are generally updated as often as the team meets to discuss a particular client. Ideally, the second team meeting should occur no later than 3 to 4 days after the first meeting. With the current trend toward shorter lengths of stay for all acute care

clients, treatment team planning needs to occur in a timely fashion to effectively address each client's specific needs.

Standardized Care Planning

One method used to plan and measure client care is known as standardized care planning (Figure 6-6). In this type of documentation, NANDA diagnoses, client outcomes, and interventions are formulated according to the identified DSM-IV-TR diagnostic categories in a standardized format. This standard format style is gaining popularity with nurses for the following reasons:

- The need to create new care plans for each client is reduced or eliminated.
- Consistency of care is encouraged through standardized guidelines.
- It requires a minimum of writing, thus freeing the nurse to spend more time interacting with clients.
- Standards of care are upheld, ensuring safe, effective treatment over time.
- It addresses managed care criteria for quality outcomes and length of stay.
- Problems are primarily initiated, evaluated, and resolved by nursing.

Standardized care plans do not preclude individualized treatment for each client, nor do they replace relevant narrative documentation.

Clinical Pathways

A **clinical pathway** (also known as a critical pathway, care path, or CareMap) is a standardized format used to provide and monitor client care and progress by way of the case management, interdisciplinary health care delivery system. Although nursing is a primary proponent of the clinical pathway method, other disciplines responsible for client care in the psychiatric mental health setting are actively involved in the development of each individualized clinical pathway. Such disciplines include social services, occupational therapy, therapeutic recreation, and dietary services, with strong collaborative input from psychiatrists. Consultations may be provided by psychologists, family practice physicians, or other professionals, depending on the special needs of the client.

A clinical pathway refers primarily to a written clinical process that identifies projected caregiver behaviors and interventions and expected client outcomes based on the client's mental disorder as defined in the DSM-IV-TR. The pathway is mapped out along a continuum that depicts chronologic milestones, generally the number of days that reflects the client's estimated length of stay for each specific diagnosis.

The pathway is a projection of the client's entire length of treatment, detailing interdisciplinary interventions or processes and client outcomes each day from admission through discharge. A pathway may be extended to include the client's transfer to home care or another type of treatment facility. The pathway would then continue for as long

Text continued on p. 107

BEHAVIORAL HEALTH INTERDISCIPLINARY TREATMENT PLAN

THIS PLAN WAS FORMULATED AT THE INTERDISCIPLINARY TREATMENT MEETING:

DATE ___1/1/03___   REVIEW DATES ___1/4/03, 1/7/03___

RECORDER ___Roseann Giordano, R.N. BSN___

ATTENDING PHYSICIAN ___Dr. Jones___

Present at Meeting: MD ___Dr. Jones___   RN ___Mary Webster, MS, RN, CS___

Social Worker ___Maggie Barker, LCSW___   Therapy
Services ___Beth Trottier, OTR___

Other ___John Clark, Student Nurse___

PRIMARY CONTACT

Name ___Jane Smith___   Relationship ___temporary conservator___   Tel. # ___123-4567___

REASON FOR ADMISSION: Striking out at   LEGAL STATUS: [√] Voluntary   [√] 72°h   Exp. Date ___
other clients and staff at Board and Care   [ ] 14 d.h.   Exp. Date ___
facility. Has refused to take meds X 3 days.   Conservator [√] Temp.   [ ] Perm.
                                                                          Date filed ___1/1/03___ Name ___Jane Smith___

PATIENT STRENGTHS
[√] Verbal   [√] Adequate Financial Resources
[√] Intelligent   [ ] Recognizes Own Problems   [ ] Supportive Family
[√] Intact Physical Health   [√] Supportive Friends   [ ] Employed
[ ] Consistent Work History   [ ] Resourceful
[ ] Compliant with Treatment [√] History of Independent Functioning [√] Other ___Cooperative and functional___
                                                                              ___when taking medications regularl___

PRELIMINARY DISCHARGE PLAN
Admission Date ___12/30/02___
Anticipated Length of Stay ___8___ days
Anticipated Services Required:
[ ] Financial Counseling   [ ] Payee   [√] Conservatorship
[√] Board & Care [ ] SNF Placement   [√] Partial Hospitalization Referral
[ ] Home Health Nurse   [ ] Psychotherapy, Marital/Family
[ ] Crisis House   [√] Medication Monitoring
[ ] Recovery Home/Sober Living   [ ] Other
[√] Self-Help Group

ADDRESSOGRAPH

Patient name: B. Brown

FIGURE 6-5 Example of an interdisciplinary treatment plan for a client with bipolar disorder. (Courtesy Tri-City Medical Center Mental Health Department, Oceanside, Calif.)

Continued

PATIENT NAME: B. Brown

PHYSICIAN:

SIGNATURE:

DIAGNOSIS

AXIS   I   Bipolar Disorder I
      II   Deferred
      III   None known

IV   mod-sev. (3-4)
V   30/60

DATE	PROBLEMS	PATIENT OUTCOME	GOAL DATE	INTERVENTION	DATE REVIEWED	DATE MET
12/30	Risk for Violence	Demonstrates absence of aggression	12/30	Provide safety by least restrictive means	12/31	12/31
12/30	Disturbed Thought Processes	Verbalizes clear realistic thoughts	1/3	Orient to reality in brief contacts	12/31	1/3
12/30	Self-Care Deficit	Demonstrates improved grooming; hygiene	1/3	Assist in grooming; hygiene as needed	1/1	1/3
12/30	Knowledge Deficient	States understanding of diagnosis	1/5	Teach signs/symptoms of diagnosis	1/3	1/6

NURSING:

SIGNATURE:

NURSING ADMISSION DATA BASE   Completed On _____

STANDARD NURSING PATIENT CARE PLAN (Title): _____

Additional Nursing Diagnosis:

1. Noncompliance, medications   4.
2. Ineffective Coping   5.
3. Chronic, low self-esteem   6.

The complete and individualized Standards of Patient Care are located in the Nursing section of the Patient Care Record.

THERAPY SERVICES

O.T. SIGNATURE:

T.R. SIGNATURE:

PROBLEMS	PATIENT OUTCOME	GOAL DATE	INTERVENTION	DATE REVIEWED	DATE MET
[√] Impaired Cognitive Skills:	OT/TR: - Demonstrates logical thought processes	1/3	[√] Task Skills Group Helps perform tasks	1/1	1/3
[√] Attention Span	Demonstrates increased attention span	1/2	[√] Living Skills Group Engages in living skills	1/2	1/5
[√] Concentration	Concentrates on unit tasks/activities	1/2	[ ] Creative Arts		
[√] Reality Testing	Tests reality appropriately	1/3	[√] Coping Skills Assists with coping skills	1/3	1/5
[√] Disorganization	Structures and organizes routine ADLs	1/4	[ ] ADL Training		
[√] Safety/Judgment	Utilizes safe judgment/behaviors	1/4	[√] Goal Setting Assists with simple goals	1/2	1/4
[ ] Orientation			[√] 1:1 Engages in 1:1 interactions	12/30	12/31
[√] Decreased Participation in Functional Activities	Increased participation in tasks/groups	1/3	[√] Leisure Education Engages in leisure ed	1/2	1/3
[√] Ineffective Coping Skills	Demonstrates effective coping skills	1/5	[√] Communication Skills Helps in group interactives	1/2	1/3
[ ] Social Withdrawal			[ ] Sensory Motor		
[√] Self-Destructive Behavior	Demonstrates absence of self-harm	12/31	[ ] Hygiene/Grooming		
[√] Low Self-Esteem	Verbalizes positive self-qualities	1/5	[√] Community Outings Accompany on outings	1/3	1/3
[ ] Other _____			[ ] Other:		
ACL Score: _____			_____ 1-2X wk _____ Frequency		
			_____ 30-45 min _____ Duration		

FIGURE 6-5—cont'd For legend see p. 103.

SOCIAL WORK

SIGNATURE: _____

PSYCHOSOCIAL DATA BASE

IDENTIFIED NEEDS/PROBLEMS	DATE REVIEWED	DATE MET
[✓] Family Dysfunction		
[ ] Placement		
[ ] Financial		
[ ] Employment		
[ ] Daily Structure		
[ ] Substance Abuse		
[✓] Limited Functioning		
[ ] Spiritual		
[✓] Inadequate Coping		
[✓] Inadequate Support System		
[ ] Other _____		

REFERRALS/INTERVENTIONS	DATE REVIEWED	DATE MET
[✓] Family Contact (Family resistant to help)		
[ ] Family Session		
[ ] Social Service Group		
[ ] CPS/APS		
[✓] Board & Care		
[ ] SNF		
✓PHP/Day Treatment (To increase support base)		
[ ] AA/NA/Alanon		
[ ] Home Health		
[ ] Clergy		
[ ] Voc. Rehabilitation		
[ ] MediCare/MediCal/SSI		
[ ] Other _____		
[✓] Extended Psychosocial Assessment (See SW notes)		

Assessment/Recommendations:

Attend all groups: interactions q shift

Appearance SL. disheveled; hyperactive; inappropriate dress for age

Age 42   Marital Status [ ] S [ ] M [✓] D [ ] W

Children (N) / Y

Status of Current Family Former spouse remarried; moved out of state; no contact
Parents elderly - unwilling or/unable to help. 0 other known family.

Religion [ ] Catholic [✓] Protestant [ ] Jewish [ ] Other

Military Service N / (Y)

Place of Birth U.S.A.

Family of Origin American

Occupation Unemployed   Employer _____

Financial Support: _____ Rep. Payee _____
_____ Manages Own Funds
____✓____ Receives Assistance   Type: SSI

Living Arrangement [ ] Home [ ] Apt. [ ] Hotel [ ] Shelter
[✓] Board & Care [ ] S.N.F. [ ] None Known [ ] Other: _____

Pt. Cooperative N / Y

Lives [ ] By Self [ ] W/Family [ ] W/Friends

Case Manager/Conservator N / (Y)   Name Jane Smith
Tel. # _____

Education: [ ] Did not complete high school   [ ] College degree
[✓] High school degree   [ ] Graduate degree
[✓] Some college

Primary Language English

Requires Interpretation Services (N) / Y

Past Psychiatric Hospitalizations N / (Y) _____
Dates _____ Locations _____

Contact: Name(s) Jane Smith, Conservator
Tel. # _____

Patient's Goal for this Admission _____

1. To maintain control over aggressive impulses
2. To comply with medication regimen
3. To utilize effective coping skills & solve problems
4. To increase self-esteem
5. To return to baseline or higher level of function

Discharge Plan: D/C to Board and Care with partial hospitalization referral

Tentative D/C Date: 1/7/03

ROOM	NAME	AGE	ADMIT DATE	DOCTOR
10-A	B. Brown	42	12/30/02	J. Jones

FIGURE 6-5—cont'd For legend see p. 103.

BEHAVIORAL HEALTH SERVICES
PATIENT CARE PLAN

TITLE:

BIPOLAR DISORDER

STANDARD OF CARE ON PATIENTS

INITIATED		NURSING DIAGNOSIS	PATIENT OUTCOMES	EVALUATION Documentation	INTERVENTIONS	RESOLVED		NOT RESOLVED	
Date	RN					Date	RN	Date	RN

12/30	RG	1. Disturbed thought processes R/T psychosis, paranoia, or delusions.	Patient will demonstrate logical, goal-directed speech and behaviors with an absence of psychosis, paranoia, or delusions.	q shift	1. Assess patient for:
					  a. Nature and content of thought processes.
					  b. Risk for harm to self or others.
					  c. Ability to participate in groups/milieu.
					  d. Ability to perform ADLs.
					
					2. Report to physician:
					  a. Actual or escalating risk for harm to self or others.
					  b. Refusal to eat/drink.
					  c. Refusal to take medication.
					
					3. Record assessments in the Progress Notes on Patient Care Record.
					
					4. Implement the following interventions:
					  a. Frequent supportive contacts with gentle reality orientation as tolerated.
					  b. Limit-setting to control inappropriate sexual, financial, or potentially harmful interpersonal behaviors.
					  c. Encourage participation in milieu groups consistent with patient's attention span.
					
					5. Implement the following protocols:
					  a. Hallucinations/Delusions Management
					  b. Lithium Management
					  c. Antipsychotic Medication Therapy Management
					
					6. Validate that outcome is met when patient has demonstrated goal-directed/logical speech and behaviors x 48°.
						1/3	RG		

12/30	MW	2. Risk for Violence: Self-directed or directed at others. Risk Factors: Delusions, hyperactivity, irritability	Patient will not harm self or others.	q shift	1. Implement the following protocols in increasing order of restrictiveness:
					  a. Agitated/Assaultive Behavior Management
					  b. Time-out
					  c. Seclusion
					  d. Restraint Management (only when it is least restrictive measure.)
					
					2. Validate that outcome is met when patient demonstrates freedom from behaviors harmful to self/others x 72°.
						12/31	MW		

FIGURE 6-6 Example of the first page of a care plan for a client with bipolar disorder mania. (Courtesy Tri-City Mental Health Department, Oceanside, Calif.)

as necessary. Clinical pathways may originate for clients in a home care situation and would then be developed by the interdisciplinary home care team.

Variances

Variances (also known as outliers) occur when a client's response to interventions is different from what is typically expected. A variance may therefore be considered an unexpected client response that "falls off" the pathway, requiring separate documentation and further investigation by the interdisciplinary team. Causes of pathway variances may be related to the client/family, caregivers, hospital, community, and payers (including insurance companies, health maintenance organizations, or managed care organizations).

A variance may be positive or negative and affect the client's length of stay and/or outcomes. An example of a positive variance would be a client who responds more rapidly to medication or other forms of treatment than expected and leaves the hospital before the estimated length of stay. An example of a negative variance would be a client who fails to achieve the desired nonmanic state or therapeutic lithium level in accordance with the time line designated on the clinical pathway continuum (generally by date of discharge), and whose length of stay is therefore prolonged.

Clinical pathways help ensure timely lengths of stay, prevention of complications, cost-effectiveness, and continued quality assurance. Also, overall coordinated management of each client's care and progress by the nurse case manager and the interdisciplinary team is ensured.

Figure 6-7 is an example of a clinical pathway describing a client with bipolar disorder mania, with a length of stay of 8 days. The upper columns list client outcomes. The larger lower columns consist of categories of care known as processes. Evaluation of client progress is measured daily along the pathway time lines. Clinical pathways continue to be developed, improved, and instituted in a variety of health care settings and are expected to reflect the changing trends and complexities of current health care delivery systems.

Electronic Methods of Documentation

New electronic methods of documentation are being introduced in many hospitals across the country. Known in some places as electronic medical records (EMRs), this progressive type of documentation can include physician orders, laboratory results, nursing orders, and progress notes. EMRs can also maintain professional and educational records of the staff. One goal is to reduce or minimize errors in communication as a result of this method. Problems identified through the use of electronic methods include reverting to paper documentation when computers are "down" or inaccessible and minimizing repetitive charting to avoid confusion and error. Many health care systems have overcome such problems and are successfully using EMRs in their facilities.

IMPLEMENTATION (STANDARD V)

In the implementation phase the nurse actually sets in motion the interventions prescribed in the planning phase. Some general nursing considerations directed toward clients and families during this phase include:

- Promote health and safety.
- Monitor medication regimen/effects.
- Provide adequate nutrition/hydration.
- Facilitate a nurturing, therapeutic environment.
- Build self-esteem, trust, and dignity.
- Engage in therapeutic groups/activities.
- Develop strengths/coping methods.
- Enhance communication/social skills.
- Use family/community support systems.
- Educate according to identified learning needs.
- Prevent relapse through effective discharge planning.

Nursing Interventions

Nursing interventions (also known as nursing orders or nursing prescriptions) are critical action components of the implementation phase and are the most powerful pieces of the nursing process. They make up the management and treatment approach to an identified health problem. Interventions are selected to achieve client outcomes and to prevent or reduce problems. Some flaws noted in nursing interventions, both in the literature and in clinical practice, are that they are often weak, vague, and nonspecific.

The **Nursing Interventions Classification (NIC)** is the first comprehensive standardized classification of treatments and interventions performed by nurses. NIC was published in 1992, 1996, and 2000. These interventions can be physiologic, such as airway suctioning and decubitus ulcer care, or psychosocial, such as anxiety reduction and assisting with coping strategies. They can prevent falls or self-harm and promote health, education, good nutrition, and stress reduction. The purpose of NIC is to identify and refine nursing actions from groups of data found throughout the literature and construct a taxonomy in which interventions are organized with clear rules and principles for the interventions selected (McCloskey and Bulechek, 2000).

For nursing interventions to be prescriptive, they must prescribe a course of action and not simply support the existing regimen. The interventions listed throughout this text reflect both actual and typical nursing responses and behaviors derived from educational preparation and a wide range of clinical experience.

In the psychiatric mental health setting, treatment frequently incorporates verbal communication skills, a major source of psychosocial interventions. Such treatments are intended to effect a change in the client's present condition, not merely to maintain the problem in its present state. Nursing interventions should explicitly describe a course of therapeutic activity that helps mobilize the client toward a

Clinical Pathway: Mania
DRG #430 - LOS - 8 Days

Interval		Day of Admit	Day 2	Day 3	Day 4
	Location				
O U T C O M E S	Physiologic	*Takes adequate nutrition, fluids with assistance *Complies with lithium level evaluation	*Demonstrates increased sleep/rest time *Demonstrates adequate elimination	*Takes adequate nutrition/fluid with reminders *Demonstrates adequate elimination	*Sleeping 4–6 hours *Demonstrates adequate elimination
	Psychologic	*Involved in stimulation-reducing activities with staff supervision	*Oriented to person and place	*Demonstrates reduction in: movement racing thoughts grandiosity/euphoria irritability	*Demonstrates increased attention span *Reality tests with staff *Oriented to person, place, time, and situation
	Functional Status/Role	*Tolerated orientation to the unit *Refrains from harming self/others with assistance	*Interacting with staff as told *Attends to hygiene/grooming needs with assistance *Refrains from harming self/others with assistance	*Engages in unit activities with staff supervision	*Maintains impulses with reminders *Complies with meds with reminders
	Family/Community Reintegration		*Identifies significant others to staff	*Attends community meetings with staff supervision	*Significant others involved in treatment/discharge planning
P R O C E S S E S	Discharge Planning	*SW Assessment *Identify DC Placement *ELOS, contact family/SO *Nursing Assessment *Identify H/O chronicity *Med compliance, strengths, needs, knowledge deficit	*Team: Involved in D/C Planning Discuss with MD *UR notify managed care ( )	*SW eval completed *Treatment Team meeting #1 ( ) *Specific D/C plans, placement facility identified ( )	*Involve family/SO in DC plans *Review DC plans with patient
	Education	*Orient to unit *Inform of patient's rights *Assess patient's and family's/SO knowledge of disorder/meds	*Assist with symptom recognition and importance of compliance *Teach family/SO as needed	*Continue with symptom recognition *Continue assessing patient and family/SO learning needs	*Assist in linking symptoms with precipitating events
	Psychosocial/ Spiritual	*Assess: Safety ( ) *Mental status ( ) Spirituality ( ) *Legal status: Vol ( ) 72 hour hold ( ) *Revise Writ ( ) Payor ( ) Conservator ( )	*Continue to assess: Safety issues Mental status Spiritual needs Legal status	*Continue to assess: Safety issues Mental status (e.g. racing thoughts, grandiosity, euphoria, irritability) Spiritual/Legal needs	*Continue to assess: Safety issues Mental status (e.g. racing thoughts, grandiosity, euphoria, irritability) Spiritual/Legal needs
	Consults	*Physical exam within 24 hours	*Other consults as needed	*Other consults as needed	*Other consults as needed
	Tests/ Procedures	*Lithium level ( ) *Tegretol level ( ) *Drug screen ( ) *Thyroid function ( ) *CBC/SMAC ( ) *Other ( )	*Tests/Procedures as ordered	*Tests/Procedures as ordered	*Tests/Procedures as ordered
	Treatment	*Monitor: I&O *Sleep/Rest patterns *Level A ( ) *Reduce milieu stimulation *S&R yes( ) no( ) *Other	*Monitor: I&O *Sleep/Rest patterns *Level A ( ) *Reduce milieu stimulation *S&R yes( ) no( ) *Other	*Move to level B ( ) *Continue with treatment plan: Monitor: I&O Sleep/Rest Other	*Move to level B ( ) *Continue with treatment plan: Monitor: I&O Sleep/Rest Other
	Medications (IV & Others)	*Medications as ordered *See relevant protocols: Lithium *Other *Monitor side effects *Toxicity	*Medications as ordered *Continue to monitor side effects/toxicity	*Medications as ordered *Continue to monitor side effects/toxicity	*Medications as ordered *Continue to monitor side effects/toxicity
	Activity	*OT assessment *1:1 brief contacts *Reality orientation *Intervene to manage impulses: prevent harm to self/others	*Engage in stimulation-reducing activities as tolerated *Assist with hygiene, grooming, ADLs *Prevent harm to self/others during activities	*OT eval completed *Encourage hygiene, grooming, ADLs with reminders *Prevent harm to self/others during activities	*Engage in 2 groups per day *Increase group stimulation as tolerated *Prevent harm to self/others during activities
	Diet/Nutrition	*Offer adequate nutrition and fluids; normal salt intake	*Provide simple meals, finger foods, easy to carry drinks	*Encourage meals in patient community as tolerated with staff supervision	*Encourage meals in patient community as tolerated with staff supervision

FIGURE 6-7 Clinical pathway for a client with bipolar disorder mania. (Courtesy Sharp HealthCare Behavioral Health Services, San Diego, Calif.)

Interval	Day 5	Day 6	Day 7	Day 8
Location				
OUTCOMES Physiologic	*Takes adequate nutrition/fluid *Sleeps 4–6 hours *Lithium level in therapeutic range *Other drug level in therapeutic range	*Sleeps 5–8 hours *Absence of drug toxicity	*Sleeps 5–8 hours	*Sleeps 5–8 hours *Able to manage food and activity requirements independently
Psychologic	*Demonstrates more reality based thoughts *Able to focus on one topic x5–10 minutes	*Demonstrates enthymic mood *Able to focus on one topic x5–10 minutes	*Able to complete activities and unit assignments	*Able to complete activities and unit assignments independently *Able to plan and structure day
Functional Status/Role	*Demonstrates less intrusive behaviors	*Able to interact with peers *Able to make simple decisions	*Demonstrates safe appropriate activities/behaviors *Independently complies with medical regimen	*Verbalizes need for ongoing medication compliance
Family/Community Reintegration	*Identifies discharge needs	*Identifies discharge needs	*Identifies discharge needs *Able to identify supports and their appropriate use	*Able to utilize supports and lists ways to access them *States specific plans to manage symptoms, comply with medications, and aftercare
PROCESSES Discharge Planning	*Assist patient/family/SO to identify discharge needs *UR contact managed care as needed ( )	*Continue to problem-solve discharge needs with patient, family/SO	*Treatment team meeting #2 ( ) *Transition to Day Treatment if indicated *Assist patient, family/SO in finalizing discharge plans	*Discharge to least restrictive environment completed *UR inform managed care as needed ( )
Education	*Teach patient/family/SO about medication effects on symptom management *Instruct in medication, diet, exercise regimen	*Emphasize importance of compliance with meds after discharge *Teach about drug-to-drug effects on symptom management	*Develop aftercare plan to manage symptoms and contact supports	*Reinforce aftercare teaching plan with patient, family/SO as needed
Psychosocial/ Spiritual	*Continue to assess: Safety issues Mental status Spirituality Voluntary status	*Continue to assess: Safety issues Mental status Spirituality Voluntary status	*Continue to assess: Safety issues Mental status Spirituality Voluntary status	*Complete assessments confirm: Safety Mental status Spirituality Legal status
Consults	*Complete consults as ordered *Arrange for aftercare consults as ordered	*Complete consults as ordered *Arrange for aftercare consults as ordered	*Complete consults as ordered *Arrange for aftercare consults as ordered	*Complete consults as ordered *Arrange for aftercare consults as ordered
Tests/ Procedures	*Check lithium level for therapeutic range *Check other drug levels for therapeutic range as needed *Tests/Procedures as needed	*Check lithium level for therapeutic range *Check other drug levels within therapeutic range as needed *Tests/Procedures as needed	*Check lithium level for therapeutic range *Check other drug levels within therapeutic range as needed *Tests/Procedures as needed	*Confirm lithium level for therapeutic range *Confirm other drug levels within therapeutic range as needed *Tests/Procedures as ordered aftercare
Treatment	*Move to level C ( ) *Continue with treatment plan I&O Sleep/Rest Other	*Move to level C ( ) *Continue with treatment plan I&O Sleep/Rest Other	*Transfer to open unit ( ) *Aftercare treatment instructions reviewed with patient, family/SO as needed	*D/C with aftercare treatment instructions
Medications (IV & Others)	*Medications as ordered *Contact managed care if any change in medication regimen	*Medications as ordered *Contact managed care if any change in medication regimen	*Medications as ordered *Review of medications with patient, family/SO as needed	*D/C with medications and instructions as ordered .
Activity	*Encourage: Independent hygiene and grooming Independent ADLs Increased participation in groups	*Engage in all unit activities and groups *Encourage independent decision-making	*Reinforce active participation in all unit activities and groups; independent decision-making	*Confirm: Ability to complete activity assignments independently Ability to make decisions independently
Diet/Nutrition	*Teach family/SO importance of adequate foods/fluids/salt intake	*Teach family/SO importance of adequate foods/fluids/salt intake	*Reinforce adequate nutrition fluids and normal salt intake	*Confirm patient/SO/family knowledge of adequate foods/fluids/salt intake

FIGURE 6-7—cont'd For legend see opposite page.

more functional state. The following are some descriptive examples:

- Gradually engage the client in interactions with other clients, beginning with individual contacts and progressing to informal gatherings and eventually to structured group activities.
- Teach the client and family/significant other that therapeutic effects of antidepressant medications may take up to 2 weeks and that uncomfortable effects may begin immediately.
- Praise the client for attempts to seek out staff and other clients for interactions and activities, and to respond to others' attempts to engage the client in interactions and activities.

Nondescriptive examples include:

- Assist the client to interact with others.
- Teach client and family about medications.
- Praise the client for socializing.

Note the clarity and substance demonstrated in the descriptive examples, as opposed to the weaker, more vague statements in the nondescriptive examples.

Nursing interventions that simply repeat physician's orders are not substantive enough to treat or manage the health problem effectively. The following are nonsubstantive examples:

- Monitor the client's progress.
- Check lithium levels.
- Notify social services.
- Obtain the client's consent form.
- Report changes in mood and affect.

Effective nursing interventions should be able to move the client to a more functional health state by virtue of their clarity, substance, and direction. In the psychiatric mental health setting, nurses constantly assess, diagnose, and treat clients' health states. Therefore the challenge for nurses is to formulate strong, effective nursing interventions that address and modify the client's health problem and are based on researched, independent nursing therapies.

The interventions in NIC are effective in the treatment of physical and psychiatric illnesses (e.g., hypertension or cognitive disorders). They are equally effective in preventing various types of trauma, such as falls or self-harm. NIC interventions are also used in health promotion and education. The purpose of NIC is to identify and refine nursing actions from groups of data found throughout the literature and construct a taxonomy such as NANDA and NOC, in which interventions are systematically organized, with clear rules and principles for the interventions selected. Table 6-5 summarizes some of the major coded classifications.

Even with the help of the nursing process and current NIC and NOC systems and the use of intuition, expertise, and critical thinking, there will be times when psychiatric nurses are unsure of which approach to take for certain client behaviors. Unlike the medical-surgical field, there are not always specific, clear-cut interventions for the complex array of behaviors manifested by clients with mental and emotional disorders. Also, clients may not always respond predictably to standard approaches, even if they have done so in the past. Clients in the psychiatric setting may be resistant to even the most carefully designed treatment plan. In such situations a variety of treatment approaches are generally applied with patience and empathy before the client responds. See Appendix C for expanded description of NIC and NOC.

Impact of Interventions on Etiologies

Interventions have the greatest impact when they are focused toward etiologies (related factors) that accompany the nursing diagnosis or, if the problem is a risk nursing diagnosis, when they are aimed at the risk factors. (Figure 6-8 illustrates the former, Figure 6-9 the latter.) This suggests that

Table 6-5	Major Coded Classifications					
	ICD-10	DSM-IV-TR	HCPCS	NANDA ICD Code	NIC	NOC
Stands for	International Statistical Classification of Diseases and Related Health Problems, Tenth Edition	Diagnostic and Statistical Manual of Mental Disorders, Fourth Edition, Text Revision	Healthcare Common Procedure Coding System	North American Nursing Diagnosis Association Translation of Taxonomy	Nursing Interventions Classification	Nursing Outcomes Classification
Published by	World Health Organization	American Psychiatric Association	Practice Management Information Corporation	North American Nursing Diagnosis Association	Mosby	Mosby
Codes for	Diseases and morbid entities	Psychiatric diagnoses	Supplies, materials, injections, and certain services and procedures in Medicare	Nursing diagnoses	Nursing interventions	Nursing outcomes

Modified from McCloskey JC, Bulechek GM: *Nursing interventions classification (NIC)*, ed 2, St Louis, 1996, Mosby.

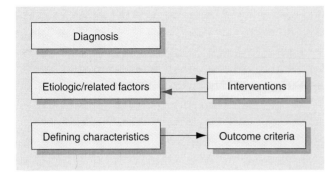

FIGURE 6-8 Developing interventions for an actual diagnosis. *Red arrow* indicates interventions for an actual diagnosis; *blue arrow* indicates impact of the interventions on etiologies.

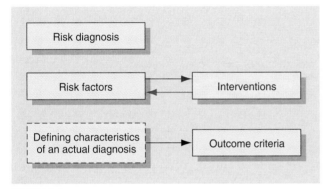

FIGURE 6-9 Developing interventions for a risk diagnosis. *Red arrow* indicates interventions for a risk diagnosis; *blue arrow* indicates impact of the interventions on risk factors.

nursing can modify or affect the etiologies of a problem, which makes sense, considering that etiologies are in some respects causal factors that greatly affect or provoke the health problem (nursing diagnosis). By the same token, risk diagnoses are less likely to become actual if interventions are aimed primarily at their accompanying risk factors. To achieve the most favorable client outcomes, etiologic factors associated with the problems (nursing diagnoses) should be examined meticulously and interventions carefully selected to modify each of them.

Interventions and Medical Actions

Interventions can include medically focused actions such as the administration of medications. However, *the major focus of nursing interventions should emphasize nursing actions, judgments, treatments, and directives.* Examples of nontherapeutic, medically focused interventions include:

- Administer antipsychotic medications as prescribed.
- Observe for extrapyramidal effects.
- Initiate benztropine (Cogentin) as ordered.

Note in the preceding examples the obvious absence of any prescribed nursing actions that would influence the client's health state.

Rationale Statements

A rationale statement is the reason for the nursing intervention. Rationales are not usually listed as part of a written care plan in clinical practice; however, they are generally part of the overall discussion of interventions in treatment team meetings. Rationales reflect nurses' accountability for their actions. Clear, descriptive rationale statements (in italics following the interventions) are provided in the disorders chapters in this text to enhance the reader's overall understanding of the selected interventions. For example:

- Actively listen, observe, and respond to the client's verbal and nonverbal expressions *to let the client know he or she is worthwhile and respected.*
- Initiate brief, frequent contacts with the client throughout the day *to let the client know he or she is an important part of the community.*
- Praise the client for attempts to interact with others and for participating in group activities *to increase self-esteem and reinforce repetition of healthy, functional behaviors.*

EVALUATION (STANDARD VI)

Evaluation of achieved expected client outcomes must occur at various intervals as designated in the outcome criteria, with the capability and health state of each client as a primary consideration. There are two steps in the evaluation phase:

1. *The nurse compares the client's current mental health state or condition with that described in the outcome criteria.* Is the client's anxiety reduced to a tolerable level? (For example, can the client sit calmly for 10 minutes, attend a simple recreational activity for 10 minutes, and engage in one-on-one interaction with staff for 5 minutes without distractions? Is there a significant reduction in pacing, fidgeting, or scanning? Were these outcomes attained within the times originally projected?) The degree to which client outcomes are achieved or not achieved is also an evaluation of the effectiveness of nursing.

2. *The nurse considers all of the possible reasons why nursing outcomes were not achieved, if this is the case.* For example, perhaps it is too soon to evaluate, and the plan of action needs further implementation. (For example, the client needed another 2 days of one-to-one interactions before attending client group activities.) Or perhaps the interventions were too forceful and frequent or too weak and infrequent. It may be that the outcomes were unattainable, impractical, or just not feasible for this client, or perhaps they were not within the client's scope and capabilities on a developmental or sociocultural level. What about the validity of the nursing diagnosis? Was it developed with a questionable or faulty database? Are more data required? What were the conditions during the assessment phase? Was it too hurried? Were conclusions drawn too quickly? Were there any language, cultural, or other communication barriers?

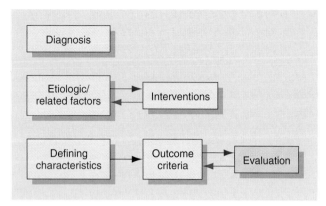

FIGURE 6-10 Evaluation process in an actual diagnosis. *Arrows* show how evaluation is determined according to identified outcomes.

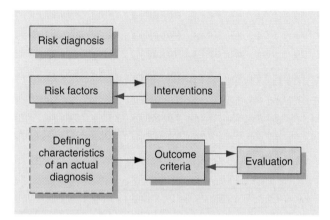

FIGURE 6-11 Evaluation process in a risk diagnosis. *Arrows* show how evaluation is determined according to identified outcomes.

Specific recommendations are then made based on conclusions drawn from the preceding questions. They include either continuing implementation of the plan of action or review of the previous phases of the nursing process (assessment, nursing diagnosis, outcome identification, planning, or implementation). Evaluation of the client's progress and the nursing activities involved in the process are critical because they require that nursing be accountable for the standards of care defined by its own discipline. Informal evaluation of the client's progress, much like that of the nursing process, takes place continuously.

Figures 6-10 and 6-11 show how evaluation is determined according to the identified outcomes and is also the measurement tool used to appraise outcome attainment for both actual and risk diagnoses, respectively.

THE NURSING PROCESS IN COMMUNITY AND HOME SETTINGS

In the past the nursing process and its multistep format have been most associated with the care of hospitalized clients. Current trends in health care delivery systems have shifted from inpatient facilities to community and home-based settings and provide yet another important avenue for use of the nursing process. Home health care is a primary alternative to hospitalization, and the nursing process continues to be a major factor in the effective management of home client care.

Psychiatric Home Health Care Case Management System

Changes in today's health care delivery system have resulted in several trends in health care reform designed to bring about cost-effective quality care. Although the case management concept has existed for years in acute care settings and public health arenas, only recently has the private home health model subscribed to total case management, and only more recently has psychiatric home care been incorporated under the case management umbrella.

Psychiatric home care case management is a method by which a client is identified as a candidate for home care and treated on a health care continuum in the familiar surroundings of the home. The interdisciplinary home care team, facilitated by a registered nurse, coordinates all available resources to meet its goals for treatment and to achieve the client's expected outcomes in a quality and cost-effective manner. At one end of the continuum is the highest degree of independent wellness within the client's capacity, and at the other end of the continuum is death, with varying levels of wellness-illness in between (Medina, 2002).

Critical to successful use of case management is the accurate placement of the client at the entry point on the continuum, and a clear understanding of the team's best estimate for the date of termination of home care services (Provancha and Hurst, 1994).

CHAPTER SUMMARY

- The nursing process is a decision-making method used by nurses for clinical care. As defined by the ANA, it has six steps: assessment, diagnosis, outcome identification, planning, implementation, and evaluation.
- The nursing process is an ongoing, multidimensional, cyclic approach in which data are continually collected, analyzed, and incorporated into a treatment plan.
- Intuition, expertise, and critical thinking are important elements in the nursing process.
- The two most common nursing assessment frameworks are the NANDA taxonomy and Gordon's Functional Health Patterns.
- NIC and NOC are two current nursing classification systems that complement NANDA and also represent taxonomies for effective interventions and outcomes.
- Nursing diagnoses provide nurses with a vocabulary that is distinctive to its own discipline and encourage nursing's theory and science-building efforts. NANDA diagnoses are the most common and accepted diagnoses used in nursing.

- Nursing diagnoses can have two formats: two-part statements that describe potential or risk problems and three-part statements that describe an actual problem.
- Outcome statements are highly specific, measurable indicators derived from nursing diagnoses and used to evaluate client progress.
- The planning phase consists of the total planning of the client's treatment regimen. Nursing interventions are selected in the planning phase.
- A clinical pathway is an interdisciplinary standardized format used to provide and monitor client care and progress.
- The implementation phase involves the actual setting into motion of the interventions that have been prescribed in the planning phase.
- Evaluation of the achieved expected client outcomes as designated by the outcome criteria should occur at various levels.
- There is a strong relationship among NANDA's nursing diagnoses, Nursing Interventions Classification (NIC), and Nursing Outcomes Classification (NOC).

REVIEW QUESTIONS

1. A 20-year-old male client walks into the hospital with a disheveled appearance and blunted affect. He is guarded on approach with no eye contact. He is restless and agitated and unable to sit still during the assessment. To assess the client's thought processes, the psychiatric nurse should ask:
   a. "Why do we have laws?"
   b. "What would you do if a fire started?"
   c. "What year is it?"
   d. "Does the TV or radio send you messages strictly for you?"

2. A 16-year-old male client is admitted to the adolescent unit. His parents observe that he has become more impulsive, irritable, and withdrawn in the last 3 months. His grades have dropped dramatically. He has lost 10 pounds and stays awake all night. The nurse demonstrates her competency in assessment skills when she asks the client:
   a. "Have you ever used alcohol or drugs?"
   b. "Have you ever been in Juvenile Hall?"
   c. "Have you ever been in therapy before?"
   d. "Do you have a family history of eating disorders?"

3. For a 40-year-old client with chronic paranoid schizophrenia, identifying discharge placement should be on which day of the clinical pathway?
   a. Day 5
   b. Day 10
   c. Day of admission
   d. Day 3

4. A 14-year-old female client with anorexia nervosa is admitted to the adolescent unit. She is 5 feet, 3 inches tall and weighs 90 pounds. She has been restricting food for the last 6 months. The best nursing outcome for the nursing diagnosis of Imbalanced nutrition: less than body requirements would be:
   a. Eats meals in the dining room
   b. Gains 1 pound per week
   c. Decreases excessive exercise
   d. Verbalizes the importance of a balanced, nutritious diet

5. A client is admitted to the detoxification unit after drinking a quart of vodka every day for the last month. The most important nursing intervention on the day of admission would be:
   a. Encourage the client to attend group therapy.
   b. Explain the addictive process.
   c. Give the client an AA meeting schedule.
   d. Monitor vital signs every hour for the first 4 to 8 hours and administer Librium according to the physician's orders.

REFERENCES

American Nurses Association: *Nursing, a social policy statement,* Kansas City, Mo, 1990, The Association.

American Nurses Association: *Standards of clinical nursing practice,* Kansas City, Mo, 2000, The Association.

Benner P: *From novice to expert: excellence and power in clinical nursing practice,* Menlo Park, Calif, 2001, Addison-Wesley.

Carnevali DL, Thomas MD: *Diagnostic reasoning and treatment decision-making in nursing,* Philadelphia, 1993, JB Lippincott.

Carpenito LJ: *Nursing diagnosis: application to clinical practice,* ed 6, Philadelphia, 1996, JB Lippincott.

Fidaleo RA: Suicide assessment and interventions: a videotaped program for nurses and physicians, San Diego, Calif, 2002, Sharp HealthCare.

Fortinash KM: Assessment of mental status. In Malasanos L, Barkauskas V, Stoltenberg-Allen K, editors: *Health assessment,* ed 4, St Louis, 1990, Mosby.

Gordon M: *Nursing diagnosis: process and application,* ed 3, St Louis, 1994, Mosby.

Gordon M: *Nursing diagnosis: process and application,* ed 2, New York, 1987, McGraw-Hill.

Johnson M, Maas ML: *Nursing outcomes classification (NOC),* St Louis, 1997, Mosby.

Kritek PB: Generation and classification of nursing diagnoses: toward a theory of nursing, *Image J Nurs Sch* 10:73, 1978.

McCloskey JC, Bulechek GM: *Nursing interventions classification,* ed 2, St Louis, 1996, Mosby.

Medina L: Clinical pathways: sharp home health, *Home Care,* October 1995, (update 2002).

Munhall PL, Oiler CJ: *Nursing research,* ed 2, New York, 1993, National League for Nursing.

North American Nursing Diagnosis Association: *Taxonomy II, NANDA, Nursing diagnoses: definitions and classification, 2001-2002,* The North American Nursing Diagnosis Association, Philadelphia, 2001, NANDA.

NANDA International (2003). Nursing Diagnoses and Classification, 2003-2004. Philadelphia: NANDA.

Olsen DP, Rickles H, Travlik K: A treatment team model of managed mental health care, *Psychiatr Serv* 46(3):252, 1995.

Provancha LE, Hurst S: Home health case management: an old approach to a new system, *NSI Home Health Newsletter* 1994.

Smith SK: An analysis of the phenomenon of deterioration in the critically ill, *Image J Nurs Sch* 20:12, 1988.

Tanner C et al: Diagnostic reasoning strategies of nurses and nursing students, *Nurs Res* 36:358, 1987.

Wescott MR: *Antecedents and consequences of intuitive thinking: final report to U.S. Department of Health, Education and Welfare,* Poughkeepsie, NY, 1968, Vassar College.

Wilkinson J: *Nursing process in action: a critical thinking approach,* Redwood City, Calif, 1992, Addison-Wesley.

Wheeler EC: The effect of the clinical nurse specialist on patient outcomes, *Crit Care Nurs Clin North Am* vol 11, 1999.

Whiteside C: A model for teaching critical thinking in the clinical setting, *Dimensions of Critical Care Nursing,* 1997.

SUGGESTED READINGS

Boomsa J, Dingemans CAJ, Dassen TWN: The nursing process in crisis-oriented home care, *J Psychiatr Ment Health Nurs* 4:295, 1997.

Kaplan H, Sadock B: *Synopsis of psychiatry: behavioral science/clinical psychiatry,* ed 8, Baltimore, 1998, Williams & Wilkins.

Southwick K et al: Strategies for health care excellence: care paths for psychiatric patients, *COR Health Care Resources* 8(2):1, 1995.

ONLINE RESOURCES

Critical Thinking: www.advancefornurses.com
Critical Thinking: www.criticalthinking.com
JCAHO Accreditation: www.ultimatenurse.com
Nursing Process and Critical Thinking:
    www.uttyler.edu/n3415/DMCthinking/DMCthinking/

7 Principles of Communication

Susan Fertig McDonald

OBJECTIVES

- Analyze the components of communication.

- Discuss factors that influence communication.

- Differentiate among social, intimate, collegial, and therapeutic communication.

- Describe the characteristics of effective helpers.

- Discuss the core qualities of the nurse and the various roles the nurse plays in interacting therapeutically with clients.

- Explain the principles of therapeutic communication.

- Compare and contrast the communication techniques that enhance and hinder therapeutic communication.

- Examine therapeutic communication in the context of the nursing process.

- Discuss three special communication challenges and their implications for the future.

ommunication is the most powerful tool a psychiatric nurse can have. It is the basic component of the therapeutic nurse-client relationship and the medium through which the nursing process occurs. **Communication** is a dynamic, two-way, circular process in which all types of information are shared between two or more people and their environment. Because we learn how to communicate at an early age, it might be thought of as quite simple. However, communication is a complex process that requires much practice to use it effectively.

Effective communication is thought to be one key factor that determines client satisfaction, treatment compliance, and recovery (Chant et al., 2002). Communication is critical to the successful outcome of nursing interventions, for without effective communication, a therapeutic nurse-client relationship would not be possible. Therefore the nurse must understand and master the general principles of communication, as well as the specific principles of therapeutic communication.

COMPONENTS OF COMMUNICATION

Communication consists of several components: the stimulus, the sender, the message, the medium, the receiver, and feedback. Usually there is a *stimulus*, a need or reason for the communication to occur. The individual who initiates the transmission of information is the **sender.** Each transmission is both verbal and nonverbal. The information being sent and received, such as feelings or ideas, is the **message.** The method by which the message is sent is the **medium,** which can be written (seen), verbal (heard), tactile (felt), or scent (smelled). For example, a note or letter is *sent;* a shout, scream, or whisper is *heard;* body odor or the scent of perfume is *smelled;* a hug or pat on the back is *felt.*

The **receiver** both receives and interprets the message that has been sent. Ideally, the receiver interprets the mes-

sage exactly as the sender meant to give it, thus producing effective communication. The **feedback** that the receiver gives back to the sender is the measure by which the effectiveness of the message is gauged. Feedback is a continual process because it is a response to the message and provides a new stimulus to the sender, whereupon the original sender then becomes the receiver. Therefore in any interaction the sender and receiver continually reverse roles. Figure 7-1 shows a model of the communication process.

FACTORS THAT INFLUENCE COMMUNICATION

Communication is a learned process influenced by several factors, including the environment, the relationship between the sender and the receiver, the content of the message, and the context in which the message takes place. Other factors include one's own attitude, values, ethnic background, socioeconomic status, family dynamics, life experience, knowledge level, and one's own ability to relate to others.

Environmental factors that control the effectiveness of communication include time, location, noise, privacy, comfort, and temperature. Timing of the interaction can be important. The phrase "counting to ten" describes a waiting or "cooling off" period necessary for some individuals to ensure that they can rationally discuss a "hot" topic or understand a critical concept. Consider the nurse who chooses to wait for a better time to begin teaching a client about medications, because the client has just experienced an emotional outburst in the medication-teaching group and is unable to concentrate in that environment. A carefully chosen time can mean the difference between successful and unsuccessful client learning.

The location of the interaction can be instrumental in conveying the sincerity or importance of communication.

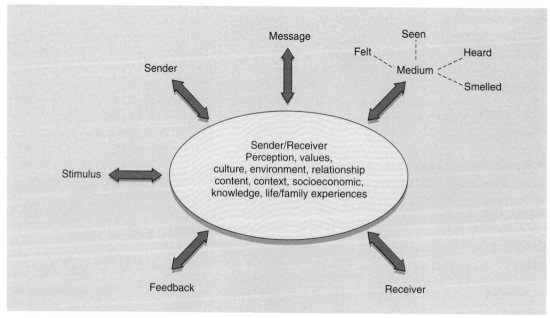

FIGURE 7-1. Model of the communication process.

Consider the man who wishes to propose marriage to a woman and chooses a mutually predetermined, romantic place in which to do it. A carefully chosen location could mean the difference between a "yes," "maybe," and "no" answer. If the location is noisy and other people are present, messages in the conversation may not be heard, resulting in ineffective communication. Therefore the type, quality, and perceived importance of the specific message conveyed depend in part on the general comfort of the environment.

The *relationship* between two people in a conversation greatly influences the communication. For example, a casual friend can give the same message to an individual as an intimate friend, but the receiver may react quite differently to each person according to the nature of each relationship.

The *context,* as well as the content, of the message also influences the receiver's response. The context, or circumstances in which the message is given, must be appropriate to the type of interaction. Individuals need to feel safe in their environment in order to disclose highly personal information.

Interaction is also affected by *attitude,* which determines how one person generally responds to another person and includes one's biases, past experiences, and levels of openness and acceptance. Also, people from one socioeconomic class, ethnic background, or family background may have difficulty communicating with individuals from a different background or class, possibly because of language, values, or knowledge barriers. For example, both eye contact and personal space may vary greatly from one culture to another.

Communication is greatly influenced by one's upbringing and those aspects of communication that were encouraged, modeled, and discouraged by significant others. Boys in traditional households taught "boys must be tough and should not cry" may grow up unable to easily express sad emotions. A teenager who is continually told to "shut up" for "talking too much" may develop a quiet or nonassertive style of communication as an adult.

Knowledge differences can create a deficiency in understanding during communication. If the sender has a greater knowledge of the subject matter than the receiver, it is the responsibility of the sender to ensure that the receiver understands the message. This is always one of the challenges in teaching students or clients important concepts. Some people have an ability to relate with ease to a variety of people and can explain complex information in simple, understandable terms. Some have a great deal of difficulty with this task and are easily intimidated by others. People can learn to communicate more easily and clearly and feel secure about it with knowledge about communication techniques, with practice, and with feedback about their efforts.

Perception is an individual's subjective experience that influences how the message is interpreted. Because misperceptions create problems in communication, the sender must be certain that the receiver has a clear understanding of the message. Thus effective communication depends on understanding what is being communicated, interpreting the message as it was meant to be given, and providing feedback that supports the correct interpretation.

MODES OF COMMUNICATION
Written Communication

Written communication is primarily used to share information. The reader reads for knowledge, pleasure, and understanding. The reader who is able to understand the written word as it appears and comprehend its meaning is prepared to absorb the meaning. It is important that the nurse be able to clearly convey ideas in written form whether it is documentation in the medical record or in the form of statistical reports. Because more and more documentation is in the form of computerized patient records, it is imperative that any form of written communication includes ability to navigate through computer systems. The ability to write legibly, spell correctly, use proper grammar, and organize ideas clearly is critical for the nurse. Although many hospitals are converting to electronic medical records, the narrative form of documentation will always be a part of the nurse's progress notes. Description of a client's behavior in the psychiatric mental health setting is an important part of effective nursing assessment and interventions and should be clearly conveyed through the written word.

Verbal Communication

Verbal communication commonly refers to the spoken words that encompass the symbols of language. Precise verbal communication is important because spoken words often mean different things to different people. Many words or phrases have slang meanings or have developed new meanings. Words or phrases may also have different meanings for different groups. Figures of speech, jokes, clichés, colloquialisms, and other terms or special phrases carry a variety of meanings. For example, "It is a blue Monday" could mean it is a sad day to a person who has the ability to think on an abstract level, but to a client with schizophrenia who interprets concretely and literally, it could mean that the sky is blue. "Don't rain on my parade" means "don't spoil my fun" to one person, but to the client with psychosis who may have loose associations, it prompts the question regarding whether a parade is actually occurring or the question, "Why would I rain on a parade?"

In interactions with individuals from different cultures, slang phrases and idioms such as "double dipping," "making good bread," "rad," "way cool," and "let's party" would not be understood and therefore would be misinterpreted. It is easy to assume that other people understand intended meanings. Thus it is necessary to periodically check their interpretation, including examining the cues obtained from their nonverbal responses.

It is increasingly important for nurses to develop a greater sensitivity to the cultural aspects of communication. It is clearly a challenge to learn how to communicate effectively with psychiatric clients who not only have difficulty communicating in a clear, logical, or reasonable manner because of their mental disorder but who are also from another culture and use English as a second language. Chapter 5 further discusses issues of communication with those from cultural groups different from one's own.

Nonverbal Communication

Nonverbal communication is believed by many communication theorists to be the most important part of any message, composing about 93% of any communication. It includes elements such as voice tone, hand and body movements, facial expressions, auditory noises that do not involve actual words, and other movements and expressions. Nonverbal cues involve all five senses. They add to the meaning of verbal messages by performing several functions such as expression of feelings, the contradiction or validation of verbal messages, and the preservation of both the ego and the relationship. As a general rule, nonverbal behavior is more revealing and truthful than verbal communication. Actions really do speak louder than words. Therefore it is important for the nurse to observe and consider the client's entire message, both verbal and nonverbal, before arriving at a conclusion.

To be an effective communicator, one's nonverbal cues should be **congruent,** or consistent, with the verbal message. An example of congruent communication follows:

Verbal: "I became very worried when you did not arrive on time."

Nonverbal: Concerned facial expression, warm, friendly, outstretched hand

An example of incongruent communication follows:

Verbal: "I would like to get to know you better."

Nonverbal: Eyes looking away, detached, arms folded across chest

Nonverbal cues are grouped into four categories: body cues (kinesics), space (proxemics), touch, and appearance (Northouse and Northouse, 1998).

Body Cues

Body cues include facial expressions, reflexes, body posture, hand gestures, eye movement, mannerisms, touch, and other body motions. Body posture and facial expressions, including eye movements, are two of the most important cues to determine how a person is responding to the message. When a client who is frowning, with clenched teeth and fists, narrowed eyes, and a red face, says "I am always glad to see my mother," there is a contradiction between verbal and nonverbal cues that needs to be addressed. A slumped or stooped posture can mean a client is depressed or, at the very least, feeling sad or dejected. A closed posture with arms folded may indicate that a client is withdrawing or possibly feeling some anger or angst. An erect posture with shoulders back can mean that the client feels more confident or may be attempting to portray confidence. The gait of an individual as it relates to posture can also indicate one's self-concept. The person who bounces along with shoulders back and head up high may be perceived as more "upbeat" than the individual who walks at a slow-moving pace with a slumped posture.

Nurses should carefully observe hand gestures, as they may also signal anger, restlessness, frustration, giving up, relaxation, or apathy. For example, the nurse needs to be aware of impending anger so that early interventions can be implemented to prevent a situation from becoming quickly out of control. The old adage, "when in doubt, observe what people do, not only what they say," is especially important when dealing with psychiatric clients, because what they say and what they do may often be incongruent.

Paralinguistic (paralanguage) behavior includes any audible sound that is not a spoken word. It includes voice tone, inflection, word spacing, rate, emphasis or intensity, groaning, coughing, laughing, crying, grunting, moaning, and other audible sounds. Along with the silent cues, these audible nonverbal cues are important in assessing clients.

Space

The use of space is another nonverbal cue. Each person has a "comfort zone" or space boundary that invisibly surrounds him or her when interacting with others. The boundary becomes larger or smaller, depending on the nature of the relationship. *Intimate space* is the closest distance between two individuals. *Personal space* is for close relationships within touching distance. *Consultive space* is farther apart than personal space, requiring louder speech. *Public space* is used for public gatherings such as speeches and is usually seen in a large hall or auditorium.

Space as a concept of boundaries and safety is important to understand because the nurse and client need to respect the distance each one needs. For example, if a client has a recent history of assault, the nurse may want to stay "a step and a kick away" from the patient for obvious safety reasons (P.A.R.T., 2002). For successful communication to occur, both parties need to feel comfortable. Some clients have problems with their boundaries and may "invade" other clients' own "safe zone." Clients who perceive this as threatening may react aggressively to such boundary violations. At such times the nurse may need to help the client understand the appropriate distance by actually stating the boundary for the client in inches or feet, as needed. When the client violates the nurse's own comfortable space, the nurse may need to set a limit for the client after the initial intrusion.

Touch

Touch is a nonverbal message that involves both action and personal space. Touch typically conveys a message to the receiver that the sender wants to connect with them. In nursing, touch has been used to convey messages of concern and empathy. The nurse must be careful when deciding whether to touch a psychiatric client. Not all clients want to be touched. They may perceive it as a threat and respond with aggression, or interpret it as an intimate move and respond by withdrawal or inappropriate sexual response. Touch as communication is discussed in more detail later in the chapter.

Appearance

Appearance communicates a particular image, as well as a clue to one's mental status. Appearance refers to the way an individual uses clothing, makeup, hairstyle, jewelry, and other items such as hats, purses, or glasses, as well as grooming and hygiene. These nonverbal cues often disclose how the person wishes to be viewed by others. For example, a female nurse who comes to work wearing a revealing blouse, tight slacks, and high-heeled shoes exhibits a look more suitable for a social engagement than one representing the profession of nursing.

Another example is an individual who comes in for a professional job interview wearing jeans, a wrinkled knit shirt, and sandals; his hair is uncombed and his beard untrimmed. On first glance, the employer wonders if the job candidate is serious about being hired, because his appearance is too casual and sloppy, and projects an unfavorable image. A third example is an elderly woman who is admitted to the hospital wearing dirty, wrinkled clothing. She was found by the home health nurse in a filthy apartment and has not bathed in several weeks. On further assessment it is revealed that her husband died 2 months ago, and she was subsequently diagnosed with depression. Therefore her appearance is one result of her obvious unresolved grief response, which has incapacitated her.

Nurses must try to interpret a client's nonverbal behavior while evaluating the verbal content, and incorporate this evaluation into the assessment of the client and their plan of care.

Finally, nurses need to be aware of their own nonverbal cues. For effective communication to occur, these nonverbal messages must be congruent with their verbal message and communicate genuine interest and respect.

TYPES OF COMMUNICATION
Intrapersonal Communication

In **intrapersonal communication** self-talk occurs, during which individuals give themselves all types of positive and negative messages. Self-talk can be helpful if the messages one gives oneself are helpful or positive. Intrapersonal communication can be functional or dysfunctional.

For example, during a session with the nurse, a client identifies several problems she needs to work on, as well as realistic goals for her hospital stay. The client then tells herself she is pleased that she has finally accomplished a useful task and is now clear about what she needs to do before she leaves the hospital. In this situation, the client gives herself positive messages that assist her in her recovery.

An example of dysfunctional self-talk occurs if this same individual persists in giving herself negative, self-defeating messages (e.g., "I can never accomplish anything," or "I will never reach my goals"). This type of self-talk can impede recovery.

In another example, a client with a diagnosis of schizophrenia continually hears many internal voices that tell him he is a "bad person," and that he must kill himself to "cleanse his soul." These internal voices, displayed through auditory hallucinations, are considered dysfunctional self-talk.

Interpersonal Communication

Interpersonal communication occurs between two or more individuals and contains both verbal and nonverbal messages. As stated previously, it is a complex process consisting of a variety of factors affecting its outcome. The nurse communicates on an interpersonal level with a variety of individuals and groups throughout the day. Emphasis is placed on *therapeutic* and *collegial communication* when the nurse is at work. *Social communication,* primarily used away from work, is discussed only briefly. The characteristics of social and therapeutic communication are listed in Table 7-1.

Social Communication

Social communication occurs in everyday situations, usually away from the work setting. This type of interaction may include discussions regarding family relationships, social activities, vacations, school, and church. Much of this interaction is superficial and light, and may not have a goal. The

Table 7-1	Characteristics of Social and Therapeutic Communication	
	Social	**Therapeutic**
Who	Friends, family, acquaintances	Nurse and client
Setting	Home, away from work, any type of setting	Clinical setting; private, quiet, confidential, safe environment
Purpose	Maintain relationships; mutual sharing of information, thoughts, beliefs, ideas, feelings	Promote growth and change in clients
Content	Social talk; focus on children, vacations, family, leisure, church, doing a favor, giving advice	Therapeutic talk; client expresses thoughts, beliefs, feelings, anxieties, fears, problems; client identifies needs
Characteristics	Superficial, light; not necessarily goal directed; spontaneous, enjoyable; two-way, focusing on both sender and receiver, giving suggestions, advice; personal or intimate relationship occurs	Learned skills; purposeful, client-focused; client sets goals; planned, difficult, intense; disclosure of personal information by client; meaningful and personal (but not intimate) relationship occurs
Skills	Uses a variety of resources during socialization	Uses specialized professional skills, primarily therapeutic interpersonal communication ▪

purpose of most social communication is to maintain relationships and for the enjoyment and mutual benefit of those involved.

Varying levels of intimacy exist in social communication. Communication between parent and child carries a level of intimacy different from communication between parent and teacher. Self-disclosure is common and occurs at varying levels, but superficiality is more the norm, as there are no real expectations of help. When help is the expected outcome of social communication, it is typically given in the form of suggestions and advice by friends and family. This type of help differs dramatically from the help given to the client by the nurse in a therapeutic relationship.

Collegial Communication

The purpose of *collegial communication* is professional collaboration. Collegial communication occurs among colleagues in the professional work setting.

The nurse may also be involved in professional nursing groups within the work setting and in the community. This type of collegial communication is called *intradisciplinary*.

When psychiatric nurses interact with members of the unit's treatment team, it is referred to as *interdisciplinary collegial communication*. The interdisciplinary team has regularly scheduled treatment team meetings designed to develop, review, and revise the client's treatment plan. It is vital that all members involved in the client's treatment attend and actively participate in the meeting. Members are assigned roles critical to the success of the treatment team process. The nurse can be the designated leader who facilitates the meeting and is expected to clearly communicate with all members of the team. The nurse can also be assigned the role of recorder, the person responsible for documenting the pertinent information discussed in the client's treatment plan. This role requires skillful written communication techniques. Within a nursing professional group, the intent of the communication is to share knowledge, collaborate on a project, or in other ways enhance or improve the profession.

Effective collaboration has the advantage of breaking through power issues and competition that arise when teams of professionals are brought together. In the collaborative process no member is more important than another member or the group as a whole. Each member's contribution is equally important to the success of the project, purpose, or goal.

The nurse therefore communicates in the collegial arena with supervisors, co-workers, physicians, consultants, and other members of the treatment team. These relationships exist within the profession of nursing and outside it. Simultaneously, the psychiatric nurse communicates on a therapeutic level with clients and their family members or significant others.

Therapeutic Communication

Therapeutic communication, the foundation in psychiatric nursing, occurs between the nurse (helper) and the client (recipient). *It is the psychiatric mental health nurse's single most important tool.* The art of interacting therapeutically is a learned skill involving both nonverbal and verbal communication; its purpose is to promote client growth. It is the medium through which health promotion interventions occur.

Therapeutic communication is client focused, whereas social communication consists of sharing information equally between two or more individuals. Even though the nurse may engage in some social interaction with the client, such as greeting the client at the beginning of the shift, the progress toward a greater level of health occurs through the therapeutic interaction between the nurse and client.

This therapeutic interaction involves the disclosure of personal information by the client. It may include hurtful memories and situations that bring up painful emotions. Sharing such feelings can be extremely beneficial for the client because it allows him or her to identify and discuss experiences and accompanying feelings in a safe, therapeutic setting. The nurse provides a confidential and quiet setting in which the interaction takes place, encourages the client to openly discuss thoughts and feelings, and practices active listening, acceptance, and empathy.

Therapeutic communication can be intimidating not only for the client but also for the nurse. Intense negative feelings are not easy to discuss. Many clients have not previously discussed them for fear of undesired responses such as a lack of understanding on the part of the listener, retaliation, feelings of being unworthy, and inadequacy in explaining them. The intensity of the client's feelings or verbal responses may frighten or catch the new nurse off guard—especially when a client openly discusses such issues as wanting to die because life is not worth living. The nurse may also feel uneasy when a client discusses an emotion or feeling similar to the nurse's personal experience. The nurse's own anxiety level may rise if she or he has not dealt with personal problems effectively.

In summary, therapeutic communication has three essential purposes: (1) to allow the client to express thoughts, feelings, behaviors, and life experiences in a meaningful way to promote healthy growth; (2) to understand the significance of the client's problem(s) and the role the client and the significant people in his or her life play in perpetuating those problems; and (3) to assist in the identification and resolution processes of the client's problem areas.

The nurse's therapeutic use of communication is the mechanism by which clients can achieve successful outcomes to the problems currently preventing them from achieving optimum health.

PRINCIPLES OF THERAPEUTIC COMMUNICATION
Personal Elements Important for Therapeutic Communication

The nurse's use of self as the primary tool in psychiatric nursing is similar to the singer's use of voice as an instrument to create music. All of the elements essential to helping another individual are within the nurse. This is both exciting and challenging.

The therapeutic use of self begins with *knowing oneself.* Nurses will not be able to help others unless they are first able to help themselves. Knowing one's self is a complex and life-long learning process. It is essential to have self-knowledge before one can use the self as a therapeutic tool to help others.

At the core of self-knowledge is the nurse's ability to correctly identify negative or unresolved issues of the self. Nurses need to know what values and beliefs they hold. It is also important for them to know and understand their own family background, including dynamic, cultural, and social issues; values; and biases and prejudices.

Nurses need to be aware of unresolved family life issues and make every effort to resolve them as soon as they are recognized. For example, consider a female nurse who has a long-held belief regarding women and alcohol dependency. She believes they can stop drinking if they really want to. Her belief developed because her maternal grandmother had died from alcohol-related liver disease. The nurse may be unaware that she holds this belief until the first alcohol-dependent female client is assigned to her. It is only when the nurse understands and resolves her issues that she can truly succeed in the necessary separation of her own issues from those of the client.

Because therapeutic communication occurs for the purpose of helping others, it is vital that nurses *understand what motivates them to help others.* Nurses' emotional needs must be recognized so that they do not interfere with the ability to relate therapeutically to clients. Because clients do not take care of nurses' emotional needs, nurses must meet their own emotional needs outside of work. A well-balanced, multifaceted lifestyle satisfies one's emotional needs. When the nurse's needs are met, he or she can better assist the client through therapeutic communication.

Nurses who are *in control of their own lives and emotions* can engage the client in effective communication while maintaining therapeutic control of the conversation, especially when a client is attempting to be intimidating, manipulative, or threatening.

Also, nurses who are comfortable with them can put the client's needs first by listening attentively and recognizing emotions in the client that may hinder a therapeutic exchange. For example, a high level of anxiety can produce "tunnel vision" in a client, which can impair communication.

Finally, the nurse needs to be able to *conduct a periodic self-evaluation of his or her responses to the client.* Questions to ask oneself may include (Shives, 2002):

- Am I open- or closed-minded regarding this issue?
- Am I accepting? Or am I rejecting?
- Am I being supportive? Or am I being nonsupportive?
- Am I being objective? Or am I allowing my biases to interfere with the interaction?
- Am I remaining calm and in control of my own feelings? Or am I allowing my anxiety, sympathy, or anger to surface?
- What are my true feelings? Do my nonverbal cues match my verbal communication?

Many employers have Employee Assistance Programs to assist employees with personal issues that arise in the workplace that may interfere with communicating effectively. Nurses should feel free to use these employee benefit services to help them deal with personal issues that may be affecting their ability to do their job well.

Roles of the Nurse in Therapeutic Communication

Nurses assume many roles during therapeutic communication with clients, such as serving as a professional role model. In the professional role the nurse acts as teacher, socializer, technician, advocate, parent, counselor, and therapist. As a *role model* the nurse is looked up to by staff, students, and the community. The nurse models therapeutic communication for clients, staff, and students. In the community, as well as in the health care setting, the nurse serves as a professional role model against which nursing, as a profession, is judged.

Clients learn about their illness and treatment modalities from the nurse as a *teacher.* As a teacher, the nurse uses excellent communication to educate other staff and clients. The nurse as a *socializer* brings clients together for activities to prevent the social isolation of the client during hospital treatment. In the *technician* role the nurse performs a glucometer test, administers medications, or takes vital signs. As an *advocate* the nurse informs the client of his or her rights and responsibilities and supports the client in decision making. The advocate nurse also serves as a liaison between the client and other members of the mental health team, ensuring that the client's rights, either legal or human, are not violated (Fontaine and Fletcher, 1995). The nurse in the *parent* role performs traditional nurturing tasks such as feeding, bathing, or comforting. As a *counselor* the nurse assists the client with personal problems such as a disagreement between the client and a family member. With advanced education the nurse can take on the role of a *therapist*, conducting individual, group, or family therapy sessions in the hospital, clinic, or community setting.

As part of the therapeutic relationship with a client, the nurse may take on part or all of these roles. The number of roles the nurse assumes varies according to the type and length of the individual nurse-client relationship, as well as the setting of the interactions.

Traits of Therapeutic Communication

The following are traits of effective therapeutic communication: genuineness, positive regard or respect, empathy, trustworthiness, clarity, responsibility, and assertiveness. These characteristics allow the nurse to influence growth and change in others. They incorporate verbal and nonverbal behaviors, as well as attitudes, beliefs, and feelings behind the communication, and are necessary for therapeutic communication to take place.

Genuineness

Genuineness is demonstrated by congruence between the nurse's verbal and nonverbal behavior. Consistent verbal and nonverbal behavior implies that the nurse is open, honest, and sincere. Genuineness is necessary for clients to develop trust in the nurse. Trust is built when the nurse does not appear "to just be doing her job" but rather responds with sincere interest. Genuine interaction does not mean that the nurse must disclose personal information or relate to the client in a social manner. Rather, the nurse remains focused on the client and responds therapeutically, using a variety of helpful responses (see Table 7-2). Nurses cannot expect a client to be open and honest if they do not display these characteristics themselves.

Positive Regard

Positive regard refers to respect and acceptance. Nurses can show that they view their clients as worthy, for example, by addressing the client by the name they prefer. Nurses accept clients for who and where they are and do not expect them to change except as it relates to their goals in treatment. Positive regard, or respect, is communicated in a variety of ways. It can be conveyed by sitting and listening to a client, by expressing concern regarding events affecting a client, by validating the client's feelings, or by effectively responding to a client's negative behavior. For example, a client who has just been admitted is found in the day room openly undressing in front of others. After assessing the situation and understanding that this activity is not harmful to others, the nurse explains to the client that this behavior needs to be done in the privacy of his or her bathroom. The nurse closes the door to allow the client to continue, but out of the view of others.

Part of positive regard is being nonjudgmental. The nurse should avoid harsh judgment of clients' behavior and feelings because both are real and cannot be argued with, discounted, or criticized. Clients must not be made to feel wrong. Labeling behaviors based on one's own value system is not useful. Instead, the nurse helps clients explore their behavior by discussing the thoughts and feelings that determine the behavior. When clients realize that they are not being judged, they may feel free to express their most intimate thoughts and feelings. A nonjudgmental attitude in the nurse relaxes clients by removing fears of being misunderstood or rejected. This open relationship can occur only when nurses identify their own thoughts and feelings regarding clients' behavior.

Empathy

Empathy, or empathic understanding, is the nurse's ability to see things from the client's viewpoint and to communicate this understanding to the client. There are two types of empathy. The first type—*natural, trait,* or *basic empathy*—implies that empathy is an inherent human trait apparent in varying degrees in everyone. Some research suggests that trait empathy is a naturally inherited potential that matures during growth. This viewpoint suggests that we all have an instinctual sensitivity that unfolds in a person, as is the case with other characteristics of human development (Alligood, 1992).

The second type, *trained* or *clinical empathy,* is said to build on the nurse's own natural level of trait empathy.

Trained empathy is a learned skill used consciously to achieve a therapeutic intervention (Pike, 1990). Some researchers suggest that nursing students should be tested for their level of basic or natural empathy before being taught the clinical empathy techniques to determine potential problematic levels that are either too low or too high (Alligood, 1992; Williams, 1990). Testing would give a baseline indicator before any empathy training to determine the effectiveness of the instruction. High levels of natural empathy may indicate that the nurse has a tendency to overidentify and thus become too involved with clients' problems. Low levels may indicate that the nurse may not be able to demonstrate enough genuine concern for clients. Knowing this information may better assist the new nurse in periodic self-assessments.

Empathy should not be confused with sympathy. Sympathy is overinvolvement and sharing one's own feelings after hearing about another person's similar experience. It is not objective, and its primary purpose is to decrease one's own personal distress.

An empathic response involves an appreciation and awareness of the client's feelings and keeps the focus on the client. For example, a client reveals to the nurse that her father died in an automobile accident 1 month before his arrival at the hospital. The nurse responds sympathetically by saying that her own father died in an automobile accident and that it had made the nurse feel sad for a year afterward. Here the focus is on the nurse, and the client may not know how to respond. An empathic response by the nurse would be: "I can understand how difficult that must be for you. Tell me how you are feeling now and how you have been coping with the loss." Now the focus is on the client, and the client is better able to reply.

The development of empathy poses a challenge for the psychiatric mental health nurse in the hospital setting, who typically has a brief time frame with clients and must primarily use crisis intervention principles. Lower levels of empathy from the nurse are healthier for clients in the beginning stage of the relationship. It has been shown through research, however, that empathy, especially if it is expressed early in a relationship, is clearly related to positive treatment outcomes.

Empathy consists of two stages. If a client shares important and uncomfortable emotions, nurses should first be receptive to understanding the client's communication by putting themselves in the client's place. This does not mean that nurses need to have had the same problem or associated feeling. Then, after stepping back into the professional role, nurses must be able to communicate understanding, which demonstrates objectivity and sensitivity to the client. This understanding mirrors the client's identity and is the process by which the client makes changes to achieve positive outcomes. The following skills help nurses develop greater empathic responses:

- Attending to the client physically, by sitting in front of the client, at a slight angle, leaning slightly forward with hands and arms in an open stance

- Attending to the client emotionally by clearing one's mind of other personal or work-related business and focusing one's full attention on the client
- Actively listening by providing a response to each of the client's verbal and nonverbal communications
- Focusing on the client's strengths
- Conveying caring, warmth, interest, and concern through nonverbal behaviors
- Choosing the most important point of what the client is trying to say
- Demonstrating congruence between one's own nonverbal and verbal communication
- Checking whether one's empathic responses are effective by looking for verbal and nonverbal clues

Closely aligned with empathy is *active listening,* because it incorporates both nonverbal and verbal behaviors necessary for therapeutic communication. Nonverbally, the nurse leans slightly forward, facing the client; uses comfortable, intermittent eye contact; nods; and uses verbal phrases such as "uh huh" or "I understand." Active listening results in articulation of the client's feelings, specifically providing the client with the knowledge that the nurse accepts how the client is feeling and attempts to understand this (Smith, 1990). A nurse who listens actively also displays interest. A client who is trying to work through problems needs to know that the nurse is there to help and wants to help.

Trustworthiness

Trustworthiness is another essential characteristic of an effective nurse. Being trustworthy means being responsible and dependable. Trustworthy nurses adhere to commitments, keep promises, and are consistent in their approach and response to clients. For example, if the nurse tells a client that he or she will meet with the client after lunch, the nurse must follow through to demonstrate dependability so that the client can increase his or her trust level. Clients need to learn they can rely on the nurse so that trust can build. Trustworthy nurses respect the client's privacy, rights, and the need for confidentiality. Clients need to be convinced that the information they share will not go beyond the health care team.

Clarity

Nurses must communicate clearly. Psychiatric clients often have difficulty processing information or thinking clearly as a result of their mental disorders. If the nurse is specific and clear, there will be less room for miscommunication. Clear communication involves selecting concise words when speaking, and asking questions to clarify meaning. Although using medical jargon is part of the nurse's work life, the nurse should remember that clients might not understand the same terminology. Everyday medical terms such as "taking your vital signs," "NPO after midnight," or "take these medications qid," can be misunderstood. Problems may arise if instructions or information is relayed in a highly technical manner because the client may be too embarrassed to ask for clarification.

A study conducted at the University of Alberta Hospital revealed that clients frequently do not understand or often misunderstand professional jargon (Cochrane et al., 1992). For 2 weeks, several nurses listened to themselves and other nurses in conversation with clients. Each time a word or phrase considered to be medical jargon was used, it was recorded. Thirty-four of the most common medical words or phrases were selected for the study. A total of 101 adult clients, both newly admitted and those on their fourth day of hospitalization, were surveyed. The results of the study showed that most of the words were defined correctly by more than half of the respondents. For example, 98% of the respondents knew what "OR" (operating room) meant; however, words that had one meaning in everyday terminology and another in the nursing profession were often misinterpreted. The newly admitted clients did not do better or worse than clients hospitalized for 4 days or those who had been hospitalized before this admission.

Thus nurses need to make a conscious effort to speak at a level the client will understand. Avoidance of abstract, lengthy explanations is also necessary. This is also true for written communication. It is strongly recommended that when educating clients using written materials, the nurse adopts a less-is-more principle, and that all instructions be written in plain language, the active voice, and be free of medical jargon (American Health Consultants, 2001). Written educational information should be printed at an eighth grade level, as 47% of all adults read at that level or below (Government Adult Literacy Survey, 1993).

Responsibility

Responsible communication involves being accountable for the outcome of one's professional interactions. When nurses communicate, they need to be responsible for their part in the interaction and ensure that all messages are received and interpreted correctly. Nurses who communicate responsibly enhance growth in others. Responsibility language involves the use of "I" statements when being assertive, as described in the following section.

Assertiveness

Assertive communication is the ability to express thoughts and feelings comfortably and confidently in a positive, honest, and open manner that demonstrates respect for self while respecting others (Balzer Riley, 2000). The nurse who communicates assertively makes a conscious choice about how to communicate with others. Communicating assertively is a style choice and can be implemented in any situation at any time. An assertive nurse should control negative feelings, which is important in communication not only with clients but also with supervisors, employees, physicians, and colleagues. Box 7-1 lists behaviors of assertive communication.

Some basic assertiveness techniques can be practiced by the nurse. First, the nurse must learn to use responsibility language by using "I" instead of "you" (e.g., "I am respon-

Box 7-1	Behaviors of Assertive Communication

Assertive

Stands up for own rights and respects those of others. Uses expressive, directive, self-enhancing speech. Chooses appropriate words and actions.

Aggressive

Stands up for own rights but abuses those of others. Speaks in demeaning or attacking manner. Fails to monitor or control words or actions.

Passive

Does not stand up for own rights and accepts the domination and bullying of others. Performs unwanted tasks and feels victimized.

Examples of Assertive Behaviors

- "I" messages (e.g., "I need," "I feel," "I will")
- Eye contact (e.g., looking directly into the eyes of the person while making or refusing a request)
- Congruent verbal and facial expressions (e.g., making certain that the facial expression matches the intent of the spoken message); a serious message accompanied by laughter could negate the credibility of the message.

Example of Assertive Plan for Change

- Target the behavior that one desires to change (e.g., how to say no and mean it).
- List approximately 10 situations in which it is difficult to say no, and order them from least to most difficult.
- Practice saying no, using the least threatening method first and working up to more challenging situations (e.g., imagery, tape recorder, feedback, role-playing), and practice in actual situations.
- Say no as the first word in the practice response, as it is a clear message without excuses or apologies.
- Follow with a clear, concise, declarative statement (e.g., "I will not rearrange my schedule. I need my day off").
- Use eye contact appropriate to the intent of the verbal message.
- Assertiveness training is most often done in small-group sessions and has been described in detail in a variety of textbooks.

Modified from Fortinash KM, Holoday Worret PA: *Psychiatric nursing care plans,* ed 4, St Louis, 2003, Mosby.

sible for the medication error," or "I feel hurt when you say that to me"). Blaming one's behavior on another takes away the personal power of the nurse to make changes. For example, the client who states, "My mother made me angry," or "God told me to hit him," indicates that he has no power or control over his behavior and takes no responsibility for his actions. Being assertive means learning how to say "no," expressing opinions and feelings, stating beliefs, and initiating conversation. Nonverbal assertive language includes giving others good eye contact when speaking to them.

Assertive messages are those in which the verbal message and nonverbal message match (congruence). Sometimes, though, clients try to cover up their true sadness by laughing or smiling while relating a painful experience that they do not know how to deal with in another way.

Responding Techniques that Enhance Therapeutic Communication

Therapeutic responding techniques are methods used to encourage clients to interact in a manner that promotes their growth and moves them toward their treatment goals. The more skilled the nurse in using these techniques, the better the nurse's ability to establish a trusting and collaborative nurse-client relationship that can efficiently and effectively accomplish mutual goals and objectives. (Schuster, 2000). These strategies create an atmosphere that promotes communication for problem solving. Table 7-2 gives examples of many of these techniques.

Silence is an important listening skill for psychiatric nurses to develop. It is not the absence of communication, but rather a useful and purposeful communication tool to give the client time to feel comfortable and respond when ready to do so. Silence must be used to serve a particular function and not to frighten or discomfort the already-anxious client. A successful interview is largely dependent on the nurse's ability to remain silent long enough to allow the client to share relevant information. Silence gives the client an opportunity to consider what is being said, weigh alternatives, and formulate an answer.

Active listening is vital to communicating effectively. It is not simply the act of hearing. Several techniques are incorporated into this skill such as paraphrasing the client's thoughts and feelings, understanding the meaning behind the words and phrases, and asking questions. Active listening involves all of the nurse's senses. It takes an incredible amount of energy, focus, and self-discipline, as well as seeing and filtering out internal and external factors and barriers that may impede communication (Antai-Otong, 1999).

Support and *reassurance* are provided in a genuine and honest manner. Clients need to be in an atmosphere where they can safely disclose information that may be of a sensitive nature. Nurses can offer both verbal and nonverbal support so that the client feels free to share thoughts and feelings, which is necessary for progress toward mental health to occur.

Sharing observations made by the nurse is important to increase the client's self-understanding. It also demonstrates to the client that the nurse is actively listening.

Acknowledging feelings is a form of client support. It is important to let the client know that his or her feelings are valid and important. There are no right or wrong answers when it comes to feelings. They cannot be taken away, argued with, or discounted.

Broad, open-ended statements allow the client to assume some control over topics to be discussed. However, the nurse should not allow the client to discuss only nonrelevant topics or engage in a conversation with a superficial or social content. The nurse should frequently ask the client questions that do not produce one-word answers. Open-ended questions result in fuller, more revealing answers, which typically stimulates further questions by the nurse.

Table 7-2	Therapeutic Responding Techniques as Related to Steps of the Nursing Process and Phases of the Therapeutic Relationship		
Therapeutic Relationship Phase	**Nursing Process Step**	**Technique**	**Examples**
Orientation	Assessment and nursing diagnosis	*Introducing self* when the client is admitted	"Hi, my name is Teresa. I will be your nurse today."
		Offering self. The nurse demonstrates an honest, open posture, making self available to demonstrate concern and interest.	"I have some information to gather. Let's sit here so we can begin your admission."
		Active listening. Practiced by using both verbal and nonverbal skills that show the nurse is giving full attention to the client.	The nurse faces the client and takes an open position, maintains eye contact, and uses verbal and nonverbal messages to demonstrate that the client has the nurse's full attention. "Go on. I am listening."
		Questioning. The nurse skillfully asks open-ended questions during the initial admission. Interviewing skills are necessary to avoid asking too many personal questions in one session. Questions are geared to achieve relevance and depth. Closed questions are used to gather factual information.	"How many children do you have?" "Has this ever happened before?" "How come you stopped taking your medication?" "What is that all about?" "Tell me how you feel now?"
		Silence is used frequently so that the client has time to verbalize thoughts and feelings. It is planned and used to draw out the client. Silence should be comfortable for both client and nurse.	Sit quietly, maintain comfortable eye contact, demonstrate interest using nonverbal nods and expressive facial movements.
		Empathizing. The nurse demonstrates warmth and acknowledges client's feelings.	"I know how hurt you must have felt. It sounds like it made you sad."
		Reality orienting/providing information. The nurse explains to the client the type of unit, gives a brief tour, and provides the client with unit information and admission paperwork.	"John, here is a copy of the unit rules. Let's go over a few important items." "You are on the locked unit now." "Today is Friday. You were admitted yesterday afternoon."
		Restating. The nurse repeats what the client says to show understanding and to review what was said.	"You say you are saddened by your friend's death." "You became depressed soon after the accident?"
		Clarifying. The nurse asks specific questions to help clear up a specific point the client makes.	"Did it help when you tried any of the techniques you mentioned?" "Which technique helped the most?" "So your mother remarried soon after you were born?"
		Offering reality. The nurse presents a realistic view to the client in a reasonable manner.	"I know you think people are out to get you. I do not think that. You are safe here, and we are here to help you. This medication will help decrease those thoughts."
		Stating observations. The nurse offers a view of what is seen or heard to increase verbalization.	"I see you are quite upset." "I noticed you had trouble sleeping last night."
		Fostering description of perceptions. The nurse requests clients to describe their situation.	"Help me to understand how this is affecting you right now." "What is the voice telling you?"
		Placing the event in time and order. The nurse asks questions to determine the relationships of events, and the nurse helps put events in perspective.	"Was the birth of your child before or after your mother died?" "Did your alcohol abuse begin immediately after your divorce?"
		Voicing doubt. The nurse discusses any uncertainty of the client's perceptions.	"I find it hard to believe that you felt no joy on hearing that she survived." "Are you sure you were in bed for one full year after that?"
		Identifying themes. The nurse voices issues that arise again and again in the course of conversation.	"It sounds like that is very important to you. You've mentioned it a few times." "When this happens over and over, how do you feel?"
		Encouraging comparisons. The nurse asks for similarities and differences among feelings, thoughts, behaviors, and various life situations.	"Was this the same way you reacted the last time it happened?"

Continued

Table 7-2	Therapeutic Responding Techniques as Related to Steps of the Nursing Process and Phases of the Therapeutic Relationship—cont'd		
Therapeutic Relationship Phase	**Nursing Process Step**	**Technique**	**Examples**
Orientation—cont'd	Assessment and nursing diagnosis—cont'd	*Summarizing.* The nurse verbalizes a compilation of what has been expressed on a particular subject or event.	"Let me see if I understand your anxiety about . . ." "From what you describe, your family seems . . ."
		Focusing. Zeroes in on a subject until the important points come into clear view for both the client and the nurse.	"You talk about loss. Tell me more about the losses you've experienced." "You mentioned his drinking. Tell me more about that."
Working	Outcome identification, planning, and implementation	*Evaluating.* The nurse encourages the client to express the importance of an event.	"What does this type of behavior mean to you?" "After thinking about it, how does it affect you now?"
		Encouraging plan formulation helps the client develop steps to make changes and solve problems.	"What are the steps you'll need to take to accomplish that?"
		Assisting in goal setting encourages client to set goals during hospitalization and after hospitalization.	"I will help you set some achievable goals during your hospital stay. Do you have some ideas?"
		Providing information offers data that will help the client in setting goals and developing a plan of action.	"This list and description of crisis houses may help you decide on which one will be best for you after discharge." "I have a problem-solving guide that helps people go through the necessary steps to follow in solving big problems."
		Offering alternatives fosters decision making by encouraging the client to work on arriving at healthy, growth-producing decisions.	"Looking over the pros and cons, which plan would be best for you?" "What would be your best alternative, given this situation?"
		Role playing. The nurse plays the part of a person the client needs to say something to, in order to help the client practice what he or she wants to say.	"Let's go over what you want to say to her." "I'll play your father, and you play yourself." "Sometimes it helps to say it in the mirror a few times before the real encounter."
		Providing feedback. The nurse provides the client with supportive comments in reaction to behaviors or statements made.	"Tell me what you want to say; I'll listen and give you my feedback." "When you walked away, I felt . . ." "You may upset some people with behavior like that."
		Confronting. The nurse supports the client but directly challenges inaction on the part of the client.	"I know this is hard to do, but I believe it will help you make the right decision." "I understand your concerns; however, you have to take some steps now."
		Setting limits. The nurse provides the client with external boundaries to an expressed thought, feeling, or behavior.	"You became very angry again. To stay in the day room, you'll need to act calmer. You can walk in the hallway if you need to get up."
Termination	Evaluation	*Evaluating actions* encourages clients to look at their behavior and the outcomes it produces.	"When you tried to do that, how well did it work?" "When you tell her to leave, how do you think she will react?" "Was that useful for you?"
		Reinforcing healthy behaviors offers positive responses to the client who is trying out new growth-producing behaviors and making helpful decisions.	"It sounds like you have made a healthy choice." "Standing up for yourself is new." "You've successfully tried it, so practicing it daily will be important." "I know you will continue to practice being assertive."
		Encouraging posthospital transition helps the client see that new thoughts and actions can be accomplished after discharge.	"What situations will you run into where you might try this new behavior?" "How can a relapse prevention plan assist you after you leave the hospital?" "Which coping skills will be useful to you after you return home?"

Information giving is an ongoing process for the nurse. Information is provided to enhance the client's knowledge about a variety of topics on his or her illness and treatment. Information may decrease fears and anxiety and increase the client's fund of resources and support for his or her problem. Examples may include information regarding the client's disorder, medication, aftercare support groups, structured living options, or treatment alternatives. Information must be given according to the client's level of understanding and willingness to receive it.

Interpretation of what is being shared by clients is useful to help them see the real meaning behind their message. The nurse must be careful when using this technique. A client may disagree with the nurse's interpretation, which may set up a roadblock. Helping clients *focus* to pursue a particular topic allows them to spend their time discussing subjects of most importance. *Identification of themes* is necessary to help clients see what they repeatedly bring up in the conversation. *Placing events in order and time* is also important to help clients develop a greater perspective on events in their lives.

Clients often need to be encouraged to *describe their perceptions* regarding their thoughts and feelings. For example, some psychiatric clients hear imaginary voices telling them to hurt themselves or others. The nurse asks such clients to tell the staff when this occurs so that the nurse can intervene and prevent clients' attempts to harm themselves or others. Treatment strategies can then be introduced to reduce this perception and therefore minimize the client's dysfunctional behavior.

To develop a sense of clients' past and current behavior, the nurse may ask clients to *compare* their present anxiety to that of their last hospitalization. Or the nurse may ask clients if they have ever experienced before what they are telling the nurse now.

Restating what clients say lets them know that the nurse heard and understands them. It is an active listening technique.

Reflecting is a technique used to turn around a question to obtain a response from the client. Coaching clients to answer a question best answered by the client helps them to accept their own ideas and feelings regarding an important event or behavior.

Clarifying is a method used to ask clients to elaborate or restate something just said. It serves to increase the nurse's understanding and to allow clients to rethink and restate their thoughts or feelings.

Confrontation in an accepting manner is necessary for the client to be more aware of incongruent thoughts, feelings, and behaviors. This helps to bring the issue into focus and should be used only after a good rapport has been established (Fortinash and Holoday Worret, 2003).

When a client is struggling to explore and solve a problem but can only see one or two solutions, the nurse may *offer alternatives*. Suggesting to the client other possible solutions to the problem is not the same as giving advice. It uses introductions such as, "What have you thought about . . .?," "Other clients have solved it using this solution," and "Other

alternatives might be . . ." The nurse avoids phrases such as "You should," and "I think you need to solve it the way I did" (giving advice).

Voicing doubt is a technique to use when the client is having difficulty relating in a way that sounds believable. Voicing some doubt may help the client to be more realistic about perceptions and conclusions of events. Voicing doubt is used cautiously, as it could set up a barrier between the client and nurse.

The nurse needs to *summarize* the information the client provides on a regular basis. Summarizing the main points of what a client has been discussing helps focus on the most important issues related to the client's life situation. After the summary is provided, the client can agree or disagree with any point, and then together the nurse and client agree on a final summary.

Role-playing provides a place for the client to act out a particular event, problem, or situation in a safe environment. The nurse can play the other part or role. He or she can also provide feedback to the client on a variety of components within the dialog, such as voice tone, use of assertive language, identification of feelings, emotion expressed, and nonverbal behavior exhibited (Fortinash and Holoday Worret, 2003).

Special Communication Techniques
Self-Disclosure

Self-disclosure is opening up oneself to another and can be an effective therapeutic skill if it is fully understood and used carefully. Experienced nurses reveal carefully selected thoughts, feelings, and life events to demonstrate to the client that they understand what the client is going through.

Disclosing one's own personal beliefs, views, and life experiences occurs in social relationships on a continual basis. In intimate relationships, what is revealed is very personal. Because a professional nurse-client therapeutic relationship exists for the purpose of helping the client, whatever the nurse discloses needs to be carefully thought out before being revealed. Because self-disclosure by the nurse is *always* for the client's benefit and *never* for the nurse's, it is important to explore the what, where, why, and when of self-disclosing to see what purpose it serves (Balzer Riley, 2000).

Criteria have been developed to help the nurse discern appropriate use of self-disclosure. The purpose of the self-disclosure should be one or more of the following (Stricker and Fisher, 1990):

- *To model and educate.* Will clients learn more about themselves and be able to deal better with the problems in their lives?
- *To build the therapeutic partnership.* Will disclosure foster a greater nurse-client alliance by obtaining a greater amount of cooperation?
- *To validate reality.* Will clients be supported in their natural feelings in response to an event?
- *To foster clients' autonomy.* Will the disclosure help clients to express previously held feelings on their own?

Table 7-3 Self-Disclosure	
Therapeutic	**Nontherapeutic**
Client: "I'm real upset that I have to leave the hospital today." *Nurse:* "I have enjoyed working with you. I realize endings can be sad. It is important for you to use the tools you have learned when you go home." *Discussion:* The nurse is using self-disclosure in the termination phase of the relationship. She is validating the client's feelings and is also validating the alliance with the purpose of encouraging the client to transfer what has been learned in treatment to life after discharge.	*Client:* "That jerk of a husband had to leave me with three children to support, and it is hard." *Nurse:* "I know how you feel because my husband was just like that, leaving me five years ago with two small children when he ran off with another woman. He gives me no support and doesn't see his children. I get angry a lot, too." *Discussion:* The nurse is using self-disclosure in the admission interview or beginning phase of the relationship, when no rapport has been established. In addition, it reveals too much personal information and is too lengthy. It seems to serve the nurse's purpose, rather than the client's, to share the incident.

The use of self-disclosure requires that the nurse and client have a therapeutic relationship. The rationale for using self-disclosure comes from the belief that in doing so, the client will in turn self-disclose. Both the amount and relevance of the nurse's own self-disclosure need to be monitored. If the self-disclosure is too lengthy, it may decrease the time the client has for disclosure and may result in a breakdown in the interaction.

If the disclosure is irrelevant to the client's problem, the client may become distracted and feel alienated from the nurse. Table 7-3 compares an example of therapeutic versus nontherapeutic self-disclosure.

Both research and literature have indicated that self-disclosure can be an important tool for client growth. The nurse must realize that not all self-disclosure is revealing personal information. It can simply be sharing a feeling. Genuine, open communication that creates a therapeutic alliance can be achieved without the use of self-disclosure. Self-disclosure can enhance that alliance only when the nurse feels comfortable with its use and when it will benefit the client.

Touch

Touch is a nonverbal method of communication that may convey many messages. Handshaking, holding hands, hugging, and kissing all demonstrate positive feelings for another human being. Nonessential touch is purposeful physical contact with the client other than the touch necessary for a procedure. Nonprocedural touches range from a light touch on the arm or a handshake to holding the hand or a full embrace. For touch to convey warmth, the nurse must be comfortable with it.

Touch carries a different meaning for each person. Several variables influence the intended message of the touch, including the length of the touch, the part of the body touched, the way in which the client is touched, and the frequency of the touch.

The nurse should use caution when touching clients in a psychiatric setting. Reactions to touch are influenced by the age and gender of the client, the client's interpretation of the gesture, the client's cultural background, and the appropriateness of the touch.

The nurse needs to take potential reactions into consideration when deciding which clients to touch and what type of

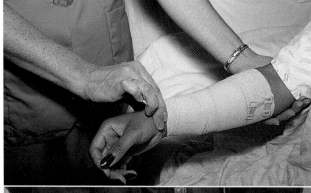

A

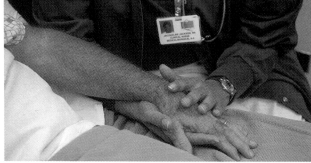

B

FIGURE 7-2. A, The nurse uses procedural touch to evaluate the client's circulation. **B,** The nurse uses nonprocedural touch to comfort the client. (From Potter PA, Perry AG: *Fundamentals of nursing,* ed 5, St Louis, 2001, Mosby.)

touch to use, if any. For example, a depressed client may respond positively to touch as a gesture of concern. An elderly, frail client or a client who is dying may also be comforted by the nurse's touch. However, a paranoid, hostile client may misinterpret touch to mean confrontation and may strike out at the nurse. An abused client may pull away and feel frightened by a hand on the shoulder.

Procedural touch may include positioning the arm of a client when taking a blood pressure or drawing blood for laboratory work, turning a client to change a dressing or diaper, lifting or assisting a client from the bed to a wheelchair, or performing a seclusion or restraint procedure on a highly agitated and hostile client (Figure 7-2, *A*). *Nonprocedural touch* may include holding an older client's hand as she is conveying sadness over her husband's death, hugging an adolescent client as he leaves the hospital, shaking the hand of a new

UNDERSTANDING and APPLYING RESEARCH

The purpose of this study was to identify and describe the ways and reasons registered nurses use nonprocedural touch in the inpatient psychiatric setting. Natural setting observation and nurse interviews were used to examine the nurses' reasons for touch.

Twenty-six incidents of nonprocedural touch initiated by 13 registered nurses with 17 psychiatric clients were recorded over 27.5 hours of observation. Observations were made on one adolescent unit and two adult psychiatric units in a large university teaching hospital.

Of the 30 nurses who agreed to participate in the study, 24 were observed. Of those 24 nurses, 13 touched clients. Several elements went into the decision to touch.

Both the client and nurse were taken into account. Client characteristics such as age, gender, needs, and the nurse's knowledge of the client were involved in the decision to touch. Also, the nurse's feelings, beliefs, intuition, style, and role expectations were acknowledged.

In all, 92% of the touches recorded were used in a purposeful, therapeutic manner. Nurses' intentions for using touch were to establish contact with the client, enhance communication, convey warmth and caring, show interest and recognition, and offer reassurance and comfort.

Nonprocedural touch can be very effective in conveying therapeutic messages, and nurses should use touch whenever therapeutically appropriate.

Tommasini NR: The use of touch with the hospitalized psychiatric patient, *Arch Psychiatr Nurs* 4(4):213, 1990.

client as they are introduced by another nurse during their transfer to the nurse's unit, or giving a back rub to a long-term, bedridden client (Figure 7-2, *B*).

The use of nonprocedural touch is an individual preference by the nurse, as not all practitioners feel comfortable touching clients. Much depends on the nurse's comfort level, the ability to correctly interpret the situation, and the appropriate use of touch. Using touch can be highly beneficial to the client's progress by enhancing the nurse-client relationship and promoting health (see Understanding and Applying Research box).

Humor

Humor can be a useful tool in psychiatric nursing. Humor is defined as the quality that makes something seem funny, amusing, or ludicrous. It is the ability to perceive, appreciate, and express what is funny, amusing, or absurd. A sense of humor including the ability to laugh with others and to laugh at oneself has often been linked to good health. Healthy humor elicits laughter between people; it encourages laughing *with* others and not *at* them. It includes others, is appropriate to the situation, respects others, and preserves their dignity. Harmful humor excludes others. It singles out people from a group and ridicules them.

A good sense of humor is considered to be a mature coping mechanism and can help the nurse adequately handle difficult situations. It also assists in gaining a different perspective on the problem by lightening a serious mood for a few moments. Appropriate humor can ease a client's concerns and communicate a sense of warmth and understanding (Bush, 2001).

Physiologically, humor has been known to improve the circulatory system, stimulate the respiratory system, and increase blood oxygen levels and heart rate. Laughter also reduces the perception of pain, as it is widely theorized that laughter stimulates the brain to release endorphins, the brain's natural painkillers (Astedt-Kurki, 1994). These changes result in a rise in the epinephrine levels, which makes one feel more alert and offers a sense of well-being. Laughing and having positive social interactions during mealtimes have been reported to aid digestion.

The psychologic benefits of laughter are well known. Laughter can function as an emotional release by decreasing anxiety; lessen negative emotions such as anger, hostility, and resentment; and decrease stress and tension (Schuster, 2000).

The nurse should assess the degree to which a client has a sense of humor. In depressed clients the outward expression of laughter and pleasure is usually missing. Clients with paranoid features are unable to laugh. In fact, they may view others' laughter as a personal attack. This is important to remember. For example, nurses in the nursing station need to be careful not to laugh and joke behind a glass partition where paranoid clients can see them and interpret the behavior as a personal affront. On the other hand, manic clients may laugh at everything, whether or not it is actually humorous. This exaggerated sense of well-being demonstrates a lack of judgment on the part of the client, and it can turn into biting sarcasm that can hurt others. Humor is nontherapeutic when a client is very ill, fearful, or anxious; is having a high level of pain; or is very depressed (Schuster, 2000).

Clinicians who have studied humor as an important indicator of a person's health believe that asking clients simple questions, such as what their favorite joke is, how often they laugh, and how their patterns of laughter have changed, offers the nurse new insights into their clients' illness (Ferguson and Campinha-Bacote, 1989).

The psychiatric mental health nurse can use humor as a therapeutic tool in a variety of ways. For example, it can be used to teach the client the difference between hurtful and healthy humor, to encourage healthy humor on the unit by role modeling, and to introduce humor in formal and informal groups and individually. The use of humor can increase the flexibility of interactions and create a more relaxed environment. It can enhance the client's insight and facilitate the type of interaction that is difficult for the client in a safe, low-keyed setting.

Obstacles to Therapeutic Communication

Certain obstacles can occur in the client-nurse relationship that affect the nature of the communication. Some obstacles are due to the client's disorder or lack of knowledge, and some have to do with the nurse's own inability to be effective because of inexperience, lack of knowledge, or personal problems. For the relationship to grow in a healthy manner, these obstacles must be overcome.

Four key therapeutic obstacles are introduced here for discussion: resistance, transference, countertransference, and boundary violations.

Resistance

Resistance occurs in clients who consciously or unconsciously maintain a lack of awareness of problems they are having in order to avoid anxiety. It can take the form of a natural and short-lived reservation about accepting a problem, or a long-term, firmly stated denial that there are problems. This resistance to change is a part of human nature but must be addressed and dealt with by both the client and the nurse for positive growth to occur. Nurses can help clients overcome resistance by pointing out their progress and strengths.

For example, a nurse can assure a client who resists impending discharge because of fear of failure, abandonment, or loneliness that such fears are not uncommon at the time of termination or discharge. The nurse can then remind the client of progress made (e.g., "You've already achieved some of your goals, and have made concrete plans to continue in treatment after you are discharged; these are accomplishments you didn't believe possible when you first arrived at this facility"). Such observations build the client's confidence and offer hope that will counteract resistance.

Transference

Transference is the unconscious response whereby clients associate the nurse with someone significant in their lives. Feelings and attitudes about the other person are transferred to the nurse. For example, a male client sees a female nurse as a mother figure because she has a mannerism that reminds him of his own mother. The client may have negative feelings about his mother and, without provocation, becomes angry or bothered by the nurse's interaction with him because of the resemblance. Often the client's intense response does not match the situation or the content of the interaction. The interaction comes to a standstill if the nurse does not address and examine the client's reasons for transference.

The nurse can deal with both resistance and transference by being prepared to hear a client's irrational and highly charged responses to the nurse. The nurse must truly listen to the client and then use the therapeutic techniques of clarifying and reflecting to begin problem solving. The goal is for the client to gain awareness and recognition of what lies behind the resistance.

Countertransference

Countertransference is initiated by the nurse's emotional response to a specific client. The response is irrational, inappropriate, highly charged, and generated by certain qualities of the client. It is simply the nurse's own transference. Nurses have a natural response to each client and likes or dislikes some more than others. Countertransference occurs when the feelings are intense—either positive or negative—and are not based on reality. Because countertransference impedes the nurse's ability to be therapeutically effective, the nurse must always observe for signs of its occurrence.

From time to time, countertransference issues are bound to surface. Even though this is natural, it can be destructive if ignored by the nurse or treated as insignificant. The nurse most often encounters countertransference when the client is displaying disruptive, aggressive, irritating, or resistive behaviors. If the nurse remains angry with the client as a result of these behaviors, the degree of objectivity needed to promote healthy change is lost. Nurses may also find themselves attracted positively to clients in excessive ways and should recognize and take steps to avoid countertransference.

To deal with countertransference, the nurse should conduct an honest self-appraisal throughout the course of the therapeutic relationship while gaining a good understanding of the client's background and issues. If the self-appraisal reveals any problems, the nurse should explore why these feelings are occurring. This work needs to be done as soon as the problem is recognized. The nurse may not be able to handle these feelings alone and may need some clinical supervision with a clinician to deal with the issues.

Boundary Violations

Boundary violations occur when the nurse goes beyond the established therapeutic relationship standards and enters into a social or personal relationship with the client. A client can also attempt to violate the boundaries of the nurse-client relationship. A client may ask the nurse, "How old are you?" or "Are you married?" or may try to touch the nurse inappropriately. Violations can also occur if the nurse treats the client at odd hours or in an unusual setting, if the nurse accepts compensation or gifts for treatment, if the nurse's language or clothing is inappropriate, or if the nurse's self-disclosure or physical contact lacks therapeutic value, for example, when the nurse discloses too much personal information to the client in order to benefit the nurse.

Responding Techniques That Hinder Therapeutic Communication

Therapeutic skills that have enhanced the communication process were presented earlier in the chapter. There are also many responses that are counterproductive to healthy outcomes and are therefore considered nontherapeutic (Table 7-4).

There are several reasons why nurses fail to interact effectively. The inexperienced nurse's insecurity is one factor. A certain amount of experience and maturity greatly helps the nurse deal effectively with the difficult and complex behaviors psychiatric clients often display.

Other explanations for nontherapeutic communication are that the nurse has allowed necessary skills to stagnate or diminish. Some nurses, who may have worked with psychiatric clients for several years, might find themselves on "automatic pilot." Their ability to begin their work each day refreshed and ready to really "be there" for the clients may be lost. Or the nurse may have developed personal problems that have not been dealt with sufficiently and are thus interfering with his or her ability to focus on the client and the client's needs.

Table 7-4   Ineffective Responses That Hinder Therapeutic Communication

Response	Discussion	Nontherapeutic Response	Therapeutic Response
Offering false reassurances	The nurse, in an effort to be supportive and to make the client's pain disappear, offers reassuring clichés. This response is not based on fact. It brushes aside the client's feelings and closes off communication. Often, it is due to the nurse's inability to listen to the client's negative emotions.	"Don't worry, everything will be fine." "Every cloud has a silver lining." "Things will be better soon; you'll see."	"I know you have a lot going on right now. Let's make a list and begin to discuss them one at a time. Working toward solutions will help you to get through this."
Not listening	The nurse is preoccupied with other work that needs to be done, is distracted by noise in the area, or is thinking about personal problems.	"I'm sorry, what did you say?" "Could you start again? I was listening to another client."	"That's interesting. Please elaborate." "I really hear what you are saying . . . it must be difficult."
Offering approval	It is most important how the client feels about what he or she said or did. The client ultimately must approve of his or her own actions.	"That's good." "I agree — I think you should have told him."	"What do you think about what you said to him?" "How do you feel about it?"
Minimizing the problem	The nurse may use this response when it is difficult to hear the enormity of a particular problem. This is used in an effort to try to make the client feel better. It cuts off communication.	"That's nothing compared to that other client's problem." "Everyone feels that way at times; it's not a big deal."	"That seems like a very difficult problem for you." "That sounds pretty important for you to deal with."
Offering advice	This response undermines clients' ability to solve their own problems. It serves to render them dependent and helpless. If the solution provided by the nurse does not work, the client may blame the outcome on the nurse. Clients do not take responsibility for developing outcomes. The nurse maintains control and at the same time devalues the client.	"I think you should put your mother into a nursing home." "In my opinion, it would be wise to . . ." "Why don't you do . . ." "The best solution is . . ."	"What do *you* think you should do?" "There can be several alternatives— let's talk about some. However, the final decision must be yours. I will listen to your problem and help you see it clearly. We can develop a pros and cons list that may assist you in solving the problem."
Giving literal responses	The nurse feeds into the client's delusions or hallucinations and denies the client the opportunity to see reality. This does not provide a healthy response toward growth.	*Client*: "That TV is talking to me." *Nurse*: "What is it saying to you?" *Client*: "There is nuclear power coming through the air ducts." *Nurse*: "I'll turn off the air conditioner for a while."	*Nurse*: "The TV is on for everyone." *Nurse*: "There is cool air blowing from the vents. It is the air conditioning system."
Changing the subject	The nurse changes the topic at a crucial time because the discussion is too uncomfortable. It negates what the client seems interested in discussing. Communication will remain superficial.	*Client:* "My mother always puts me down." *Nurse*: "That's interesting, but let's talk about . . ."	*Nurse:* "Tell me about that."
Belittling	The nurse puts down the client's expressed feelings to avoid having to deal with painful feelings.	*Client:* "I don't want to live anymore now that my child is gone." *Nurse*: "You shouldn't feel that way."	*Nurse*: "The death must be very difficult for you. Tell me more about how you are feeling."
Disagreeing	The nurse criticizes the client who is seeking support.	"I definitely do not agree with your view." "I really don't support that."	"Let's talk about the way you see that."
Judging	The nurse's responses are filled with his or her own values and judgments. This demonstrates a lack of acceptance of the client's differences. It provides a barrier to further disclosures.	"You are not married. Do you think having this baby will solve your problems?" "This is certainly not the Christian thing to do." "You are thinking about divorce when you have three children?"	"It seems hard to believe. Please explain further." "What will having this baby provide for you?" "What do you think about what you are attempting to do?" "Let's discuss this option," or "Let's discuss other options."

Continued

Table 7-4	Ineffective Responses That Hinder Therapeutic Communication—cont'd		
Response	**Discussion**	**Nontherapeutic Response**	**Therapeutic Response**
Excessive probing	This serves to control the nature of the client's responses. The nurse asks many questions of clients before they are ready to provide the information. This is self-protective to the nurse by avoiding the anxiety of uncomfortable silences. The client feels over-whelmed and may withdraw. The use of the "why" question places the client in a defensive position and may block further communication.	"Why do you do this?" "What do you think was the real reason?" "Why do you feel this way?" "Why do you think that way?"	"Tell me how this is upsetting to you." "Tell me what you believe to be the cause." "Tell me how you feel when that happens." "Explain your thinking on this if you can."
Challenging	This stems from the nurse's belief that if clients are challenged regarding their unrealistic beliefs, they will be coerced into seeing reality. This client may feel threatened when challenged, holding onto the beliefs even more strongly.	"You are not the Prince of Peace." "If your leg is missing, then why can you walk up and down this hall?"	"You sound like you want to be important." "It seems like you are missing a leg. Tell me more about that."
Superficial comments	The nurse gives simple or meaningless responses to clients. It suggests a lack of understanding regarding the client as an individual. The interactions remain superficial, maintaining distance between the nurse and client. Nothing of significance gets communicated.	"Great day, huh!" "You should be feeling good; you are being discharged today." "Keep the faith; your doctor should be coming anytime now."	"What kind of day are you having?" "How are you feeling about leaving the hospital today?" "You look worried. Your doctor called and said he would be here within the hour."
Defending	The nurse may believe that he or she must defend herself or himself, the staff, or the hospital. The nurse may not take the time to listen to the client's concerns. Efforts need to be made to explore the client's thoughts and feelings.	"Your doctor is a good doctor. He would never say that." "We have a very experienced staff here. They would never do that."	"What has you so upset about your doctor?" "Tell me what happened last night."
Self-focusing	The nurse focuses attention away from the client by thinking about sharing his or her own thoughts, feelings, or problems. The focus is taken away from the client, who is seeking help. The nurse is more interested in what to say next instead of actively listening to the client.	"That may have happened to you last year, but it happened to me twice this month, which hurt me a great deal and . . ." "Excuse me but could you say that again? I have a response to make, but I want to be sure of what you just said."	"Tell me about your incident and how it might relate to your sadness now." "If I heard you accurately, you said . . ."
Criticism of others	The nurse puts others down in his or her communication with the client.	*Client*: "The staff members on the evening shift let me smoke two cigarettes." *Nurse*: "The evening shift is always breaking the rules. On this shift we follow the one cigarette per break policy." *Client*: "My daughter is hateful to me." *Nurse*: "She must be just awful to live with."	*Nurse*: "The policy is one cigarette, which we will follow." *Nurse*: "It sounds like you are having a rough time right now with your daughter."
Premature interpretation	The nurse does not wait until the client fully expresses thoughts and feelings related to a particular problem. This rushes the client and disregards his or her input. The nurse may miss what the client wants to explain.	"I think this is what you really mean." "You may think that way consciously, but unconsciously you believe . . ."	"What do you think this means?" "So you think . . .?"

It is important that nurses build on the knowledge they possess by continually practicing and perfecting skills and attending skills-building classes and therapeutic communication in-service workshops to refresh and enhance skills they already possess. It is also important that they know when to obtain outside help for their own life problems so that those problems do not interfere with work, and to enjoy their time away from work with friends, family, and alone doing the things they enjoy.

There are other potential instances for a nurse's ineffective responses. A nurse may display anger toward the client for not behaving in a socially acceptable manner or for not doing what is asked. Or the nurse may take personally what the client says. A client may be angry or delusional and display out-of-control behavior. The client may say something to the nurse that hurts the nurse's feelings. For example, a client may say to the overweight nurse placing him in seclusion, "Get out of here, you big fat . . ." The nurse, upset by the client's statement, may respond angrily or defensively if the nurse is not able to detach from the statement and realize that the client is angry at his or her own behavior, and is projecting it to the nurse in the form of a personal statement.

COMMUNICATION AND THE NURSING PROCESS

There are many opportunities to communicate therapeutically throughout the nursing process. Each step of the nursing process—assessment, nursing diagnosis, outcome identification, implementation, planning, and evaluation—corresponds with the three phases of the therapeutic relationship—beginning, working, and termination. Therapeutic responding techniques unique to each step and phase are used throughout.

The nurse's first communication task is to greet the client on admission. The nurse communicates the nature of his or her role. This orientation or beginning phase begins with the initial contact, continues with the admission interview and assessment, and ends with the formulation of a nursing diagnosis. This phase can last one or more sessions because much of highly personal data must be collected, and it occurs when the client is in the most need of help and may be displaying highly dysfunctional behavior.

In the working phase of the relationship when the care plan is being developed and implemented with the client and treatment team, many therapeutic responding techniques can be used. The therapeutic communication skills the nurse uses during this phase are designed to help clients deal with the issues that brought them into the hospital.

During the termination phase both evaluation and discharge planning are predominant. The nurse uses communication techniques associated with assisting the client toward discharge and aftercare. Throughout the nurse-client relationship, the nurse must avoid responding in ways that hinder therapeutic communication (see Table 7-4). The phases of the therapeutic relationship are discussed in greater detail in Chapters 6 and 19.

CHALLENGES IN COMMUNICATION
Legal Issues

Confidentiality, legal status, patient's rights, and informed consent are legal issues that impact nurse-client communication. They are discussed briefly here as they relate to the therapeutic relationship. They are discussed in detail in Chapter 4.

All client information the nurse obtains is protected by the client's right to privacy, or **confidentiality.** Information can be shared with the health care team so that the most effective plan of care can be developed. However, the nurse must fiercely protect the client's right to privacy and the right to keep that information from individuals outside the health care team.

All communication therefore is considered confidential or privileged. In the initial interview the nurse has the responsibility to inform the client of the confidential nature of the disclosure. The client also has the right to know with whom the nurse will share the disclosed information. The nurse needs to explain that the information may be shared with team members such as the social worker, physician, and other nursing staff, but not the client's family members or friends, unless the client has given written permission to reveal specific information. If information is to be shared with family, it is usually done by their physician.

Often clients with mental illness have difficulty trusting others. To encourage clients to confide in the nurse, the nurse must gain the client's trust through honest, open, and congruent communication and by doing what he or she says will be done; however, the client may wish to confide something that the nurse needs to share. It is the nurse's responsibility to tell the client that secrets cannot be kept, and that shared information critical to the client's own or others' safety or treatment plan will be discussed with the members of the health care team.

For example, a client shares with a nursing student that he has a sharp object in which to cut himself when everyone has gone to bed because he is feeling even more and more depressed and suicidal. The student explains that this type of disclosure must be shared with the charge nurse. The client then begs the student not to tell the physician. The student replies that the charge nurse must communicate to the client's physician all disclosures that reveal behavior harmful to the client.

There is much opportunity for the nurse to communicate with clients regarding their legal status. For example, a client is brought into the hospital by the police, who have placed the client on a legal "hold." A client may not understand this term, which can seem confusing. It is often the nurse who communicates to the client the exact nature of his or her legal status, explaining the implications and patient rights associated with the status. Clients' specific legal rights are discussed in Chapter 4.

Informed consent is a legal document outlining a procedure to be conducted or specific types of medication to be given to the client. The client must be informed fully by his or her physician in an understandable manner so that he or she can decide whether to have the procedure or take the specific medication considered helpful to treatment. The nurse often assists the physician with communication regarding informed consent. The nurse must work with the physician to verify that the client has a basic understanding of the informed consent regarding treatment, medication, alternative therapies, and/or the client's prognosis with or without treatment.

Effective nurse-client communication is extremely helpful in processing legal paperwork, especially with clients who have difficulty trusting, understanding legal terms, or knowing their legal rights. The nurse must be honest, open, congruent, and clear in all messages given to the client regarding all communication of a legal nature, thus preparing a client to be well informed and to consent to treatment.

Length of Stay

Another communication challenge comes with brief hospital stays. For the chemically dependent client, for example, the length of stay could be as short as 1 to 3 days. For the client with schizophrenia, it could be a 3- to 7-day stay. Communication must then be geared toward a crisis intervention style of relating, where the initial phase of the relationship takes on a new meaning. Gathering data and initiating the treatment plan must be accomplished within hours. Thus the nurse needs to establish rapport quickly. If the client's behavior is not conducive to working quickly, then rest and medication can be provided to calm the client so that the preliminary interview and data gathering can occur.

Physical Impairments

Other issues affecting communication are special client care needs. Consider, for example, the client with hearing impairment. If the client reads lips or the nurse "signs," then communication is possible. The nurse should sit in a manner that facilitates the communication. The nurse may wish to inform the other clients what is being done and why. This is especially helpful in a group setting.

The older client may have both visual and hearing impairments, as well as cognitive deficits. The nurse needs to carefully assess each client to determine his or her special needs when communicating. With clients who are visually challenged, the nurse must physically assist the clients to and from activities, groups, and their rooms. These actions communicate caring and concern, as does sitting near the client when speaking. When approaching the visually impaired client, the nurse must proceed slowly and speak in soft tones to avoid startling the client. Communicating is challenging, but it can be effective with the help of the client and the nurse's own sensitivity.

Communicating With Children and Adolescents

Communicating with children and adolescents presents unique challenges. Often the nurse is in a position of caring for infants, children, and adolescents through the age of 18

years. In caring for patients in these age groups, the nurse needs to adapt his or her communication level to the developmental age of the child or adolescent to match the young client's ability to comprehend. In today's health care environment, children need to be informed and should participate in their own health care decisions. It is crucial that the nurse have effective communication skills in dealing with children of all ages. It is also important for the nurse to understand the developmental age of the child with whom he or she is trying to communicate so that not only the language but also the examples and educational materials can be adapted to basic concepts that the young client can easily grasp. Generally several techniques can be used to build rapport with children, including taking a personal interest in them by asking them about school, hobbies, and interests; being a skillful listener; using simple language; being nonjudgmental; appearing relaxed; sitting at eye level and establishing good eye contact; communicating directly with the child to demonstrate interest; using broad, open-ended questions; and welcoming the child's thoughts and feelings. Keen observation of the parent-child interaction can assist nurses in their assessment of the home environment (O'Neill, 2002).

Because the child's capacity to grasp language does not begin until the second year of life, the nurse needs to rely on nonverbal skills in very young children, using kind and gentle facial expressions and a nurturing and caring attitude, with soothing voice tones. Having the parents participate in the child's care can be helpful and may reduce their anxiety. Between the ages of 2 and 6 years, the child is in the beginning stage of language development and the nurse can begin to communicate verbally with the child, using simple explanations and instructions and keeping the interactions in the here and now. The nurse may use pictures or storybooks to provide information and clarify meanings.

The nurse usually experiences less difficulty when communicating with the young school-age child between 6 and 10 years, because the child is accustomed to adults other than the parents, such as teachers and coaches, giving instruction and assistance. By this time the child has developed a more mature mode of communication and has a need for close relationships, both of which are helpful when interacting with the child. However, the nurse must immediately establish a rapport and trust, with both the child and parent. The use of concrete examples, as well as simple videotapes and books suitable for the child's age, can be used with success.

During preadolescence, from the ages of 10 to 12 or 13 years, when the onset of puberty begins, the preadolescent remains receptive to adults and their influence. The nurse may begin to use some of the preadolescent's own language to communicate more effectively. Keeping explanations relevant, brief, and at a level commensurate with the preteen's understanding may help the process.

The adolescent stage begins with puberty, ordinarily ages 12 or 13 years through ages 18 or 19 years. During the early adolescent years, the child is trying to form a self-identity and feel comfortable with himself or herself. The adolescent may be self-conscious, self-absorbed with their body image, and easily embarrassed. The nurse needs to respect the adolescent's privacy, as confidentiality is important in this age group. The nurse also needs to relate more directly with the adolescent and less through the parents, as the adolescent is trying to separate emotionally from the parents and become independent, a significant characteristic of adolescence. The early-age adolescent begins to develop abstract thinking and can now not only grasp past and present events but also think about and discuss future events. The nurse can use these skills in his or her interactions with the early-age adolescent. As the adolescent reaches 14 or 15 years, the nurse may find that doing an activity with the adolescent while communicating allows the adolescent to feel more comfortable with the adult. That the nurse is not the adolescent's parent is an advantage and assists in the communication process. Regardless of the child's age, the nurse needs to present a verbal and nonverbal environment in which the child feels comfortable. The degree of success that the nurse has in communicating with a child or adolescent greatly depends on the nurse's understanding of both the developmental and chronologic age of the child.

Language and Cultural Differences

Because the United States is one of the most diverse societies in the world and part of a rapidly changing and growing multicultural world, it is imperative that nurses become culturally competent to best deal with the diverse cultures and multicultural patients. Cultural competence is defined as the ability of a system, agency, or individual to respond to the unique needs of populations whose cultures are different from that of the dominant or mainstream society (Lester, 1998a). Demographers state that there were 12 million new arrivals to the United States in the past 10 years, the largest number since the period between 1905 and 1914, when 10 million immigrants came to the United States (Leininger, 1997).

Communication is one of six areas of cultural uniqueness that needs to be assessed in the initial nursing assessment because communication and culture are intertwined. Oral and written language, gestures, facial expressions, and body language are the means by which culture is conveyed and preserved.

Cultural patterns of communication are set early in life and affect the way in which a person communicates ideas and feelings. It also affects decision making and communication methods (Lester, 1998a). Even though a cultural group shares the same communication pattern, the nurse should not assume that all members of the cultural group use the same method of expression. Cultural competence does not suggest that the nurse needs to know everything about every culture. Rather, it is thought of as the ability to develop working relationships with those who are different from the nurse. Cultural competence encompasses self-awareness, cultural knowledge about illness and healing practices, intercultural communication skills, and behavioral flexibility (Lester, 1998b).

The nurse needs to be aware of the potential language barriers to effective intercultural communication. As in any attempt to establish a good nurse-client relationship, the nurse should try to understand the client's point of view and frame of reference. Respecting and allowing a free exchange of the client's and family's ideas, thoughts, and feelings can facilitate effective intercultural communication.

For clients who are not native English speakers, verbal and nonverbal barriers to effective communication can inhibit:

- An accurate understanding of their diagnosis, progress, and prognosis
- The assurance of knowing what is going on and what procedures will be done
- The assurance of the expertise of the nurse and other health care providers
- The ability to explain their symptoms to the nurse, to assist in their diagnosis and treatment

Therefore nurses need to make a special effort to provide these essentials to clients, such as locating an interpreter who can not only speak the client's language but also translate at the level required. Most hospitals have lists of local interpreters who offer their services and who can communicate technical terminology to the client. For nontechnical, uncomplicated translation, the nurse can usually locate a hospital staff member who communicates in the client's own language. Chapter 5 discusses this issue in greater detail.

Difficult Clients

Nurses may find it difficult to communicate with clients who are aggressive, unpopular, or distressed. Clients who exhibit *aggressive* behaviors are hostile and may be verbally or physically abusive, rejecting, and manipulative. They may have a violent past history with jail or prison time for egregious offenses related to their aggressive behavior. These are unpleasant behaviors that are difficult to be around. This attacking style of behavior demonstrates a general lack of consideration and respect for others, and the natural response is to protect the self and reject the client. Even though the nurse's self-esteem and personal safety are under attack, the nurse must meet the aggression assertively by setting firm limits that do not embarrass himself or herself or the client. A specific behavioral treatment plan and a united team approach are critical to treatment success. Most facilities offer assault response training and education to help staff members manage these behaviors.

Unpopular clients have a variety of characteristics. They may be unreasonably demanding, possess unacceptable personal habits, or may be sexually inappropriate. Nurses naturally have likes and dislikes regarding client behaviors. The behavior that one nurse enjoys working with may be another nurse's displeasure. Some general characteristics of unpopular clients are shown in Box 7-2.

When dealing with unpopular clients, nurses often feel frustrated, angry, or fearful. These clients may be ignored, la-

Box 7-2	General Characteristics of Unpopular Clients

Clients who:
- Claim they are more ill than nurses believe
- Express their dislike of the hospital
- Take up much of the nurse's time and attention
- Misuse hospitalization
- Are uncooperative and argumentative
- Are very aggressive or assaultive
- Have severe, complicated problems and a poor prognosis
- Have problems brought on by themselves (e.g., alcohol-related disease)
- Have low morals or social stigmas
- Produce feelings of incompetence in the nurse

beled as troublemakers or problems, medicated more often, admonished, and generally given less care than other clients.

Distressed clients express their physical or emotional pain both verbally and nonverbally, and sometimes continuously. Becoming too involved with a client's distress can overwhelm the nurse and interfere with effective communication. Often the nurse feels inadequate dealing with severe emotional or physical distress. It is important for the nurse to remain clearheaded and to responsibly communicate understanding and concern without becoming judgmental or diminishing the patient's perceptions and related feelings.

Difficult Co-Workers

Not only must the nurse deal effectively with clients who are distressed, aggressive, and unpopular, but there are also times when the nurse must deal with health care professionals who exhibit this same behavior. Health care can be emotionally and physically demanding, which produces stress and conflict in the health care environment. There are times when colleagues become irritated, angry, argumentative, and occasionally even verbally abusive.

The nurse can use similar effective communication techniques when dealing with conflict in professional relationships. Conflict in health care settings has to do with the level of stress in the work environment, responsibility, conflicts, role differences and uncertainty, power issues, and value differences. Effective communication skills are necessary to deal with a variety of conflicting professional relationships. Win-win solutions are necessary for a growth-producing outcome. Thus both parties must use creative problem-solving techniques. Communication efforts are geared toward understanding the other person and the issues involved, using compromise and collaboration, and avoiding competition. In these situations, nurses must communicate both assertively and responsibly, owning their part of the conflict (Northouse and Northouse, 1998).

The nurse should have the skills necessary to communicate therapeutically with clients and their families. They also have the responsibility to communicate effectively with other health care professionals and with those throughout the health care setting using some of these same learned skills.

CHAPTER SUMMARY

- The components of communication are the stimulus (reason), the sender, the message, the medium, the receiver, and feedback.
- Communication can be influenced by environmental factors, the relationship between the sender and the receiver, the context of the communication, and the individual's attitudes and beliefs, knowledge, and perception. Nonverbal communication cues involve all five senses. Ninety percent of communication is thought to be nonverbal. Verbal and nonverbal communication must be congruent for the communication to be effective.
- Interpersonal communication—communication between two or more people—can be collegial, social, or therapeutic.
- The three purposes of therapeutic communication are to allow the client self-expression to promote healthy growth, to understand the significance of the client's problems, and to assist in the identification and resolution of the problems.
- Empathy is an important quality of therapeutic communication and is necessary to the success of the nurse-client relationship.
- Some responding techniques that enhance therapeutic communication are silence, active listening, support and reassurance, giving information, restating, reflecting, clarifying, and role-playing.
- Self-disclosure by the nurse can be an effective technique if used for the right reasons.
- Resistance, transference, countertransference, and boundary violations can be obstacles to therapeutic communication.
- Certain therapeutic responding techniques correspond to specific steps of the nursing process and phases of the nurse-client relationship.
- Effective communication can be challenged by issues relating to the nurse's skill and self-awareness levels, the client's length of stay in treatment, the client's physical and emotional impairments, the client's age, or language and cultural differences.

REVIEW QUESTIONS

1. A client arrives for her therapy appointment. The nurse observes that the client's clothes are baggy and unkempt. She has no makeup and avoids eye contact. While she waits for her appointment, the client stares at the floor, not interacting with anyone or reading any magazines. Based on these body cues, the psychiatric nurse determines that the client is:
   a. Psychotic
   b. Depressed
   c. Bipolar
   d. Obsessive-compulsive

2. A 15-year-old male is admitted to the adolescent unit after attempting suicide. He verbalizes to the psychiatric unit staff that he felt he was worthless, that he couldn't do anything right, and that no one would care if he was gone. The psychiatric nurse demonstrates therapeutic communication when she responds:

a. "I'm a mother and I know that I would be devastated if my child committed suicide."

b. "Do you realize that it's a sin to commit suicide?"

c. "Tell me more about why you feel worthless and not worthy of living."

d. "I appreciate you trusting me with your feelings. I will keep what you tell me just between us."

3. A child's mother entered the nurse's station yelling, "What is wrong with you people? My daughter cut herself and you allowed it to happen. I put her in here to be safe." The nurse is demonstrating assertive communication when she responds:

a. "She is not my patient."

b. "Mrs. Hall, I can't hear you when you're screaming. Let's sit down and talk about this."

c. "Why are you always yelling when you come to visit?"

d. "I'm sorry. Please don't tell my supervisor."

4. The psychiatric nurse assesses that a 15-year-old client who is anorexic is resistant to treatment when:

a. Peggy states, "I feel so fat after gaining 2 pounds this week."

b. The nurse discovers that Peggy hid her food in a napkin.

c. Peggy refuses to attend cognitive therapy.

d. Peggy tells her roommate, "I'm only in this hospital because my parents admitted me. I only lost weight after my friend said that I was fat. I've reached my goal weight."

5. A 46-year-old client yells at a male staff person after he reminded her that it was group time. The staff person reminded her of her controlling father. This is an example of:

a. Transference

b. Countertransference

c. Resistance

d. Boundary violation

REFERENCES

Alligood MR: Empathy: the importance of recognizing two types, *J Psychosoc Nurs* 30:3, 1992.

American Health Consultants: Patient Education Management 8:9, Sept 2001.

Antai-Otong D: It's not what you say, it's how you say it, *Am J Nurs*, vol 99, no 8, 1999.

Balzer Riley J: *Communication in Nursing,* ed 4, St Louis, 2000, Mosby.

Bush K: Do you really listen to patients? *RN* vol 64, no 3, March 2001.

Chant S et al: Communication skills: some problems in nursing education and practice, *J Clin Nurs* 11(1):12-21, 2002.

Cochrane DA et al: Do they really understand us? *Am J Nurs* 92(7):19-20, 1992.

Ferguson MS, Campinha-Bacote J: Humor in nursing, *J Psychosoc Nurs* 26(4):29, 1989.

Fontaine KL, Fletcher JS: *Essentials of mental health nursing,* ed 2, Reading, Mass, 1995, Addison-Wesley.

Fortinash KM, Holoday Worret PA: *Psychiatric nursing care plans,* ed 4, St Louis, 2003, Mosby.

Leininger M: Overview of the theory of culture care with the ethnonursing research method, *J Transcult Nurs* 8(2):32, 1997.

Lester N: Cultural competence: a nursing dialogue, part I, *Am J Nurs* 98(8):26, 1998a.

Lester N: Cultural competence: a nursing dialogue, part II, *Am J Nurs* 98(9):36, 1998b.

Northouse PG, Northouse LL: *Health communication: strategies for health professionals,* ed 3, East Norwalk, Conn, 1998, Appleton & Lange.

O'Neill K: Kids speak: effective communication with school-aged, adolescent patient, *Pediatr Emerg Care* 18(2):137-140, 2002.

Pike AW: On the nature and place of empathy in clinical nursing practice, *J Prof Nurs* 6(4):235, 1990.

Professional Assault Response Training (PART), a Sharp HealthCare program manual for assaultive behaviors, San Diego, Calif, 2002, Sharp HealthCare.

Schuster PM: *Communication: the key to the therapeutic relationship,* Philadelphia, 2000, FA Davis.

Shives LR: *Basic concepts of psychiatric mental health nursing,* ed 5, Philadelphia, 2002, JB Lippincott.

Stricker G, Fisher M: *Self-disclosure in the therapeutic relationship,* New York, 1990, Plenum Press.

Tommasini NR: The use of touch with the hospitalized psychiatric patient, *Arch Psychiatr Nurs* 4(4):213, 1990.

Trossman S: Diversity: a continuing challenge, *Am Nurse* 30(1)P24-25, 1998.

Williams C: Biopsychosocial elements of empathy: a multidimensional model, *Issues Mental Health Nurs* 11:155, 1990.

SUGGESTED READINGS

Armstrong MA, Kelly AE: Enhancing staff nurses' interpersonal skills: theory to practice, *Clin Nurse Spec* 7:6, 1993.

Eckroth-Bucher M: Philosophical basis and practice of self-awareness in psychiatric nursing, *J Psychosoc Nurs* 39:2, 2001.

Kemper BJ: Therapeutic listening: developing the concept, *J Psychosoc Nurs* 30:7, 1992.

Kirkham S: Nurses' descriptions of caring for culturally diverse clients, *Clin Nurs Res* 7:125, 1998.

Morse J et al: Exploring empathy: a conceptual fit for nursing practice? *Image: J Nurs Sch* 24:4, 1992.

Rowland-Morin PA, Carroll JG: Verbal communication skills and the patient satisfaction survey, *Evaluation Health Prof* 13:2, 1990.

Stern SB: Privileged communication: an ethical and legal right of psychiatric clients, *Perspect Psychiatr Care* 26(4):22-25, 1990.

Stewart M: Nurses need to strengthen cultural competence for next century to ensure quality patient care, *Am Nurse* 30(1):26-27, 1998.

8

Growth and Development Across the Life Span

Linda Hollinger-Smith

OBJECTIVES

- Identify factors that impact development across the life span.
- Compare and contrast developmental theories and the driving forces that influence human development.
- Describe the development theories that take a life span perspective.
- Discuss life span transitions and their biologic, psychologic, and social aspects.
- Distinguish between normal and abnormal physical and psychosocial processes of aging.
- Explore the meaning of health and wellness for older adults.
- Compare the developmental tasks of aging with tasks of younger cohorts.

From birth to death, human development follows a pathway of transition, change, and evolution marked by key milestones. In many cases, mental health problems arise at particular points along this pathway and are affected by developmental factors. Understanding human development is important for psychiatric-mental health nurses in order to identify and apply psychosocial interventions appropriate to particular phases of the life span.

Continuing advances in health care, genetics, and medical technology have ensured that a larger proportion of people will be living longer. To facilitate a better quality of life throughout extended years, discerning the factors that affect human development is key to helping individuals achieve optimal physical and mental health across the life span.

The process of aging, described as a series of physical and psychosocial changes, begins at the moment of birth. Developmental theorists have differentiated these aging changes according to **life stages** or periods. The greatest emphasis and achievements in the study of human development have focused on children and adolescents because areas such as intellect, cognition, personality, and social abilities are acquired at early ages.

More recently, researchers have supported the contention that development extends well beyond adolescence into adulthood and even into old age. The relatively new fields of social gerontology and cognitive aging contend that human development is not limited to internal processes, but may be highly influenced by a host of external, social, and environmental factors that may be modifiable through psychosocial interventions. To understand these factors and apply this knowledge to psychiatric-mental health nursing, this chapter begins with a discussion of developmental theories applied across the life span.

OVERVIEW OF DEVELOPMENT ACROSS THE LIFE SPAN

How individuals adapt and respond within dynamic environments is at the core of development theories. Human development occurs as a result of mechanisms involving heredity-environment interactions that are not yet completely understood. Stroufe, Cooper, and DeHart (1992) noted that development is affected by (1) a predetermined plan genetically built into the individual, (2) one's past developmental history, and (3) accommodating environmental circumstances.

The links among heredity, environment, and human development have a philosophic foundation. Rousseau viewed human development as a natural process of evolution or change, regardless of the influence of external factors. On the other hand, John Locke's philosophy of human development is derived from a **social learning** model stating that life experiences frame and shape an individual's development. The degree to which "nature versus nurture" influences human development continues to be debated.

CHILD AND ADOLESCENT DEVELOPMENT

PSYCHOSEXUAL THEORY

Sigmund Freud (1856-1939) developed **psychosexual theory,** which views the child's development as a biologically driven series of conflicts and gratifying internal needs. According to his theory, the infant is primarily focused on meeting its own internal needs. Through parental interactions, the infant experiences conflict between its own selfish desires and parental controls. The child must learn to reduce tensions from these conflicting situations in socially acceptable ways.

Freud (1923) described a child's development as a series of psychosocial stages. Each stage is characterized by confrontation of two forces, the id (representing primitive drives for pleasure) and the superego (representing morals and principles). During the early years of life, a person's sense of reality, or ego, begins to develop and serves as mediator between the id and superego.

The individual learns from past conflicts and implements defensive processes (ego defense mechanisms) to maintain balance in life. Unlike several subsequent child development theories, Freud believed that "who you are" and "everything you become" is formed during the first few years of life. Further development is based on managing asocial thoughts and impulses in socially acceptable ways. At each psychosocial stage, the individual increases the ability to tolerate clashes between the id and superego because of past childhood experiences.

Freud supposed that one's ability to deal successfully with life's conflicts and challenges was influenced by libido, or one's sexual energy. Everyone has a set amount of libido to respond to frustrations during developmental stages. If an individual cannot successfully handle problems, he or she may experience fixation or reaction formation. Fixation occurs when the individual experiences persistent needs for pleasure from the source dominating that particular development stage. Reaction formation results in the opposite reaction (i.e., repugnance of the pleasure source).

Freud identified five stages of development: oral, anal, phallic, latency, and genital (Table 8-1). From birth to about 1 year of age, libido focuses on the mouth as a source of nurturance and pleasure. Later in life, oral fixation may be characterized by overeating or smoking. From age 2 to 3 years of age, the anal stage is prominent as children begin to contend with rules and regulations for the first time with toilet training. As an adult, anal fixation may be displayed as being overly tidy or miserly.

The phallic stage begins around ages 4 to 5 years. A boy may experience the Oedipus conflict, which consists of sexual longings for his mother and perceptions of his father as a rival figure. The boy may fear that his father discovers these feelings for his mother, and subsequently

Table 8-1	Psychosexual Theory—Freud

Development results from sexual aim or biologic need for tension reduction. The goal of development is maximizing need gratification while minimizing punishment and guilt, using defenses to control anxiety.

Stage	Age (Yr)	Basic Concepts	Developmental Issues
Oral	0-1	Id	Internalized, selfish, unable to delay gratification of needs. Primary activities: receiving and taking; major conflict: feeding.
Anal	2-3	Ego	Develops ability to delay gratification of impulses and self-control; responds to external limits. Primary activity: giving and withholding; major conflict: bowel training.
Phallic	3-5	Superego	Learns values and rules from parents; development of guilt and self-esteem. Primary activity: heterosexual interactions; major conflicts: Oedipus/Electra in boys and girls, respectively.
Latency	6-12	Sexually repressed	Mastery of learning: focus is on relationship with same-sex peers.
Genital	13	Mature sexuality	Combines learning of pregenital stages; develops ability to love and work.

wants to punish his son through castration. The fear becomes overwhelming such that the boy forsakes his thoughts of his mother and begins to identify more with his father. Freud believed that the phallic stage for girls is somewhat different. Girls develop penis envy when they realize they do not have a penis, and subsequently become attracted to their fathers. Similar to boys, when girls fear their mothers discover this attraction, they refocus their attention on their mothers. The latency stage is from age 7 years to puberty and represents a period of no particular developmental trials. The final stage, the genital stage, begins at puberty and reflects sexual feelings for the opposite sex. Freud stated that these feelings bring up anxieties, as the child recalls feelings for parents during the phallic stage.

Critics of Freud's theory point to some inherent weaknesses in the initial development and testing of the theory's basic premises. The psychosexual theory of development was not generated from studying children; rather Freud developed his principles based on his adult patients' recall of childhood memories, dreams, and free associations. Difficulties in observing and studying components of the theory are also cited. Pennebaker (1999) stated that effect of releasing negative or socially unacceptable thoughts leads to positive well-being. He believes that Freud may have correctly identified an important link between releasing unacceptable thoughts or actions and feeling better about oneself. However, the source of those thoughts or behaviors may not be sexual in nature.

PSYCHOSOCIAL THEORY

A student of Freud, Erik Erikson (1902-1994) disagreed with his mentor on factors that drive human development and behavior. In contrast to Freud's focus on biologic instincts, Erikson saw social interaction as the driving source influencing human development. Erikson also believed that human development extends across the entire life span, rather than being limited to the first 5 years of life as purported by Freud. Combining the effects of the social environment on biologic maturation, Erikson formulated the **psychosocial theory** of human development entitled, "The Eight Stages of Man" (Erikson, 1963). Each stage builds on

the previous stages influenced by past experiences. Erikson's stages are summarized in Table 8-2.

Each of the eight stages represented a particular psychosocial crisis that must be resolved by the ego, either successfully or unsuccessfully, before the individual moves to the next stage. The source of the crisis may be internal (biologic) or external (social). Each stage is represented by a dyad of specific traits, one positive and one negative. For example, at infancy, the first stage represents traits of *trust versus mistrust*. To successfully resolve the psychosocial crises experienced at this stage, the infant develops the belief or trust that the social environment may be relied on to meet basic physiologic or psychologic needs. Resolution of these crises is typically not an "all or nothing" situation. In some cases, future experiences may cause the individual to mistrust the social environment. Overall an individual's psychosocial development is considered successful if he or she is comfortable trusting the social environment in most situations, and thus one trait dominates the other.

The second stage is represented by *autonomy versus doubt* at the age of toddlerhood. Once toddlers realize they can trust their social environment, they begin to see their behaviors as their own and to develop a sense of independence and self-confidence with encouragement of their parents. On the other hand, if parents overprotect or overly disapprove of the toddler's expression of independence, he or she may develop feelings of self-doubt or shame. The third stage (early childhood or preschool years) is characterized by *initiative versus guilt*. At this stage, children are exposed to a larger social world and must learn to take responsibility for demonstrating more socially acceptable behavior. Accepting more responsibility for themselves and their possessions results in expressions of initiative. Again, if parents are inconsistent or strict disciplinarians, children may develop feelings of guilt regarding their behaviors.

The fourth stage, *competence versus inferiority,* begins during the elementary and middle school years (ages 6 to 12 years). In the school years, children's social environment continues to expand as they make new friends and develop

Table 8-2 Psychosocial Theory—Erikson

Development results from social aims or conflicts arising from feelings, parent-child interactions, and social relationships.

Stage	Age (Yr)	Virtue	Developmental Issues
Trust vs. mistrust	0-1	Sense of hope	Care that satisfies basic oral and sensory needs (feeding, cuddling, and bowel relaxation) develops trust in self and world. Inconsistent, unpredictable, discontinuous care develops mistrust in self and world.
Autonomy vs. shame and doubt	1-3	Sense of willpower	Satisfying needs for autonomy and free choice results in child's developing impulse control and mastery of toileting, dressing, feeding, and separation from parents. Undercontrolling or overcontrolling parental behavior results in shame and doubt in abilities.
Initiative vs. guilt	3-6	Sense of purpose	Learns to plan tasks and join with others in cooperation and pretend play. Accepts responsibility and is enthusiastic about helping. If desire to show initiative causes excessive conflict in family, guilt results.
Industry vs. inferiority	7-11	Sense of competence	Focus on learning and mastery of skills. Success in peer interactions leads to self-assurance. Failure to master academic and social pursuits leads to inferiority and hinders attempts to try new things.
Identity vs. role confusion	12-18	Sense of self	Concerned with how others view him or her. Begins to make occupational choices and fit in society. Development of self-identity leads to making long-term goals, self-esteem, and emotional stability. Failure to develop self-identity leads to role confusion, poor self-confidence, alienation, acting out, and no occupational choice.
Intimacy vs. isolation	18-21 to 40	Sense of belonging	Task is to develop close, sharing relationship that may include sexual partner. Person unable or unwilling to share or unsure of self-identity may have difficulty developing relationships and may be lonely.
Generativity vs. stagnation	40-65	Focus is on concern for next generation and nurturance	Guiding younger generation and giving back to the world brings pleasure. Self-preoccupied person will stagnate.
Ego integrity vs. despair	65-death	Sense of satisfaction and acceptance	Older adult can look back with acceptance of life and death. If person is unable to resolve inevitable death issue, despair and crises will result.

new relationships. Children gain new knowledge, learn new skills, and grow more competent. If children do not experience successes in learning or productivity, they will develop a sense of inferiority. The fifth stage, *identity versus role confusion,* occurs around ages 12 to 18 years. Entering the adolescent years, children begin to develop social identity. Adolescents consider how they appear to their peers, and they begin to think about what sort of occupational roles they will be seeking in the future. An emerging sense of identity is also important in the development of self-esteem and self-concept. Adolescents who experience difficulties "fitting" in with their peers and who suffer from low self-esteem are in Erikson's stage of "role confusion." Erikson's final three stages are discussed in the next section addressing adult developmental theory.

Compared to Freud's view of the ego, Erikson's theory places more importance on the ego in resolving conflict situations independent of the id and superego (Erikson, 1982). Erikson's focus on personality development was broader, encompassing the impact of social, cultural, and environmental factors, rather than just the effects of sexuality. Similar to Freud's theory of development, critics also note that Erikson's *Stages of Man* was not developed through empiric testing, nor are its constructs consistently valid. But Erikson's model still stands as one of the most important

contributions to human development theory across the life span.

INTERPERSONAL THEORY

The **interpersonal theory** of human development developed by Harry Stack Sullivan (1882-1949) highlights interpersonal behaviors and relationships as the central factor influencing child and adolescent development across six "eras," from infancy to late adolescence (Table 8-3). There are two dimensions to interpersonal behaviors: (1) the need to satisfy social attachments and (2) the longing to meet biologic and psychologic needs. Interpersonal behaviors also invite social reactions that can either complement or discredit the behaviors (Sullivan, 1953). For example, children learn that behaviors that result in praise from parents are more preferred than behaviors that result in discipline from parents, which may increase the child's anxieties. Overreactions to negative behaviors, such as a parent's extreme reactions or punitive responses to their child's occasional "accident" during toilet training, may produce intense anxieties in the child, interfering with the child's ability to separate the mood and reactions from parents to the biologic act of excretion.

The *infancy era,* the first 2 years of life, represents a phase of dependency on parents to meet all biologic or survival needs. Parents empathetically communicate their moods to the child such that the child feels comforted when parents communicate tenderness, and the child feels anxiety when parents communicate frustration. During the first several months of life, infants are in what is termed the *prototaxic mode* in which they cannot distinguish themselves from the external environment. Gradually infants begin to separate themselves from others and realize that the source of comfort or discomfort originates with parents (*parataxic mode*). At this point, infants begin to develop coping responses to deal with anxiety, mostly through trial-and-error processing. Sullivan identified the development of the infant's "good me" when gratification needs are met and parents react positively and the converse "bad me" when needs are not met, parents react negatively, and anxiety is heightened. If the parents' reactions are continuously extreme or punitive in nature, the "not me" sense develops to cope with the high level of anxiety the child is facing in response to the parents' mood.

The *childhood era* (ages 2 to 6 years) extends from the inception of language development to beginning social relationships with peers. Development moves from a trial-and-error system of training to actual learning through education. Children's coping mechanisms ("good me," "bad me") continue to be shaped from the interpersonal interactions with parents, teachers, and other caregivers. One such defense mechanism, *sublimation*, or the expression of desires in socially acceptable manners, is a positive development during this era. On the other hand, continuous punitive or extreme disapproval ("not me") may result in what Sullivan termed *malevolent transformation* (feeling that one is living among enemies). The child's anxieties may develop into fears of disapproval from all authority figures and inability to respond to positive feedback from others (Maddi, 1972). Parents who role-model malevolence educate their children to become malicious. In many cases, these children become known as the class "bullies," behaving abusively to fellow students.

Ages 6 to 10 years represent the *juvenile era* during which juveniles begin to develop friendships with peers, representing a widening of social circles. Juveniles are learning to develop elements of their conscience and personalities that will help them succeed in society. They begin to learn the importance of being members of a group, as well as gaining experience in competitive, rivalry, and compromising situations. Along with group membership, juveniles learn various ways to ostracize individuals from the "in group" to the "out group," forming stereotypes about these individuals that often have cultural roots. Juveniles are also learning to distinguish fantasy from reality in this stage. In addition, they continue to develop aspects of their self-system in their ability to participate in a more mature form of communication, that of *syntaxis*, in which they are able to perceive the interrelationships between their own behaviors and the reactions or responses of others. The self-system is

Table 8-3   Interpersonal Theory—Sullivan

Development results from interpersonal relationships with others in maximizing satisfaction of needs while minimizing insecurity.

Era	Age (Yr)	Basic Concept	Developmental Issues
Infancy	0-2	Trial-and-error learning from parental interactions of tenderness or annoyance molds development; ends with language development	Infant learns to differentiate self from others and that comfort and discomfort are connected to caregiver: parataxic mode. Develops self-system: "good me" from positive paternal mood, "bad me" from negative paternal mood with mild anxiety, and "not me" from extreme parental disapproval with severe anxiety and emotional withdrawal.
Childhood	2-6	Language development allows child to be educated, not trained	Language takes on symbolic function of communication. Self-system continues to develop with sublimation (expression of impulses in socially acceptable ways) or develops malevolent transformation (a feeling of living among enemies).
Juvenile	6-10	Relations with peers allow children to see themselves objectively	Increased peer interactions help to give child feedback from others and widen sphere of interactions to include society. Develops conscience. Self-system develops internalized reputation and cultural stereotypes. Able to distinguish fantasy and reality and develop syntaxic communication (a mature method of communicating): their own behavior is connected to others' opinions of them.
Preadolescent	10-13	Develops same-sex chums	Transition from egocentrism to love. Development of chumships helps to validate personal worth through collaboration and mutual satisfaction of needs. Able to work with peers toward a common goal and develop sense of oneness. All for one and one for all.
Adolescent	13-17	Lust: interest in sexual activity	Sexual attractions allow adolescent to test the waters of intimacy. If attractions are severely discouraged or thwarted by adults, the adolescent will feel insecure and lonely.
Late adolescent	17-19	Personality integration	Able to become genuinely intimate with others by integrating needs of society without excessive insecurity or anxiety. Inability to achieve personality integration results in regression and egocentrism for life.

also developing and internalizing personality patterns that Sullivan termed *supervisory patterns* that develop during the juvenile era, refine over the subsequent years, and remain with the person throughout life.

In contrast to Erikson's single stage of adolescence, Sullivan divides adolescence into three eras: preadolescence (ages 10 to 13 years), adolescence (ages 13 to 17 years), and late adolescence (ages 17 to 19 years). During *preadolescence*, friendships of same-sex friends deepen because of the need for alliances in meeting mutual needs (Maddi, 1972). Social groups continue to evolve their self-identity and become goal-focused. Preadolescents learn the importance of reciprocity and equality in interpersonal relationships. The *adolescent era* begins at puberty and is hallmarked by sexual attraction and feelings of lust. Low self-esteem, insecurity, anxiety, and loneliness may develop if the adolescent is constantly berated or disciplined by parents for sexual thoughts or behaviors. The *late adolescent era* is characterized by the adolescent's ability to be comfortable with his or her own intimate relationships while meeting the socially acceptable expectations of society. Adolescents who have not learned to develop intimate relationships may revert to the juvenile era and remain with an egocentric personality throughout life, unable to develop satisfying interpersonal relationships.

COGNITIVE THEORY

Jean Piaget (1896-1980), a Swiss philosopher and psychologist who had his doctorate in zoology, dedicated his life work to observing and interacting with children to determine how their thinking processes differed from adults. His prolific work established several new areas of science including cognitive theory, developmental psychology, and genetic epistemology. The application of his work on cognitive learning influenced generations of educators who applied his constructivist learning concepts to elementary level education, focusing on the child's abilities to continuously create and test new knowledge (Gallagher and Reid, 1981). This was in stark contrast to the more traditional pedagogic theory of childhood learning that viewed children as "empty vessels" who needed to be filled with knowledge by educators.

Cognitive theory explains how thought processes are structured, how they develop, and their influence on behavior. Structuring of thought processes occurs through the development of *schema* (i.e., mental images or cognitive structures). Thought processes develop through assimilation and accommodation. When the child encounters new information that is recognized and understood within existing schema, *assimilation* of that new information occurs. If new information cannot be linked to existing schema, the child must learn to develop new mental images or patterns through the process of *accommodation*. As long as the child is able to assimilate or accommodate adequately to new knowledge, the child is able to achieve *equilibrium* or mental balance. When schemas are inadequate to facilitate learning, *disequilibrium* may occur.

Piaget viewed the development of thought processes as progressing over four stages (Piaget, 1970; Piaget and Inhelder, 1969). At each stage, the child's behavior is influenced by the development of cognitive images or structures. The child must successfully achieve goals of each stage before moving onto the next. These stages are summarized in Table 8-4. During the first stage, the *sensorimotor period* (birth to 2 years of age), the infant learns about the environ-

Table 8-4   Cognitive Development—Piaget

Development results from a tendency to organize and adapt to the environment. Intelligence development allows children to have increasingly effective and more organized interactions with the environment.

Stage	Age (Yr)	Basic Concepts	Developmental Issues
Sensorimotor	0-2	In-the-moment thinking: ability to differentiate self from objects	Child moves from reflexive action to instrumentability: actions lead to outcomes through trial and error. Develops decentering: ability to differentiate self from objects. Develops object permanence: ability to hold mental representations when objects or people are out of sight.
Preoperational	2-7	Here-and-now thinking: uses symbols and words to represent objects, actions, people, and places not present	Engages in pretend (symbolic) play. Remains egocentric: unable to take another's point of view. Cannot distinguish reality from fantasy. Acquires language. Only intuitively guesses about cause and effect. Time is oriented in present only. Can focus on only one emotion at a time. Beginning development of self-system. Noncontested respect for authority.
Concrete operational	7-11	Past and present thinking	Able to conserve: understands that physical properties such as volume and length remain the same when there are changes in shape, group, or position. Able to reverse operations. Able to decenter: relates two classifications at one time. Able to think about past and present events but not future. Begins to appreciate perspective of others.
Formal operational	11-16	Future thinking	Able to think in abstract and hypothetical terms. Able to ponder what might be rather than just what is. Can think of future events and develop strategies for solving complex problems.

ment through the senses in a trial and error fashion that Piaget termed *instrumentality*. Gradually the infant begins to recognize the difference between the self and others in the environment, or the process of *decentering*. It was originally believed that *object permanence*, or the ability to recognize that an object or person is in a given area or continues to exist even outside of the infant's field of vision, begins to develop toward the end of the sensorimotor period (around age 2 years). More recent research has shown that the infant gains this ability much earlier, around 6 months of age.

The *preoperational period* (ages 2 to 7 years) is characterized by the use of verbal and mental symbols to represent persons, objects, and actions that may or may not be present. The child also begins to exhibit pretend play, has difficulty distinguishing real from fantasy, and focuses only on the present. Thought processes are egocentric in nature such that the child considers only his or her viewpoint, and aspects of one's self-esteem begin to show. The child's emotional state is in constant fluctuation, and he or she is able to focus only on one emotion at a time. Later in this period, unconditional acceptance of authority begins to develop.

The *concrete operations period* (ages 7 to 11 years) is exemplified by thought processes that are only concrete in character, which fosters the ability to sort objects and place them in some order. Thoughts about the past and present are recognized, but not thoughts about the future. The child is also able to understand conservation, or the principle that an object can change shape but retain the same volume. The child is also able to acknowledge the viewpoints of others and appreciate feelings such as camaraderie, truthfulness, and integrity.

The final period, the *formal operations period* (ages 11 to 16 years), is distinguished by the development of systematic ways to think about and solve problems. The individual is able to think in abstract (i.e., explaining metaphors) or hypothetical terms (i.e., "what if" statements). Thinking in terms of the future and solving or debating problems in a logical manner are also characteristic of this period.

Cognitive development represents human's constant attempts to adapt to and make sense of their environment. Piaget's stages of cognitive development are associated with particular age spans, but typically vary among individuals. In addition, each period is also made up of distinct structures. For example, the concrete operational period consists of more than 40 structures that deal with relationships, movements, time and space, conservation, and measurement (Brainerd, 1978). Examination of these structures has been of great value to scientists studying the development of intelligence and to educators applying Piaget's theory to learning activities at specific elementary school grades. Although more recent research has confirmed that Piaget may have underestimated cognitive development, particularly during the sensorimotor period, his body of work has been a major influence on those who followed in the study of human development.

Attachment Theory

John Bowlby (1908-1990) recognized the importance of maternal bonding in child development, a consistent phenomenon across all cultures. From initial animal studies, Bowlby saw bonding as a type of "protective" response by the youngster in a dangerous situation (Bowlby, 1988). Ainsworth (1989) expanded the concept of attachment to include all caregivers or "primary attachment figures" and found that infants from all cultures showed the same distress (although to different degrees) in all cultures of the world. Positive interactions with caregivers facilitate growth of secure attachments, whereas negative interactions result in insecure attachments. Bowlby viewed attachment as the core of all human development. Responses of the caregiver to the infant's distress over time result in what Bowlby called "internal working models of self and parent." These formed models influence the development of social interactions (Stroufe, Cooper, and DeHart, 1992). Children who experienced secure attachments develop into resilient, happy, and capable individuals, whereas those who faced insecure attachments tended to become antisocial, helpless, passive, or needing attention.

Bowlby further recognized that a child's development may be influenced by other figures as their social circle expands. For example, a child experiencing helpless or passive behaviors may be positively affected by a caring elementary school teacher who encourages, supports, and nurtures the child toward a more positive developmental process. On the other hand, a child who is greatly affected by the loss of a parent may face a more negative developmental pathway. Bowlby explained these experiences as a process of **adaptation**. Later theorists continued to build and refine on a theory of adaptation relative to human development.

BEHAVIORAL THEORIES

Behavioral theories, or learning theories, focus on the basic relationship between a stimulus and a response and involve the study of situations in which responses may be accurately predicted. For the psychologists concerned with developing behavioral theories, it was also a way to break with the biologists and psychiatrists who believed instincts drive all human behavior and that patterns of behavior were determined at early ages. It is probably not a coincidence that the early behavioral scientists were also American, in contrast to the domination of European scientists involved in the previously discussed development theories.

Classical and Operant Conditioning

The early influences on what has come to be social learning theory were the scientific works of John B. Watson (1878-1958) and B.F. Skinner (1904-1990). Using the research techniques designed by Ivan Pavlov, Watson showed that humans learn new behaviors through the process of *classical conditioning*. He demonstrated that a conditioned stimulus could be paired with an unconditioned stimulus to elicit a conditioned response or behavior change. When the un-conditioned stimulus was removed, the conditioned stimulus continued to result in the same conditioned response.

Skinner expanded on Watson's work stating that learning does not only involve an association between a stimulus and response. He believed that learning occurred through association of a behavior with a particular consequence. Skinner referred to this process as *operant conditioning*. He identified three basic consequences or responses to learning situations: reinforcement, extinction, and punishment. *Reinforcement* may be a positive response, which then increases a particular behavior, or it may be a negative response, also termed *extinction*, which removes or eliminates the behavior. *Punishment*, or an unpleasant response, reduces the frequency of the behavior.

Social Learning Theory

Social learning theory is considered to be a general theory to explain human behavior. The term *social learning theory* was first seen in a 1941 publication by Miller and Dollard entitled *Social Learning and Imitation*. They outlined the concepts that formed the foundation of several versions of social learning theory. From their early work, behaviorists were able to empirically test and validate their hypotheses.

One of the pioneers of social learning theory, Julian Rotter (1916-?), questioned Freudian theory that biologic motives determined human behavior. Instead, he selected the *empiric law of effect* as the motivating factor that drives human behavior. Basically, individuals are motivated to search for positive stimulants, or *reinforcers*, and to shun negative stimulants. He went further to say that an individual's personality is inherently linked to his or her environment. His approach to clinical psychology included study of not just one's life history, personality, and experiences, but also of one's awareness of and response to the environment. Changing either one's personality or environment affects the other. In contrast to other child development theorists, Rotter also believed that personality can continue to evolve based on new life experiences or new learning opportunities, although, as one ages, the stimulants must be more intense to effect the same degree of personality change.

Rotter's social learning theory (1982) has four main components:

1. *Behavior potential* is the degree of probability that the individual will engage in a specific behavior in a particular situation. For each specific behavior, there is a corresponding behavior potential. Rotter believed that the person seeks the behavior with the greatest potential.
2. *Expectancy* is the degree of likelihood that a behavior will lead to a certain outcome and is based on past experiences. As the person is more liable to seek a positive outcome, or reinforcer, he or she would select the behavior with the highest expectancy of achieving a positive outcome. Expectancy is subjective, as some individuals may experience unrealistic

expectations that have no basis in reality (e.g., irrational expectations).

3. *Reinforcement value* is the desirability of behavior outcomes, such that those outcomes that one rates highest have the greatest reinforcement value. Again, reinforcement value is subjective, being affected by past experiences. For example, for most children parental punishment is a negative outcome with low reinforcement value. But for some children who suffer from neglect, parental punishment may have a high reinforcement value, as it is more desirable than abandonment.
4. *Psychologic situation* represents how different individuals have different elucidations of the same circumstances. How individuals behave is affected by their subjective analyses of the environment.

Rotter's work on social learning theory formed the basis for the concept he is better recognized for, that of *locus of control* (Rotter, 1992). Locus of control is concerned with a person's belief of who is in control of the reinforcers—self or some outside force. Some mistakenly have attempted to categorize people with "internal" locus of control or "external" locus of control personalities. Rotter explained that under specific situations "internals" may function more like "externals" or vice versa, based on past experiences, again reinforcing the interaction of individual and environment.

Albert Bandura's (1971) addition to social learning theory emphasized the importance of observation and *modeling* actions, emotions, and attitudes of others. By copying the behaviors of others, information is encoded and forms the basis for new behaviors. For example, children are often observed imitating other children or even adults. By role playing and dressing up as the mother and father, children are programming their own future behaviors. Cognitive, environmental, and behavioral factors interact during observational learning processes that have four basic components:

1. Attention to the modeled behavior
2. Retention or coding of the behavior
3. Motor reproduction of the behavior
4. Motivation and reinforcement of the reproduced behavior

Modeled behaviors are more likely to be implemented by individuals if they perceive the outcomes to be functionally valuable or result in positive reinforcement. If the consequence of the modeled behavior is recognized and rewarded, the new behavior is further strengthened.

Interestingly, Bandura's work with social and observational learning began from his focus on how children learn aggression (Bandura, 1986). In fact, Bandura cautioned parents and educators that television and movie violence influenced aggressive and violent behaviors in children. Although he did not claim that the media are the sole source of learned aggression, he did note that they are a key ingredient. Television network and film executives were so concerned that Bandura's warnings would result in a climate of fear among parents (and were probably more fearful of not making money) that they petitioned his removal from an expert panel to develop the 1972 Surgeon General's Report on Violence (Liebert and Sprafkin, 1988).

Bandura expanded his social learning theory to include the concept of self-reflection as a way for persons to examine their experiences, consider their own thinking processes, and adjust their thinking as a result. Self-efficacy is a form of self-reflection that affects one's behaviors; it was a central focus for Bandura's research (Bandura, 1989). Basically, individuals develop perceptions about their own effectiveness that in turn guide their behavior. Self-efficacy determines what individuals attempt to achieve and the amount of effort their give to achieve their goals.

Social learning theory has greatly contributed to many fields including education, health care, and behavior therapy. Most recently, social learning theory has been applied to the study of how children internalize morals and values of society. Concepts of social learning theory have also been used successfully in psychomotor skill training.

MORAL DEVELOPMENT

Moral development encompasses moral judgment or reasoning processes and involves making decisions about right or wrong actions in a particular situation (Stroufe, Cooper, and DeHart, 1992). Piaget examined the concept of moral development and determined there were two stages of development. Before the ages of 10 or 11 years, children considered moral dilemmas differently from older children. These dichotomous views are based on how children view "rules." For younger children, rules are absolute, coming from an authority figure. Older children learn that rules are sometimes able to be changed in given situations. According to Piaget, moral judgment is first based on consequences and later on motives. For example, if a child is asked to select which situation represents the greater wrong—the child who steals food everyday to feed his poor family, or the child who steals money once to buy a toy—the younger child would say the child who steals food daily is doing the greater wrong, based on the consequences or amount of harm. In contrast, the older child judges wrongness according to motives in the situation.

Lawrence Kohlberg built on Piaget's work in the area of moral development. Kohlberg (1973) completed his doctorate in psychology at University of Chicago focusing his research on moral issues faced by children and adolescents. Following Piaget's schema, Kohlberg identified seven stages of moral development that are categorized into three levels (Table 8-5). Kohlberg's model was based on a core sample of 72 boys, ages 10, 13, and 16 years, from lower and middle class families in Chicago. He asked the boys to reason out a series of moral dilemmas, and he then classified their responses according to six stages.

The first level, *preconventional morality,* consists of three stages:

1. *Egocentric judgment* in which children make decisions based what they like or wish with no obligations to obey authority figures.
2. *Punishment and obedience orientation* when children realize there are physical consequences in the form of punishment for bad behaviors. In this stage, children learn the authority role.
3. *Instrumental relativist orientation* stage when children focus on satisfying their own instrumental needs and occasionally the needs of others. Moral judgment is based on, "What do I get out of this decision?"

Table 8-5 Moral Development—Kohlberg

Moral development is influenced by the child's motivation or need, the child's opportunity to learn social roles, and the forms of justice the child encounters in the social institutions where he or she lives.

Level	Age (Yr)	Stage	Developmental Issues
I. Preconventional (self-centered orientation)	4-10	1. Punishment-obedience orientation	Moral decisions are based on avoidance of punishment.
		2. Hedonistic and instrumental orientation	Moral decisions are motivated by desire for rewards rather than avoiding punishment, and belief that by helping others they will get help in return.
II. Conventional (able to see victim's perspective)	10-13 but can go into adolescence	3. Good boy/girl orientation	Moral decisions are based on desire for approval from others and on avoiding guilt experienced by not doing the right thing.
		4. Law-and-order orientation	Moral decisions are defined by rights, assigned duty, rules of the community, and respect for authority.
III. Postconventional (underlying ethical principles are considered that take into account societal needs)	13-death	5. Social contract orientation	Moral decisions are based on a sense of community respect and disrespect. Rules should be followed to maintain community harmony.
		6. Hierarchy of principles orientation	Moral judgments are based on principles of justice, the reciprocity and quality of human rights, and respect for the dignity of human beings as individual persons: Golden rule: do to others as you would have them do to you.

The second level, the *conventional level*, seeks conformity and loyalty as key behaviors and consists of two stages:

1. *Interpersonal concordance* deals with the reciprocal nature of helping or good behaviors. Children receive approval by others for doing good works. Intent is also taken into account and grows in importance, such as "she means well" in her attempt to assist others.

2. *Law and order orientation,* which is a stage of doing good in respect of authority or because of duty to maintain "social order."

The third level, the *postconventional* or *principled level*, seeks to define moral judgment and values in terms of the universal good and consists of two stages.

1. *Social-contract legalist orientation* that focuses on "the legal point of view" but is also open to considering what is moral and good for society.

2. *Universal ethical-principle orientation* deals with abstract and ethical moral values, rather than concrete moral rules. These include universal principles such as equality, justice, and beneficence.

Kohlberg's continued work on his stages of moral development has combined the two stages of the final level, as responses to his moral dilemma examples do not yield differentiation between these two stages. Critics of his model view his work as culturally and sexually biased. His theories are based on Western views of moral development and do not reflect other cultural views.

Carol Gilligan, an associate of Kohlberg, agreed that his premises may be sexually biased. Along with his sample consisting of all males, Gilligan felt that the stages connoted a male orientation geared toward moral rules and responsibilities. She saw female moral values as being based in interpersonal relationships and reality situations rather than in abstract concepts. Gilligan (1982) raised another possibility to explain gender differences in forming moral values. She suggested that moral development may progress along more than one pathway: one focused on ethics, justice, and other abstract concepts and the other course focused on interpersonal relationships. At some point, each gender tends toward making one of these paths becoming dominant.

ADULT DEVELOPMENT

Since the time of the Chinese philosopher Confucius (511-479 BC), adult development has been viewed as contiguous, with child and adolescent development at one end of a continuum and old age at the other end.

There is a dearth of adult development research in comparison to study of infancy, childhood, and adolescence. Stevens-Long (1992) attributed this gap to social, psychologic, and economic issues. Much of the emphasis on child development was in the fields of education, biology, and psychology. With the implementation of compulsory education, teachers wanted to develop and test optimal teaching methodologies. Biologists and psychologists studied child development to understand human evolution.

It is important for psychiatric-mental health nurses to recognize that many mental health problems develop or are identified at certain ages. For instance, schizophrenia is most often diagnosed in late adolescence or early adulthood, but is uncommon after age 50 years. Certain forms of dementia are also more commonly identified at particular ages. For example, symptoms of Pick's disease may be evident by middle age, but symptoms of Alzheimer's disease are typically observed by age 75 years.

As human development theories expanded in their attempts to explain concepts of personality, cognition, motivation, emotions, and intellect, it soon became apparent that values, cognitive abilities, mental and physical health, and many other factors continue to evolve throughout adulthood. Child and adolescent development theories with finite stages seemed inadequate to explain the dynamics of human development past 18 years of age. Many life experiences are achieved only during adulthood (i.e., marriage, raising children, starting or ending a career) that will significantly affect growth and development during those years. Arnold Van Gennep was one of the pioneers of adult development theory. In his book, *The Rites of Passage* (1909), he described **rites of passage** as the significant and meaningful rituals that mark and celebrate milestones and transitions in life.

LIFE STAGE THEORIES

Several life stage theories have been advanced over the last several years. These theories divide the life span into a series of sequential transitions. Individuals who are adjusted and happy are able to achieve age-appropriate developmental tasks at each stage.

Jung's life stage theory (1971) was based on psychoanalytic theory that states that as one goes through life, one develops inner exploratory abilities that add meaning to life. He also postulated that personality differences between males and females become less distinct as people age. The final life stage deals with maintaining a balance between wisdom and senility in old age. The older person who is successful in life does not attempt to compete with youth but rather is able to deal with age changes.

Jung considered adult development on a continuum across the life cycle. He found that adults, ages 20 to 35 years, continue to develop their individuality and other personality patterns while they are establishing their families. Jung was one of the first to describe midlife transition, a period of growing awareness of masculine and feminine aspects of personality present in each individual.

Erikson was the most well known of the life stage theorists and identified eight stages of psychologic development (see Table 8-2). Each stage of development involves maintaining a balance between the *syntonic* (state of stability) and *dystonic* (state of disorder) (Erikson, Erikson, and Kiunick, 1986) to adjust and move forward to the next level. The first five stages focused on children and adolescents.

The remaining three stages followed adulthood from young to old age. During young adulthood individuals struggle with *intimacy versus isolation.* They develop the abilities to reciprocate loving relationships and begin to establish long-term commitments in their relationships. Some individuals retain a sense of self-absorption and find it difficult to make and keep intimate relationships; therefore they tend toward isolation (Colarusso and Nemiroff, 1981).

The stage of *generativity versus stagnation* occurs during middle adulthood and is characterized by an interest of individuals in wanting to guide development of the next generation. As the children of adults grow more independent, their aging parents become more dependent. Therefore those at middle adulthood are faced with new roles, responsibilities, and challenges. Generativity also includes the ability to evaluate and appreciate past life experiences, embrace the future, assume new relationships and responsibilities, and develop creativity. For adults who cannot achieve such outcomes and who view their lives at this point as boring or unfulfilling, their existence feels to be in a period of stagnation.

The final stage, *ego integrity versus despair,* occurs in late life. Older adults develop a sense of acceptance of how they lived their lives and the importance of relationships they acquired throughout their lives. This stage may be considered the culmination of the previous seven stages. The possessor of ego integrity is prepared to defend the dignity of one's own lifestyle and life choices. Individuals who have not successfully accomplished development tasks of earlier stages may lack the accumulated ego integration and thus feel despair about a lack of life fulfillment and impending death. In describing the final stage of life, Erickson stated that "the process of bringing into balance feelings of integrity and despair involves a review of and a coming to terms with the life one has lived thus far" (Erikson, Erikson, and Kiunick, 1986).

More recently, a psychologic model encompassing life span development, called *selective optimization with com-*pensation, has been developed (Baltes, Smith, and Staudinger, 1992). This theoretic framework focuses on managing age-related gains and losses for successful aging. Individuals who age successfully are those who select and modify activities that enrich their lives despite energy declines.

Human Motivation and Development Theory

Maslow's motivation and development theory (1962) is widely viewed as a valuable framework to understand human needs and values from a holistic point of reference. Maslow's theoretic construct is described as a hierarchy of needs and is diagrammed in the form of a pyramid (see Figure 2-2). Five levels of needs are identified, the most basic representing the base of the pyramid. From the most basic (1) to the highest (5) level, these needs include:

1. Biologic and physiologic
2. Safety and security
3. Affiliation or sense of belonging
4. Self-esteem
5. **Self-actualization**

Ebersole and Hess (1999) conceptualized Maslow's hierarchy of needs and applied his theory to identification of special needs of older adults at each level. Table 8-6 identifies some of these specific needs of the older adult and potential strategies to meet those needs.

CONTEMPORARY THEORISTS

During adulthood development focuses on the ability to interact with transitional aspects of the life experiences and the environment. Integral to adult development is recognition and acceptance of finiteness of time and the inevitability of death.

Daniel Levinson, a psychosocial theorist, examined life stages from early through late adulthood (1986), broadly based on Erikson's work. In contrast to Erikson, Levinson focused less on changes within the person, but more on the

Table 8-6 Special Needs of Older Adults According to Maslow's Hierarchy of Needs		
Needs of Older Adults	**Maslow's Hierarchy of Needs**	**Strategies to Meet Needs**
Finding meaning in life and death	Self-actualization	Identify value and contributions of individual
Transcendence over aging process		Encourage continuity of participation in decision-making processes
Creativity and mastery		Reminisce about past in relation to present and future
Responsible roles	Self-esteem	Maintain aspects of roles important to individual
Social supports		Facilitate socialization
Locus of control		Promote physical appearance
Cognitive awareness		Facilitate decision making
Relationships	Belonging	Identify impact of loss on individual
Intimacy		Support needs for intimacy and sexuality
Affiliations		Facilitate changes in lifestyle
Sensory awareness	Safety and security	Obtain necessary equipment or supplies for home independence
Environmental safety		Assist with obtaining legal or financial help
Legal and economic issues		Educate older person and family regarding home safety
Biologic needs	Biologic integrity	Provide for physical comfort
Comfort needs		Provide for nutritional needs

From Ebersole P, Hess P: *Toward healthy aging: human needs and nursing responses*, ed 5, St Louis, 1998, Mosby.

interface between the self and the interpersonal world. His psychosocial theory of adult development addressed assessment of one's self within the world, functioning of the individual self, and relationship between the self and environment (Newton and Levinson, 1979). Psychosocial theory focuses on one's connection to the self and the environment, living life's experiences, and the creative potential of human variability.

Levinson proposed a universal life cycle consisting of specific eras sequenced from birth to old age. The "era" is the basic unit of the life cycle and lasts about 20 years (e.g., preadulthood from 0 to 20 years; early adulthood from 20 to 40 years; middle adulthood from 40 to 60 years; late adulthood from 60 to 80 years to death) (Figure 8-1). Stable periods of 6 to 7 years are followed by transitional periods of 4 to 5 years. Each period consists of specific tasks to be en-

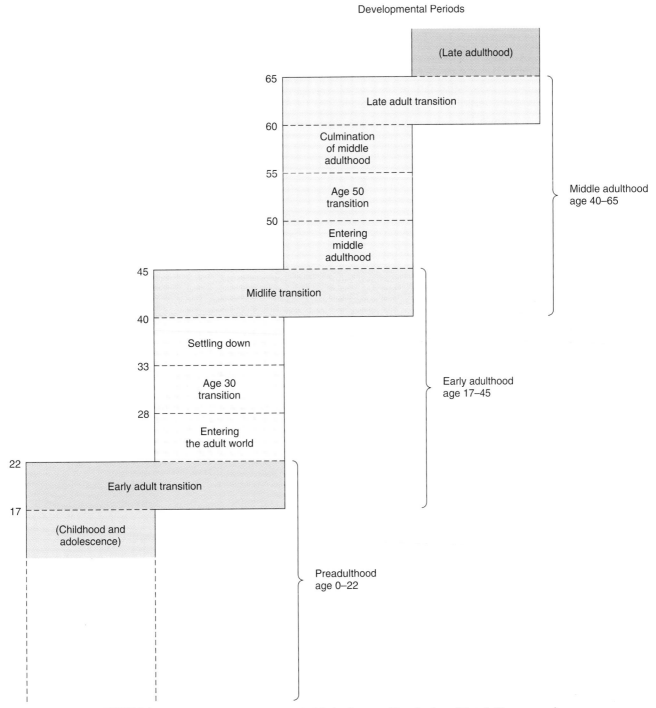

FIGURE 8-1. Levinson's psychosocial theory of adult development. (From Levinson DJ et al: *The seasons of a man's life*, New York, 1986, Ballantine Books.)

countered and achieved. From a clinical viewpoint, therapists found this framework useful in identifying transitional periods that were often times of internal conflict and thus an impetus for seeking treatments (Myers, 1998). The following summarizes key events during Levinson's stages and transitions:

- Preadulthood lasts up to about age 17 years, and early adult transition occurs from ages 17 to 22 years, during which individuals begin to modify their relationships with family and friends.
- Early adulthood stage is between 17 and 45 years, characterized by periods of vitality, contradiction, and stress. Individuals are faced with major life tasks, including following aspirations, raising families, and establishing their position in society.
- Midlife transition is between ages 40 and 45 years. Individuals face the realization that failure to accomplish all of life's goals leads first to disappointment and then to reformulation of earlier goals.
- Middle adulthood lasts from ages 40 to 65 years. During these years adults have the greatest potential to have a positive impact on society.
- Late adult transition occurs between 60 and 65 years of age, and individuals experience some anxiety over physical decline.
- Late adulthood era is characterized by an acceptance of realities of the past, present, and future.

The Harvard Study of Adult Development, the longest and most thorough study of aging ever attempted, has followed the life course of 268 undergraduate students from 1938 to the present. Current director of the study, George Vaillant, is studying adult adaptation related to ego defense mechanisms. His book published in 2002, *Aging Well: Surprising Guideposts to a Happier Life from the Landmark Harvard Study of Adult Development,* identifies behaviors that promote adaptation as well as maladaptation.

Using a series of interviews and questionnaires, the study followed three groups of men and women for the last six to eight decades. The first group consists of a sample of 268 socially advantaged Harvard graduates born about 1920. The second group is a sample of 456 socially disadvantaged urban-dwelling men born about 1930. The third group is a sample of 90 middle-class, intellectually gifted women born about 1910.

Vaillant identified six factors in middle adulthood that promotes longevity:
1. Experiencing a warm, caring marriage
2. Having effective adaptive or coping strategies
3. Not smoking heavily
4. Not abusing alcohol
5. Getting adequate exercise
6. Being at recommended weight

Vaillant's study built on the intrapsychic styles of adaptation first described by Freud. The ego mechanisms of defense are the major channels towards managing instinct and affect. Ego defense mechanisms may be adaptive or patho-

Box 8-1   Vaillant's Hierarchy of Adaptive Mechanisms

Level I: Psychotic Mechanisms (Common in Psychosis, Dreams, Childhood)
Denial (of external reality)
Distortion
Delusional projection

Level II: Immature Mechanisms (Common in Severe Depression, Personality Disorders, and Adolescence)
Fantasy (schizoid withdrawal, denial through fantasy)
Projection
Hypochondriasis
Passive-aggressive behavior
Masochism, turning against the self
Acting out (compulsive delinquency, perversion)

Level III: Neurotic Mechanisms (Common in Everyone)
Intellectualization (isolation, obsessive behavior, undoing, rationalization)
Repression
Reaction formation
Displacement (conversion, phobias, wit)
Dissociation (neurotic denial)

Level IV: Mature Mechanisms (Common in "Healthy" Adults)
Altruism
Suppression
Anticipation
Humor

From Vaillant GE: *Adaptation to life,* Boston, 1977, Little, Brown.

logic in nature. Vaillant (1977) was able to develop a theoretic hierarchy of ego defenses, grouping them according to their relative maturity and pathology (Box 8-1). As ego defense mechanisms are dynamic and mature throughout the life cycle, individuals who successfully adapt are able to select from a range of defense mechanisms to deal with problems. In healthy adults these successful mechanisms include altruism, suppression, anticipation, and humor.

The adaptation theory as described by Vaillant (1977) is more of a conceptual model that categorizes the changes brought about by aging. Vaillant identified a series of shifts and trade-offs that occur during the aging process. What is critical to successful adaptation is the ability of the individual to let go of parts of the past while pursuing quality-of-life components. For example, the older person often experiences sensory losses, especially in the areas of vision and hearing, and adapts to such losses by facilitating the quality of the remaining sensory perceptions. For example, the use of large-print books, direct lighting, or hearing aids would enhance the older person's remaining sight and hearing. Encouraging the use of other sensory perceptual systems such as touch or taste would be another way for the older individual to gather pertinent information from the environment (see Understanding and Applying Research box).

LIFE SPAN TRANSITIONS

Many young adults anxiously anticipate a "mid-life transition" as they enter middle adulthood. As previously discussed, Levinson noted that, for many, this "transition" is a period of struggle or crisis (Myers, 1998). Levinson believed that up to 80% of persons experience such a period of crisis. Recent research has examined the possibility of a possible mid-life crisis and whether it is universal throughout cultures and genders.

Midlife Transitions

Middle age is typically characterized by physical changes and new responsibilities of taking care of children, grandchildren, and older parents. Also, middle-age adults may assume new work responsibilities and subsequently feel a need to reappraise their life situations and make changes while they still have the time (Huyck, 1997). The term *midlife crisis* (Jaques, 1970) described a point in time when individuals experience a life crisis as their own mortality becomes real (Shek, 1996). These realizations often result in negative outcomes such as perceptions that health is deteriorating, bad feelings about marital relations or work, inability to enjoy leisure time, and stress from caring for aging parents (Shek, 1996). The focus shifts from, "How long have I lived?" to "How many years do I have left?"

Daniel Shek examined the concept of mid-life crisis among adults from Chinese descent. He found that some of the participants were unhappy with work and personal achievements, but most did not indicate dissatisfaction that would be considered at crisis level. Other studies (McCrae, 1984) also support the view that mid-life crisis is not a universal phenomenon, nor does it cluster around any particular age group.

The work of Arnold Kruger (1994) also focused on the presence of a mid-life crisis in middle-age adults. He con-

cluded that the "symptoms" of a mid-life crisis are reflected by criteria in the DSM-IV for adjustment disorders. Adjustment disorders are described as "problematic responses to life events" (see Chapter 18). Myers (1998) further challenged the idea of adult stages of development, noting that particular life events (working, getting married, having children, retiring) vary among cultures. For example, 40% of Jordanian women marry in their teens; that number is about 3% in Hong Kong. Regarding retirement, six times the number of men over the age of 65 years in Mexico continue to work compared with men in the United States or Europe (Myers, 1998).

Role of Stress in Adult Development

The negative effects of stress on aging are well documented. A growing body of research confirms that stress plays a part in hastening cognitive and memory decline, and it may even speed aging changes in the very structure of the brain (Aldwin, 1994). The effects of stress on adult development are complex. Some researchers are examining the possibility that stress may actually have a positive benefit to adult development. In many cases, individuals who have experienced a very stressful life event find that they have "learned from the experience" in the long run, gaining new coping skills, increasing their self-knowledge, or enhancing social networks. These persons often feel that these stressful experiences "made them a better person." Further research needs to be done in this area, as it is difficult to generalize these findings across all adult populations.

Gender Differences in Adult Development

As research in adult development has evolved, particularly in the areas of adult personality and adult learning concepts, gender differences have become apparent. Some studies focused on a *trait approach* to adult personality that suggests personality is constant or stable over time. These studies also highlight gender differences in their approaches to adult development.

Personality is continuous for the most part, but there are some gender and age-related differences. The most stable aspects of personality include coping styles, life satisfaction factors, and goal-directed behaviors. Neugarten (1979) noted the following changes with aging:

- From ages 40 to 60 years, there is a shift from feeling in control over one's environment to perceiving the environment as more threatening, referred to as a change from *active* to *passive mastery*.
- Older adults become more *introspective and self-reflective* as they age.
- There are shifts in *sex-role expressiveness* between men and women. Men take on a more nurturing role, and women become more accepting of their aggressive tendencies.
- Older adults tend to become more *introverted*.

The Baltimore Longitudinal Study began in the 1950s and focused on the conceptualization of personality according to the *Five-Factor Model of Personality* (McCrae, 1984). Differences in personality were found; for example, men became less masculine and demonstrated a lower activity level with increased age.

Life Events Framework

The life events framework proposes that major life events result in stressful circumstances that individuals respond to by changing their personalities (Miller, 1997). The model recognizes individual differences, unlike the stage theories such as Levinson's, which focus on similarities among individuals. The author noted that life events may or may not necessarily be age linked, particularly those that are not biologically driven such as menopause or death. Critics note that the life events framework:

- Places too great an emphasis on change
- Fails to recognize stability of personality characteristics
- Focuses to a great extent on the impact on major life events, but does not recognize the impact of daily annoyances or aggravations that may have additive effects.

Optimum Growth

Erikson (1974a, 1974b) described what is necessary to sustain a person's opportunity and ability to grow and mature. He noted that vital individual strengths arise from the stages of life. These strengths include faith, willpower, purposefulness, competence, fidelity, love, care, and wisdom. Slowly, there is a paradigm shift occurring with increasing longevity. Growth and maturity are being looked on as dynamic processes, many of which are under the control of individuals, that lead to new opportunities and rewards in later life.

ADULT DEVELOPMENT IN LATER LIFE

Advances in health care sciences have ensured that a larger proportion of people will be living longer with a better quality of life. More than ever as we enter the twenty-first century, aging is viewed as an evolutionary process. Aging is a complex process involving biologic, psychologic, social, and environmental factors. How a person adapts to aging is very individualized, and no single theory adequately explains the effects of aging from a developmental perspective. New theories of aging are attempting to integrate biologic and behavioral changes to view aging as a series of life events.

The process of aging is described as a series of physiologic and psychosocial changes. It is important that psychiatric nurses understand normal and abnormal aging changes and their impact on such factors as activities of daily living (ADLs), mental processes, social supports, sexuality, and role development. For older adults, their physical and mental health represents the summation of health care beliefs and practices across the years. The psychiatric mental health nurse needs to consider the older person's perceptions of health and wellness as key information in the assessment and management of care.

Changing attitudes and images of aging have important implications for the psychiatric mental health nurse. Jung stated that we would not grow to be 70 or 80 years old if this longevity had no meaning for the species. Two decades ago that concept was poetically stated as follows: "The afternoon of human life must also have a significance of its own and cannot be merely a pitiful appendage to life's morning" (Campbell, 1979). This is even more significant in the new millennium. Scientists are beginning to heed those words, focusing on successful aging processes as reality rather than an ideal.

Overview of the Older Adult Population

Because more than 70% of all health care resources are used by those age 65 years and older, it is imperative for all health care professionals to understand basic gerontology (U.S. Bureau of the Census, 2000). *Gerontology* is defined as the study of the aging process across multiple disciplines and settings. Gerontologists who receive specialized training and education in the field of aging may be found in many disciplines including nursing, medicine, psychiatry, social services, pharmacology, biology, and the humanities. The term *geriatrics* broadly refers to the health care and human services that are provided to older adults (Eliopoulos, 2001).

Demographics

During the last 100 years the average growth rate of the population age 65 years and older has greatly surpassed the overall population rate according to the U.S. Census Bureau (2000). From 1900 to 2000 the older population increased more than 11-fold, from 3 million to 35 million. In comparison, the total population tripled during that same period. By 2050, projections show a marked increased in the older population to more than 80 million persons. With the aging of the baby boomers, one in five individuals will be over 65 years in 2030. Older adult minority groups, including African Americans, Asians and Pacific Islanders, Native Americans, and Hispanics, will see substantial population growth into the middle of the twenty-first century.

The most rapidly growing group of the older population are those age 85 years and older, termed the *oldest old*. Currently 1.3% of the U.S. population is in this age cohort. By 2050 this group will grow to 19 million, or almost one fourth of the entire older population (U.S. Bureau of the Census, 2000). Table 8-7 presents findings from the recent report, "Sixty-five Plus in the United States," showing several important characteristics of the older population now and in the future.

Health Status

Overall older adults report that their health is good to excellent (Rowe and Kahn, 1998). Socioeconomic status and availability of social support have direct effects on reports of health. Minority groups and those with low incomes consistently report poorer health, even when age is controlled. Be-

Table 8-7	Profile of the Older US Population: 1990 and 2050 Comparisons	
Ethnic Group	Older Population in 1994 (%)	Older Population in 2050 (%)
Caucasian	87	67
African American	7	10
Native American	<1	<1
Asian, Pacific Islander	3	7
Hispanic	3	16

Other Facts

Sex ratios will continue to decline (number of males per 100 females) as age increases:
- Ratio of 82 males 65-69 years old
- Ratio of 44 for males 85-89 years old
- Ratio of 26 for males 95-99 years old

Eight states will double their older population by 2020: Nevada, Arizona, Georgia, Washington, Alaska, Utah, Colorado, and California.

Increasing numbers of older women live in poverty compared with older men:
- Currently 16% of older women are at or below poverty level, compared with 9% of men.
- 2 million of the 2.3 million older poor living alone are women.
- Poverty rates are higher for older minorities.

Modified from U.S. Bureau of the Census: Sixty-five plus in the United States. In *Current Population Reports*, P23-190, No. 178RV, special studies, Washington, DC, 1996, US Department of Commerce, Economics and Statistics Administration.

cause both males and females are living longer, a greater proportion of couples are surviving into old age. Older adults of today are more educated, with a greater portion having completed some college. More than 22% of persons age 65 years and older completed at least 1 year of college, compared with 12.5% in 1970. Older adults also maintain better health care practices than some of their younger-age cohorts. The most recent data from the U.S. Department of Health and Human Services (1993) reported that older persons had better dietary habits and smoked and consumed alcohol to a lesser extent than those less than 65 years old. Only in the area of physical exercise did older adults report less activity than younger age groups.

Although a majority of older adults across all settings suffer from at least one chronic condition, illness in itself does not appear to influence individual perception of health status if functional abilities are not impaired. Functional ability is categorized as ADLs and instrumental ADLs (IADLs). Physical and psychosocial functions are included in a functional assessment. Assessing functional abilities of older adults is discussed later in this chapter.

A LIFE SPAN PERSPECTIVE OF AGING

Gerontologists in a variety of scientific fields have attempted to explain the developmental processes of aging from biologic and behavioral perspectives. A variety of theories on aging exist because scientists do not agree on a single definition of aging. Chronologic, biologic, psychologic, and so-

cial definitions of aging have been described extensively in the literature but they do not adequately describe the process of aging. Therefore scientists and philosophers have developed theories to explain the meaning, causes, and factors related to the aging process.

Biologic Theories of Aging

Biologic theories of aging are classified into various categories based on causative factors. Most biologic theories view the process of aging as either a normal, gradual wearing down of all systems or an abnormal series of cellular damage or mutations eventually leading to the body's inability to make repairs (Schneider and Rowe, 1990).

One method of classifying biologic theories of aging relates to categorizing predisposing factors as intrinsic or extrinsic to the organism. Intrinsic, or genetic, theories focus on the process of aging as internal to the organism. It is estimated that up to 30% of one's life expectancy is genetically determined, with lifestyle and environmental influences having more profound effects on aging than what was earlier believed (Finch and Tanzi, 1997). Certain genetic diseases, including several types of cancers and high cholesterol syndromes that lead to heart disease, have a negative impact on life expectancy (Rowe and Kahn, 1998).

Extrinsic or nongenetic theories propose that aging occurs as a result of environmental factors acting on the organism, such as radiation, ozone, drugs, and toxic substances, which have been theorized to damage cellular structures, leading to aging and death.

Researchers have not agreed on any single biologic theory to explain the aging process. A combination of genetic and environmental factors may best explain why individuals age differently. Four biologic theories of aging most examined by researchers follow.

Genetic Theory

The genetic theory of aging represents a group of intrinsic aging theories, all of which focus on an internal genetic code that drives the aging process. The premise of the theory is that genes are categorized as juvenescent or senescent. *Juvenescent* genes promote and maintain growth and vigor through the adult years, whereas *senescent* genes become active in middle adult and later years and initiate a process of decline and deterioration. Empiric evidence to support the theory of this "aging" gene is lacking.

Another popular genetic theory is known as the *biologic clock theory* (Schneider and Rowe, 1990) and suggests that an organism's development and subsequent decline are regulated by some programmed internal genetic clock. This internal clock runs down over a predetermined length of time. Supporters of this theory point to certain normal physiologic changes in humans that appear to be correlated with time, such as hair graying and menopause.

Although the biologic clock theory gives dramatic evidence for boundaries of the human life span, there are limitations to this theory. One limitation is the inability to generalize in vitro studies to in vivo studies. Second, the theory does not explain what factor triggers the end of cellular replication and the beginning of cellular degeneration. Finally, the theory does not explain extreme cases of longevity.

A final genetic theory, *error theory,* has been suggested to explain the development of harmful genes that interfere with biologic processes such as protein synthesis (Hayflick, 1985). Damage to biologic synthesis results in the development of damaged cells that interfere with normal biologic functions. The proliferation of cancerous cells is an example of a process in which normal cells become aberrant through some error process.

Immunologic Theory

Most biologists agree that changes in the immunologic system after puberty influence the process of aging. Antibody production declines, and autoimmune responses change in response to the decline. The result is that the body's ability to differentiate normal and abnormal or foreign substances fails. This response is sometimes seen in cases of tissue rejection in organ transplantation.

Immune function significantly declines with aging. By age 85 years an individual's immune system functions at 5% to 10% of the system's level at puberty. Rheumatoid arthritis and mature-onset diabetes are two diseases commonly experienced in older age that are caused by alterations to the immune system. Although it is not exactly known how or why the immune system exhibits a functional decline with aging, the appearance of autoantibodies in the serum of older persons is common. Autoantibodies are antibodies particular to an individual's own normal serum or tissue. It is hypothesized that their appearance signals declines in immune system function (Mille, 1996).

Cross-Linkage Theory

Collagen tissue, an important component of connective tissue that maintains the structure of cells, tissues, and organs, undergoes changes with aging. Collagen provides the elasticity necessary in many types of tissue such as cardiac and muscle. With age the combination of chemical changes and external stimuli causes the formation of molecular bonds in collagen, or cross-links that tend to stabilize the collagen fibers, resulting in rigid, fragile tissue. Scientists do not understand the mechanism that triggers the formation of cross-links, but it is believed that the most active period of cross-link development is between age 30 and 50 years.

Cross-links also form in elastin in connective tissue. Elastin is similar to collagen in that it maintains tissue flexibility and permeability. The effects of cross-linking in elastin fibers are most pronounced in the changes in facial skin with aging. Skin becomes brittle, dry, saggy, and appears translucent. The formation of cross-links is probably not the sole cause of aging, but structural and functional changes associated with aging are affected by collagen alterations at the cellular level.

Free Radical Theory

Biologists theorize that some environmental stimuli, such as radiation, ozone, and certain chemicals, interfere with cellular activity, resulting in the production of free radicals, which are compounds produced in cells as a result of environmental stimuli. They may interact with various cellular structures, causing damage to normal cellular function. Free radicals are also formed during the normal process of cellular oxygenation when the cell removes waste products. Although the cell is capable of neutralizing and removing such by-products, it is theorized that over time the cell loses its capacity to eliminate waste and repair itself. Researchers are continuing to study the potential effectiveness of antioxidants such as vitamins A, C, and E, in protecting cellular structures.

Sociologic Theories of Aging

Sociologists have observed that an individual's role, relationships, and social experiences change as he or she ages. Sociologic theories of aging attempt to explain the social aspects of the aging process. Three of the earliest theories were developed in the 1960s. These three theories— *disengagement, continuity,* and *activity*—all take a different approach to the social aspects of aging. Common to the three theories is the focus on action and adaptation by the individual (i.e., the aging person needs to change or adjust to new situations). Relocation to a nursing home is often traumatic for the older person who cannot adjust to the highly structured institutional routines. Social theories that focus more on the interaction between the aging individual and the environment have evolved.

Disengagement Theory

The **disengagement theory** was the first sociologic aging theory developed by social gerontologists. In 1961 Cumming and Henry published the results of their exploratory study of 275 healthy, financially stable persons, ages 50 to 95 years, who lived in Kansas City. They theorized that a process of mutual withdrawal naturally occurs between the aging individual and society that is inevitable and universal in its occurrence. The retirement process is an example of this disengagement. Society clearly identifies the age of 65 years as the time for retirement. Identifying a retirement marker, or target, is also a mechanism for society to open the opportunity for a young person to enter the workforce. According to Cumming and Henry (1961), if the older person is prepared for retirement, he or she will have an easier time "disengaging" from society. The older person's social ties continue to shrink, perpetuating the individual's further withdrawal into self.

The disengagement theory has been the most controversial of the social aging theories. Most of the criticism focuses on its presumed universality and on the fact that it does not allow for biologic or personality differences between individuals. In addition, it presumes that the individual will see disengagement as an obligation to society. How ready and accepting older persons are to change roles determines their ability to adjust and, subsequently, their life satisfaction.

Havighurst, Neugarten, and Tobin (1968) reexamined the original data used to formulate the disengagement theory and arrived at different conclusions in support of disengagement. For example, they found that individual personality traits and past experiences influence how an individual in society adapts to aging. A person who is withdrawn early in life will probably continue to withdraw and adapt if his or her social ties also support withdrawal behaviors. Society today is less insistent that older adults completely disengage. For example, some industries are hiring retired persons on a part-time or per diem basis or using them as expert consultants. It is a combination of one's personal preferences and the needs of society, rather than personal preference or societal needs alone, that dictates the degree and pattern of disengagement.

Continuity Theory

The **continuity theory** was developed out of Havighurst, Neugarten, and Tobin's reformulation of the disengagement theory (1968). The basic premise behind the continuity theory is that people adapt best when they are allowed to be who they are and that, with aging, people become "more like themselves" (i.e., as an individual ages, he or she attempts to maintain continuity and consistency of habits, beliefs, norms, values, and other aspects of the personality). If a person is having difficulties adjusting to changes such as retirement or relocation, the continuity theory holds that it is not the process of aging that interferes with adaptation, but rather personality factors or the individual's social environment that influences adaptation. The continuity theory allows for individual differences in the aging process and theorizes that each individual's personality contains a self-maintaining component, meaning that the individual's longstanding behavior patterns enhance coping and adjustments to new situations across the life span (Atchley, 1989).

Activity Theory

The supporters of the **activity theory** believe that maintaining an active lifestyle and social roles offsets the negative effects of aging (Figure 8-2). Activity theorists postulated that, by retaining a high level of participation in his or her socioenvironment, the older individual would report a higher level of overall life satisfaction and a more positive self-concept. Four propositions were initially identified in the conceptualization of the activity theory (Lemon, Bengston, and Peterson, 1972):

- The greater the loss in social roles (both formal and informal), the less the activity participation.
- The more activity maintained, the greater the social role support for the older person.
- Maintaining stability of social roles supports a person's positive self-concept.
- The more positive a person's self-concept, the greater the degree of life satisfaction experienced.

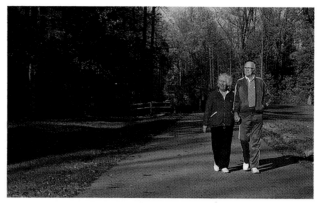

FIGURE 8-2. Physical exercise is good for the older population, as it is for any age group, and would be viewed by an activity theorist as possibly offsetting the negative effects of aging. (From Sorrentino SA: *Mosby's textbook for nursing assistants,* ed 4, St Louis, 1996, Mosby.)

Wider acceptance of the activity theory is hindered by the lack of empiric evidence to support these postulates. The importance, type, and availability of a particular activity as perceived by the older person is an important consideration affecting self-concept and life satisfaction. The activity theory may apply only to older persons who enjoy and have the opportunity to participate in meaningful activities and social interactions.

Psychologic Theories of Aging

Studying human behavior and attempting to explain why persons act the way they do have been the focus of developmental psychologists since Freud, the founder of psychoanalysis. Because in many cases older adults do not exhibit the same patterns of behavior as their younger counterparts, theorists developed psychologic theories and models of aging. Whereas sociologic theories of aging focus more on the interaction between the aging individual and his or her socioenvironment within an age *cohort* (group with one or more factors in common) or a culture, developmental psychologists examine human development from an *intrapsychic* or mental viewpoint. Few of the human development theories address characteristics of developmental change in older adults. Most of the developmental theories focus on a single area of one's *psyche*, or the center of thought processes, emotions, and behavior. For example, Freud's theory and practice focused on sexual aspects across the human life span. A focus on cycles or stages during which key developmental tasks or events are carried out is apparent in most of the developmental theories.

New Theories of Aging

In the realm of theory, theories of aging are considered to be in their infancy. This is especially true with psychologic theories, most of which were developed after World War II. New theories of aging include behavioral genetics, gerotranscendence, and gerodynamics theories.

Behavioral genetics theory examines the relevant impact of genetic and environmental factors on biologic and behavioral differences among individuals across the life span (Pedersen, 1996). *Gerotranscendence theory* looks at aging from three levels: cosmic, the self, and social relations. The theory implies that aging brings on changes such as (1) changes in time perception, (2) acceptance of the mysteries of life and death, (3) altruistic behavior, and (4) increased need for solitude and reflection (Tornstam, 1994). *Gerodynamics theory* is based on several physics theories, including general systems theory and chaos theory. Gerodynamics postulates that individuals pass through a series of transformations, or life events, and are thereby changed in some way (Schroots, 1995). Individuals respond differently and are either weakened or strengthened by the events. Those who age successfully have the ability to cope with traumatic events and maintain healthy lifestyles. As yet, these theories need additional empiric testing to support the concepts.

PROCESS OF AGING

The process of aging incorporates physiologic and psychosocial changes within the individual. As described in several of the biologic and psychosocial theories of aging, external or environmental factors affect aging in many ways. The physiologic changes that come with aging are universal. Because the changes that characterize normal physiologic aging mirror pathologic changes, normal and abnormal aging processes are often confused. Although aging is ultimately irreversible, disease and disability can be significantly delayed even into very old age (Rowe and Kahn, 1998).

Psychosocial changes during aging in the areas of cognition, personality, social interactions, sexuality, and roles are even less distinct. Personality and socioenvironmental factors play a huge role in determining psychosocial aging changes. Particular aspects of such processes as cognition and memory may decline with aging, whereas other aspects may remain the same or even be enhanced with advanced age.

Physiologic Aging

The physiologic aging changes considered part of normal aging affect all body systems, but not necessarily at the same rates. It is important to have an understanding of the common physiologic aging changes, as some of these changes may indicate the development of pathologic conditions. Many of these changes begin as early as the fourth and fifth decades of life. There are also individual differences in the rates of aging of some biologic systems because of factors such as heredity, environment, lifestyle, and nutrition (Steinberg, 1983).

Musculoskeletal System

Aging changes occur in bone and muscle mass, tendon and joint flexibility, and cartilage structure. It appears that bone continues to grow up to the eighth decade in some bony structures, but the resorption of the interior of flat and long bones occurs at a greater rate than bone growth. Also, bone minerals and proteins are lost from the bone matrix. Osteoporosis, or loss of bone mass, and loss of minerals, especially calcium, increase the possibility of fractures and subsequent immobility. Women are affected by osteoporosis twice as often as men.

Changes in joints begin about the third decade and continue throughout the remainder of the life span. With severe loss of cartilage and fluids, bones may begin to rub together, resulting in painful, slow movements. Changes in the vertebral column combined with osteoporosis cause a loss of sitting height with aging.

Cardiovascular System

Changes in the cardiovascular system as a result of aging are complex. Some of the changes that have been attributed to disease may be part of normal aging; thus it is difficult for researchers to separate normal from abnormal cardiovascular changes to a great extent (Lakatta, 1988).

With normal aging the size of the heart may decrease slightly as a result of loss of muscle cells. In the heart, muscle cells are replaced with fat cells and connective tissue that cause rigidity in the heart muscle. This results in a slower heart rate and decreased cardiac output. A decrease in oxygen consumption by the heart reflects decreased effectiveness of the heart. Changes in the structure of the heart muscle fibers may result in changes in the heart rhythm. Atrial dysrhythmias, including atrial fibrillation and atrial flutter, are common.

Blood pressure may increase to compensate for changes in atrial circulation. The structure of arteries changes with aging. Collagen fibers, lipids, and minerals increase in the walls of arteries and veins. These arterial changes also affect the baroreceptors that are important in moderating blood pressure during postural changes. This is reflected in the older person's complaint of dizziness when standing quickly.

Respiratory System

The respiratory system exhibits changes in its structure and function with aging (Kumpe et al., 1985). The diameter of the chest wall increases with age as a result of loss of lung resiliency and muscle strength, giving the appearance of a "barrel" chest. Lung compliance increases with aging, but the work of breathing increases because the chest wall compliance decreases. The ability to remove secretions through ciliary movement and coughing decreases with aging. The lungs of older adults stay partially inflated at rest as a result of an increase in residual volume. It is believed that changes in lung tissue with aging decrease pulmonary diffusion capacity, which results in decreased oxygen saturation. Under normal circumstances the older person puts less stress on the lungs; thus a slight decrease in oxygen use balances out the decrease in oxygen availability.

Gastrointestinal System

Changes in the gastrointestinal system with aging are not well understood. Most of the gastrointestinal changes are due primarily to disease rather than to aging alone.

Decreased motility of the esophagus may lead to spasm and reflux. Delayed emptying of stomach contents may occur as a result of decreased motility and acid secretion. Decreased absorption of vitamins, nutrients, and water also results from diminished muscle tone and changes in vascular perfusion (Bowman and Rosenberg, 1983).

The size of the liver decreases with age and results in decreased blood flow, protein synthesis, and metabolism of some drugs. The potential for serious toxic effects of drugs that are metabolized in the liver should be closely monitored through blood levels.

The formation of stones in the gallbladder increases with aging. It is believed that the absorption of cholesterol is less efficient as one ages, resulting in stone production. Changes in the pancreas with aging primarily affect enzyme production, but not to a degree that significantly affects normal digestive processes in the absence of disease.

Integumentary System

Changes in the skin, hair, and nails are most pronounced with advancing age. A loss of subcutaneous fat, thinning of the dermis and epidermis, and loss of elastin flexibility are responsible for the wrinkling and saggy appearance of the skin. Fragility of the dermal vasculature causes *senile purpura,* a condition that appears as bruises under the skin.

Sometimes the loss of skin turgor in older adults is mistaken for dehydration. Decreased skin turgor results from a combination of less body water and subcutaneous fat and a loss of flexibility of the skin's elastin. Dryness of the skin also increases with aging as a result of a decrease in the number and size of sweat glands and reduced hormonal levels.

Changes in hair production and appearance occur with aging. Decreased melanin production results in the appearance of gray hair. Genetics influence the onset of gray hair. Hair also grows more slowly with aging and becomes coarse and thick in such areas as the nose, ears, and eyebrows, whereas general body hair thins.

The growth of nail tissue also decreases with aging. Years of use or injury may cause changes in the appearance of nails. Yellowing, the formation of ridges, or thickening of the nails may be observed in older individuals.

Immune System

The ability of the body to form antibodies to some antigens such as pneumococcal and influenza vaccines is greatly reduced in older adults. Delays in hypersensitive reactions also come with aging. Across the life span, the older individual's immune system was required to fight off exposure to many pathogens, with the additive effect resulting in more frequent and severe infections in older adults.

The thymus, a small organ above the heart, is important to the development of the immune system. The thymus produces hormones that assist with the maturation of T lymphocytes, which are one type of lymph cell that may ward off cancer cells. The actual number of T lymphocytes does not decline with aging, but the ability of T lymphocytes to proliferate in the presence of particular viruses decreases significantly. Therefore the older person has a more difficult time developing defense mechanisms to infections such as pneumonia, bronchitis, and bloodstream infections.

CLINICAL ALERT

Because many drugs are excreted through the kidneys, it is important to test creatinine clearance, which is an indicator of the proportion of muscle mass. Reduced creatinine clearance indicates a decrease in muscle mass, so dosages of medication that are absorbed by the kidneys may need to be reduced for older clients.

Renal System

The renal system is critical in the removal of a variety of waste products and drugs and in the regulation of fluid volume in extracellular space. With normal aging, the functioning of the renal system decreases significantly, although the remaining kidney functions are usually adequate. Changes to the kidney as a result of aging include loss of glomeruli, loss of total kidney tissue mass, and a decreased glomerular filtration rate. Glomeruli are small structures in the kidney made up of clusters of blood capillaries. The rate and degree of changes to the kidneys are highly variable; therefore researchers believe that aging is not the chief cause of the structural and functional changes. Because cardiac output decreases as a result of aging, the elimination of waste products is affected.

Nervous System

Unlike cells of other body systems, the cells of the nervous system do not reproduce. There is a loss of nerve cells with normal aging, but the degree of loss differs, depending on the structure of the nervous system. The aging pigment, lipofuscin, is deposited in nerve cells, and neurofibrillary plaques and tangles form in the aging brain. These plaques and tangles may indicate Alzheimer's disease but are found in normal aging brains in the absence of dementia (also see Chapter 14).

The amount of neurotransmitters also decreases with normal aging. Changes in cognitive functioning such as memory storage may be affected by a decrease in acetylcholine and epinephrine. Because of the redundancy of nerve cells, it is impossible to generalize that all older persons have diminished memory or cognitive abilities. Decreases in another neurotransmitter, serotonin, is also part of normal aging. Serotonin is important in the regulation of activities such as sleeping, drinking, and breathing. Serotonin also affects temperature regulation, heart rate, and affect. Reductions in the amount of serotonin result in the older person's inability to respond to physical and psychologic stressors in an appropriate manner (see Chapters 3 and 10).

The sleep cycle is influenced as a result of the normal aging process. Older adults usually complain of frequent periods of restlessness or insomnia. They may go to the bathroom often during the night and, as a result, they may nap during the day to make up for the loss of night sleep. Periods of rapid eye movement (REM) sleep are also decreased with aging.

CLINICAL ALERT

The use of sedatives over an extended time should be discouraged because the older person's normal pattern of sleep usually recurs after only a few nights of sedative use. Frequent periods of sleeplessness should be monitored because the possibility of an underlying physiologic or psychologic problem may be a precipitating factor.

UNDERSTANDING and APPLYING RESEARCH

How women with breast cancer adapt to the illness and its effects is influenced by personal history, psychosocial stage, and life concerns. Breast cancer is experienced differently by women at different psychosocial life stages. This review of the literature presents an overview of how breast cancer affects women across the life span. With extended life span, older women are beginning to experience some of the same dramatic alterations that younger women have typically faced, as many continue in the workforce, are raising children at older ages, and may be caring for parents themselves. Implications for nursing practice and research are discussed. Nurses need to consider interventions for women with breast cancer in the context of psychosocial life stages, as women of different ages may have distinct views of their illnesses. Researchers need to consider developmental stages of women with breast cancer related to examining quality of life issues. Along with age, the effects of ethnicity and social status need to be examined from a life-stage perspective.

Sammarco A: Psychosocial stages and quality of life of women with breast cancer, *Cancer Nurs* 24:272-277, 2001.

Reproductive System

In females, menopause, or the permanent cessation of menses, occurs at around age 51 years. Ovarian estrogen ceases to be produced, but adrenal estrogens continue to be manufactured. Menopausal women commonly complain of hot flashes, or intermittent sensations of warmth and palpitations in the upper body. Hot flashes lessen in frequency with aging. There is a narrowing of the vagina and a decrease in vaginal secretions. The uterus, ovaries, and cervix also decrease in size as a result of vascular and muscular changes (see Understanding and Applying Research box).

In males the production of androgen hormones decreases with aging. The consequences of reductions in androgen to aging are not yet known. Androgens may affect the libido and nocturnal erections, but they do not appear to influence erections resulting from the presence of erotic stimuli. The changes in testosterone levels with aging are not agreed on at this time. Although not well studied, the production of sperm, or spermatogenesis, seems to be sustained well into old age in the absence of disease. Physically the testes and penis may decrease in size, and the scrotal sac becomes pendulous.

Many health care providers erroneously believe that the physiologic changes to the reproductive system resulting from aging mean that the older person's sexuality is also impaired. This has become a self-fulfilling prophecy for some older individuals who think that sexual pleasures are taboo in the later years. Many older persons do enjoy various forms and degrees of intimacy, and caregivers need to encourage such feelings.

Endocrine System

Changes in the endocrine organs and the hormones they secrete vary with aging. The endocrine organs are highly interrelated; thus a change in one system usually affects the others. Researchers believe that focusing on preventing some endocrine changes may hold the greatest promise for reducing the occurrence of disabilities and disorders of older adults. The endocrine system is composed of the following organs:

- Adrenal glands
- Thyroid gland
- Parathyroid glands
- Pancreas
- Pituitary gland

The adrenal glands appear to decrease in size with aging. The major hormones secreted by the adrenal glands (i.e., cortisol, aldosterone, and the adrenal androgens) decrease in amounts, but the functional implications of these reductions are not well understood.

The thyroid gland atrophies with aging and undergoes some structural changes such as the development of fibrotic tissue and nodules. Thyroid hormonal production decreases with aging, but the impact appears to be minimal, as there is less need for these hormones into old age. The parathyroid hormone may decrease or increase with aging. It appears that the parathyroid hormone increases in the presence of osteoporosis, as it is a factor stimulating bone demineralization.

The secretion of the hormone insulin by the pancreas appears to decrease with aging, resulting in a decreased ability of older adults to metabolize glucose. Insulin is necessary to the metabolism of blood glucose and for maintenance of normal blood glucose levels in the body. Recent studies have demonstrated that the amount of total insulin produced by the body remains the same across the life span; thus the problem for older adults may be that release of the available insulin is delayed in some still unknown manner.

The pituitary gland, which secretes several hormones, undergoes structural changes with aging in its cellular and vascular components. With aging there is a decline in growth hormone and an increase in levels of follicle-stimulating and luteinizing hormones. Alterations in mechanisms that regulate the secretion of thyroid-stimulating hormones, adrenocorticotropic hormones, and antidiuretic hormones are believed to occur with aging, but further research is needed before the significance of these changes for older adults can be determined.

Sensory System

The senses of vision and hearing decline with aging. Everyone experiences some visual changes as a part of the normal aging process. The lens of the eye continues to grow throughout aging, but the appearance of the lens changes. The lens becomes rigid and transparent and loses the ability to accommodate or adjust to changing distances—a condition commonly known as *presbyopia*. The pupil decreases in size and becomes less responsive to light. The ability to discriminate color in the blue, green, and violet hues becomes less distinct (Carter, 1982). Decreases in the lacrimal secretions result in feelings of dryness in the eyes. *Arcus senilis*, a condition that appears as a white circle around the iris, is due to lipid deposits and is considered a definite normal result of aging.

Hearing loss is gradual with aging and occurs in about one third of individuals age 75 years and older (Olsho, Harkins, and Harmon, 1985). Diminished ability in hearing acuity related to perception of tones is known as presbycusis. Increases in earwax in the ear canal and external noise also contribute to presbycusis.

It is believed that taste sensation is not markedly changed as a result of normal aging and that changes in taste sensation may be due to individual perceptions. The sense of smell appears to have minor decreases with aging, although environmental exposures to smoke or chemicals influence changes in the sense of smell over the life span.

Changes in the sense of touch during aging are complex and highly individualized. There are few changes to tactile nerve endings, but dermal changes may decrease touch sensation acuity in older adults. Although some older persons experience a decreased pain threshold, others experience an increased pain threshold, and it appears that past experiences with pain are an influential factor in pain perception.

The sense of proprioception, or kinesthetics, refers to the individual's sense of balance and orientation in space. As a result of skeletal and inner ear structural changes with aging, the person's sense of orientation, and especially of balance, may be severely compromised. The older person also has difficulty regaining a sense of balance.

Functional Assessment

In view of all of the physiologic changes older adults experience throughout the life span, most individuals are able to cope with the minor aches and pains attributed to normal aging. It is when the older person's ability to function and carry out ADLs independently is hindered that coping mechanisms may fail. Most situations that bring the older person to the primary care practitioner involve an inability to carry out specific functional tasks. Therefore it is important to assess the older person's functional status and its effect on the person's daily life (Table 8-8).

Functional assessment usually consists of evaluating two areas. The first area, ADLs, includes categories of personal care such as bathing, grooming, toileting, and transferring. The second area, IADLs, addresses activities important for the individual to function in the community. IADLs include shopping, preparing meals, and getting around. Box 8-2 highlights the major categories of ADL and IADL assessment.

Box 8-2	ADL and IADL Functional Assessment Categories
ADL Categories	**IADL Categories**
Bathing	Shopping
Dressing	Meal preparation
Hair care	Transportation
Mouth care	Use of telephone
Nutrition/assist with feeding	Medication usage
Ambulation/mobility	Housekeeping
Mental status	Laundry
Elimination	Financial management

Activities of Daily Living

ADLs focus on the physical skills necessary to function from day to day. A recent study by the U.S. Department of Health and Human Services (1993) reported that 12.9% of the total population age 65 years or older reported having at least one ADL problem. Older African Americans and Hispanics tended to have more difficulties with ADLs (Federal Interagency Forum on Aging Related Statistics, 2000). Older adults reported having the greatest amount of difficulty bathing, walking, and transferring between the bed and chair.

Several ADL assessment instruments are available. A good ADL instrument should be able to discriminate between physical and cognitive sources of the limitations. ADL scales typically categorize activity limitations in one of two ways. One type of ADL scale classifies limitations as present or absent. This scale fails to differentiate degrees of ADL limitations. The value of an ADL assessment tool is in its ability to identify areas for interventions. The Katz Index of ADL (Katz et al., 1963) is a valid, objective tool that measures six areas of function: (1) bathing, (2) dressing, (3) toileting, (4) transferring, (5) continence, and (6) feeding. The degree of limitation in each category is measurable. For example, in assessing transfer ability, the caregiver selects from one of the following three choices:

1. Moves in and out of bed or chair without assistance (may be using an object for support such as a cane or walker)
2. Moves in or out of bed or chair with assistance
3. Does not get out of bed

The Katz Index of ADLs was developed and tested with older subjects across a variety of settings and is considered a reliable measure of function in the older population.

Instrumental Activities of Daily Living

The ability of the individual to function in the community is an important aspect of the functional assessment. Approximately 17.5% of older adults report difficulty with at least one IADL (U.S. Department of Health and Human Services, 1993). Transportation, or getting around in the community, was most often identified as a problem area, followed by difficulty with shopping and light household chores.

Table 8-8 Functional Assessment of Common Physiologic Aging Changes

System	Normal Aging Changes	Areas for Functional Assessment
Musculoskeletal	↓Muscle strength ↓Body mass ↑Fat deposit ↓Bone mass ↓Joint mobility ↓Sitting height	Activity/exercise tolerance Joint pain on movement Gait, balance, and posture Susceptibility to falls Ability to perform ADLs and IADLs
Cardiovascular	↓Cardiac output ↓Basal metabolic rate ↓Cardiac performance ↓Arterial circulation ↑Peripheral resistance ↑Systolic blood pressure	Adaptation to stress Activity/exercise tolerance Orthostatic hypotension
Respiratory	↓Elasticity of chest walls ↑Anteroposterior diameter of chest ↓Intercostal muscle strength ↑Rigidity of lung tissue ↑Residual capacity ↓Cough reflex	Cough reflex Ability to blow out candle with open mouth Use of accessory muscles
Gastrointestinal	↓Saliva production ↓Motility ↓Gastric acid production ↓Absorption of nutrients ↓Drug metabolism	Condition of teeth/denture fit Dental hygiene Swallow reflex Frequency/size of meals Pattern of elimination Drug blood levels (metabolized by liver) History of constipation
Integument	↑Wrinkling of skin ↑Dryness of skin ↓Skin turgor ↑Thinning, graying body hair ↓Nail growth ↑Nails thicken, yellow	Assess for skin breakdown, especially over bony prominences Assess hydration status Susceptibility to infection
Immune	↓Size of thymus gland ↓Antibodies ↑Healing time	Assess for secondary infections History of allergies
Renal	↓Mass of kidney ↓Nephrons ↓Glomerular filtration rate ↓Nitrogen waste removal	Criterion for renal function is creatinine clearance Maintain adequate hydration Assess for incontinence
Nervous	↓Nerve cells ↓Neurotransmitters ↓Blood flow to central nervous system ↑Lipofuscin ↑Plaques and tangles ↓REM sleep	Response to pain is highly individualized Diminished deep tendon reflexes Complaint of restlessness/frequently go to bathroom May have memory changes
Reproductive	↓Estrogen production ↓Size of clitoris, cervix, uterus, and ovaries ↓Free testosterone ↓Size of penis and testes	Support need for intimacy/sexuality Hormonal replacement
Endocrine	↓Production of adrenal gland hormones ↓Insulin release ↓Thyroid structure ↓↑Mixed changes to pituitary hormones	Response to stressors may be diminished
Sensory	↓Vision (loss of depth perception, accommodation, and visual acuity; increased glare) ↓Hearing (loss of sound conduction) ↓Odor recognition ↓↑Changes in pain threshold ↓Sense of balance	Need for increased illumination Need for corrective appliances Avoidance of night driving Assess tolerance to pain Assess thresholds for hot/cold Safety precautions

ADLs, Activities of daily living; *IADLs,* instrumental activities of daily living; *REM,* rapid eye movement.

There is a subjective, as well as objective, component of IADLs. Assessing the ability of the older person to perform daily skills needed to function in the community is important. In addition, the meaning of the activity to the individual needs to be assessed. For example, taking care of shopping needs may not be as important to an individual as housekeeping or meal preparation. An older individual who fears going out into the community because of safety issues may essentially become isolated. Another older person may have difficulty with chewing and swallowing, so that meal preparation seems like a difficult task.

Both aspects of the functional assessment, ADLs and IADLs, are relevant indicators for identifying outcomes of illness, both physical and mental. Often changes in ADLs and IADLs may be the forerunner of a new illness. Individuals respond differently to physical aging changes, so the ability to function independently is more predictive of outcomes of aging than physical aging changes alone.

Psychosocial Aging

Psychosocial aging changes typically focus on an individual's responses to particular events across the life span. Past coping mechanisms may not be effective in adjusting to stressful events in later life. The reason adaptation may be more difficult for older adults is that the life events of old age differ from those of younger ages. Miller (1990) distinguished the life events of older adults as follows:

- They are viewed as losses, rather than gains.
- They are most likely to occur close together with less time to adjust to each event.
- They are more intense and demand greater energy than is available for the coping process.
- They are longer lasting and often become chronic problems.
- They are inevitable and evoke a feeling of powerlessness.

Preparing for some life events may facilitate adjustment in old age. For instance, some employers offer preretirement counseling for older employees in preparation for retirement. Psychosocial aging changes are reflected in several areas, including cognition and memory, personality, social support, sexuality, and role status. From a developmental perspective, the meaningfulness of life events is important in determining patterns of psychosocial aging in these particular areas. A great deal of research is needed before any conclusion can be drawn regarding normal versus abnormal psychosocial aging. The following section explores the current state of knowledge on psychosocial aging from a developmental perspective.

Cognition and Memory

Probably no other area of aging research has been studied to such an extent as cognition, especially in the areas of intelligence and memory. Evidence on the development of cognitive functions into old age is coming to light with studies that have followed older subjects over time. It is now apparent that cognitive functioning shows as much variability in aging as do physiologic indicators (Christensen et al., 1994).

Several factors may contribute to the variability in cognitive functioning observed in older adults. These factors include health status, genetic profile, socioeconomic status, education, and lifestyle behaviors (Herzog and Wallace, 1997). In turn, cognitive losses often result in functional impairment and physical disabilities, causing a spiraling decline for the older person.

Cognitive behaviors are divided into several interrelated processes including intelligence, memory, attention, reaction time, and problem solving. These divisions are arbitrary and are based on the ways researchers typically study cognitive behaviors.

Studies of intelligence during the 1940s reported that older adults experience declines in all aspects of intelligence including knowledge acquisition, calculating, vocabulary, and abstract thought. The problem with these early studies was that the cross-sectional method was used to collect the data, with younger-age cohorts being compared with older cohorts in these studies. The younger-age cohorts consistently had higher intelligence scores on the various tests, prompting researchers to conclude that intelligence declines with aging (Woodruff, 1983). Later longitudinal studies, which followed the same older subjects over a period of time, found that intelligence showed little or no decline in healthy aging persons. Declines that occurred were in the oldest age cohorts (Schaie and Willis, 1991).

Horn and Cattell (1967) theorized that age-related differences in intelligence may be due to distinctions between two types of intelligence that seem to develop from birth. *Crystallized intelligence* develops from knowledge gained through the accumulation of experience and education. Crystallized intelligence may decline slightly, remain the same, or even increase with aging, depending on one's life experiences. On the other hand, *fluid intelligence* is affected by neurophysiologic processes across the life span. Declines in the nervous system with aging that affect one's attention span or reaction time reflect a loss of fluid intelligence. Instruments that measure intelligence using performance standards show declines in intelligence with aging (Birren and Schaie, 1985), and even these conclusions have been questioned by some gerontologists. Older adults may have shown an increased time in completing intelligence performance tests because they are more cautious and take additional time to make correct choices.

Much aging research is devoted to the study of memory processes during aging. It is unfortunate that society equates aging with memory loss. Older persons are often portrayed on television or in movies as forgetful. A common joke is, "There are three telltale signs you are getting old. The first is loss of memory, and the other two . . . I forget." There is much that is still unknown about the process of memory perception, storage, and retrieval.

Most of the early theories of memory focused on the three components of memory (i.e., perception or encoding, storage, and retrieval). Memory was categorized as short or long term, or as primary, secondary, or tertiary. These categorizations were based on the length of storage time and the process of retrieval.

Other memory theories focused on the encoding processes, which yield different types of information in various ways. For instance, information that is processed in a more complex manner, such as algebraic equations, is stored in a deeper area of memory and will last longer. Information that is easily recognized requires less attention; thus tasks such as starting a car are performed almost automatically. It is believed that automatic processing of information does not change with aging (Botwinick, 1984). Offering cues to older adults may help them recall information stored in deeper areas of memory.

Contextual theory of memory was developed from the information-processing model. This theory expands the information-processing model by including individual factors that may impact memory, such as learning behaviors, past experiences, personality, degree of motivation, physical health, and socioeconomic status (Perlmutter et al., 1987).

Certain types of memory decline as a part of normal aging. *Explicit memory,* the ability to recall a specific name or place, tends to decline in aging (Rowe and Kahn, 1998). *Working memory,* the type of memory needed to perform daily activities, does not show an aging decline. Because older adults may take longer to process information (also normal to aging) and have some specific recall problems, they often fear that this is a harbinger of Alzheimer's disease. It is important to dispel this myth and to encourage older adults to seek ways to improve cognitive functioning through training and practice.

Self-perception of memory changes and self-efficacy also influence memory performance (Ryan, 1992; Ryan and See, 1993). The concept of *metamemory* refers to one's self-perceptions of memory changes and their effect on memory processes (Hertzog, Dixon, and Hultsch, 1990). For example, an older person may falsely believe that memory loss is part of aging and perceive that forgetfulness indicates the start of memory decline. In reality, forgetting information may be due to a lack of attention to detail in a particular situation. Further study is needed to determine whether an individual can mentally control or influence the development of memory across the life span.

Attention span refers to the ability to concentrate throughout the performance of some task. With aging, the ability to maintain the attention span through completion of complex tasks diminishes because complex tasks require dividing one's attention among several tasks at the same time. Some of these normal aging changes with the attention span are misinterpreted as dementia. Two other segments of attention also show some decrements in aging. *Vigilance,* or the ability to sustain attention over longer periods of time, and *selective attention,* or the ability to discriminate and focus on relevant information, are less acute in older adults.

Increased reaction time/decreased speed of performance on intelligence tests is one of the most agreed on changes in normal aging, but its mechanism is not well understood. Unfamiliarity with performance tests or increased cautiousness caused by fear of failure and resulting in test anxiety may affect reaction time in older adults.

Problem-solving ability is considered a higher cognitive function. The complexity of the problem, past experiences, the amount of information that is irrelevant to a situation, and the individual's level of education are factors that influence problem solving. There is little known about normal changes in higher cognitive functioning during aging. Most older persons are able to live and function effectively in the community.

Personality

Personality traits develop over the life span and are influenced by internal and external environmental factors. Personality is molded by an individual's ability to cope with stress and adapt to change. It is reflected in how individuals perceive themselves in what is referred to as *self-concept.* In general, most personality traits remain stable during the aging process. Personality influences how an individual interacts and reacts within the socioenvironment (see Chapter 12).

Personality theorists have attempted to identify specific traits that predict successful aging. Individuals described as introverted are more self-centered and internalize behaviors and responses. Extroverted personalities focus more on the outside world and are described as outgoing. Certain personality traits may assist individuals in adapting to aging better than others. Successful aging is determined more by the individual's ability to adapt to change than by a particular category of personality traits.

Some traits may intensify with aging, such as that of cautiousness, which may be an effective safety mechanism for older adults. For example, the older person may tend to drive a car with more caution, drive only in daylight hours, or avoid high speeds. In unfamiliar situations or when several choices are available, older adults tend to act more cautiously. They also tend to prefer familiar tasks, places, or situations.

Locus of control is another aspect of personality that remains stable over time (Reid, Haas, and Hawkings, 1977). Individuals with an *internal locus of control* perceive that they actively control their own destiny. On the other hand, individuals with an *external locus of control* believe they have no control over their destiny and think that their behaviors have no effect on any outcomes. Another phenomenon, that of *secondary locus of control,* describes individuals with an external locus of control who learn to adapt to their beliefs. This has also been termed *learned helplessness.* These individuals learn dependency and prefer others to decide for them.

Social Support and Interactions

In an extensive review of the literature, Broadhead et al. (1983) presented Kahn and Antonucci's comprehensive definition of social support as interpersonal transactions that include one or more of the following behaviors: (1) expression of positive affect between individuals, (2) affirmation or endorsement of another person's behaviors, and (3) providing direct aid or assistance to another. Different individuals within one's social network may provide different types of support.

Hyde (1988) suggested that the quality, rather than the quantity, of social relationships is significantly related to life satisfaction among older adults. The quality of social support is a key area for interventions in the training of health care providers. Social support has been conceptualized as a communication process in which facilitation of communication skills improves the quality of support (Albrecht and Adelman, 1984).

Social networks are generally viewed as the web of social ties that surround a person and include several characteristics important in the study of health and well-being of older adults, including:

- Size of the social network
- Frequency of social contacts
- Density of the interactions
- Intimacy or closeness among members
- Durability of ties
- Geographic dispersion of members
- Reciprocity of assistance

Social networks and social supports are different concepts. Considering the network as the web or structure, social support refers to the emotional or tangible assistance obtained from the social resource network. Not all social ties are supportive, and not all social supports come from the closest social network such as a son or daughter living near older parents. Oxman and Berkman (1990) proposed a three-component model of social relationships that incorporates the quantitative and qualitative nature of social relationships. Because social relationships have been associated with subsequent physical and mental illness in older adults, an assessment tool that addresses the multidimensional aspects of social relationships is important. An example of some of the questions according to the dimensions being assessed is presented in Table 8-9 (Oxman and Berkman, 1990).

Sexuality and Intimacy

Physical aging changes related to the reproductive system occur in men and women. Psychologic aspects of sexuality and intimacy in older adults are influenced by several factors, including past experiences, attitudes toward intimacy, societal views about sexuality in older adults, and functional status.

Many older adults feel a newfound freedom in their sexual behaviors because they no longer need to focus on concerns regarding pregnancy. Hindering such feelings may be the unavailability of an acceptable partner, stereotypes that older adults are asexual, or fears of inability to initiate and maintain sexual performance. Older women probably experience the greatest effects because many become widowed or suffer from the effects of long-standing values about sexual taboos.

It has only been in recent years that older persons, and especially those over 80 years, have been subjects of studies of sexuality. Bretschneider and McCoy (1988) reviewed the available studies of psychosocial aspects of sexuality and aging. The following summarizes some of their findings:

- The frequency of sexual activity decreases with aging, but the interest and ability in sexual function do not necessarily decline with aging.
- Older individuals who are in normal health and functioning have the ability to maintain sexual activity.
- Declines in sexual activity are mostly related to lack of a partner, especially for women.
- Psychosocial factors that may impede sexual activity by older adults include stereotypic beliefs, attitudes, and personality factors.
- Sexual behaviors and beliefs generally remain stable across the life span.
- Men remain more sexually active than women across the life span.

Table 8-9	Social Relationship Components and Characteristics	
Components	**Characteristics**	**Sample Questions**
Social network	Marital status/confidant	Are you married? Is there any one special person that you feel very close and intimate with?
Structure and composition	Number, kinship	How many children/close family members do you have?
	Proximity	How many live within an hour's drive?
	Frequency and type of contact	How many do you have phone or letter contact with at least once per month?
Type and amount of social support and function	Emotional	How frequently did someone try to make you feel better about your illness in the past month?
	Tangible aid	How frequently did someone help you get your medication in the past month?
	Guidance	How frequently did someone suggest that you call the doctor in the past month?
Perceived adequacy of social support	General	In the past year could you have used more help with daily tasks than you received?
	Specific	How helpful was it for your children to try to make you feel better about your illness?

From Oxman T, Berkman L: Assessment of social relationships in elderly patients, *Int J Psychiatr Med* 20:65, 1990.

Role Transitions

Accompanying changes of aging are changes in roles for the older person. Some of these role changes are more obvious than others, and individuals adapt to role changes in different ways. The degree of importance attributed to a particular role by the individual influences how well the older person is able to cope with a role transition. From a developmental perspective, roles contain various tasks one must carry out in life. Each role carries with it different life tasks. Some tasks may be new to the person if the role is a completely new one, and other tasks may be similar to ones carried out early in life, as in role reversals.

Retirement. Retirement implies a major role transition for many individuals. Because individuals live longer and retire earlier, the retirement period may last for 30 to 40 years. Only recently have researchers begun to explore gender differences in adaptation to retirement. Adaptation to retirement appears to be affected more by the life events surrounding retirement than by the retirement process itself (Szinovacz and Washo, 1992). Particular life events may even precipitate retirement. For instance, a middle-age woman may take an early retirement because she needs to care for her older mother at home who has Alzheimer's disease. This individual's adjustment to retirement may be negatively affected because of a conflict between the woman's role in the workforce and her caregiver role.

Loss of a Spouse. A major role transition occurs after loss of one's spouse, when adaptation requires the survivor to assume tasks previously performed by the partner. Couples who have shared responsibilities across the life span have less difficulty with the role changes. Personality traits seem to influence adjustment to widowhood. For example, a widow may have deferred to her husband concerning finances, or the husband who lost his wife may not have learned how to cook or clean. If the surviving spouse can adapt to change, he or she will rapidly adjust and learn these tasks. The widower may also find himself the center of attention by family members who want to assist him, as well as by widows looking for male companionship.

Grandparent Role. The role of the grandparent is another transition. The grandparent who adjusts successfully can provide grandchildren with a viewpoint that may differ from that of the parents but be equally positive. Many grandparents take on the role of full- or part-time surrogate parents.

Role Reversal. When physical or mental deterioration is present, the roles of the parent and child may be reversed. Most often the oldest female child, on reaching middle age, may need to provide care for the incapacitated older parent. This is an especially difficult transition for the female middle-age child who has just completed raising her own children and who was planning her own retirement in a few years. If the caregiver is a middle-age man, it is often an awkward situation because his wife must adapt to a role for which she may have no emotional connection (i.e., caring for the older parent-in-law). Supporting the caregiver is as important as supporting the care receiver under these circumstances. Table 8-10 summarizes some normal aging changes discussed in this section and areas for functional assessment.

Mental Assessment

Gerontologists are attempting to develop adequate standardized tests designed specifically for older adults to assess their mental status and cognitive functioning. Designing reliable instruments for older adults continues to be a challenge because of the interrelationships among several factors including health status, physical/mental aging changes, socioenvironmental variables, and life events. Thus the context of what is considered normal development for an older individual should be the focus of any mental status assessment.

Several mental status assessment instruments have been designed to evaluate mental and cognitive functions. Most instruments examine mental status in view of the individual's ability to function in daily living activities. However, the mental status assessment is not sufficient to provide a diagnosis of a disorder. Other sources of information, such as the health history, physical examination, diagnostic/laboratory tests, and psychosocial factors, are required for diagnosing.

The mental status assessment of older adults includes the following areas: appearance, mood, communication, thought processes, perceptual motor abilities, attention, memory, consciousness, and orientation. Appearance, behaviors, and responses of the older client should be areas for attention by the health care provider performing the assessment. For instance, the older person may state that he or she has no suicidal ideations, but appearance may indicate self-neglect and behaviors may include withdrawing from social networks and accumulating drugs. Such discrepancies are important to identify.

Several screening instruments are available for the health care provider to provide a quick assessment of mental status. Each instrument addresses different areas of the mental status examination. Often these brief instruments provide an initial baseline of cognitive functioning to be used for further in-depth assessment and screening for diagnosis and subsequent interventions.

The Mini-Mental State Examination (MMSE) continues to be one of the most commonly used instruments to screen for cognitive disorders in older adults (Folstein, Folstein, and McHugh, 1975). Several dimensions of cognitive function are assessed, including orientation, memory, attention, and speech. Out of a total score of 30, normal persons score 25 and above, whereas individuals diagnosed with dementia score lower than 20 points.

Table 8-10 Functional Assessment of Common Psychosocial Aging Changes

Area	Normal Aging Changes	Areas for Functional Assessment
Cognition and memory	Normal crystallized intelligence ↓Fluid intelligence (slight, gradual) ↑Reaction time ↓Divided attention ↓Vigilance ↓Selected attention ↑Information-processing time ↑Cautiousness	Degree of external stimulation Environmental distraction Assess barriers to learning (e.g., sensory impairments, relevancy/level of information, learning environment) Assess factors influencing memory process (e.g., education level, learning style, past experiences, physical/mental health, motivation)
Personality	Stability of most personality traits ↑Cautiousness ↑Rigidity (slight)	Adaptive coping mechanisms Decision-making processes Adjustment to change (e.g., retirement, relocation, loss)
Social support and interactions	Perceived social support affected by several factors (personality, health status, past experiences, coping style) Changes in social network (size, intimacy, geographic dispersion, reciprocity of assistance) Changes in source of social support with aging	Attitude/perception of social support Past experience with social support Social network ties Types of social support needed Sources of social support
Sexuality and intimacy	Sexual behaviors/interests maintained across life span in absence of physical/mental disorders ↓Sexual activity in males ↓Intensity of sexual responses Lack of partner is greatest factor affecting sexual activity	Attitudes toward expressions of sexuality and intimacy Means to maintain sexual behaviors/interests Availability of privacy in environment Risk factors impeding sexual behaviors
Role transitions	Retirement Widowhood Grandparenting	Importance of past roles/tasks Responses to retirement Relation of life events to retirement Effects of retirement on spouses Impact of loss of spouse Ability to take on new tasks in ADLs/IADLs Social supports/network Relationships with children/grandchildren Parenting role

ADLs, Activities of daily living; *IADLs,* instrumental activities of daily living.

Another commonly used instrument is the Short Portable Mental Status Questionnaire (SPMSQ) (Pfeiffer, 1975). Although it is not adequate to provide a diagnosis of dementia, this tool provides a rapid assessment of mental status. Areas of cognitive function assessed by the SPMSQ include orientation, immediate and remote memory, thought processes, and attention span. The scoring also allows for differences in education and race (Figure 8-3).

HUMAN DEVELOPMENT IN THE TWENTY-FIRST CENTURY

Something historic will occur on January 1, 2011: the date that the first "baby boomer" will turn 65 years old. Society's entire perception of aging will continue to evolve over the next 20 to 30 years as the older adult population experiences unprecedented growth during that time frame. Images of aging and attitudes toward older persons are gradually changing for the better. As the aging society also grows more ethnically and racially diverse, cultural values about aging will

need to be reexamined. In fact, the entire body of knowledge on human development may need to be rewritten, as research in aging has begun to refocus efforts to understand successful aging. In particular, scientists are examining health, learning, and creativity as areas to promote quality of life for older adults.

Images of Aging

Images of aging and attitudes of society toward older adults have been changing over the last several years. Unfortunately, society has usually focused on the negative aspects of aging. The term **ageism** has been used to describe the stereotypic views of older adults (Butler, 1987). The myth of the "burden of the elderly" has been gradually dispelled with the growing body of scientific evidence disproving that "to be old is to be sick" (Rowe and Kahn, 1998).

In 1995 the American Association of Retired Persons (AARP) published a study entitled *Images of Aging in America* (Speas and Obenshain, 1995). The purpose of this

Short Portable Mental Status
Questionnaire

Instructions:

Ask questions 1–10 in this list, and record all answers. Ask question 4A only if patient does not have a telephone. Record total number of errors based on ten questions.

1. What is the date today? (month, day, year)

2. What day of the week is it?

3. What is the name of this place?

4. What is your telephone number?

4a. What is your street address? (Ask only if patient does not have a telephone.)

5. What is your street address?

6. When were you born? (month, day, year)

7. Who is the president of the United States now? (last name)

8. Who was president just before him? (last name)

9. What was your mother's maiden name?

10. Subtract 3 from 20 and keep subtracting 3 from each new number, all the way down.

Scoring

For Caucasian subjects with at least some high school education, but not more than high school education, the following criteria have been established:

0–2 errors	Intact intellectual functioning
3–4 errors	Mild intellectual impairment
5–7 errors	Moderate intellectual impairment
8–10 errors	Severe intellectual impairment

Allow one more error if subject has only grade school education.

Allow one more error for African-American subjects, using identical education criteria.

Allow one less error if subject has education beyond high school.

FIGURE 8-3. Short portable mental status questionnaire (SPMSQ). (From Pfeiffer E: A short portable mental status questionnaire for the assessment of organic brain deficit in elderly patients, *J Am Geriatr Soc* 23:433, 1975.)

report was to examine knowledge, perceptions, and attitudes about aging. Key results of this study are listed in Table 8-11. One's personal experience with older adults was the strongest predictor of perceptions and attitudes toward aging. Most Americans had misconceptions about older adults, reflecting a lack of knowledge about aging. On a positive note, respondents showed a lack of stereotypes and myths about aging. These findings have important implications for health care professionals who work with older adults.

Cultural Impact

Cultural beliefs also influence one's attitudes toward older adults. Culture influences the responses of older adults to health, illness, and treatment. Some cultures subscribe to health care practices or home remedies that may be in direct

Table 8-11	AARP Report on Knowledge, Perceptions, and Attitudes Toward Aging
Area	**Key Findings From Respondents**
Knowledge of aging	Most answered correctly 50% of the items from the Facts on Aging Quiz.
	Misconceptions related to the financial status of older adults, perceptions that most older adults are lonely or bored, that 10% of all older persons are institutionalized, and that the overall health of older adults will decline in the future.
	Respondents with more incorrect answers held more negative views of older persons; those with more correct answers held more positive views of older adults.
	A low level of knowledge was related to a low socioeconomic status and high anxiety about aging.
Stereotypes of the older adults	Poor health, disabilities, isolation, and financial problems were most often identified as problems for older adults.
	Younger respondents thought older adults did not receive the respect they deserved; older respondents thought they received the right amount of respect.
	Younger respondents overestimated the number of serious problems experienced by older adults.
	Personal experience with older adults had the greatest impact on perceived images of aging.
	Younger respondents described old age in chronologic years; older respondents saw old age in terms of health, attitudes, and level of activity.
	Respondents with less education and high anxiety about aging held more negative stereotypes about older adults.
Perceptions of the aging process	Physical dependency was the number one cause for anxiety related to aging for younger respondents.
	Minorities and low-income persons tended to be more anxious about aging.
	At least one half of respondents had some anxiety about health, independence, and finances in their future.

Modified from Spear K, Obenshain B: *Images of aging in America: final report, American Association of Retired Persons*, Chapel Hill, NC, 1995, FGI Integrated Marketing.

opposition to modern health care practices. The health care professional needs to examine his or her own feelings toward differing cultural beliefs and health care practices of older clients. The incorporation of some home remedies into the older client's care plan may increase compliance, given that these remedies are not in conflict with treatment.

Various cultures hold different views regarding aging. Since ancient times, the contributions of older adults to a so-ciety affect the status of older adults within a particular cultural group. For example, Far Eastern cultures value the wisdom of their elders and thus hold the older population in high esteem. In contrast, some primitive cultures may have considered older adults a burden, unable to hunt and provide for the tribe. Such cultures have been known to banish older adults from the tribe.

In the current Western culture there is greater support for views of successful aging. The focus on age has presented the public with issues relating to functional, economic, and political aspects of aging that future older persons will experience. The situation of today's older population may be the most optimistic in terms of availability of social and economic resources, but future generations of older persons may face difficult resource issues (Conrad, 1992). The costs may outweigh the contributions by future older persons in society, and cultural values toward older adults may change.

Refocusing on Healthy Aging

Perceptions of health and wellness develop across the life span and affect attitudes and behaviors related to health care practices. For older adults, their physical and mental health represent the summation of health care beliefs and practices across the years. The majority of older persons consider their health to be good to excellent (74.3% of those ages 65 to 74 years and 66.8% of those ages 75 years and older) (Federal Interagency Forum on Aging Related Statistics, 2000). Perceived health has been shown to affect disease and disability among older adults. Rogers (1995) found that in older persons suffering from multiple chronic conditions and disability, those who perceived their overall health as very good to excellent lived longer than persons who considered themselves to be in poor health.

The MacArthur Foundation Study (Rowe and Kahn, 1998) has brought together 10 years of scientific knowledge and expertise related to aging. They identify three components necessary for successful aging:

1. Avoidance of disease and risk factors
2. Maintaining high cognitive and physical abilities
3. Engagement with life through productive relationships and behaviors

Early identification of risk factors and disease prevention/health promotion behaviors can have a significant impact on the development and progress of several chronic diseases. For example, exercise is beneficial to older adults in prevention of heart disease, hypertension, and diabetes. A regular, moderate program of aerobic and strength training for older adults is both safe and effective in improving function.

Challenging the mind as well as the body is important to maintain mental capabilities. Not all cognitive processes decline in aging, and most of these changes occur very late in life. Older persons who maintain a high level of self-efficacy, a measure of one's self-esteem, appear to manage well both mentally and physically.

Maintaining social relationships and continuing some sort of meaningful activities contribute positively to aging.

Social networks often shrink for older adults who outlive their peers and relatives. Older persons find support in reciprocal relationships with friends or family members. Grandparents find joy in having their grandchildren visit for extended periods, offering a respite to the parents. In terms of productive activities, many older retirees remark that they are much busier after retirement, with new projects and volunteer work. With the aging of the baby boomers over the next 30 years, the focus on successful aging may be more of a reality than an ideal.

Refocusing on Learning and Aging

A large body of literature has focused on adult learning theory. In contrast to children, adults prefer self-directed learning and incorporate past experiences in new opportunities. Adults also prefer to learn about things that have application to their daily lives. Older adults can continue to learn well into their seventies or eighties. Physical limitations may affect speed of learning, so teaching methods need to be adapted for older learners. Older adults also should be given a choice as to how they best learn materials (i.e., auditory, visual, or tactile).

As much as possible, new learning by older adults should be linked to experiences or activities they are familiar with or have enjoyed, particularly those with a social component. For example, older adults who enjoyed the years raising their own children may join a foster grandparent program or a senior volunteer program where they can develop new relationships and learn about new resources. Intergenerational programs are also growing in popularity. Elementary and high schools are joining with senior communities to share learning experiences. Retired persons may teach young people about skills such as woodcrafting. In turn, young people would reciprocate and teach the older persons about computers and the Internet.

Refocusing on Creativity and Aging

In his book, *The Creative Age: Awakening Human Potential in the Second Half of Life* (2000), Gene D. Cohen provided striking evidence that the human potential for creativity continues well into old age. He found that although information processing slows down as one ages, older persons can go on to learn new information by modifying how they process this information through slowly digesting bits of data or thoughtfully asking questions to clarify key points. Studies on computer training of persons over the age of 65 years reported that practicing increased both the speed and accuracy of their computing.

In another example, older persons tend to have difficulty bringing up certain words. In contrast, persons in their eighties who keep on challenging themselves reading, writing, or doing crossword and word game puzzles have continued to grow their vocabularies. Recent research has even demonstrated links between creative activities and the consequential positive feelings with increased production of protective immune cells. Creativity may also be linked to delaying the onset of Alzheimer's disease. Continually challenging oneself mentally may be a way to build up "reserves" of neurologic structures and connections.

CHAPTER SUMMARY

- Whatever the directions and results of future studies on aging and human development, it is clear that human development cannot occur in isolation. The constant impact of biologic, psychosocial, and environmental factors creates a dynamic system in which human development occurs across the life span.
- Human development also begins at a much earlier age than was believed, and it continues into much later years than was ever anticipated.
- It is important for the psychiatric mental health nurse to consider that development is a continuous process. Although there are common "markers" of human development at particular ages, there is a great degree of human variation.
- External factors such as culture or traditions may also have a significant impact on human development, so the nurse must be aware of and take these factors into account in caring for clients.
- Understanding that many aspects of human development continue to evolve well into old age provides the nurse additional opportunities to promote and stimulate successful aging.

REVIEW QUESTIONS

1. To assess that a 4-year-old child is in the initiative versus guilt developmental stage according to Erikson, the nurse asks the mother:
   a. "Can she put on her socks?"
   b. "Does she participate in any activities with other children?"
   c. "Does she get upset when you leave the room?"
   d. "Does she do any chores to help you out at home such as making her bed or picking up her toys?"

2. A 3-year-old child who experiences intense anxiety during bowel training because the child's parents expressed extreme disapproval and frustration is an example of which theory:
   a. Freud's psychosexual—anal stage
   b. Erikson's psychosocial—autonomy versus shame and doubt stage
   c. Sullivan's interpersonal—childhood era
   d. Piaget's cognitive—preoperational stage

3. A 45-year-old female is admitted to the hospital for the first time. She complains of increased feelings of hopelessness, helplessness, and social withdrawal. She sleeps 10 to 12 hours a day and has lost 10 pounds. She complains of anhedonia and lethargy. She is diagnosed with major depression. Because of her age, the psychiatric nurse must consider the following as a causative factor:
   a. Midlife transition
   b. Hormonal imbalance
   c. Fear of death
   d. Postpartum depression

4. A 65-year-old male is admitted to the geriatric unit with confusion and disorientation. He was found by a neighbor to be wondering down the street without any clothes on. He was irritable on admission. This was his first psychiatric hospitalization. The psychiatric nurse must consider biologic causative factors for the symptoms to include:
   a. Dehydration
   b. Medication noncompliance
   c. Hypotension
   d. Hypothyroidism

5. Which statement by a 70-year-old client reflects adaptation to the aging process:
   a. "My wife passed away five years ago. I'm nothing without her."
   b. "I'm enjoying my free time and being able to spend time with my kids."
   c. "I can't get around like I used to since my hip replacement. I don't want to live like this anymore."
   d. "I worked all my life to support my family and my kids never come to see me. I wasted my life."

REFERENCES

Ainsworth M: Attachments beyond infancy, *Am Psychol* 44:709, 1989.

Albrecht T, Adelman M: Social support and life stress: new directions for communication research, *Hum Communication Res* 11:3, 1984.

Aldwin C: *Stress, coping, and development: an integrative approach*, New York, 1994, Guilford.

Atchley R: A continuity theory of normal aging, *Gerontologist* 29:183, 1989.

Baltes P, Smith J, Staudinger U: Life-span developmental psychology, *Annu Rev Psychol* 23:65, 1992.

Bandura A: *Social learning theory*, New York, 1971, General Learning Press.

Bandura A: *Social foundations of thought and action: a social cognitive theory*, Englewood Cliffs, NJ, 1986, Prentice-Hall.

Bandura A: Human agency in social cognitive theory, *Am Psychol* 44:1175, 1989.

Birren J, Schaie K: *Handbook of the psychology of aging*, ed 2, New York, 1985, Van Nostrand Reinhold.

Botwinick J: *Aging and behavior*, ed 3, New York, 1984, Springer.

Bowlby J: *A secure base: clinical applications of attachment theory*, London, 1988, Routledge.

Bowman B, Rosenberg I: Digestive function and aging, *Human Nutr Clin Nutr* 27C:75, 1983.

Brainerd, C: *Piaget's theory of intelligence*, Englewood Cliffs, 1978, Prentice-Hall.

Bretschneider J, McCoy N: Sexual interest and behavior in healthy 80 to 102 year olds, *Arch Sex Behav* 17:109, 1988.

Broadhead W et al: The epidemiologic evidence for a relationship between social support and health, *Am J Epidemiol* 117:521, 1983.

Butler R: Ageism. In Maddox G, editor: *The encyclopedia of aging*, New York, 1987, Springer.

Campbell J: *The portable Jung*, New York, 1979, Penguin Books.

Carter J: The effects of aging upon selected visual functions: color vision, glare sensitivity, field of vision, and accommodation. In Sekuler R, Kline D, Dismukes K, editors: *Aging and human visual function*, New York, 1982, Oxford University Press.

Christiansen H et al: Age differences and interindividual variation in cognition in community-dwelling elderly, *Psychol Aging* 9:381, 1994.

Cohen G: *The creative age: awakening human potential in the second half of life*, New York, 2000, Avon Books.

Colarusso CA, Nemiroff RA: *Adult development*, New York, 1981, Plenum Press.

Conrad C: Old age in the modern and postmodern western world. In Cole T, Van Tassel D, Kastenbaum R, editors: *Handbook of the humanities and aging*, New York, 1992, Springer.

Cumming E, Henry W: *Growing old: the process of disengagement*, New York, 1961, Basic Books.

Ebersole P, Hess P: *Toward healthy aging: human needs and nursing responses*, ed 5, St Louis, 1999, Mosby.

Eliopoulos C: *Gerontological nursing*, ed 5, Philadelphia, 2001, JB Lippincott.

Erikson EH: *Eight stages of man in childhood and society*, New York, 1963, WW Norton.

Erikson EH: *Childhood and society*, ed 2, New York, 1974a, WW Norton.

Erikson EH: *Dimensions of a new identity: Jefferson lectures*, New York, 1974b, WW Norton.

Erikson E: *The life cycle completed*, New York, 1982, WW Norton.

Erikson E, Erikson J, Kiunick H: *Vital involvement in old age: the experience of old age in our time*, New York, 1986, WW Norton.

Federal Interagency Forum on Aging Related Statistics: *Older Americans 2000: key indicators of well-being*, website: www.agingstats.gov, 2000.

Finch C, Tanzi R: Genetics of aging, *Science* 278:407, 1997.

Folstein M, Folstein S, McHugh P: "Mini-mental state": a practical method of grading the cognitive state of patients for the clinician, *J Psychiatr Res* 12:189, 1975.

Freud S: *The ego and the id*, New York, 1923, WW Norton.

Gallagher J, Reid D: *The learning theory of Piaget and Inhelder*, Monterey, 1981, Brooks/Cole.

Gilligan C: *In a different voice*, Cambridge, Mass, 1982, Harvard University Press.

Havighurst R, Neugarten B, Tobin S: Disengagement and patterns of aging. In Neugarten B, editor: *Middle age and aging*, Chicago, 1968, University of Chicago Press.

Hayflick L: Theories of biological aging. In Andres R, Bierman E, Hazzard W, editors: *Principles of geriatric medicine*, New York, 1985, McGraw-Hill.

Herzog A, Wallace R: Measures of cognitive functioning in the AHEAD study, *J Gerontol* 52B:37, 1997.

Hertzog C, Dixon R, Hultsch D: Relationships between metamemory, memory predictions, and memory task performance in adults, *Psychol Aging* 5:215, 1990.

Horn J, Cattell R: Age differences in fluid and crystallized intelligence, *Acta Psychol* 26:107, 1967.

Huyck M: Middle age, *Acad Am Encyclopedia* 13:390, 1997.

Hyde R: Facilitative communication skills training: social support for elderly people, *Gerontologist* 28:418, 1988.

Jaques E: Death and the mid-life crisis. In Jaques E: *Work, creativity, and social justice,* London, 1970, Heinemann.

Jung C: The stages of life. In Campbell J, editor: *The portable Jung,* New York, 1971, Viking Press.

Katz S et al: Studies of illness in the aged: the Index of ADL, a standardized measure of biological and psychological function, *JAMA* 185:914, 1963.

Kohlberg L: Stages and aging in moral development: some speculations, *Gerontologist* 13:497, 1973.

Kohlberg L: The development of children's orientations toward a moral order. In Damon W, editor: *Social and personality development essays on the growth of the child,* New York, 1983, WW Norton.

Kruger A: The mid-life transition, crisis or chimera? *Psychol Rep* 75:1299, 1994.

Kumpe P et al: The aging respiratory system, *Clin Geriatr Med* 1:143, 1985.

Lakatta E: Cardiovascular system aging. In Kent B, Butler R, editors: *Human aging research: concepts and techniques,* New York, 1988, Raven Press.

Lemon B, Bengston V, Peterson J: An exploration of the activity theory of aging: activity types and life satisfaction among inmovers to a retirement community, *J Gerontol* 27:511, 1972.

Levinson DJ et al: *The seasons of a man's life,* New York, 1986, Ballantine Books.

Maddi S: *Personality theories: a comparative analysis,* Homewood, Ill, 1972, Dorsey Press.

Maslow A: *Toward a psychology of being,* New York, 1962, Van Nostrand.

McCrae R: Situational determinants of coping responses: loss, threat, and challenge, *J Pers Soc Psychol* 46:919, 1984.

Mille R: The aging immune system: primer and prospectus, *Science* 273:70, 1996.

Miller C: *Nursing care of older adults: theory and practice,* Glenview, Ill, 1990, Scott, Foresman.

Miller M: Life changes scaling for the 1990s, *J Psychosom Res* 43:279, 1997.

Miller N, Dollard J: *Social learning and imitation,* New Haven, 1941, Yale University Press.

Myers D: Adulthood's ages and stages, *Psychology* 5:196, 1998.

Neugarten BL: Time, age, and the life cycle, *Am J Psychiatry* 136:887, 1979.

Newton PM, Levinson DJ: Crisis in adult development. In Lazare A, editor: *Outpatient psychiatry: diagnosis and treatment,* Baltimore, 1979, Williams & Wilkins.

Olsho L, Harkins S, Harmon B: Aging and the auditory system. In Birren J, Schaie K, editors: *Handbook of the psychology of aging,* ed 2, New York, 1985, Van Nostrand Reinhold.

Oxman T, Berkman L: Assessment of social relationships in elderly patients, *Int J Psychiatr Med* 20:65, 1990.

Pederson N: Gerontological behavior genetics. In Birren JE, Schaie K, editors: *Handbook of the psychology of aging,* ed 3, San Diego, 1996, Academic Press.

Pennebaker J: The effects of traumatic disclosure on physical and mental health: the values of writing and talking about upsetting events, *Int J Emerg Ment Health* 1:9, 1999.

Perlmutter M et al: Aging and memory, *Annu Rev Gerontol Geriatr* 7:57, 1987.

Pfeiffer E: A short portable mental status questionnaire for the assessment of organic brain deficit in elderly patients, *J Am Geriatr Soc* 23:433, 1975.

Piaget J: *The science of education and the psychology of the child,* New York, 1970, Grossman.

Piaget J, Inhelder B: *The psychology of the child,* New York, 1969, Basic Books.

Reid D, Haas G, Hawkings D: Locus of desired control and positive self-concept of the elderly, *J Gerontol* 32:441, 1977.

Rogers R: Sociodemographic characteristics of long-lived and healthy individuals, *Popul Dev Rev* 21:33, 1995.

Rotter J: *The development and application of social learning theory,* New York, 1982, Praegor.

Rotter J: Cognates of personal control: locus of control, self-efficacy, and explanatory style: comment, *Appl Prevent Psychol* 1:127, 1992.

Rowe J, Kahn R: *Successful aging: the MacArthur Foundation study,* New York, 1998, Pantheon Books.

Ryan E: Beliefs about memory changes across the adult life span, *J Gerontol* 47:41, 1992.

Ryan E, See S: Age-based beliefs about memory changes for self and others across adulthood, *J Gerontol* 48:199, 1993.

Schaie K, Willis S: *Adult development and aging,* Boston, 1991, Little, Brown.

Schneider E, Rowe J: *Handbook of the biology of aging,* ed 3, San Diego, 1990, Academic Press.

Schroots J: Gerodynamics: toward a branching theory of aging, *Can J Aging* 14:74, 1995.

Shek D: Mid-life crisis in Chinese men and women, *J Psychol* 130:109, 1996.

Speas K, Obenshain B: *Images of aging in America: final report,* American Association of Retired Persons, Chapel Hill, NC, 1995, FGI Integrated Marketing.

Steinberg F: The aging of organs and organ systems. In Steinberg F, editor: *Care of the geriatric patient,* ed 6, St Louis, 1983, Mosby.

Stevens-Long J: *Adult life: developmental processes,* ed 4, Palo Alto, Calif, 1992, Mayfield.

Stroufe A, Cooper R, DeHart G: *Child development: its nature and course,* New York, 1992, McGraw-Hill.

Sullivan H: *The interpersonal theory of psychiatry,* New York, 1953, WW Norton.

Szinovacz M, Washo C: Gender differences in exposure to life events and adaptation to retirement, *J Gerontol* 47:191, 1992.

Tornstam H: Gero-transcendence: a theoretical and empirical exploration. In Thomas L, Eisenhandler S, editors: *Aging and the religious dimension,* Westport, Conn, 1994, Auburn House.

U.S. Bureau of the Census: Sixty-five plus in the United States. In *Current Population Reports,* P23-190, No. 178RV, special studies, Washington, DC, 1996, U.S. Department of Commerce, Economics and Statistics Administration.

U.S. Bureau of the Census: *Census of population: general population characterisics (2000),* Washington, DC, 2000, U.S. Department of Commerce, Economics and Statistics Administration.

Vaillant GE: *Adaptation to life,* Boston, 1977, Little, Brown.

Vaillant G: *Aging well: surprising guideposts to a happier life from the landmark Harvard study of adult development,* New York, 2002, Little, Brown.

Van Gennep A: *The rites of passage,* Chicago, 1909, University of Chicago Press.

Woodruff D: A review of aging and cognitive processes, *Res Aging* 5:139, 1983.

SUGGESTED READINGS

Campbell M: Study of the attitudes of nursing personnel toward the geriatric patient, *Nurs Res* 20:127, 1971.

Miller RA: The aging immune system: primer and prospectus, *Science* 273:70, 1996.

PART II   PSYCHIATRIC DISORDERS

9

Anxiety and Related Disorders

Pamela E. Marcus

KEY TERMS

agoraphobia (p. 179)
anxiety (p. 172)
anxiolytic (p. 191)
compulsions (p. 181)
defense mechanisms
  (p. 172)
denial (p. 175)
depersonalization (p. 180)
dissociation (p. 180)
humanistic nursing (p. 174)
obsessions (p. 180)
panic (p. 178)
panic attacks (p. 178)
phobias (p. 178)
repression (p. 180)
stress (p. 175)

OBJECTIVES

- Discuss two etiologic paradigms to explain the four stages of anxiety.

- Describe the defining characteristics of anxiety in the NANDA classification to differentiate between circumscribed and pervasive anxiety disorders.

- Design a teaching plan for family members of clients with agoraphobia.

- Appraise the coping mechanisms of trauma victims to evaluate risk for posttraumatic stress disorder.

- Apply a cost-benefit approach to weigh the advantages of inpatient and outpatient treatment of dissociative identity disorder (formerly multiple personality disorder).

- Apply the nursing process in managing clients with anxiety disorders.

- Evaluate the advantages of the humanistic nursing model in providing care to clients experiencing varying levels of anxiety.

- Discuss the usefulness of clinical rating scales in evaluating collaborative treatment outcomes of inpatients with anxiety disorders and obsessive-compulsive disorder.

- Relate the biologic paradigm to target symptoms and therapeutic agents for psychopharmacologic intervention in anxiety and related disorders.

Anxiety is an integral part of the universal human experience. For most people, most of the time, it is a vague, subjective, nonspecific feeling of uneasiness with no identifiable object, resulting from an external threat to one's integrity. The function of **anxiety** is to warn the individual of impending threat, conflict, or danger. Anxiety is also a state of tension, dread, or impending doom, arising from external influences that threaten to be overwhelming. When an individual receives a signal of approaching danger, he or she is motivated to action: flee the threatening situation or control dangerous impulses. The person may even freeze to the spot, immobilized.

Defense mechanisms (see Box 1-3) are the primary methods the ego uses in an attempt to control or manage anxiety. Defenses protect the individual from threats to the biologic, psychologic, and social aspects of the self. The consequence of ignoring anxiety signals is the threat of being destroyed, or of no longer existing. Anxiety responses exist on a continuum (Table 9-1), and individuals are more or less successful at using various methods to control their own anxiety experiences. Those who are less successful, or who rely primarily on less adaptive defense mechanisms, such as dissociation in the case of dissociative identity disorder or projection in the case of an individual with an antisocial personality disorder, develop the defining characteristics of anxiety disorders.

HISTORICAL AND THEORETIC PERSPECTIVES

In *Interpersonal Relations in Nursing,* Hildegard Peplau (1952), a pioneer of psychiatric mental health nursing, identifies four stages of anxiety on a continuum. Her work illustrates the view of anxiety and tension developed by Harry Stack Sullivan (1882-1949), an early, prominent, American-born psychiatrist and expert in developmental theory. These stages of anxiety—mild, moderate, severe, and panic—are described and expanded on in Figure 9-1. Optimally functioning people generally function in the mild range of anxiety. This stage of anxiety facilitates learning, creativity, and personal growth, an important point for nursing students and other learners to acknowledge as they strive to excel in their work. Occasional movement to the moderate stage may also be an adaptive mechanism to cope with stressful situations, whether pleasant or unpleasant. A nursing student who is giving an important oral presentation or who is involved in a challenging situation with a client may be experiencing moderate anxiety. When the stressor is managed, the adapted person moves back along the continuum to mild anxiety. Moderate and severe anxiety can be acute or chronic. In severe anxiety, energy is focused primarily on reducing the pain and discomfort of anxiety, rather than on coping with the environment. Consequently, the individual's level of function is impaired, and the person may need help

Table 9-1	Responses to Anxiety		
Anxiety Level	**Physiologic**	**Cognitive/Perceptual**	**Emotional/Behavioral**
Mild	Vital signs normal. Minimal muscle tension. Pupils normal, constricted.	Perceptual field is broad. Awareness of multiple environmental and internal stimuli. Thoughts may be random but controlled.	Feelings of relative comfort and safety. Relaxed, calm, appearance, and voice. Performance automatic; habitual behaviors occur.
Moderate	Vital signs normal or slightly elevated. Tension experienced; may be uncomfortable or pleasurable (labeled as "tense" or "excited").	Alert; perception narrowed, focused. Optimum state for problem solving and learning. Attentive.	Feelings of readiness and challenge; energized. Engage in competitive activity and learn new skills. Voice, facial expression interested or concerned.
Severe	"Fight or flight" response. Autonomic nervous system excessively stimulated (vital signs increased, diaphoresis increased, urinary urgency and frequency, diarrhea, dry mouth, appetite decreased, pupils dilated). Muscles rigid, tense. Sense affected; hearing decreased, pain sensation decreased.	Perceptual field greatly narrowed. Problem solving difficult. Selective attention (focus on one detail). Selective inattention (block out threatening stimuli). Distortion of time (things seem faster or slower than actual). Dissociative tendencies; vigilambulism (automatic behavior).	Feels threatened, startles with new stimuli; feels on "overload." Activity may increase or decrease (may pace, run away, wring hands, moan, shake, stutter, become very disorganized or withdrawn, freeze in position/be unable to move). May appear and feel depressed. Demonstrates denial; may complain of aches or pains; may be agitated or irritable. Need for space increased. Eyes may dart around room, or gaze may be fixed. May close eyes to shut out environment.
Panic	Above symptoms escalate until sympathetic nervous system release occurs. Person may become pale; blood pressure decreases; hypotension. Muscle coordination poor. Pain, hearing sensations minimal.	Perception totally scattered or closed. Unable to take in stimuli. Problem solving and logical thinking highly improbable. Perception or unreality about self, environment, or event. Dissociation may occur.	Feels helpless with total loss of control. May be angry, terrified; may become combative or totally withdrawn, cry, or run. Completely disorganized. Behavior is usually extremely active or inactive.

From Fortinash K, Holoday Worret P: *Psychiatric nursing care plans,* ed 4, St Louis, 2003, Mosby.

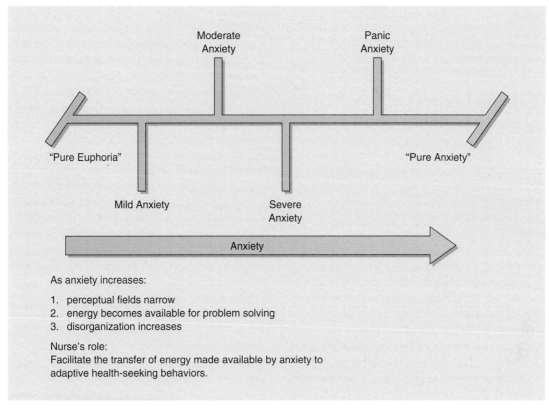

FIGURE 9-1. Hildegard Peplau's construction of the anxiety continuum. (Modified from Peplau H: *Interpersonal relations in nursing: a conceptual frame of reference for psychodynamic nursing,* New York, 1991, Springer.)

to reverse the situation. In panic anxiety the individual is disorganized, with increased motor activity, a distorted visual-perceptual field, loss of rational thought, and decreased ability to relate to others. Responses to the stages of anxiety are more fully explained in Table 9-1.

In *The Meaning of Anxiety,* Rollo May (1979) distinguishes between fear and anxiety by differentiating anxiety from all other affects. According to May, fear is a threat to the periphery of an individual existence, but anxiety is a threat to the foundation and center of existence.

In addition to describing anxiety by degree, anxiety can also be differentiated by type. Signal anxiety is the type of anxiety experienced when a precipitant is identified. It is important to note that although signal anxiety is learned, it results from situations that have been successfully repressed, or coped with, by using another defense mechanism. Consequently, the precipitant is successfully excluded from one's consciousness. Signal anxiety is the predominant etiologic factor in phobic disorders.

Trait anxiety is a function of personality structure. As a part of the developmental processes or events, some individuals have more traumatic experiences or have less success in coping with these events, resulting in unresolved conflict or confusion. These individuals are described as having an anxiety diathesis, or predisposition to anxiety when stressed. Situations that re-create or represent the original conflict or experience evoke a more severe anxiety response in persons with a higher level of trait anxiety. For example, a woman whose mother was chronically ill for much of her childhood may worry excessively about her own children being injured or catching colds. As a result, she limits their activity and is anxious and overprotective.

State anxiety develops in situations identified as conflictual or stressful and in which the individual experiences limited control. This is often perceived as anxiety that has occurred before. The "butterflies" in the stomach experienced by a student before an important examination is an example of mild state anxiety. An increased heart rate that a person who has been bitten by a dog in the past may experience when seeing a large dog walking down the street without a leash is a more moderate form of state anxiety. A woman with a strong family history of cancer who delays making an appointment with her primary health care provider after noticing a lump in her breast demonstrates severe and maladaptive state anxiety. Free-floating anxiety is characterized by a pervasive sense of dread or doom that cannot be attached to any idea or event. This type of anxiety may result in a panic state if stressors exceed the person's ability to cope.

State and trait anxiety are important concepts for nurses because they can be differentiated and estimated by a rating scale known as the State-Trait Anxiety Inventory. Persons with high levels of trait anxiety are likely to experience higher levels of state anxiety when confronted with significant stressors. Nurses who are able to estimate their clients' levels of trait anxiety during the assessment process are better able to promptly institute interventions directed at helping clients cope with high state anxiety responses to identified stressors.

Anxiety in the Context of Psychiatric Mental Health Nursing

The term *anxiety* is used in such a variety of contexts that it is important to be precise in its use. One definition of anxiety is "the inability to choose among potentials" (May, 1979). Inherent in all nurse-client relationships is the nurse's role in facilitating meaning and becoming within the relationship. Another important nursing goal is to facilitate choices through the relationship. Although all relationships are not nursing, the basis for all nursing is a relationship. The phenomenon of a relationship as applied to nursing does not imply equal participation or responsibility on the part of the nurse and the client but rather the nurse's intention to establish a connection. Caring for an unconscious, anesthetized client or for an individual experiencing psychosis or dementia establishes a connection; therefore it is a relationship. For psychiatric mental health nurses, the primary goal of the nurse-client relationship is to become available to the individual. Through establishing a relationship, both the client and the nurse have the opportunity to develop their potentials as human beings, with the understanding that the focus of therapy is the client. Recognizing and managing anxiety and making appropriate choices are critical for both the client and the nurse in the relationship.

Influence of Hildegard Peplau

In the 1950s Peplau described the nurse in a relationship as a person who is "to" the client rather than "with" the client. She presented the phases of the nurse-client relationship in a social learning model that today appears maternalistic but was nonetheless consistent with the meaning of developmental theory and mental health nursing practice at the time. In fact, Peplau is considered by both seasoned and novice colleagues as the "matriarch" of psychiatric mental health nursing.

According to Peplau, it is critical that nurses recognize the choices or potentials that exist in the emerging relationship between the client and the nurse. In *Interpersonal Relations in Nursing,* Peplau (1952) addressed the term *unexplained discomfort,* which includes the needs, frustrations, and conflicts that arise within the relationship. She considers them to be experiences that influence behavior by providing energy to the relationship. According to Peplau, anxiety needs to be examined as it occurs in nurses and clients and in the communication of the interpersonal relationship.

Peplau also presented a method for the nurse to examine the relationship between the nurse and the client. This method is known as process recording. Process recording helps nurses develop self-awareness about the way they relate to clients and underscores the value of the nurse-client relationship. This method is currently widely used in educating nurses, despite the technologic advances of videotape. In process recording, the nurse simply "records" or writes the interaction that occurred between nurse and client as the nurse remembers it. It is best to record the words directly after the interaction so that the recalled information is as valid as possible. The nurse then "processes" the interaction with a professor or clinical supervisor so as to analyze the responses of the nurse and client, the intent of the client's statements, and the overall effectiveness of the nurse in interacting with the client. It is important to note that recording always takes place after the interaction and not with the client present. However, as part of developing a relationship with the client, the nurse recorder and the client need to agree that the client is part of a valuable learning experience and that confidentiality outside of the learning experience will be protected. It is important to observe the protocols of the individual facilities. The defining purpose of process recording is to provide a practical vehicle for nurses to reflect on the content of the interaction in a safe, effective manner. As nurses review their responses to clients or "the nursed," Peplau's position is that nurses will develop a growing awareness of their responses, which is a critical factor in helping clients to achieve their goals and to function optimally. Peplau's anxiety continuum is a theory that is widely used in the treatment of anxiety disorders.

Humanistic Nursing Theory

Humanistic nursing theory can also be applied in treating anxiety and anxiety disorders. Patterson and Zderad (1976) developed a theory of **humanistic nursing** based on existential theory and the phenomenologic method. The cornerstone of their theory is an interactive process that occurs between two persons: one needing help and one willing to give help. Nurses and clients interact; the client "calls," and the nurse "responds." Humanistic nursing differs from Peplau's interpersonal nursing in that in humanistic theory the nurse is clearly identified as a participant in the process. The nurse strives to be fully present in the process and is described in relationship "with" the client, rather than "to" the client, as defined in Peplau's theory. In humanistic theory the nurse's availability to the client is critical to the process of nursing.

Anxiety in Psychiatric Practice

Descriptions of anxiety as a phenomenon of concern in mental health are relatively recent. Psychiatry as a medical specialty had its origins in France in the late eighteenth century. Before that time, care for the insane (lunatics) fell to the law or to the church. Foucault (1988) has asserted that "madness" replaced death as a major theme in human experience. During the Age of Reason and into the nineteenth century, early psychiatric practitioners concerned themselves with the psychoses, those mental disorders believed to pose the greatest risk to society. However, in the second half of the nineteenth century, as the roots of psychoanalytic theory developed, anxiety (or "neuroses") emerged as a source of a variety of emotional and behavioral disturbances.

Philosophic Roots of Anxiety

The philosophers most commonly associated with the concept of anxiety are the existentialists. However, Kierkegaard, a Danish philosopher (1813-1855), antedated the existentialists, and his work influenced them profoundly in some instances. His concept of anxiety is a seminal work on the subject from a theologic perspective. Kierkegaard was supportive of the phenomenologic method from the standpoint of *te unum noris omnes*, meaning "if you know one, you know all, and hold fast to the one that actually is all." Kierkegaard went on to write from his own experience: "The one that actually is all, is the self" (Kierkegaard, 1980). His philosophic discussion of anxiety begins by considering innocence and, through a dialectic, develops the idea that anxiety is the qualitative leap (i.e., the "nothingness") between innocence and guilt. Kierkegaard viewed anxiety as the questioning of one's existence—the potential **denial** of self.

Martin Heidegger, a German phenomenologist and existentialist (1889-1976), stated that existential being (self-relatedness) is the only door to *being* itself. To Heidegger, being in the world projects itself entirely on possibilities. He viewed anxiety as "not being at home; therefore it is a state of discomfort; but nonetheless, anxiety is a condition of being" (Heidegger, 1962).

ETIOLOGY
Biologic Model

Roots of the biologic model for anxiety disorders date back to the nineteenth-century writings of Charles Darwin. Darwin postulated that emotional expression and anatomic structures both changed in the course of evolution to enable the species to adapt to its environment. Darwin further identified certain emotions as being universally demonstrated through expression, using motor and postural changes. In the early part of the twentieth century, investigators linked the endocrine system with emotions, first through establishing the relationship of the adrenal medulla in the production of epinephrine, resulting in the "fight or flight" response.

Selye (1956) built on this work after World War II, using observations of stress and anxiety demonstrated by soldiers who served in combat. A new conceptualization of **stress** replaced the former "psychic trauma." Selye expanded on the notion that the endocrine system and the central nervous system, particularly the hypothalamus and pituitary gland, have a reciprocal relationship. At the same time, important investigations were conducted regarding the neuropharmacology of the autonomic nervous system (ANS) in regulating cardiovascular, gastrointestinal, and motor responses. The ANS, particularly the sympathetic nervous system, was shown to be responsive to environmental stimuli, including emotional states.

As the ability to understand the physiologic state by observing the living brain in imaging techniques such as positron emission tomography (PET) and the functional magnetic resonance imaging, the role of stress and the brain functioning has become more apparent. The amygdala is particularly important to understand as it relates to fear responses, particularly in posttraumatic stress disorder (PTSD). The amygdala is involved in the fight or flight response. It is hypothesized that the different anxiety disorders affect different parts of the amygdala (NIMH, 2002). The medial prefrontal cortex organizes the response to a traumatic episode, and the hippocampus has the spatial and contextual memory of the trauma. Chronic stress can cause changes in the hippocampus (Korn, 2002; NIMH, 2002).

Genetic considerations are important when assessing individuals with anxiety disorders. In one genetic study of panic disorder, Heun and Maier (1995) showed an 8% to 17% risk in first-degree relatives. NIMH is studying the genetic impact on most major psychiatric disorders in the NIMH Human Genetics Initiative (NIMH, 2002).

By studying and understanding brain functioning and genetics, new advances can be made in the use of pharmaceutic agents to assist patients with anxiety-related disorders (see Chapter 20).

Psychodynamic Model

In psychoanalytic terms anxiety is conceptualized as a warning to the ego that it is in peril from either an internal or external threat. Anxiety is involved in the development of personality and personality functioning and in the development and treatment of neuroses and psychoses. Freud's work is the basis for anxiety neurosis existing as a separate classification.

Three types of anxiety are identified in psychoanalytic theory: reality anxiety, moral anxiety, and neurotic anxiety. Reality anxiety is a painful emotional experience resulting from the perception of danger in the external world. Fear is the response to external danger; consequently, anxiety parallels fear. Moral anxiety is the ego's experience of guilt or shame. Neurotic anxiety is the perception of a threat according to one's instincts (Hall, 1954). According to Freud's theory of "signal anxiety," anxiety is a signal of impending emergence of threatening, unconscious mental content. Neurotic symptoms develop in an attempt to defend against anxiety—including hysterical symptoms, obsessions, compulsions, and phobias.

Interpersonal Model

Both the interpersonal and the social psychiatry models view anxiety as a response to the individual's external environment, rather than the relatively simple psychoanalytic view of a response to instinctual drives. Interpersonal theorists, particularly Sullivan, regarded symptom formation as a result of expectations, insecurities, frustrations, and conflicts between individuals and primary groups. Primary groups include families, work colleagues, and social associates.

Like psychoanalytic theorists, interpersonal theorists place a great deal of emphasis on early development and experiences in relation to future mental health. According to Sullivan, the individual's first experience of anxiety is the infant's perception of the anxiety of the mothering person. The self system develops in the context of approval or disapproval from significant others. Disapproval results in a threat to the self system, a fear of rejection—in other words, anxiety.

Interpersonal theorists define anxiety broadly. According to Sullivan, anxiety is the first great educative experience in living. Also according to Sullivan, one of the great tasks of psychology is to discover the basic vulnerabilities to anxiety in interpersonal relations, rather than to try to deal with the symptoms of anxiety.

Environmental Model: Social Psychiatry

Social theorists emphasize the role of social conditions in deviant behavior and assert that symptoms, including anxiety and its manifestations, result from the dynamic relationship between individuals and their environment. Social psychiatry evolved after World War II and began to be defined by the large number of community and epidemiologic surveys designed to develop a model for understanding the role of vulnerability, predisposition, and stressors in symptom formation. Social psychiatry views factors such as socioeconomic status, racial inequalities, and migration as stressors equivalent to combat in the military. Individuals respond to the environment on a continuum, either adaptively or with symptom formation—mental illness or physical illness. The mediating factor in this response is the individual's ability to manage anxiety. Social psychiatric influences, particularly with respect to sampling methodology and the use of standardized questionnaires and scales, have contributed significantly to the current research base for the anxiety disorders.

Behavioral Model

Behavioral models in psychiatry and psychology were proposed by clinicians who were stimulated by the shortcomings of the psychoanalytic model and methods. They identified experimental psychology as a resource for ideas from which to develop new treatments. In behavioral models, based on learning theory, the etiology of anxiety symptoms is a generalization from an earlier traumatic experience to a benign setting or object. An example is an awkward child who was ridiculed by parents while bowling. As a result he associates embarrassment and shame with sports events in indoor facilities and develops panic attacks during basketball games. The same kinds of cognitive operations that link embarrassment with sporting events link cognitions of the expectation of embarrassment with the idea of a sporting event, and the individual begins to experience panic attacks while reading the sports page. Consequently, in this model, anxiety occurs when an individual encounters a signal that "predicts" a painful or feared event.

Early behavioral therapists directed their efforts at the anxiety disorders. In 1958 Wolpe, a South African physician working with soldiers experiencing symptoms of what is now classified as posttraumatic stress disorder (PTSD), reported success using systematic desensitization applied to simple phobias (Wolpe, 1973). Systematic desensitization is

Table 9-2	Clinical Manifestations of Anxiety: Symptoms and Responses
Manifestation	**Symptom/Response**
Physiologic	
Cardiovascular system	Palpitations, racing heart, increased blood pressure, fainting, decreased pulse, decreased blood pressure
Respiratory system	Rapid, shallow breathing, pressure in chest, shortness of breath, gasping, lump in throat
Gastrointestinal system	Loss of appetite or increased appetite, abdominal discomfort or feeling of fullness, nausea, heartburn, diarrhea
Neuromuscular system	Hyperreflexia, insomnia, tremors, pacing, clumsiness, restlessness, flushing, sweating, muscle tension
Genitourinary system	Decreased libido, frequency or urgency of urination
Cognitive	Decreased attention, inability to concentrate, forgetfulness, impaired judgment, thought blocking, fear of injury or death
Behavioral	Rapid speech, muscle tension, fine hand tremors, restlessness, pacing, hyperventilation
Affective	Irritability, impatience, nervousness, fear, uneasiness

a method derived from learning theory in which the deeply relaxed client is exposed to a graded hierarchy of phobic stimuli. This method has been refined further into a method termed *in vivo desensitization,* whereby the individual is exposed to progressively more anxiety-provoking situations, often accompanied by a therapist. These live exposure treatments can take a variety of forms, including graded practice, participant modeling, and prolonged or brief duration. In 1981 behaviorists demonstrated that 60% to 79% of patients with agoraphobia experienced clinically significant improvement by using the methods of systematic desensitization.

Table 9-2 demonstrates the clinical manifestations of anxiety, which take into account the biologic, cognitive, behavioral, and affective patterns of behavior. This table is a good tool to help nurses recognize the manifestation anxiety has on the body systems, as well as on thought patterns and behavior.

EPIDEMIOLOGY

A 12-month study conducted to determine the extent of anxiety disorders in the population showed that 20% of individuals in the United States have a type of anxiety disorder (Kessler et al., 1994). The NIMH research on anxiety disorders reports that more than 19 million adult Americans have anxiety disorders. A number of anxiety disorders such as obsessive-compulsive disorder (OCD), social phobia, and body dysmorphic disorder begin in childhood and continue into adulthood.

Almost all clients presenting with agoraphobia in clinical samples have a current diagnosis or history of panic disorder. In contrast, epidemiologic samples identify more clients with agoraphobia without a history of panic disorder. Agoraphobia is diagnosed more often in women than in men.

Simple phobia is common in the general population, with reported lifetime prevalence rates of 10% to 12% (APA, 2000). Overall, the prevalence of simple phobia is higher for women than for men. However, with fear of heights and blood injection injury, the percentage of males is higher, from 30% to 45%, as compared with 10% to 25% in other categories.

In contrast to other anxiety disorders, in clinical samples equal numbers of men and women seek treatment for social phobia. In community-based samples, however, social phobia is more common among women. Lifetime prevalence rates vary from 3% to 13% (APA, 2000). In outpatient treatment settings, rates of social phobia range from 10% to 20% of persons seeking treatment for anxiety disorders. Similarly, OCD is equally common in men and women; the lifetime prevalence is estimated at 2.5% (APA, 2000).

Estimates for the prevalence of PTSD range from 3% to 58% of at-risk individuals. This wide variability is due to both sampling methods and the population assessed. Community-based samples for prevalence range from 1% to 14% (APA, 2000).

The prevalence of dissociative disorders is difficult to estimate. The diagnosis is usually made after an individual seeks treatment. There is still substantial controversy surrounding dissociative disorders. The lack of epidemiologic data reflects both case-finding difficulty and clinician bias. The disorder is more commonly diagnosed in women than in men.

Age of Onset

In general, anxiety disorders develop during adolescence and early adulthood. The typical age of onset for panic disorder varies from late adolescence to the mid-thirties. Rare cases have an onset in childhood, and a small number develop symptoms after age 45 years. Acute and posttraumatic stress disorders can develop at any age.

The age of onset for specific phobias, situational type, is bimodally distributed. There is a peak of onset in childhood and another peak in early adulthood. Other types of phobias usually have an onset in childhood.

Cultural Variance

Most research supporting the development of the DSM-IV-TR classification was done in the United States; consequently, symptoms defining disorders are representative of that culture. However, care should be taken to establish cultural norms when evaluating clients for anxiety and related disorders. For example, some cultures restrict women's par-

ticipation in public activities; thus agoraphobia is less commonly diagnosed. Fears of magic or spirits are present in many cultures and should be considered pathologic only when the fear is excessive in the context of that culture. Many cultures prescribe rituals to mark important events in peoples' lives. The observation of these rituals is not considered indicative of OCD unless it exceeds norms for that culture, is exhibited at times or places inappropriate for that culture, or interferes with social functioning.

It seems that with the exception of OCD and social phobia, anxiety and related disorders exhibit a higher prevalence among women than among men. This observation may represent a cultural variation. Overall, women are more likely than men to present for treatment or come in contact with health care providers.

Comorbidity

Anxiety disorders do not exist in a clinical vacuum. Understanding the comorbidity of different anxiety disorders with other Axis I disorders is helpful in providing comprehensive treatment. There is a high comorbid rate of anxiety and depression. Often patients with these disorders are at a 15-fold increased risk of suicidal ideation than patients who have neither disorder (Goodwin et al., 2001). Clients with major depression were found to have an 18.8% increased risk of panic and a 15.3% increased risk of agoraphobia. There is substantial comorbidity between substance abuse disorders and anxiety disorders.

OCD exists with other anxiety disorders, as well as substance abuse, major depression, and eating disorders. In Tourette's syndrome 30% to 50% of clients also have OCD; however, the rate of Tourette's syndrome among OCD clients is lower, with estimates ranging from 5% to 7%.

Acute and posttraumatic stress disorders are associated with increased risk for major depression, other anxiety disorders, somatization disorder, and substance abuse disorders. Because of the nature of the disorder and its presentation after a significant event, it is difficult to determine whether the comorbid condition developed before the stress disorder or as a consequence of it.

CLINICAL DESCRIPTIONS
Anxiety Disorders
Panic

In the nineteenth century clinical syndromes similar to those we now label panic disorder and agoraphobia began to appear in the literature. In 1871 an American physician, Da Costa, described panic attacks occurring in soldiers who served in the Civil War. Around the same time, Westphal, a German physician, presented clinical data on four patients with classic agoraphobic syndromes. Freud first named panic attacks as occurring when "the connection between anxiety and threatened danger is entirely lost from view . . . spontaneous attacks . . . represented by intensely developed symptoms . . . tremor, vertigo, palpitations of the heart"

(Freud, 1963). Freud also noted the comorbidity of the anxiety disorders and depression.

World Wars I and II contributed to the development of the knowledge base of the anxiety disorders, as did the work of the noted cardiologist Paul Dudley White. He and his colleagues collected data on a number of patients referred to them at Massachusetts General Hospital who did not have organic heart disease, and they named the clinical syndrome *neurocirculatory asthenia*. In the same institution neuropsychiatrists identified a similar symptom complex and named it *anxiety neurosis*. Both the cardiologists and the neuropsychiatrists were describing what today we call *panic disorder*.

Panic anxiety refers to anxiety symptoms that occur during panic attacks. Panic anxiety is differentiated from generalized anxiety by the sudden onset of distressing physical symptoms combined with thoughts of dread, impending doom, death, and fear of being trapped.

Panic Attack.

It is important to note that in and of themselves, panic attacks are not listed in the DSM-IV-TR classification as psychiatric illnesses. Rather, **panic attacks** are symptoms, potentially meeting some of the defining characteristics of many of the disorders described in this chapter. Panic attacks are sudden, spontaneous episodes accompanied by symptoms such as a racing heart or palpitations, dizziness, dyspnea, and a feeling that death is imminent.

Panic attacks occur in a variety of anxiety disorders, including panic disorder, social phobia, simple phobia, and PTSD. Panic attacks can occur in specific, cued situations (as with simple phobias) or be unexpected (uncued) (APA, 2000). The DSM-IV-TR Criteria box lists the symptoms of a panic attack.

DSM-IV-TR CRITERIA
Panic Attack

A discrete period of intense fear or discomfort in which four or more of the following symptoms developed abruptly and reached a peak within 10 minutes:
1. Palpitations, pounding heart, accelerated heart rate
2. Sweating
3. Trembling or shaking
4. Sensations of shortness of breath or smothering
5. Feeling of choking
6. Chest pain or discomfort
7. Nausea or abdominal distress
8. Feeling dizzy, unsteady, lightheaded, or faint
9. Derealization (feelings of unreality) or depersonalization (being detached from oneself)
10. Fear of losing control or going crazy
11. Fear of dying
12. Paresthesias (numbness or tingling sensations)
13. Chills or hot flushes

From American Psychiatric Association: *Diagnostic and Statistical Manual of Mental Disorders,* Fourth Edition, Text Revision. Washington, DC, American Psychiatric Association, 2000.

Panic Disorder.

An individual may be diagnosed with panic disorder if the following two criteria are met: (1) recent and unexpected panic attacks are present, and (2) at least one of the attacks has been followed for 1 or more months by (a) persistent concern about having additional attacks, (b) worry about the implications of the attack or its consequences (e.g., losing control, having a heart attack, "going crazy"), or (c) a significant change in behavior related to the attacks.

In panic disorder without agoraphobia, the individual is free from agoraphobic symptoms, the panic attacks are not related to direct effects of a substance (illicit drugs, medication), and the attacks are not due to a physiologic condition (e.g., hyperthyroidism). In addition, the anxiety is not better accounted for by another mental disorder, such as OCD (for example, a fear of contamination) or PTSD (e.g., in response to stimuli associated with a severe stressor).

To be diagnosed with panic disorder with agoraphobia, the individual must meet the criteria for panic disorder, as well as experience debilitating agoraphobic symptoms. These agoraphobic symptoms are feeling anxiety about being in areas where it would be difficult to escape or where there is no assistance available, such as being in a crowd, being on a bridge, or traveling in a subway train. The individual with agoraphobia avoids these situations or stays homebound if the agoraphobia involves fear of being outside the house alone.

Panic disorder is primarily seen in ambulatory settings. Nurses are among the first health care providers that clients with new-onset panic disorder come in contact with, either in a clinic or physician's office or, more typically, in a hospital emergency department. The sudden onset of physical symptoms and the pervasive feelings of impending doom are frightening, and the client often responds by seeking reassurance from a caregiver. However, it is not uncommon for clients with panic disorder to have been ill for 8 to 10 years before presenting for treatment and to have experienced one or two attacks per week. In addition, clients have learned to avoid those situations that trigger attacks. The attack may begin with a feeling of general unease that is quickly followed (in a few seconds to minutes) by the onset of physical symptoms.

Phobias

The prominent features of phobic disorders, or **phobias,** are that the patient experiences panic attacks in response to particular situations or learns to avoid the situations that evoke panic attacks.

Agoraphobia.

To meet the first DSM-IV-TR criterion for panic disorder with agoraphobia, the person must experience recurrent, unexpected panic attacks, with at least one attack followed by one of the following for a month: (1) persistent concern about having additional attacks, (2) worry about the implications or its consequences, or (3) a significant change in behavior related to the attacks. The second criterion is that the individual experiences **agora-phobia** (i.e., anxiety about being in places or situations from which escape may be difficult [or embarrassing] or in which help might not be readily available in the event of an unexpected or situationally predisposed panic attack). Agoraphobic fears typically involve characteristic clusters of situations that include being outside the home alone, being in a crowd or standing in line, being on a bridge, and traveling in a bus, train, or car. The third criterion is that agoraphobic situations are avoided or endured with distress or anxiety about having a panic attack, or the individual requires the presence of a companion. The fourth criterion stipulates that panic attacks are not due to the direct effects of a substance or a general medical condition. Finally, the anxiety or phobic avoidance is not better accounted for by another mental disorder, as described in the panic disorder section (APA, 2000).

Agoraphobia can exist apart from panic disorder according to DSM-IV-TR criteria. The individual with agoraphobia without a history of panic disorder meets the criteria for agoraphobia as just described but has no history of panic attacks. The description of agoraphobia is expanded to include "in the event of suddenly developing paniclike symptoms that the individual fears could be incapacitating or extremely embarrassing, for example, fear of going outside because of fear of having a sudden episode of dizziness or a sudden attack of diarrhea." If the individual has a comorbid medical condition, the fear described is clearly in excess of the fear usually associated with that disorder.

Specific Phobias. The DSM-IV-TR criteria define a specific phobia as a marked and persistent fear that is excessive or unreasonable, cued by the presence or anticipation of a specific object or situation, such as animals, insects, heights, flying, or seeing blood. Exposure to the phobic stimulus invariably provokes an anxiety response, which may take the form of a cued panic attack (i.e., the individual experiences symptoms listed in the DSM-IV-TR Criteria box). Children with a specific phobia may express their anxiety by crying, throwing tantrums, freezing, or clinging. Persons with a simple phobia (except children) recognize that their fear is excessive or unreasonable. Phobic situations are avoided or endured with distress. The avoidance, anticipatory anxiety, or distress interferes significantly with the person's routine, occupational, or social functioning; or there is marked distress about having the phobia. Finally, as with panic disorder and agoraphobia, the condition cannot be better accounted for by another Axis I mental disorder (APA, 2000).

Social Phobia. Social phobia, or social anxiety disorder, is characterized by a marked and persistent fear of one or more social or performance situations in which the person is exposed to unfamiliar people or to possible scrutiny by others. The individual fears that he or she will act in a way (or show anxiety symptoms) that will be humiliating or embarrassing. To make this diagnosis in a child, the child must demonstrate the capacity for social relationships with familiar people, and the anxiety must occur in interactions with peers. In addition, exposure to the feared social situation almost invariably provokes anxiety, which may take the form of a situationally bound panic attack. Children may express their fear by crying or exhibiting tantrumlike behavior. Adults acknowledge that their fear is excessive or unreasonable. Individuals with social phobia avoid social or performance situations or endure them with intense anxiety or distress (APA, 2000).

Individuals with social phobia are compromised when working in groups. If an individual is in the psychiatric hospital for a comorbid disorder, such as substance abuse, using the group format causes undo anxiety and would be countertherapeutic. The individual is able to work on problem areas with individual attention and medication such as the selective serotonin reuptake inhibitor (SSRI) antidepressant, paroxetine (Paxil) (see Case Study).

CASE STUDY

Neil is a 19-year-old freshman at a local college. He is brought to the Emergency Department from a fraternity party one Saturday night with acute alcohol intoxication. He is referred to the college health service.

During his initial evaluation, the nurse asks Neil about his patterns of drinking. He reports that he began drinking at age 14 when one of his friends suggested having a beer or two before attending a school dance. He reported that ever since he started school, he was unable to participate in the easy banter, the "social chit-chat" common among fellow students. However, he did not have the same experience with family members. He was afraid that he wouldn't have anything to contribute to the conversation. He began to worry about his appearance and his tendency to trip over his own feet.

When Neil reached high school, he found that this uneasiness was beginning to isolate him from others in his age group. At home his parents usually began dinner parties with a glass of wine or a cocktail, so when his friend suggested a beer before the dance, Neil eagerly accepted. To his surprise, he found that once he arrived at the dance, he was relaxed and able to interact. He was even able to ask two girls to dance!

He continued to drink before arriving at parties, dances, football games, and just about any other social activity. He was worried that he was an alcoholic. The clinical specialist at the health service talked with Neil at length about social phobia and prescribed the antidepressant paroxetine (Paxil). Neil also began attending a group focused on behavioral strategies to cope with anxiety (see Chapter 19).

Critical Thinking
1. What cues does Neil offer that will lead to the most appropriate nursing diagnoses for him?
2. What are two beliefs Neil may have formed that led to his experience at the fraternity party?
3. Using information in this chapter and information in Chapter 13, what would be the prognosis for Neil?
4. What is an alternative pharmacologic choice for Neil? (See Chapter 20.)
5. How would you describe the advantages of group therapy to Neil?

Posttraumatic Stress Disorder

PTSD was first defined as a diagnostic category in DSM-III. Before that time, the pattern of responses after traumatic events was most commonly found in soldiers and the syndrome was called "shell shock" or "combat fatigue." Psychiatric diagnosis currently relies on a simple description of predictable symptoms to define a disorder.

PTSD is a model diagnostic category for psychiatric disorders from a theoretic perspective: the causal factors are identifiable. Recently investigators have begun to adapt the PTSD model to traumatic events in human experience beyond combat, including the experiences of adult and child survivors of sexual abuse, physical abuse, disasters, and the grieving process. Controversy still exists in refining the level of intensity required of an event or an experience to meet the definition of trauma and in separating PTSD symptoms from other comorbid disorders, including substance abuse, depression, and anxiety.

To be diagnosed with PTSD, the individual must have experienced a traumatic event before the onset of symptoms. The individual must have either experienced the event, witnessed the event, or been confronted with an event that involved actual or threatened death or serious injury, or a threat to the physical integrity of self or others. The individual's response must have involved intense fear, helplessness, or horror. Children may express their response with agitated or disorganized behavior.

The second group of defining criteria for PTSD involves various mechanisms of reexperiencing the event. One of the following must be present: recurrent and intrusive disturbing recollections of the event, including thoughts, images, or perceptions; recurrent dreams of the event; acting or feeling as though the event were recurring; the experience of psychologic distress when internal or external cues resemble the event; and/or physiologic reactivity on exposure to internal or external cues that resemble the event.

Furthermore, the individual avoids stimuli associated with the trauma and experiences a numbing of general responsiveness (that was not present before the trauma). Numbing and avoidance are marked by at least three of the following: efforts to avoid thoughts, feelings, or conversations about the trauma; efforts to avoid persons or places that evoke memories of the trauma; inability to remember an important aspect of the trauma (**repression**); diminished interest or participation in significant activities; a feeling of estrangement or detachment from others; restricted range of affect; and/or a sense of a foreshortened future (no expectation of a career or normal life span).

The fourth criterion is concerned with symptoms of increased arousal that were not present before the trauma. Two of the following must be present: sleep disturbances, irritability or angry outbursts, difficulty concentrating, hypervigilance, and exaggerated startle response. Symptoms must persist for more than 1 month and cause significant impairment in social or occupational or other significant areas of functioning.

PTSD can be further defined as acute if symptoms have occurred for 1 to 3 months or as chronic if the symptoms have persisted for at least 3 months. When the onset of symptoms is more than 6 months after the traumatic event, the further definition of delayed onset is specified (APA, 2000).

Acute Stress Disorder

Acute stress disorder is differentiated from PTSD in three ways: the individual experiences at least three symptoms indicating dissociation, the time frame of development and duration of symptoms is shorter, and the dissociative symptoms may prevent the individual from adaptively coping with the trauma. Three of the following indications of **dissociation** must be present: subjective sense of numbing or detachment, reduced awareness of surroundings (being in a daze), derealization, **depersonalization,** and dissociative amnesia. In terms of time, the symptoms may last from 2 days to a month. The onset of the dissociative experience may occur during the traumatic experience or develop immediately afterward. The defining characteristic of causing significant distress or impairment in social and occupational functioning is that the individual is prevented from pursuing some necessary task, such as obtaining necessary medical or legal assistance or mobilizing personal resources.

Generalized Anxiety Disorder

Generalized anxiety disorder (GAD) is characterized by excessive anxiety and worry (apprehensive expectation) that occurs more days than not, for at least 6 months. This anxiety involves concerns about a number of events and activities. The individual finds it difficult to control the worry. Three of the following six symptoms must be present to some degree for at least 6 months. These symptoms include restlessness or feeling on edge, being easily fatigued, difficulties with concentration, irritability, muscle tension, and sleep disturbance. The focus of the anxiety and worry is not confined to features of another Axis I disorder (worry about having a panic attack, as in panic disorder, or fear of contamination, as in OCD) and is not a part of PTSD. The anxiety or worry interferes with normal social or occupational functioning and is not due to the direct effects of a substance or a general medical condition, and it does not occur exclusively in the presence of another Axis I disorder (mood disorder, psychotic disorder, or pervasive developmental disorder).

An interesting paper and pencil test is shown in Box 9-1.

Obsessive-Compulsive Disorder

OCD is characterized by the presence of either obsessions or compulsions. DSM-IV-TR defines **obsessions** as recurrent and persistent thoughts, impulses, or images that are experienced at some time during the disturbance as intrusive and inappropriate and cause marked anxiety or distress. The thoughts, impulses, and images are not simply excessive worry about real problems. The individual attempts to sup-

Box 9-1   Generalized Anxiety Disorder Self-Test

The following questions can help you determine if you are experiencing symptoms of generalized anxiety disorder (GAD). Simply answer "yes" or "no," then take this to your health care professional to see if further evaluation and treatment are necessary.

Yes or No?   Are you troubled by:

Y N   Excessive worry, occurring more days than not, for at least 6 months?

Y N   Unreasonable worry about a number of different situations, such as work, school, and/or health?

Y N   Your inability to "shut off" your worry?

Yes or No?   Are you bothered by at least three of the following:

Y N   Restlessness, feeling keyed-up or on edge?

Y N   Being easily tired?

Y N   Concentration problems?

Y N   Irritability?

Y N   Muscle tension?

Y N   Trouble falling asleep, trouble staying asleep, or restless/unsatisfying sleep?

Y N   Anxiety that interferes with your daily life?

Having more than one illness at the same time can make it difficult to diagnose and treat the different conditions. Conditions that sometimes complicate anxiety disorders include depression and substance abuse, among others. The following information will help your health care professional in evaluating you for GAD.

Yes or No?   In the last year, have you experienced:

Y N   Changes in sleeping or eating habits?

Y N   Feeling sad or depressed more days than not?

Y N   A disinterest in life more days than not?

Y N   A feeling of worthlessness or guilt more days than not?

Y N   An inability to fulfill responsibilities at work/school or family because of alcohol or drug use?

Y N   Being arrested because of alcohol or drugs?

Y N   The need to continue using alcohol or drugs despite their causing problems for you and/or your loved ones?

Modified from the Anxiety Disorders Association of America, website: http://www.adaa.org.

CASE STUDY

Darren is a 31-year-old accountant who has been disabled from his job with a national firm for 8 months. He reports that he has been hospitalized for treatment of depression, which he has experienced since college. Despite his depression, he graduated with honors, obtained certification as a public accountant, and finished graduate school.

Darren first was treated for OCD 2 years after graduate school when he began experiencing trouble with his supervisor. A number of the firm's clients had complained that Darren was unable to either give them completed tax forms or file for the necessary extensions in a timely manner.

Darren received some relief from his counting and checking behaviors with treatment with paroxetine but presently spends his time preoccupied with thoughts about killing himself. He is unable to decide on a method of suicide that will not endanger his family's entitlement to his accidental death insurance policies; however, he has plans to have an automobile accident that would be fatal. After relating this lethal suicidal plan to his nurse psychotherapist, Darren is admitted to an inpatient facility to prevent a suicidal gesture and to stabilize the medication regimen.

Critical Thinking

1. What type of treatment plan is indicated for Darren, using safety as a priority?
2. What are three collaborative treatment approaches that are important in Darren's long-term therapy?
3. Which methods can be used to measure outcomes achieved as a result of Darren's treatment?

press or ignore these thoughts and impulses or to neutralize them with some other thought or action. Finally, the individual recognizes that the obsessional thoughts are a product of his or her own mind (not imposed from without, as in thought insertion).

Compulsions are repetitive behaviors that the person feels driven to perform in response to an obsession. Examples are repeated hand washing in response to thoughts of contamination and checking over and over again to ensure that appliances are unplugged before leaving the house (see Case Study). The behaviors or mental acts are an attempt to prevent or reduce the distress invoked by the obsession or to prevent some dreaded threatening situation (such as a fire in the example of checking appliances). However, these behaviors or mental processes are either not connected in a realistic way with what they are designed to prevent or are clearly excessive.

Except in children, individuals recognize that the obsessions or compulsions are excessive or unreasonable at some point in the disorder. The obsessions or compulsions cause marked distress, are time consuming, or significantly interfere with the person's normal routine or occupational functioning. If another Axis I disorder is present, the content of obsessions or compulsions is not restricted to it (e.g., food rituals in anorexia, hair pulling in trichotillomania). Finally, the disorder is not due to the direct effects of a substance or a general medical condition (see Client and Family Teaching Guidelines box on p. 182).

The etiology of OCD has been investigated. It is thought to result from a trauma to the basal ganglia or cortical connections (Blackman, 1997). There may be a genetic predisposition that could be triggered by an infection or environment stressors (Blackman, 1997). In 1989 PET scan studies demonstrated differences in functioning of the caudate nucleus of the basal ganglia and parts of the frontal lobe. This finding has implication for treatment, including identifying the most effective medication, as well as cognitive behavioral psychotherapy. The SSRI medications of fluoxetine, fluvoxamine, paroxetine, and sertraline are indicated (Fredman and

Obsessive-Compulsive Disorder

TEACH THE CLIENT'S FAMILY:

Obsessive-compulsive disorder is a chronic anxiety disorder that responds to different treatment strategies.

The client experiences recurrent thoughts that intrude in his/her day to day functioning. To decrease the overwhelming anxiety felt as a result of the thought pattern, the client manifests compulsions or behavior patterns. Some of the thoughts are counting, checking (to see if the stove is off or the door is locked), and concern about germs.

Thoughts, impulses, and images are involuntary and may worsen with stress.

TEACH THE CLIENT:

Behavioral and cognitive strategies to manage the anxiety and reduce the symptoms of the disorder by attending to them when the thought patterns are more pervasive and the compulsions most disruptive.

Medication management is an effective treatment modality and usually involves treatment with a drug in the antidepressant category.

Different classes of drugs have different side effect profiles; recognizing and reporting side effects are an important part of managing the client's drug therapy.

Achieving symptom control through pharmacotherapy may take months.

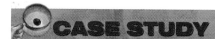

CASE STUDY

Terry is a 28-year-old executive secretary. She was referred to a mental health practice group by the fourth plastic surgeon with whom she had consulted regarding dermabrasion surgery to remove three 2-cm flat scars from her right upper arm. Although she lives in a coastal Florida city, Terry wears only long-sleeved jackets, blouses, and dresses. The garments are always loosely fitted. Terry is certain that people notice her "lumpy" arm and make comments about it; therefore she goes to extreme lengths to prevent this embarrassment and bears the consequences of an extremely hot climate. She refuses to go to the beach with friends or swim in front of anyone because of her preoccupation with her scars.

Critical Thinking

1. What type of plan would assist Terry to become aware of her preoccupation?
2. What are three outcome strategies Terry can perform that would help reduce her exaggerated perceptions?
3. What are two verbal outcome statements that would illustrate Terry's progress in managing her problem?
4. How could Terry be helped to understand the role medication plays in decreasing her symptoms?
5. What are two behavioral outcomes that would indicate Terry's ability to better cope with her disorder?

Korn, 2002). Developing a nursing care plan with the aim of understanding the symptoms and the difficulty they impose on the client is important.

Somatoform Disorders

The common focus of somatoform disorders is physical symptoms in the absence of clinically significant organic disease.

Body Dysmorphic Disorder

Body dysmorphic disorder is characterized by a preoccupation with an imagined defect in appearance. If the individual has a slight physical anomaly, the person's concern is markedly excessive. This preoccupation causes clinically significant distress or impairment in social or occupational functioning. Finally, the preoccupation is not better accounted for by another mental disorder (see Case Study above).

Pain Disorder

The predominant focus of the clinical presentation in pain disorder is pain in one or more anatomic sites. The pain is of sufficient severity to warrant clinical attention and causes clinically significant impairment in one or more areas of functioning. Psychologic factors are judged to have an important role in the onset, severity, exacerbation, or maintenance of the pain. Finally, the pain is not better accounted for by a mood, anxiety, or psychotic disorder and does not meet the criteria for dyspareunia. The disorder can be further defined as a pain disorder associated with psychologic factors if an associated medical condition does not play a major role in the onset, severity, and maintenance of symptoms. If a general medical condition plays a major role in the maintenance of the syndrome, the disorder is termed *pain disorder associated with both psychologic factors and a general medical condition*. Both disorders can be specified as acute (if the duration is less than 6 months) or chronic.

Somatization Disorder

The characteristic pattern of clients presenting with somatization disorder is one of frequently seeking and obtaining medical treatment for multiple, clinically significant somatic complaints. To meet DSM-IV-TR criteria, the complaints must begin before age 30 years, and the complaints cannot be adequately explained by any general medical disorder or the direct effects of a substance. For example, patients with multiple sclerosis, systemic lupus erythematosus, or other chronic debilitating diseases that have an onset in early adulthood frequently present with multisystem complaints but are not also diagnosed as having somatization disorder because a general medical condition better explains their symptom complex.

Distribution of symptoms in somatization disorder requires that symptoms have a distinct pattern that can be differentiated from general medical conditions if the following three criteria are met: (1) there is involvement of multiple organ systems (gastrointestinal, sexual/reproductive, and/or neurologic), (2) the symptoms exhibit an early onset and chronic course without development of physical signs or structural abnormalities (e.g., degenerative changes in bones and joints associated with complaints of pain), and (3) clin-

DSM-IV-TR CRITERIA
Somatization Disorder

A. A history of many physical complaints beginning before age 30 that occur over several years and result in treatment being sought or significant impairment in social, occupational, or other important areas of functioning.

B. Each of the following criteria must have been met, with individual symptoms occurring at any time during the course of the disturbance:
1. *Four pain symptoms*: a history of pain related to at least four different sites or functions (e.g., head, abdomen, back, joints, extremities, chest, rectum, during menstruation, during sexual intercourse, or during urination)
2. *Two gastrointestinal symptoms*: a history of at least two gastrointestinal symptoms other than pain (e.g., nausea, bloating, vomiting other than during pregnancy, diarrhea, or intolerance of several different foods)
3. *One sexual symptom*: a history of at least one sexual or reproductive symptom other than pain (e.g., sexual indifference, erectile or ejaculatory dysfunction, irregular menses, excessive menstrual bleeding, vomiting throughout pregnancy)
4. *One pseudoneurologic symptom*: a history of at least one symptom or deficit suggesting a neurologic condition not limited to pain (conversion symptoms such as impaired coordination or balance, paralysis, or localized weakness; difficulty swallowing or lump in throat; aphonia; urinary retention; hallucinations; loss of touch or pain sensation; double vision; blindness; deafness; seizures; dissociative symptoms such as amnesia; or loss of consciousness other than fainting)

C. Either 1 or 2:
1. After appropriate investigation, each of the symptoms in Criterion B cannot be fully explained by a known general medical condition or the direct effects of a substance (e.g., a drug of abuse, a medication).
2. When there is a related general medical condition, the physical complaints or resulting social or occupational impairment is in excess of what would be expected from the history, physical examination, or laboratory findings.

D. The symptoms are not intentionally produced or feigned (as in factitious disorder or malingering).

From American Psychiatric Association: *Diagnostic and Statistical Manual of Mental Disorders*, Fourth Edition, Text Revision. Washington, DC, American Psychiatric Association, 2000.

ical laboratory abnormalities commonly associated with general medical conditions are absent. The specific diagnostic criteria are detailed in the DSM-IV-TR Criteria box. Nurses in general hospital or clinic practices are more likely to encounter clients with somatization disorder than those working in inpatient psychiatric units.

Conversion Disorder

Clients who present with conversion symptoms exhibit one or more symptoms or deficits that affect voluntary motor or sensory function that appear to be related to a neurologic or general medical condition. As in somatization disorder, however, the symptom or deficit cannot be fully accounted for by a general medical condition, the direct effects of a substance, or as a culturally sanctioned behavior or experi-

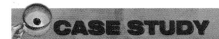
CASE STUDY

Juan is a 34-year-old client on a neurologic unit in a Department of Veterans Administration medical center. He has been treated on the psychiatric service in this facility for a number of years and was diagnosed with schizophrenia, based primarily on his prominent and constant visual and auditory hallucinations regarding his drill sergeant. In the past he has been treated with the antipsychotic medication haloperidol (Haldol).

Juan was born in Puerto Rico and joined the Marines in San Juan when he turned 18. He was unable to complete basic training because he experienced a psychotic episode during which he assaulted his drill sergeant. Juan was admitted to the Neurology Department when one morning he told his family he was unable to walk. Juan had no recent falls or other injuries. No abnormalities were found on his physical examination or CT scan. During a mental status examination he reported that he no longer heard any voices. His assessment was also remarkable for his lack of concern about his paralysis, a seemingly serious problem. The psychiatric mental health nurse specialist was consulted and learned from Juan's family that about a month before his admission, his appeal for a service-related disability was turned down. His family was depending on that financial supplement to help them obtain better housing, a goal they had voiced on many occasions.

Critical Thinking
1. What are two symptoms that indicate Juan may be experiencing a conversion disorder?
2. How does the recent behavior of Juan's family play a role in his current symptomatology?
3. Which symptom experienced by Juan might be labeled *la belle indifference* (beautiful indifference)?
4. How does Juan's assaultive behavior during his psychotic episode influence his perceived paralysis?

ence. The symptom is not intentionally produced or feigned and is not limited to pain or sexual dysfunction; nor does it occur exclusively in the context of somatization disorder. As in other somatization disorders, the symptom causes clinically significant distress or impairment in social, occupational, or other important areas of functioning (see Case Study above).

The critical defining characteristics of conversion disorder are as follows: (1) psychologic factors are identified as being related to the onset or exacerbation of the symptom; (2) specific, identifiable conflicts or stressors precede the development of the conversion symptoms; and (3) the person demonstrates an obvious lack of concern about the seriousness of the symptoms, which is incongruent with the problem. This lack of concern is known as *la belle indifference*, or "beautiful indifference."

Hypochondriasis

"Don't be such a hypochondriac!" is a common theme in American culture and perhaps other cultures as well. Parents say it to children who complain of stomachaches before school on the day of an important test. Sometimes even nursing students say it to each other as they worry about potential signs and symptoms while learning and acquiring knowledge related to medical, surgical, or psychiatric mental health nursing. However, such instances probably do not reflect true hypochondriasis as defined in the DSM-IV-TR.

Six major criteria are associated with this diagnosis. First, the individual is preoccupied with fears of having—or the idea of having—a serious medical disorder based on the individual's misinterpretation of bodily symptoms. Second, this misinterpretation of symptoms persists despite appropriate medical evaluation and reassurance. Third, the individual's preoccupation with symptoms is not as intense or distorted as in delusional disorder, nor is it as restricted as in body dysmorphic disorder. The fourth criterion is, as in the other somatoform disorders, that the preoccupation causes clinically significant distress or impairment in social, occupational, or other major areas of functioning. To meet the fifth criterion, the duration of the disturbance must be at least 6 months. Finally, as in other Axis I diagnoses, the condition is not better accounted for by another anxiety disorder, somatoform disorder, or major depressive episode.

Dissociative Disorders
Dissociative Amnesia

In persons with dissociative amnesia, the defining symptom is one or more episodes of inability to recall important personal information, usually of a traumatic or stressful nature, that is too extensive to be explained by ordinary forgetting. In addition, the disturbance does not occur exclusively during the course of dissociative identity disorder and is not due to the effects of a substance (blackouts during ethyl alcohol intoxication) or as a result of a general medical condition (amnesia after head trauma).

Dissociative Fugue

Dissociative fugue is characterized by sudden, unexpected travel away from home or one's customary place of work, with an inability to recall one's past (or where one has been). The individual demonstrates confusion about personal identity or assumes a new identity, which may be partial ("filling in the blanks"). As in dissociative amnesia, the disturbance does not occur in the context of a dissociative identity disorder and is not due to the effects of a substance or to a general medical condition.

Dissociative Identity Disorder

No other disorder in current psychiatric nosology (classification) has aroused as much controversy as dissociative identity disorder (DID).

DSM-IV-TR criteria for DID are straightforward. The first criterion is that the individual must demonstrate two or more distinct identities or personality states, each with its own relatively enduring pattern of perceiving, relating to, and thinking about the environment and self. Second, at least two of these personality states recurrently take control of the person's behavior. The individual is unable to recall important personal information that is too extensive to be accounted for by ordinary forgetting. Finally, these phenomena are not due to the effects of a substance (e.g., blackouts or chaotic behavior during alcohol intoxication) or a general medical condition (complex partial seizures). In children the symptoms are not attributable to imaginary playmates or other fantasy play.

PROGNOSIS

The prognosis for anxiety and associated disorders is related to factors specific to the disorder, the client, and the clinician. Clients treated for panic disorder with or without agoraphobia are typically described as chronic. Follow-up studies indicate that 6 to 10 years after treatment, 30% of clients are well, 40% to 50% are improved but still symptomatic, and 20% to 30% are the same or slightly worse (APA, 2000).

Specific phobias that persist into adulthood generally do not remit. The course of social phobia is often continuous, with onset or reemergence after stressful or humiliating experiences. The prognosis for OCD is similar to the other anxiety disorders, with waxing and waning symptoms related to stressors. However, 15% of clients demonstrate a chronically deteriorating course with progressive compromise of social and occupational functioning.

For acute and posttraumatic stress disorders, the prognosis is closely related to individuals' exposure to the stressful event, as well as their premorbid functioning and support systems. Persons with acute stress disorder by definition either recover in 4 weeks or are diagnosed with PTSD. Approximately half of those diagnosed with PTSD recover in 3 months; half continue to experience symptoms persisting for longer than a year after the trauma.

The somatoform disorders, with the exception of conversion disorder, are chronic and fluctuating and rarely remit fully. Conversion disorders usually remit within 2 weeks; however, there is recurrence in 20% to 25% of cases. A single recurrence of symptoms is predictive of future episodes. Factors that have been identified with a good prognosis are identifiable stressors at the time that symptoms develop, early treatment, and above average intelligence.

The dissociative disorders have varying prognoses, ranging from a rapid, complete recovery (fugue) to both episodic and continuous chronic courses (dissociative identity disorder). Dissociative identity disorder frequently reemerges during periods of stress or relapse of substance abuse (APA, 2000).

DISCHARGE CRITERIA
Client will:
- Identify situations and events that trigger anxiety and select ways to prevent or manage them.
- Describe anxiety symptoms and levels of anxiety.
- Discuss the connection between anxiety-provoking situations or events and anxiety symptoms.
- Explain relief behaviors openly.
- Identify adaptive, positive techniques and strategies that relieve anxiety.

- Demonstrate behaviors that represent reduced anxiety symptoms.
- Use learned anxiety-reducing strategies.
- Demonstrate ability to problem solve, concentrate, and make decisions.
- Verbalize feeling relaxed.
- Sleep through the night.
- Use appropriate supports from the nursing and medical community, family, and friends.
- Acknowledge the inevitability of occurrence of anxiety.
- Discuss ability to tolerate manageable levels of anxiety.
- Seek help from appropriate sources when anxiety is not manageable.
- List the medication used to control the symptoms as well as the appropriate dosage and scheduled times.
- Continue postdischarge anxiety management including medication and therapy.

THE NURSING PROCESS

ASSESSMENT

New treatment modalities have markedly improved the quality of life and level of participation in activities for people with anxiety disorders. Nurses no longer expect to encounter clients with psychiatric disorders only in traditional psychiatric settings. It is important for all nurses to identify dysfunctional manifestations of anxiety so that treatment can be implemented promptly.

Panic disorders are primarily seen in ambulatory settings. Nurses are among the first health care providers to come in contact with clients who are experiencing their first symptoms of panic disorder, either in a clinic or physician's office or, more typically, in a hospital Emergency Department. The sudden onset of physical symptoms and the pervasive feelings of impending doom are frightening, and the client often responds by seeking reassurance from a caregiver. It is these physical symptoms that bring clients to the Emergency Department with the concern that they may be experiencing a heart attack and impending death.

The client with agoraphobia may come to the attention of a nurse when preparing a client for diagnostic testing that includes a computed tomography (CT) scan or magnetic resonance imaging (MRI). The client who becomes visibly anxious at the prospect of entering a confined space when the nurse describes the procedure and the equipment may be agoraphobic.

Most often clients with anxiety symptoms do not present with anxiety as their reason for seeking treatment. Anxiety by definition is a vague, nonspecific feeling of discomfort. Nurses who use an assessment tool that addresses each identified human response pattern will obtain cues from the client experiencing anxiety that indicate further assessment is needed. The guidelines for a comprehensive nursing assessment, listed in Box 9-2, are adaptable for any practice

setting. When thought of as a list of questions, an "admission interview" becomes a task for nurses and consequently an ordeal for clients. As the nurse becomes more experienced, assessment is integrated into the continuing nursing process, and inquiring about human response patterns evolves into a less threatening interaction between client and nurse.

NURSING DIAGNOSIS

To determine which nursing diagnoses will most effectively guide treatment for clients with anxiety and related disorders, the nurse relies on information obtained in the assessment process. The nurse identifies defining characteristics for the target diagnoses from the client, and the nurse and client jointly identify etiologic factors.

Etiologic factors influence selection of intervention. It is impossible to anticipate each potential diagnosis for all of the disorders discussed in this chapter. Typical diagnoses for clients with anxiety and related disorders are listed here.

Nursing Diagnoses for Anxiety and Related Disorders

- Activity intolerance
- Impaired adjustment
- Anxiety
- Death anxiety
- Disturbed body image
- Ineffective coping
- Defensive coping
- Decisional conflict
- Compromised family coping
- Ineffective denial
- Interrupted family process
- Fatigue
- Fear
- Health-seeking behaviors (somatoform disorders)
- Hopelessness
- Deficient knowledge
- Risk for loneliness
- Impaired memory
- Impaired physical mobility
- Noncompliance
- Imbalanced nutrition: less than body requirements
- Imbalanced nutrition: more than body requirements
- Chronic pain
- Post-trauma syndrome
- Risk for post-trauma syndrome
- Powerlessness
- Risk for powerlessness
- Rape-trauma syndrome
- Rape-trauma syndrome: compound reaction
- Rape-trauma syndrome: silent reaction
- Relocation stress syndrome
- Ineffective role performance
- Chronic low self-esteem
- Self-mutilation

Box 9-2   Nursing Assessment Guidelines According to Human Response Patterns

Exchanging: A Pattern Involving Mutual Giving and Receiving

Assess eating and elimination patterns. *Clients with anxiety disorders and somatization disorders have frequent appetite disturbances and such gastrointestinal complaints as gas, constipation, and diarrhea. Urinary frequency is another associated symptom.*

Communicating: A Pattern Involving Sending Messages

Observe for tics, stuttering, or other unusual speech patterns. Note whether the client maintains eye contact throughout the interview, and whether there are any instances of blushing. *There is comorbidity between Tourette's syndrome and obsessive-compulsive disorder; blushing and difficulty communicating with those the client perceives as having authority are common in social phobia.*

Relating: A Pattern Involving Established Bonds

In taking a social history, be particularly attentive to the client's affect in describing roles and role-related problems including occupational function, financial issues, and role in the home. Ask about the client's role satisfaction and what contributes to it. Note whether the client presented alone for the appointment with the provider. If the client was accompanied, what is the client's relationship to the accompanying individual? *Clients with multiple roles are at risk for role strain, and role strain is often characterized by anxiety symptoms. Alternatively, if the individual describes an isolated existence, probe gently for contributing factors to this isolation. Clients with severe obsessive-compulsive disorder are isolated in part because their degree of involvement with rituals is a competing demand on their time available for social and occupational functioning. Clients with dissociative identity disorder also have poor role functioning, or one of the personality states may be unable to articulate its role functioning. Chronic worry about children or parents as a defining characteristic of anxiety disorders also may be expressed in exploring this pattern.*

Valuing: A Pattern Involving the Assigning of Relative Worth

Inquire about cultural background and values. *Be particularly attentive when assessing a client with a cultural experience different from your own. In addition to various culture-bound syndromes that are related to anxiety, somatization, and dissociative disorders, clients may exhibit behaviors and cognitive patterns that are adaptive and syntonic in one culture, yet labeled pathologic in another.*

Choosing: A Pattern Involving the Selection of Alternatives

Assess client's usual methods of coping with stressors. What aspects of the client's life are stressful? If the individual is part of a family unit, how does the family cope with change? Does the individual use alcohol to cope with stressful situations or public appearances? *Social phobia is often diagnosed only after a maladaptive substance use disorder is identified.*

What is the client's usual method of decision making? Does the individual usually follow recommendations? What strategies does the person use to enhance success? *Clients with obsessive-compulsive disorder most often experience a disturbance in this pattern. Obsessional thinking and ritualistic behaviors are developed to cope with perceived threats (that range from intrusive thoughts to adaptive motor responses that become overgeneralized). If the nurse suspects symptoms of obsessive-compulsive disorder, the client should be asked quite frankly if she or he has any particular ways that tasks should be performed and if interruptions during the performance of these are stressful. Clients with other anxiety disorders, particularly generalized anxiety disorder, often express difficulties in coping and making choices, fearing they will make the wrong decision.*

Moving: A Pattern Involving Activity

In inquiring about an individual's history of physical disability, remember to ask about any episodes of motor dysfunction that may indicate conversion symptoms. If the client indicates past traumatic injury, ask about the circumstances. *Although posttraumatic stress disorder develops after combat situations, sexual abuse, and disasters, it also can follow less dramatic events, such as automobile accidents, and may be related to grief or bereavement as well.* Questions about traveling, sports activities, and hobbies may yield content suggesting agoraphobic symptoms.

Perceiving: A Pattern Involving the Reception of Information; and Knowing: A Pattern Involving the Meaning Associated With Information

These two patterns together compose the traditional mental status examination, formerly a touchstone for psychiatric mental health nurses. Orientation and memory questions are key to identifying anxiety, somatization, and dissociative disorders. *Look for signs of hesitation in answering questions about an individual's history that may indicate periods of dissociation. Listen carefully as the client describes past medical treatment for clusters of illnesses that suggest somatization disorder.* When asking about self-perception and self-concept, be alert for responses that indicate a negative body image. *Clients with body dysmorphic disorder may seek reassurance about a perceived defect if offered the opportunity and the subject is opened in a nonthreatening manner.*

Feeling: A Pattern Involving the Subjective Awareness of Information

Ask directly about experience of pain and fears. Anxiety symptoms are more easily identified if the nurse prompts the client for actual phenomena (e.g., "Are your muscles tight from time to time, is your mouth dry, do you perspire a lot—particularly when you're expecting something unpleasant?" "Have you had more difficulty concentrating lately?" "Have you ever had these feelings come out of nowhere?") *Endorsement of several of the defining characteristics of panic attack warrants a more thorough evaluation for panic disorder and agoraphobia.* Explore the client's experiences of guilt and shame for signs of social phobia.

- Risk for self-mutilation
- Disturbed sensory perception
- Sexual dysfunction
- Risk for impaired skin integrity
- Disturbed sleep pattern
- Impaired social interaction

- Social isolation
- Spiritual distress
- Risk for suicide
- Disturbed thought processes
- Risk for other-directed violence
- Risk for self-directed violence

NURSING CARE PLAN

Sarah, a 47-year-old woman, presented to the employee health department of a teaching hospital after walking there from her office. She was complaining of chest pain and shortness of breath. The staff instituted the standard cardiac workup for clients with new-onset chest pain. Sarah's medical history included psoriasis. Her vital signs were remarkable for a pulse of 116; her electrocardiogram and laboratory work were within normal limits.

Sarah mentioned to the staff that her son had died 3 months ago. She was referred to a research team conducting a study on panic disorder and was seen by a clinical specialist in psychiatric mental health nursing. Sarah participated in the research protocol after giving informed consent. During the course of the interview, she revealed that her deceased son, an only child, had been an alcoholic whose death was a suicide. She was presently considering separating from her husband of 27 years who was involved in a long-term extramarital affair. Her screening was positive for limited-symptom panic attacks that were increasing in frequency. She agreed to an extended evaluation after her initial interview.

During her evaluation, Sarah and the nurse explored her symptoms of anxiety and depression, the exacerbation of her psoriasis, and her chronic headaches, which had become worse since her son's death. On moving back from the West Coast, Sarah had obtained her first job in 24 years. In addition to concern about financial matters and her son's alcoholism, she now worried frequently about her performance at work. She revealed that her husband's extramarital affair had been ongoing for several years and related his behavior to their sexual difficulties. The nurse recommended a medication trial. Sarah refused medication because of her fears of addiction and loss of control.

DSM-IV-TR Diagnoses

Axis I	Generalized anxiety disorder (with limited-symptom panic attacks)
	Bereavement
	Partner relational problem
Axis II	Deferred
Axis III	Psoriasis
	Headaches
Axis IV	Problems with primary support system
Axis V	GAF = 60 (current)
	GAF = 75 (past year)

NURSING DIAGNOSIS: Anxiety related to change in role functioning, recent loss of son (dysfunctional grieving), threat to socioeconomic status, and stressors exceeding ability to cope, as evidenced by uncertainty, intermittent sympathetic nervous system stimulation, restlessness, and exacerbation of medical condition (psoriasis).

CLIENT OUTCOMES	NURSING INTERVENTIONS	EVALUATION
Sarah will identify common situations that provoke anxiety.	Assign "homework" to client (e.g., keeping a panic attack and headache diary). *Documenting anxiety responses helps client link symptoms with precipitating events.* During weekly sessions, review with Sarah, her log of panic symptoms. *Discussing the linking of events/situations with anxiety symptoms teaches Sarah which stressor events provoke anxiety, so she can learn to manage/avoid them.*	Sarah identifies returning home after work as a critical time for symptoms to develop. She reports that she visits her mother or does errands daily.
Sarah will describe early warning symptoms of anxiety.	Assist Sarah in associating her panic attack symptoms with thoughts about separation from her husband. *This will help illustrate to Sarah specific situations in her life that result in panic anxiety.*	Sarah reports that she does not experience headaches when her husband is traveling.
Sarah will report willingness to tolerate mild to moderate levels of anxiety.	In weekly sessions, explore with Sarah the advantages and disadvantages of separation and divorce. *These discussions will help Sarah problem solve viable options that may offer some control over her anxiety.*	Sarah reveals unwillingness to live alone.
Sarah will demonstrate adaptive coping mechanisms.	During weekly sessions discuss options that will allow Sarah maximum control over her choices. *Increased choices over life situations tend to minimize anxiety responses to some degree.*	Sarah informs her husband that she wants a trial separation. The husband moves into their son's former room.

Continued

NURSING CARE PLAN—cont'd

NURSING DIAGNOSIS: Dysfunctional grieving related to ineffective coping response to son's death, as evidenced by anxiety on returning home; disturbed sleep pattern; expression of guilt, sadness, and crying; and difficulty with concentration.

CLIENT OUTCOMES	NURSING INTERVENTIONS	EVALUATION
Sarah will return to her home directly after work, without going immediately to bed.	Explore with Sarah her usual patterns of behavior before her son's death. Identify possible modifications of those behaviors. *These discussions will help Sarah to focus on alternative activities/behaviors that would minimize dysfunctional grieving patterns and increase coping skills.*	Sarah describes cooking dinner for her son. She identifies other constructive activities she could perform to modify that routine.
Sarah will be able to talk with family and significant others about her son's death.	Promote recognition that others also experience the loss of Sarah's son. *This may help Sarah recognize that others share her grief, which can be comforting during critical times.*	Sarah is able to visit with her mother and talk about her son without experiencing panic symptoms.
Sarah will be able to use her son's former bedroom as a functional part of the house.	Initiate discussion of ways Sarah and her husband can plan for disposal of some of their son's possessions without feeling disloyal to his memory. *Discussing difficult topics at appropriate time with a trusted nurse may help feelings emerge and expedite functional grieving.*	As part of their trial separation agreement, Sarah's husband moves into their son's room.

NURSING DIAGNOSIS: Decisional conflict related to unclear personal values and beliefs, as evidenced by delayed decision making and physical signs of distress.

CLIENT OUTCOMES	NURSING INTERVENTIONS	EVALUATION
Sarah will make an informed decision about her relationship with her husband.	During weekly sessions explore with Sarah her expectations of marriage, how her relationship with her husband has changed over the course of their marriage, and what part she played in the changes. *This type of exploration may help Sarah to clarify values and expectations about her role in the marriage, which can assist her in making critical life choices.*	Sarah describes increasing involvement with her son as his substance abuse worsened and the consequent discord in an already strained marriage. She reports frequent conflict with her husband over his own drinking.
Sarah will identify potential outcomes of separation and divorce and prioritize them according to social, financial, and interpersonal values.	Review with Sarah some of the important relationships in her life. Support her considerations in the values clarification process. *It is critical that the nurse be aware of his or her own values and choices and maintain clear distinctions between his or her worldview and that of the client.*	Sarah describes her parental relationships as conflict ridden, with her father frequently abusing alcohol. She is critical of her mother's domination of her father. She acknowledges long-standing differences with her husband over sexual issues and feelings of disgust toward her husband when he smells of beer.

NURSING DIAGNOSIS: Chronic low self-esteem related to unresolved developmental issues, as evidenced by self-negating verbalizations, evaluation of self as unable to deal with decisions, and passive dependence on marital partner.

CLIENT OUTCOMES	NURSING INTERVENTIONS	EVALUATION
Sarah will exhibit a more positive self-evaluation.	Suggest the use of a diary. *Putting things in writing, will help Sarah to record interactions with her husband that result in anxiety symptoms.* During weekly sessions, role-play other responses that seem more satisfactory to Sarah. *This will help Sarah to distinguish anxiety-producing interactions and modify responses through role playing and other teaching strategies.*	Sarah reports fewer episodes of headaches and limited-symptom panic attacks. Sarah frequently describes reinitiating discussions with her husband that she previously identified as being unsatisfactory.
Sarah will demonstrate assertive behaviors and a positive interpersonal relationship.	Provide feedback to Sarah about behaviors observed. *This will give Sarah information about her responses/behaviors so she can begin to modify/manage them.* Help Sarah identify and label angry feelings. *This will help Sarah to begin processing her feelings more accurately and not misinterpret feelings or their meaning.*	Sarah initiates the subject of marital therapy with the nurse. Sarah requests that her husband join her in weekly sessions to deal with issues involving the husband's use of alcohol, his extramarital affair, and their sexual difficulties.

NURSING CARE PLAN—cont'd

NURSING DIAGNOSIS: Sexual dysfunction related to values regarding sexual intimacy conflict, as evidenced by ineffective role performance with husband and inability to achieve desired satisfaction.

CLIENT OUTCOMES	NURSING INTERVENTIONS	EVALUATION
Sarah will demonstrate ability to attain an ongoing intimate relationship with her husband.	Provide an open, neutral atmosphere where Sarah and her husband can discuss their differences regarding the level of interest in intimate relations and achievement of satisfaction. *This will encourage sound discussion in a nonthreatening environment.*	Sarah and her husband report increased mutually satisfying sexual encounters.

OUTCOME IDENTIFICATION

Outcome criteria differ according to the characteristics that define each client's nursing diagnoses and collaborative (DSM-IV-TR) diagnoses (see Collaborative Diagnoses table). Determining outcomes before implementation of the plan will guide both nursing interventions and evaluation. Nursing diagnoses are associated with outcomes (goals) to serve as a guide in outcome development. In practice, outcomes are generally determined by the patient's presentation of clinical manifestations.

Outcome Identification for Generalized Anxiety Disorder

Client will:
- Demonstrate significant decrease in physiologic, cognitive, behavioral, and emotional symptoms of anxiety.
- Demonstrate effective coping skills.
- Exhibit enhanced ability to make decisions and problem solve.
- Demonstrate ability to function adaptively in mild anxiety states.
- Discuss the medication regimen and take the medications per the prescription.
- Identify when to call the therapist for more visits when a crisis occurs.

Outcome Identification for Obsessive-Compulsive Disorder

Client will:
- Participate actively in learned strategies to manage anxiety and decrease obsessive-compulsive behaviors.
- Describe increasing sense of control over intrusive thoughts and ritualistic behaviors.
- Demonstrate ability to cope effectively when ruminations or rituals are interrupted.
- Spend less time involved in anxiety-binding activities and instead use time gained to complete activities of daily living and participate in social/recreational activities.

COLLABORATIVE DIAGNOSES

DSM-IV-TR Diagnoses*	NANDA Diagnoses†
Dissociative identity disorder	Disturbed personal identity Ineffective role performance Impaired social interaction Risk for other-directed violence
Obsessive-compulsive disorder	Impaired social interaction Social isolation Risk for other-directed violence Risk for self-directed violence
Posttraumatic stress disorder	Risk for suicide Post-trauma syndrome Rape-trauma syndrome
Somatization disorder	Risk for self-directed violence Ineffective role performance Impaired social interaction Fatigue

*From American Psychiatric Association: *Diagnostic and Statistical Manual of Mental Disorders,* Fourth Edition, Text Revision. Washington, DC, American Psychiatric Association, 2000.
†NANDA International (2003). NANDA Nursing Diagnoses: Definitions and Classification 2003-2004. Philadelphia: NANDA.

- Successfully manage times of increased stress by integrating knowledge that thoughts, impulses, and images are involuntary, thus reducing sense of responsibility and consequent anxiety.
- Be able to discuss the medication regimen and take the medications as per the prescription.
- Identify when to call the therapist for more visits when a crisis occurs.

Outcome Identification for Posttraumatic Stress Disorder

Client will:

- Demonstrate concern for personal safety by beginning to verbalize worries.
- Participate actively in support group.
- Identify and involve significant support system.
- Assume decision-making role for own health care needs.
- Acquire and practice strategies for coping with anxiety symptoms such as breathing techniques; progressive relaxation exercises; thought, image and memory substitution; and assertive behaviors (see Chapter 19).
- Discuss the medication regimen and take the medications as prescribed.
- Contact the therapist for immediate help when a crisis occurs.
- Identify the need for increase in visits if there is an increase in symptoms.

Outcome Identification for Somatization Disorder

Client will:

- Construct an exercise program.
- Address two positive somatic responses (e.g., massage therapy, the satisfied feeling after a successful exercise session).
- Keep an intake log to document somatic preoccupation and stressors (including intrusive thoughts or concerns).
- Assist the therapist to coordinate the information from the primary care provider and any other involved specialists.
- Take the medication as prescribed and be able to identify the rationale for the medication.
- Contact the therapist for increase in visits if there is an increase in somatization.

Outcome Identification for Dissociative Identity Disorder

Client will:

- Respond to name when addressed by a member of the treatment team.
- Refer to self in the first-person pronoun form: "I think."
- Identify periods of increasing anxiety.
- Inform others of dissatisfaction in a nonthreatening manner.
- Use assertive-response behaviors to meet needs (see Chapter 19).
- Keep a written journal to identify stressors and when the dissociation occurs.
- Alert the therapist and/or use a hot line of 1-800-SUICIDE when feeling suicidal.
- Take medications as prescribed.
- Contact the therapist if there is an increase in symptoms.

PLANNING

Treatment planning for the client with anxiety and related disorders in the current health care environment is complex and varied. Clients with severe OCD were formerly hospitalized for structured behavioral programs. Treatment for dissociative identity disorder also occurred in special units with a prolonged hospitalization.

Today both clinicians and administrators in inpatient facilities are struggling to balance effective treatment with the high costs associated with these specialty units. Increasingly, inpatient hospitalization is available only for short periods of time for clients at imminent risk to themselves or others. Rather than assuming their traditional roles of providing direct care to clients in inpatient facilities, nurses are increasingly involved as case managers. As case managers, nurses provide information on treatment alternatives to clients and families.

IMPLEMENTATION

The role of a nurse in the implementation of a care plan for clients with anxiety and related disorders depends on the setting in which the client is treated. The following interventions are useful for clients with anxiety symptoms, regardless of diagnosis or treatment setting. Specific issues community nurses may face are found in the Nursing Care in the Community box.

Nursing Interventions

1. Assess own level of anxiety and make a conscious effort to remain calm. *Anxiety is readily transferable from one person to another.*
2. Recognize the client's use of relief behaviors (pacing, wringing of hands) as indicators of anxiety. *Early interventions help to manage anxiety before symptoms escalate to more serious levels.*
3. Inform the client of the importance of limiting caffeine, nicotine, and other central nervous system stimulants. *Limiting these substances, prevents/minimizes physical symptoms of anxiety, such as rapid heart rate and jitteriness.*
4. Teach the client to distinguish between anxiety that can be connected to identifiable objects or sources (illness, prognosis, hospitalization, known stressors) and anxiety for which there is no immediate identifiable object or source. *Knowledge of anxiety and its related components increases the client's control over the disorder.*
5. Instruct the client in the following anxiety-reducing strategies, *which help reduce anxiety in a variety of ways and distract the client from focusing on the anxiety* (see Chapter 19):
   a. Progressive relaxation technique
   b. Slow deep-breathing exercises
   c. Focusing on a single object in the room
   d. Listening to soothing music or relaxation tapes
   e. Visual imagery

NURSING CARE IN THE COMMUNITY   Anxiety and Related Disorders

Anxiety disorders are seldom found in a pure form. Clients who seek help or who are found at home in a highly anxious state are usually reacting to a situational crisis that may be physical or psychologic. They may benefit from a brief intervention such as reassurance or reorientation to the environment.

Older adults may often become extremely anxious about somatic complaints, ranging from worries about constipation to sensations of having a heart attack. Community mental health nurses may have responded to a client's repeated complaints, but these complaints should be investigated medically before psychiatric intervention is attempted. After a medical condition has been ruled out, these types of anxious persons will usually respond to cognitive interventions and/or medication. They may benefit from increased unsolicited attention and involvement of a community-based support system, such as the family, visiting nurse, and/or social worker.

The older client with progressive dementia also presents with increased anxiety or paranoia as a result of the confusional state of the disease itself. In some cases antipsychotic or antianxiety medications are prescribed, and the older client must be monitored closely for hypotension and the increased risk of accidental falls.

A client with a chronic mental disorder such as paranoid schizophrenia may often seek reassurance from the nurse. Kindness and simple self-care suggestions for stress reduction are usually enough to return the client's attention to normal functioning, but an adjustment in medication may also be indicated.

Occasionally the nurse encounters a person who cannot identify a current stressor but is experiencing severe anxiety verging on panic. Daily functions are seriously impaired, and a family member or friend must intervene to call for help or deliver the client to a care site. Such individuals may respond to anxiolytic medications but are not generally capable of processing cognitive therapy. They usually continue to experience overwhelming apprehension despite reassurance and reality testing.

It is essential to recognize that the client's sensations are beyond rationality and to maintain a calm presence until the appropriate medications act to decrease pathologic activity in the brain and allow resumption of functional response patterns. The client should not be expected to supply information, and if feasible, it can be obtained from a significant other. As the client becomes calmer, the nurse may establish a therapeutic relationship, and gaps in the history may be filled and validated by the client.

If the intensity of the anxiety is not mitigated by a standard dose of medication within a reasonable time, the nurse working in the community must consider hospitalizing the client. Hospitalization will relieve the client of the pressures of family and daily maintenance behaviors until rational abilities are restored. The hospital offers a safe environment with reduced stress and therapeutic suggestions for more positive coping activities.

6. Help the client build on coping methods that helped to manage anxiety in the past. *Coping methods that were previously successful will generally be effective in subsequent situations.*

7. Help the client identify support persons who can help him or her perform personal tasks and activities that current circumstances make difficult (such as hospitalization). *A strong support system can help circumvent anxiety-provoking situations/activities.*

8. Help the client gain control of overwhelming feelings and impulses through brief, directive verbal interactions. *Individual interactions executed at appropriate intervals can help reduce/manage client's anxious feelings/impulses.*

9. Help the client structure the environment so that it is less noisy. *A less stimulating environment can create a calming, stress-free atmosphere that reduces anxiety.*

10. Assess the presence and degree of depression and suicidal ideation in all clients with anxiety and related disorders. *A thorough assessment results in early intervention that can prevent self-harm.*

11. Administer **anxiolytic** (antianxiety) medication as a least restrictive measure. *Medication may be the first appropriate method to reduce debilitation anxiety.*

12. Assist the client to understand the importance of the medication regimen and to take it as prescribed. *Medication may be an effective adjunct to other psychosocial therapeutic interventions when necessary.*

Additional Treatment Modalities
Biologic Interventions

Pharmacologic Interventions. Pharmacologic interventions alone or in combination with cognitive behavioral interventions are among the most successful treatments for anxiety and related disorders. Since the early 1960s, benzodiazepines have been widely used in the treatment of anxiety disorders. They are relatively safe and effective for short-term use in controlling debilitating symptoms of anxiety. Longer term treatment of these drugs raises issues of tolerance, abuse, and dependence.

SSRIs, antidepressants now widely used to treat anxiety disorders, are particularly effective in treating OCD and panic disorders. Fluoxetine and fluvoxamine are indicated for OCD, paroxetine is indicated for GAD, OCD, panic disorder, PTSD, and social phobia. Sertraline is indicated for OCD, panic disorder, and PTSD; and venlafaxine is indicated for GAD (Fredman and Korn, 2002).

Pharmacologic treatment for PTSD and DID is largely symptomatic. Varying combinations of antidepressants, antipsychotics, and to a lesser extent benzodiazepines are used. Research is currently being done on the best medication regimen for individuals with somatoform disorders. For example, clomipramine versus desipramine was recently studied for individuals with body dysmorphic disorder. Clomipramine was more effective for individuals with this disorder than desipramine. The medication improved the individual's ability to function, including the clients who have delusions accompanying the body dysmorphic disorder (Hollander et al., 1999). (For more specific information about dosages and side effect profiles, see Chapter 20.)

Electroconvulsive Therapy. The primary indication for electroconvulsive therapy (ECT) is depression. However, ECT may be used for anxiety disorders when other treatments are too high a risk or have failed. For example, in clients with OCD who have only a partial response to clomipramine and who are suicidal, ECT is a reasonable treatment alternative. The mechanism of ECT is unknown, but it is thought to be related to improving transmission of dopamine, norepinephrine, and serotonin and release of hypothalamic and pituitary hormones (Keltner and Folks, 1997) (see Chapter 19).

Psychotherapy

Psychotherapeutic intervention can take place in group or individual settings. One advantage of group therapy is the opportunity for the client to learn from the successes and failures of others with similar symptoms. Behavioral and cognitive behavioral therapies have proved to be widely effective in treating a variety of anxiety disorders (see Chapter 19).

Behavioral Therapy. Behavioral treatments, including systematic desensitization, are among the most effective treatments for panic disorder with agoraphobia. First, the phobic stimulus is defined. Clients are assisted in defining a hierarchy for the phobic stimulus. The client and therapist then expose the client to events on the hierarchy that increase the client's degree of anxiety. As the client and therapist move through the hierarchy, the client experiences progressive mastery of increasing levels of anxiety until the phobic stimulus is encountered (see Chapter 19).

Cognitive Behavioral Therapy. Cognitive behavioral therapy is widely used in the treatment of anxiety disorders. The success of this approach centers on the client's understanding that symptoms are a learned response to thoughts or feelings about behaviors that occur in daily life. The client and therapist identify the target symptoms and then examine circumstances associated with the symptoms. Together they devise strategies to change either the cognitions or the behaviors. Cognitive behavioral therapy is short term and demands active participation on the part of both client and therapist (see Chapter 19).

Additional treatment modalities and collaborative interventions may include consultation with occupational therapists, vocational rehabilitation counselors, and psychologists, depending on the particular treatment needs of a client. A summary of additional treatment modalities appears in the Additional Treatment Modalities box and is explored in depth in Chapter 19.

Additional Treatment Modalities
For Clients With Anxiety and Related Disorders

Biologic
- Pharmacologic
  - Benzodiazepines
  - Selective serotonin reuptake inhibitors
  - Tricyclic antidepressants
  - Monoamine oxidase inhibitors
- Electroconvulsive therapy
Psychotherapy
- Behavioral therapy
- Cognitive behavioral therapy

EVALUATION

One of the most difficult aspects of applying the nursing process to psychiatric mental health nursing, in particular, nursing care of clients with anxiety and related disorders, is generating measurable outcomes. Outcome criteria for clients with the more concrete nursing diagnoses, such as hyperthermia, decreased cardiac output, or even disturbed thought processes as evidenced by auditory hallucinations, seem clear and straightforward when compared with the more vague concept of anxiety. Fortunately, a number of valid, time-tested tools are available that yield reliable information for anxiety-related disorders. Although not developed by and for nurses specifically, clinical rating scales offer a method to track changes in symptoms over time with a numeric value. These changes can be correlated with discrete interventions (such as instituting a behavioral program or a change in medication). Two rating scales commonly used with clients exhibiting anxiety disorders are the Yale-Brown Obsessive-Compulsive Scale (Y-BOCS) and the Hamilton Anxiety (HAM-A) Scale.

Ideally the nurse evaluates client progress toward the identified outcomes at every interaction with the client. If satisfactory progress is not made, the nurse either modifies the expected outcomes or the interventions. The nurse examines all factors that relate to the outcomes, including what occurred in the previous phases of the nursing process, the role of the nurse in setting client and clinician expectations, the clarity of communicating client goals with the client, and other intervening events that may have occurred since the outcomes were set.

CHAPTER SUMMARY

- Anxiety and related disorders encompass a wide variety of illnesses that share the common symptoms of anxiety.
- Etiologic models for anxiety include biologic, psychosocial, psychodynamic, and social theories.

- Anxiety disorders have high comorbidity with depression and substance abuse.
- Anxiety disorders are more commonly diagnosed and treated among women, although obsessive-compulsive disorder is equally common in both men and women.
- Treatment of anxiety and related disorders is multidisciplinary and usually involves more than one treatment modality.
- Inpatient treatment of anxiety disorders is increasingly rare and is generally confined to managing acute exacerbations if the person becomes a danger to self or others, or if the symptoms are so severe that self-care functions are greatly reduced.
- The nursing role in the treatment of clients with anxiety symptoms varies. Common to all treatment settings is the nurse's role in client and family education about the disorders and their treatment.
- Nursing care plans for clients with symptoms of anxiety reflect the understanding that managing anxiety effectively is part of daily living.
- Nurses actively participate in behavioral interventions structured to decrease phobic responses.
- Rating scales are an effective means for nurses to measure success of strategies implemented to reduce anxiety.

REVIEW QUESTIONS

1. A 30-year-old client walks into the clinic. She is restless, pacing, and having difficulty concentrating. She complains of insomnia and fatigue. She verbalizes that she worries about her children to the point that she doesn't want them to play outside for fear that they will get hurt. The nurse determines that client is experiencing:
   a. Panic disorder
   b. Obsessive-compulsive disorder
   c. Generalized anxiety disorder
   d. Posttraumatic stress disorder

2. A 10-year-old boy arrives for his therapy appointment. He is diagnosed with obsessive-compulsive disorder. He is plagued with obsessive thoughts that every time he steps on a crack he hurts his mother and experiences anxiety every time he does step on a crack. An appropriate nursing intervention would be:
   a. Explain to his parents the symptoms and treatment of the disorder.
   b. Explain how irrational his thoughts are.
   c. Have him avoid stepping on cracks because it causes him such increased anxiety.
   d. Teach cognitive strategies to deal with anxiety.

3. A 24-year-old client seeks outpatient therapy after being raped 2 weeks earlier. She complains of insomnia, decreased appetite, depression, and anxiety when she is outside of her home. The most appropriate initial nursing intervention would be:
   a. Refer her to a support group for victims of rape.
   b. Suggest that she attend a self-defense class.
   c. Validate her feelings, use active listening, and ensure that she is safe to build a trusting relationship.
   d. Teach her relaxation techniques.

4. A 28-year-old client is admitted to the psychiatric unit for the fourth time after she cut her wrists, requiring sutures. She does not remember cutting herself. She is diagnosed with dissociative identity disorder. The best nursing short-term outcome would be:
   The client will:
   a. Inform staff when she has the urge to harm herself.
   b. Not "switch" personalities within 7 days.
   c. Discuss her childhood issues that relate to her anxiety.
   d. Assume a decision-making role for her own health care needs.

5. A 20-year-old client is admitted to the Emergency Department with complaints of severe abdominal pain. The nurse obtains her old record and discovers that she has had numerous surgeries, including surgery to rule out bowel obstruction, appendicitis, and gallstones. All the surgeries revealed no abnormalities or obstructions. She was also seen in the Emergency Department for complaints of back pain, migraine headaches, and chest pain. An appropriate nursing diagnosis for this client would be:
   a. Deficient knowledge
   b. Health-seeking behaviors
   c. Noncompliance
   d. Acute pain

REFERENCES

American Psychiatric Association: *Diagnostic and Statistical Manual of Mental Disorders,* Fourth Edition, Text Revision. Washington, DC, American Psychiatric Association, 2000.
Anxiety Disorder Research at the National Institute of Mental Health. Fact Sheet. June 27, 2002, website:www.nimh.nih.gov/publicat/anxresfact.cfm.
Blackman S: OCD: past, present and future, *Psychiatric Times* XIV:5-14, 1997.
Fortinash K, Holoday Worret P: *Psychiatric nursing care plans,* ed 4, St Louis, 2003, Mosby.
Foucault M: *Madness and civilization,* New York, 1988, Vantage.
Fredman S, Korn, ML: Anxiety disorders and related conditions, *Medscape* June 20, 2002, website: www.medscape.com/viewprogram/1917-pnt.
Freud S: Introductory lectures on psychoanalysis. In *The standard edition of the complete psychological works,* London, 1963, Hogarth Press (originally published in 1917). (classic)
Freud S: *The standard edition of the complete psychological works,* London, 1963, Hogarth Press. (classic)
Goodwin R et al: Panic and suicidal ideation in primary care, *Depress Anxiety* 14:244-246, 2001.
Hall CS: *A primer of Freudian psychology,* Cleveland, 1954, World. (classic)
Heidegger M: *Being and time,* New York, 1962, Harper & Row.
Heun R, Maier W: Relation of schizophrenia and panic disorder: evidence from a controlled family study, *Am J Med Genet* 60:127-132, 1995.

Hollander E et al: Clomipramine vs desipramine crossover trail in body dysmorphic disorder, *Arch Gen Psychiatry* 56:1033-1044, 1999.

Keltner NL, Folks DG: *Psychotropic drugs,* ed 2, St Louis, 1997, Mosby.

Kessler RC et al: Lifetime and 12 month prevalence of DSM III-R psychiatric disorders in the United States. Results from the National Comorbidity Survey, *Arch Gen Psychiatry* 51:8-19, 1994.

Kierkegaard S: *The concept of anxiety,* Princeton, 1980, Princeton University Press.

Korn M: Recent developments in the science and treatment of PTSD, *Medscape* June 20, 2002, website: www.medscape.com/viewprogram/1917-pnt.

May R: *The meaning of anxiety,* New York, 1979, Pocket Books. (classic)

National Institutes of Mental Health, *Effects of chronic stress on the hippocampus,* Korn, 2002.

NANDA International (2003). NANDA Nursing Diagnoses: Definitions and Classifications 2003-2004. Philadelphia: NANDA.

Patterson JG, Zderad LT: *Humanistic nursing,* New York, 1976, Wiley.

Peplau H: *Interpersonal relations in nursing,* New York, 1952, Putnam. (classic)

Peplau H: *Interpersonal relations in nursing: a conceptual frame of reference for psychodynamic nursing,* New York, 1991, Springer.

Selye H: *The stress of life,* New York, 1956, McGraw-Hill. (classic)

Wolpe J: *The practice of behavior therapy,* ed 2, New York, 1973, Pergamon Press. (classic)

SUGGESTED READINGS

Bailey K, Glod CA: Post-traumatic stress disorder; a role for psychopharmacology, *J Psychosoc Nurs Ment Health Serv* 29(9):42, 1991.

Kluft RP: Enhancing the hospital treatment of dissociative disorder patients by developing nursing expertise in the application of hypnotic techniques without formal trance induction, *Am J Clin Hypnosis* 34(3):158, 1992.

Lederman C: Worry: how much is too much? Generalized anxiety disorder, *ADAA Reporter* 8 (October 2002): 1, 13-14, website: www.adaa.org.

Neziroglu FA, Yaryura-Tobias JA: A review of cognitive-behavioral and pharmacological treatment of body dysmorphic disorder, *Behav Modif* 21:324, 1997.

Roy-Byrne PP: Generalized anxiety and mixed anxiety-depression: association with disability and health care utilization, *J Clin Psychol* 57(7):86, 1996.

ONLINE RESOURCES

Anxiety Disorders (NIMH): www.nimh.nih.gov/anxiety/anxietymenu.cfm

National Center for PTSD: www.ncptsd.org

Obsessive Compulsive Foundation: www.ocfoundation.org

10

Mood Disorders: Depression and Mania

Bonnie Hagerty and Kathleen L. Patusky

OBJECTIVES

- Describe neurobiologic, ethologic, and psychosocial theories about the etiology of mood disorders.

- Compare and contrast the DSM-IV-TR groupings of depressive disorders and bipolar disorders.

- Discuss the epidemiology and life course of depressive and bipolar disorders.

- Apply the nursing process for clients with mood disorders.

- Describe independent and collaborative interventions used by nurses and other mental health professionals for clients with mood disorders.

- Examine personal feelings, thoughts, and reactions to clients with mood disorders that may affect the therapeutic relationship and management of client care.

- Examine issues in the health care system that affect the care of persons with mood disorders.

Mood disorders, sometimes known as affective disorders, are a group of common psychiatric disorders characterized by dysregulation of emotion. Persons exhibiting mood disorders may demonstrate a range of emotions from intense elation or irritability to severe depression. Mood disorders are also characterized by a constellation of symptoms including impaired cognition, physiologic disturbances such as sleep and appetite problems, and lowered self-esteem. Mood disorders have serious consequences that result in personal and family suffering, interpersonal and occupational impairment, and expensive social costs. In recent years mood disorders, including their recurrent and cyclic nature and the disabling outcomes associated with repeated episodes, are better understood. Mood disorders are now viewed as major public health problems in terms of both economic costs and personal suffering. Depression alone has been identified as the fourth-ranked illness in the world, causing "burden," morbidity, and mortality throughout multiple countries (DHHS, 1999; Murray and Lopez, 1996).

Although most people experience mood fluctuations of depression and elation, normal variations tend not to be prolonged or incapacitating. Mood fluctuation is often a normal response to life experiences and events that influence the human capacity for feeling. Grief and sadness in response to loss of a loved one or excitement at the thought of a long-awaited vacation are normal, adaptive responses. Most people experience sadness and depression with losses (e.g., of loved ones, jobs, status, possessions). This sadness may persist for days, weeks, or longer as the individual grieves the loss (see Chapter 25). When mood states become maladaptive, however, they persist, are pervasive, incorporate additional symptoms such as impaired sleep and cognition, and interfere with usual functioning. At that point the mood dysregulation, accompanied by a pattern of signs and symptoms, affects cognitive, behavioral, spiritual, social, and physiologic functioning.

HISTORICAL AND THEORETIC PERSPECTIVES

Disturbances in mood have been recognized for many years. It is thought that the term *melancholia* was first coined by Hippocrates when he described changing temperament. In 1896 Kraepelin distinguished between dementia praecox (now known as schizophrenia) and manic depression. He described dementia praecox as a chronic illness with progressive deterioration in the client's functioning. Kraepelin (1913, 1921) saw manic depression as cyclic abnormalities of mood, marked by a family history of similar disorders and caused by innate physical factors. This differentiation served as a primary underpinning for modern approaches to understanding and diagnosing mood disorders.

Since Kraepelin, attempts have been made to describe nuances of both **depression** and **mania**. Freud (1957) differentiated between maladaptive depression and grief in his famous article "Mourning and Melancholia," which described the psychodynamic genesis of depression. Leonhard (1974), a German psychiatrist, proposed the separation of manic-depressive illness into two types: bipolar (history of depression and mania) and monopolar (history of depression only). This differentiation is the basis for the current clinical depiction of bipolar disorder and unipolar disorders.

Throughout much of the twentieth century, various forms of bipolar and unipolar disorders have been described. Unipolar depression, for example, has been considered to be one of two types: reactive (exogenous) depression or endogenous depression. Reactive depression was believed to be caused by external stressors and was considered less severe than endogenous depression, which was believed to be due to physiologic dysregulation. Mental health professionals currently recognize various forms of bipolar disorders and unipolar depression. Researchers and clinicians continue to document a broad spectrum of mood disorders with varied features and clinical characteristics.

In recent years mood disorders have commanded more public attention as a result of their pervasiveness. New treatments, including use of drugs such as fluoxetine (Prozac), have created social controversy. Famous persons, including Patty Duke, William Styron, and Dick Cavett, have publicly acknowledged their struggles with mood disorders; and it is now recognized that many other prominent persons, including Abraham Lincoln, Winston Churchill, Vincent Van Gogh, Ernest Hemingway, Sylvia Plath, and Herman Melville, experienced a mood disorder.

ETIOLOGY

Various theories have been presented to explain the development of mood disorders, but their exact cause remains unknown. Many researchers and clinicians support the premise that mood disorders have multicausal origins, in which neurobiologic, ethologic, psychosocial, and cognitive factors converge to promote the development of depression and mania. Others contend that specific types of mood disorders may be related more to certain specific etiologic factors. Research findings suggest that depression, for example, includes several distinct syndromes that can be differentiated clinically and over time (Kendler et al., 1996). Each theoretic perspective helps to explain some aspect of mood disorders, but none fully accounts for their development. In general, these etiologic factors can be grouped primarily as neurobiologic, ethologic, or psychosocial. These factors are summarized in Box 10-1.

Neurobiologic Factors

Over the last decade, research on the etiology of mood disorders has focused on the biologic mechanisms that may be related to their onset and clinical course. Although this research has been able to identify physiologic correlates of depression and mania, direct cause-and-effect relationships have not been established. The more common biologic theories include those related to altered neurotransmission, neuroendocrine dysregulation, and genetic transmission.

Box 10-1 Etiologic Factors Related to Mood Disorders

Neurobiologic Factors
Altered neurotransmission
Neuroendocrine dysregulation
Genetic transmission

Ethologic Factors
Evolutionary
Psychobiology/Biology

Psychosocial Factors

PSYCHOANALYTIC THEORY
Depression is a result of loss.
Mania is a defense against depression.

COGNITIVE THEORY
Depression is a result of negative processing of thoughts.

LEARNED HELPLESSNESS
Depression is a result of a perceived lack of control over events.

LIFE EVENTS AND STRESS THEORY
Significant life events cause stress, which results in depression or mania.

PERSONALITY THEORY
Personality characteristics predispose an individual to mood disorders.

Neurotransmission

Research on the biology of mood disorders has emphasized investigation of neurotransmitter disturbances. Interest in **neurotransmission** was sparked initially by investigations of the action of antidepressant drugs. In 1954 it was discovered that clients treated with reserpine for hypertension developed depression. Several years later, isoniazid was found to have an antidepressant effect on persons being treated for tuberculosis. Imipramine was introduced as an antidepressant in 1958, and research began on its mechanisms of action in the brain. The discoveries resulting from this line of research became the basis for the monoamine hypothesis of mood disorders.

Monoamine or biogenic amine neurotransmitters are crucial for sending electrical signals throughout the brain. Although there are hundreds of neurotransmitters in the brain, the biogenic amine neurotransmitters include the catecholamines of epinephrine, norepinephrine, dopamine, and acetylcholine, and the indolamine serotonin. To accomplish neurotransmission, these chemicals are released from the presynaptic neuronal terminal into the synaptic cleft. Once in the synaptic cleft, the neurotransmitter diffuses until it reaches its specific receptors on the postsynaptic membrane of the adjacent neuron or is resorbed through special autoreceptors on the presynaptic membrane The neurotransmitter may also be degraded by another chemical, such as the enzyme monoamine oxidase, within the neuron. When the neurotransmitter locks into its receptors on the postsynaptic membrane of an adjacent neuron, it opens an ion channel. The opening of the channel triggers a series of chemical actions that electrically depolarize the cell and sends an electrical impulse throughout that neuron, thus continuing the process of transmission of nerve impulses. Specialized neurons of each of the neurotransmitters project to various parts of the brain that control a wide range of functions, including appetite, sleep, and arousal.

It is believed that monoamine neurotransmitter systems, especially those of norepinephrine and serotonin, their metabolites, and their receptors, are somehow altered during episodes of depression and mania. Research on neurotransmission has focused on the altered sensitivity of neuronal receptors and properties of neuronal membranes. In response to a decrease or increase in availability of neurotransmitters, it appears that, over time, there is a change in the sensitivity or density of presynaptic and postsynaptic receptors specific to a particular neurotransmitter. This results in delayed postsynaptic receptor-mediated responses.

Availability and receptor change theories propose that there is an underactivity of neurotransmission in depression and an overactivity in mania. Support for this comes from the administration of monoamine oxidase inhibitors (MAOIs) to clients with depression. MAOIs inhibit the monoamine oxidase enzyme from breaking down neurotransmitters, thus resulting in an increased supply of neurotransmitters and an accompanying decrease in clinical depression. Additional support is evident through research that demonstrates how medications such as fluoxetine, paroxetine (Paxil), and sertraline (Zoloft) (selective serotonin reuptake inhibitors [SSRIs]) selectively block serotonin reuptake in their presynaptic neuronal receptors, thus increasing the supply of serotonin in the synaptic cleft (Struder and Weicker, 2001). Newer antidepressants, selective norepinephrine reuptake inhibitors such as reboxetine, increase the supply of norepinephrine in the synaptic cleft by blocking its reuptake (Frazer, 2000). It can be argued that therapeutic responses to most antidepressant medications usually take several weeks, possibly because of the delayed sensitization or change in quantity of receptors.

Post (1992) has postulated that a phenomenon called **kindling** occurs, in which neurotransmission is altered initially by stress, resulting in a first episode of depression. This initial episode creates an electrophysiologic sensitivity to future stress, requiring less stress to evoke another depressive or manic episode. In essence, kindling creates new "hardwiring" of the brain or long-lasting alterations of neuronal functioning. Research with rats has shown that maternal deprivation may lead to decreases in neurotrophic factors in the hippocampus, ultimately damaging brain functioning by causing early cell death (Post, 1997). It appears as though these alterations influence many cellular processes and structures, including changes in cell dendrites, and changes in cellular metabolism through second- and third-messenger systems that ultimately influence the

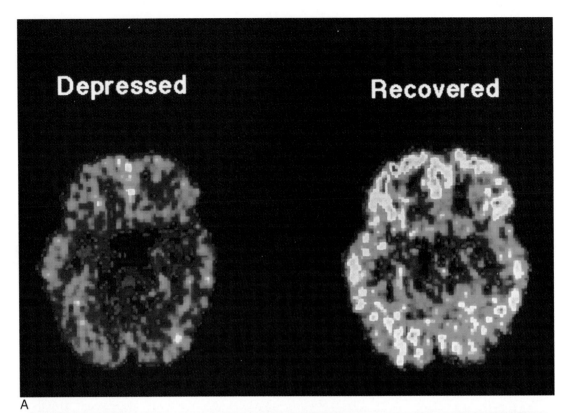

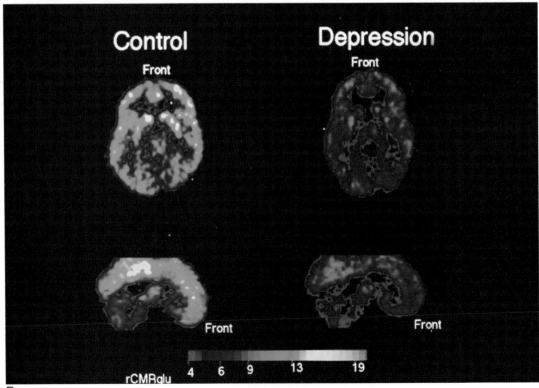

FIGURE 10-1. **A,** Positron emission tomography (PET) scans of the brain in the same individual during depression *(left)* and after recovery through treatment with medication *(right).* Several brain areas, particularly the prefrontal cortex *(at top),* show diminished activity *(darker colors)* during depression. **B,** PET scans of a normal subject *(left)* and a depressed subject *(right)* reveal reduced brain activity *(darker colors)* during depression, especially in the prefrontal cortex. A form of radioactively tagged glucose was used as a tracer to visualize levels of brain activity. (Courtesy Mark George, MD, National Institute of Mental Health Biological Psychiatry Branch, U.S. Department of Health and Human Services.)

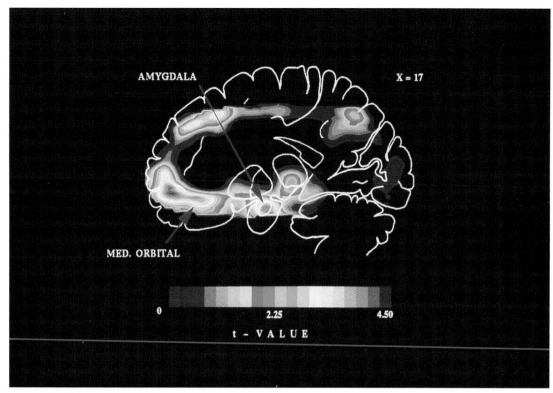

FIGURE 10-2. PET scan indicates increased blood flow in the amygdala and prefrontal cortex in persons with major depression of the familial pure depressive disease subtype. The scan is a composite of images of 13 individuals. (Courtesy Wayne C. Drevets, MD, Department of Psychiatry, Washington University School of Medicine, St Louis.)

expression of selected genes. The kindling model is consistent with the cyclic and progressive nature of mood disorders and suggests that clients be treated early for their mood episodes and remain on medication for extended periods to avoid physiologic deterioration over time.

Recent technologic advances in studying the brain provide additional support for the theory of disturbances in brain functioning during depression. The positron emission tomography (PET) scanner enables researchers to examine brain physiology of depressed persons as compared with normal control subjects, as well as compare brain functioning in individuals both during depression and after recovery. Magnetic resonance imaging (MRI) and single photon emission computed tomography (SPECT) are also used to produce images of the functioning of the brain (Renshaw and Rauch, 1999). Figure 10-1 depicts the differences that are apparent using PET scanning of depressed, recovered, and normal control brains. Figure 10-2 indicates increased blood flow in components of the brains of persons with major depression. PET scanning has shown that the prefrontal cerebral cortex and the limbic system (including the amygdala) appear to have physiologic disruptions in the brains of persons experiencing depression.

Although research continues on these biochemical theories, the complexity of the biologic structural and physiologic changes occurring with mood disorders continues to pose challenges for investigation. In addition, the research is hampered by inconsistent definitions and criteria for depression and mania, as well as the difficulties of measuring concentrations of specific neurotransmitters in selected sites in the brain and removing selected brain structures for analysis. Peripheral indicators of neurotransmitters and their metabolites, such as those in the blood, urine, or central spinal fluid, may not be related to their amounts or mechanisms of action in various parts of the brain. In addition, neurotransmission, as a complex activity, encompasses multiple processes such as neurotransmitter synthesis and release, receptor site function and change, interactions among the various neurotransmitters and hormones, and the action of these transmitters and hormones on genetic material via second- and third-messenger systems.

Neuroendocrine Dysregulation

Another area of research on the biologic basis of mood disorders is the role of the endocrine system. Studies indicate that dysregulation of the hypothalamic-pituitary-adrenal (HPA) axis is associated with depression. The HPA axis comprises the hypothalamus, pituitary, and adrenal glands and controls physiologic responses to stress. The hypothalamus regulates endocrine functions and the autonomic nervous system and is involved in behaviors related to fight, flight, feeding, and mating. In response to stress, the hypothalamus releases corticotropin-releasing hormone (CRH), which stimulates the anterior pituitary to secrete corticotropin. In turn, corticotropin causes the adrenal cortex to release cortisol into the blood. Through an elaborate feedback mechanism, levels of cortisol signal the hypothalamus via the hippocampus to increase or decrease CRH production. The specific physiologic ways that stress signals for this process to begin are not well understood, although stress-input signals may come from the brainstem, autonomic nervous system, or cerebral cortex (Young et al., 1993).

Hyperactivity of the HPA axis is often evident in depression. As many as 50% of clients with moderate to severe depression exhibit elevated serum cortisol levels. This phenomenon led to the creation of the dexamethasone suppression test (DST), which was hoped to be a potential biologic diagnostic indicator of endogenous depression. The DST is based on the premise that when clients are given dexamethasone (synthetic cortisol) at night, a signal is sent to the hypothalamus to shut down production of CRH, leading to decreased output of corticotropin and, subsequently, cortisol by the next morning. For many clients with severe depression, measurement of the blood cortisol level the next morning revealed continued excessive amounts of cortisol production. Subsequent research regarding the DST has revealed problems with its selectivity and specificity. It is not consistent with regard to its results in persons with depression, may be affected by other variables (e.g., age, gender), and is evident in other disorders such as alcoholism and anorexia nervosa (Zimmerman, Coryell, and Pfohl, 1986).

Chronobiology

The functioning of the HPA axis is related to the 24-hour cycle of circadian rhythms that control physiologic processes. With mood disorders, many normal, cyclic patterns are disrupted. Blood cortisol is normally at a low level in the early morning and highest in late afternoon, although constant increases are often apparent in depression. Sleep-wake cycles are disrupted in mood disorders, and during depression clients experience decreased rapid eye movement (REM) latency and decreased shallow, slow delta wave sleep, thus fragmenting the sleep-wake cycle. Even seasonal patterns appear to have some relationship to mood disorders, with episodes of depression often occurring during periods of decreased light.

Over time high levels of cortisol may damage the hippocampus. There is evidence that decreased hippocampal volume is associated with recurrrent and chronic depression. Consequences include cognitive impairment, particularly memory difficulties (Sapolsky, 2000). Research on HPA axis dysfunction continues, with special interest in the relationships among mood disorders, stress, and neuroendocrine functioning.

Genetic Transmission

Mood disorders tend to run in families, and it is commonly believed that, to some extent, genetic transmission is responsible for their manifestation. Data regarding the genetic transmission of mood disorders are derived from family, twin, and adoption studies.

In family studies families who exhibit mood disorders are selected, and the morbid risk for developing these disorders in relatives is compared with the general population. Results of these studies consistently demonstrate that first-degree relatives of persons with bipolar disorder and unipolar depression have a greater risk for developing a mood disorder. This risk is particularly high for relatives of persons with bipolar disorder, possibly indicating a greater genetic component than that for unipolar depression (McGriffin and Katz, 1989).

Twin studies are based on the assumption that monozygotic twins share the same genes and that dizygotic twins have about 50% of their genes in common. Results of twin research provide additional evidence for the genetic transmission of mood disorders. If one monozygotic twin suffers from bipolar disorder, there is a high rate of concordance, ranging to 100% in some studies, whereby the other twin will also develop a mood disorder, usually bipolar illness. Although there are high rates of concordance for dizygotic twins, they tend to be less than those for monozygotic twins. For unipolar disorders the concordance rates continue to be higher for monozygotic twins, and both twin types have a higher concordance than the general population (Kendler, 2001).

Using adoption studies, researchers can examine the contributions of both the environment and genetic transmission. In general, adoption studies also support the role of genetic factors in mood disorders. Most studies have focused specifically on bipolar disorder and have found that the biologic parents of adult adoptees diagnosed with bipolar disorder have a much higher incidence of the disorder than parents of adoptees with no mood disorder.

Although all of the preceding information supports the role of genetics in the development of mood disorders, particularly bipolar disorders, the research does not reveal the specific genes or genetic mechanisms involved in transmission. Early scientific reports describing the location of genetic markers on specific genes have not been replicated, although this type of research is evolving with advances in DNA and genetic analysis. The search for the specific genetic basis of mood disorders continues, with special emphasis on genetic location and genetic processes, including the role of **selective gene expression** and neuromodulation (Barondes, 1998). Many researchers agree that genetic expressions and genetic transmission of mood disorders may hold the key to future major advances in understanding, diagnosing, and treating depression and bipolar disorders (Sullivan, Neale, and Kendler, 2000).

Ethologic Factors

Ethologic theories of human development look to evolutionary concepts as explanations of mood disorders. Human behavior serves the survival of the species and helps individuals adapt to their environments. For example, psychiatrist

John Bowlby (1969) concluded that bonding and attachment between mothers and their infants evolved as a means of ensuring that helpless infants would have adequate protection for continued development. Ethologic approaches to development and biology have existed since the time of Charles Darwin, but renewed interest in the field has extended these approaches to offer a different perspective on the occurrence of mood disorders.

Evolutionary Psychology/Biology

Evolutionary psychology is a way of thinking about any topic within psychology. The basic idea is that the human mind was designed by natural selection to solve problems of adaptation. All human minds develop reasoning and regulatory mechanisms that organize the interpretation of experiences, account for recurrent concepts and motivations, and provide universal meaning structures that help us understand the behavior of others (Cosmides and Tooby, 2002). Evolutionary biology is a related field that examines the selective advantage of human traits and biology (Nesse, 2002). Both areas want to understand how human beings have adapted and are adapting still to changes in the environment, and to identify defenses that may seem like diseases but are actually evolved protective mechanisms. In exploring mood disorders the focus can be on proximate explanations such as brain chemistry, past experiences, or personality. From an evolutionary perspective the focus can be on the purpose of a mood disorder, and why it persists in the present.

The evolutionary function of bipolar disorder has not been examined, but much has been considered about the function of depression. On the surface, depression and its main symptoms (lack of energy, fearfulness, loss of interest, sleep and eating disorders) would not seem to promote survival; however, a number of possible functions have been suggested (Watson and Andrews, 2002). Depression may serve as a cry for help, may force the loser of a social conflict to accept defeat and thus stop oppressive behavior by the winner, or may force greater involvement by a partner. Depression may serve a social rumination function; that is, the symptoms may permit the individual to focus on and analyze social problems. Depression may have a social motivation function; that is, the severity of symptoms may influence reluctant social partners to provide help or withdraw demands. Nesse (2002) suggested also that depression prevents wasted effort by allowing the individual to disengage from unreachable goals.

One ethologic perspective suggests a number of treatment approaches. Assessment should consider social factors that are limiting the individual's ability to function in all areas of life. The social system is an important element in ethology; therefore group and family therapies are supported, as well as multidisciplinary teamwork. The ethologic perspective calls into question the use of antidepressant medications, as they might interfere with the client's ability to address issues within the social environment. If medications are used, they should not replace work on the social problems. In any event, medications should not be used to remove the very suffering that provides motivation for life change in an adaptive depressive episode (Watson and Andrews, 2002).

Psychosocial Factors

Psychosocial explanations for the development of mood disorders represent a range of theoretic positions, including psychoanalytic theory, learned helplessness, cognitive theory, life events (stress) theory, and personality theory.

Psychoanalytic Theory

The basic premise of psychoanalytic theory is that unconscious processes result in expression of symptoms, including depression and mania. Freud (1957) distinguished between depression and normal grief, citing both as a response to real or symbolic loss. According to Freud, in depression the loss generates intense, hostile feelings toward the lost object that are turned inward onto the self (anger turned inward), creating guilt and loss of self-esteem. Thus depression is viewed together with loss and aggression.

Psychodynamically, mania is explained as a defense against depression. The client denies feelings of anger, low self-esteem, and worthlessness and reverses the affect such that there is a triumphant feeling of self-confidence. Mania represents a conquered superego with little inclination to control id impulses. Yet, over time this distorted view of reality waivers, and the client demonstrates outward hostility toward others, often focusing on the weaknesses of others that are similar to the internal weaknesses being avoided.

Few data support the psychodynamic theories of depression and mania, but there is some evidence that clients with depression have experienced more early childhood loss and deprivation than persons without depression (Bowlby, 1969; Brown and Harris, 1978). Clinicians also note that anger is often associated with depression, although the relationship between anger and depression remains obscure. Many people who experience early childhood loss and anger never experience depression, whereas many who do not experience a visible or acknowledged loss do experience depression. The psychoanalytic theory is only one of many explanations that attempt to explain the internal dynamics of depression and mania. The relevance of this theoretic perspective may be in its references to the early childhood environment in which loss, disruption, or chaos may trigger stress that in turn triggers the physiologic mechanisms described previously (Goodman, 2002).

Cognitive Theory

The cognitive model of depression points to errors of logical thinking as causative factors for depression. It assumes that mood is influenced by underlying cognitive structures, some of which are not fully conscious. These cognitive structures, or schemata, may be shaped by early life experiences and are predisposed to negative processing of information. In a diatheses-stress model, when persons predisposed to depression with negative schemata encounter stress, the negative processing is activated, resulting in depressive thinking (Beck, 1967).

Beck (1967) differentiated among levels of cognition that influence depression: automatic thoughts, schemata or assumptions, and cognitive distortions. Automatic thoughts are those that can be brought into awareness, although they appear fleetingly and are usually unrecognized. They form the person's perception of a situation, and it is this perception, rather than the objective facts about the situation, that results in emotional and behavioral responses. If the perceptions are distorted, inferences and responses will be maladaptive. For example, a college student who was very bright was never invited to join a class study group. She interpreted this as personal rejection and was convinced that no one in the class liked her. On discussing this with some other members of the class, she learned that no one invited her to a study group because they perceived her as so smart, that she did not need to study with others.

Schemata are internal representations of the self and the world. They facilitate information processing because they are used to understand, code, and recall information. Beck (1967) proposed a triad of thinking (schemata) that gives rise to the development of depression:

1. Negative, self-deprecating views of self
2. Pessimistic views of the world, so that life experiences are interpreted in a negative way
3. The belief that negativity will continue into the future, promoting a negative view of future events

These mind-sets result in the misinterpretation of events and situations, so that the client's cognitive schema of self as worthless and the world and future as hopeless are supported. This faulty cognitive processing leads to assumptions and continued errors of logic that result in depressive symptoms and an ongoing negative view of life. This was evidenced by a client who began each meeting with the nurse by saying, "There is no point to this. I know things will never be better."

Cognitive distortions link schemata and automatic thoughts. Faulty information processing includes cognitive distortions, such as *overgeneralization* (drawing general conclusions based on isolated incidents), *dichotomous thinking* (perceiving events and experiences in only one of two opposite categories), and *magnification* (placing a distorted emphasis on a single event or error). The following example illustrates each of these types of distortion. A 55-year-old factory worker was recently passed over for promotion. He concluded that his supervisors hated all of the work he was doing (overgeneralization). He was convinced that his competitors for the promotion were either those who went along with everything done by administration or those who tended to think very independently (dichotomous thinking). He is irate with factory managers since he learned from the bulletin board that someone else had gotten the promotion and was convinced that the company was trying to get rid of him (magnification).

There is considerable research support for the cognitive model of depression (Robins and Hayes, 1993; Scott, 1996). It has led to the development of specific treatment for depression using cognitive techniques. These techniques are short term and focus on changing the client's faulty negative cognition.

Hopelessness/Learned Helplessness Theory

Cognitive theory traced the determinants of depression to altered cognition. One such altered cognition was termed **learned helplessness**, demonstrated by the lack of motivation exhibited by dogs subjected to laboratory shocks that they were unable to control. According to the original theory as stated by Seligman (1975), stressful events that are experienced as uncontrollable result in the development of helplessness, apathy, powerlessness, and depression.

Learned helplessness theory was modified to specify that, in the face of current events and past experiences, persons have the expectation (cognition) that external events are uncontrollable (Abramson, Seligman, and Teasdale, 1978). This in turn results in helplessness, passivity, and sadness, which leads to other symptoms of depression, such as decreased appetite and low self-esteem.

Further reformulation of the theory resulted in the *hopelessness theory of depression* (Abramson, Metalsky, and Alloy, 1989). In this theory revision hopelessness is a sufficient cause of depression, with the individual's inferred negative outcomes and negativity about self as key elements of depression. Helplessness is viewed as one component of hopelessness. With the occurrence of an unpleasant event, persons prone to depression (having negative expectations) attribute stability (versus instability), globalization (versus specific), and importance (versus unimportance) to those events. This is exemplified by a client who perceived that she would not be able to recover from divorce (stability), that her entire life had been ruined (globalization), and that her former marriage had been the major focus of her life (importance).

More recently, researchers have posited that cognitive vulnerability, represented by a person's negative cognitive style (Just, Abramson, and Alloy, 2001), in the presence of negative life events leads to hopelessness, which results in the valid and distinct subtype of *hopelessness depression* (Joiner et al., 2001). Symptoms of this type of depression include slow initiation of voluntary behavior, apathy, lack of energy, and psychomotor retardation. Studies provide some support for hopelessness depression as a cohesive entity, but additional testing needs to be done with more general client populations.

Abramson et al. (1989) hypothesized that a lack of social support during times of negative life events may lead to increased hopelessness and thereby to hopelessness depression. Research with human immunodeficiency virus (HIV) clients has supported this model, with hopelessness rather than low social support as the key contributor to depression. The influence of low social support on hopelessness was necessary to account for depression (Johnson et al., 2001). More research is needed to identify other mechanisms that may lead to the specific symptom pattern of hopelessness depression.

Life Events and Stress Theory

The relationship of life events and stress to mood disorders has been widely acknowledged, and is the focus of much research. In studying depression, researchers have been interested in the quantity and nature of life events, and in the size and perceived supportiveness of the client's social network. In an enduring study, Brown and Harris (1978) reported that stressful social factors (e.g., lack of an intimate, confiding relationship with a significant other; having three or more children at home; being unemployed; and loss of one's mother before age 11 years) contributed significantly to vulnerability for depression. All life events are considered to evoke various degrees of stress. Thus a joyous wedding can be as stressful as the death of a loved one.

The client's perception or emotional evaluation of an event is as important as the change in daily life caused by the event. The effect of an event is influenced also by mechanisms such as social support, and the person's perception of that support as wanted or unwanted, sufficient or insufficient. Life events most likely influence the development and recurrence of depression through the psychologic and ultimately biologic experiences of stress.

Ravindran et al. (2002) noted that depressive illness has been associated with increased stress perception, reduced perception of uplifting events, reliance on coping styles that express or contain emotional expression rather than cognitive styles, and impaired aspects of quality of life. In a study of clients with varying degrees of depression, researchers found that hassles, coping styles, and quality of life were related to the severity of the depression. Increased perception of daily hassles was the most pronounced factor, especially with treatment-resistant clients. However, the researchers maintained that, although life events might contribute to the recurrence of depressive illness, the influence decreased with an increasing number of depressive episodes (Ravindran et al., 2002; Kendler, Thornton, and Gardner, 2000).

The occurrence of stressful life events and depression has been examined with regard to gender differences. Stressful life events have shown a causal relationship with episodes of depression in women, mediated by genetic risk factors (Kendler, Karkowski, and Prescott, 1999). A comparison of men and women revealed that women reported more interpersonal stressors, whereas men reported more legal and work-related stressful life events. At the same time, most life events influenced the risk for depression in men and women in a similar fashion. Researchers concluded that the greater prevalence of depression in women versus men was not due to differences in the rate of reported stressful life events nor to a greater sensitivity of women to the harmful influences of stressful life events (Kendler, Thornton, and Prescott, 2001).

Hankin and Abramson (2001) have proposed an integrative model of depression that combines elements of hopelessness theory and life stress theory. Termed the *cognitive vulnerability-transactional stress theory,* the model is developmental in nature, attempting to explain gender differences in the emergence of depression. Negative life events are seen as contributing to a general negative affect. Cognitive vulnerability factors then influence the likelihood that depression will emerge. Other vulnerability factors include genetic risk, personality, and environmental adversity. Increases in depression can lead to negative life events that feed into a causal cycle of depression.

Less has been known about the relationship between stressful life events and bipolar disorder, although studies have suggested a role of disrupted social routines or circadian rhythms. Malkoff-Schwartz et al. (2000) studied the influence of social rhythm disruption as a stressful life event on clients with pure mania, pure depression, cycling episodes, and recurrent unipolar depression. The researchers found that the onset of manic episodes was influenced by stressful life events, especially those involving social rhythm disruption. The onset of bipolar cycling or depression, however, was relatively unaffected by severe life events or social rhythm disruption. The authors suggested that interventions to minimize stress and social rhythm disruption in clients with a history of mania might help prevent the onset of manic episodes.

Personality Theory

For many years psychiatric clinicians have debated the role of personality in relation to mood disorders, particularly depression. A number of possible relationships may be supposed.

- The term *depressive personality* has been used to describe personality traits believed to predispose to a depressive disorder.
- Depressive disorders have been linked with certain personality traits, including interpersonal dependency or sensitivity to rejection, and it has been unclear whether depressive disorders lead to the expression of these personality traits or vice versa.
- There may exist a distinct *depressive personality disorder.*
- Other personality disorders may be linked with mood disorders.

Researchers have tried to identify personality characteristics that tend to occur concurrently with depression. It is not always clear if depression emerges because the person possesses these personality characteristics, or if the characteristics emerge because of the depression. In an examination of temperament and character (Marijnissen et al., 2002), depressed clients showed higher tendency to avoid harm (harm avoidance) and lower self-directedness compared with normal control subjects. No association was shown between harm avoidance and severity of depression, and harm avoidance did not change with successful antidepressant treatment. Thus harm avoidance behaved as a more enduring personality trait. These findings were supported in a similar study of personality characteristics in clients with depression (Luty et al., 2002). Two constructs were particularly relevant in describing the clients with depression. The first consisted of separation anxiety, fragile inner self, interpersonal awareness, harm avoidance, and negative self-directedness. The second consisted of need for approval, timidity, reward dependence, and cooperativeness. Further study showed that improvements in personality dimensions were associated with favorable depression outcomes, whereas little personality change was seen in clients with poor depression outcomes (Corruble et al., 2002).

Does a distinct depressive personality disorder exist? By nature a personality disorder is composed of consistent behaviors that recur across situations and across most of the life course. Many perspectives have been used to describe the etiology of personality disorders, including intrapsychic, interpersonal, or ethologic theories. Neurobiologic theories have looked at the influence of temperament or the possibility that patterns of neurotransmitter activity define personality types. By contrast, mood disorders are considered pathologic states that can be defined by pathology occurring within a limited time frame.

At present, the category of depressive personality on Axis II is a research diagnosis in the DSM-IV-TR. This means that empiric studies of the category are being considered to determine if it is a distinct phenomenon for inclusion in future editions of the manual. Arguing against the inclusion is the conceptual overlap of criteria for depressive personality with already identified disorders, particularly dysthymia. Arguments for inclusion emphasize the uniqueness of a personality disorder from other disorders. The debate continues and will need to address how personality disorders should relate to other disorders (Dolan-Sewell, Krueger, and Shea, 2001). For example, is there a continuum of mood disorders, with depressive personality at one end and major depressive disorder at the other end? Or does depressive personality exist separate and apart from any mood disorder that appears?

Criteria being considered for depressive personality disorder include a pervasive pattern of depressive cognitions and behaviors that begin by early adulthood; that are not better explained as major depressive episodes or dysthymic disorder; and that exist before, during, and after a depressive episode. The individual's mood is usually dejected, gloomy, cheerless, joyless, or unhappy. The self-concept may revolve around beliefs of inadequacy, worthlessness, and low self-esteem. The person may be critical, blaming, and derogatory toward the self and negativistic, critical, and judgmental toward others. The person may be seen as pessimistic, brooding, tending to worry, and prone to feeling guilty or remorseful. Personality characteristics associated with depressive personality disorder may include introversion, passivity, and unassertiveness, preferring to follow rather than lead. Unlike major depressive disorder, depressive personality disorder is seen equally in men and women, and may predispose to developing dysthymic disorder or major depressive disorder (APA, 2000).

Other personality disorders have been associated with mood disorders. The suggestion is that the functional and occupational difficulties encountered as a result of the maladaptive behaviors that are part of personality disorders create an atmosphere conducive to mood disorders. In one study of hospitalized clients (Rossi et al., 2001), proportions of clients with depression were also found to have avoidant (31.6%), borderline (30.8%), and obsessive-compulsive (30.8%) personality disorders. Proportions of clients with bipolar disorder were also found to have obsessive-compulsive (32.4%), borderline (29.6%), and avoidant (19.7%) personality disorders. It may be important to consider the presence of personality disorder side by side with depression, because there has been a suggestion that this concurrence influences treatment outcomes. For example, when clients having major depression were compared at 6 months after treatment with clients having a Cluster C personality disorder and major depression (Viinamaki et al., 2002), 54% of the major depression group had recovered from their depression, but only 16% of those with Cluster C personality disorder and major depression had recovered. The authors concluded that the presence of a Cluster C personality disorder hindered treatment effectiveness. However, an analysis of articles that reported treatment outcomes with depression and personality disorders disputed the finding (Mulder, 2002). Mulder concluded that study design influenced many of the findings, and that depressed clients with personality disorder might be less likely to receive adequate treatment in uncontrolled studies. Overall the strongest studies reported the least effect on treatment outcome.

The fact that the preceding studies contradict each other means that research on the relationship between personality and depressive disorders certainly will continue, particularly with regard to treatment outcomes. Greater attention is also being paid to the association of personality disorders with bipolar disorders. In any case, the experience of depression or mania can shape behavioral characteristics or strengthen preexisting personality features.

EPIDEMIOLOGY

Mood disorders, particularly depression, are common. Data suggest that the lifetime prevalence of developing any affective disorder is 19.3%: 14.7% for men and 23.9% for women (Kessler et al., 1994). Because the lifetime prevalence of bipolar disorder is about equal for men and women (1.4% and 1.3%, respectively), much of this difference is due to unipolar depression. Women have a lifetime prevalence of 21.3% for major depression and 8.0% for dysthymia, whereas men have a lifetime prevalence of only 12.7% for major depression and 4.8% for dysthymia. A number of theories have been proposed to account for gender differences in the rates of depression, including hormonal or biologic differences, social roles, and cognitive processing (Nolen-

Hoeksema, 1987, 2000). However, these gender differences for depression have not been adequately explained, and additional research is needed to determine why women are at higher risk for depression.

The first episode of a mood disorder seems to be occurring at younger ages. The average age for onset of bipolar illness is the mid to late twenties. Although the average age of onset for unipolar depression has been considered the middle thirties, there is some evidence that onset is occurring in younger cohorts (Lewinsohn et al., 1993). Although the most frequent age of onset for depression is the 25- to 44-year age group, people in younger age groups have an ever-increasing risk of developing depression. Data indicate that the onset of depression at an early age (teens or early twenties) or at age 55 years or over predicts a more protracted, chronic course (Klerman and Weissman, 1992; Greden, 2001). Rates of depression do not significantly increase during menopause. The risk of developing depression and mania is increased if there is a positive family history for mood disorders (Akiskal, 1989).

Sociocultural factors may be related to the onset of depression and mania. Depression seems to occur less frequently in African-Americans than in either Caucasian or Hispanic groups in the United States. It also appears that depression may be more frequent in lower socioeconomic groups, whereas bipolar disorders are more frequent in higher socioeconomic groups. Although depression and mania occur throughout the world, the expression of symptoms is influenced by ethnicity and culture. Asians, for example, describe more somatic symptoms of depression, whereas people from Western cultures describe more mood and cognitive changes.

In an increasingly stressful society characterized by mobility, family disruptions, and economic stressors, women and younger persons are manifesting depression more than in previous generations. Persons with depression often seek help for physiologic symptoms such as fatigue. Ultimately less than half of those with depression are diagnosed and treated properly (Greden, 2001). Unfortunately, the relationships among biologic, psychologic, developmental, and sociocultural factors and their influence on the development of mood disorders remain unclear. Epidemiology data for mood disorders are summarized in Box 10-2.

Box 10-2   Epidemiology of Mood Disorders

19.3% of the general population develop a mood disorder.
21.3% of women and 12.7% of men develop major depression.
Average age of onset for bipolar illness is mid- to late-twenties.
Average age of onset of depression is mid-thirties.
Depression occurs more frequently in Caucasians and Hispanics than in African-Americans.
Depression occurs more frequently in lower socioeconomic groups.
Bipolar disorders occur more frequently in higher socioeconomic groups.

Mood Disorders Across the Life Span

Unless the focus is on child, adolescent, or geriatric clients, most information presented in textbooks and literature addresses the average adult, generally covering ages between 18 and 65 years. There has been growing concern in recent years, however, with the increase in mood disorders among children and adolescents. At the same time, there have been changes in the way mood disorders are perceived with older adults. It is important to recognize that new variables may be introduced when mood disorders, particularly depression, are discussed at either end of the life span.

Mood Disorders in the Young

Mood disorders presenting in childhood or adolescence are significant for three reasons: (1) they generate extraordinary pain and distress for young individuals who are not prepared to understand or deal with the resulting emotions and behaviors, (2) they initiate major difficulties during a period of time essential to development and therefore influence the rest of the life span, and (3) they produce tremendous stress and concern for the entire family unit. Assessment of children and adolescents should address not only symptomatology of the current illness episode, but also the influence a mood disorder may be having on normal development and social learning, as well as the impact of the disorder on family dynamics and coping status.

Concerns with childhood psychiatric disorders begin during infancy, addressed by the relatively new specialty of *infant mental health*. The focus within this specialty is generally on the influence of parenting and parent-infant relationships. Research on the emergence of mood disorders in children places greater emphasis on inborn and environmental issues. Temperament is an inborn factor that has been receiving increased attention across the life span. In one study of young children, the temperamental trait of behavioral disinhibition was associated with higher rates of mood disorders (Hirshfeld-Becker et al., 2002). Familial relationships form an environmental factor that has been explored at length. For example, attachment relationships have been associated with depression from infancy through adolescence. The specific nature of the association is still being investigated, particularly with regard to those factors that moderate and mediate the connection (Sexson, Glanville, and Kaslow, 2001). Most recently the diagnosis of early-onset bipolar disorder (EOBD) has become a controversial addition to child psychiatry. Bipolar disorder was once thought to emerge by early adulthood, but in recent years the diagnosis has been made as early as age 5 years. The symptom profile of EOBD overlaps with that of other childhood psychiatric disorders, some of which may be comorbid. The main differential characteristic seems to be that EOBD symptoms show a cyclical pattern not evident in other disorders. Because of the difficulty separating EOBD from other possible diagnoses, the role of the school nurse has been identified as important in documenting behaviors that can aid in clarifying the diagnosis (St. Dennis and Synoground, 1998).

Mood disorders in adolescents have received a good deal of attention. Depression may appear as irritable hostility and is often comorbid with anxiety and personality disorders, as well as illicit drug use (Parker and Roy, 2001). Multiple studies have shown long-term consequences of adolescent depression, but some of the studies may not have been adequately controlled for social factors. A longitudinal study of more than 900 children of a birth cohort revealed that 13% of the cohort developed depression between ages 14 and 16 years. At age 21 the depressed individuals were three times more likely than nondepressed adolescents to have a subsequent depression and twice as likely to have an anxiety disorder. Other consequences that appeared to be related to early depression, including suicidal behaviors, academic and employment difficulties, and early parenthood, could not be directly related to early depression once social factors were controlled for (Fergusson and Woodward, 2002). Bipolar disorder in adolescents may present initially as recurrent depressive episodes, developing into bipolar I disorder in 10% to 15% of cases. When manic episodes occur during adolescence, they may be associated with psychotic symptoms, school truancy, antisocial behavior, or substance abuse (APA, 2000).

Mood Disorders in the Elderly

Just as the picture of mood disorders has changed for children and adolescents, new information has emerged for mood disorders in older adults. Researchers have suggested that late-life depression can be categorized into three subtypes, each with a different etiologic pathway: (1) early-onset depression with lifelong vulnerability, (2) late-onset depression in reaction to severe life stress, and (3) late-onset depression with vascular risk factors. Early-onset depression was found to be associated with greater parental history of depression and higher levels of the personality trait of neuroticism. Late-onset depression could be broken down between disorders caused by social distress and those mediated by cerebral deterioration. Vascular depression, as this last type has been called, has been associated with physical findings of white matter hyperintensities apparent during MRI. The presence of this physical finding has been connected with poor treatment results (van den Berg et al., 2001). The existence of the third type of depression has gained support in growing efforts to identify criteria for depression in Alzheimer's disease (Olin et al., 2002) and for vascular depression (Provinciali and Coccia, 2002).

Although rates of major depression among older adults have been estimated from 5% to 10%, researchers have noted that much of late-life depression is subthreshold, meaning that symptomatology may not meet stringent DSM-IV-TR criteria for major depressive disorder. Such minor depression is seen frequently in primary care rather than psychiatric treatment settings and may be underestimated with regard to functional impairment, mortality risk especially among men, and treatment needs (Beekman et al., 2002; Travis and Lyness, 2002). However, both major and minor depression respond well to treatment, especially when pharmacotherapy and psychotherapy are combined (Beekman et al., 2002; Lenze et al., 2002).

Social considerations take on different characterizations in addressing treatment needs of older adults. The availability of a support network may be decreased, as peers of the older adult may no longer be present through lack of mobility for visits, cognitive disability, nursing home placement, or death. Familial supports may be more necessary but may be more variable because they depend on lifelong patterns of relationship. Those patterns may prompt the provision of needed assistance, or they may lead to greater stress. Family members may view the older adult's symptomatology as a normal part of aging and would require instruction on the nature of depression to recognize the need for and positive prognosis of treatment. Further, the values and attitudes of the older adult may influence treatment participation. Generational differences in the acceptance of psychiatric treatment may lead the older adult to refuse care or deny the need for care. When asked if they are depressed, older adults may say they are not. However, asking about the specific DSM-IV-TR criteria (e.g., What activities do you enjoy these days? Are you participating in the same activities as you would have a few months ago?) may provide a clearer picture of depressive symptoms.

Apart from direct effects of depression in older adults, findings that depression may have a relationship with cognitive disorders are of particular concern. The relationship may be that depression is an early prodrome of dementia, that depression is a risk factor of dementia, or that depression initiates a physiologic cascade effect that results in damage to the hippocampus and dementia (Jorm, 2001). The effects of depression on cognitive function in older adults led to the proposal of a *depressive-executive dysfunction (DED) syndrome*. Clinical manifestations of DED have been described as reduced fluency, impaired visual naming, paranoia, loss of interest in activities, psychomotor retardation, and a mild vegetative syndrome. DED was associated with disability, poor treatment response, relapse, and recurrence (Alexopoulos et al., 2002).

Ultimately depression is of particular concern with older adults because the symptoms can result in life-threatening situations within a rather short time. For example, vegetative symptoms can lead to dehydration and electrolyte imbalance, and can compromise any existing medical conditions. Higher mortality in older adults with depression has been attributed to suicide, comorbid medical illness, and impairment of physical functioning. In one study late-onset depression was associated with mortality for both men and women. With men mortality was also associated with severity of depression; with women mortality was associated with self-rated vascular and cardiac conditions. Researchers concluded that older women with depression could require closer follow-up monitoring of vascular conditions (Steffens et al., 2002). In particular, older women with depression who are taking psychotropic medications have also demonstrated lower health-related quality of life (Stein and Barrett-Connor, 2002).

Mood disorders at either end of the life span are just as responsive to treatment as mood disorders during midlife. The important idea to keep in mind is that the features and considerations may be somewhat different. Research is providing new knowledge on child, adolescent, and older adult mood disorders. The challenge is to keep up with changes in the characterizations of illness and the progress in available treatments.

CLINICAL DESCRIPTION

Although mood disorders are considered to be primarily changes in mood, cognitive, physiologic, and behavioral changes are also evident. Mood disorders are defined by a pattern of episodes over time and by a pattern of symptoms in each episode. Mood disorders are classified in the DSM-IV-TR as depressive disorders, bipolar disorders, or other mood disorders. Signs and symptoms of these disorders are described in the following sections.

Depressive Disorders

Persons diagnosed with a depressive disorder have experienced only episodes of depression with no manic or hypomanic episodes. This is also referred to as **unipolar depression**. The DSM-IV-TR Criteria box lists criteria for a major depressive episode. The clinical symptoms of depressive disorders are summarized in the Clinical Symptoms box on p. 208.

Major Depressive Episode, Single or Recurrent

An episode of major depression can be indicative of a first episode or of a recurrent episode of depression. Symptoms occur as a result of the disorder and not from the effects of a substance, medical condition, or loss of a loved one within the previous 2 months.

Emotional Symptoms. Two primary symptoms of major depression are depressed mood and **anhedonia,** or loss of interest and pleasure in activities. For clients to be diagnosed with major depression, one of these symptoms must be present most of the day, nearly every day, for at least 2 weeks. Clients may describe their mood as depressed, sad, empty, or numb. They may report difficulty receiving pleasure or satisfaction from their usual activities, including eating, sex, or going out with friends. Although clients may describe feelings of sadness or frequent crying, some persons with depression are unable to describe feelings and report disinterest, disconnection, or an inability to feel emotion. Anxiety, irritability, or anger may also be present. Clients may also report feelings of loneliness, helplessness, or hopelessness. The affect of a person with depression may be flat and constricted, with minimal expression, or may appear rather normal as the person attempts to camouflage his or her inner struggles.

DSM-IV-TR CRITERIA
Major Depressive Episode

A. Five (or more) of the following symptoms have been present during the same 2-week period and represent a change from previous functioning; at least one of the symptoms is either (1) depressed mood or (2) loss of interest or pleasure.
  NOTE: Do not include symptoms that are clearly due to a general medical condition, or mood-incongruent delusions or hallucinations.
  1. Depressed mood most of the day, nearly every day, as indicated by either subjective report (e.g., feels sad or empty) or observation made by others (e.g., appears tearful). NOTE: In children and adolescents, can be irritable mood.
  2. Markedly diminished interest or pleasure in all, or almost all, activities most of the day, nearly every day (as indicated by either subjective account or observation made by others).
  3. Significant weight loss when not dieting or weight gain (e.g., a change of more than 5% of body weight in month), or decrease or increase in appetite nearly every day. NOTE: In children, consider failure to make expected weight gains.
  4. Insomnia or hypersomnia nearly every day.
  5. Psychomotor agitation or retardation nearly every day (observable by others, not merely subjective feelings of restlessness or being slowed down).
  6. Fatigue or loss of energy nearly every day.
  7. Feelings of worthlessness or excessive or inappropriate guilt (which may be delusional) nearly every day (not merely self-reproach or guilt about being sick).
  8. Diminished ability to think or concentrate, or indecisiveness, nearly every day (either by subjective account or as observed by others).
  9. Recurrent thoughts of death (not just fear of dying), recurrent suicidal ideation without a specific plan, or a suicide attempt or a specific plan for committing suicide.
B. The symptoms do not meet criteria for a mixed episode.
C. The symptoms cause clinically significant distress or impairment in social, occupational, or other important areas of functioning.
D. The symptoms are not due to the direct physiologic effects of a substance (e.g., a drug of abuse, a medication) or a general medical condition (e.g., hypothyroidism).
E. The symptoms are not better accounted for by bereavement (i.e., after the loss of a loved one, the symptoms persist for longer than 2 months or are characterized by marked functional impairment, morbid preoccupation with worthlessness, suicidal ideation, psychotic symptoms, or psychomotor retardation).

From American Psychiatric Association: *Diagnostic and Statistical Manual of Mental Disorders*, Fourth Edition, Text Revision. Washington, DC, American Psychiatric Association, 2000.

Cognitive Symptoms. Cognitive criteria for major depression include a diminished ability to think, concentrate, or make decisions; recurrent thoughts of death; and an excessive focus on self-worthlessness and guilt. Many clients describe difficulty attending to and concentrating on a task or conversation. Reading a newspaper or following the train of thought in a lecture may be overwhelming. Clients may be unable to make decisions about routine concerns, such as what clothing to put on in the morning or what to buy at the grocery store. Recurrent thoughts of death are often evident,

CLINICAL SYMPTOMS

Depressive Disorders

Major Depression

EMOTIONAL
Anhedonia
Depressed mood
Irritability

COGNITIVE
Diminished ability to think, concentrate, or make decisions
Recurrent thoughts of death
Excessive focus on self-worthlessness and guilt

BEHAVIORAL
Significant weight loss or gain; change in appetite
Insomnia or hypersomnia
Psychomotor agitation or retardation
Fatigue

SOCIAL
Withdrawal from family and social interactions
Problems at work in organizing, initiating, and completing work

Dysthymic Disorder

EMOTIONAL
Depressed mood
Anhedonia
Irritability or angry mood

COGNITIVE
Feelings of low self-esteem and inadequacy
Feelings of guilt and brooding about the past
Difficulty with concentration, memory, and decision making
Attitudes of pessimism, despair, and hopelessness

BEHAVIORAL
Chronic fatigue

SOCIAL
Social withdrawal

CLINICAL ALERT

The nurse must be alert to suicidal ideation and intent with clients with depression and clients with mania who are cycling into depression or whose insight and judgment are impaired. A particularly high-risk time is 1 to 6 weeks after the initiation of antidepressant therapy, before it reaches its full therapeutic effect.

when it represents a 5% change in body weight in 1 month. Sometimes the weight change is not apparent, but the client reports a major change in appetite. Sleep disturbances are common, and clients report not being able to sleep or sleeping too much. **Psychomotor agitation** is evident when the client appears to be restless, paces, fidgets, or is irritable. With **psychomotor retardation** the client appears to be slowed down in movement and in speech. Persons with depression may appear listless and disheveled. They may not carefully attend to their dress, appearance, or hygiene. They may exhibit a stooped posture and make little eye contact. Many clients report feelings of fatigue and loss of energy, citing an inability to accomplish tasks and an increased need for naps. They may even appear very tired. Fatigue may cause many clients to visit their family physician or nurse practitioner, believing that the fatigue is indicative of a physical problem. Thus depression is often diagnosed first during a visit to the primary care provider.

Social Symptoms. For major depression to be diagnosed, the convergence of symptoms must cause personal distress and significant impairment in social and occupational functioning. Clients may withdraw from family and social interactions. They may have problems at their job, including problems with executive functions originating in the frontal lobe of the brain, resulting in an inability to organize, begin, and complete their work. Although some people are able to function at work with relatively little impairment, this often comes at great personal and family expense as their energy for social interaction is depleted. Family members begin to feel confused, angry, guilty, abandoned, and sad.

Marital distress is often a cited stressor at least 6 months before the onset of a depressive episode (Schmaling and Becker, 1991). During an episode the client's erratic behavior, mood, and cognition can alienate a loved one, who may become frustrated with how to help the partner. Unfortunately, it appears as though marital distress continues even after the acute episode subsides. Continued marital strain has been cited as a factor in episode recurrence (Schmaling and Becker, 1991).

Dysthymic Disorder

Dysthymia differs from major depression in that it is a chronic, low-level depression. To receive this diagnosis, the client must have had depressed mood and at least three of the following symptoms for most of the day, nearly every

including thoughts of suicide, death from natural causes, or existential thoughts about dying. At times, these thoughts may occupy a large portion of the client's waking hours. Negative thinking is often apparent, with feelings of worthlessness and excessive guilt. Clients ruminate about past deeds and their negative view of themselves and the world. Clients with severe depression can become delusional with fixed beliefs that cannot be changed by logic; they may focus on persecution, punishment, **nihilism,** or somatic concerns.

Behavioral Symptoms. Behavioral symptoms that are criteria for major depression are significant weight loss or gain or change in appetite, insomnia or hypersomnia, psychomotor agitation or psychomotor retardation, and fatigue. Weight gain or weight loss is considered to be significant day, for at least 2 years (1 year for children and adolescents): poor appetite or overeating, insomnia or hypersomnia, low energy, low self-esteem, poor concentration or difficulty making decisions, and feelings of hopelessness. There cannot have been a manic or hypomanic episode. The client may have experienced an episode of major depression before the onset of dysthymia, provided there were at least 6 months with no signs or symptoms of depression. After 2 years of dysthymia, the client may be diagnosed with major depression superimposed on dysthymia if symptoms increase in severity. The dysthymic disorder is not due to the effects of a substance or medical condition. Psychotic features are usually not present in this disorder.

Emotional Symptoms. The predominant symptom that must be present for the diagnosis of dysthymia is depressed mood. Clients report feeling chronically "down, gloomy, sad." Many are unable to remember a time when they felt good or their usual self. Another symptom indicative of dysthymia is a generalized loss of interest or pleasure in activities, but unlike major depression, anhedonia is not a primary emotional symptom. Another symptom is irritability or angry mood. Clients may find themselves feeling impatient with family members or co-workers and demonstrating angry outbursts. Many feel bad about their irritable state but find themselves unable to control it.

Cognitive Symptoms. Cognitive symptoms of dysthymia include low self-esteem and inadequacy; guilt and brooding about the past; difficulty with concentration, memory, and decision making; and negative thinking evidenced by pessimism, despair, and hopelessness. Clients with dysthymia often have little regard for themselves and are plagued by a sense of inadequacy and a lack of self-confidence. They reflect on past actions and attribute personal guilt to their circumstances. Negativity pervades much of what they do and say; life seems hopeless, and situations are bounded by pessimism and despair. Clients often report poor memory and decreased concentration on tasks. They may have problems making decisions, but the impairment is usually not as severe as impaired decision making during major depression.

Behavioral Symptoms. Clients with dysthymia commonly complain of chronic fatigue. They are exhausted from usual activities and often believe that they have a physical illness or chronic fatigue syndrome. Clients may make repeated visits to their health care provider, hoping to determine the cause of their fatigue. In conjunction with the fatigue, clients display decreased activity and productivity. Everything becomes a chore, and it becomes difficult to complete tasks in the usual amount of time.

Social Symptoms. Social withdrawal is common with dysthymia. Clients are tired, irritable, and depressed and no longer get satisfaction from outings or activities with family and friends. Clients' mood states and negativity may prevent

DSM-IV-TR CRITERIA
Bipolar I and Bipolar II Disorders

Type	Characteristics
BIPOLAR I DISORDER	
Single manic episode	Only one manic episode
	No past major depressive episodes
Most recent episode: hypomanic	Current hypomania
	At least one previous manic episode
Most recent episode: manic	Current mania
	At least one previous depressive, manic, or mixed episode
Most recent episode: mixed	Meets criteria for both manic and depressive current episode
	At least one past major depressive or mixed episode
Most recent episode: depressed	Current depressive episode
	At least one past manic or mixed episode
BIPOLAR II DISORDER	No previous full manic episode
	At least one past major depressive episode and past or current hypomanic episode

Modified from American Psychiatric Association: *Diagnostic and Statistical Manual of Mental Disorders,* Fourth Edition, Text Revision. Washington, DC, American Psychiatric Association, 2000.

people from wanting to be with them, increasing their isolation from others.

Depressive Disorders Not Otherwise Specified
There are types of depression that do not meet the criteria for the depressive disorders presented thus far or that may be found to be disorders in their own right. Some of these include premenstrual dysphoric disorder, minor depressive disorder, recurrent brief depressive disorder, and the postpsychotic depression of schizophrenia. *Dysphoria* refers to a depressed, sad mood. The reader is referred to the DSM-IV-TR classification for more extensive descriptions of these diagnoses.

Bipolar Disorders
A **bipolar disorder** occurs when the client experiences episodes of depression and episodes of mania or hypomania over time. Bipolar disorders are defined by the pattern of manic, hypomanic, and depressed episodes over time. The depressed and manic episodes are not due to the effects of a substance, including antidepressant medication, electroconvulsive therapy, or light therapy. Clients may be diagnosed with a bipolar I or a bipolar II disorder (see the DSM-IV-TR Criteria box). Although the public continues to refer to bipolar disorders as manic depression, that term connotes a single, polarized disorder. A bipolar disorder encompasses the range of possible disturbances in mood. The clinical symptoms of bipolar disorders are summarized in the Clinical Symptoms box on p. 210.

CLINICAL SYMPTOMS

Bipolar Disorders

Manic Episode

EMOTIONAL
Abnormally and persistently elevated, expansive, or irritable mood

COGNITIVE
Thoughts of inflated self-esteem and grandiosity
Thought-flow disturbance with racing thoughts and flight of ideas

BEHAVIORAL
Increased talkativeness
Increased goal-directed behavior or agitation
Excessive involvement in activities thought to be pleasurable

SOCIAL
Increased sociability
Intrusive, interruptive, and disruptive during conversations or activities
Fluctuations between euphoria and anger

PERCEPTUAL
Distractibility
Hallucinations

Cyclothymic Disorder

BEHAVIORAL
Periods of hypomania
Periods of depressed mood and anhedonia
Irritability or angry mood
Chronic fatigue

COGNITIVE
Feelings of low self-esteem and inadequacy
Feelings of guilt and brooding about the past
Difficulty with concentration, memory, and decision making
Attitudes of pessimism, despair, and hopelessness

SOCIAL
Social withdrawal

Manic Episode

Manic episodes occur when there is an abnormally and persistently elevated, expansive, or irritable mood for at least 1 week. At least three of the following symptoms must also be present: inflated self-esteem, decreased need for sleep, more than usual talkativeness, racing thoughts, distractibility, increase in goal-directed activity, and excessive involvement in pleasurable activities (see the DSM-IV-TR Criteria box).

Mixed episodes occur when both manic and major depressive criteria are met nearly every day for 1 week (see the DSM-IV-TR Criteria box).

Emotional Symptoms. To be diagnosed as having a manic episode, the client must exhibit an abnormally and persistently elevated, expansive, or irritable mood for at least 1 week. The client appears euphoric, with periods punctuated by irritability and anger. Some clients report minimal euphoria but describe irritability as their primary mood. Emotional lability, fluctuating between euphoria and anger, is common.

Cognitive Symptoms. Inflated self-esteem and grandiosity are common symptoms of mania. Clients report that they are confident, capable, and can do things better than others. As the mania becomes more intense, clients describe themselves in glowing terms and may believe that they are capable of amazing feats and achievements. Delusions of grandeur may be evident during severe episodes of mania as clients believe that they possess extraordinary gifts and talents, that they are famous, or that they personally know someone famous. These delusions of inflated self-worth and ability represent mood-congruent psychotic features of mania. Cognitively, clients with mania also experience thought-flow disturbance with racing thoughts and flight of ideas. **Flight of ideas** is a type of thought disorder in which somewhat connected thoughts occur quickly, resulting in little elaboration and rapid changing of subjects. It becomes difficult to block out incoming stimuli, and the client becomes distractible, responding to irrelevant stimuli. Clients with mania often deny the seriousness of their status and lack judgment regarding personal, social, and occupational needs and activities.

Behavioral Symptoms. Increased talkativeness, increased goal-directed behavior or agitation, and excessive involvement in pleasurable activities are notable symptoms of mania. As the mania progresses, clients become more talkative and their speech is pressured (delivered with urgency). The rate of speech may increase and become rapid. Clients may exhibit extremes in appearance, wearing bright colors, unusual dress, and heavy makeup. Clients begin and engage in more activities, taking on additional tasks and initiating new projects. Productivity may appear to increase as the client delves into more tasks, but as the mania becomes more intense, actual productivity decreases as clients become more distractible, disorganized, and agitated. They begin to physically move faster—pacing, fidgeting, rarely letting their body stay still. As insight and judgment become more impaired, clients become involved in activities that they perceive as pleasurable, but that may carry a high risk for harm or negative consequences. Clients often report engaging in extramarital affairs, promiscuity, spending sprees, gambling, wild driving, and unwise business deals.

Social Symptoms. At first, mania seems to promote sociability, and clients become more outgoing and active; however, before long, insight and judgment fail, and these same clients become intrusive—interrupting others' conversations and activities, fluctuating from euphoria to anger, and disrupting social interactions. Clients with mania find it difficult to set both physical and emotional boundaries, in-

DSM-IV-TR CRITERIA
Manic, Mixed, and Hypomanic Episodes

Manic Episode

A. A distinct period of abnormally and persistently elevated, expansive, or irritable mood, lasting at least 1 week (or any duration if hospitalization is necessary).

B. During the period of mood disturbance, three (or more) of the following symptoms have persisted (four if the mood is only irritable) and have been present to a significant degree:
    1. Inflated self-esteem or grandiosity
    2. Decreased need for sleep (e.g., feels rested after only 3 hours of sleep)
    3. More talkative than usual or pressure to keep talking
    4. Flight of ideas or subjective experience that thoughts are racing
    5. Distractibility (i.e., attention too easily drawn to unimportant or irrelevant external stimuli)
    6. Increase in goal-directed activity (either socially, at work or school, or sexually) or psychomotor agitation
    7. Excessive involvement in pleasurable activities that have a high potential for painful consequences (e.g., engaging in unrestrained buying sprees, sexual indiscretions, or foolish business investments)

C. The symptoms do not meet criteria for a mixed episode.

D. The mood disturbance is sufficiently severe to cause marked impairment in occupational functioning or in usual social activities or relationships with others, or to necessitate hospitalization to prevent harm to self or others, or there are psychotic features.

E. The symptoms are not due to the direct physiological effects of a substance (e.g., a drug of abuse, a medication, or other treatment) or a general medical condition (e.g., hyperthyroidism).

    NOTE: Manic-like episodes that are clearly caused by somatic antidepressant treatment (e.g., medication, electroconvulsive therapy, light therapy) should not count toward a diagnosis of bipolar I disorder.

Mixed Episode

A. The criteria are met both for a manic episode and for a major depressive episode (except for duration) nearly every day during at least a 1-week period.

B. The mood disturbance is sufficiently severe to cause marked impairment in occupational functioning or in usual social activities or relationships with others, or to necessitate hospitalization to prevent harm to self or others, or there are psychotic features.

C. The symptoms are not due to the direct physiological effects of a substance (e.g., a drug of abuse, a medication, or other treatment) or a general medical condition (e.g., hyperthyroidism).

    NOTE: Manic-like episodes that are clearly caused by somatic antidepressant treatment (e.g., medication, electroconvulsive therapy, light therapy) should not count toward a diagnosis of bipolar I disorder.

Hypomanic Episode

A. A distinct period of abnormally and persistently elevated, expansive, or irritable mood, lasting throughout at least 4 days, that is clearly different from the usual nondepressed mood.

B. During the period of mood disturbance, three (or more) of the following symptoms have persisted (four if the mood is only irritable) and have been present to a significant degree:
    1. Inflated self-esteem or grandiosity
    2. Decreased need for sleep (e.g., feels rested after only 3 hours of sleep)
    3. More talkative than usual or pressure to keep talking
    4. Flight of ideas or subjective experience that thoughts are racing
    5. Distractibility (i.e., attention too easily drawn to unimportant or irrelevant external stimuli)
    6. Increase in goal-directed activity (either socially, at work or school, or sexually) or psychomotor agitation
    7. Excessive involvement in pleasurable activities that have a high potential for painful consequences (e.g., engaging in unrestrained buying sprees, sexual indiscretions, or foolish business investments)

C. The episode is associated with an unequivocal change in functioning that is uncharacteristic of the person when not symptomatic.

D. The disturbance in mood and the change in functioning are observable by others.

E. The episode is not severe enough to cause marked impairment in social or occupational functioning, or to necessitate hospitalization, and there are no psychotic features.

F. The symptoms are not due to the direct physiological effects of a substance (e.g., a drug of abuse, a medication, or other treatment) or a general medical condition (e.g., hyperthyroidism).

    NOTE: Hypomanic-like episodes that are clearly caused by somatic antidepressant treatment (e.g., medication, electroconvulsive therapy, light therapy) should not count toward a diagnosis of bipolar II disorder.

From American Psychiatric Association: *Diagnostic and Statistical Manual of Mental Disorders*, Fourth Edition, Text Revision. Washington, DC, American Psychiatric Association, 2000.

fringing on the physical space and personal issues of others. The funny, witty client becomes angry and isolated as the mood escalates and intensifies.

Perceptual Symptoms. One symptom of mania is distractibility, in which attention is easily and frequently drawn to irrelevant external stimuli. Clients appear unable to screen out peripheral stimuli (e.g., noises, other voices, and visual attractions) that are not necessary or relevant to the task at hand. Distractibility interferes with attention, concentration, and memory. Perceptual disturbances can also occur in the form of hallucinations. Manic hallucinations can occur in any sensory mode but are usually auditory, with themes that pertain to grandiosity, power, and, occasionally, paranoia. These indicate manic psychosis.

Hypomanic Episode

Manic and hypomanic episodes share symptom criteria and are differentiated primarily by their severity and duration. Hypomanic episodes are not severe enough to cause significant impairment in social and occupational functioning or to require hospitalization. However, it must be evident that the mood and behavioral disturbances of **hypomania** represent a definite change in the person's usual functioning for at least 4 days. During a hypomanic phase, clients may appear extremely happy and congenial, at ease with social conversation, and offer humorous input. Although the moments of elevated mood appear to be desirable, they represent dysfunctional affective states during which the client is not fully in control of moods and accompanying behavior. The criteria for hypomanic episodes are presented in the DSM-IV-TR Criteria box on p. 211.

Cyclothymic Disorder

Cyclothymic disorder is a chronic mood disturbance of at least 2 years' duration (1 year for children and adolescents), with many periods of hypomanic symptoms, depressed mood, and anhedonia. Clients with cyclothymic disorder have not been without the symptoms for more than 2 months over a period of 2 or more years; however, these symptoms are less severe or intense than those in major depressive or manic episodes.

Additonal Types of Mood Disorders

The DSM-IV-TR also provides diagnostic criteria for mood disorders resulting from general medical conditions and from substance use. In these instances the depressed or elevated mood and accompanying symptoms can be attributed to some general medical condition or to the ingestion of or withdrawal from medications or other substances. Box 10-3 lists examples of the types of medical conditions and substances commonly associated with the development of mood disorders.

Box 10-3   Medical Conditions and Substances Associated with the Development of a Mood Disorder

Medical Conditions
Hypothyroidism/hyperthyroidism
Mononucleosis
Diabetes mellitus
Cushing's disease
Pernicious anemia
Pancreatitis
Hepatitis
Human immunodeficiency virus
Multiple sclerosis

Substances
Digitalis
Thiazide diuretics
Reserpine
Propranolol
Anabolic steroids
Oral contraceptives
Disulfiram
Sulfonamides
Alcohol
Marijuana

Medical Conditions and Mood Disorders

When mood disorders and medical conditions are concurrent, the presentation, treatment, and prognosis of both can be complicated and compromised. Comorbidity can arise from a number of possible scenarios:

- A medical client may develop a mood disorder as a stress response to a serious medical condition.
- A medical client may develop a mood disorder as a physiologic response to either medical pathology or medications.
- A psychiatric client with a persistent mood disorder may develop common medical disorders.
- A psychiatric client with a persistent mood disorder may have an exacerbation of symptoms as a result of medical pathology or treatment.
- Previously unrecognized relationships between mood and medical disorders may be identified.

Medical conditions can be stressful and frightening, and may result in a depressive reaction to the situation or a major depression. A variety of medical disorders have been associated with depression. In one study of 176 consecutive clients between ages 20 and 60 years admitted to medical units, 32% met criteria for a major depression. Most episodes were mild to moderate rather than severe, and all types of medical problems apart from malignancies or neurologic illnesses were included. The rates of depression were similar for acute and chronic illnesses (Sharma et al., 2002). Another study of more than 2500 community residents concluded that the prevalence of major depression was elevated in individuals who reported one or more chronic medical conditions (Gagnon and Patten, 2002). Medical illnesses can introduce insecurity and powerlessness into the lives of individuals who are already physically vulnerable. For example, the uncertainty of awaiting organ transplant has been associated with depression and other coping problems (Crone and Wise, 1999). After heart transplant surgery, the lack of a sense of personal control has been associated with depression (Bohachick et al., 2002).

The pathophysiology of a medical condition, or a response to the medications given for a medical condition, can result in a mood disorder. Research has implicated disorders in nearly every body system with comorbid mood disorders. *Cardiovascular disorders* have been associated with major depression to a great extent. Major depression and depressive symptomatology have been noted as common in clients with coronary artery disease and have been found to significantly increase risk and complicate recovery from a range of cardiac events (Lavoie and Fleet, 2000). Depression after myocardial infarction (MI) has been reported to increase mortality, especially during the first 18 months after the MI (Strik et al., 2001). More recently, the association of cardiac events with vessel inflammation has resulted in the description of a possible causal pathway. One theory is that the inflammatory process of cardiac disease results in lower tryptophan levels. Because tryptophan is associated with serotonin availability, the decrease in both levels may predispose to mood disturbances and depression (Murr, Ledochowski, and Fuchs, 2002).

Neurologic disorders are closely associated with depression. Depression after stroke is particularly common. Estimates suggest that an average 20% of poststroke clients are diagnosed with major depression, and another 21% meeting criteria for minor depression. When onset of major depression occurred shortly after a stroke, vegetative symptoms were found to be more frequent than if the onset appeared later (12 to 24 months poststroke). Late-onset depression was more frequently associated with poor social functioning. Both early- and late-onset depression were attributed to etiology provoked by brain injury (Tateno, Kimura, and Robinson, 2002). Researchers have suggested that early treatment of poststroke depression would have a significant influence on the rehabilitation and recovery of ADL function of stroke clients (Chemerinski, Robinson, and Kosier, 2001). Parkinson's disease (PD) has long been noted in connection with depression. A review of MEDLINE literature reported the prevalence of depression among clients with PD as 31%. Clinical manifestations included apathy, psychomotor retardation, memory impairment, pessimism, irrationality, and suicidal ideation without suicidal behavior (Slaughter et al., 2001). In one study 52.5% of clients with PD were severely depressed, and 37.5% were mildly to moderately depressed. The depression was associated with stage of disease and functional capacity, with significantly higher depression among clients in the severe stage of PD (Gupta and Bhatia, 2000).

Endocrine disorders have been implicated in the emergence of psychiatric disorders. In one study, researchers suggested that there is a relationship between type 2 diabetes mellitus and bipolar I disorder, separate and apart from effects of age, race, gender, medication, and body mass (Regenold et al., 2002).

Additional disorders can result in mood disturbances and continue to be the focus of much research. For example, cancer and thyroid disease have long been studied with regard to mood disorders. Alternatively, a number of medical conditions have been identified that can mimic psychiatric illness. The problem lies in determining the root cause of symptoms, whether they are the result of medical, psychiatric, or psychologic pathology. In the process of treatment, care must be taken to ensure that illnesses are not further complicated by the medications being administered. Many of the medical drugs used today have been associated with the emergence of mood disorders. At the same time, many side effects of psychotropic drugs may be initially assessed as medical in nature (e.g., cardiac or blood pressure changes seen with certain antidepressant drugs). Ultimately the assessment of medical clients must include the psychiatric component.

Psychiatric clients are at least as likely as individuals without psychiatric disorders to develop medical problems ranging from the common cold to serious medical disorders. This is particularly problematic because psychiatric clients have not always received timely or adequate medical care. Consequently psychiatric clients may tend to present at more advanced stages of illness, with more complicated psychosocial factors influencing care. Clients with a preexisting psychiatric disorder may well be present for treatment on any hospital inpatient unit. Unless the treatment plan considers the psychiatric disorder along with the medical illness, problems may arise with medication compatibility, accurate interpretation by staff of client behavior, client cooperation with and involvement in care, or client ability to follow treatment instructions after hospitalization. For example, major depression and bipolar disorder have been identified as increasing the risk for HIV and increasing the morbidity of HIV-related illnesses by impeding treatment. Poor client adherence to antiretroviral therapies has been related to mental illness, whereas treatment of mood disorders has improved adherence to treatment and clinical outcomes of HIV infection (Angelino and Treisman, 2001).

Among psychiatric clients the pathophysiology of, or treatment received for, a medical disorder may promote the return of psychiatric symptoms or the emergence of a new disorder. For example, when clients are admitted to the hospital, a complete history of previous medications may not be available. If psychotropic medications are not continued, the symptoms of a preexisting mood disorder may return, or the client may experience a withdrawal response from medications.

Comorbidity

Current research is expanding our awareness of medical and psychiatric comorbidity, with new knowledge and new questions available every day. Psychiatric clients are living longer than they did in previous generations. Consequently, clinics are seeing an increase in clients with comorbid medical and psychiatric disorders who are also showing signs of

CLINICAL ALERT

Rapid discontinuation of some antidepressants can result in withdrawal symptoms. *Tricyclic antidepressant discontinuation syndrome* can result in gastrointestinal symptoms (nausea, vomiting, abdominal cramps, diarrhea), general distress (headaches, lethargy, sweating), sleep disturbances (insomnia, excessive dreaming, nightmares), affective symptoms (anxiety, agitation, low mood, mania, hypomania), movement disorders, or cardiac arrhythmias. *SSRI discontinuation syndrome* can manifest as gastrointestinal (GI) symptoms (nausea, GI distress), general distress (flulike symptoms, lethargy, sweating), sleep disturbance, affective symptoms (anxiety, irritability, crying spells, agitation, confusion), problems with balance (dizziness, light-headedness, vertigo, ataxia), or sensory abnormalities (paresthesias, numbness, tremor). SSRI discontinuation syndrome is especially likely with the shorter lasting SSRIs, and is most problematic with fluvoxamine (Luvox), nefazodone (Serzone), paroxetine (Paxil), and venlafaxine (Effexor). The nurse should instruct patients to avoid missing doses of antidepressants, reassure patients that withdrawal symptoms are usually mild and short lived, and anticipate that most antidepressants will need to be tapered gradually.

dementia. Epidemiologic data indicate that from 30% to 50% of clients with Alzheimer's disease (AD) have significant depressive symptoms. As a result, discussion is underway to develop criteria that will define the course of depression in AD (Olin et al., 2002). Similar efforts are being made to identify criteria for vascular depression, a subtype occurring within acute and chronic cerebrovascular pathology (Provinciali and Coccia, 2002). Thus two new diagnostic categories may become available, separate from existing depressive disorders. In the end the comorbidity of mood and medical disorders must be acknowledged in all treatment settings.

Additional Symptom Features of Mood Disorders

The DSM-IV-TR recognizes that there are features of mood disorders that may indicate various subtypes of unipolar and bipolar disorders. Persons experiencing an episode of major depression, whether it is part of a unipolar or bipolar pattern, may demonstrate melancholic, atypical, or seasonal features. Postpartum onset represents another type of mood disorder.

Features of **melancholic depression** include anhedonia and a lack of reactivity to any pleasurable stimulus, a distinct quality of mood in which the depression is perceived as different from the feeling felt after the death of a loved one, depression that is worse in the morning, sleep disturbance of early morning, awakening at least 2 hours before the usual time, marked psychomotor retardation or agitation, significant weight loss or loss of appetite, and excessive guilt.

Features of **atypical depression** include mood reactivity, loss of the ability to react to positive stimuli, significant weight gain or increase in appetite, hypersomnia, leaden paralysis or a heavy feeling in the arms and legs, and a longstanding pattern of being sensitive to interpersonal rejection.

A seasonal pattern occurs when there is a regular, temporal relationship between the onset and the remission of an episode of major depression (unipolar or bipolar) at a particular time of the year. This pattern must be evident for 2 consecutive years with no intervening, nonseasonal episodes. Seasonal episodes of altered mood must outnumber any nonseasonal episodes over a lifetime. This pattern is commonly called **seasonal affective disorder (SAD).** Clients with SAD often develop depression during October or November and find it remitting in March or April. Atypical features may also be associated with SAD. A seasonal pattern can also occur with bipolar disorder, particularly bipolar II disorder, in which increased light triggers manic or hypomanic episodes.

Women may experience a *postpartum mood disorder*, including depression or mania, after the birth of a child. About 10% to 15% of new mothers have postpartum depression (Righetti-Veltema et al., 2002). This usually occurs within 4 weeks of the birth and consists of symptoms of depression or mania described earlier. New mothers who are depressed may have a great deal of difficulty providing childcare; in fact, the child may be at risk for neglect or injury.

CLINICAL SYMPTOMS

Additional Mood Disorders

Melancholic Depression
EMOTIONAL
Anhedonia
Increased depression in the morning

COGNITIVE
Excessive feelings of guilt

BEHAVIORAL
Waking at least 2 hours before normal and being unable to fall back to sleep
Psychomotor retardation or agitation
Significant weight loss

Atypical Depression
EMOTIONAL
Mood reactivity
Ability to react to positive stimuli

COGNITIVE
Sensitivity to interpersonal rejection

BEHAVIORAL
Significant weight gain or increase in appetite
Hypersomnia
Leaden paralysis

Seasonal Affective Disorder
EMOTIONAL
Depression between October/November and March/April

Postpartum Depression
BEHAVIORAL
Difficulty caring for child

A summary of clinical symptoms of these additional types of mood disorders is given in the Clinical Symptoms box.

PROGNOSIS AND CLINICAL COURSE

Recently more attention has been given to understanding the life course of persons with mood disorders. The bipolar disorders have historically been perceived as recurrent, with cycles of mania and depression interspersed with periods of **euthymia.** The pattern of cycles varies from person to person, with episodes of depression, mania, and euthymia varying widely in duration. The bipolar disorders have a high rate of recurrence and relapse. Factors that contribute to relapse include the number of and recovery from previous episodes, a family history of bipolar disorder, functional incapacity associated with episodes, past psychotic episodes, and past suicide attempts (Consensus Development Panel, 1985). However, many recurrences can be controlled with proper treatment and monitoring (Keller, 1988).

Major depression is a serious, recurrent disorder for the majority of persons with the disorder (Greden, 2001). Research indicates that 50% to 85% of clients with unipolar depression experience a subsequent episode and that recurrent episodes tend to be increasingly intense with shorter time periods between episodes (Angst, 1988; Greden, 2001). Data suggest that nearly two thirds of people who experience major depression will suffer at least one recurrence within 10 years. Adverse long-term effects impair self-care, productivity, social functioning, occupational functioning, and physical health (Greden, 2001). Fifteen percent of people with depression eventually commit suicide (Hirschfeld et al., 1997).

These data depict the need for education, lifetime monitoring, and maintenance treatment for many persons with depression. The prognosis for major depressive disorder is good; it can be well controlled with medications, psychotherapy, and self-help strategies. However, clients need to be made aware of the recurrent nature of their disorder and educated about the importance of recognizing symptoms and seeking help early when depression begins. Unfortunately, many persons do not recognize the onset of their recurrences (Hagerty, Williams, and Liken, 1997), and less than a third of the people who experience depression seek help, putting them at risk for future, more severe depression.

Dysthymia often continues for years before individuals seek assistance for their symptoms. Many people are unaware that the chronic, low-level depression that is depleting their energy is indeed a form of depression and can be treated. Unfortunately, more than 50% of persons with dysthymia go on to develop major depression (Horwath et al., 1992).

With proper treatment the prognosis for maintaining individual functioning with a mood disorder is favorable. Inevitably, failure to seek help, lack of education regarding the disorder, lack of adherence to treatment, or resistance of the symptoms to usual treatments means that some persons will become so impaired that their daily functioning will diminish for long periods.

DISCHARGE CRITERIA

Most clients with a mood disorder are not hospitalized. They generally receive outpatient treatment. Because of insurance constraints, both settings have become increasingly limited in the amount of time available to clients for treatment. Inpatient stays may range from 4 to 7 days unless symptoms are documented as severe. Outpatient visits may be limited to 20 per year, unless the client pays privately for care. Consequently, the goals of treatment may be quite different for hospital versus outpatient treatment, and realistic outcomes to be expected within the available time frame may be different from ideal expectations. When clients are discharged from the hospital, it is hoped that they will be linked with outpatient treatment so that progress can continue. Clients require attention to ensure that they meet the following realistic criteria for each setting before discharge, whereas continued improvements in delivery of care aim for the ideal criteria.

Hospital Discharge Criteria
Realistic
Client will:
- Verbalize plans for the future, including absence of imminent suicidal intent or behavior.
- Verbalize plan for seeking help (a contract) if suicidal thoughts become intensified or if thoughts progress to plans.
- Demonstrate ability to manage basic self-care needs, such as personal hygiene, or verbalize strategies to acquire assistance.
- Identify psychosocial or physical stressors that may have negative influences on mood and thinking.
- State positive and helpful strategies to cope with threats, concerns, and stressors.
- Identify signs and symptoms of the mood disorder, including prodromal (early) signs that might indicate the need to seek help.
- Describe how to contact appropriate sources for validation and/or intervention when necessary.
- Verbalize knowledge about medication treatment and necessary self-care strategies.

Ideal
Client will:
- Describe mood state and demonstrate ability to identify changes from euthymic mood.
- Verbalize realistic perceptions of self and abilities that are positive and hopeful.
- Verbalize realistic expectations for self and others.
- Use learned techniques and strategies to prevent or minimize symptoms.
- Engage family or significant other as a source of support.
- Structure life to include appropriate activities that promote social support, minimize stress, and facilitate healthy living (e.g., diet, exercise).

Outpatient Discharge Criteria
Realistic
Client will:
- Verbalize plans for the future, including absence of imminent suicidal intent or behavior.
- Verbalize plan for seeking help (a contract) if suicidal thoughts become intensified or if thoughts progress to plans.
- Demonstrate ability to manage basic self-care needs, such as personal hygiene, or verbalize strategies to acquire assistance.
- Describe mood state and demonstrate ability to identify changes from euthymic mood.
- Identify psychosocial or physical stressors that may have negative influences on mood and thinking.
- State positive and helpful strategies to cope with threats, concerns, and stressors.
- Identify signs and symptoms of the mood disorder, including prodromal (early) signs that might indicate the need to seek help.

- Describe how to contact appropriate sources for validation and/or intervention when necessary.
- Use learned techniques and strategies to prevent or minimize symptoms.
- Verbalize knowledge about medication treatment and necessary self-care strategies.

Ideal

Client will:

- Verbalize realistic perceptions of self and abilities that are positive and hopeful.
- Verbalize realistic expectations for self and others.
- Engage family or significant other as a source of support.
- Structure life to include appropriate activities that promote social support, minimize stress, and facilitate healthy living (e.g., diet, exercise).

THE NURSING PROCESS

ASSESSMENT

Mood is the key variant in mood disorders. In the performance of a mental status examination by the nurse, the assessment of mood is enhanced by consideration of related phenomena. **Mood** is defined as a feeling state reported by the client that can vary with external and internal changes. A prolonged time course of the state is implied, and the identification of a specific cause can be difficult. **Affect** is defined as the expression of a client's feeling state that can be observed by others. The expression can be highly changeable. **Temperament** is defined as observable differences in the strength and duration of a client's tendency to respond to circumstances and degree of emotionalism expressed. It is generally thought to be a product of a person's biologic constitution. The term is generally applied when speaking of infants or children, but it should be considered that temperament patterns have been shown to influence a variety of phenomena that extend into adulthood, including impulse control and attachment. *Emotion* is the client's experience of a feeling state, and antecedents often can be identified in what may be, for the client, highly intense and variable experiences. *Emotional* or *affective reactivity* is the degree to which a client tends to respond to external and internal changes with feeling states. This may be noted in terms of how the client responds to questions. *Emotional regulation* refers to the client's ability to control or modify the occurrence and intensity of feeling states. *Range of affect* is the breadth of emotional expression the client shows. Limitations of range may be described as restricted, blunted, or flat (Box 10-4).

The prevalence and incidence of mood disorders demand that nurses be alert for symptoms of depression and mania. Most persons experiencing a mood disorder, particularly depression, never seek psychiatric care. More often, these individuals visit family practitioners, clinics, or Emergency

Box 10-4   Mental Status Phenomena
Mood: the psychologic manifestation of subjective feeling
Affect: the objective manifestation of a feeling state
Temperament: objective differences in the intensity and duration of arousal and emotionality
Emotion: the experience of a feeling state
Emotional reactivity: the tendency to respond to internal or external events with emotion
Emotional regulation: the ability to control or modify the occurrence and intensity of feeling states
Range of affect: the breadth of emotional expression displayed

Departments reporting symptoms of fatigue, lack of activity, or vague physical complaints. Many do not realize that they are experiencing a mood disorder.

Clients with mood disorders pose a challenge because their primary symptom is one of depression or emotional elation. Their affective dysregulation often evokes emotional responses in nurses, who find themselves feeling depressed, anxious, or angry while caring for the individual. The negativity of depression or the expansive euphoria, hyperactivity, and grandiosity of mania may also promote fatigue, irritability, and negativity in the nurse. Therefore when caring for clients with mood disorders, nurses must maintain awareness of their own personal reactions to the client and the ways in which these reactions can affect the nurse-client relationship and subsequent care.

Clients experiencing mood disorders are in emotional pain. They are unable to change their emotional state at will. Yet, many have heard people close to them make comments such as, "Pull yourself together . . . get a hold of yourself." These clients need validation that their emotional state is not their fault, that they are experiencing a psychiatric disorder. They should be approached with acceptance and respect.

It is important that nurses appear confident, straightforward, and hopeful. Reassuring comments such as, "I know you'll feel better soon," are usually not helpful, because they may be false reassurance. It is appropriate to convey hope with comments such as, "I've known many clients with depression, and they have felt better within several weeks of starting on their medications."

Communication with the person with depression depends on the severity of the depression. Clients with severe depression may be physically and cognitively slowed down and have problems with attention, concentration, and decision making. Simple, clear communication is most helpful in this situation. The nurse may need to be more directive if the person is having a difficult time making decisions (e.g., "It's time for lunch. I'll go with you," rather than, "Would you like to go to lunch?"). As clients' conditions improve, they can cognitively process more complex information and make decisions more easily.

Communication with clients experiencing mania can also be difficult. Their hyperactivity, expansive or irritable mood, and inability to filter stimuli are barriers to effective communication. Nurses need to be simple, clear, direct, and firm. Clients need to know that the nurse cares about them and is concerned about their behavior. Acute episodes of mania are not appropriate times for the nurse to delve into the client's feelings and motives. Interactions should be brief and direct, with minimization of unnecessary stimuli. It is also important not to threaten or challenge a client in the turmoil of a manic episode, because the client might respond with rage.

Information from the client may be minimal or inaccurate because of their cognitive impairment, altered mood, or behavioral disturbances. A significant other can be an important source of information when the client is not reliable. Interviews may need to be short and more directive if the client is having behavioral or cognitive difficulty.

Assessment of the client with depression or mania includes information about his or her presenting problem and mental status, past psychiatric history, social and developmental history, family history, and physical health history. Assessment instruments can assist with the specificity of data collection. These instruments include the Beck Depression Inventory (BDI), Carroll Rating Scale for Depression (CRSD), and Zung Self-Rating Depression Scale. Nurses can also ask clients to assess their own level of depression or mania by having them rate it on a 10-point scale (e.g., "If zero represents feeling fine and 10 represents the worst depression you have ever experienced, how would you rate your depression now?"). This allows for daily comparisons of mood.

Physiologic Disturbances

Body physiology is altered during episodes of depression and mania. During moderate or severe depression, body processes frequently slow down. The client with depression may report and exhibit neurovegetative signs of depression, which include psychomotor retardation, fatigue, constipation, anorexia (loss of appetite), weight loss, decreased libido (sex drive), and sleep disturbances. These symptoms relate to changes in body processes that cause disruption and slowing of normal physiology. Clients may also describe vague physical symptoms such as headache, backache, gastrointestinal pain, and nausea. Clients may seek assistance from their family health care provider, thinking that they are experiencing some physical illness that is causing fatigue and loss of energy. Sleep disturbance is a common problem. Clients describe initial insomnia (the inability to fall asleep after going to bed), middle insomnia (waking up in the middle of the night and being unable to return to sleep easily), and terminal, or late, insomnia (waking up in the early hours of the morning and being unable to return to sleep). Another type of sleep disturbance seen in depression is hypersomnia, in which the client sleeps excessively but never feels rested. Clients with depression may have a decreased or increased appetite with corresponding changes in weight. Food is often described as tasteless (see Case Study, top right).

The client experiencing mania also has difficulty sleeping. Not feeling the need for sleep, the client may sleep

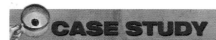

CASE STUDY

Ed is a 42-year-old male who has been unable to go to work for more than a month. He reports extreme fatigue, lack of energy, loss of appetite, and inability to fall asleep, and speaks in a monotone. He has an appointment with a family nurse practitioner and is concerned that he has some form of cancer. His wife states that he has been sullen and quiet. You are assessing Ed before the nurse practitioner enters the examination room.

Critical Thinking

1. What are important questions for the nurse to ask Ed at his appointment?
2. What laboratory tests might be appropriate?
3. What specific signs and symptoms suggest that Ed might be depressed?
4. If you had the symptoms exhibited by Ed, would you be able to seek help immediately? How long would you wait? Would you consider that you might be depressed?

CASE STUDY

Sandra is a 38-year-old mother of three. She was brought to the hospital by her husband, who was concerned that she had lost 20 pounds within the past several weeks and lay on the sofa, crying much of the day. The house had not been cleaned for weeks, and the children were making their own meals and doing the laundry. Sandra was dressed casually in wrinkled clothes. Her movements and verbalizations were slow. Sandra had told her husband that she thought they should buy a cemetery plot but could not explain why.

Critical Thinking

1. What additional information would be helpful for the nurse to know about Sandra to develop nursing diagnoses and goals?
2. Which nursing diagnoses would be relevant for Sandra?
3. What long- and short-term outcomes, based on the nursing diagnoses, might be established with Sandra?

only a few hours a night or not at all and yet feel rested afterward. Hyperactive behavior and the inability to attend to tasks often preclude the client from eating properly, resulting in dehydration and inadequate nutrition. As the client becomes increasingly stimulated, metabolic activity increases, and vital signs may become elevated. Without proper intervention, clients with mania may be at physical risk for dehydration, hypertension, and cardiac arrest, which can lead to death.

NURSING DIAGNOSIS

The nurse uses objective and subjective data obtained during the assessment of clients with mood disorders to arrive at relevant nursing diagnoses. Data from all sources, including the client, significant others, and other professionals, are organized into a pattern of relationships that reflect the client's major areas of health care needs (see Case Study above and

NURSING ASSESSMENT QUESTIONS
Mood Disorders

1. How would you describe your mood? *To assess client's insight into feeling state*
2. Have you noticed a change in your behavior within the past month? *To determine client's awareness of behavioral changes*
3. Do you feel that people are noticing a change in your behavior, such as irritability or hyperactivity? *To determine client's sensitivity to others' observations of behavioral changes*
4. What activities have you found enjoyable over the past month? Did you enjoy them as much as you previously did? Can you imagine an event or situation that would give you pleasure? Have you been able to enjoy food and/or sex over the past month? *To determine client's current quality of life*
5. When did you first begin to feel depressed or elated? Did others comment that your mood seemed more depressed (or higher) than usual? Have you ever felt this way before? When? What was it like? *To establish behavioral patterns*
6. How has your sleep been? Are you able to fall asleep at night? Stay asleep? Do you find yourself waking up early and being unable to return to sleep? Are you sleeping more than usual in a 24-hour period? How much? Are you sleeping less than usual? How much? *To determine sleep patterns*
7. How has your appetite been in the past month? How much weight have you lost or gained in the past month? *To determine nutritional/metabolic status*
8. How has your energy level been? Do you feel tired every day? Do you ever feel as though your limbs are heavy? Do you have more energy than usual? *To assess fatigability*
9. How has your concentration been? Are you able to attend to things such as reading the newspaper? Can you concentrate on projects or activities to finish them? What has your decision making been like? Have you had racing thoughts? *To evaluate cognitive abilities*
10. How have you felt about yourself lately? Have you felt guilty more than usual about things you have done? *To determine client's level of self-worth/self-esteem*
11. Have you felt particularly slowed down, or have others told you that you seemed to move or speak more slowly than usual? *To determine presence of sensorimotor retardation*
12. Have you felt particularly "speeded up" to the point where you noticed it or someone told you this? *To evaluate presence of mania/hypomania*
13. Have you had thoughts of death or suicide? How often? What specifically have you thought about doing to harm yourself? What prevented you from committing suicide? Have you had thoughts of harming or killing someone else? How often? What specifically have you thought about doing to harm someone else? *To determine suicidal/homicidal intent/plans*
14. What have you been doing lately to manage your feelings? Has it helped? *To assess for effective coping mechanisms/strategies*
15. How has your mood affected your job? Your family? Your social life? Your interpersonal relationships? *To assess pervasiveness of client's present mood state*
16. Have your received treatment from a mental health professional in the past? What kind of treatment? Did it help? *To determine presence and effectiveness of any past treatment*

Nursing Assessment Questions box). Box 10-5 lists nursing diagnoses relevant to clients experiencing a mood disorder.

OUTCOME IDENTIFICATION

Outcome criteria for clients with mood disorders include short- and long-term client behaviors and responses that indicate improved functioning. These criteria are based on nursing diagnoses and are achieved through implementation of planned nursing care. Outcome criteria provide the nurse with direction for evaluating client response to treatment.

Client will:
- Remain safe and free from harm.
- Verbalize suicidal ideations and contract not to harm self or others.
- Verbalize absence of suicidal or homicidal intent or plans.
- Express desire to live and not harm others.
- Make plans for self for the future, verbalizing feelings of hopefulness.
- Engage in self-care activities in accordance with ability, health status, and developmental stage.
- Develop a plan to manage inadequate sleep.
- Establish a pattern of rest/activity that enables fulfillment of role and self-care demands.
- Make decisions based on examination of options and problem solving.
- Report absence of hallucinations/delusions.
- Initiate satisfying social interactions with significant others or peers.
- Demonstrate participation in milieu, group, and community activities.
- Report increased communication and problem solving among family members regarding issues related to the disorder.
- Describe alternative coping strategies for responses to stressors, strengths, and limitations.
- Report increased feelings of self-worth and confidence.
- Engage in activities and behaviors that promote confidence, belonging, and acceptance.
- Describe information about the disorder, including the course of illness and personal symptom patterns, as well as resources.
- Identify medications, including action, dosage, side effects, therapeutic effects, and self-care issues.
- Adhere to prescribed professional and self-care treatment strategies.

Box 10-5	Nursing Diagnoses for Depression and Mania

Depression	Mania
Activity intolerance	Impaired adjustment
Adult failure to thrive	Caregiver role strain
Anxiety	Impaired verbal communication
Constipation	Compromised family coping
Ineffective individual coping	Defensive coping
Death anxiety	Ineffective individual coping
Deficient diversional activity	Ineffective denial
Disturbed energy field	Disturbed energy field
Fatigue	Impaired environmental interpretation syndrome
Dysfunctional grieving	Dysfunctional family processes
Delayed growth and development	Risk for deficient fluid volume
Ineffective health maintenance	Delayed growth and development
Hopelessness	Ineffective health maintenance
Deficient knowledge	Deficient knowledge
Risk for loneliness	Risk for loneliness
Noncompliance	Noncompliance
Imbalanced nutrition: less than body requirements	Imbalanced nutrition: less than body requirements
Imbalanced nutrition: more than body requirements	Imbalanced nutrition: more than body requirements
Risk for impaired parenting	Risk for impaired parenting
Powerlessness	Ineffective role performance
Ineffective role performance	Self-care deficit, bathing/hygiene
Self-care deficit, bathing/hygiene	Self-care deficit, dressing/grooming
Self-care deficit, dressing/grooming	Self-care deficit, feeding
Self-care deficit, feeding	Disturbed sensory perception
Chronic low self-esteem	Sexual dysfunction
Sexual dysfunction	Disturbed sleep pattern
Disturbed sleep pattern	Sleep deprivation
Impaired social interaction	Impaired social interaction
Social isolation	Spiritual distress
Chronic sorrow	Risk for suicide
Spiritual distress	Ineffective therapeutic regimen management
Risk for suicide	Ineffective family therapeutic regimen management
Ineffective therapeutic regimen management	Disturbed thought processes
Risk for self-directed violence	Risk for other-directed violence
	Risk for self-directed violence

From NANDA International (2003). NANDA Nursing Diagnoses: Definitions and Classification 2003-2004. Philadelphia: NANDA.

PLANNING

Recent information about the epidemiology and recurrent course of depression and mania provides the basis for caring for clients with mood disorders in the hospital and in the community. Nursing care addresses the acute episodes of the disorder and the client's risk for recurrent episodes. Interventions during the acute depressive or manic episodes can be effective, but too often the client is left with little understanding of the importance of long-term management and self-care strategies. Interventions must be planned for each client based on his or her particular behaviors and concerns. Planning care not only involves the client but may also include the client's significant others and additional health care providers. Using nursing diagnoses derived from assessment data, interventions that facilitate achievement of desired client outcomes are planned (see Collaborative Diagnoses table).

IMPLEMENTATION

The plan of action for clients with mood disorders varies depending on whether the client is depressed or manic. In the short term nursing and collaborative interventions are available that are effective in reducing the acuity of the episode and promoting more optimal functioning. With the current trend of short-term hospitalizations, nurses in the hospital setting do not have the opportunity to observe the client's recovery from the episode. Projected treatment responses, however, should be documented and communicated to the client and to nurses, other mental health professionals, and significant others who will care for the client in the commu-

COLLABORATIVE DIAGNOSES

DSM-IV-TR Diagnoses*	NANDA Diagnoses†	
Bipolar I disorder, manic or hypomanic	Activity intolerance	Imbalanced nutrition: less than body requirements
Bipolar II disorder	Impaired adjustment	Imbalanced nutrition: more than body requirements
Cyclothymic disorder	Adult failure to thrive	Risk for impaired parenting
Dysthymic disorder	Anxiety	Powerlessness
Major depressive episode	Death anxiety	Ineffective role performance
Mood disorder due to a general medical condition	Caregiver role strain	Self-care deficit, bathing/hygiene
	Impaired verbal communication	Self-care deficit, dressing/grooming
Substance-induced mood disorder	Constipation	Self-care deficit, feeding
	Compromised family coping	Chronic low self-esteem
	Defensive coping	Disturbed sensory perception
	Ineffective individual coping	Sexual dysfunction
	Ineffective denial	Disturbed sleep pattern
	Deficient diversional activity	Sleep deprivation
	Disturbed energy field	Impaired social interaction
	Impaired environmental interpretation syndrome	Social isolation
	Interrupted family processes	Chronic sorrow
	Fatigue	Spiritual distress
	Risk for deficient fluid volume	Risk for suicide
	Dysfunctional grieving	Ineffective therapeutic regimen management
	Delayed growth and development	Ineffective family therapeutic regimen management
	Ineffective health maintenance	
	Hopelessness	Disturbed thought processes
	Deficient knowledge	Risk for other-directed violence
	Risk for loneliness	Risk for self-directed violence
	Noncompliance	

*From American Psychiatric Association: *Diagnostic and Statistical Manual of Mental Disorders,* Fourth Edition, Text Revision. Washington, DC, American Psychiatric Association, 2000.
†From NANDA International (2002). NANDA Nursing Diagnoses: Definitions and Classification 2003-2004. Philadelphia: NANDA.

nity. Nurses who work with clients in the community are able to see treatment responses over time (see Nursing Care in the Community box).

Mood disorders, although primarily disturbances in emotional regulation, affect the whole person—physically, cognitively, socially, and spiritually. Short-term interventions in the hospital or community address priority issues such as preventing self-harm, promoting physical health (e.g., adequate nutrition, bathing, grooming, sleep), monitoring effects of medications, and assisting with altered thought flow and impaired communication. Other concerns to be addressed include promoting social interaction, self-esteem, understanding of the disorder and its treatment, treatment compliance, and planning for discharge and continuation or discontinuation of services. Because episodes of depression and mania affect the entire family, involving the client's significant others provides an opportunity for them to understand the disorder and to support clients in their recovery. Clinical pathways, which specify collaborative interventions relevant to mood disorders, can be found on pp. 222 to 224.

Nursing interventions for clients with mood disorders span a wide range of biopsychosocial areas, with consideration of the effects of depression and mania on the physiologic, cognitive, psychologic, behavioral, and social spheres. Intervention for clients experiencing depression and mania requires that nurses maintain self-awareness and boundaries regarding their own reactions to clients, because client depression, irritability, anger, negativity, euphoria, and hyperactivity can influence nursing response. It is potentially difficult and exhausting to interact with clients who provoke personal feelings and reactions during highly emotional encounters. Initiating and maintaining a therapeutic connection with clients are accomplished through consistency, caring, concern, empathy, and genuineness on the part of the nurse. Clients with mood disorders may have a difficult time developing a therapeutic alliance and avoid interpersonal connection with others. A knowledgeable, consistent, and matter-of-fact (but genuine and caring) presentation is reassuring to clients and promotes their confidence in the nurse.

NURSING CARE IN THE COMMUNITY — Mood Disorders

Working with persons experiencing mood disorders can be challenging for the community mental health nurse. The nurse must deal with a wide range of behaviors and may find recommendations to be minimized by the client, if not negated entirely. A person manifesting a manic episode is often grandiose, expresses pleasure in his or her increased activity level, and becomes irritable when confronted about problematic behavior. In contrast, a person suffering from depression also often rejects help, because nothing seems meaningful and change appears impossible. In either case the client may see the process of assessment as intrusive, and efforts toward engagement may be rejected. The nurse must work carefully through the evaluation process to decide whether hospitalization is indicated.

Context and timing are significant when evaluating the mood-disordered individual in the community. The nurse should consider the following questions:

Have situational stressors caused the sadness or elation?
Has a grief process evolved into a depressed state?
Have vegetative signs developed? (Have the person's sleeping and eating patterns changed?)
Are nonverbal signs such as posture and affect consistent with expressed emotion?
Is there a history of suicidal or homicidal behavior, current suicidality or homicidality, or a plan for suicide or homicide?
Has the person ever been treated for depression or bipolar disorder successfully?
Is the person willing to accept treatment now?

The nurse remains unbiased, neither trying to superficially cheer the client nor offering situational advice. The nurse may suggest treatment options and assess the client's response. Screening tests for depression may be used to facilitate diagnosis. Some facilities offer free screening for depression in the community.

Assessing the person experiencing a manic episode is often dramatic and can be frustrating for the nurse. The manic individual reiterates that he or she is fine, does not need help from anyone, and resents the "interrogation." It is best to enlist the help of members of the client's support system, as well as the client, to identify a developing manic episode on the basis of behavioral changes. The client may be experiencing increases in spending patterns, sexual activity, or erratic sleep patterns. It is easier to influence the client to seek help early, rather than waiting until sleep deprivation and increased tension have made the client so irritable or fatigued that he or she experiences psychosis, requiring involuntary hospitalization.

Monitoring medication levels and effectiveness is another critical element for the nurse caring for clients with mood disorders in the community. Antidepressants may cause clients to feel stronger but still depressed enough to be at high risk for suicide. Antimanic medications such as lithium carbonate and carbamazepine (Tegretol) can be life threatening if excesses build up in the client's system. These medications require periodic blood tests to verify medication compliance and discriminate between toxic and therapeutic levels. Symptoms of toxicity may resemble an increasing disease process, and higher doses of medication may be administered if evaluation is not timely and insightful. The nurse must encourage the client to discriminate among feeling states and pathologic or physiologic symptoms so that he or she can seek assistance if out of control.

Nursing Interventions

1. Conduct a suicide assessment as necessary *to ensure the client's safety and prevent harm to self or others.*
2. Maintain a safe, harm-free environment through close and frequent observations *to minimize the risk of violence.*
3. Establish rapport and demonstrate respect for the client *to facilitate the client's willingness to communicate thoughts and feelings.*
4. Assist the client in verbalizing feelings *to promote a healthy, expressive form of communication.*
5. Identify the client's social support system and encourage the client to use it *to minimize isolation and loneliness as possible precursors to hopelessness.*
6. Praise the client for attempts at alternate activities and interactions with others *to encourage socialization.*
7. Gently refuse to be pulled into secrecy agreements with the client, instead encouraging the client to share important and relevant information with staff *to promote the client's participation in care and responsibility for own actions.*
8. Monitor the client's fluid intake and output, food intake, and weight *to ensure adequate nutrition and hydration and adequate weight for body size and metabolic need.*
9. Promote self-care activities, such as bathing, dressing, feeding, and grooming, *to ascertain the client's level of functioning and increase self-esteem.*
10. Assist the client in establishing daily goals and expectations *to promote structure and minimize confusion/anxiety.*
11. Plan self-care activities around those times when the client may have more energy *to increase activity tolerance and minimize fatigue.*
12. Reduce choices of clothing and tasks *to make decision making easier, increasing choices as the client improves cognitively.*
13. Assess the client's cognitive/perceptual process *to ascertain the existence of hallucinations/delusions that may be troubling or harmful for the client.*
14. Assist the client in identifying negative, self-defeating thoughts and modifying them with realistic thoughts *to promote more accurate, positive thoughts about self.*
15. Encourage the client to attend therapeutic groups that provide feedback regarding thinking *to reframe thinking with the support of others* (see Chapter 19).
16. Provide simple, clear directives/communication in a low-stimulus environment *to assist with focus, attention, and concentration with minimal distractions.*

ST. JOSEPH HOSPITAL

DRG Number :
Primary Physician :
Physician(s) in Consult :
Anticipated Discharge Date :
Actual Discharge Date :
Financial :

MAJOR DEPRESSION CLINICAL PATHWAY©

CARE NEEDS	DAY OF ADMIT	LEVEL 1	LEVEL 2	LEVEL 3	LEVEL 4	LEVEL 5
CONSULTS/ ASSESSMENTS:	MD. CM. SW. RN. OT. Consults? Medical? Other?	Psy eval? Fam mtg? Complete all assess.	Complete family mtg. Complete psy testing if ordered.	SW/CM process family mtg w/pt. Complete psy consult if ordered.	OT reassess? Transfer summaries.	Send results of assess to out-pt Tx.
HEALTH MAINTENANCE Sleep Disturbance. ADL's. Diet. Med Dx	Chem 19. CBC. UA. Tox? T_3T_2Tsh? Pg? TCA/Li/Other? Sleep? ADL? Medical (below)? Nutri? VS ___ Ortho? ---->	Lab results? Nutri? Sleep? ADL? Review prot? Medical? VS ___ ------>	Nutri? Sleep? ADL? Review prot? Medical? VS ___ ------>	Nutri? Sleep? ADL? Review prot? Medical? VS ___ ------>	Nutri? Sleep? ADL? Review prot? Medical? Med refer to med f/u. VS ___ ------>	VS ___
PROGRAM: Target Sx

Meds. Teaching needs. Stressors. Compliancy. Tx | Orientation Prot. Rest 24"? Sx? Groups? Med orders? Consent form? Teaching needs? Stressors?

Tx compliancy? | Shift Assess Prot. Multidis Tx plan mtg. Assess need for alt pathway. Groups per prot. Comm mtg:

Meds/SE? Chart to target Sx. Tx compliancy? | Shift Assess Prot. Groups per prot. ___

Tx compliancy? Med/SE? Chart to target Sx. Prov med sheets. | Shift Assess Prot. Groups per prot. ___ Med group. D/C planning

Tx compliancy? Med/SE? Chart to target Sx. 1 unit resp. | Shift Assess Prot. Multidis Tx plan? Groups per prot. ___

Chart to target Sx. Med/SE? Tx compl? | Daily Assess Prot. D/C Prot. |
| SAFETY - Harm to self, others, and destruction of property. Elopement. Potential for falls. Sexually acting out. | Suicide Prot.? Safety Prot.? SFC? Verbal contract? Mental status? E? | Suicide Prot.? Mental status? SFC? E? OW Prot.? | Suicide Prot.? Mental status? Safety Prot.? SFC? E? OW Prot.? | Suicide Prot.? Mental status? Safety Prot.? SFC? E? OW Prot.? | Suicide Prot.? Mental status? Safety Prot.? SFC? E? SI review opt if ref. OW Prot.? | Review opt if SI reoccurs. Use of support systems. |
| DISCHARGE PLANNING: Compliancy. F/u. Teaching. MHC

Financial | CM/SW 1 data - family? placement? Support system? Release of info. LOS expectation.

DSHS form? Insurance? | Housing? LOS. F/up resources? Support system? Contact fam. Assign fam. grp. Contact MHC/out-pt Tx. | Placement? MHC call liaison? Formulate f/up plan. Fam. attend sup/ed group. LOS. | Finalize f/up plan. LOS. Arrange for trans on day of D/C. Assess for therapeutic pass. | Liaison from MHC to see. Review Sx & cues to reoccurrence. Consider long-term care. Resources for meds. Coord D/C w/fam. | Check transportation & meds by 8 am for D/C by 11 am. |

MAJORDEP.PIH 2/28/92

Axis I _____   Axis II _____   Axis III _____   Axis IV _____   Axis V _____

PERMANENT PART OF THE PATIENT RECORD

NOTE: This is not a Physician Order

Barnes and Jewish Hospitals
Department of Nursing
Patient Clinical Management Path

Admission _____
D/C Date _____
Estimated LOS _____
Case Manager _____

Case Type & Number **(DRG – 430) Bipolar Affective Disorder**

	Day 1/Adm. Loc ( )	Var. n/d m u	Day 2 – 3 Loc ( )	Var. n/d m u	Day 4 – 6 Loc ( )	Var. n/d m u	Day 7 – 9 Loc ( )	Var. n/d m u
Date								
Procedure/Test	Organic Workup (MD), EEG (MD), CT (MD), MRI (MD), EKG (MD), CXR (MD), Electrolytes (MD), Lithium Level (MD), Drug Screen (MD), Thyroid Studies (MD), Routine Labs (MD), Other _____ (MD)		Lab Results (ID abnormals)		– – – – – > Psych Testing complete		Labs _____ Tests _____ Med. Blood Levels _____	
Consults	Medical (MD) Behavior Med. (MD) Psych Testing (MD) Other _____ (MD)		ID additional consults		– – – – – >		– – – – – >	
Meds/Tx	Meds ordered per MD including PRN to control behavior. ECT (MD) – permits (Nsg) – teaching (Nsg) – team notified (Nsg)		Monitor antidepressant, lithium, tegretol, valproic acid, PRN Meds. Other anti-psychotic meds; if mania DC antidepressant – – – – – >		– – – – – > – – – – – >		– – – – – > – – – – – >	
Activity	Voluntary/Involuntary SP/EP (MD, Nsg) Fall precautions (MS, Nsg)		Assess ADL's – – – – – > – – – – – > Integrate into milieu Participate in groups Individual therapy		– – – – – > Assess precautions – – – – – > – – – – – > – – – – – >		– – – – – > – – – – – > – – – – – > – – – – – >	
Nutrition	Assess appetite (MD, Nsg) Assess elimination patterns (MD, Nsg)		– – – – – > – – – – – > Teaching diet		– – – – – > – – – – – > – – – – – >		– – – – – > – – – – – > – – – – – >	
Discharge Planning	Legal Guardian ID (Nsg) Assess support system (Nsg, MD, SW, AT) Initial Plan (MD/Nsg)		SW Acknowl. note Placement issues MTP signed (MD/Nsg/SW)		Family Mtg		Plans discussed with patient (MD) – – – – – > Weekly Progress Note (MD, SW, Nsg, TR) Completes SW assess Referrals Resources MTP developed	
INTERVENTIONS: Assessment Functional Assessment	H+P & Psych orders (MD) Nsg Assessment and ADB SW notified – pt/family Proper envir. assessed Mini Mental (Nsg) Assess LOF (Nsg, SW, AT) Assess methods to control behavior (Nsg) Remove ext. stimuli (Nsg)		Ongoing assess & treatment (MD, Nsg, SW, TR) BM initial Assess. Assess for dystonia If ADL assess needed OT referral		– – – – – > Assess: – thought patterns – orientation – cog. skills – task completion		– – – – – > Assess task completion Encourage incr. LOF – – – – – > Assess lifestyle changes – – – – – >	
Patient Teaching	Orient pt/family to unit (Nsg) Bill of Rights Given (Nsg)		Ed. Pt/family to various therapies MED Educ. Primary Nurse (Nsg)		– – – – – > – – – – – >		– – – – – > – – – – – >	

Signature & Initials   Refer to Nurses Notes for documentation regarding variances.

_____ _____ _____
_____ _____ _____
_____ _____ _____
_____ _____ _____

	Day 10 – 12 Loc ( )	Var. n/d m u	Day 13 – 14 Loc ( )	Var. n/d m u	Day 15 Loc ( )	Var. n/d m u	Discharge Expected Outcome
Date							
Procedure/Test	Labs _____ Tests _____ Med. Blood Levels _____		Labs _____ Tests _____ Chart copied if appropriate		DC Orders Written		
Consults	– – – – >		F/u appts made		– – – – >		
Meds/Tx	– – – – > – – – – > Begin ECT outpt. arrangements		– – – – > – – – – > – – – – >		Perscriptions written		Pt will verbalize/ demonstrate imp. of medication +/or other therapies in maintaining optimal level of fcn after DC as evidenced by _____
Activity	– – – – > – – – – > – – – – > – – – – > – – – – >		Do teaching r/t follow up therapy		Plans finalized r/t outpt therapy		
Nutrition	– – – – > – – – – > – – – – >		DC teaching r/t nutrition		– – – – >		
Discharge Planning			DC teaching w/family Weekly progress notes (MD, SW, TR, Nsg) DC teaching on utilization of skills learned while in hosp and how to integrate to home. Written information r/t resource given.		MTP closed or remains ongoing Final DC instructions given to pt/family F/U appt finalized		Pt will return to least restrictive/most supportive environment after DC with improved coping skills and identified resources as demonstrated by _____ _____.
INTERVENTIONS: Assessment	– – – – > – – – – >		– – – – > – – – – >		Final assessments & DC summary written.		
Functional Assessment	MMSE (Neg) – – – – > – – – – > – – – – > – – – – >		– – – – >		– – – – >		
Patient Teaching	– – – – > – – – – >		– – – – > – – – – > DC teaching		Final DC teaching to patient. Patient's responses to teaching documented		

*SW works M – F

Teaching (initial and date when complete)
1. Medication Education _____
2. Education on illness _____
3. Social Skills _____
4. Coping Skills _____
5. ADL's _____
6. Self-Esteem _____
7. Dealing with Anger _____
8. Communication Skills _____
9. Dealing with Sadness _____
10. Decision Making _____
11. Other _____
∗Document patient response in progress notes

Addressograph:

17. Teach the client and significant others about the disorder and treatment *to minimize guilt and remorse in clients and families about the disorder.*

18. Gradually increase levels of activity and exercise *to minimize fatigue and increase activity tolerance.*

19. Identify sources of external stress and assist the client in coping with them in a more effective manner *to minimize stressors and promote adaptive coping mechanisms.*

20. Educate the client with depression about the disorder and symptoms as appropriate *to lessen feelings of inadequacy, minimize guilt, and increase the knowledge base about the effects of the illness.*

21. Educate the client with mania about the disorder and symptoms as appropriate *to lessen feelings of inadequacy, minimize guilt, and increase the knowledge base about the effects of the illness.*

Additional Treatment Modalities
Psychopharmacology

During the last 40 years there have been major advances in the use of medications to treat symptoms of mood disorders. Investigation of the neurobiology of depression and mania has provided directions for development of these new medications. These are discussed in Chapter 20. Because there are multiple types of medications that seem to work with various individuals and their types of depression and mania, selecting the drug and the dosage that is effective for any individual is often a difficult process. Clients who do not respond to one type of medication may do well with another.

Various types of antidepressant medications are used to treat persons with episodes of major depression and some persons with dysthymia. These include tricyclics, heterocyclics, MAOIs, SSRIs, and most recently joint serotonin and norepinephrine reuptake inhibitors. These medications exert powerful effects not only on mood but also on the entire syndrome of depression symptoms, including the neurovegetative symptoms. Not surprisingly, medications also cause side effects that can create discomfort and even danger. Taken in large quantities, many are toxic or even lethal. In addition, these medications usually have a lag period of 1 to 6 weeks for initiation of therapeutic effects, during which time the side effects are often the most pronounced. As the medication begins to exert its therapeutic effect, the side effects often diminish. In view of recent data regarding the recurrent nature of depression and how it impairs functioning over time, many clients are now taking these medications for years, or for an entire lifetime.

Mood stabilizers have been shown to be effective in treating mania in clients with bipolar disorders. The primary, most widely used mood stabilizer is lithium, although anticonvulsants (e.g., carbamazepine, valproate, lamotrigine, gabapentin) also appear to promote mood stabilization. Lithium acts as a salt within the body, and its blood levels are closely linked to the client's hydration and sodium intake. Side effects of lithium include neuromuscular and central nervous system effects (tremor, forgetfulness, slowed cognition), gastrointestinal effects (nausea, diarrhea), weight gain and hypothyroidism, and renal effects (polyuria). Blood lev-

CLINICAL ALERT

Serotonin syndrome is an idiosyncratic medication reaction with a fairly rapid onset that can occur with excessive accumulation of serotonin (5HT1A). In depressed clients, serotonin syndrome can result from high doses or concurrent use of such medications as serotonin reuptake inhibitors (including tricyclic antidepressants), serotonin precursors (e.g., L-tryptophan), serotonin agonists (e.g., buspirone), MAOIs, or other medications that influence serotonin levels (e.g., cold or allergy preparations, cocaine, lithium, ginseng, or St. John's Wort). Risk factors include genetic predisposition (MAO activity), acquired disorders (liver, pulmonary, or cardiovascular disease), or iatrogenic situation (medications). At least three of the following symptoms contribute to the diagnosis: mental status changes, agitation, myoclonus, hyperreflexia, fever, diaphoresis, ataxia, or diarrhea. Symptoms may also include abdominal pain, elevated blood pressure, tachycardia, irritability, hostility, increased motor activity, or mood change. Severe reactions may manifest as high fever, cardiovascular shock, or death. Early identification is important. The nurse will obtain a full history of all medications being taken (including over the counter); instruct patients and families to report immediately any subtle changes of confusion, unusual behavior, or agitation; and monitor vital signs carefully. If serotonin syndrome is suspected, the contributing agents should be discontinued and the physician notified.

CLINICAL ALERT

Foods containing tyramine must be avoided while taking MAOI antidepressants. These include avocados; yogurt; aged cheese; smoked or pickled fish, meat, or poultry; processed meats; yeast; overripe fruit; chicken or beef liver pate; red wine; beer; liqueurs; and fava beans. Foods to use in moderation include caffeine beverages, cottage and cream cheese, soy sauce, chocolate, and sour cream. *Medications* to avoid include over-the-counter cough and cold medicines, appetite suppressants, muscle relaxants, allergy remedies, hay fever remedies, narcotics, analgesics, and several prescription medications. The nurse should ask the client to contact the physician or nurse *before* taking any over-the-counter medication.

CLINICAL ALERT

Lithium toxicity is a potentially dangerous medication effect detailed in Chapter 20. The nurse should be aware that target blood levels for children are lower than levels for adults.

els are monitored to ensure an adequate, but not toxic, level. Usually, blood levels of 0.5 to 1 mEq/L are appropriate for maintenance therapy, whereas in the treatment of acute mania, levels of up to 1.5 mEq/L are required. The therapeutic-range blood level for lithium is narrow; toxicity can occur quickly and is marked by vomiting, oversedation, ataxia, and, finally, seizures. Lithium blood levels approaching 2 mEq/L are considered toxic. Lithium is excreted through the kidneys and should be used with caution in clients with renal disease. Clients taking lithium should use diuretics only with extreme caution and under close supervision, because diuretics can elevate lithium blood levels quickly.

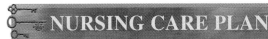

NURSING CARE PLAN

Maria is a 39-year-old Hispanic female who has lived in the United States for 3 years and whose primary language is Spanish. She is the mother of four children, ages 6 months, 3 years, 5 years, and 7 years. She had a difficult time after the birth of each child, including depressed mood, crying spells, weight loss, apathy, and difficulty concentrating. After her 3-year-old was born, Maria's husband, Juan, took her to their family physician who prescribed Prozac, 20 mg once a day. Maria was breastfeeding her baby and did not fill the prescription. Within a year, Maria felt better. Her current depressive episode began after the birth of her last child. Maria has been lying on the sofa, refusing most food, crying, and often unable to attend to her children, although she is still breastfeeding her infant. Maria appears disheveled and has a body odor. Maria's mother has moved into their home to care for the children. Juan has brought Maria to your clinic for a psychiatric evaluation after Maria told him she did not want to live anymore because she was a "bad mother." After her evaluation, Maria is brought to the inpatient unit.

DSM-IV-TR Diagnoses

Axis I	Major Depressive Disorder: With Postpartum Onset
Axis II	Deferred
Axis III	Recent childbirth
Axis IV	Parenting stress
Axis V	GAF = 30 (current)
	GAF = 70 (past year)

NURSING DIAGNOSIS: Risk for self-directed violence and risk for other-directed violence related to depressed mood (postpartum); depleted coping ability and skills; history of depression; stopped taking medications as evidenced by crying; refusing food; neglecting children; verbalizing not wanting to live; states that she is a "bad mother."

CLIENT OUTCOMES	NURSING INTERVENTIONS	EVALUATION
Maria will remain free of harm to self or children.	Conduct suicide and homicide risk assessments with Maria while hospitalized and initially at home. *Early comprehensive assessment of self-harm or assault risk may prevent harm or injury.*	Maria refrained from any attempt to harm self or children.
	Maintain safe hospital environment by removing dangerous objects and frequent observation. *Safety is the highest priority in client care.*	
Maria will agree to have other adults with her at all times while caring for her children.	Monitor family visits while Maria is hospitalized, and plan for monitoring if interactions with Maria and children until depression improves. *Reinforces client and family sense of security and maintains safety.*	Maria expressed feeling safer with the involvement of other adults.
Maria will contract to verbalize any suicidal or homicidal thoughts to either adult family members or professional health care providers.	Encourage Maria to verbalize all suicidal or homicidal thoughts to health care provider or to adult family member. Assist Maria to sign a contract to refrain from hurting self or others. *Outward verbal and written expression of intent to remain safe; reinforces client commitment to safety.*	Maria voiced and wrote commitment to safety and remained safe while saying she was anxious about her role as mother.
Maria will describe reasons for living and hopefulness about the future.	Encourage Maria to express feelings and thoughts. *Expression provides relief from pent-up feelings or guilt and assists her to problem solve.*	Maria to discuss her thoughts and feelings with nurses and family. She expressed relief that family still cared about her.
	Assist Maria to verbalize reasons for living. *Helps client focus on healthy aspects of her life.*	
Maria will use cognitive restructuring techniques to increase positive-thinking pattern.	Role play thought stopping and thought substitution techniques with Maria. *Cognitive restructuring techniques help client to change negative thought patterns.*	Maria used techniques and voiced relief when gaining control over thoughts and impulses.
Maria will take medications.	Describe benefits and action of medications to Maria and family. *Client compliance increases when they understand benefits of medications.*	Maria agreed to follow medication and bottle-feed the baby.
	Encourage family to assist Maria to take medication when at home. *Family involvement increases success of medication regimen.*	

NURSING CARE PLAN—cont'd

NURSING DIAGNOSIS: Ineffective coping related to depressed mood, inability to care for self and family as evidenced by lying on couch, refusing food, neglecting to bathe or provide for needs of family.

CLIENT OUTCOMES	NURSING INTERVENTIONS	EVALUATION
Maria will verbalize acceptance of professional help.	Assess cultural expectations and language barriers. *Barriers are blocks to compliance with program.*	Maria understood English and said she was a bad mother.
	Encourage Maria to verbalize her thoughts and feelings. *Expression provides relief and beginning of problem solving.*	Maria expressed concern over inability to take care of family and was beginning to welcome the assistance.
Maria will participate in therapeutic program.	Administer medications and monitor compliance. *Assistance by nurse reinforces importance of regimen.*	Day 1: Maria reluctantly took medications.
	Assist Maria to:	Day 10: Taking all medications, expressed feeling better.
	Establish realistic goals	Maria engaged in program slowly but willingly.
	Break down complex goals into small manageable steps	Maria attended group and was relieved to find other mothers that help each other.
	Do relaxation techniques	
	Identify and develop strengths	
	Discuss strategies to manage parenting responsibilities	
	Ask for help when needed	
	Techniques and strategies are tools that guide progress toward wellness.	
	Encourage Maria to attend postpartum support group. *Group provides affiliation, education, and empathy.*	

NURSING DIAGNOSIS: Self-care deficit related to depressed mood and fatigue secondary to major depression, as evidenced by disheveled appearance, body odor, and lack of attention to grooming.

CLIENT OUTCOMES	NURSING INTERVENTIONS	EVALUATION
Maria will bathe daily and dress herself in clean clothes.	Offer assistance until able to wash and dress on own. Provide articles to facilitate grooming (soap, shampoo, deodorant). *Clients frequently require help with grooming when severely depressed.*	Day 1: Maria required assistance with grooming. Day 5: Maria initiated own grooming in AM.
Maria will report adequate amount of sleep.	Discuss sleep hygiene strategies with client. *Use of simple methods promotes sleep (e.g., relaxation techniques, warm bath, warm milk before bedtime)*	Maria reported adequate sleep and appeared rested.

Other medications prescribed for clients during episodes of depression or mania may include benzodiazepines for associated anxiety symptoms, sedative-hypnotics for sleep regulation, and antipsychotics for relief from hallucinations, delusions, and extremely agitated behavior. Although antidepressants and mood stabilizers can assist with minimizing and regulating symptoms related to anxiety and sleep, their therapeutic effects take longer to occur than those of the other medications mentioned here.

Although medications are prescribed by physicians or advanced practice nurses, the nursing care related to administration of psychopharmacologic agents is extensive. The nurse needs to understand the mechanisms of action, dosages (therapeutic), side effects, and self-care considerations of each medication. This enables the nurse to explain the medication to clients and observe for intended and unintended effects. Through teaching clients more about their medications, the nurse promotes and encourages adherence to the treatment regimen and the minimization of negative effects. Clients are able to discuss their concerns and to make informed decisions about their treatments.

Many of these medications require special considerations that clients must understand to ensure efficacy and safety. Nurses teach clients specific self-care activities associated with medication, such as the required dietary restrictions for MAOIs, precautions regarding hydration and salt intake for lithium, and management of anticholinergic effects of the tricyclics. The Client and Family Teaching Guidelines boxes present teaching plans for clients taking SSRIs and lithium, respectively.

Serotonin Selective Reuptake Inhibitors

TEACH THE CLIENT:

The purpose of SSRIs is to treat depression. The medication alters brain nerve cells, thus increasing the availability of serotonin. A deficiency of serotonin in the brain is believed to be related to the onset of depression.

It is important to take the medication as prescribed; changing the dosage or missing a dose can prevent it from helping the depression.

Common side effects of SSRIs include nausea, increased anxiety, and insomnia. These side effects often diminish once the medication begins to exert its therapeutic effect.

Sexual side effects, including delayed ejaculation, impotence, or anorgasmia are not uncommon. You should discuss any such difficulties with your health care provider before making any medication changes on your own.

The medication usually does not immediately improve symptoms of depression. It may take 1 to 6 weeks before you feel the effects of the medication. At first, you may still feel depressed but have more energy and look less depressed. These medications often work "from the outside inward."

Biologic Intervention

Electroconvulsive Therapy. Electroconvulsive therapy (ECT) involves the use of electrically induced seizures to treat severe depression or, less frequently, intense mania not controlled with lithium or antipsychotics. Research has demonstrated it to be the most effective treatment for psychotic depression (Depression Guideline Panel, 1993). Although ECT was introduced in the 1930s, its use decreased after the discovery of antidepressants and lithium. In recent years procedures have been developed for ECT that make it a safe and effective treatment for many individuals who have not achieved a treatment response with medication or other types of treatment. The exact mechanism by which ECT alleviates depression and mania is unknown, but it is believed to be related to alteration of neurotransmission. A more complete discussion of ECT is presented in Chapter 19.

Transcranial Magnetic Stimulation. Transcranial magnetic stimulation is an intervention currently being investigated for its antidepressant effects. It is a noninvasive procedure in which an electromagnet is placed on the scalp. Electrical current is generated by rapid oscillations in the magnetic field, causing the cortical neurons to depolarize. Although the specific mechanisms involved in its antidepressant effect remain unclear, this intervention may increase monoamine concentrations in the brain when used repetitively. Initial research has been encouraging with respect to its effects with unipolar depression (George et al., 1997; George, Lisanby, and Sackeim, 1999).

Vagal Nerve Stimulation. Vagal nerve stimulation is a recent development for the treatment of depression. A device called the vagal nerve stimulator is implanted under the

Lithium

TEACH THE CLIENT:

Lithium is a mood stabilizer for persons with mania and depression.

Lithium alters brain neurotransmission, changes cell membrane function, and inhibits release of thyroid hormone. It is not clear how lithium specifically stabilizes mood.

Before lithium is started, laboratory tests are done to ensure adequate functioning of the heart, kidneys, thyroid gland, and electrolytes.

It is important to take lithium daily as prescribed to maintain a steady blood level of the medication. Do not take extra doses to make up for missed doses.

Lithium may take a week to begin working and to develop a steady blood level. Your health care provider will have you get your blood drawn to check lithium blood levels. Blood for the lithium level must be drawn about 12 hours after the last dose of lithium (e.g., if you take your dose at 8 PM, your blood level must be drawn at 8 AM).

Common side effects of lithium include increased urine output, increased thirst, fine tremors, muscle weakness, nausea, weight gain, and diarrhea.

Lithium levels can be increased rapidly, leading to toxicity. Signs of toxicity include nausea and vomiting, marked tremors, muscle weakness, muscle twitching, lack of coordination, sluggishness and drowsiness, confusion, seizures, and coma. Toxicity can occur as blood levels approach 2 mEq/L.

It is important to maintain a stable blood level of lithium. You should not change the amount of sodium (salt) in your diet, because decreasing salt may increase the amount of lithium in the blood.

Any activity or situation that can affect your fluid and salt intake or output can change the level of lithium in your blood. Exercise, sunbathing, and the flu are examples of situations in which you may perspire and lose salt and fluid, increasing your lithium level. It is important to contact your health care provider if you believe that your lithium level may be changed or if you experience any side effects or early toxic signs.

Other drugs can affect your lithium level. Medications (e.g., diuretics, ibuprofen, verapamil) can raise lithium levels. Be sure to check with your health care provider before taking any new prescribed or over-the-counter medications.

Lithium can cause birth defects if taken during the first trimester of pregnancy. Tell your health care provider if you intend to become pregnant or are pregnant.

collarbone and electrically stimulates the vagus nerve in the neck. Research is currently underway to determine the effectiveness of this treatment for major depressive disorder (Prater, 2001; Hammerly, 2001).

Phototherapy. Seasonal affective disorder (SAD) has been identified as a type of mood disorder, and its features are recognized in the DSM-IV-TR classification. Phototherapy is one type of treatment that has effectively lessened symptoms of this recurrent, seasonal disorder. The exact mechanism of action remains unclear, although it is believed that exposure to morning light causes a circadian rhythm shift (phase advance) that regulates the normal relationships between sleep and circadian rhythms.

NURSING CARE PLAN

Mark is a 43-year-old male who was diagnosed with bipolar disorder when he was 21 years old. Over the last 2 months Mark has been increasingly hyperactive, starting new projects every day such as painting the garage, setting up a mail order business, and writing songs he sends to Celine Dion. He is now sleeping only 2 hours a night and is unable to sit still for a full meal or even stand still to drink a beverage. Mark exhibits flight of ideas; his thoughts come quickly with minimal connection between them. His verbalization is difficult to follow. His insurance business is in financial trouble, and he has not been attending to his job. His wife left him 3 months ago, citing his irritability, angry outbursts, and lack of financial responsibility. Mark is distraught about the separation but has been cruising bars, picking up women, and having unprotected sex.

Mark's 22-year-old son brought him to the Emergency Department because he was concerned that his dad is increasingly unable to care for himself or his apartment.

DSM-IV-TR Diagnoses

Axis I	Bipolar I Disorder: Manic episode
Axis II	Deferred
Axis III	None
Axis IV	Marital stress due to recent separation from spouse, financial difficulty due to neglect of business
Axis V	GAF = 25 (current)
	GAF = 65 (past year)

NURSING DIAGNOSIS: Disturbed thought processes related to neurobiologic alterations, ineffective processing and synthesis of stimuli, multiple psychosocial stressors, secondary to bipolar mania as evidenced by flight of ideas, grandiosity, starting multiple simultaneous projects and unable to complete tasks, poor judgment.

CLIENT OUTCOMES	NURSING INTERVENTIONS	EVALUATION
Mark will communicate using logical and appropriate language and control of speech (rate, tone, amount).	Actively listen and calmly respond to Mark. *Signifies respect for client and encourages him to express concerns in interactive process.*	Day 1: Mark's speech was rapid, pressured, and demanding.
	Demonstrate appropriate role modeling. *Helps to promote change by examples.*	Day 3: Mark quietly and appropriately communicated with clients and staff.
Mark will refrain from being intrusive and grandiose.	Encourage Mark to think before interrupting. *Assists client to curb impulsivity.*	Mark responded to staff approach by controlling outbursts and speaking appropriately by the end of the second day.
	Redirect behaviors in calm, firm, nondefensive manner by suggesting a walk, physical activity. *Provides healthy channel for excess energy and prevents escalation of behavior.*	Mark used suggestions for engaging in activities and demonstrated control by second day.
	Praise client for all attempts to use socially appropriate language and behaviors. *Provides positive feedback, promotes expected behaviors, increases self esteem.*	Mark apologized for being out of control and thanked staff for helping him maintain his behavior.
Mark will demonstrate accurate interpretation of self and environment.	Assist Mark to correct misinterpretations using problem solving and recalling actual events. *Encourages client's reality orientation.*	Day 1: Mark continued to express grandiose delusions.
	Convey acceptance of need to hold onto false beliefs while not agreeing with delusions. *Builds trust and maintains client's dignity.*	Day 3: Mark engages staff in discussions about his thinking and is increasingly logical.
	Tell Mark to notify staff when troubling thoughts occur. *Helps keep client to break illogical thought patterns. Assistance from staff reinforces client's efforts.*	Day 5: Absence of delusional thinking. Mark engage in milieu activities.
	Encourage Mark to stay involved in the milieu and real events. *Reinforces reality.*	
Mark will participate in treatment plan.	Administer mood stabilizing medications and monitor symptoms. *Maintenance of effective medication regime helps to reduce manic symptoms.*	Day 1: Mark reluctantly took medications stating he "didn't need anything but himself."
	Encourage Mark to attend scheduled activities and groups.	Day 3: Mark displays calmer speech and behavior.
	Engage family in client's care. *Family awareness of client's problems results in more effective responses and interactions.*	Day 1: Mark stated he didn't need any help.
		Day 5: Mark attended all groups, stating logical goal and directed thoughts.

Clients are referred for phototherapy after a careful and complete psychiatric history that documents the occurrence of SAD. Phototherapy consisting of a minimum of 2500 lux is usually administered on waking in the morning. Clients sit or lie in front of the light box for 30 minutes to several hours, depending on the strength of the light source. An antidepressant effect is usually seen within 2 to 4 days and is complete after 2 weeks. Maintenance therapy consists of sitting in front of the lights for about 30 minutes each day. Side effects are rare, although some clients do report irritability, headaches, or insomnia. Phototherapy is not effective for everyone with a diagnosis of SAD; some fail to respond, and others experience only a partial response. Because phototherapy requires a large amount of time each day, research is in progress that examines alternative methods to acquire the additional light, including the use of light visors and lights that shine onto the bed in early morning before awakening (Hammerly, 2001).

Alternative and Complementary Therapies

Natural and alternative remedies for illness have become popular. Persons frequently turn to health food stores for vitamins and supplements, yet there is minimal evidence about the effects of these products on depression and mania. St. John's Wort, believed to change serotonin levels, has been heralded for its antidepressant effects. Research has not consistently supported this result. In fact, St. John's Wort is not recommended for severe depression or bipolar disorder and may cause serotonin syndrome when taken with other medications that increase serotonin levels (Hammerly, 2001). SAMe (S-adenosylmethionine) may also be a natural antidepressant, making brain cells more responsive to neurotransmitters and showing clinical effectiveness in alleviating postpartum depression. However, SAMe may trigger manic episodes in individuals with bipolar disorder (Hammerly, 2001; Murray, 2002). Fish oils, also known as omega-3 fatty acids, do appear to affect health, including alleviating depressive symptoms and promoting cardiovascular health (Murray, 2002). Much more research must be done on the effectiveness, long-term effects, and drug interactions of these natural supplements. Because these substances are available over the counter as food products rather than medications, concern also exists about quality control in their preparation, purity, and dosing accuracy. It is important that nurses ask clients about their use of such products, as natural supplements may interact with prescribed medications and influence medication response.

Family Intervention

Mood disorders affect the entire family, not just the client who is experiencing the depression or mania. Most often the family or significant others become known to the nurse during the client's acute episode of depression or mania. Conflicts and communication problems, which may have existed in the family network before the onset of the episode, become intensified, and the usual role functioning is disrupted.

Nurses in both the hospital and community interact with the client's family, who often appreciate the opportunity to vent feelings of confusion, anger, concern, or frustration. Teaching family members about the client's disorder, especially the biologic nature of the disorder, allows them to reframe the situation and minimize blame on the client. Many are relieved to hear that their loved one's behavior has an explanation and can be managed. They also find it helpful to know that the client's behavior (e.g., irritability, inability to accept love, and negativity) is not a personal affront to other family members but may be part of the symptomatology of depression or mania. Nurses run family education groups in the hospital and in the community, inviting family and clients to learn more about the disorder and its impact on the family.

Nurses also collaborate with other mental health professionals, including advanced practice nurses, regarding assessing the need for family therapy. Nurses observe client-family interactions, listen to their concerns, and identify potential problem areas. Referrals are made for marital therapy or family therapy that also includes the children.

Interventions that include preparing the family for a client's discharge from the hospital can facilitate the client's return to functioning in the community. Data suggest that even after abatement of symptoms, the client who has experienced affective episodes continues to have difficulty in his or her interpersonal and occupational functioning (Klerman and Weissman, 1992; Greden, 2001).

Group Intervention

Group intervention can provide multiple benefits to clients with mood disorders, including socialization, education about their disorder and more useful coping mechanisms, the opportunity to vent feelings, the establishment of personal goals, and the realization that others have similar problems, thus reducing isolation and hopelessness. Nurses assess clients' ability to participate in groups based on their behavior, mental status, psychologic readiness in view of the nature of the particular group, and physiologic status. For example, clients with mania who are hyperactive and extremely agitated are not able to attend to the group discussion and may become overstimulated and disruptive in the group. Clients with severe depression with psychomotor retardation and cognitive impairment may have a difficult time and become overwhelmed by a formal group. Certain types of groups (e.g., a unit community meeting or activities groups) may be less structured and less imposing to clients than formal group therapy.

In addition to assessing clients' readiness for groups, nurses encourage their attendance at the appropriate functions. Some clients may need to be directed with statements such as, "It's time for group now. I'll walk there with you." Others require only encouragement or reminders.

Nurses who are qualified may conduct groups in conjunction with other nurses or therapists. Nurses may initiate and lead groups such as social skills training and educational groups. Clients often need to debrief or discuss their experiences and reactions after the completion of a group. Nurses listen, allow ventilation of feelings, and reinforce new insights or perceptions experienced by the clients.

Psychotherapeutic Intervention

Although the effectiveness of antidepressant and mood-stabilizing medications is undisputed, psychotherapeutic interventions are also important in the treatment of mood disorders. Psychopharmacologic agents pose a number of problems for many clients. These medications have major side effects that create discomfort, interfere with usual functioning, and promote noncompliance. Alternative treatment is required for the 20% to 30% of persons with mood disorders who do not respond to medications. Also, although mood disorders represent alterations in neurobiologic functioning, numerous psychologic, social, and interpersonal issues that warrant psychotherapeutic intervention are associated with episodes of depression and mania.

Types of psychotherapy that have been used to treat mood disorders and associated psychosocial issues include cognitive therapy, behavioral therapy, interpersonal relationship therapy, and psychodynamic therapy. Although each of these differs with respect to the underlying theoretic framework, goals, and approach, there are some commonalities. Therapeutic success is related to several factors: the nature of the relationship between the therapist and client; the provision of understanding, support, help, and hope; the establishment of a framework for understanding and interpreting clients' problems; and the provision of an opportunity to explore and try out new coping strategies.

Cognitive Therapy. Cognitive therapy, as outlined by Beck (1967), addresses systematic errors in the client's thinking that maintain negative cognitive processing. The goal of the therapy is to identify underlying cognitive schemata and specific cognitive distortions. Schemata are internal models of the self and the world that individuals use to perceive, code, and recall information. Clients are asked to identify their automatic thoughts, silent assumptions, and arbitrary inferences so that negative thoughts and assumptions can be examined logically, challenged against realistic attributes, and subsequently validated or refuted.

Cognitive therapy has been shown to be effective in treating outpatients with unipolar mild to moderate depression. In studies that have investigated the effectiveness of medication versus cognitive therapy, findings indicate that both appear to be equally effective for outpatients with depression and may provide some modest gain when used in com-

bination (Gloaguen et al., 1998; Scott, 1996). In addition, use of cognitive therapy also may increase the rate of symptom improvement in depression, although longer term follow-up studies fail to find differences over time. The use of cognitive therapy with inpatients experiencing severe depression has not been extensively explored, although there are indications that it may be useful for symptom reduction (Stravynski and Greenberg, 1992; Hollon, Haman, and Brown, 2002).

Behavioral Therapy. Behavioral therapy, often used in conjunction with cognitive therapy for treating mild to moderately depressed outpatients, is an effective treatment for depression, comparing favorably with medication and cognitive therapy (Stravynski and Greenberg, 1992). There is less information about its usefulness with persons experiencing mania (Freeman et al., 1990).

The behavioral approach is based on learning theory. Abnormal behaviors such as the symptoms of depression and mania represent behaviors acquired as a result of aversive (negative) environmental events. These are reinforced by positive environmental responses to the maladaptive behaviors or by avoidance of negative consequences. The behavioral therapist works with clients to determine specific behaviors to be modified and to identify the factors that evoke and reinforce these behaviors. Using role modeling, role playing, and situational analysis, clients are assisted in learning and practicing different adaptive behaviors that elicit positive environmental reinforcement. The therapy is not concerned with understanding underlying issues or pathopsychology; it is concerned only with those discrete behaviors that can be modified. Behavioral therapy has several advantages (e.g., shorter treatment duration than other types of therapy, focus on specific behaviors that can be modified) and is applicable to various types of clients.

Interpersonal Therapy. The therapist using interpersonal therapy views depression as developing from pathologic, early interpersonal relationship patterns that continue to be repeated in adulthood. The emphasis is on social functioning and interpersonal relationships, with particular emphasis on the milieu. Life events, including change, loss, and relationship conflict, trigger earlier relationship patterns; and the client experiences a sense of failure, decreased importance, and loss. The goal of the therapy is to understand the social context of current problems based on earlier relationships and to provide symptomatic relief by solving or managing current interpersonal problems. The client and therapist select one or two current interpersonal problems and examine new communication and interpersonal strategies for more effective management of relationships.

Interpersonal therapy has been shown to be effective for clients with mild to moderate depression, although not more so than other types of psychotherapy. Some research suggests that when used in combination with medications, interpersonal therapy may help clients adhere to medication treatment and may lengthen the time between the recovery period and recurrence of a major depression episode (Frank et al., 1991; Klerman, 1990).

Psychodynamic Therapy. Psychodynamic therapy is derived from Freud's psychoanalytic model (see Chapter 19). Depression is viewed as a result of early childhood loss of a love object and ambivalence about the object; introjection of anger onto the ego, resulting in blockage of the libido; and unresolved intrapsychic conflict during the oral or anal stage of psychosexual development. Thus self-esteem is damaged and eroded, with repetition of the primary loss pattern occurring throughout life. Through the relationship with the therapist, the client is helped to uncover repressed experiences, experience catharsis of feelings, confront defenses, interpret current behavior, and work through early loss and cravings for love.

There has been little research on the effect of psychodynamic psychotherapy on depression or mania. Techniques used in this therapy have been modified over time, and there have been problems with standardizing the approach for research purposes. For some clients psychodynamic psychotherapy assists in developing insights that promote behavioral change. However, many clients, including those with severe depression, may be unable or unmotivated to participate in this type of therapy. For these clients problems such as self-care deficits, psychomotor retardation, and fatigue assume priority.

Self-Management Intervention

In the current health care environment with fewer financial resources and difficulty with access to health care, more and more clients must fend by self-managing their chronic illnesses. Self-management approaches for chronic illnesses such as asthma and cardiac disease have resulted in reduced health care costs and improved longer term health outcomes (Lorig et al., 1999; Clark, Gong, and Kaciroti, 2001). There is little documentation of specific interventions to teach and assist clients and their families to better manage their mood disorder on an on-going, daily basis. Related research has shown that depression management and relapse prevention strategies, including extra visits with a depression specialist and telephone follow-up calls, result in greater adherence to antidepressant medication and fewer depressive symptoms (Katon, et al., 2001). Pollack (1996) described the ways in which persons with bipolar disorder self-manage their illness and noted that professionals need to better understand these strategies to assist clients in using them and preventing relapse.

Nurses have a major role in educating clients with mood disorders about their illness and assisting them to develop strategies for on-going management of the disorder and its impact on their lives. Clients can be taught self-management

UNDERSTANDING and APPLYING RESEARCH

Hagerty, Williams, and Liken (1997) conducted a qualitative study to determine clients' experiences with onset of symptoms in recurrent depression. They conducted four focus groups with 16 persons who had at least three well-documented episodes of major depression. The focus groups were audiotaped and videotaped, and results were transcribed for analysis. Using phenomenologic analysis, the researchers identified themes embedded in the focus group content. Results showed that participants experienced distinct phases as they were entering a recurrent episode of depression. These phases were termed, "Something's not right," "Something's really wrong," "the Crash," and "Connection." Participants reported that sometimes these phases occurred over a short period of time (days), whereas sometimes they were more insidious. Participants agreed that once they experienced "the crash," descending into the acute depressive episode, it was too late to initiate activities that could prevent the episode. All participants reported a "prodromal" phase of symptom onset in which specific signs and symptoms in patterns unique to them occurred. Many of these early signs and symptoms were different than those listed as DSM criteria for diagnosing depression. Based on study results, the researchers posited that persons with recurrent depression often did have a prodromal phase in which early signs and symptoms could be identified; clients could learn to monitor for and recognize these early signs, make judgments about their depression, and initiate strategies to prevent or minimize the oncoming episodes.

Hagerty BM, Williams RA, Liken M: Prodromal symptoms of recurrent major depressive episodes: a qualitative analysis, *Am J Orthopsychiatry* 67:308, 1997.

strategies such as identifying prodromal symptoms of recurrence (see Understanding and Applying Research box), problem solving about potential options for intervention, and building a repertoire of self-management strategies that can be used during times of increased stress and potential recurrence.

EVALUATION

Nurses evaluate clients' progress by measuring their achievement of identified outcomes. Data that support or refute achievement of outcomes are collected from personal observations, clients, clients' family and friends, and other health care providers. Evaluation occurs throughout hospitalization and may be continued by community mental health providers after clients have been discharged. Nurses working in community settings, such as psychiatric home care, may be evaluating outcomes for clients who have never been admitted to an inpatient setting.

With decreasing lengths of stay in hospitals, nurses in inpatient psychiatric units may not see dramatic changes in clients' symptoms. However, they must see some clear progress related to priority short-term outcomes such as absence of imminent suicidal intent, a plan for addressing the potential return of suicidal ideation after discharge, the ability to conduct self-care activities, some alleviation of the neurovegetative symptoms of depression (sleep, loss of appetite, fatigue, psychomotor retardation), alleviation of the severe hyperactive behavior of mania, improvement in cognitive functioning and communication, and initial understanding of the disorder and its treatment, including necessary self-care management. Referrals are made to therapists, psychiatrists, home care and community mental health agencies, and partial hospitalization programs for continued care in the community.

Nurses working with clients in the community see improvement in longer term outcomes such as improved socialization, return to usual activities, reduction in negative thinking, increased self-esteem, use of new coping strategies, resumption of family/work roles, continued improvement in cognitive processes (e.g., attention and concentration), decreased or absence of fatigue, and adherence to regimens. For some clients, these outcomes become evident within weeks of starting psychotherapy or somatic treatment regimens. For others, improvement may require months before longer term outcomes are achieved. Data suggest that return to previous levels of functioning after an episode of depression takes longer than previously thought, particularly if clients have had multiple episodes (Klerman and Weissman, 1992; Greden, 2001).

Clients with mania present a unique evaluative situation, because episodes of mania may be followed by episodes of depression. Therefore, although clients may have returned to a hypomanic or euthymic state at the time of hospital discharge, the nurse should be alert to any indications of depression. Careful follow-up monitoring after discharge into the community is imperative for clients with bipolar disorders.

CHAPTER SUMMARY

- Mood disorders are a major public health problem, and depression has been identified as the fourth leading cause of "burden," including morbidity and mortality, in the world.
- Major depression is currently occurring at younger ages, and those most at risk are women with a family history of mood disorders.
- Mood disorders are usually recurrent and require lifelong management. Manifestations and treatment concerns may vary across the life span.
- Two broad types of mood disorders include unipolar depressive and bipolar disorders.
- Mood disorders are explained by multiple theories, including biologic, ethologic, cognitive, psychodynamic, and personality theories. Theories for etiology of mood disorders are multiple, including a genetic, biologic predisposition for risk.
- Mania and depression are manifested by symptoms involving the affective, cognitive, physical, social, and spiritual aspects of the individual.
- The occurrence of mania and depression is not limited to psychiatric units.
- Comorbidity between medical and mood disorders is high.

- The nursing care of persons experiencing depression or mania consists of thorough assessment and subsequent planning and interventions for an array of nursing diagnoses related to physical, psychosocial, and spiritual needs.
- Nurses collaborate with other mental health care providers for care related to somatic, family, and group interventions.

REVIEW QUESTIONS

1. To assess for symptoms of depression the nurse will ask the client:
   a. "Do you believe you have special powers?"
   b. "You look really sad right now. Have you ever thought of harming yourself?"
   c. "Your husband states you never stop and that you have so much energy. How many hours of sleep do you average each night?"
   d. "Do you ever lose lapses of time when you can't remember where you've been or what you've done?"

2. A 43-year-old female client was admitted to the psychiatric unit 1 week ago for depressed mood with suicidal ideation. Which response from the client reflects an improvement in her depression?
   a. "I'm still having trouble sleeping."
   b. "I don't feel up to going to group therapy today."
   c. "I'm thinking about going back to school."
   d. "I don't deserve to have my husband."

3. The client who was admitted to the psychiatric unit 3 days before is exhibiting increased restlessness and hyperverbal speech and is wearing excessive make-up and multicolored clothes. The night shift staff has reported that the client sleeps 2 hours per night. The psychiatric nurse's intervention will be:
   a. Explain to the client the proper way to apply make-up.
   b. Continue to monitor her sleeping patterns.
   c. Discourage her from attending groups because her behavior may be disruptive.
   d. Discuss with the attending physician the need to obtain a lithium level because the client may be "cheeking" her lithium.

4. A 30-year-old client diagnosed with bipolar disorder is preparing for discharge. A priority nursing intervention is:
   a. Teach the importance of medication compliance, including regular blood draws or lithium levels.
   b. Teach relaxation techniques.
   c. Teach anger management techniques.
   d. Explain the psychologic testing process.

5. A 19-year-old male was admitted to the psychiatric unit with major depression and suicidal ideation. He had a his-

tory of attempted suicide by cutting his wrists 3 years ago. For the first 2 days of hospitalization the client ate 20% to 30% of his meals, stayed in his room in between groups, and refused to participate in groups. On the fourth day of admission, the nurse observed that the client was more sociable with peers, eating his meals and exhibiting a bright affect. The nurse must consider that the client:

a. Is showing improvement and may be ready for discharge.
b. Has decided to commit suicide and the nurse must place him on suicide precautions.
c. Is feeling rested and less depressed.
d. Is benefiting from the antidepressant he's been taking for the past 3 days.

REFERENCES

Abramson LY, Metalsky GI, Alloy LB: Hopelessness depression: a theory-based type of depression, *Psychol Rev* 93:358, 1989.

Abramson LY, Seligman MEP, Teasdale JD: Learned helplessness in humans: critique and reformulation, *Abnorm Psychol* 87:49, 1978.

Ackley BJ, Ladwig GB: *Nursing diagnosis handbook. A guide to planning care,* ed 5, Philadelphia, 2002, Mosby.

Akiskal HS: New insights into the nature and heterogeneity of mood disorders, *J Clin Psychiatry* 50:6, 1989.

Alexopoulos GS et al: Clinical presentation of the "depression-executive dysfunction syndrome" of late life, *Am J Geriatric Psychiatry* 10:98, 2002.

American Psychiatric Association: *Diagnostic and Statistical Manual of Mental Disorders,* Fourth Edition, Text Revision. Washington, DC, American Psychiatric Association, 2000.

Angelino AF, Treisman GJ: Management of psychiatric disorders in patients infected with human immunodeficiency virus, *Clin Infect Dis* 33:847, 2001.

Angst J: Clinical course of affective disorders. In Helgason T, Daly R, editors: *Depressive illness: prediction of course and outcome,* Berlin, Germany, 1988, Springer-Verlag.

Barondes S: *Mood genes: hunting for the origins of mania and depression,* New York, 1998, WH Freeman.

Beck AT: *Depression: clinical, experiential, and theoretical aspects,* New York, 1967, Hober.

Beekman AT et al: The natural history of late-life depression: a 6-year prospective study in the community, *Arch Gen Psychiatry* 59:605, 2002.

Bohachick P et al: Social support, personal control, and psychosocial recovery following heart transplantation, *Clin Nurs Res* 11:34, 2002.

Bowlby J: *Attachment and loss.* vol. 1: *Attachment,* New York, 1969, Basic Books.

Brown GW, Harris T: *Social origins of depression,* New York, 1978, The Free Press.

Chemerinski E, Robinson RG, Kosier JT: Improved recovery in activities of daily living associated with remission of poststroke depression, *Stroke* 32:113, 2001.

Clark NM, Gong M, Kaciroti N: A model of self-regulation for control of chronic disease, *Health Educ Behav* 24:28, 2001.

Consensus Development Panel: Mood disorders: pharmacological prevention of recurrences, *Am J Psychiatry* 142:469, 1985.

Corruble E et al: Early and delayed personality changes associated with depression recover: a one-year follow-up study, *Psychiatr Res* 109:17, 2002.

Cosmides L, Tooby J: *Evolutionary psychology: a primer,* Retrieved September 13, 2002, from University of California Santa Barbara, Center for Evolutionary Psychology website: www.psych.ucsb.edu/research/cep/primer.html, 2002.

Crone CC, Wise TN: Psychiatric aspects of transplantation, II. Preoperative issues, *Crit Care Nurse* 19:51, 1999.

Department of Health and Human Services: *Mental health: a report of the Surgeon General,* Rockville, Md, 1999, Department of Health and Human Resources.

Depression Guideline Panel: *Depression in primary care,* vol 1, *Detection and diagnosis,* Washington, DC, 1993, U.S. Department of Health and Human Services, Agency for Health Care Policy and Research.

Dolan-Sewell RT, Krueger RF, Shea MT: Co-occurrence with syndrome disorders. In Livesley, WJ, editor: *Handbook of personality disorders. Theory, research, and treatment,* New York, 2001, Guilford Press.

Fergusson DM, Woodward LJ: Mental health, educational, and social role outcomes of adolescents with depression, *Arch Gen Psychiatry* 59:225, 2002.

Fortinash K, Holoday Worret P: *Psychiatric nursing care plans,* ed 4, St Louis, 2003, Mosby.

Frank E et al: Efficacy of interpersonal psychotherapy as a maintenance treatment of recurrent depression, *Arch Gen Psychiatry* 48:1053, 1991.

Frazer A: Norepinephrine involvement in antidepressant action, *J Clin Psychiatry* 61(Suppl 10):25, 2000.

Freeman A et al: *Clinical applications of cognitive therapy,* New York, 1990, Plenum Press.

Freud S: Mourning and melancholia. In *The complete psychological works of Sigmund Freud,* London, 1957, Hogarth Press.

Gagnon LM, Patten SB: Major depression and its association with long-term medical conditions, *Can J Psychiatry* 47:149, 2002.

George MS et al: Mood improvement following daily left prefrontal repetitive transcranial magnetic stimulation in patients with depression: a placebo-controlled crossover trial, *Am J Psychiatry* 154:1752, 1997.

George MS, Lisanby SH, Sackeim HA: Transcranial magnetic stimulation: applications in neuropsychiatry, *Arch Gen Psychiatry* 56:300, 1999.

Gloaguen V et al: A meta-analysis of the effects of cognitive therapy in depressed patients, *J Affect Disord* 49:59, 1998.

Goodman SH: Depression and early adverse experiences. In Gotlib IH, Hammen CL, editors: *Handbook of depression,* New York, 2002, Guilford Press.

Greden JF: *Recurrent depression,* Washington, DC, 2001, American Psychiatric Publishing.

Gupta A, Bhatia S: Depression in Parkinson's disease, *Clin Gerontol* 22:59, 2000.

Hagerty BM, Williams RA, Liken S: Prodromal symptoms of recurrent major depressive episodes: a qualitative analysis, *Am J Orthopsychiatry* 67:308, 1997.

Hammerly M: *Depression. How to combine the best of traditional and alternative therapies,* Avon, Mass, 2001, Adams Media.

Hankin BL, Abramson LY: Development of gender differences in depression: an elaborated cognitive vulnerability-transactional stress theory, *Psychol Bull* 127:773, 2001.

Hirschfeld RMA et al: The National Depressive and Manic-Depressive Association consensus statement on the undertreatment of depression, *JAMA* 277:333, 1997.

Hirshfeld-Becker DR et al: Temperamental correlates of disruptive behavior disorders in young children: preliminary findings, *Biol Psychiatry* 51:563, 2002.

Hollon SD, Haman KL, Brown LL: Cognitive-behavioral treatment of depression. In Gotlib IH, Hammen CL, editors: *Handbook of depression,* New York, 2002, Guilford Press.

Horwath E et al: Depressive symptoms as relative and attributable risk factors for first onset major depression, *Arch Gen Psychiatry* 49:817, 1992.

Johnson JG et al: Hopelessness as a mediator of the association between social support and depressive symptoms. Findings of a study of men with HIV, *J Consult Clin Psychol* 69:1056, 2001.

Joiner TE et al: Hopelessness depression as a distinct dimension of depressive symptoms among clinical and non-clinical samples, *Behav Res Ther* 39:523, 2001.

Jorm AF: History of depression as a risk factor for dementia: an updated review, *Aust N Z J Psychiatry* 35:776, 2001.

Just N, Abramson LY, Alloy LB: Remitted depression studies as tests of the cognitive vulnerability hypotheses of depression onset: a critique and conceptual analysis, *Clin Psychol Rev* 21:63, 2001.

Katon W et al: A randomized trial of relapse prevention of depression in primary care, *Arch Gen Psychiatry* 58:241, 2001.

Keller MB: The course of manic-depressive illness, *Clin Psychiatry* 49:4, 1988.

Kendler KS: Twin studies of psychiatric illness: an update, *Arch Gen Psychiatry* 58:1005, 2001.

Kendler KS et al: The identification and validation of distinct depressive syndromes in a population-based sample of female twins, *Arch Gen Psychiatry* 53:391, 1996.

Kendler KS, Karkowski LM, Prescott CA: Causal relationship between stressful life events and the onset of major depression, *Am J Psychiatry* 156:837, 1999.

Kendler KS, Thornton LM, Gardner CO: Stressful life events and previous episodes in the etiology of major depression in women: an evaluation of the "kindling" hypothesis, *Am J Psychiatry* 157:1243, 2000.

Kendler KS, Thornton LM, Prescott CA: Gender differences in the rates of exposure to stressful life events and sensitivity to their depressogenic effects, *Am J Psychiatry* 158:587, 2001.

Kessler RC et al: Lifetime and 12-month prevalence of DSM-IIIR psychiatric disorders in the U.S., *Arch Gen Psychiatry* 51:8, 1994.

Klerman GL: Treatment of recurrent unipolar major depressive disorder, *Arch Gen Psychiatry* 47:1158-1162, 1990.

Klerman GL, Weissman MM: The course, morbidity, and costs of depression, *Arch Gen Psychiatry* 49:831, 1992.

Kraepelin E: *Lectures in clinical psychiatry,* London, 1913, Baillière, Tindall, & Cox.

Kraepelin E: *Manic-depressive insanity and paranoia,* Edinburgh, UK, 1921, E&S Livingstone.

Lavoie KL, Fleet RP: The impact of depression on the course and outcome of coronary artery disease: review for cardiologists, *Can J Cardiol* 16:653, 2000.

Lenze EJ et al: Combined pharmacotherapy and psychotherapy as maintenance treatment for late-life depression: effects on social adjustment, *Am J Psychiatry* 159:466, 2002.

Leonhard K: Aufteilung der endogenen Psychosen. Cited in Buher J: *Depression: theory and research,* New York, 1974, Winston Wiley.

Lewinsohn PM et al: Age cohort changes in the lifetime occurrence of depression and other mental disorders, *J Abnorm Psychiatry* 102:110, 1993.

Lorig KR et al: Evidence suggesting that a chronic disease self-management program can improve health status while reducing hospitalization, *Med Care* 37:5, 1999.

Luty SE et al: The interpersonal sensitivity measure in depression: associations with temperament and character, *J Affect Disord* 70:307, 2002.

Malkoff-Schwartz S et al: Social rhythm disruption and stressful life events in the onset of bipolar and unipolar episodes, *Psychol Med* 30:1005, 2000.

Marijnissen G et al: The temperament and character inventory in major depression, *J Affect Disord* 70:219, 2002.

McGriffin P, Katz R: The genetics of depression: current approaches, *Br J Psychiatry* 155:18, 1989.

Mulder RT: Personality pathology and treatment outcome in major depression: a review, *Am J Psychiatry* 159:359, 2002.

Murr C, Ledochowski M, Fuchs D: Chronic immune stimulation may link ischemic heart disease with depression, *Circulation* 105:83, 2002.

Murray CJL, Lopez AD: *The global burden of disease: a comprehensive assessment of mortality and disability from diseases, injuries, and risk factors in 1990 and projected,* Boston, 1996, Harvard University Press.

Murray M: *The pill book guide to natural medicines,* New York, 2002, Bantam.

Nesse RM: Evolutionary biology: a basic science for psychiatry, *World Psychiatry* 1:7, 2002.

Nolen-Hoeksema S: Sex differences in unipolar women: evidence and theory, *Psychol Bull* 101(2):259, 1987.

Nolen-Hoeksema S: The role of rumination in depressive disorders and mixed anxiety/depressive symptoms, *J Abnorm Psychol* 109:504, 2000.

Olin JT et al: Provisional diagnostic criteria for depression of Alzheimer disease: rationale and background, *Am J Geriatr Psychiatry* 10:129, 2002.

Parker G, Roy K: Adolescent depression: a review, *Austr N Z J Psychiatry* 35:572, 2001.

Pollack LE: Inpatient self-management of bipolar disorder, *Appl Nurs Res* 9:71, 1996.

Post RM: Transduction of psychosocial stress in the neurobiology of recurrent affective disorders, *Am J Psychiatry* 149:999, 1992.

Post RM: Molecular biology of behavior, *Arch Gen Psychiatry* 54:607, 1997.

Prater JF: Recurrent depression with vagus nerve stimulation, *Am J Psychiatry* 158:816, 2001.

Provinciali L, Coccia M: Post-stroke and vascular depression: a critical review, *Neuro Sci* 22:417, 2002.

Ravindran AV et al: Stress, coping, uplifts, and quality of life in subtypes of depression: a conceptual frame and emerging data, *J Affect Disord* 71:121, 2002.

Regenold WT et al: Increased prevalence of type 2 diabetes mellitus among psychiatric inpatients with bipolar I affective and schizoaffective disorders independent of psychotropic drug use, *J Affect Disord* 70:19, 2002.

Renshaw PF, Rauch SL: Neuroimaging in clinical psychiatry. In Nicholi AM, editor: *The Harvard guide to psychiatry,* Cambridge, Mass, 1999, Belknap Press.

Righette-Veltema M et al: Postpartum depression and mother-infant relationship at 3 months old, *J Affect Disord* 70:291, 2002.

Robins CJ, Hayes AM: An appraisal of cognitive therapy, *J Consult Clin Psychol* 61:205, 1993.

Rossi A et al: Personality disorders in bipolar and depressive disorders, *J Affect Disord* 65:3, 2001.

Sapolsky RM: Glucocorticoids and hippocampal atrophy in neuropsychiatric disorders, *Arch Gen Psychiatry* 57:925, 2000.

Schmaling K, Becker J: Empirical studies of the interpersonal relations of adult depressives. In Becker J, Kleinman D, editors: *Psychosocial aspects of depression,* Hillsdale, NJ, 1991, Lawrence Erlbaum.

Scott J: Cognitive therapy of affective disorders: a review, *J Affect Disord* 37:1, 1996.

Seligman MEP: *Helplessness: on depression development and death,* New York, 1975, WH Freeman.

Sexson SB, Glanville DN, Kaslow NJ: Attachment and depression: implications for family therapy, *Child Adolesc Psychiatr Clin N Am* 10:465, 2001.

Sharma P et al: Depression among hospitalized medically ill patients: a two-stage screening study, *J Affect Disord* 70:205, 2002.

Slaughter JR et al: Prevalence, clinical manifestations, etiology, and treatment of depression in Parkinson's disease, *J Neuropsychiatry Clin Neurosci* 13:187, 2001.

St. Dennis C, Synoground G: Pharmacology update. Medications for early onset bipolar illness: new drug update, *Image J Nurs Schol* 14:29, 1998.

Steffens DC et al: Sociodemographic and clinical predictors of mortality in geriatric depression, *Am J Geriatr Psychiatry* 10:531, 2002.

Stein MB, Barrett-Connor E: Quality of life in older adults receiving medications for anxiety, depression, or insomnia: findings from a community-based study, *Am J Geriatr Psychiatry* 10:568, 2002.

Stravynski A, Greenberg D: The psychological management of depression, *Acta Psychiatr Scand* 85:407, 1992.

Strik JJM et al: Clinical correlates of depression following myocardial infarction, *Int J Psychiatry Med* 31:255, 2001.

Struder HK, Weicker H: Physiology and pathophysiology of the serotonin system and its implications on mental and physical performance. Part I, *Int J Sports Med* 22:467, 2001.

Sullivan PF, Neale MC, Kendler KS: Genetic epidemiology of major depression: review and meta-analysis, *Am J Psychiatry* 157:1552, 2000.

Tateno A, Kimura M, Robinson RG: Phenomenological characteristics of poststroke depression, *Am J Geriatr Psychiatry* 10:575, 2002.

Travis LA, Lyness JM: Minor depression: diagnosis and management in primary care, *Geriatrics* 57:65, 2002.

Van den Berg MD et al: Depression in later life: three etiologically different subgroups, *J Affect Disord* 65:19, 2001.

Viinamaki H et al: Cluster C personality disorder impedes alleviation of symptoms of major depression, *J Affect Disord* 71:35, 2002.

Watson PJ, Andrews PW: Toward a revised evolutionary adaptationist analysis of depression: the social navigation hypothesis, *J Affect Disord* 72:1, 2002.

Young EA et al: Dissociation between pituitary and adrenal suppression to dexamethasone in depression, *Arch Gen Psychiatry* 50:395, 1993.

Zimmerman M, Coryell W, Pfohl B: The validity of the DST as a maker for endogenous depression, *Arch Gen Psychiatry* 43:347, 1986.

11 The Schizophrenias

Katherine M. Fortinash

Key Terms

affect (p. 238)
ambivalence (p. 238)
autistic thinking (p. 238)
cognitive symptoms
  (p. 249)
delusion (p. 237)
dereism (p. 237)
double-bind (p. 245)
hallucination (p. 237)
loosening of associations
  (LOA) (p. 238)
negative symptoms
  (p. 237)
perseveration (p. 257)
positive symptoms
  (p. 237)
poverty of thought (p. 257)
premorbid (p. 247)
primary process thinking
  (p. 249)
prodromal symptoms
  (p. 250)
psychosis (p. 237)
residual symptoms
  (p. 250)
schizoaffective disorder
  (p. 254)
thought blocking (p. 237)

Objectives

- Analyze the various theories and models explaining schizophrenia that have evolved over time.

- Relate the significance of the biologic theory and its current role in the development of schizophrenia.

- Discuss the role of heredity/genetics in the development of schizophrenia according to twin studies and other familial research.

- Explain the dopamine hypothesis and the research that distinguishes dopamine as a critical neurotransmitter in the development of schizophrenia.

- Describe the effects of typical antipsychotics (haloperidol) on the dopamine receptors in the brain in treating positive symptoms of acute schizophrenia (hallucinations, delusions).

- Explain the effects of atypical antipsychotics (clozapine, risperidone) on the negative symptoms of chronic schizophrenia such as apathy, impaired social skills, avolition, and decreased motivation.

- Define dopamine (D2) and serotonin (5-HT2) receptors, and how they are impacted by typical and atypical antipsychotics.

- Describe the assessment tools and data currently available for medical and nursing diagnoses of schizophrenia.

- Apply the nursing process to clients experiencing the positive and negative symptoms of schizophrenia.

- Differentiate the nursing responsibilities and approaches in caring for clients with schizophrenia from those of other disciplines.

- Assess the situation of persons with schizophrenia and their families in the community, developing nursing care plans for prevention, aftercare, and education.

- Compare and contrast the course of illness, symptoms, and nursing interventions for the subtypes of schizophrenia and for associated disorders such as schizoaffective disorder.

- Evaluate the effectiveness of the various treatment modalities for schizophrenia in the clinical setting.

Schizophrenia is a condition that exists in all cultures and in all socioeconomic groups (Betemps and Ragiel, 1994; Kaplan and Sadock, 1998). It is an illness that "ebbs and flows," meaning there are acute periods called *relapses* in which clients experience sensations in addition to their usual feelings. These additional sensations are known as **positive symptoms**, although they are far from positive in the sense of being wanted. Positive symptoms are the hallucinations, delusions, and confused thoughts that seem to return periodically, most likely triggered from a variety of stressors. They usually respond favorably to hospitalization, medication, reduced stimuli, and interactive therapy. During nonacute periods, clients often experience **negative symptoms.** Examples of negative symptoms are apathy, lack of motivation, blunted affect, and loss of warmth. Negative symptoms are more complex and difficult to treat (Thornton et al., 2001a). See Table 11-3 for a complete list of positive and negative symptoms and a more detailed explanation later in the chapter.

In the United States a person can drive down any number of streets and identify people who may be experiencing schizophrenia. What does schizophrenia look like? How is it manifested? Although not everyone with schizophrenia exhibits signs of the disorder, there are behaviors that may indicate its presence. Perhaps the middle-age woman with an unkempt appearance who is talking to herself while pushing a shopping cart filled with mismatched items has schizophrenia. Or possibly the young man with a disheveled look, cursing to himself and frantically searching for cigarettes in the gutter has schizophrenia (Maguire, 2002). These individuals may have other problems as well, including drug or alcohol abuse, mood symptoms, and malnutrition. However, many of them are also struggling with untreated schizophrenia, and they represent the disenfranchised, mentally ill people of the streets. They are generally left alone to wander aimlessly, with no purpose, until they commit a crime or social injustice that brings them to the attention of the psychiatric or legal system. Then they may be hospitalized or jailed for a time, receiving sporadic treatment, until they are once again released to the streets. Their families and friends have long since abandoned them, and with no support system and no insurance, prospects for recovery seem dim (see Chapter 28).

For other more fortunate individuals who receive treatment early in the course of schizophrenia and have a strong support network, there is now new hope, if not yet a cure. An example is the young first-year college student with a strong familial history of schizophrenia experiencing his first psychotic break, who tried to kill both parents with a knife, believing they were out to get him. With newer medications and early interventions, this young adult can likely be helped to manage his symptoms of *paranoid schizophrenia* and possibly finish college. This is a very different outcome from what might have happened 10 years ago when he may have been institutionalized for the rest of his life.

Despite their prevalence, chronicity, and pervasive symptoms, the schizophrenias did not have the benefit of a scientific, biologic approach until the mid-nineteenth century.

Research supporting the relationship of these complex disorders with the structure and function of the brain cautiously offers hope for more effective treatments and outcomes in the years ahead.

HISTORICAL AND THEORETIC PERSPECTIVES

From a historical perspective, schizophrenia was described as a complex, multifaceted disorder that goes beyond the hallucinations, delusions, or decreased motivation and drive that are most commonly associated with it (Kaplan and Sadock 1998; Maguire, 2002). Until recently little was known about the cognitive function of the brain. The term *schizophrenia* has been used to describe this type of mental disorder only since the 1800s (Kaplan and Sadock, 1998).

In the late 1800s prominent psychiatrist Emil Kraepelin (1856-1926) identified the cognitive impairment of schizophrenia (memory impairment); at the same time, he labeled the disorder *dementia praecox*, which is defined as "precocious madness" (Kaplan and Sadock, 1998). Dementia praecox is associated with two hallmark symptoms: (1) **hallucination**, a subjective sensory-perceptual disorder involving all of the five senses, most commonly the auditory type; for example, a person may be hearing voices belittling him or commanding him to act when no actual presence exists; and (2) **delusion**, a fixed belief held by the individual that is not changed by logic or reason (APA, 2000); for example, a person may believe he is being followed by the CIA, or that he is a famous, historical figure, or a fictional, omnipotent character. These hallmark symptoms are often preceded by a condition known as **dereism,** a loss of connection with reality and logic, where thoughts become private and idiosyncratic (odd or peculiar). The person may also experience **thought blocking,** which is an abrupt blocking of the flow of thoughts or ideas.

At about the same time, renowned Swiss psychiatrist, Eugene Bleuler (1857-1939) identified the four As of schizophrenia as disturbances in *affect, autism, ambivalence,* and *associations* (loosening of associations [LOA]) (Kaplan and Sadock, 1998; Maguire, 2002) (Box 11-1). Bleuler named delusions and hallucinations as *accessory symptoms* to the syndrome (Kaplan and Sadock, 1998). Bleuler also was the first to coin the term *schizophrenia*, which means "split mindedness." According to historical sources, the word was derived from the Greek *skhizo* (split) and *phren* (mind). It is this meaning that may be responsible for confusing the disorder of schizophrenia with *dissociative identity disorder*, formerly multiple personality disorder, in which the personality "splits" off into different parts (see Chapter 12). In schizophrenia Bleuler saw the split as an inconsistency between emotion, thought, and behavior, with the personality remaining intact. Bleuler was also the first to redefine schizophrenia as a thought disorder, which is a more refined and accurate description (Maguire, 2002).

At critical times throughout the illness, clients with schizophrenia experience episodes of **psychosis,** which

> **Box 11-1   Bleuler's Four As: Fundamental Symptoms of the Thought Disorder**
>
> **Loosening of associations (LOA):** Thought disturbance in which the speaker rapidly changes from one subject to another in an unrelated fragmented manner.
> **Affect:** Observable, outward, bodily expression of emotions such as joy, sorrow, and anger. *Blunted affect:* Restricted expression of emotions. *Flat affect:* Lack of expression of emotions. *Inappropriate affect:* Affect that is not congruent with the emotion being felt (e.g., laughing when sad). *Labile affect:* Rapid changes in emotional expression.
> **Ambivalence:** Simultaneously holding two different attitudes, emotions, thoughts, or feelings about a person, object, or situation.
> **Autistic thinking:** Disturbances in thought resulting from the intrusion of a private fantasy world that is internally stimulated, resulting in abnormal responses to people and events in the real world.

From Kaplan HI, Sadock BJ: *Synopsis of psychiatry: behavioral sciences, clinical psychiatry,* ed 8, Baltimore, 1998, Williams & Wilkins.

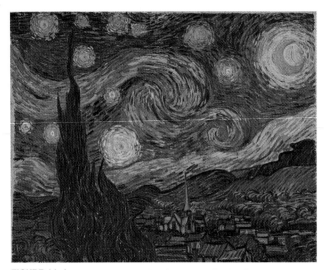

FIGURE 11-1. *The Starry Night* by Vincent van Gogh. (Courtesy The Museum of Modern Art, New York, NY, USA. Digital Image© The Museum of Modern Art/Licensed by SCALA/Art Resource, NY.)

means their capacity to recognize reality is limited or absent. During psychotic episodes, clients may be particularly troubling to society because of their impaired ability to cope with life's demands. Hallucinations and delusions are symptoms of psychotic behavior, as clients who are experiencing these symptoms have limited or absent capacity to recognize reality. Throughout the ages, however, persons with severe mental illness have had great influences on the world. For example, the famous Dutch painter, Vincent van Gogh (1853-1890), went on to create one of his most noted paintings, *The Starry Night*, while institutionalized with a mental illness (Figure 11-1).

The earliest knowledge about recognition and treatment of psychotic disorders comes from artifacts and cave drawings from the Stone Age, a half million years ago. The earliest writings on the subject can be traced to Sanskrit (an an-

cient Indo-European language) of 1400 BC. The belief of possession by demons persisted as early civilizations developed, as noted in the early writings of the Hebrews, Egyptians, Chinese, and Greeks (Bendik, 1996).

Harry Stack Sullivan (1882-1949), a psychiatrist and social learning theorist, emphasized the importance of interpersonal relationships and believed that social isolation was the key in schizophrenia (Sullivan, 1953). Kurt Schneider described various delusional and hallucinatory experiences as first-rank symptoms, currently known as *positive symptoms*, and labeled the less decisive symptoms, such as perceptual disturbances, confusion, mood changes, and emotional impoverishment, as second-rank symptoms, most of which are now called *negative symptoms*. His explanation goes beyond the DSM-IV-TR definition (Kaplan and Sadock, 1998; Maguire, 2002).

ETIOLOGY

Schizophrenia is a no-fault illness. No one is to blame for its causation. Expert opinion is that culture, family environment, or stress cannot cause schizophrenia (Amenson, 1999). By the same token, these elements may influence the way an individual who has schizophrenia or is predisposed to the illness responds to life stressors. The search for the etiology of schizophrenia continues to focus on the biologic perspective. This includes not only the traditional medical model that stresses medication management to alter brain chemistry for symptom relief; but also genetic influences; the role of neuroanatomy, endocrinology, and immunology in producing symptoms; as well as trauma, disease, and the stress diathesis model and its relation to genetic redisposition. As the brain continues to be the focus of both diagnosis and treatment, the research being generated in the new millennium continues to challenge nurses who treat the person with schizophrenia as a whole human being, integrating the biologic sciences with the caring, interpersonal concepts of the psychosocial models (Box 11-2).

Genetic/Heredity Factors

There is a strong genetic component to schizophrenia as demonstrated by a 50% concordance rate in identical or single-egg twins, whether they are raised in the same household or far apart. In nonidentical or fraternal twins, the concordance rate drops to 12% (Maguire, 2002). Complex genetic patterns account for 50% of the cause of schizophrenia. Research shows that combinations of genes from parents can result in an individual inheriting schizophrenia even if no one else in the family has ever experienced it (Amenson, 1999).

Adoptive studies show that schizophrenia is related to the genes inherited from the biologic parents and not to the upbringing of the adoptive parents. Genetic risks are shown in Table 11-1 and vary slightly depending on the study (Amenson, 1999).

Since the renowned twin study in 1953, researchers agree that the incidence of developing schizophrenia is much

Box 11-2   Etiologic Factors

Biologic Factors
Heredity and genetics
Neuroanatomics and neurochemicals
    Structure and function of the nervous system
    Teratogenic drug exposure
    Neuroanatomic differences in the brain
Neurotransmitter function
    Abnormal neurotransmitter-endocrine interactions
Immunologic factors
    Viral exposure in pregnancy
High arousal levels from stress, disease, trauma, and drugs
    Stress such as a bombardment of stimuli from life events
    Diseases such as prenatal virus exposure and encephalitis
    Trauma from obstetric complications, head trauma, and childhood
        accidents
    Drugs such as cannabis and cocaine

Psychoanalytic and Developmental Factors
Distortions in the mother-child relationship
Ego disorganization
Faulty reality interpretation

Familial Factors
Repressed unhappiness
Double-bind patterns
Marital schism of parents
Destructive, expressed emotion communication patterns

Cultural and Environmental Theories
Low socioeconomic status
Lessened social support of family and community; changes in social roles

Learning Theories and Behavioral Models
Irrational problem-solving methods, distorted thinking, and deficient
    communication patterns learned from parents
Generalized social interactions

Theories of Psychophysiologic Effects of the Environment
Toxic substances (selenium) in the atmospheric pollution

Table 11-1   Schizophrenia and Genetic Risks

Relationships to Person with Schizophrenia	Genetic Risk of Developing Schizophrenia
Identical twin	46%
Child (both parents have schizophrenia)	50%
Child (one parent has schizophrenia)	12%
Brother, sister, or parent	12%
Nephew, niece, or grandchild	5%
First cousin	2%

From Amenson CS: The family's role in recovery: *Pacific Clinics Institute: The Journal*, 1999 and Guest Speaker, Schizophrenia: *Grand Rounds Conference, Sharp HealthCare*, San Diego, CA, 2001.

more genetic avenues to explore before the etiology or etiologies of this elusive disorder is revealed.

Stress-Diathesis Model and Genetic Influences

The stress-diathesis model claims that something in the environment may influence a person to succumb to schizophrenia if he or she is already genetically exposed (Amenson, 1999; Maguire, 2002). The following factors are thought to activate a genetic vulnerability, which may contribute to the cause of schizophrenia; however, it is important to note that *95% of persons who experience these factors do not develop schizophrenia* (Amenson, 1999):

- Winter birth (during flu season)
- Viral infection during the twentieth to thirtieth week of pregnancy
- Incompatibility of the Rh factors between the blood of mother and fetus
- Starvation during pregnancy
- Complications at birth, especially oxygen deprivation

Dopamine Hypothesis

Dopamine, a catecholamine type neurotransmitter, is thought to act within certain brain cells and nerve tracts to help regulate movement as well as emotions. Dopamine, therefore, affects mood, affect, thoughts, and motor behavior. The *dopamine hypothesis*, a major hypothesis in the etiology of schizophrenia, suggests that schizophrenia is associated with an increased level of dopamine in certain areas of the brain such as the nigrostriatal tract, which runs from the substantia nigra to the basal ganglia (Figure 11-3). This is a main dopamine tract responsible for normal execution of motor and cognitive functions. A certain amount of dopamine is thus necessary for smooth motor movements and clear thought processes. Excess dopamine, however, is believed to cause symptoms of psychosis, such as hallucinations and delusions, as it disrupts cognition and thought. This theory is supported by postmortem data showing that the numbers of dopamine receptors are increased by two thirds in persons with schizophrenia. It is thought that schizophrenia, or symptoms that resemble schizophrenia, may result from too much dopamine-dependent neuronal activity in the brain. This means

higher when one has a parent, identical twin, or sibling with schizophrenia (46% for an identical twin and 12% for a sibling), than in the general population (1% for an unrelated person) (Figure 11-2).

It is obvious that if genetics were the only cause of schizophrenia, there would be a 100% concordance rate (Maguire, 2002). Yet scientists continue to explore the genetic possibilities. The search for a major gene or gene site led one researcher to locate an anomaly on chromosome 5. The findings were controversial because further study could not link the causation of this complex disorder to a single gene (Tsuang, 1994). Evidence shows that there are multiple risk factors important in susceptibility, and inheritance is considered the most critical one. There obviously remains

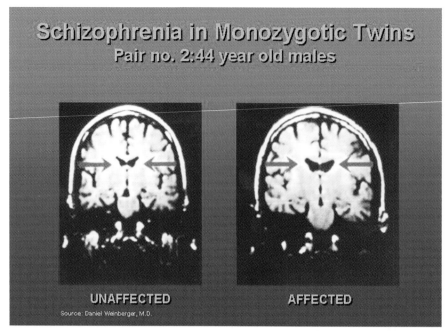

FIGURE 11-2. Loss of brain volume associated with schizophrenia is clearly shown by magnetic resonance imaging (MRI) scans comparing the size of ventricles (butterfly-shaped, fluid-filled spaces in the midbrain) of identical twins, one of whom has schizophrenia *(right).* The ventricles of the person with schizophrenia are larger, suggesting structural brain changes associated with the illness. Note that such MRI scans cannot be used to diagnose schizophrenia in the general population because of normal genetic variation in ventricle size; many unaffected people have large ventricles. (Daniel Weinberger, MD, Clinical Brain Disorders Branch, Division of Intramural Research Program, NIMH, 1990, Updated, December 11, 2000.)

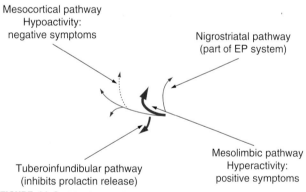

FIGURE 11-3. The four main dopaminergic tracts. (Courtesy David G. Daniel, MD, Bioniche Development, Inc., 2001.)

that there may be an abundance of nerve cells that "crave" dopamine and overreact in a way that produces psychotic symptoms. There may also be an excess in the production or release of dopamine at nerve endings, increased receptor sensitivity, or decreased activity of dopamine antagonists (drug or substance that blocks or counteracts dopamine).

Dopamine Hypothesis and Typical Antipsychotic Effect

The positive effects of the older, typical antipsychotics, such as haloperidol (Haldol) or fluphenazine (Prolixin), are their actions as dopamine antagonists, blocking the dopamine receptors (D2), so that less dopamine is available. This will re-

duce the client's psychosis, but may also disrupt execution of smooth motor function by the nigrostriatum, resulting in many troubling movement disorders (Figure 11-4). Briefly stated, too much dopamine can cause psychosis, and not enough dopamine can lead to movement disorders, also known *as extrapyramidal symptoms*, or *extrapyramidal side effects.* Extrapyramidal nerve tracts lie outside the pyramidal tracts and are part of the central nervous system (Maguire, 2002; Boyd, 2002) (see Chapter 20 for description of extrapyramidal symptoms).

Dopamine Hypothesis and Illicit Drugs

Cocaine and amphetamines are *dopaminergic compounds* (meaning their chemical structure is dopamine-like; therefore, they are dopamine agonists). They are also known to increase psychosis, which supports the dopamine hypothesis (too much dopamine produces psychosis). Psychosis can also be induced in individuals with Parkinson's disease who take levodopa (a type of dopamine) to replace the reduced levels of dopamine that is a feature in Parkinson's disease. These reduced levels of dopamine are responsible for the tremors and shuffling gait noted in clients with Parkinson's disease. The dopamine hypothesis is further supported by clients who develop a drug-induced pseudo-parkinsonism as a result of the dopamine-blocking effects of antipsychotic medication, specifically the older generation types. The client experiencing this phenomenon resembles a client with Parkinson's disease, with shuffling gait and an expression-

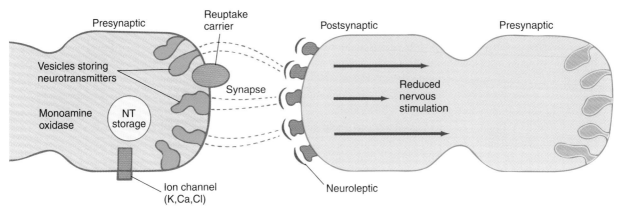

FIGURE 11-4. Neuroleptic (antipsychotic) action. Neurotransmitter action at the synapse is modified by neuroleptics, which block postsynaptic receptor sites to reduce nervous stimulation (reducing symptoms of schizophrenia).

Table 11-2	Neurotransmitters in Schizophrenia: Type and Function	
Neurotransmitter	**Type**	**Function**
Dopamine	Catecholamine	Regulates motor behavior in extrapyramidal nerve tracts and also transmits in the cortex. Increases vigilance and may increase aggression. Too much may produce psychosis; too little may cause movement disorders (EPS).
Serotonin	Indolamine	Brainstem transmitter; modulates mood; lowers aggressive tendencies. A deficiency may be responsible for some forms of schizophrenia.
Acetylcholine	Cholinergic	Transmits at nerve-muscle connections (central nervous system and autonomic nervous system). A deficiency may increase confusion and acting out behavior. Controls extrapyramidal symptoms (EPS).
Norepinephrine	Catecholamine	Transmits in the sympathetic nervous system. Induces the "flight or fight" syndrome (hypervigilance). May be insufficient in clients with schizophrenia who display anhedonia (loss of pleasure).
Cholecystokinin	Peptide	Excites the limbic neurons. A deficiency is related to avolition (lack of motivation) and a flat affect.
Glutamate	Amino acid	Excitatory neurotransmitter. Impairment in the *N*-methyl-D-aspartate or NMDA affects glutamate, which can lead to problems in cognition, delusions, and possibly some negative symptoms of schizophrenia (Maguire, 2002).
γ-Aminobutyric acid (GABA)	Amino acid	Inhibitory neurotransmitter; predominantly a brain transmitter. Promotes a balance between dopamine and glutamate and thus inhibits impulsive behaviors.

less face, also known as *masked facies* (Kapan and Sadock, 1998) (see Chapter 20).

Another hypothesis states that lysergic acid diethylamide (LSD) can cause or increase hallucinations by its effects on serotonin. This indicates that the newer generation antipsychotics may achieve a synergistic, therapeutic effect by blocking both dopamine and serotonin (Maguire, 2002). Persons with schizophrenia who take "street drugs" are at risk because of the unpredictable effects caused by these illicit substances. Conscious-altering drugs, such as marijuana, tend to counteract the effects of antipsychotic medications by inducing the effects of the illness again (Thornton et al., 2001b).

Other Neurotransmitters Associated With Schizophrenia

Six other neurotransmitters that may also be relevant by themselves or in conjunction with dopamine are *serotonin, acetylcholine, norepinephrine, cholecystokinin, glutamate,* and *γ-aminobutyric acid (GABA)* (Table 11-2).

New Research on Atypical Effect on Serotonin

New research reveals that although the atypical antipsychotics are the current standard of care, they are not all equal. For atypical drugs to sustain a low risk for extrapyramidal effects, they must block serotonin type 2A and serotonin type 2C receptors. This causes a release of dopamine in the nigrostriatal pathways of the brain, which can combat some of the extrapyramidal symptoms and improve negative symptoms as well. Haloperidol lacks this property (Maguire, 2002). It was also found that effective outcomes for atypical therapy are often dose related (Kapur and Seeman, 2001).

Other new research into the way antipsychotics work shows that increased activity of dopamine in the brain explains only the positive symptoms of schizophrenia (delusions, hallucinations), whereas increased serotonin activity explains most of the negative symptoms such as affective flattening and lack of motivation. There are other considerations as well, such as cognitive impairment, mood symptoms, socializing problems, and comorbid conditions such as substance abuse (Maguire, 2002).

Studies indicate a paucity of dopamine in the frontal lobe of the brain (prefrontal cortex), which is the area of the brain that is responsible for cognition, volition, and motivation. Typical antipsychotics such as haloperidol depress dopamine activity in the frontal lobe, thereby "shutting down" these critical cognitive functions. Atypical agents can help increase dopamine in this area of the brain by blocking serotonin, as a decrease in serotonin will release dopamine, thereby making it more available to improve cognitive symptoms.

Aripiprazole (Abilify), a new atypical antipsychotic now in clinical trials, is reported to be both a dopamine and a serotonin system stabilizer, with both agonistic and antagonistic effects. Only time will prove its efficacy.

Atypical Effect on *N*-Methyl-D-Aspartate, Glutamate, and Acetylcholine
Impact on Cognition, Mood Symptoms, and Dyskinesias. It has been suggested that impairment in the *N*-methyl-D-aspartate (NMDA) or glutamate system explains more of the problems in cognition, delusions, and perhaps even some of the negative symptoms of schizophrenia. Newer, atypical drugs such as olanzapine, quetiapine, and clozapine have been shown to be selective for the A-10 neurolimbic system pathway and the NMDA system, where they influence glutamate. Similar research has shown that these atypical agents increase acetylcholine and thus improve cognition (concentration, memory, and learning), as well as depression. They also block oral dyskinesias (tongue thrusting and lip smacking) and improve tardive dyskinesia (TD), a serious movement disorder generally occurring late in treatment with older, typical antipsychotics that may be irreversible (see Chapter 20). Olanzapine and clozapine have been noted to decrease the delusions and hallucinations in animal studies, which may be valuable in treating clients who are high on phencyclidine hydrochloride (PCP) or ketamine. Agents such as risperidone and haloperidol, however, do not help in this situation, and they have also been linked to depression in clients who are prone to depression (Maguire, 2002).

Other Biologic Research
Hans Selye (Medical Model)
Several early twentieth-century theorists favored biologic factors as causes for schizophrenia and other illnesses based on their research. Hans Selye (1907-1982), physician and medical educator, was a successful pioneer with his work on the general adaptation syndrome (GAS). In 1936, Selye showed that the effects of alarm, resistance, and exhaustion after stress were related in a causal manner to several physiologic disease states (e.g., hypertension and peptic ulcer) and wrote about it extensively (Selye, 1978; McCain and Smith, 1994).

Extensive research on the neuroendocrine mechanisms underlying the stress response also influenced psychiatrists to view these mechanisms as a possible explanation for several forms of psychotic states. This foundation remains a part of the theoretic framework explaining psychopathology even today, as well as a part of the stress and adaptation theories used in psychiatric nursing such as the Roy Adaptation Model described in the following paragraph.

Callista Roy (Nursing Model)
Sister Callista Roy, theorist and nursing educator, developed the Roy Adaptation Model in 1976. Her theory stresses the need for human beings to continually adapt to internal and external stimuli that she labeled *focal, contextual,* and *residual.* Roy determined that the ways in which people adapt include both physiologic (biologic) and psychologic and social modes of adaptation. She clearly relates the importance of viewing people as holistic, biologic, and social beings in a constant state of flux with their internal states and the environment (Roy, 1976).

Neuroanatomic and Neurochemical Factors
There have been many recent advances in the study of neuroanatomic and neurochemical factors as they relate to schizophrenia. Starting with the work of Plum (1972), Crow (1980), and others, the field has expanded to include the study of the human nervous system from the perspectives of physiology, chemistry, and endocrinology (Hemsley et al., 1993; Joseph, 1993). Also, the immune system may be involved in schizophrenia (Lieberman and Koreen, 1993; Tsuang, 1994).

Neurotransmitter-Endocrine Interactions
Human behavior, thoughts, and feelings are also influenced by the much larger and more complex endocrine system. Schizophrenia has been linked to abnormal neurotransmitter and neuroendocrine interactions (Benes, 1993; Hemsley et al., 1993; Lieberman and Koreen, 1993; Malone, 1990). For example, although direct evidence of serotonin dysfunction has not been obtained, the antipsychotic drugs clozapine and risperidone owe their unique therapeutic effects to their influence on dopamine and the serotonin receptors in the frontal cortex. The role of GABA in schizophrenia promotes a balance of dopamine and glutamate and thus inhibits impulsive behaviors.

Several studies have examined the neurotransmitter interactions in schizophrenia, as well as the effect of interactions between hormones and neurotransmitters. Patterns of dopamine-thyroid interactions and dopamine-pituitary hormone secretions were found to be consistent with schizophrenia symptoms. Other patterns involved β-endorphins and other opioid compounds, cholecystokinin and other neuropeptides, in interaction with dopamine. Also, abnormal composition and structure of neuronal membranes may also contribute to symptoms of schizophrenia (Lieberman and Koreen, 1993).

Drugs that have high dopamine-blocking activity, such as haloperidol, can cause elevated serum prolactin levels because dopamine acts as an inhibitory neurotransmitter in the hypopituitary axis, resulting in increased levels of prolactin, as noted previously.

Currently the studies of neurochemistry and neuroendocrinology are fragmentary but promising. It is clear that the patterns and balance between the neurotransmitter and neuroendocrine systems in schizophrenia are distinctly different from those of unaffected individuals.

Immunologic Factors

Viral exposure, particularly exposure to influenza during pregnancy, is a risk factor for developing schizophrenia. It is theorized that the influenza virus may create maternal antibodies. In the fetus, these become autoantibodies, which are an external source of developmental change. The mother's exposure to a virus during pregnancy may explain why some siblings develop schizophrenia, and others do not (Takei et al., 1994; Maguire, 2002). There are few immunologic studies of schizophrenia, and they depend on epidemiologic data for their hypotheses.

Structural and Functional Factors

This theory states that the structure of the nervous system includes both gross and microanatomic defects, possibly resulting from a congenital developmental condition (Benes, 1993; Bogerts, 1993; Cannon and Marco, 1994). Other researchers have cited that drug exposure to the fetus in the uterus, or birth trauma, may lead to a gradual deterioration that seems to affect many clients with chronic schizophrenia. Both of these ideas suggest a faulty developmental pattern. Complications at birth, mentioned earlier in the stress-diathesis model, may play a role in subsequent developmental impairment that may affect clients with chronic schizophrenia (Amenson, 1999). Studies used to examine structural and functional impairment of the brain are described next.

Magnetic Resonance Imaging. Magnetic resonance imaging (MRI), a brain imaging techniques available today, can be used at the time of diagnosis to rule out structural causes of psychosis in clients with schizophrenia (Maguire, 2002). MRIs are internal snapshots of the brain taken slice by slice over time. MRI examinations can reveal ventricular enlargement, prominence of cortical sulci, defects in limbic brain structures, and cortical atrophy, which, when present, are usually more pronounced in the left hemisphere of the brain. Smaller cerebrums and frontal lobes are noted in clients with chronic schizophrenia. Specifically, there are subtle neuroanatomic differences in parts of the thalamus, septum, hypothalamus, hippocampus, amygdala, and cingulate gyrus in the brains of clients with schizophrenia when compared with the brains of unaffected persons (Bogerts, 1993; Cannon and Marco, 1994; Joseph, 1993) (see Figure 11-2).

New research using functional MRIs to study the brains of persons with schizophrenia is being conducted by several major medical institutions across the country. Functional MRIs take snapshots of the brain over time to produce a moment-by-moment three-dimensional movie of the *energy pathway* inside the brain. Subjects involved in the study (clients and healthy control subjects) will perform certain tasks while lying inside the bores of MRI machines to see how the brain responses of clients with schizophrenia compare with those of healthy individuals. Information will be shared among researchers nationwide via computerized brain images through high-speed Internet connections. Research like this offers new hope for clients with various types of schizophrenia.

Electroencephalogram. Physiologically electroencephalograms reveal a decrease in metabolic activity and slower brain waves in the frontal lobes of persons with schizophrenia (Malone, 1990). At the microlevel, changes in neurotransmitter activity at the synaptic junctions between the nerve cells lead to abnormalities in the brain circuits (Benes, 1993; Cannon and Marco, 1994). It is difficult to establish the relationship between neuronal damage and functional impairment, but Previc (1993) maintains that the visual-perceptual and visual-motor functions of the brain, located in the posterior parietal lobes, are affected in individuals with schizophrenia. Consequently, these clients manifest poor audiovisual integration, spatial orientation difficulties, prolonged reaction time responses, accommodation problems, and distortions in perceived body image. Some clients with schizophrenia cannot tell whether or not a person is looking at them because of eye tracking dysfunctions (Clementz, McDowell, and Zisook, 1994).

To cite another specific relationship, Hemsley et al. (1993) believe that hippocampal lesions can cause learning failure and an inability to differentiate between meaningless and meaningful information. These are only two examples of the functional difficulties encountered by clients as a result of damage in neuron structures.

Positron Emission Tomography. A recent positron emission tomography (PET) study, an imaging technique using cross-sectional single computerized photographs of a select area in the brain, illustrated the clinical responses of haloperidol, olanzapine, and risperidone in relation to their occupancy of dopamine (D2) receptors, which affects the positive symptoms of schizophrenia, and their occupancy of serotonin (5-HT2) receptors, which affects the negative symptoms. Results of the study support the hypothesis of variable brain activity by both typical and atypical antipsychotics, possibly as a result of the different manner in which these drugs occupy the receptor sites. This may explain the different treatment outcomes of these drugs, even by drugs within the same category (Kapur and Seeman, 2001).

Stress, Disease, Trauma, and Drug Abuse

In Selye's stress model, described earlier, the individual was seen as interacting with the environment and being bombarded by various stimuli in the form of life events. This created stress that differed in magnitude and meaning for each individual and that was capable of producing disease states. In Roy's adaptation model, explained previously, the person was viewed as continually adapting to internal and external stimuli (some of which may be stress-producing), using both physiologic (biologic) and psychosocial modes of adaptation.

For clients with chronic schizophrenia, environmental stress-producing events and situations are always present. They increase dopaminergic transmission and precipitate a high level of arousal, leading to episodic recurrences of the disease. The high level of arousal results in intense hallucinatory experiences (Kaplan and Sadock, 1998). Several of the nursing theories (i.e., King's, Levine's, and Neuman's) examined the relationship between stress and illness (physical or mental), using this theory.

Some recent studies support the idea that schizophrenia may be developmentally related to disease and trauma occurring during the prenatal period or in early childhood (Amenson, 1999; Maguire, 2002). As cited earlier, Takei et al. (1994) studied the effect of prenatal exposure to the influenza virus and concluded that exposure in the second trimester of pregnancy was a significant risk for adult schizophrenia, especially for females, This indicated that there may be gender differences in the presentation of the disease. Maguire (2002) states that it is more common for babies carried in the uterus in winter months (and born in winter and spring) to have schizophrenia. He says that some theories suggest that the mother may be infected in the second trimester with a virus that affects the cortical development in the child.

Studies of childhood indicated that encephalitis was found to be a risk factor for schizophrenia. Also, studies of head trauma requiring hospitalization for the child less than 10 years old revealed a significant difference in the later occurrence of schizophrenia between persons who had suffered prenatal or childhood head trauma and a comparison group. Injuries included hemorrhage into the ventricles and ischemic damage to the cortex in areas commonly associated with schizophrenia (Gureje et al., 1994).

Several comorbid conditions tend to be more prevalent in persons with schizophrenia; for example, substance abuse is common in this population. More than 75% are addicted to nicotine, 30% to 50% are addicted to alcohol, 15% to 25% are addicted to cannabis, and 5% to 10% are addicted to cocaine and amphetamines (Maguire, 2002). The relationship between drugs of abuse and schizophrenia has also been studied. According to Linszen et al. (1994), cannabis abuse may be a precipitant of schizophrenia or may promote relapse. Also, the extreme stimulating effect of cocaine (a dopamine agonist that generates impulsivity) induces relapse in persons with schizophrenia (Stirling et al., 1994). Cocaine initiates neurochemical changes in the brain by substituting for the natural endorphins, creating an intense craving for the drug. Eventually the long-term user experiences apathy, depression, and anhedonia, as often seen in clients with chronic schizophrenia.

Maguire (2002) notes that persons with schizophrenia may indulge in substances such as nicotine, caffeine, and cocaine to self-medicate and perhaps help improve their attention span, as they attempt to deal with competing stimuli that is a constant disruption in their lives. In addition, there is accumulating evidence that certain drugs used in pregnancy are linked with later schizotypal illnesses in childhood and adolescence. For example, cocaine used by a pregnant woman is linked to later schizotypal illness in the affected child (Scherling, 1994).

It is interesting to note that diabetes mellitus is two to four times more common in clients with schizophrenia than in the general population (Maguire, 2002). Guthrie (2002) states that some of the newer, atypical antipsychotics have been associated with diabetes mellitus, but this may be because today's practitioners are more watchful for diabetes mellitus in their clients rather than the result of the medication.

Psychodynamic Theories

Many biologic factors can predispose an individual to schizophrenia; however, psychosocial considerations are significant as well. Most causative models stipulate that a person's vulnerability interacts with stressful environmental influences to produce the symptoms of schizophrenia (Kaplan and Sadock, 1998). The theories that deal with psychosocial and environmental factors are psychoanalytic, family, and sociocultural/environmental. *Systems theory* also has been used to explain the reciprocal interactions among the theories. Systems attempt to achieve *homeostasis* or balance within a system, whether it is a family, a group, or different theories (see Chapter 19).

Psychoanalytic and Developmental Theories

Psychoanalytic theory, which has been viewed much less favorably in recent times, states that there are distortions in the mother-child relationship, brought on by anxious mothering, so that the child is unable to progress beyond dependence. This affects the ego organization (sense of self), and the interpretation of reality in the developing child. Being unable to interpret reality, the individual is susceptible to a fantasy world in which hallucinations and delusions attempt to create a reality of wishful thinking or to express inner fears. Inner drives, such as sex and aggression, are not brought under the person's control, and self-object differentiation is not achieved (person cannot distinguish self from the environment). The person's sense of identity is therefore weakened, and his or her personality is vulnerable to stress (Kaplan and Sadock, 1998) (see Chapters 8 and 12).

Family Theory Model

According to the family theory model, the child is assumed to have been raised in an atmosphere of unhappiness and tension, which may not be apparent to others or even to the family members themselves. Families make great attempts to conceal or repress unhappiness, resulting in psychologic insensitivity. However, no studies have demonstrated that family attributes are *causally* related to schizophrenia. Considering the reciprocal nature of interactions, one cannot say whether stressful relationships would precede or follow an episode of schizophrenia.

Several family patterns have been cited as being particularly damaging to the developing child. The first pattern is the **double-bind**, in which the child is forced to make a choice between two unreasonable perceptions, thus producing confusion, anxiety, and fear in the child's mind. For example, a verbal message may differ from a nonverbal one; a parent may insist that he or she is not angry at the child's behavior but expresses obvious anger in aggressive, hostile, and destructive behavior toward the child.

The second family pattern seen as destructive involves marital problems between the parents. This pattern results in the children being asked to support one parent against the other. Such a situation causes guilt feelings in the children because of divided loyalties. Often a power struggle begins between the parents, with one parent emerging as dominant and authoritative. This authoritative stand is likely to suppress the child's drive toward independence. In addition, the spouse forced into submissiveness may displace his or her anger onto the children or make one child a scapegoat.

The third serious family disturbance arises from emotions that are expressed in family communication patterns that are destructive. At times, there is a false agreement about family rules that is not communicated directly but produces explosive behaviors from one or more members when violated. There is also an air of pseudohostility that forces some family members into emotional isolation. The constant criticism and hostility destroy the family functions of support and protection (see Chapter 19).

Many recent studies conclude that low-key families, where there is little criticism and anger, where emotional bonds are relatively distant, and where family members interact less, create a climate that is conducive to better outcomes for the member with schizophrenia. Outcomes related to family climate studies, however, have been defined only in terms of rehospitalization frequency and symptom intensity (Thornton et al., 2001c).

Cultural and Environmental Theories

Although schizophrenia exists in all socioeconomic groups, it is disproportionately represented in the lower socioeconomic group. Various explanations have been reported for this condition, one having to do with a "downward drift hypothesis" (Kaplan and Sadock, 1998). According to this hypothesis, the client with schizophrenia who possesses low social skills either moves into a lower socioeconomic group or fails to rise to a higher group (Maguire, 2002).

On the other hand, some social scientists believe that the stress of living in a lower socioeconomic group is often enough to trigger schizophrenia in the vulnerable popula-

tion. Individuals with schizophrenia who are under psychologic stress manifest low levels of self-esteem and self-efficacy perception (view of self as a normally functioning, partially functioning, or low functioning member of society), and may have limited resources to cope with their situation. In addition, the family networks of mentally ill persons are often unable to be supportive, and clients may resort to homelessness (Bendik, 1992) (see Chapter 28).

Low socioeconomic status affects not only the psychologic but also the biologic functioning of an individual, adding to chronic symptom profiles (Cohen, 1993). For example, clients with schizophrenia are more likely than other persons in the lower socioeconomic group to get an infectious disease, particularly tuberculosis. Living in heavily populated rural areas, in poverty, adversity, and fear, because of rising crime rates, is conducive to psychopathology (Betemps and Ragiel, 1994) (see Chapter 27).

Studies have also looked at the physical environment and its relationship to schizophrenia. Because people may be exposed to toxic substances that cause a variety of illnesses through atmospheric pollution or a contaminated food chain (e.g., lead and mercury), researchers have compared the geographic distribution of selenium and other trace elements with the prevalence of schizophrenia in the same locations. The hypotheses were formulated according to an assumption that either an excess or a deficiency of certain substances in the environment can cause the disease (Brown, 1994).

Learning Theory

According to the learning theory, the irrational ways of handling situations, the distorted thinking, and the impaired communication of persons with schizophrenia are a result of poor parental models in early childhood. Children learn the things they are exposed to on a daily basis from parents who have their own significant emotional problems. Therefore the child does not develop skill in forming good interpersonal relationships (Kaplan and Sadock, 1998).

Sullivan, cited earlier, was a principal proponent of the learning theory, believing that the developing individual was shaped by social interactions. The complexity of feelings, thoughts, and behavioral expressions, therefore, grew out of the individual's experiences with those closest to him or her. For example, if the child's father was perceived as mean and dictatorial, this perception may have generalized to other men in positions of authority, such as teachers, policemen, and employers, and shaded the individual's interpersonal relationships with these individuals. Or, if the child's mother coped with problems by projecting blame to others, the child learned this pattern of behavior and alienated others by putting it into practice (see Chapter 19).

EPIDEMIOLOGY

In the United States schizophrenia has a lifetime prevalence of 0.7 years and affects 1% of the general population (Csernansky, Mahmoud, and Brenner, 2002) (Box 11-3). The prevalence

Box 11-3	Epidemiology

New diagnoses of schizophrenia occur between 0.3% and 0.6% per 1000 persons per year in the United States.

1.5% of the US population has been diagnosed with schizophrenia.

The age of onset is greater in females than in males.

Paranoid-type schizophrenia occurs earlier in males than in females.

Disorganized-type schizophrenia occurs earlier in females than in males.

Prevalence is equal for males and females.

The oldest age-of-onset group is between 66 and 77 years old.

A female fetus exposed to influenza has a higher risk for schizophrenia than a male fetus.

Males show significantly more structural brain abnormalities from perinatal or early childhood trauma than females.

50% of persons with schizophrenia attempt suicide.

of schizophrenia is equal in both men and women, and the peak age of onset is usually 15 to 25 years for men, and 25 to 35 years for women (Maguire, 2002). The incidence of schizophrenia, or the frequency of newly diagnosed cases in a specified population during a certain time period, is between 0.3% and 0.6% per 1000 persons per year in the United States. The prevalence and prognosis of the disease vary according to socioeconomic, geographic, and cultural factors; schizophrenia presents itself in different ways, depending on the clients' situations and demographic characteristics (Betemps and Ragiel, 1994; Kaplan and Sadock, 1998). Schizophrenia accounts for 20% of all hospital bed-days, and 50% of all psychiatric beds in the United States. One percent of the gross U.S. domestic product goes toward treating schizophrenia. The economic burden of schizophrenia on society was estimated in 1990 to be $33 billion in the United States. Much of this cost was attributed to relapse of psychosis and rehospitalization, as most clients experience a chronic course even though it varies from client to client (Csernansky et al., 2002). Loss of work and productivity is also attributed to the cost. Family, twin, and adoption studies have consistently found varying rates of inheritance patterns according to the closeness of the genetic relationship (Kendler and Diehl, 1993; Kaplan and Sadock, 1998; Amenson, 1999; Maguire, 2002) (see Genetic/Heredity Factors earlier in this chapter).

Later-Onset, Premorbid Functioning, and Outcomes

Persons who first experience schizophrenia later in life have better outcomes in all areas. This may be related to the amount of time they lived before the onset of schizophrenia, during which they had more opportunities to be productive and acquire coping skills. This depends, in part, on their **premorbid** functioning (how they functioned before the illness). For example, if a client developed good social skills, had a satisfying sex life, and succeeded in academic or vocational achievements before the onset of schizophrenia, the chances for a successful outcome after the illness is significantly improved (Thornton et al., 2001a).

Age, Gender, and Outcomes

Two demographic characteristics that have been extensively studied with regard to schizophrenia are age and gender. These variables have an interactive effect. For example, the age of onset of the disease in females is significantly greater than the age of onset in males (about 10 years). Also, women tend to be rehospitalized less often, to respond better to antipsychotic medication, and to be less aggressive and less self-destructive than men (Thornton et al., 2001c).

Subtypes of schizophrenia tend to appear at different times. The paranoid type, in which prominent delusions or auditory hallucinations of a persecutory nature are present, appears earlier in males. On the other hand, the disorganized type, which features confusion in speech, disorganization in behavior, and inappropriate affect, appears earlier in females (Castle and Murray, 1993; APA, 2000). However, over the course of time there is no difference in the prevalence of schizophrenia between males and females (Kaplan and Sadock, 1998).

Older-Adult Onset. In a well-known incidence study of the age of onset for schizophrenia, the oldest group range was 66 to 77 years, and accounted for about one third of the prevalence rate. This is contrary to earlier beliefs that schizophrenia rarely occurs after age 50 years. Clients in the oldest age-of-onset group tended to be women exhibiting paranoid symptoms (Castle and Murray, 1993).

Fetal Exposure to Disease and Trauma. When the fetus is exposed to influenza from the mother during the second trimester, the female child appears to be at greater risk for developing schizophrenia in her adult years (Takei et al., 1994). However, males show significantly more structural brain abnormalities than females as a result of perinatal or early childhood trauma (Gureje et al., 1994). Overall, gender differences in the age of onset, physiologic deficits, prognosis, and response to treatment show evidence of a gender difference in the way schizophrenia is expressed.

Marital Status, Rates of Reproduction, and Mortality

Since the introduction of psychotherapeutic drugs, people with schizophrenia have been freed from ongoing care in a state mental institution. Without the burden of many of their symptoms and with easier access to rehabilitation programs where available, many individuals with schizophrenia have gone on to live reasonably normal and even productive lives, including marrying and having a family. Thus, the marriage and fertility rates that were once low among people with schizophrenia are now in closer proximity to the larger population aggregate (Fortinash and Holoday Worret, 2003; Kaplan and Sadock, 1998).

Schizophrenia continues to manifest high rates of suicide in those who cannot cope with the demands of society. Despite the relief of some of their symptoms, many people with schizophrenia are prone to episodic decompensation during exacerbation of the disorder. At these times, they may attempt suicide, become accident prone, or neglect their health. It is estimated that between 10% and 15% of persons with schizophrenia commit suicide, usually before age 30 years. It is often difficult to predict the type of client who will attempt suicide. The intelligent high achiever with good social support may become frustrated with the inability to meet expectations and may decide that suicide is a better option than living with a debilitating mental illness (Thornton et al., 2001a).

Relapse Prevention and Research

Maguire (2002) suggests that relapse may be part of the natural course of schizophrenia and may also result from a variety of reasons such as poor insight leading to denial of the illness, nonadherence to treatment, lack of family support, inability to cope with the complex mental health system, or the failure of certain medications to maintain their efficacy in the long term.

Research is currently focused on long-term treatment and relapse prevention for clients with schizophrenia. A recent study identified clozapine and olanzapine as cost-effective antipsychotics that showed favorable response rates in preventing relapse. Csernansky et al. (2002) conducted a study involving adult outpatients with clinically stable schizophrenia or schizoaffective disorder. They found a lower risk of relapse in clients treated with risperidone than in clients treated with haloperidol.

Cramer and Rosenheck (1998) also studied client adherence to taking prescribed antipsychotics and antidepressants. Relapse was identified as one of many factors affecting adherence (see Understanding and Applying Research box).

Socioeconomic Class

The portion of schizophrenia that is attributed to the social problems of the underprivileged class remains controversial (Betemps and Ragiel, 1994; Kaplan and Sadock, 1998; Fortinash and Holoday Worret, 2003). The overcrowded poor neighborhoods and the homeless mentally ill persons receiving inadequate follow-up care are added burdens on this vulnerable population and on society. In economic terms, schizophrenia is the costliest of all mental disorders (see Chapter 28). Thornton et al. (2001c) suggest that schizophrenia ap-

pears to be a milder illness in developing countries than it does in industrialized societies. Although the reasons for this are not clear, factors such as lower expectations and more extensive family networks may contribute to this phenomenon.

Culture, Geography, and Seasonal Influences

The manifestations of schizophrenia and its prognosis vary in different cultures. In less-developed nations the prognosis for schizophrenia is better than in the technologically advanced cultures. Clients in developing countries tend to have a more acute onset, fewer episodic occurrences, and less frequent problems with affect. Severe cognitive impairment is rare in Western nations. However, after an acute episode, the person with schizophrenia in developing countries is more readily reintegrated into the family and community (Betemps and Ragiel, 1994; Kaplan and Sadock, 1998). This last statement concurs with the finding of Thornton et al. (2001c) and their look at developing countries.

Variations in the prevalence of schizophrenia in different geographic regions have been studied. In some climates, the

DSM-IV-TR CRITERIA
Schizophrenia

A. *Characteristic symptoms*: Two (or more) of the following, each present for a significant portion of time during a 1-month period (or less if successfully treated):
1. Delusions
2. Hallucinations
3. Disorganized speech (e.g., frequent derailment or incoherence)
4. Grossly disorganized or catatonic behavior
5. Negative symptoms (i.e., affective flattening, alogia, or avolition)
NOTE: Only one Criterion A symptom is required if delusions are bizarre or hallucinations consist of a voice keeping up a running commentary on the person's behavior or thoughts, or two or more voices conversing with each other.

B. *Social/occupational dysfunction*: For a significant portion of the time since the onset of the disturbance, one or more major areas of functioning, such as work, interpersonal relations, or self-care, are markedly below the level achieved before the onset (or when the onset is in childhood or adolescence, failure to achieve expected level of interpersonal, academic, or occupational achievement).

C. *Duration*: Continuous signs of the disturbance persist for at least 6 months. This 6-month period must include at least 1 month of symptoms (or less if successfully treated) that meet Criterion A (i.e., active-phase symptoms) and may include periods of prodromal or residual symptoms. During these prodromal or residual periods, the signs of the disturbance may be manifested by only negative symptoms or two or more symptoms listed in Criterion A present in an attenuated form (e.g., odd beliefs, unusual perceptual experiences).

D. *Schizoaffective and mood disorder exclusion*: Schizoaffective disorder and mood disorder with psychotic features have been ruled out because either (1) no major depressive, manic, or mixed episodes have occurred concurrently with the active-phase symptoms; or (2) if mood episodes have occurred during active-phase symptoms, their total duration has been brief relative to the duration of the active and residual periods.

    Substance/general medical condition exclusion: The disturbance is not due to the direct physiologic effects of a substance (e.g., a drug of abuse, a medication) or a general medical condition.

E. *Relationship to a pervasive developmental disorder*: If there is a history of autistic disorder or another pervasive developmental disorder, the additional diagnosis of schizophrenia is made only if prominent delusions or hallucinations are also present for at least a month (or less if successfully treated).

F. *Classification of longitudinal course* (can be applied only after at least 1 year has elapsed since the initial onset of active-phase symptoms):
Episodic with interepisode residual symptoms (episodes are defined by the reemergence of prominent psychotic symptoms); *also specify if*: **with prominent negative symptoms**
Episodic with no interepisode residual symptoms
Continuous (prominent psychotic symptoms are present throughout the period of observation); *also specify if*: **with prominent negative symptoms**
Single episode in partial remission; *also specify if*: **with prominent negative symptoms**
Single episode in full remission
Other or unspecified pattern

season of birth appears to be a factor. More babies who later become schizophrenic are born in the winter months (Amenson, 1999). There are two possible explanations for this phenomenon. One is that schizophrenia may be related to prenatal exposure to viral infections. The other is that there is a seasonal release of overripe ova in the winter, which results in consequent anomalies in the fetus at fertilization (Kaplan and Sadock, 1998).

CLINICAL DESCRIPTION

According to the DSM-IV-TR classification, a diagnosis of schizophrenia must meet the following criteria: (1) it lasts at least 6 months, at least 1 month of which includes "active-phase symptoms," and (2) the active-phase symptoms include at least two of the following manifestations: hallucinations, delusions, disorganized or catatonic behavior, or disorganized speech (see DSM-IV-TR Criteria box).

There are five major subtypes of schizophrenia and eleven closely related disorders. The five subtypes of schizophrenia are:
1. Paranoid
2. Disorganized (formerly called hebephrenic)
3. Catatonic
4. Undifferentiated
5. Residual

The closely related disorders are:
1. Schizophreniform disorder
2. Schizoaffective disorder
3. Delusional disorder
4. Brief psychotic disorder
5. Shared psychotic disorder (*folie a deux*)
6. Psychotic disorder due to a general medical condition
7. Substance-induced psychotic disorder
8. Pervasive developmental disorder (autism and others) (NOTE: The additional diagnosis of schizophrenia is warranted only if prominent delusions or hallucinations are present for at least 1 month.)
9. Simple deteriorative disorder (simple schizophrenia)
10. Postpsychotic depressive disorder of schizophrenia
11. Psychotic disorder not otherwise specified (NOS)

Paranoid Schizophrenia

Paranoid schizophrenia results in less neurologic and cognitive impairment and a better prognosis for the individual. However, in the active phase of the disorder, the afflicted individual is extremely ill, and the symptoms may constitute a danger to self or others.

Delusions tend to be persecutory or grandiose and have a coherent theme. The persecutory delusions may generate anxiety, suspiciousness, anger, hostility, and violent behavior. Auditory hallucinations are common and are related to the delusionary theme. Interactions with others are rigid, intense, and controlled (APA, 2000; Fortinash and Holoday Worret, 2003; Kaplan and Sadock, 1998).

According to the DSM-IV-TR criteria for schizophrenia, a diagnosis of paranoid schizophrenia must meet two of the symptoms in criterion A: the presence of delusions and hallucinations. The other diagnostic criteria for paranoid schizophrenia—disorganized speech, behavior, and other negative symptoms—are not prominent. The delusions and hallucinations must be present for a significant portion of time over a period of 1 month. This period can be shorter if the condition is successfully treated. Also, if delusions are unusually bizarre or if the hallucinations involve commanding or commenting voices, only one of the criteria needs to be met. Paranoid schizophrenia often has a sudden onset, sometimes triggered by severe stressors (APA, 2000; Fortinash and Holoday Worret, 2003). The individual with paranoid schizophrenia is sometimes referred to as a type I, productive client, with positive symptoms.

Crow (1980) proposed that symptoms in schizophrenia could be classified as positive symptoms (the syndrome includes hallucinations, increased speech production with loose associations, and bizarre behavior) or negative symptoms (the syndrome includes flat affect, poverty of speech, poor grooming, withdrawal, and disturbance in volition) as a guide to establishing the prognosis (Andreasen and Carpenter, 1993). Table 11-3 defines positive and negative symptoms.

Prognosis

The course of paranoid schizophrenia is varied but tends to be more hopeful than the courses of other subtypes. Of all the schizophrenias, paranoid schizophrenia is the most responsive to proper treatment and the most likely to qualify for the course of a single episode in full remission (APA, 2000; Kaplan and Sadock, 1998).

Disorganized Schizophrenia

The *disorganized* type of schizophrenia, formerly known as hebephrenic schizophrenia because of its early, insidious onset and silly, childish affect, is characterized by a severe disintegration of the personality. Speech is disorganized and may include word salad (communication that includes both real and imaginary words in no logical order), incoherent speech, and clanging (rhyming). Behavior is odd, encompassing grimacing, grunting, sniffing, posturing, rocking, stereotyped behaviors, and uninhibited sexual behaviors such as masturbating in public. Socially the client with disorganized schizophrenia is withdrawn and inept. There may be many cognitive and psychomotor defects, such as concrete thinking, the literal interpretation and use of language or inability to abstract; **primary process thinking**, prelogical thought that aims for wish fulfillment and is associated with the pleasure principle characteristic of the id portion of the personality; and poor coordination (APA, 2000; Fortinash and Holoday Worret, 2003).

The client with disorganized schizophrenia has poor personal grooming and is often unable to complete activities of

Table 11-3	Symptoms of Schizophrenia Classified According to Type I (Positive) or Type II (Negative)
Type I	**Type II**
Delusions, persecutory or grandiose	Flat or inappropriate affect
Delusions of being controlled	Poor eye contact
Mind reading or thought insertion ideas	Anhedonic attitude and asocial behavior; withdrawal
Hallucinations, auditory or other sensory modes	Poverty of speech; blocking and lack of inflection
Bizarre dress and behavior	Poor grooming and hygiene
Thought disorganization and tangential speech	Decreased spontaneity in behavior
Aggressive, agitated behavior	Lack of expressive gestures
Pressured speech	Avolition (lack of motivation); apathy
Suicidal ideation may be present	Severely disturbed relationships with family, friends, peers
Ideas of reference	Inattentiveness

daily living (ADLs) without constant structural reminders, because the behavior is aimless and without goals (Kaplan and Sadock, 1998). Many type II symptoms are present. Development seems to have been impaired and held to approximately age 7 or 8 years.

Prognosis

Prognosis for the client with disorganized schizophrenia is poor, stemming from an early premorbid history of impaired adjustment that continues after the active phase of the disorder. As mentioned earlier, premorbid refers to the period just preceding the onset of the mental illness. This individual may or may not hallucinate or have delusions, but if they exist, they are disorganized and fragmented.

Of all the subtypes, paranoid schizophrenia and disorganized schizophrenia have the most clearly defined clinical criteria and have been studied the most. Recent studies have indicated a wide interest in the **cognitive symptoms** of schizophrenia, which include memory impairment and lack of problem-solving skills. Negative symptoms, such as emotional blunting, apathy, withdrawal, and avolition, also remain a focus of concern. After all, it is the residual negative symptoms and the cognitive impairment that prevent individuals with this type of schizophrenia from holding jobs and forming lasting, satisfying relationships. Continued research, new medications, and innovations in therapy all offer hope for a brighter prognosis.

Catatonic Schizophrenia

Catatonic schizophrenia has, as its predominant feature, intense psychomotor disturbance. This disturbance may take the form of stupor (psychomotor retardation) or excitement (psychomotor excitation). Manifestations of psychomotor disturbance include posturing, immobility, catalepsy (waxy flexibility), mutism, and negativism. There may be automatic obedience on the one hand and excessive and purposeless movement on the other. Other symptoms include echopraxia (imitating the movements of others), echolalia (repeating what was said by another), grimacing, and stereotypic movements. Often there is rapid alteration between these extremes (APA, 2000; Fortinash and Holoday Worret, 2003; Kaplan and Sadock, 1998).

The onset of catatonic schizophrenia often occurs with dramatic suddenness. Catatonic stupor may be preceded by an earlier withdrawal, carried to the extreme. It reflects the individual's reduced neurologic ability to filter out stimuli. There is no significant difference in age, sex, or education in the incidence of catatonic schizophrenia. To meet the DSM-IV-TR criteria for catatonic schizophrenia, the client must exhibit two of the following behaviors: motor immobility or excessive motor activity; extreme negativism (resistance to all instructions and attempts to be moved); peculiar voluntary movements such as grimacing, stereotyped movements, or posturing; and echolalia or echopraxia (APA, 2000).

The person with catatonic schizophrenia presents a nursing challenge. While in a state of psychomotor excitement, the client may develop hyperpyrexia or collapse from extreme exhaustion. Close watch is indicated to prevent harm to self or others. Conversely, while in a stuporous state, the disease can be life threatening because the person approaches a vegetative condition, will not eat, and is in danger of malnutrition or even starvation. Other complications may include decubitus ulcers (pressure sores) from lack of mobility or strange posturing, constipation, or even stasis pneumonia in the older client.

Delusions often persist throughout the withdrawn state. For example, a client may believe that he has to hold his hand out flat in front of him because the forces of good and evil are warring on the palm of his hand and he will upset the balance of good and evil if he moves his hand. Oddly enough, although this individual may seem not to be attending to the environment around him, when he later returns to a normal state of consciousness, he will remember in detail what has occurred. Nurses need to be aware of this factor and not say or do anything within the stuporous client's hearing that they would not say or do when the client is in a normal state of consciousness.

Prognosis

The prognosis for catatonic schizophrenia varies depending on the age of onset, which is often in the early twenties to thirties. It tends to begin with an acute episode having an identifiable precipitating factor. If the client has developed a good support system before the illness, he or she will probably recover from the acute phase and have a partial or complete remission. More research is indicated for this particu-

lar type of illness, especially as it seems to have subsided in Western nations but is more prevalent in developing nations, where remission is usually complete.

Undifferentiated Schizophrenia

Undifferentiated schizophrenia meets criterion A for schizophrenia but cannot be classified as paranoid, disorganized, or catatonic. It does not clearly meet the criteria necessary for a diagnosis in any of these conditions, but it has some aspects of each type. The psychotic manifestations are extreme, including fragmented delusions, vague hallucinations, bizarre and disorganized behavior, disorientation, and incoherence (Fortinash and Holoday Worret, 2003; Kaplan and Sadock, 1998). Affect is usually inappropriate rather than flat, and catatonic symptoms are not present. A clinical pathway for a client presenting with psychosis is shown in Figure 11-5.

The onset can be acute, with excited behaviors such as aggressive hitting or biting. Or the client may have chronic schizophrenia, with behavior that no longer fits a specific type but is a mixture of positive and negative symptoms. Usually the **prodromal symptoms** have developed over a period of years. Growth and development milestones may have been delayed. Thought processes are fragmented and have a high fantasy content (primary process thinking). The individual has few or no friends, and family relationships are strained because of odd and restless behaviors. Dress and grooming are careless, and the individual seems bored with life. Sleep patterns are disturbed by nightmares and early morning awakening.

Prognosis

The prognosis for the client with undifferentiated schizophrenia is generally poor, and the course is usually chronic. There are periods of exacerbation and remission where many negative symptoms prevent the patient from doing productive work, pursuing normal relationships, or enjoying life (Kaplan and Sadock, 1998).

Residual Schizophrenia

If an individual has had at least one acute episode of schizophrenia and is now free of prominent positive symptoms but has some negative symptoms, he or she is diagnosed with *residual schizophrenia*, or **residual symptoms.** In some clients, this pattern may persist for years, with or without exacerbations. In others it seems to taper down to a complete remission. The usual signs of the illness that may persist for the chronic or subchronic individual are mild loosening of associations, illogical thinking, emotional blunting, social withdrawal, and eccentric behavior. Diagnostic criteria for the client with residual schizophrenia are (1) absence of prominent delusions, hallucinations, disorganized speech, and disorganized or catatonic behavior; and (2) continuing evidence of the presence of negative symptoms or attenuated positive symptoms.

Psychosis

Interval / Location	Day of Admit	Day 2	Day 3	Day 4	Day 5	Day 6	Day 7	Day 8
Physiologic	*Takes adequate fluid/nutrition with assistance *Tolerates meds	*Takes adequate fluid/nutrition with assistance *Increased sleep/rest time *Adequate elimination	*Adequate nutrition with reminders *Adequate elimination	*Sleeps 3-6 hours *Adequate elimination	*Takes adequate nutrition/fluids *Drug levels therapeutic range	*Sleeps 5-8 hours *Absence drug toxicity side effects	*Sleeps 5-8 hours	*Sleeps 5-8 hours *Able to manage food/activity requirements independently
Psychologic	*Tolerates orientation to unit within capacity	*Oriented ×2	*Oriented ×3 *Demonstrates reduction in hallucinations and delusions	*Oriented ×4 *Reality testing with staff *Increased trust demonstrated	*Demonstrates more reality-based thoughts	*Able to focus on one topic 5-10 minutes	*Able to complete unit assignments and activities	*Able to complete unit assignment and activities independently *Able to plan/structure day
Functional Status/Role	*Refrains from harming self or others with assistance	*Refrains from harming self *Attends to basic ADLs *Seeks staff when anxious	*Refrains from harming self *Increased trust demonstrated *Increased ADLs *Complies with meds with reminders	*Increased ADLs *Controls impulses with assistance *Utilizing basic stress management techniques with assistance	*Demonstrates less psychosis and intrusive behavior	*Interacts with peers *Able to make decisions	*Able to maintain safety *Demonstrates safe behaviors	*Able to maintain safety *Independently complies with medical regime
Family/Community Reintegration	*Family/significant other aware of treatment program goals *Family/significant other provide history including meds	*Identifies family/significant other to staff	*Attends community meetings/milieu activities with staff supervision *Identifies family/significant other *Communicates with SW for increased understanding of Treatment goals/DC plans	*Family/significant other included in treatment/DC plans	*Identifies DC needs	*Identifies DC needs	*Identifies DC needs *Able to identify supports and how to use them	*Able to utilize supports and list ways to access them *State specific plans to manage symptoms, comply with meds and aftercare

(Left margin vertical label: OUTCOMES)

Note: This Clinical Pathway is a tool to assist health care providers in achieving quality patient outcomes by providing appropriate and timely patient care. It is not intended to establish a community standard of care, replace a clinician's medical judgment, establish a protocol for all patients, or exclude alternative therapies. (See Variances at end of figure.)

Abbreviations: *CBC,* complete blood chemistry; *DC,* discharge; *ELOS,* estimated length of stay; *etal,* evaluation; *H/O,* history of; *I&O,* intake and output; milieu, therapeutic patient environment; *OT,* occupational therapist; *Résieurit, Résieurit,* hearing to determine if patient is cognitively able to make a decision to refuse psychotropic medication; *S&R,* seclusion and restraint; *SW,* social worker; *UR,* utilization review.

Continued

FIGURE 11-5. Clinical pathway for psychosis.

Interval / Location	Day of Admit	Day 2	Day 3	Day 4	Day 5	Day 6	Day 7	Day 8
Discharge Planning	*(SW) initiate assessment *Identify DC placement ELOS contact family/significant other (nursing) initiates assessment *Identify H/O med compliance knowledge deficit and chronicity	*Team involved in DC planning *Discussed with MD *UR notify managed care	*SW evaluation completed *Specific DC plan identified *Treatment team meeting #1	*Involve family/ significant other in DC plan *Review with patient	*Patient, family/ significant other communicate understanding DC plan and follow-up *UR contact manage care	*Reinforce patient, family/significant other understanding DC plan and follow-up	*Transition to day treatment if indicated *Continue to identify/ reinforce support system	*DC to least restrictive environment
Education	*Orient to unit *Patient's rights *Assess patient/ significant other *Assess knowledge of meds and chronicity	*Assist with symptom recognition and importance of compliance *Include family/ significant other as necessary	*Continue with symptom recognition *Continue to assess level of knowledge re: disorder and meds	*Assist in linking symptoms with precipitating event	*Assist in linking symptoms with precipitating events (noncompliance, drug abuse)	*Reinforce med education *Importance of compliance	*Develop aftercare plan to manage symptoms *Contact supports	*Develop aftercare plan to manage symptoms and contact supports
Psychosocial/ Spiritual/Legal	*Assess: Safety issues Mental status Spirituality Voluntary status	*Continue to assess: Safety issues Mental status Spirituality Voluntary status	*Continue to assess: Safety issues Mental status Spirituality Voluntary status	*Complete assessments and confirm: Safety Mental status Spirituality Legal status	*Continue to assess: Safety issues Mental status Spiritual Voluntary status	*Continue to assess: Safety issues Mental status Spiritual Voluntary status	*Continue to assess: Safety issues Mental status Spirituality Voluntary status	*Legal, psychosocial, spiritual eval completed
Consults	*Physical exam within 24 hours ( )	*Other consults as needed	*Other consults as needed	*Other consults as needed	*Other consults as needed	*Other consults as needed	*Arrange aftercare consults as ordered	*Complete all consults
Tests/Procedures	*Med levels ( ) *Drug screen ( ) *CBC ( ) *Thyroid function ( ) *SMAC ( )	*Other test/ procedures as ordered	*Other test/ procedures as ordered	*Other test/ procedures as ordered	*Other test/ procedures as ordered	*Other test/ procedures as ordered *Check drug levels in therapeutic range	*Other test/ procedures as ordered	*Test procedures as ordered outpatient
Treatment	*Monitor I&O *Monitor sleep/rest patterns *Level of observation 1:1 ( ); every 15 min ( ); every 30 min ( ) *Reduce milieu stimulation *Treatment as ordered *S&R ( ) yes ( ) no ( )	*Monitor I&O *Monitor sleep/rest patterns *Level of observation 1:1 ( ); every 15 min ( ); every 30 min ( ) *Treatment as ordered	*Monitor I&O *Monitor sleep/rest patterns *Level of observation 1:1 ( ); every 15 min ( ); every 30 min ( ) *Treatment as ordered	*Monitor I&O *Monitor sleep/rest patterns *Level of observation 1:1 ( ); every 15 min ( ); every 30 min ( ) *Continue treatment plan as ordered	*Level of observation: 1:1 ( ); every 15 min ( ); every 30 min ( ) *Treatment plan as ordered *Monitor sleep/rest pattern	*Level of observation: 1:1 ( ); every 15 min ( ); every 30 min ( ) *Treatment plan as ordered *Monitor sleep/rest pattern	*Level of observation: 1:1 ( ); every 15 min ( ); every 30 min ( ) *Treatment plan as ordered *Monitor sleep/rest pattern	*Discharge with specified treatment confirmed for aftercare

PROCESSES

PROCESSES								
Medications (IV & Others)	*Meds as ordered *Protocols for antipsychotic med management *Monitor side effects *Toxicity	*Meds as ordered *Protocols for antipsychotic med management *Monitor side effects *Toxicity	*Meds as ordered *Protocols for antipsychotic med management *Monitor side effects *Toxicity	*Meds as ordered *Protocols for antipsychotic med management *Monitor side effects *Toxicity	*Meds as ordered *Contact managed care with med changes *Protocols for antipsychotic med management *Monitor side effects *Toxicity	*Meds as ordered *Protocols for antipsychotic med management *Monitor side effects *Toxicity *Review meds with family/significant other	*Meds as ordered *Protocols for antipsychotic med management *Monitor side effects *Toxicity	*Discharge with meds and instructions as ordered
Activity	*OT assessment *1:1 reality orient/brief contact *Assist with ADLs *Interventions to control self/other harm/impulses	*Continue OT eval *Engage in groups as tolerated *Assist with ADLs *Interventions to control self/other harm/impulses	*OT eval *Engage in groups as tolerated *ADLs with reminders *Interventions to control self/other harm/impulses	*Engage in 2 groups as tolerated *Interventions to control self/other harm/impulses	*Independent ADLs *Engage in 2 groups per day *Provide opportunity for simple decision making	*Independent ADLs *Engage in all unit activities *Provide opportunity for simple decision making	*Independent ADLs *Engage in all unit activities *Encourage independent decision making	*Independent ADLs *Engage in all unit activities *Confirm decision making *Confirm safety
Diet/Nutrition	*Nutritional screening *Elicit food preference *Offer adequate nutrition/fluids *Baseline weight (weekly unless otherwise ordered)	*Offer adequate nutrition/fluids *Provide simple meals: Finger foods Room-temperature drinks	*Offer adequate nutrition/fluids *Encourage meals in milieu as tolerated with staff supervision	*Offer adequate nutrition/fluids *Encourage meals in milieu as tolerated with staff supervision	*Offer adequate nutrition/fluids *Teach family/significant other importance of adequate nutrition/fluids	*Offer adequate nutrition/fluids *Teach family/significant other importance of adequate nutrition/fluids	*Reinforce adequate nutrition/fluids *Weekly weight	*Confirm patient family/significant other knowledge adequate nutrition/fluids *Confirm adequate nutrition/fluids

Pathway Variances: P1. CP completed early   P2. Patient off CP   P3. Pathway Completed & Patient Not Discharged   P4. Initial Interval Not Appropriate

Element Variances:

1. Patient/Family:
1. Patient physiologic status
2. Patient psychologic status
3. Patient/family refusal
4. Patient/family unavailable
5. Patient/family other
6. Patient/family communication barrier
7. Element met early

2. Clinician:
1. Order differs from CP
2. Action differs from CP
3. Response time
4. Clinician other
5. Court/guardianship

3. Operating Unit
1. Bed/appointment not available
2. Lack of data
3. Supplies/equipment not available
4. Department overbooked/closed
5. Court/guardianship
6. Operating unit other

4. Community
1. Placement not available
2. Home care not available
3. Ambulance delay
4. Transportation not available
5. Community other

5. Payer
1. Delayed giving authorization number
2. Payer limitations
3. Payer other

FIGURE 11-5—cont'd. Clinical pathway for psychosis.

Prognosis

Prognosis is varied and unpredictable. It depends largely on premorbid history and the adequacy of support systems (APA, 2000; Kaplan and Sadock, 1998).

Schizophreniform Disorder

The defining characteristics of *schizophreniform disorder* are the same as for schizophrenia, with two exceptions. The first is the duration, and the second is impairment of function. The duration is at least 1 month but less than 6 months. If symptoms persist for 6 months or longer, the diagnosis is changed to schizophrenia. Social or occupational functioning may or may not occur in this disorder, unlike the diagnosis of schizophrenia, where functional disturbance (relationships, school or work, self-care) will be present. It is estimated that one third of these individuals recover completely, and two thirds are likely to develop schizophrenia.

Prognosis

It is estimated that one third of these individuals recover completely, whereas two thirds are likely to develop schizophrenia.

Schizoaffective Disorder

Schizoaffective disorder is a closely related disorder of schizophrenia, but the onset of illness generally occurs later in life. It presents with severe mood swings of either mania or depression and also with some of the psychotic symptoms. Most of the time, mania or depression coexists with the psychotic symptoms, but there must be at least one 2-week period in which there are only psychotic episodes. The cause of schizoaffective disorder is still unknown, but most researchers believe that the etiology is related to a combination of biologic, genetic, and environmental factors.

Symptoms

Symptoms that may occur during the depressed phase include:
- Poor appetite
- Weight loss
- Inability to sleep
- Agitation
- General slowing down
- Loss of interest in usual activities (anhedonia)
- Lack of energy or fatigue
- Feelings of worthlessness
- Self-reproach
- Excessive guilt
- Inability to think or concentrate, or thoughts of death or suicide

Symptoms that may occur during the manic phase include:
- Increase in social, work, or sexual activity
- Increased talkativeness
- Rapid or racing thoughts
- Grandiosity
- Decreased need for sleep
- Increased goal-directed activity
- Agitation
- Inflated self-esteem
- Distractibility
- Involvement in self-destructive activities

Symptoms that may occur during psychotic episodes include:
- Delusions (fixed beliefs—altered thought processes)
- Hallucinations (sensory/perceptual alterations)
- Incoherence
- Severely disorganized speech or thinking
- Grossly disorganized behavior
- Total immobility
- Lack of facial emotional expression (flattened or blunted affect)
- Lack of speech or motivation

Treatment

- *Psychotherapy*. It is recommended that the nurse and client work together to establish goals.
- *Medications*. Antipsychotics, antidepressants, lithium, and/or other mood stabilizers. Often several medications are used in combination.
- *Skills training*. Focuses on interpersonal skills, grooming and hygiene, budgeting, grocery shopping, job seeking, cooking, etc.

Self-Management

The following instructions may be given to the client regarding measures that may maximize the prognosis:
- Accept the fact that this is a prolonged illness.
- Identify strengths and limitations.
- Set clear, realistic goals.
- After a relapse, slowly and gradually return to responsibilities.
- Plan a regular, consistent, predictable, daily routine.
- Make home a quiet, calm, relaxed place (as possible).
- Identify and reduce stress (as possible).
- Make only one change in life at a time.
- Work toward an active, trusting relationship with nurses and treatment staff.
- Take medication regularly, as prescribed.
- Identify early signs of relapse and develop an early warning list.
- Become involved with people with whom you feel comfortable.
- Avoid street drugs.
- Discuss intake of alcoholic beverages with your physician.
- Eat a well-balanced diet.
- Get sufficient rest.
- Exercise regularly.
- Check reality with a trusted individual if you are unsure of the nature of your thoughts or feelings.
- Contrast your behavior with others if you are unsure of the nature of your actions.
- Accept that there may be occasional setbacks.

Managing Relapse

The following instructions may be given to the client for managing a relapse:

- Develop a plan of action with your nurse or therapist if relapse signs appear. (This is best done during well periods.)
- Involve a friend, family member, or other trusted individual to help in times of relapse.
- Your plan should include specific warning signs of relapse, an agreement to notify the nurse or therapist as soon as relapse warning signs appear, an agreement to contact those individuals who can help reduce stress and stimulation, and a list of specific ways to decrease stress and stimulation and increase structure.

Prognosis

This disorder often has a better prognosis than schizophrenia but a less positive prognosis than depression. It is a lifelong illness for most individuals, although the precise course of illness differs for each person. Symptoms tend to worsen during times of stress and may limit functioning, resulting in hospitalization.

Symptom Profiles of the Schizophrenias

Neuropsychiatrists have tried to find common threads that link the schizophrenias or areas of differentiation that separate them. There is a common underlying theme in schizophrenic disorders that gives rise to certain symptom profiles of a perceptual, cognitive, emotional, behavioral, or social nature (Table 11-4).

Perceptual Disturbances

Hallucinations can occur in any of the five receptive senses (auditory, visual, tactile, olfactory, or gustatory), but the most common are auditory. It is believed that a left hemisphere brain abnormality may precipitate hallucinations because the left hemisphere contains Broca's area, the language-processing center. From assessment procedures, it was determined that the left hemisphere responded to hallucinations as if it were hearing real voices. There is an indication that the hallucinations are a reflection of the actual delusional thinking of the person with schizophrenia (Green et al., 1994; Lewandowski, 1991).

Another aspect of perception that has been explored in the individual with schizophrenia is self-perception. One way in which the nurse can assess the severity of perceptual disturbances is by using art forms that indicate how the person with schizophrenia perceives the world or the self. Because of their tendency to generalize, individuals with schizophrenia often report an overall negative self-perception (Evans et al., 1994). It has been noted in the literature, however, that clients with schizophrenia who lived in a satisfactory setting saw themselves as mentally well, although they were disabled to the extent that they were not able to live independently.

Clients and families must recognize that hallucinations are symptoms of the illness and are real to the client. As such, family attempts to force the objective truth or plausibility are not therapeutic and may even be demeaning. Hallucinations respond to a reduction of stress and an increase in antipsychotic medication. They can often be made less troubling by time-proven distractions such as keeping the client busy, using competing stimuli to "drown out" the voices (whistling, clapping, shouting the word "stop"), and teaching the client not to "wait" for the voices to occur, but instead occupy the mind with some other activity (Thornton et al., 2001c).

Thought Disturbances

According to D'Angelo (1993), thought disorders can begin in children at risk for schizophrenia as a result of their heredity. Children of parents with schizophrenia tend to be conceptually disorganized, possibly because they do not correctly categorize information as other children do in the childhood learning process. Also, children are normally very distractable, so it may be difficult to determine the onset of a thought disorder at such an early age (Smothergill and Kraut, 1993).

Even as adults there is a tendency to personalize and misinterpret events, most notably in times of stress or fatigue. It is self-fulfilling to occasionally escape from reality and imagine ourselves as more powerful or successful than we really are. For those of us without schizophrenia, however, these periods of fantasy are generally short-lived and well within our control. What is different in the client with schizophrenia who is experiencing a delusion during an acute period is that the conviction is fixed, and any attempt by well-meaning individuals to explain reality during this time is rejected out of hand. Arguing with a client experiencing a delusion leads to further mistrust or anger. Families and friends must realize that delusions are a result of the illness and not stubbornness or stupidity on the part of the client. Emotional reactions, sarcasm, or threats should be avoided. There is always something about the delusion or conviction that can invoke an empathetic response.

For example, if the client believes he or she is at the center of a government plot and cannot sleep at night, there may be underlying feelings of worthlessness or fear, and the delusion fills the need to be important and protected. An empathetic response might be: "It must be difficult not to be able to get some sleep at night and to feel afraid. You are safe here in the hospital, and the care you get will help you feel better." This type of response builds trust, rapport, and, it is hoped, adherence to the treatment plan that will help the client improve (Thornton et al., 2001c). Implications for the psychoeducation of persons with schizophrenia include:

- Teaching at times when symptoms are relatively stable
- Simplifying instructions and reducing distractions (or providing distractions to offset symptoms as necessary)
- Providing both visual and verbal information
- Using direct, clear terms versus abstractions or concepts
- Teaching in small segments with frequent reinforcement
- Not offering choices that often confuse the individual, yet offering simple choices as client improves

Table 11-4   Clinical Symptoms of Schizophrenia

Perceptual	Cognitive	Emotional	Behavioral	Social
Hallucinations: **Auditory:** May be commanding; content matches delusions Visual **Tactile** (e.g., may feel like being surrounded by spiderwebs) **Olfactory and gustatory:** Client may refuse to eat because food seems to smell or taste bad **Illusions:** False perceptions due to misinterpretations of real objects **Altered internal sensations:** **Formication:** Sensation of worms crawling around inside one **Chill:** Feeling of chills in the marrow of one's bones **Agnosia:** Perceptual failure to recognize familiar environmental stimuli, such as sounds or objects seen or felt; sometimes called "negative hallucinations" **Distortion of body image:** With respect to size, facial expression, activity, amount and nature of detail, exaggeration or diminution of body parts **Negative self-perception:** With respect to ability and competence	**Delusions:** Unusual ideas, not reality based: Omnipotence Persecution Controlling or being controlled **Derealizaiton:** Loss of ego boundaries; cannot tell where own body ends and environment begins; feeling that the world around one is not real or distorted **Ideas of reference:** Notion that other people or the media are talking to or about one **Errors in recall of memory:** Due to incorrect categorization **Difficulty sustaining attention:** Unable to complete tasks Errors of omission **Incorrect use of language:** Neologisms (invented words) Incoherence Echolalia and word salad Concrete, restricted vocabulary Comprehension difficulties Looseness of associations **Flight of ideas:** Abrupt change of topic in a rapid flow of speech	**Labile affect: range of emotions:** Apathy, dulled response Flattened affect Reduced responsiveness Exaggerated euphoria Rage **Inappropriate affect:** Laughing at sad events, crying over joyous ones **Disruption in limbic functioning:** Inability to screen out disruptive stimuli and loss of voluntary control of response	**Little impulse control:** Sudden scream as a protest of frustration Self-mutilation, to substitute physical for emotional pain Injury to a body part believed to be offensive Response to command hallucinations **Inability to cope with depression:** Depressed client has a 50% risk for suicide Frequent exacerbations and remissions in one who has insight Lack of social support to help **Inability to manage anger:** Anger and lack of impulse control lead to violence—verbal aggression, destruction of property, injury to others, homicide **Substance abuse as coping:** Dulls painful psychologic symptoms **Noncompliance with medication:** May feel it is not needed or has too many side effects	**Poor peer relationships:** Few friends as a child or adolescent Preference for solitude **Low interest in hobbies and activities:** Daydreamer Not functioning well in social or occupational areas Preoccupied and detached Behavioral autism **Loss of interest in appearance:** Careless grooming Introversion **Not competitive in sports or academics:** Poor adjustment to school Withdrawal from activities **May suffer from:** Attention deficit disorder Somatic symptoms

As a result of thought disturbance, speech is affected. Subtle forms of speech disorders are *circumstantiality,* in which the person digresses to unnecessary details, and *tangentiality,* or responding in a manner irrelevant to the topic at hand. If the person is less impaired, listening for themes may help to identify client concerns (Hoffman, 1994; Kaplan and Sadock, 1998).

Thought processes in schizophrenia fluctuate with the individual's clinical status. As clinical status worsens, thoughts may evolve into a world of fantasy or be expressed as autistic thinking (internally stimulated thoughts not based in reality), **perseveration** (persistent repetition of the same idea in response to different questions), **poverty of thought** (lack of ability to produce thoughts), and loosening of associations (LOA) (fragmented, incoherent thoughts) (Gundel and Rudolf, 1993; Kaplan and Sadock, 1998).

It is difficult to communicate with the client during these acute phases, which is frustrating to family and friends. Communicating nonverbally such as through the written word may work, as thoughts tend to be more organized in writing. Do not force yourself to listen, as it will only frustrate both the client and the listener. Also, do not speak to others about the client as if the client were not there. Determine where the client's interests and talents are, and use music, art, exercise, or movement to communicate during this period. Even if the language side of the brain is not functioning, the client may still be able to focus on other activities. In the client with chronic disease, there is a general decline in intellectual functioning over the years, which presents a real challenge to nurses, families, and caregivers (Thornton et al., 2001c).

Memory in adult-onset schizophrenia is usually intact, but in persons with chronic schizophrenia it is affected by emotion; the client remembers less and forgets rapidly over time. Negative emotional experiences and concepts, however, are remembered more readily than positive ones, perhaps reflecting a depressed and negative outlook on the world (Calev and Edelist, 1993). Clients with chronic schizophrenia have little insight into their illness and, as such, experience impaired judgment. Patience, empathy, and understanding are critical factors in caring for clients with chronic schizophrenia. As in clients with dementia who also suffer from memory loss, group sing-a-longs in which long-term memory stores are invoked may be helpful.

Emotional Disturbances

Although emotional disturbance is a primary sign of all forms of schizophrenia, affect flattening and poor eye contact are most associated with undifferentiated schizophrenia. Persons with schizophrenia cannot adapt their thinking to the common reality; they block whatever does not fit into their own inner reality (Gundel and Rudolf, 1993).

Biologically the individual with schizophrenia may be unable to screen out disruptive stimuli because of an imbalance in neurotransmitters. A deficiency in GABA, for example, may result in a rush of conflicting stimuli and labile or inappropriate emotional expression, whereas a deficiency in cholecystokinin is related to avolition and flat affect (see Table 11-2). Developmentally, it was found that in children at risk for schizophrenia, neuromotor dysfunction resulting from trauma or other causes indicated the later appearance of flat affect (Dworkin et al., 1993).

Behavioral Disturbances

The behavioral disturbance of greatest concern that is seen in schizophrenia is the possibility of violence. The incidence and type of violence largely depend on certain factors: diagnostic type of schizophrenia, degree of psychopathology, history of violent behavior in the past, abuse of substances, and noncompliance with medications (Kennedy, 1993; Mulvey, 1994). In terms of diagnostic type, there is a significant difference between paranoid schizophrenia and other types of schizophrenia with regard to aggression. Clients with paranoid schizophrenia exhibit physical aggression toward others more often than clients with other types (Kennedy, 1993; Mulvey, 1994).

However, although the *relative risk* for violence is higher in the mentally ill population (of any diagnosis) than in the general population, the *absolute risk* is very small (Mulvey, 1994). Whether or not the inclination for violence is expressed depends on other factors, as indicated previously.

Social Competence Profiles

Typically the individual with schizophrenia has a history of a schizoid or schizotypal personality. According to Dworkin et al. (1994), poor social competence may be important in the development of schizophrenia. Once again, the issue of nature versus nurture arises, and there is speculation that children raised by parents with schizophrenia may emulate their parents in socialization behavior (Turner, 1993). There is a detachment from the environment and an autistic relationship to reality (Gundel and Rudolf, 1993; Kaplan and Sadock, 1998).

Of all of the diagnostic profiles, however, the two still most commonly used to describe schizophrenia were derived from the early work of Bleuler and Schneider, as presented in Table 11-5 (Kaplan and Sadock, 1998).

Biologic Profiles

Symptom profiles are supported by neurologic examinations, neuropsychologic tests, and various brain-scanning techniques (neuroimaging) relevant for clients with schizophrenia. Some of these examinations are presented in Table 11-6. In general, the tests verify findings that schizophrenia has diffuse, nonlocalizable areas of dysfunction. Evidence of generalized impairment can be found in persons with a first episode, as well as chronic schizophrenia, although the degree of impairment may differ with subtypes. Individuals with schizophrenia seem to have impairments in the stimulus inhibition (gating) circuitry of the brain, sometimes leading to stimulus overload. Thus they are handicapped in sorting out and paying attention to the information necessary to solve a problem.

Table 11-5	Diagnostic Profiles of Bleuler and Schneider
Bleuler	Schneider
Characteristics of schizophrenia:	First-rank symptoms of schizophrenia:
Incongruence between feelings and thoughts	Hallucinations
Incongruence in the behavioral expression of feelings and thoughts	Thought withdrawal (belief that one's thoughts have been removed from one's head)
Four primary symptoms of schizophrenia:	Thought broadcasting (belief that one's thoughts are broadcast from one's head)
Affect is disturbed	Delusions
Autism is present	Somatic experiences
Ambivalence is common	Second-rank symptoms of schizophrenia:
Associations are loosened	
Accessory symptoms:	Perceptual disorders
Hallucinations	Perplexity
Delusions	Mood changes
	Feelings of emotional impoverishment

Table 11-6	Biologic Profiles in Schizophrenia	
Neurologic Examinations		
Test	*Function*	
Apgar rating of the newborn	To rate functioning of the newborn nervous system	
Physiologic and anatomic testing of the nervous system (general)	To discover infections, lesions, or metabolic problems that may affect the nervous system	
Neuropsychologic Tests		
Test	*Function*	
Halstead-Reitan battery	To test higher cortical functioning	
	To detect early signs of memory and cognitive dysfunction	
	To design and evaluate remediation programs (Osmon, 1991)	
Luria-Nebraska test battery	To predict behavior by examining neurologic functioning (Meador and Nichols, 1991)	
	To assess client progress in various areas	
Eye-tracking and auditory tests	To discover information-processing deficits (Perry and Braff, 1994)	
Electrical Impulse Testing		
Test	*Function*	
Electrodermal activity (EDA) test	To indicate the extent of negative symptomatology present in the client with schizophrenia (Fuentes et al., 1993)	
Electroencephalogram (EEG)	To detect electrical activity in seizure disorders, sometimes associated with schizophrenia	
Neuroimaging Studies		
Test	*Function*	
Magnetic resonance imaging (MRI)	To determine structural and functional changes in the brain, which may confirm specific anomalies in the brains of individuals diagnosed with schizophrenia	
Positron emission tomography (PET)	To determine effects of antipsychotic medications on certain neurotransmitter receptor sites and their various rates of occupancy by studying sections of the brain	
Bioelectron activity measure (BEAM)	To measure activity of the brain in clients with schizophrenia by using colorized topography	

Modern brain-scanning technology has enabled scientists to assemble not only a structural image of the brain, active or inert, but also a functional image that indicates activity in various areas (Figure 11-6). Forthcoming functional MRI studies, mentioned earlier (see Figure 11-2), may improve this contemporary area of research, as modern technology will enable information to be transmitted more rapidly via the Internet.

PROGNOSIS

In addition to the general statements about the expected prognosis for each subtype of schizophrenia, there has been evidence for specific relationships between symptom profiles and prognostic predictions. For example, Goldman et al. (1993) looked at the interrelationship between neuropsychologic functioning and treatment response, and found that the ability to encode, process information, and interact with the environment depends on being able to attend, focus, and remember. When these abilities are compromised by frontal lobe impairment, partly as a a result of a paucity of dopamine in the frontal lobe areas, negative symptoms (apathy, avolition, withdrawal, blunted affect) tend to remain and interfere with daily living.

Fortunately, newer, atypical antipsychotics show promise in treating the negative symptoms of schizophrenia, which may improve the prognosis for clients who respond favorably to these medications. As mentioned earlier, increased dopamine results from the blocking effects of atypical agents on serotonin, thereby increasing dopamine in the frontal lobes and improving cognitive functioning. Also significant is that clients taking atypical agents are at much less

risk for developing extrapyramidal symptoms, which has been a major deterrent in medication adherence. Clozapine, discovered in 1958 in Switzerland and given limited approval in 1989, is currently viewed by many psychiatrists as the "gold standard" atypical agent, in that it relieves negative symptoms and also reduces suicidality (10% to 15% of persons with schizophrenia are suicidal). Atypical agents such

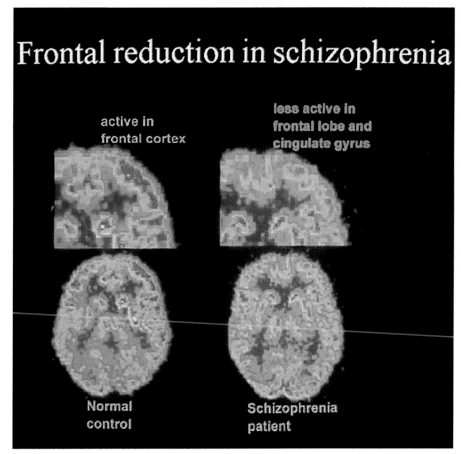

FIGURE 11-6. Positron emission tomography (PET) scan with 18F-deoxyglucose shows metabolic activity in a horizontal section of the brain in a control subject *(left)* and in an unmedicated client with schizophrenia *(right)*. Red and yellow indicate lower activity in the white matter areas of the brain. The frontal lobe is magnified to show reduced frontal activity in the prefrontal cortex of the client with schizophrenia. (Courtesy Monte S. Buchsbaum, MD, Mt. Sinai School of Medicine, New York, NY.)

as aripiprazole (Abilify), now in clinical trials, may pave the way for improved treatment outcomes and a brighter prognosis because of its synergistic effect on both dopamine and serotonin systems.

The use of technology such as PET scans, MRI, and BEAM allows researchers to probe into the structure and function of the brain to a greater extent than ever before.

Finally, schizophrenia is similar to other medical conditions. It has a range of courses and outcomes. Contrary to many misconceptions contained in the older literature, five long-term studies exceeding 20 years' duration confirm that approximately 60% of people with schizophrenia achieve an outcome of full recovery or significant improvement. Unfortunately, those who have successfully overcome this complex disorder are reluctant to talk about it, and the group who are among the 40% who do not fare as well receive more attention. Even in this group, however, the likelihood of improvement remains positive (Thornton et al., 2001a).

As we think about how far research has come since the beginning of the "decade of the brain," there is a new optimism that researchers will find the key to the multiple causes of this complex disorder, so that its sufferers can re-turn to the community with confidence and hope. While we wait for a cure, people with schizophrenia still need care and treatment, whether they are clients in a hospital setting or struggling to exist in the community neighborhoods. Specific issues that challenge a community health nurse are discussed in the Nursing Care in the Community box.

DISCHARGE CRITERIA

For the client with schizophrenia to be discharged to the community, the following criteria need to be met.

Client will:
- Demonstrate absence of suicidality.
- Verbalize absence or control of hallucinations.
- Identify events or episodes of increased anxiety that promote hallucinations.
- Have family or a significant other willing to serve as a support network.
- Accept referral of self or a significant other to a physician, therapist, or agency for help and monitoring.
- Accept responsibility for own actions and self-care.
- Verbalize ways of coping with anxiety, stress, and problems encountered in the community.

NURSING CARE IN THE COMMUNITY   The Schizophrenias

The community mental health nurse often works with a continuum of clients with schizophrenia. This clientele includes young persons newly diagnosed and mature adults with schizophrenic illnesses who have been functioning adequately for several years with antipsychotic medications.

The nurse must also help older adults, who are often socially isolated because their support systems have been exhausted, as friends and family members have withdrawn, moved away, or died. Their most important contacts may be either in mental health agencies or in peripheral support systems, such as board-and-care operators, hotel managers, store owners in the proximate community, or employers. They may need not only monitoring regarding medications but also help with financial management and basic activities of daily living, such as those involving nutrition, clothing, and cleanliness. Sometimes, planning a periodic special outing promotes increased interest in appearance and behavior.

When a young person who has been hospitalized and received a diagnosis of schizophrenia returns to the community, the family has already been disrupted by bizarre behavior. Parents and siblings may need increased help in adjusting to this disturbing diagnosis. The community mental health nurse is an essential liaison to the medical establishment and may also provide a reality check when family interactions seem out of control. The nurse may make referrals to community service organizations and support groups while serving as the liaison with the hospital.

For the adult client who carries a diagnosis of schizophrenia, the community mental health nurse is also an important contact. The nurse can help with problems of medication management, give support when stressful situations arise, and advise the psychiatrist when the client's behavior indicates that the current medication regimen is not effective. The goal is to maintain the client at an optimal, satisfying level of life activities.

The problem of street drug abuse and homelessness is also a concern of mental health nurses in the community. Many socially isolated individuals with a diagnosis of schizophrenia find the society of the streets to be a tolerant environment and the use of street drugs an acceptable alternative to prescribed medications. The mental health nurse who attempts to intervene in this cycle may encounter immense resistance from the client and the community. Often it requires the support of a trained mental health team, as well as the education and participation of the entire community, to break this destructive cycle. Mental health nurses must be prepared to collaborate with the community to help clients reach their potential.

- Have access to a safe living environment in the community: own home, board-and-care facility, or halfway house.
- Use known community resources, such as support groups, day care centers, and vocational or rehabilitation programs.
- Explain the following about medication: importance, expected effects, adverse effects, prescribed dose and time of taking the medication, and effects of the interaction of the medication with other substances such as food or alcohol.

THE NURSING PROCESS

ASSESSMENT

Assessment of the individual with schizophrenia is complicated because of the different symptom profiles for the various subtypes of the condition. Subjective data are obtained through symptom reporting and by the behavioral descriptions of significant others. Objective assessment is done by observation, by using rating scales, and by checking biologic indicators, as described in earlier sections. For psychiatric mental health nurses, it is important not to lose sight of the biologic focus so prevalent in the other specialties. For example, ataxia may indicate extrapyramidal side effects of medication. Also, just as with any other patient, vital signs, nutrition, exercise, and sleep assessment are important (Trygstad, 1994).

Although the nursing assessment includes certain biologic indicators, it relies largely on psychologic data and may use the Mental Status Examination rating scale to organize the data (see Chapter 6). The Mental Status Examination considers the categories of appearance, behavior, orientation, memory, thought processes, perceptual processes, intellectual functioning, feelings (mood) and affect, insight, and judgment. Four of these categories are particularly important in schizophrenia: disturbances in perception, thought, feelings, and behavior (see Nursing Assessment Questions box on p. 261).

For children and adolescents the assessment of positive and negative symptoms must take into consideration the developmental status of the individual. Measures of thought disturbances in children must consider that their normal patterns of thinking are concrete; abstract thought is not a part of normal thinking in the child. Likewise, because impulse control is developmental in the adolescent, the measures of impulse control must be adjusted in consideration of the client's age (Fields et al., 1994).

NURSING DIAGNOSIS

Nursing diagnoses are formulated from the information obtained during the assessment phase of the nursing process. The accuracy of the diagnosis depends on a careful in-depth assessment. The following is a listing of some of the more common diagnoses applicable to schizophrenia (Collaborative Diagnoses table).

Nursing Diagnoses for Schizophrenia
- Disturbed sensory perception
- Disturbed thought processes
- Impaired verbal communication
- Ineffective coping
- Interrupted family processes
- Risk for self-directed violence

NURSING ASSESSMENT QUESTIONS
The Schizophrenias

1. What problems have you been having recently? How do you feel differently now than before? *To determine the client's perception of the problem.*
2. Do you now or have you ever in the past used alcohol or drugs? If so, when and how often? *To determine the client's use of substances.*
3. Have you heard (sounds, voices, messages), seen (lights, figures), smelled (strange, bad, good odors), tasted (strange, bad, good tastes), or felt (touching, warm, cold sensation) anything that others who were present did not? *To determine if the client is having hallucinations.*
4. What are the voices like that you hear? What do they say? Are they troubling for you? *To determine if they instruct the client to harm self or others.*

Questions to Determine if the Client Is Experiencing Delusions

1. Do you feel that someone or something outside of you is controlling you in some way? Are you able to control other people?
2. Do you feel you are being watched? Followed?

3. Are people talking about you? If yes, explain how you know this.
4. Are you experiencing guilt? Do you have anything to feel guilty about? Do you think you are a bad person? If yes, what makes you believe this?

Things to Observe for During Assessment

- Cognitive changes (e.g., concrete thinking, delusions, fantasies, or autistic communication)
- Hallucinations
- Depersonalization
- Somatization
- Unusual gestures, posture, tone of voice, mannerisms
- Flat affect
- Disheveled, unkempt physical appearance
- Reaction to the interviewer (receptive, distant, resistant)

COLLABORATIVE DIAGNOSES

DSM-IV-TR Diagnoses*	NANDA Diagnoses†
Catatonic schizophrenia	Impaired verbal communication
Disorganized schizophrenia	Ineffective coping
Paranoid schizophrenia	Interrupted family processes
Residual schizophrenia	Disturbed sensory perception
Undifferentiated schizophrenia	Disturbed thought processes
	Risk for self-directed violence
	Risk for other-directed violence

*From American Psychiatric Association: *Diagnostic and Statistical Manual of Mental Disorders,* Fourth Edition, Text Revision. Washington, DC, American Psychiatric Association, 2000.
†From NANDA International (2003). NANDA Nursing Diagnoses: Definitions and Classification 2003-2004. Philadelphia: NANDA.

- Risk for other-directed violence
- Self-care deficit (bathing/hygiene, dressing/grooming, feeding, toileting)
- Social isolation

OUTCOME IDENTIFICATION

Outcome identification is an estimate of the behavioral changes anticipated after interventions and is influenced by the severity of the symptoms, the cultural milieu, and the prognosis for the particular diagnosis. The outcomes of schizophrenia therefore may reflect complex interactions.

Client will:
- Demonstrate significant reduction in hallucinations and delusions.
- Demonstrate absence of self-mutilating, violent, or aggressive behaviors.
- Demonstrate reality-based thinking and behavior.
- Engage in own hygiene, grooming, and ADL skills.
- Socialize with peers and staff and participate in all groups.
- Adhere to medication regimen and verbalize an understanding of the role of medications in reducing psychotic symptoms.
- Demonstrate more functional coping and problem-solving methods.
- Participate in discharge planning with family/significant others.

PLANNING

Planning nursing interventions and treatment geared to the whole person and his or her social environment, including the family, is challenging. Because behavioral problems come from many sources and may range from less serious to extremely serious, interventions at a variety of levels also need to be considered. Medical interventions generally are focused on underlying biologic factors and involve diagnostic procedures such as neuroimaging, somatic strategies, and treatment with medication. The nurse's role at this level is to prepare the client and family by explaining the rationale for the interventions and assisting with treatment adherence. The nurse also uses nursing measures at this level based on his or her knowledge of basic biologic functions and needs.

Interpersonally and socially, clients with schizophrenia are disadvantaged by being unable to view things from the

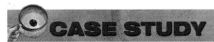

CASE STUDY

Kevin, a 45-year-old male with chronic schizophrenia, was living in a single room in a downtown hotel that houses people with mental illness. Kevin was never able to budget his meager income to last the whole month. He had a fixed delusion that he owned the hotel where he lived, but that the manager and the city government were defrauding him of his rent money. When Kevin was short of cash at the end of the month, he became abusive and aggressive. Fearing assault, the manager would call the police, and Kevin would be readmitted to the psychiatric hospital. In about 10 days he would be discharged to the same hotel where he lived quietly for a while, helping the manager with tasks until the next delusional episode. This was a repetitive pattern for Kevin who had no support from relatives or friends.

Critical Thinking

1. What is the significance of Kevin's delusion, given his low socio-economic status?
2. Kevin received good care at the psychiatric hospital. Standard outcome criteria for discharge were always met. If this pattern continued, what would the chances be that Kevin would hold onto his delusion?
3. Why might a nurse's attempt to challenge the delusion be risky? What are some teaching strategies that nurses could use with Kevin? In what form would they best be implemented?
4. If you were a community mental health nurse, how would you do follow-up care for Kevin?
5. What signs of escalating anxiety would you look for in Kevin's behavior? How would you manage the anxiety?

Box 11-4 The Four Ss of Schizophrenia

Stimulation. Introducing, slowly and gradually, new routines, people, events, and situations to the client.
Structure. Providing daily routine and expectations for every part of the day; waking, dressing, eating, activity.
Socialization. Getting people in their lives to help with finances, health, food, socializing.
Support. Offering encouragement to try new tasks; accompanying client to new places until they make friends.

From Thornton JF et al: *Schizophrenia: symptoms and management at home,* Internet Mental Health, Jan 2, 2001.

perspective of others. Because of the inability to abstract and correctly interpret, the individual with schizophrenia sees others as unpredictable, as being competitors for attention, and as being in control of what is "right" or "wrong" in an absolute sense. Role-playing scenarios, which help clients to see things from another person's perspective, are helpful. Socialization should be a focus of the treatment plan by including the clients in activities that are supportive and nonthreatening and that provide helpful feedback on how the client presents to others. Activities that do not include competition are useful in quelling or preventing aggressive tendencies. Nurses must be alert to avoid power struggles (see Case Study).

Family interactions may be particularly difficult for the client with schizophrenia. If the family (or foster family) does not understand what the treatment team is trying to accomplish and how they are structuring the treatment plan, clients who have been discharged from the hospital after an acute psychotic episode are more likely to experience recidivism. The closer the kinship, the stronger the tension created by ambivalent emotions, which often confuse the client whose insight may be poor (McEnvoy et al., 1993).

IMPLEMENTATION

First and most important is the involvement of the client and family in the treatment process, with explanations and rationales given for all interventions. Interventions may be well

planned but still be challenging for the nurse if there are misunderstandings about what is expected; resistance from client, family, or others; or financial or environmental constraints. As much as possible, clients should set their own goals and pace for treatment and progress.

In the beginning a client may be so ill that he or she cannot understand or accept an appropriate effort to help. In that case, the nurse may need to work on establishing a therapeutic relationship first before the well-meaning interventions will be accepted.

An existing therapeutic relationship between the client and nurse will be expanded later to include the client's family or significant others for lasting effectiveness of the proposed interventions. In some cases the interventions will need to be made at yet another level, the level of the school or the workplace. All involved must be made aware of the what, why, and how of the therapeutic plan so that they can work as a team. The client's cultural background should also be considered when planning interventions.

The family's economic situation also deserves attention. Health care personnel are not usually thinking of the cost of implementing a care plan, which may involve psychotherapy, medication, diet, transportation access to outpatient care, or other factors creating unplanned expenses. It is important to assess for such expenses, problem solve the issues, and include the solutions with the plan.

Thornton et al. (2001c) identifies four important Ss of schizophrenia—stimulation, structure, socialization, and support—to help families and caregivers assist clients to overcome negative symptoms (apathy, lack of motivation, lack of interest, lack of energy) (Box 11-4).

Nursing Interventions

1. Assess and monitor risk factors. *This prevents violence and promotes safety of the client and others.*
2. Reduce/minimize environmental stimulation. *This promotes a quiet, soothing milieu that may lessen the client's impulsivity and agitation and prevent accident or injury.*
3. Provide frequent "time-outs" and/or brief, low-key interactions. *This will calm the client by providing opportunities for rest, relaxation, and ventilation of impulsive feelings, which will reduce the risk of acting-out behaviors.*

4. Support and monitor prescribed medical and psychosocial interventions. *This will encourage the client and family to participate in the treatment plan and prevent the client's behavior from escalating to violence.*

5. Use clear, concrete statements versus abstract, general statements. *The client may not be able to understand complex messages, and, as such, the client may exacerbate misperceptions and/or hallucinations. Individuals with schizophrenia generally respond better to concrete messages during the acute phase.*

6. Attempt to determine precipitating factors that may exacerbate the client's hallucinatory experiences (e.g., stressors that may trigger sensory-perceptual disturbances). *Although hallucinations may have a biochemical etiology, they may be exacerbated by outside stressors in a vulnerable client, and identifying such stressors may help to prevent the severity of the hallucinatory experience.*

7. Praise the client for reality-based perceptions, reduction/cessation in aggressive/acting-out behaviors, and appropriate social interaction and group participation. *Warranted praise reinforces repetition of functional behaviors when given at appropriate times during the treatment regimen, such as when medication has begun to take effect.*

8. Educate the client and family/significant others about the client's symptoms, the importance of medication compliance, and continued use of therapeutic support services after discharge. *This will facilitate learning and increase the client and family/significant other knowledge base, ensure the client's continued therapeutic support, and possibly prevent relapse after discharge from the hospital.*

9. Distract the client from delusions that tend to exacerbate aggressive or potentially violent episodes. *Engaging the client in more functional, less anxiety-provoking activities increases the reality base and decreases the risk for violent episodes that may be provoked by troubling delusions.*

10. Focus on the meaning or feeling engendered by the client's delusional system rather than focusing on the delusional content itself. *This will help to meet the client's needs, reinforce reality, and discourage the false belief without challenging or threatening the client.*

11. Accompany the client to group activities, beginning with the more structured, less threatening ones first, and gradually incorporating more informal, spontaneous activities. *This will promote the client's socialization skills and expand the reality base in a nonthreatening way.*

12. Assist with personal hygiene, appropriate dress, and grooming until the client can function independently. *This will help to prevent physical complications and preserve self-esteem.*

13. Establish routine times and goals for self-care and add more complex tasks as the client's condition improves. *Routine and structure tend to organize and promote reality in the client's world.*

14. Spend intervals of time with the client each day, engaging in nonchallenging interactions. *This will help to ease the client out into the community by first developing trust, rapport, and respect.*

15. Assess the client's self-concept. *A low self-concept may result from or perpetuate social isolation.*

16. Act as a role model for social behaviors in interactions by maintaining good eye contact, appropriate social distance, and a calm demeanor. *This will help the client to identify appropriate social behavior.*

17. Keep all appointments for interactions with the client. *This will promote client trust and self-esteem.*

18. Listen actively to the client's family/significant others, allowing them to express fears and anxieties about mental illness, giving them support and empathy, and emphasizing client's strengths. *This will provide ventilation of pent-up emotions and calm irrational fears while acknowledging realistic concerns, and will promote hope and bonding between the family/significant others and the client.*

Additional Treatment Modalities

It is important that the mental health interdisciplinary treatment team work together to manage each client's mental and emotional disorder and symptoms. Consequently, team meetings are common on the psychiatric unit, where psychiatric mental health nurses, psychiatrists, psychologists, social workers, occupational therapists, recreational therapists, pharmacologists, special education teachers (for children and adolescents), and other support staff come together to communicate their expertise regarding the client's diagnosis, problems, and treatment plans. Briefly described next are the various goals and activities of these collaborative professionals in their respective disciplines (see Additional Treatment Modalities box on p. 264).

Psychopharmacology

Psychopharmacology is the somatic treatment of choice for schizophrenia. The pharmacist dispenses medications for clients with psychiatric disorders according to the physician's prescription, keeps informed on new developments in psychotropic drugs, and, in collaboration with the physician and advanced practice nurses, educates the staff regarding the actions and side effects of the newer neuroleptic drugs. The pharmacist also consults with the psychiatrist regarding chemical properties of the medications and their interactions with food and other drugs. In many institutions the pharmacist also takes some responsibility, along with physicians and nurses, for client and family education.

Psychotropic drugs often have serious side effects. Three of the most serious are akathisia, tardive dyskinesia, and neuroleptic malignant syndrome (NMS) (see Chapter 20 for descriptions).

Additional Treatment Modalities
For Clients With Schizophrenia

Psychopharmacology
Somatic therapy
Milieu therapy
Psychosocial rehabilitation
Individual psychotherapy
    Supportive therapy
    Reeducation therapy
    Reconstructive therapy
Group therapy
Family therapy
Behavior modification
    Operant conditioning
Cognitive-behavioral therapy
Guided imagery
Assertiveness training
Exercise, movement therapy, and dance therapy
Occupational and recreational therapy
Community client-family programs
Therapies to prevent acting out or assault

Atypical Antipsychotic Effect on Serotonin and Dopamine. Results of recent short-term studies indicate that all available atypical antipsychotics, such as clozapine (Clozaril), risperidone (Risperdal), olanzapine (Zyprexa), quetiapine (Seroquel), and ziprasidone (Geodon), are more effective than the typical or conventional antipsychotic haloperidol (Haldol) in blocking serotonin (5-HT2) receptors. This means that the atypical agents are better able to treat the negative symptoms of schizophrenia (apathy, lack of motivation, blunted affect, loss of warmth, loss of humor), with little or no risk of movement disorders. Long-term treatment of schizophrenia is more difficult because of its chronicity and frequent relapse rates. Some studies show that risperidone may be superior to haloperidol in reducing the risk of relapse in chronic schizophrenia (Csernansky, Mahmoud, and Brenner, 2002). Although all antipsychotics block dopamine receptors, research shows that some atypical drugs *dissociate*, or detach, from the receptors more quickly than others, and that fast dissociation from the dopamine (D2) receptors leads to the *atypical antipsychotic effect*.

The term *atypical* currently refers to drugs that have two main effects: (1) they produce no or low extrapyramidal side effects, reducing the risk for movement disorders; and (2) they have the ability to avoid sustained hyperprolactinemia, which is desirable, as there may be some correlation between reduced serum levels of the hormone prolactin and schizophrenia. Many side effects have been attributed to hyperprolactinemia such as galactorrhea, gynecomastia, amenorrhea, decreased libido, ejaculatory problems, and decreased bone density (Kapur and Seeman, 2001). Elevated serum prolactin is related to the antagonism of dopamine receptors and is more common with typical antipsychotics than with atypical antipsychotics (Kapur et al., 2000).

Clozapine (Clozaril) was one of the first drugs to be recognized as atypical and is regarded by many as the "gold standard" of atypical drugs, as it has been shown to reduce negative symptoms as well as suicide risk. The risk of agranulocytosis can be an issue with clozapine, especially for clients who are resistant to medications and frequent blood tests. In such instances a strong support network may increase the client's adherence to medication and laboratory tests that are critical in clozapine therapy (see Chapter 20).

Although these newer antipsychotics have reduced or in some cases eliminated serious side effects such as extrapyramidal symptoms, tardive dyskinesia, and NMS, unpredicted side effects and problems have been documented and may also arise in the future. Thus keen nursing observations and ongoing assessment are critical factors in medication therapy.

Atypical Impact on Anticholinergic Effects

Research shows that *anticholinergic effects*, such as constipation, dry eyes, and urinary retention, which are especially troubling in older adult clients, can be minimized. Recent research conducted in older clients with dementia showed much less incidence of anticholinergic effects in clients treated with risperidone than in clients treated with olanzapine. All of these features affect the person's ability to work, maintain a job, and live a more independent, satisfying life (Maguire, 2002; Boyd, 2002).

Clinical Trials Comparing Typical and Atypical Emergency Medication

An open-label randomized trial was conducted using ziprasidone (Geodon) IM in one group of clients and haloperidol (Haldol) IM in another group. Results yielded significant reduction in baseline client agitation in the ziprasidone group versus the haloperidol group according to the Brief Psychiatric Rating Scale (BPRS) total score and individual agitation items (Brook, Lucey, and Gunn, for the Ziprasidone IM Study Group, 2000). Two clients in the ziprasidone group experienced tachycardia (Brook et al., 2000). This finding is important because the drug has been known to prolong the QTc interval (Glassman and Bigger, 2001); therefore ziprasidone should be used cautiously in clients with cardiac conditions, and individuals admitted to emergency departments who qualify for this treatment must be thoroughly evaluated (Boyd, 2002).

The Role of the Nurse in Pharmacotherapy. The role of the nurse, in collaboration with the physician and pharmacist, is to support or participate in drug research that leads to effective treatment outcomes for clients with schizophrenia, with minimal or no dibilitating side effects. Although the newer, atypical antipsychotics show promise in improving positive symptoms and an even geater advantage in improving negative symptoms, there are still many challenges in treating clients with schizophrenia and helping their families to understand and cope with the illness. These challenges include ongoing adherence to drug therapy, promot-

CLIENT AND FAMILY TEACHING GUIDELINES

Medications

TEACH THE CLIENT AND FAMILY	STRATEGIES	RATIONALE
Right to informed consent and disclosure regarding benefits, side effects, anticipated prognosis with and without medication, alternatives	Initially and any time the medication or dosage is changed, written permission is obtained from the client. Items in the left column are discussed with the client. The nurse consults with the physician regarding disclosure beneficial to the client versus disclosure that may be harmful.	The client has the right to choose the extent to which society may intervene. The client experiences autonomy, self-esteem, and self-control. The client develops trust because of others' regard for his or her concerns.
Correct storage and administration of medications	Explain, demonstrate, and request return demonstration on handling and administration of medications. Work with the client to prepare a check chart on medication, dosage, and times. Gain control of the environment: reduce distractions, simplify instructions, teach in small segments, reinforce often.	Safety of client and others is ensured. The client who is involved develops ownership of process and adherence to treatment regimen. The client will be able to better focus, minimize frustration, and feel successful.
Symptoms that may be reduced or eliminated by the use of medication, action of medication	Encourage the client's own desire to prevent relapse; explain in a matter-of-fact way that many people have various illnesses and take medication for them.	Offers the client hope and reinforcement. Shares the rationale for treatment.
Side effects that may be experienced	Show the client how to use a journal to record feelings, thoughts, and behaviors over time.	Helps the client to assume responsibility for self-care; documents treatment effect.
Food and drug interactions to be avoided	Inform the client about symptoms and events that must be reported, and to whom.	Keeps side effects from getting out of control and causing complications.
How to use the support of family and friends	Include significant others in teaching sessions. Offer thorough education, answer questions, and engage in discussion.	Elicits the support of significant others, decreases family anxiety, and allows the nurse to be a client advocate.

ing medication education, and providing lifelong skills for reintegration into community (Guthrie, 2002; Boyd, 2002).

Quality of life issues are also important in the long-term drug treatment of clients with schizophrenia. Potential adverse effects such as weight gain, diabetes mellitus, sexual dysfunction, cardiac effects, cognitive impairment, and risk for suicide must all be considered and managed by nurses and the health care team, including the client and family (Boyd, 2002). As drug research continues to evolve, most nurses, clinicians, and researchers agree that best treatment practice consists of medication in combination with individual, group and family therapies, and ongoing community involvement.

When a client is discharged to the family and community, one important criterion is that he or she accept responsibility for self-care, particularly with respect to medication. This has important implications for health teaching by nurses (see Client and Family Teaching Guidelines box).

Interventions for Agitation Symptoms. For clients demonstrating agitated or combative behaviors, the "gold standard" of treatment has been the use of intramuscular (IM) antipsychotics (haloperidol) and benzodiazepines (lorazepam) (Osser and Sigadel, 2001). Recent research indicates that rapid control of acute agitation in schizophrenia can be achieved through use of certain atypical antipsy-

chotics, with low incidence of extrapyramidal symptoms. However, researchers also indicate that more clinical experience is needed to ensure safety and efficacy, especially with the older population and clients with renal or hepatic impairment (Murphy, 2002).

Pharmacotherapy may be used in conjunction with physical or behavioral restraints for assaultive or combative clients when verbal interventions fail and client refuses to take oral medications). Restraints are applied according to guidelines set forth by the Joint Commission on Accreditation of Health Care Organizations (JCAHO) in conjunction with other accrediting bodies such as the Department of Health Services (DHS) and the Centers for Medicare and Medicaid Services (CMMS) (Murphy, 2002) (see Chapter 4).

Somatic Therapy

Somatic therapy had its origin in the concept of the sanitarium, a place where persons with mental illness could go for rest and healthy physical treatment. The idea of the sanitarium was to offer the clients fresh air, vitamins, a healthy diet, and rest and relaxation. Although this is still a good idea, more than just palliative treatment is available today.

Somatic therapies are infrequently used today, except for electroconvulsive therapy (ECT), which is used most often for severe depression and for some schizophrenic syndromes that are short term and have affective symptoms (Valente, 1991). ECT is also useful for the client with catatonic schizophrenia. A course of treatment usually consists of 6 to 12 episodes. Nursing implications for the client receiving therapy are clear explanation of the procedure, client and family education, renegotiation of the client's consent, nurturance, monitoring, orientation, support, and analgesics for headache after treatment. ECT is discussed in detail in Chapter 19.

Other somatic therapies that have fallen into disuse are psychosurgery (lobotomy), insulin coma therapy, hydrotherapy, and narcotherapy. Therapeutic use of seclusion, restraints, and jackets (walking restraints) is a means for the client to gain self-control of escalating aggressive behavior that may pose a danger to self or others (Table 11-7).

Milieu Therapy

Milieu therapy is a 24-hour environment that shelters, protects, supports, and enhances the client with mental illness. This is the model currently in use on psychiatric units today. It is characterized by individualized treatment programs, self-governance, humanistic attitudes, an enhancing environment, and links to the family and community. The purpose of milieu therapy is to assist the client in learning to manage and cope with stress, as well as to correct maladaptive behaviors (see Chapter 19).

Psychosocial Rehabilitation

As clients move toward community living, a similar model, the psychosocial rehabilitation model, helps them readjust to community living (Boyd, 1994; Olfson et al., 1993). This model, with the assistance of community services, encourages clients to participate with others in the community. This enables clients to develop skills and talents that have lain dormant during their illnesses. The model differs from the hospital-based program in that there is more focus on independence and fewer constrictions. Psychosocial rehabilitation is coordinated by psychiatric mental health nurses who assess physical problems, oversee the functioning of the client in the environment, dispense medications, meet with families, and refer clients to job training and to appropriate service providers in the community. With the loss of hospital beds, future trends point toward case management and psychosocial rehabilitation (Thompson and Strand, 1994).

Table 11-7	Deescalation of Aggressive Behavior	
Concept	**Behavior**	**Rationale**
Managing the environment	Persuade the agitated/angry client to move to another area. Enlist help from colleagues to remove other clients, but have one colleague near you.	Prevents anxiety transference and protects others.
Showing confidence and leadership	(Hold regular drills with staff to practice strategies.) Give clear instructions. Be brief. Be assertive. Negotiate options. If the client has a weapon, instruct him/her to put it on the floor.	Prevents panic when crises occur. Avoids misunderstandings and not knowing what to do. Allows the client to feel that he or she has some room in exercising options.
Maintaining safety	Give signal to staff to call/phone assault team or police per policy (if verbal negotiations fail).	Protects client and others from harm or injury as a result of possible lethal attack.
Encouraging verbalization	Ask questions that are open ended and nonthreatening. Use "How?" "What?" "When?" to get details, but not "Why?" Keep voice calm and modulated.	Refocuses on the client's problem and not on his or her intent to act out the anger. Stops anger from escalating. (Why questions may challenge client.)
Using nonverbal expression	Allow the client body space; do not stand closer than about 8 feet. Keep your body at a 45-degree angle. Assume an open posture; hands at sides, palms outward.	Conveys nonthreatening message, willingness to listen and accommodate the client.
Personalizing yourself and showing concern	Remind the client who you are; the world may seem terrible now, but you haven't done any harm to him or her. Use words such as "we" or "us." Show that you are listening; use general leads such as "go on." Shows empathy.	Encourages and reflects cooperation.
Using disengagement breakaways	Manage hair pulls, choke holds, grabs, and hugs according to safety instructions, videos, and return demonstrations.	Prevents injury to self, the client, and others.
Using removal, seclusion, and restraints	Rehearse these procedures regularly.	Allows the client to regain self-control.
Accurately documenting the event; holding a debriefing session with staff	Keep a detailed record: time, place, circumstances. Review and discuss the event.	Keeps an accurate account (e.g., for legal aspects). Helps staff to deescalate, talk about feelings and learn what went right and how to improve.

Data from Turnbull J et al: Turn it around: short-term management for aggression and anger, *J Psychosoc Nurs* 28(6):6, 1990; *Assault response training and education manual*, Sharp HealthCare, 2002.

In recent years rehabilitative efforts have become increasingly important in the management of long-term schizophrenia. Individuals who are well controlled on their medications but have difficulty with daily activities are excellent candidates for rehabilitative interventions. When these interventions are properly timed in the course of the illness, they can mean the difference between a good and a poor outcome (Thornton et al., 2001a).

Individual Psychotherapy

Individual psychotherapy may be given by a psychiatrist, psychologist, psychiatric social worker, psychiatric clinical nurse specialist, or specialist in family and child counseling, all of whom are educationally prepared at the master's or doctorate level and work autonomously with their clients. The purpose of psychotherapy is to effect a positive change in the client by helping him or her develop effective coping patterns and overcome the feeling of helplessness most clients experience. There are many types of therapy, as described in Chapter 19. The choice of therapy depends on the client's condition and symptoms, as well as the therapist's area of expertise. The levels of therapy are:

- *Supportive therapy:* allows the person to express feelings and reinforces effective coping mechanisms. It is particularly effective for clients with schizophrenia (Olfson et al., 1993).
- *Reeducative therapy:* is useful for the higher-functioning client. It is a cognitive technique that uses role-playing to explore new ways of perceiving and behaving.
- *Reconstructive therapy:* is not considered helpful for clients with schizophrenia (Olfson et al., 1993). It consists of psychoanalysis or intensive therapy groups and delves into all aspects of the client's life (Weiden and Havens, 1994).

Group Therapy

The type of group therapy suitable for clients with schizophrenia varies according to their level of functioning. Nurses generally use the Rogerian Model, also known as Client-Centered Therapy, developed by Carl Rogers (1902-1987), an American psychiatrist, in the 1940s. This is a humanistic therapy that helps clients to express and clarify feelings and promotes acceptance by the therapist. This therapy uses the technique of reflection, is evocative, is not confrontative, and may allow behavioral tryouts by the client (Rogers, 1951) (see Chapter 19).

Family Therapy

For the client with schizophrenia, especially one with paranoia, it may be necessary to begin with individual family therapy in which each family member has a therapist. This type of family therapy is also recommended as a first step for extremely disturbed families. Later, the family may progress to conjoint (nuclear) family therapy, in which communication patterns are emphasized among family members and the integrity of each family member is supported. According to Bellack and Mueser (1993), intervention programs that include educating families through family therapy have helped families to cope with the client's illness, resulting in positive effects on the course of the schizophrenia (see Chapter 19).

Behavior Modification

Behavior modification is a precise approach to bringing about behavioral change. Several types of behavior modification are used for schizophrenia. For example, *operant conditioning* is widely used in child and adolescent units, and is useful for anyone needing to control the behavior of other individuals. It operates on the principle of reinforcing desirable behaviors so that they will recur, and ignoring negative behaviors. Techniques include relaxation and self-control procedures. Results from using this form of therapy indicate that intolerable behaviors such as withdrawal, screaming, incontinence, and incoherence lessen. In some cases it has then been possible to prepare chronically ill, hospitalized persons to live in the community, as both positive and negative symptoms of schizophrenia have improved (Liberman et al., 1994).

Cognitive-Behavioral Therapy

Cognitive-behaviorial therapy explores the connection between distorted thinking and negative behavior. For example, the client who engages in all-or-nothing thinking may not be participating in a craft session because "I can never do anything right." For high-functioning patients, "homework" is assigned to separate out negative thoughts from negative feelings. Intensive cognitive behavior therapy has been used in connection with reduction of neuroleptic dosages in clients who have negative symptoms, suffer medication side effects, and are minimally responsive to medication.

Guided Imagery

Guided imagery is a therapy in which the client pictures past pleasant memories. It is often combined with relaxation therapy and may be used in conjunction with role playing. However, it is not recommended for clients who are experiencing psychosis because it may confuse the client who is out of touch with reality and further compound the client's perceptual or thought disorder.

Assertiveness Training

Assertiveness training deconditions the anxiety arising from interpersonal relationships, which are usually a problem for the client with schizophrenia. This training promotes expressive, spontaneous, goal-directed, self-enhancing behavior.

Exercise, Movement Therapy, and Dance Therapy

These physically oriented therapies help promote identification of the body image through kinesthetic stimulation and provide a form of coping with stress (see Chapter 19).

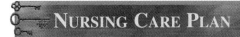

NURSING CARE PLAN

Tyler, a 29-year-old male, was estranged from his family (parents) at age 19 years, when he was diagnosed with chronic undifferentiated schizophrenia, which resulted in his unpredictable and disruptive behavior at home that finally became intolerable. He was sent to live in a board-and-care facility where he was maintained if he took his medications and complied with the program at the day treatment center he attended. The day treatment program provided Tyler with the predictable structure, support, and guidance from staff that he needed, as well as some affiliation and socialization with other clients. Because of his disorder, Tyler was easily influenced by the other clients. One day he was persuaded by a group of clients he considered his "friends" to take the government assistance check he had just received to "go party." He stopped taking his medications, took various street drugs, and failed to return to the board-and-care facility or the day treatment center for a week. He showed up at the center one morning disheveled, dirty, incoherent, and frightened, stating "I am really scared. Everybody left me. I'm hearing voices saying that I'm stupid and hopeless, and no one would help me because I'm not worth saving." Tyler was admitted to the acute care unit in a psychiatric hospital.

DSM-IV-TR Diagnoses

Axis I	Chronic, undifferentiated schizophrenia
Axis II	None
Axis III	None
Axis IV	Moderate to severe = 6 to 7
	Negative influence of "friends"
	Rejection by peers
	Ingestion of illicit drugs
	Lack of adequate support system (family, friends)
	Economic issues (misuse of government assistance check)
Axis V	GAF = 10 (current)
	GAF = 30 (past year)

NURSING DIAGNOSIS: Disturbed sensory perception (auditory hallucinations) related to client stopped taking medications, substance use, inability to process information (biologic factors) secondary to diagnosis of schizophrenia, rejection by peers, isolation and loneliness, low self-esteem, negative self-image/self-concept, and lack of adequate supports as evidenced by verbalization that he hears derogatory voices, fear that no one will help, anxiety; frustration, self-deprecation, and self-care deficit.

CLIENT OUTCOMES	NURSING INTERVENTIONS	EVALUATION
Tyler will demonstrate a reduction in symptoms and an absence of behavior that is harmful to self or others.	Focus on modification and management of symptoms versus elimination of symptoms. *Hallucinations may not be helped by interventions initially. In the meantime, client needs coping skills to manage his symptoms and the environment.*	Tyler remains safe on the unit even though the voices are troubling to him.
	Continually assess Tyler for risk of harm to self or others, even though past history is negative. *Frustration, anger, inability to cope, and derogatory hallucinations could result in violence.*	
Tyler will verbalize that voices are under control ("The voices don't bother me" or "I don't hear the voices").	Assess Tyler's hallucinatory activity, and observe for verbal and nonverbal behaviors associated with hallucinations (talking to self; bolting and running out of the room). *Assessment gives the nurse the opportunity to observe for behaviors that may be associated with hallucinations, and to intervene early in the disturbance, which can often prevent aggression and violence.*	Tyler continues to respond to the "voices."
	Identify, whenever possible, the need filled by hallucinations (dependency, loneliness, rejection, loss of control). *Hallucinations may fill the void created by lack of human contact. Once the need is identified, the client experiences relief and anxiety reduction, and the nurse may then use the therapeutic alliance to assist the client with strategies for growth and change.*	Hallucinations increase when Tyler is rejected by peers, but brief, frequent discussions with nursing staff reduce his anxiety.
	Explore auditory hallucinations for violent content (command hallucinations to harm self or others), and intervene to promote safety for the client and others in the environment. *Immediate intervention is required if the client is a threat to self or others. Otherwise, discussions of content serve only to fix negative beliefs.*	No threatening content is voiced by Tyler.
Tyler will focus on real events and people in the environment.	Orient Tyler to actual activities and events in the therapeutic milieu. *Presenting reality in a nonthreatening way may distract Tyler from his hallucinatory experience by focusing on actual events.*	Tyler is better able to focus on events when rested and not under stress.
	Address Tyler, other clients, and staff by name. *Using the real names of people in Tyler's environment helps to orient Tyler and reinforces reality.*	Tyler responds to own name when addressed.
Tyler will participate in relevant conversations with staff and other clients.	Use simple, concrete, specific language (versus abstract, global language). *The client's misperceptions and altered perceptions may influence the message and interfere with his understanding.*	Tyler responds coherently when conversation is simple and undemanding.
	Use direct verbal responses versus unclear gestures (nodding head yes or no). *Gestures may confuse the client and provide distorted perception or misinterpretation of reality.*	Tyler misinterprets any subtle conversations or gestures by staff or peers.
	Help Tyler to speak slowly and clearly if his speech is incoherent. *This will help Tyler to organize his thought processes and increase his ability to be understood.*	Tyler can slow down and make himself understood when encouraged.

NURSING CARE PLAN—cont'd

CLIENT OUTCOMES	NURSING INTERVENTIONS	EVALUATION
Tyler will participate in planned treatment to decrease or eliminate hallucinations.	Assist Tyler in stopping or managing hallucinations *to give him some control and increase his self-esteem.* Teach techniques that will help control hallucinations: Instruct Tyler to sing, whistle, or clap hands over voices; describe disbelief in messages; contact staff when voices are bothersome; engage in an activity, exercise, or a project when voices begin. *Providing strategies and alternatives to hallucinations gives the client some control and reduces fear and anxiety.* Describe the hallucinatory behavior when the client appears to be hallucinating. "Tyler, you seem distracted. Are you hearing voices?" *By reflecting on the client's behavior in an accepting way, the nurse facilitates disclosure and promotes trust.*	Tyler begins to practice strategies to interrupt hallucinations, with prompting by staff as necessary. Tyler accepts the nurse's observations and continues to use strategies to interrupt hallucinations.
Tyler will engage in more reality-based dialog with staff.	Refrain from arguing or discussing details of content. *When the nurse disagrees, the client will defend the content, which reinforces the importance of the hallucinations.* Voice the nurse's reality about Tyler's hallucinations (e.g., "I don't hear the voices you describe, Tyler. The only voices I hear are those of the people in this room. I know you hear the voices, but with time they may stop.") Don't deny the client's experience. *A realistic, yet nonthreatening, accepting response helps the client to distinguish actual voices from internal stimulation and increases trust.* Refrain from using a judgmental attitude when interacting with Tyler. *A nonjudgmental attitude will avoid diminishing the client's self-esteem and enhances rapport.* Support the medical regimen, including medications. *Medication assists in managing the biologic factors related to hallucination, and often makes it easier to engage the client in psychosocial and interactive therapies.* Discuss with Tyler that sometimes voices do not completely go away, but that he can learn to manage them. *This type of information will help the client to tolerate persistent, unremitting hallucinations and continue techniques that relieve them (whistling, singing, clapping).*	Tyler is beginning to discuss real events more often each day, as staff focus on reality and show acceptance of Tyler. Tyler states he hears the voices less when engaged with staff. Tyler says he appreciates "not being ridiculed" during this troubling time. Tyler takes all prescribed medications; symptoms are remitting. Tyler expresses hope that he can continue strategies when discharged.
Tyler will name two precipitating events occurring just before the onset of hallucinations (e.g., frustration, fear).	Help the client to name precipitants (stressors that trigger hallucinations). *Example:* "What happened just before you heard the voices?" *Anxiety-provoking situations may precede hallucinations. When situations are identified, the client understands the connection and begins to manage, avoid, reduce, or eliminate them.* Continue to explore the content of the hallucinations for violence (command hallucinations to harm self or others). *Immediate intervention is required if this problem arises to protect the client and/or environment from harm. When it is determined that the client is not harmful to self or others, the nurse proceeds to use other therapeutic interventions relevant to the client's needs.*	Tyler is able to reduce the frequency and intensity of hallucinations by using learned techniques (whistling, singing, clapping).
Tyler will express feelings of fear, anxiety, isolation, and rejection.	Continue the nurse-client relationship to encourage sharing of areas that are problematic for the client. *Focusing on the client's immediate needs first relieves client tension, fosters feelings of being understood and accepted, and encourages client to remain engaged with staff.*	Tyler states that he feels understood and helped by staff.
Tyler will engage in milieu schedule and activities.	Provide environmental opportunities (groups and activities) to increase social contact and skills learning. *Involving client in milieu and group activities promotes feeling of belonging, reduces feelings of fear and isolation, and increases self-esteem and mastery of social skills.* Encourage Tyler to attend to self-care (showers, mouth care, grooming). *Attention to self-care promotes acceptance by peers, enhances physical well-being, and increases self-esteem.*	Tyler engages in the same types of groups. He avoids discussion groups but likes occupational therapy. He states that the voices decrease when he is involved in activities or conversations with others. He says he will try harder to get more involved. Tyler's self-care deficit continues, along with other "negative symptoms" such as apathy and withdrawal (he stays in bed much of the time).

Occupational and Recreational Therapy

Occupational therapy is a diagnostic tool that assesses the functional level and progress of the client with schizophrenia. The occupational therapist uses crafts as a tool to check hand-eye coordination, perception, and fine muscle tone. Some visit the client's home to provide special equipment or needed therapy. In fact, today's psychosocial rehabilitation programs depend on active-directive learning principles designed to help the client regain or improve skills, or to develop alternate, compensatory skills useful for community living (Boyd, 1994).

The recreational therapist's emphasis is on body kinesics, movement therapy, and resocialization through recreation. The emphasis is on cooperation rather than competition, especially for the client with schizophrenia. The therapist works on client motivation, planning trips and outings. For a more detailed description of occupational and recreational therapy, see Chapter 19.

Community Client-Family Programs

The National Alliance for the Mentally Ill (NAMI) is an example of an effective community organization that conducts family-to-family and peer-to-peer education programs that train members to teach others about mental illness and its effects on day-to-day living. NAMI also offers strategies for moving forward while coping with mental illness (NAMI Advocate, 2001).

Therapeutic Methods To Prevent and Manage Violence

Given that there is a possibility for violent behaviors in seriously ill clients with schizophrenia, nurses and other clinicians need to be aware of the ways that anger, aggression, and violence are reinforced, and take steps to prevent impending assault. The expression of aggressive behavior may be influenced by defective functioning of the central nervous system (Harper-Jaques and Reimer, 1992). Generally violence occurs as a result of emotional stress, attitude, or behavior of others toward the client with schizophrenia (Vincent and White, 1994). Violence in interpersonal relationships may arise as a result of differing expectations regarding therapeutic rules and their enforcement. Because of the nature of the illness, a client may misinterpret another person's intent, which may provoke a violent response. A person in the acute stages of schizophrenia may exaggerate another's irritation and misread it as fury, or he or she may misinterpret laughter as ridicule and strike out in defense. Violence may also be triggered by substance abuse (Thornton et al., 2001c).

Negative reinforcement may also play a part, in that violent behavior intimidates people and drives them away from the aggressor, who then gains a feeling of self-control (Morrison, 1994). When aggression or violence occurs, it is important to intervene early and use deescalation skills and/or physical methods to contain it in order to protect the client and others in the environment (Turnbull et al., 1990).

Deescalation skills are effective techniques that can be used in interpersonal relationships in any context, but are especially important for the psychiatric mental health nurse. Deescalation may consist of less intrusive interventions such as using nonthreatening verbal and nonverbal messages, or it may require a more hands-on method to safely disengage and control the aggressor physically. The choice to use the techniques set forth in Table 11-7 depends on the stage of the threat, the speed of escalation of the impending violence, and the feedback received from the client, which illustrates the effectiveness of the technique.

However, sometimes strategies fail and medication may be the most effective treatment of choice to manage the emergency situation. A panel of experts have identified the oral types as the preferred alternate medications for acutely aggressive or agitated clients because of the traumatic effects of involuntary medication, especially when coupled with restraint. The oral medication risperidone was preferred to the oral medication olanzapine (48% to 21%, respectively), whereas quetiapine was less preferred (Allen et al., 2001). However, practitioners and regulatory standards concur that, if it is not possible to administer oral medications and the imminent danger of the emergency situation exceeds the client's ability to demonstrate safe behaviors, IM medications used in a limited manner (only for the emergency) may be the safest choice. IM formulations of the newer, atypical drugs are still under investigation. Drugs such as olanzapine and ziprasidone may offer lower risk of side effects compared with the older, typical drugs such a haloperidol (Murphy, 2002). The expert panel identified the risk of side effects as the most important factor in the use of IM medications. Mental trauma experienced by the client and the risk of compromising the client-physician relationship were also important (Allen et al., 2001).

To prevent violence, it is important to try to avoid blame, ridicule, confrontation, teasing, or insult. Give the individual privacy and respect emotional boundaries. Be aware of your feelings and emotions and try to keep them in check, as clients are generally sensitive to others' emotional turmoil. Maintain a calm, moderate demeanor, with a nonthreatening physical stance with arms unfolded, and remain a reasonable distance from the client. Keep your voice tone low to moderate, and refrain from whispering or laughing with others in the milieu, especially within view of a client with paranoid tendencies.

Do not allow yourself to be cornered in the room of a client with a known history of violence or with one who has threatened others; always have another staff member with you, making sure there is an easy exit. Try not to be intimidated by violent outbursts, but take whatever measures necessary to secure the safety of everyone concerned. In the hospital this may involve calling the assault response team, hospital security, or the local police department. In the community, try to secure help from friends or neighbors, and call the police if needed. The best way to prevent dangerous situations is to anticipate them and be prepared with an effective plan of action per hospital or community protocol (Thornton et al., 2001c; Flowers, 2002). See Chapter 23 for more information about violence.

EVALUATION

Evaluation follows specific intervention statements and behavioral objectives, incorporating the concepts of quality, quantity, and time. For example, if a goal is to resocialize a client who has been isolating herself while on the unit, an intervention might consist of having the client join the community meeting along with other clients on the unit. To evaluate the effectiveness of this intervention, specific behavioral client outcomes to be accomplished are stated in measurable terms. For example, a beginning behavioral objective might be: "On her second day on the unit, Kayla will accompany the nurse to the community meeting, and she will remain with the group for 15 minutes."

Note that the outcome is criteria specific as to time (on the second day), quality of experience (going to the community meeting with the nurse), and quantity (for 15 minutes). These criteria can be seen and measured. If all criteria are met, the minimal acceptable level of performance will progress, so that by the third day, the client outcome might read, "Kayla will go to the community meeting on her own, remain for 30 minutes, and make at least one comment."

The nursing process is not a static concept. It is an ongoing design for interaction with the environment and is evaluated as such. If the criteria were evaluated and found not to be met on the second day, for instance, the client outcomes and nursing interventions would have to be reconsidered and perhaps rewritten at a level closer to the client's ability to perform. If outcomes are revised and are still not met, the rest of the nursing process will need to be examined in total. Thus eventual success with the nursing process demands patience and persistence, as gains are made in small increments, especially in clients with chronic schizophrenia (see Chapter 6).

CHAPTER SUMMARY

- The schizophrenias are the largest group of mental disorders.
- Biologic factors are the primary focus in the research on etiology and treatment of schizophrenia.
- Five biologic models currently considered are heredity/genetic, neuroanatomic/neurochemical, neurotransmitter function (specifically the dopamine hypothesis), immunologic, and stress/disease/trauma/drug abuse.
- The five major subtypes of schizophrenia are paranoid, disorganized, catatonic, undifferentiated, and residual. Diagnostic criteria for schizophrenia include two or more symptoms of hallucinations, delusions, disorga-

nized or catatonic behavior, or disorganized speech that are evident for at least 1 month.
- Involving the client with schizophrenia and the client's family or significant others in the client's treatment plan, as appropriate, is important and contributes to more effective treatment.
- Psychopharmacology is a widely used intervention for many symptoms of schizophrenia. New medications with fewer side effects are being used or researched and offer hope and more effective treatment outcomes for the complex symptoms of schizophrenia.
- Milieu therapy, psychosocial rehabilitation, psychotherapy, and behavior modification techniques are some treatments used with clients with schizophrenia.
- Community resources are critical in rehabilitating clients and reintegrating them back into the community.
- Family groups help family members cope more effectively with the complexities of schizophrenia.
- Client and family education by nurses, physicians, and others is critical to the overall understanding of schizophrenia and its management.

REVIEW QUESTIONS

1. A 24-year-old male client was admitted to the Emergency Department with a laceration of the finger. While waiting to be sutured the nurse assesses him. He states that he works as a research assistant. The nurse notices that he smiles inappropriately in between questions and cocks his head to one side at times. He also has poor eye contact and disheveled clothes. The client states that he's been doing work for the government but he's discovered some government secrets and "they" have been chasing him for the past month. The appropriate diagnosis would be:
   a. Paranoid schizophrenia
   b. Bipolar disorder
   c. Schizophreniform disorder
   d. Schizoaffective disorder

2. A 17-year-old male is admitted to the adolescent unit. He has suffered his first psychotic break. His parents are confused and filled with despair and guilt. An appropriate nursing response would be:
   a. "No one knows the cause of schizophrenia, but it is not your fault or because of anything you did in the past. The important thing is to understand the illness and treatment and to support your son and to find support for yourselves."
   b. "Is there anyone in your family that has mental illness because schizophrenia is genetic."
   c. "Consider yourself lucky. At least he doesn't have cancer."
   d. "They have some great websites to learn about mental illness."

3. A 200-lb, 40-year-old male client is restless, agitated, pacing the hallways, and muttering to himself. The nurse's best intervention at this time would be:
   a. Call a team together to seclude the client.
   b. Ask that the client go to his room and lie quietly.
   c. Redirect the client to go to group therapy.
   d. Give the client a prn of Zyprexa and observe the client closely.

4. The nurse determines that the client understands his medication regimen when he states:
   a. "I will stop taking my Clozaril when I'm feeling better."
   b. "I don't see the need to have a psychiatrist. My own doctor can give me the medication I need."
   c. "I know I need to monitor my blood levels every 2 weeks."
   d. "I won't take the medication if I have any side effects."

5. A 21-year-old female client diagnosed with chronic paranoid schizophrenia is admitted to the partial hospitalization program after spending 4 days in the inpatient unit. An appropriate outcome for the first week would be that the client will:
   a. Know all other clients by name.
   b. Attend all groups.
   c. Verbalize an absence of hallucinations and delusions.
   d. Verbalize events that make her anxious.

REFERENCES

Allen MH et al: *The expert consensus guideline series: treatment of behavioral emergencies, a postgraduate medicine special report,* New York, 2001, McGraw Hill.

Amenson CS: The family's role in recovery, *Pacific Clinics Institute: the Journal,* 1999 and Guest Speaker, Schizophrenia: *Grand Rounds Conference, Sharp HealthCare,* San Diego, Calif, 2001.

American Psychiatric Association: *Diagnostic and Statistical Manual of Mental Disorders,* Fourth Edition, Text Revision. Washington, DC, American Psychiatric Association, 2000.

Andreasen N, Carpenter W: Diagnosis and classification of schizophrenia, *Schizophr Bull* 9(2):199, 1993.

Bellack A, Mueser K: Psychosocial treatment for schizophrenia, *Schizophr Bull* 19(2):317, 1993.

Bendik M: Reaching the breaking point: dangers of mistreatment in elder caregiving situations, *J Elder Abuse Neglect* 4(3):39, 1996.

Benes F: Neurobiological investigations in cingulate cortex of schizophrenic brain, *Schizophr Bull* 19(3):537, 1993.

Betemps E, Ragiel C: Psychiatric epidemiology: facts and myths on mental health and illness, *J Psychosoc Nurs* 32(5):23, 1994.

Bogerts B: Recent advances in the neuropathology of schizophrenia, *Schizophr Bull* 19(2):431, 1993.

Boyd M: Integration of psychosocial rehabilitation into psychiatric nursing practice, *Issues Ment Health Nurs* 15:13, 1994.

Boyd M: Considerations for antipsychotic therapy: Implications for the safe and appropriate management of patients, *J Am Psychiatric Nurses Association,* Aug, 2002, website: www.apna.org

Brook S, Lucey, JV, Gunn, KP, for the Ziprasidone IM Study Group: Intramuscular ziprasidone compared with intramuscular haloperidol in the treatment of acute psychosis, *J Clin Psychiatry* 61:933-944, 2000.

Brown J: Role of selenium and other trace elements in the geography of schizophrenia, *Schizophr Bull* 20(2):387, 1994.

Calev A, Edelist S: Affect and memory in schizophrenia: negative emotion words are forgotten less rapidly than other words by long-hospitalized schizophrenics, *Psychopathology* 26:229, 1993.

Cannon J, Marco E: Structural brain abnormalities as indicators of vulnerability to schizophrenia, *Schizophr Bull* 20(1):89, 1994.

Castle D, Murray R: The epidemiology of late-onset schizophrenia, *Schizophr Bull* 19(4):691, 1993.

Clementz B, McDowell J, Zisook S: Saccadic system fixing among schizophrenic patients and their first-degree biological relatives, *J Abnorm Psychol* 130(2):277, 1994.

Cohen C: Poverty and the course of schizophrenia: implications for research and policy, *Hosp Community Psychiatry* 44(10):951, 1993.

Cramer JA, Rosenheck R: Compliance with medication regimens for mental and physical disorders, *Psychiatric Services* 49:196-201, 1998.

Crow T: Molecular pathology of schizophrenia: more than one disease process, *BMJ* 12:66, 1980.

Csernansky R, Mahmoud R, Brenner R: A comparison of risperidone and haloperidol for the prevention of relapse in patients with schizophrenia, *N Engl J Med* 346:16-22, 2002.

D'Angelo E: Conceptual disorganization in children at risk for schizophrenia, *Psychopathology* 26:195, 1993.

Dworkin R et al: Childhood precursors of affective vs. social deficits in adolescents at risk for schizophrenia, *Schizophr Bull* 19(3):563, 1993.

Dworkin R et al: Social competence deficits in adolescents at risk for schizophrenia, *J Nerv Ment Dis* 182(2):103, 1994.

Evans D et al: Self perception and adolescent psychopathology: a clinical developmental perspective, *Am J Orthopsychiatry* 64(3):293, 1994.

Fields J et al: Assessing positive and negative symptoms in children and adolescents, *Am J Psychiatry* 151(2):249, 1994.

Flowers CJ: Antipsychotic polypharmacy in schizophrenia: *Eighth Annual Psychopharmacology Update,* Sponsored by Sharp HealthCare, San Diego, CA, September 21, 2002.

Fortinash KM, Holoday Worret PA: *Psychiatric nursing care plans,* ed 4, St Louis, 2003, Mosby.

Fuentes I et al: Relationships between electroderms activity and symptomatology in schizophrenia, *Psychopathology* 26:47, 1993.

Glassman AH, Bigger JT: Antipsychotic drugs: prolonged QTc interval, torsade de pointes and sudden death, *Am J Psychiatry* 158:1774-1782, 2001.

Goldman R et al: Neuropsychological prediction of treatment efficacy and one-year outcome in schizophrenia, *Psychopathology* 26:122, 1993.

Green M et al: Dichotic listening during auditory hallucinations in patients with schizophrenia, *Am J Psychiatry* 151(3):357, 1994.

Gundel H, Rudolf G: Schizophrenic autism: proposal for a nomothetic definition, *Psychopathology* 26:304, 1993.

Gureje O et al: Early brain trauma and schizophrenia in Nigerian patients, *Am J Psychiatry* 151(3):368, 1994.

Guthrie SK: Managing psychiatric drug therapy across the continuum of care: focus on the schizophrenic patient: introduction, *Am J Health System Pharmacists* vol 59, 2002.

Harper-Jaques S, Reimer M: Aggressive behavior and the brain: a different perspective for the mental health nurse, *Arch Psychiatr Nurs* 6(5):312, 1992.

Hemsley D et al: The neuropsychology of schizophrenia: act 3, *BBS* 16(1):209, 1993.

Hoffman R: Commentary: dissecting psychotic speech, *J Nerv Ment Dis* 182(4):212, 1994.

Joseph M: The neuropsychology of schizophrenia: beyond the dopamine hypothesis to behavioral function, *BBS* 16(1):203, 1993.

Kaplan HI, Sadock BJ: *Synopsis of psychiatry: behavioral sciences, clinical psychiatry,* ed 8, Baltimore, 1998, Williams & Wilkins.

Kapur S, Seeman P: Does fast dissociation from the dopamine D2 receptor explain the action of atypical antipsychotics?: a new hypothesis, *Am J Psychiatry* 158:3, 2001.

Kapur S et al: A positron emission tomography study of quetiapine in schizophrenia: a preliminary finding of an antipsychotic effect with only transiently high dopamine D2 receptor occupancy, *Arch Gen Psychiatry* 57:553-559, 2000.

Kendler K, Diehl S: The genetics of schizophrenia: a current, genetic-epidemiologic perspective, *Schizophr Bull* 19(2):261, 1993.

Kennedy M: Relationship between psychiatric diagnosis and patient aggression, *Issues Ment Health Nurs* 14:263, 1993.

Lewandowski L: Brain-behavior relationships. In Hartlage L et al, editors: *Essentials of neuropsychological assessment,* New York, 1991, Springer.

Lieberman J, Koreen: Neurochemistry and neuroendocrinology of schizophrenia: a selective review, *Schizophr Bull* 19(2):371, 1993.

Liberman R et al: Optimal drug and behavior therapy for treatment-refractory schizophrenic patients, *Am J Psychiatry* 151(5):756, 1994.

Linszen D et al: Cannabis abuse and the course of recent-onset schizophrenic disorders, *Arch Gen Psychiatry* 51(4):273, 1994.

Maguire GA: Comprehensive understanding of schizophrenia and its treatment, *Am J Health Syst Pharm* vol 59, 2002.

Malone J: Schizophrenia research update: implications for nursing, *Psychosocial Nurs* 28(8):4, 1990.

McCain N, Smith J: Stress and coping in the context of psychoneuroimmunology: a holistic framework for nursing practice and research, *Arch Psychiatr Nurs* 8(4):221, 1994.

McEnvoy J et al: Insight about psychosis among outpatients with schizophrenia, *Hosp Community Psychiatry* 44(9):883, 1993.

Meador K, Nichols F: The neurological examination as it relates to neuropsychological issues. In Hartlage L et al, editors: *Essentials of neuropsychological assessment,* New York, 1991, Springer.

Morrison E: The evolution of a concept: aggression and violence in psychiatric settings, *Arch Psychiatr Nurs* 8(4):245, 1994.

Mulvey E: Assessing the evidence of a link between mental illness and violence, *Hosp Community Psychiatry* 45(7):663, 1994.

Murphy MC: The agitated, psychotic patient: guidelines to ensure staff and patient safety, *J Am Psychiatric Nurses Association* vol 8, 2002.

NAMI's New Department of Education and Training: Advancing peer education and training, *NAMI Advocate,* Spring, 2001.

NANDA International (2003). NANDA Nursing Diagnosis: Definitions and Classification 2003-2004. Philadelphia: NANDA.

Olfson M et al: Inpatient treatment of schizophrenia in general hospitals, *Hosp Community Psychiatry* 44(1):40, 1993.

Orrison WW et al: *Functional brain imaging,* St Louis, 1995, Mosby.

Osmon D: The neuropsychological examination. In Hartlage L et al, editor: *Essentials of neuropsychological assessment,* New York, 1991, Springer.

Osser DN, Sigadel R: Short term inpatient pharmacotherapy of schizophrenia, *Harvard Rev Psychiatry* 9:89-104, 2001.

Perry W, Braff D: Information-processing deficits and thought disorder in schizophrenia, *Am J Psychiatry* 151(3):363, 1994.

Plum F: Prospects for research in schizophrenia. III. Neuropsychology: neuropathological findings, *Neurosci Res Prog Bull* 10:348, 1972.

Previc F: A neuropsychology of schizophrenia without vision, *BBS* 16(1):207, 1993.

Rogers CP: *Client-centered therapy,* Boston, 1951, Houghton Mifflin (classic).

Roy C: *Introduction to nursing: an adaptation model,* New Jersey, 1976, Prentice-Hall.

Scherling D: Prenatal cocaine exposure and childhood psychopathology, *Am J Orthopsychiatry* 64(1):9, 1994.

Selye, H: *Stress of life,* ed 2, New York, 1978, McGraw Hill (classic).

Smothergill D, Kraut A: Toward the more direct study of attention in schizophrenia: alertness decrement and encoding facilitation, *BBS* 16(1):208, 1993.

Stirling J et al: Expressed emotion and schizophrenia: the ontogeny of EE during an 18-month follow-up, *Psychiatr Nurs* 1(1):40, 1994.

Sullivan H: *The interpersonal theory of psychiatry,* New York, 1953, WW Norton (classic).

Takei N et al: Prenatal exposure to influenza and the development of schizophrenia: is the effect confined to females? *Am J Psychiatry* 151(1):117, 1994.

Thompson J, Strand K: Psychiatric nursing in a psychosocial setting, *J Psychosoc Nurs* 32(2):25, 1994.

Thornton JF et al: Schizophrenia: Course and Outcome, Internet Mental Health, Jan 2, 2001a, website: www.mentalhealth.com.

Thornton JF et al: Schizophrenia: The Medications, Internet Mental Health, Jan 2, 2001b.

Thornton JF et al: Schizophrenia: Symptoms and Management at Home, Internet Mental Health, Jan 2, 2001c.

Torrey EF: *Surviving schizophrenia,* ed 3, New York, 1995, Harper Perennial.

Trygstad L: The need to know: biological learning needs identified by practicing psychiatric nurses, *J Psychosoc Nurs* 32(2):13, 1994.

Tsuang M: Genetics, epidemiology, and the search for causes of schizophrenia, *Am J Psychiatry* 151(1):3, 1994.

Turnbull J et al: Turn it around: short-term management for aggression and anger, *J Psychosoc Nurs* 28(6):6, 1990.

Turner B: First-person account: the children of madness, *Schizophrenia Bull* 19(3):649, 1993.

Valente S: Electroconvulsive therapy, *Arch Psychiatr Nurse* 5(4):223, 1991.

Vincent M, White K: Patient violence toward a nurse: predictable and preventable? *J Psychosoc Nurs* 32(2):30, 1994.

Weiden P, Havens L: Psychotherapeutic management techniques in the treatment of outpatients with schizophrenia, *Hosp Community Psychiatry* 45(6):549, 1994.

SUGGESTED READINGS

Arieti S: *Interpretation of schizophrenia,* ed 2, New York, 1974, Basic Books (classic).

Arieti S: Schizophrenia: the manifest symptomatology, the psychodynamic and formal mechanisms. In Arieti S, editor: *American handbook of psychiatry,* vol 1, New York, 1959, Basic Books (classic).

Breier A et al: Effects of clozapine on positive and negative symptoms in outpatients with schizophrenia, *Am J Psychiatry* 151(1):20, 1994.

Conley R, Mahmoud R: A randomized double-blind study of risperidone and olanzapine in the treatment of schizophrenia or schizoaffective disorder, *Am J Psychiatry* 158:5, 2001.

Daniel DG et al: Intramuscular (IM) zisprasidone 20 mg is effective in reducing acute agitation associated with psychosis: a double-blind randomized trial, *Psychopharmacology* 155:128-134, 2001.

Joint Commission on Accreditation of Health Care Organizations: *1999-2000 Comprehensive accreditation manual for behavioral health care,* Washington, DC, 2000, Author.

Peplau H: Future directions in psychiatric nursing from the perspective of history, *J Psychosoc Nurs* 27(2):18-28, 1989.

Peplau H: Principles of psychiatric nursing. In Arieti S, editor: *American handbook of psychiatry,* vol 2, New York, 1959, Basic Books (classic).

Weiden PJ, Midder AL: Which side effects really matter? Screening for common and distressing side effects of antipsychotic medications, *J Psychiatr Practice* 7:41-47, 2001.

ONLINE RESOURCES

Find Articles: www.findarticles.com
Internet Mental Health: www.mentalhealth.com
National Alliance for the Mentally Ill: www.nami.org
National Institutes of Mental Health: www.nimh.nih.gov
National Center for Biotechnology Information: www.ncbi.nlm.nih.gov
Nursing Library: www.nursingcenter.com

12 Personality Disorders

Pamela E. Marcus

OBJECTIVES

- Identify three elements of personality development as described by Freud in the psychosexual stages of development.

- Discuss two contributions made by Margaret Mahler and Otto Kernberg to object relations theory.

- Name two biologic indices that are often abnormal in clients with a personality disorder.

- Explain one behavior, in one or two words, that differentiates Clusters A, B, and C of Axis II in the DSM-IV-TR.

- Recognize two nursing diagnoses for each cluster of the personality disorders.

- Define splitting behaviors, and list two nursing interventions that effectively challenge the client's "black or white" view of the world.

- Apply the nursing process in managing clients with personality disorders.

- Identify a plan of care for two different personality disorders, including two treatment modalities that are collaborative and two outcome criteria relevant to the client's DSM-IV-TR diagnosis.

DEFINITION OF PERSONALITY DISORDERS

The definition of personality disorders, as classified by the DSM-IV-TR, are long-standing, pervasive, maladaptive patterns of behavior relating to others that are not caused by Axis I disorders. According to the DSM-IV-TR, a personality disorder is an "enduring pattern of inner experience and behavior that deviates markedly from the expectations of the individual's culture, is pervasive and inflexible, has an onset in adolescence or early adulthood, is stable over time, and leads to distress or impairment" (APA, 2000). All human beings have a personality made up of one's definition of self, skills used to relate to others, and a defense structure. When studying personality disorders, one has to determine to what degree these qualities are compromised. One can determine these behaviors by observing how individuals relate to others, their perception of surroundings, and their ability to problem solve. According to Manfield (1992):

> The term personality disorder, also called a "disorder of the self," refers to a lack of a genuine sense of "self" and a consequent impairment of self-regulating abilities. Instead of looking within themselves to locate feelings or to make decisions, persons with personality disorders look outside themselves for evaluations, directions, rules, or opinions to guide them.

Definition of Axis II in DSM-IV-TR

When reviewing the diagnostic criteria for the various personality disorders (Axis II), it is important to differentiate personality traits from personality disorders. DSM-IV-TR has defined six general diagnostic criteria for a personality disorder as listed in the DSM-IV-TR Criteria box.

Personality traits are those behaviors, patterns of perceiving, relating to others, and thinking about the environment and oneself that are exhibited in a wide range of social and personal contexts (APA, 2000). These traits may be adaptive or maladaptive **trait disorders,** depending on whether the trait is inflexible or causes significant functional impairment or subjective distress. When this occurs, one is said to have a personality disorder. The symptoms of a personality disorder are neither time limited nor do they occur only in a time of crisis (APA, 2000). Behaviors are long-standing, enduring, and not responsive to short-term psychotherapy or pharmacologic measures.

Diagnoses made on Axis I are considered **state disorders.** These diagnoses constitute behavior patterns that are not as long in duration. Often the symptoms of these disorders can be alleviated through the use of medication, psychotherapy, and milieu therapy for severe symptoms. Personality disorder diagnoses are classified on Axis II of the DSM-IV-TR in a cluster format as follows:

Cluster A: Paranoid, schizoid, and schizotypal are described as the odd and/or eccentric cluster. These diagnoses are more likely to be **comorbid** (i.e., both diagnoses may be present in the same individual with psychotic disorders).

DSM-IV-TR CRITERIA
Personality Disorder

A. An enduring pattern of inner experience and behavior that deviates markedly from the expectations of the individual's culture. This pattern is manifested in two (or more) of the following areas:
   1. Cognition (i.e., ways of perceiving and interpreting self, other people, and events)
   2. Affectivity (i.e., the range, intensity, lability, and appropriateness of emotional response)
   3. Interpersonal functioning
   4. Impulse control
B. The enduring pattern is inflexible and pervasive across a broad range of personal and social situations.
C. The enduring pattern leads to clinically significant distress or impairment in social, occupational, or other important areas of functioning.
D. The pattern is stable and of long duration, and its onset can be traced back at least to adolescence or early adulthood.
E. The enduring pattern is not better accounted for as a manifestation or consequence of another mental disorder.
F. The enduring pattern is not due to the direct physiologic effects of a substance (e.g., a drug of abuse, a medication) or a general medical condition (e.g., head trauma).

From American Psychiatric Association: *Diagnostic and Statistical Manual of Mental Disorders,* Fourth Edition, Text Revision. Washington, DC, American Psychiatric Association, 2000.

Cluster B: Antisocial, borderline, histrionic, and narcissistic are described as the dramatic and emotional cluster. The Cluster B group is often comorbid with affective disorders.

Cluster C: Avoidant, dependent, and obsessive-compulsive compose the anxious and fearful cluster. These diagnoses are often affiliated with anxiety disorders (APA, 2000).

Individuals with personality disorder diagnoses in each cluster may be predisposed to developing a comorbidity with specific Axis I diagnoses. However, this is not a hard-and-fast rule, and there are no consistent research findings that bear this out (APA, 2000; Oldham and Skodol, 1992; Widiger and Rogers, 1989).

THEORIES OF PERSONALITY DEVELOPMENT
Freudian Theories

Sigmund Freud was one of the early published students of human development and inner psychologic conflict. The two areas that are covered in this chapter are (1) his structural theory, often referred to as the tripartite model of the hypothetical psychic structures of the id, ego, and superego, and (2) his psychosexual stages of development.

The psychosexual stages of development are described by Freud (1905) in his "Three Essays on the Theory of Sexuality." The first stage described by Freud is the oral stage. The traits associated with successful completion of this stage include the ability to relate to others without excessive dependency or jealously. Trust begins to develop, and with trust comes a sense of self-reliance and trust of self. Individuals who have difficulty with this stage often lack trust and are self-centered, dependent, and jealous (Tyson and Tyson, 1990).

The anal stage is the second stage described by Freud. This stage takes place during the time when the child begins to develop enough sphincter control to be able to control excretion of feces. This takes place approximately from ages 1 to 3 years. Successful completion of this stage is demonstrated in adult functioning by the individual's ability to deal with ambivalence in such a manner that decisions are made without shame or self-doubt; there is a sense of self-autonomy. A person who has difficulty with successful completion of this stage of development is unable to make decisions, withholds friendships or cannot share with others, is rageful, is stubborn, and has sadomasochistic tendencies (Tyson and Tyson, 1990).

The phallic stage is the next stage identified by Freud. It is the period of development when the child becomes interested in his or her genitals. Freud understood this stage in terms of male development; according to his theory, the phallus is the principal organ of concern for both boys and girls. This stage occurs during the ages of 3 through 6 or 7 years. Successful completion of this stage assists the child in achieving mastery over his or her internal processes and impulses, as well as in gaining a beginning sense of relating to other people in the environment. Individuals who are unable to resolve the conflict inherent in the phallic stage have multiple psychiatric disorders, particularly those that involve the superego function of guilt (i.e., the individual with an antisocial personality disorder does not have a well-developed superego).

According to Freud, the antisocial, borderline, histrionic, and narcissistic personality disorders involve individuals who experienced problems identifying with their sexual identity during the critical phallic stage. For example, an individual with a histrionic personality disorder who acts sexually provocative but denies that this behavior is sexually driven may have experienced an internal conflict with his or her sexual identity.

The next stage of psychosexual development is the latency stage. During this stage the child represses the libidinal (sexual) drives, and attention is turned toward learning and industry. At this time there is further development of the ego in an effort to gain control over instinctual impulses. This stage takes place from the sixth or seventh year of life until puberty.

With this stage comes the exploration of the environment and play, when the child learns how to do things, to enjoy life and have fun, and continues to develop inner control over instinctive drives and emotions. This stage is important for later adult functioning, because the child with a sense of industry is able to delay gratification, which helps in areas of learning, work, and relating to others. Problems in suc-

cessful completion of this stage are seen with individuals who either have too much or too little ability to develop inner control. Those who lack inner control have difficulty relating to others, because their emotions rule their interactions and problem-solving abilities. Individuals who have an excess of inner control have isolated their emotions and are more regulated, using repetition of thoughts or behavior to relate or problem solve.

The genital stage is the last stage described by Freud in an individual's psychosexual development. This stage takes place during puberty. The importance of this stage is that there is an opportunity to rework earlier issues that have not been resolved, in the service of achieving a healthy, mature sense of sexual and adult identity. With the ability to work and learn, individuals can establish goals and values within the context of their own unique personal identities.

If individuals have difficulty during the genital stage, their sense of self and ability to relate to others will be compromised. They will therefore be unable to attain their identified goals or form values. They will also experience difficulty in identifying their strengths and weaknesses, likes and dislikes, and types of skills they want to acquire. Individuals who have difficulty resolving the genital stage can manifest symptoms and behaviors that are described within the whole range of personality disorders.

Object Relations

As theorists studied human behavior further, particularly observing development of personality structure and relatedness, the theory of **object relations** began to be developed. This theory has many contributors and is being reevaluated and expanded as the study of human relations and personality development and disorders is more clearly understood. Tyson and Tyson (1990) have clarified the difference between interpersonal relations and object relations in the following manner:

> The first (interpersonal relations) has to do with the actual interactions between people. Object relations (or "internalized" object relations) refers to the intrapsychic dimensions of experiences with others—that is, to the mental representations of the self and of the other and of the role of each in their interactions.
>
> Object relations, then, is the stability and depth of an individual's relations with significant others as manifested by warmth, dedication, concern, and tactfulness.

Separation-Individuation Phase

When studying object relations from a developmental standpoint, Margaret Mahler identified and studied the separation-individuation phase of development occurring between ages 3 and 25 months. Mahler's theory of separation and individuation evolved from a longitudinal study where she observed normal mothers and their babies during the child's first 3 years of life. The term *separation* in this context refers to the child's gradually developing an intrapsychic self-representation that is distinct and separate from the representation of the mother. The term *individuation* is used in

Box 12-1	Mahler's Stages of Separation-Individuation

1. *Differentiation.* Occurs when the child is between 3 and 8 months old. During this stage, the child begins to differentiate his or her own image from that of the mother or significant nurturer.

2. *Practicing.* Occurs when the child is between 8 and 15 months old. The task of this stage is for the child to actively explore his or her world in a manner in which the child seems oblivious to the mother. This occurs when the child begins to walk and is able to explore the environment around him or her, as locomotion becomes more stabilized.

3. *Rapprochement.* Occurs when the child is between 15 and 22 months old. The child begins to return to the mother for emotional needs when the exploration of the surroundings (which is done during the practicing phase) is completed. During this time the toddler becomes moody and in distress with temper tantrums, even when the mother is with the child. The child wishes to have things his or her way, which may not be what the mother had planned. The task is for the child to deal with the conflict between his or her wish for independence and individuation, and with wanting to be loved and comforted by the mother.

4. *The beginning of object constancy.* Occurs around 25 months. Object constancy involves the ability to maintain a relationship regardless of frustration and changes in the relationship. The toddler at 25 months can think about the mother even when the mother is not close to the child and can therefore comfort himself or herself by the mother's representation. This comfort may include a blanket or stuffed toy that may remind the child of the mother.

Modified from Mahler MS: Thoughts about development and individuation, *Psychoanal Study Child* 18:307, 1963; Mahler MS: On the first three subphases of the separation-individuation process, *Int J Psychoanal* 53:333, 1972.

this context to recognize the infant's attempts to form a distinctive identity and to develop characteristics that are unique to that individual (Mahler, 1963).

Mahler (1963, 1972a) described four stages of the process of separation-individuation: differentiation, practicing, rapprochement, and object constancy. These stages are explained in Box 12-1.

Kernberg's Theories

Otto Kernberg studied individuals with severe personality disorders and formulated some ideas about these disorders and their development, primarily with borderline and narcissistic personality disorders. According to Kernberg (1984), a person who is emotionally healthy has an integrated working structure of the id, superego, and ego. This means that the ego is intact, with sufficient ability to determine reality from fantasy and to separate self from another object. The superego is functional, not too rigid or punishing, but a filter for the ego. The id is integrated and not in conflict with the other two structures.

Kernberg identified two essential tasks that the early ego must accomplish for the internalization of object relations. The first task involves the ability of the child to distinguish between self and other people to formulate healthy feelings about self and identification with the other person. This is similar to Mahler's differentiation stage. The second task

that Kernberg discussed in relation to the internalization of object relations is that there is an integration of "good" and "bad" self-images, as well as an integration of "good" and "bad" object (the other person's) images. This consolidation of images leads to total self and object representations that are differentiated from one another and realistic in that both structures have good and bad, satisfaction and frustration, in their systems.

In the borderline personality disorder, or what Kernberg has called the "borderline personality organization," this is a particularly important aspect. Kernberg identified splitting as a primary defense of the individual with borderline personality disorder. **Splitting** is the inability to synthesize the positive and negative aspects of self and others. The person with borderline personality disorder exhibits splitting by his or her difficulty in perceiving that he or she and other people have both good and bad aspects. There is a tendency to idealize persons or groups when those persons meet the needs of the individual with borderline personality disorder. This process is called **idealization.** At the other extreme, a person with borderline personality disorder can devalue persons or groups when needs are not perceived to be met. This process is called **devaluation.** The person with borderline personality disorder views self and others as either all good or all bad and is unable to reach a state of **object constancy,** which means that one is unable to hold the memory of significant others in mind. This individual is unable to use **transitional objects** that represent the significant other person and that help the individual remember the other person. For example, an individual with object constancy can think of his or her loved one when experiencing something that may remind him or her of the other person, such as a favorite song or a tangible object. An individual who is unable to obtain object constancy cannot picture his or her loved one when that individual is away from him or her. Therefore the person views the absence of the significant other as an abandonment.

Masterson (1976) identified four defenses that block the client's developmental growth from the stages of individuation-separation to autonomy: projection, clinging, denial, and avoidance. According to Masterson, the client with borderline personality disorder becomes stuck in the subphases of the individuation-separation stage. This leads to the client's failure to achieve object constancy.

A client with borderline personality disorder does not relate to people as wholes but as parts. He or she is unable to sustain a relationship through the frustration of everyday living and tends to experience anger and rage when feeling rejected or ignored. This individual is unable to evoke the image of the other when the other is not present. If a significant person in the client's life dies, the client with borderline personality disorder cannot mourn but may exhibit one or more of the six constituent states: depression, anger and rage, fear, guilt, passivity and helplessness, and emptiness and void.

Another defense against the client's anxiety that is important in understanding the individual with a Cluster B personality disorder is **projective identification.** This defense is a primitive type of projection. Kernberg (1984) described this defense as having the following characteristics:

- The tendency to continue to experience the impulse that is simultaneously being projected onto the other person
- Fear of the other person under influence of that projected impulse
- The need to control the other person under the influence of this mechanism

BIOLOGIC CONTRIBUTIONS TO PERSONALITY DISORDERS

As researchers in the biologic aspects of behaviors began to study some of the physiologic markers consistent with the Axis I diagnoses, some of the same studies were used with individuals with personality disorders, with consistent results. There have been family studies, including twin studies, that demonstrate a strong genetic influence, thus suggesting some ties between biologic factors and personality organization (Coryell and Zimmerman, 1989; Kavoussi and Siever, 1991; Marin et al., 1989; Siever, 1992; Siever and Davis, 1991).

One interesting aspect of this research is noted in the studies done on individuals with schizotypal personality disorder who demonstrate impaired eye-tracking behavior. Impaired eye-tracking behavior is described as "the inability to track a smoothly moving target" (Siever, 1992). This is important for cognitive interpretation of information in the environment. Individuals with schizophrenia demonstrate difficulty with smooth-pursuit eye movements, and this is thought to reflect disrupted neurointegrative functioning of the frontal lobes (Siever, 1992). The impaired eye-tracking studies are associated with the "deficit" traits of schizophrenia, namely the social isolation, detachment, and inability to relate to others.

Another biologic test indicative of cognitive-perceptual difficulties that is often seen in clients who have schizotypal personality disorder is *backward masking.* This test of neurointegrative functioning involves a "process in which a visual stimulus is rapidly followed by another visual stimulus and the subject is asked to identify the original stimulus" (Kavoussi and Siever, 1991). Siever (1985) found individuals with this personality disorder to have results similar to those noted in individuals with schizophrenia, but not as severe.

The ability to pay attention to stimuli is a biologic/cognitive marker that can be used to predict schizophrenia. The Continuous Performance Test, Identical Pairs Version, tests the ability to attend to stimuli. In their study of the schizotypal personality disorder, Roitman et al. (1997) reported that individuals demonstrated a verbal and spatial deficit when tested with the Continuous Performance Test, Identical Pairs Version, as compared with normal subjects and individuals who had other types of personality disorders. The test results were similar to the pattern usually seen with individuals with schizophrenia.

There are some neurochemical measures that are important indicators of biologic manifestations of the schizotypal personality disorder. Siever (1992) reported that cerebrospinal fluid homovanillic acid was increased in preliminary studies of schizotypal clients and correlated with positive psychotic-like criteria for schizotypal personality but without the negative or deficit symptoms. He also reported that plasma homovanillic acid was increased in clients with schizotypal personality disorder, as compared with client controls (Kavoussi and Siever, 1991). In 1988 researchers found that clients with borderline personality disorder who also had schizotypal personality disorder demonstrated evidence of a worsening of psychotic-like symptoms in response to an infusion of amphetamines.

In clients who have difficulty with affective regulation (mood), some biologic indices are important to consider. The dexamethasone suppression test (DST), the thyrotropin-releasing hormone test (TRH), and electroencephalographic (EEG) sleep studies have been used in research as biologic markers of affective disorders. Abnormal DST and TRH results were found in clients with borderline personality disorder, prompting researchers to question whether these clients have a variant of mood disorders. However, in studies that separated clients with borderline personality disorder into groups with and without depression, it was reported that the nondepressed subjects had a higher percentage of normal DST and TRH results. Marin et al. (1989) have suggested that these results may be related to depression rather than to the personality disorder.

Several studies demonstrate disturbances in central serotonergic neurotransmission, indicating that aggressive and suicidal behaviors in individuals with a personality disorder correlate with reduced levels of the cerebrospinal fluid 5-hydroxyindoleacetic acid (5-HIAA), a major metabolite of serotonin, which indicates a reduction in serotonin activity (Brown et al., 1982). Mann et al. (1986) found increased postsynaptic serotonergic receptors in suicide victims. Stanley and Stanley (1990) demonstrated information on both presynaptic and postsynaptic serotonergic "markers," which suggests that a reduction in serotonin neurotransmission is an underlying biochemical "risk factor" for suicide. Marin et al. (1989) and Kavoussi and Siever (1991) surveyed several studies involving serotonin and its metabolites and found that there seems to be serotonergic reduction in behaviors such as impulsiveness, motor aggression, and suicidal tendencies. Brown and Linnoila (1990) studied the cerebrospinal fluid metabolites of serotonin (5-HIAA), which indicated a relationship between reduced serotonergic activity and aggressive and impulsive behavior. Layton et al. (2001) studied the relationship of 5-HT (serotonin) and brain regional alpha [11 C] methyl-L-tryptophan trapping in impulsive individuals. They found that individuals who have borderline personality disorder made more punishment-reward commission errors on a psychological test called the "go/no go task." This correlates with the behavior patterns of difficulty inhibiting or delaying responses and relates to the impulsive behavior seen in this population. Low 5-HT synthesis capacity was seen in the corticostriatal pathways, which may be a factor to the development of impulsive behaviors seen in individuals with borderline personality disorder.

There may also be a dysfunction of the brain system's ability to modulate and inhibit aggressive responses to environmental stimuli (Siever and Davis, 1991). Some data indicate that EEG slow-wave activity and a low threshold for sedation discriminate individuals with antisocial personality disorder from individuals with long-term depression (Siever and Davis, 1991).

That individuals with personality disorders manifest some biologic markers is exciting for researchers and clinicians, as this information provides some suggestions that may be useful when treating this population. There is a need for future research in this area as the functions of the brain and the neurotransmitters become better known and understood.

CLINICAL DESCRIPTION AND EPIDEMIOLOGY
Cluster A Personality Disorders

Cluster A, often described as the "odd" or "eccentric" cluster, consists of the following personality disorders: paranoid, schizoid, and schizotypal. Clients in this cluster all have difficulty relating to others, isolate themselves, and are unable to socialize comfortably. The Clinical Symptoms box at right and Box 12-2 provide summaries of the key clinical symptoms and epidemiology of each disorder.

Cluster B Personality Disorders

Cluster B personality disorders have components of dramatic behavior, a description widely used when describing individuals with a Cluster B personality disorder. The four diagnostic categories that make up this cluster are antisocial, borderline, histrionic, and narcissistic. Each personality disorder has unique features; each shares a dramatic quality in the way the individual lives his or her life. The Clinical Symptoms box on p. 280 and Box 12-3 summarize the key clinical symptoms and epidemiology of each of these disorders.

Cluster C Personality Disorders

Cluster C personality disorders are described as the anxious or fearful cluster. They include avoidant personality disorder, dependent personality disorder, and obsessive-compulsive personality disorder. The Clinical Symptoms box on p. 281 and Box 12-4 summarize the key clinical symptoms and epidemiology of these disorders.

Unspecified Personality Disorders

The category of unspecified personality disorders describes individuals whose personality pattern meets the general criteria for a personality disorder but not the criteria for any specific personality disorder. It is also used for

CLINICAL SYMPTOMS

Cluster A Personality Disorders

Paranoid Personality Disorder
Distrust, suspicion
Difficulty adjusting to change
Sensitivity, argumentation
Feelings of irreversible injury by others—often without evidence
Anxiety, difficulty relaxing
Short temper
Difficulty with problem solving
Lack of tender feelings toward others
Unwillingness to forgive even minor events
Jealousy of spouse or significant other—often without evidence

Schizoid Personality Disorder
Lack of desire to socialize; enjoys solitude
Lacks strong emotions
Detached, self-absorbed affect
Lacks trust in others
Brief psychotic episodes in response to stressful events
Difficulty expressing anger
Passive reactions to crises

Schizotypal Personality Disorder
Incorrect interpretation of external events/belief that all events refer to self
Superstition, preoccupation with paranormal phenomena
Belief in possession of magical control over others
Constricted or inappropriate affect
Anxiety in social situations

Box 12-2	Epidemiology of Cluster A Personality Disorders

Paranoid Personality Disorder
Diagnosed in 0.5% to 2.5% of the general population.
10% to 30% of the paranoid population is in inpatient psychiatric settings.
2% to 10% are in outpatient mental health clinics.
Families who have one or more members already diagnosed with paranoid personality disorder are at increased risk.
Males are diagnosed more often than females.
Substance abuse is common.

Schizoid Personality Disorder
Males are diagnosed slightly more often than females.
Families with members who have schizophrenia or schizotypal personality disorder have increased prevalence.

Schizotypal Personality Disorder
Diagnosed in 3% of the general population.
30% to 50% also have major depression.
Individuals with schizotypal personality disorder seek treatment for anxiety and/or depression, not for the personality disorder features.
First-degree relatives of individuals with schizophrenia are at increased risk.
Males are diagnosed slightly more often than females.

CLINICAL SYMPTOMS

Cluster B Personality Disorders

Antisocial Personality Disorder

Irresponsibility
Failure to honor financial obligations, plan ahead, provide children with basic needs
Involvement in illegal activities
Lack of guilt
Difficulty learning from mistakes
Initial charm dissolves to coldness, manipulation, blaming others
Lacks empathy
Irritability
Abuse of substances

Borderline Personality Disorder

Intense, stormy relationships
Sees people as "all good" or "all bad"
Impulsivity
Self-mutilation
Difficulty identifying self
Negative or angry affect
Feelings of emptiness and boredom
Difficulty being alone, feeling of abandonment
Engages in impulsive acts (e.g., bingeing, spending money, reckless driving, unsafe sex)
Suicidal ideations

Histrionic Personality Disorder

Fluctuation in emotions
Attention-seeking, self-centered attitude
Sexual seduction and flamboyance
Attentiveness to own physical appearance
Dramatic, impressionistic speech style
Vague logic—lack of conviction in arguments, often switching sides
Shallow emotional expression
Craving for immediate satisfaction
Complaints of physical illness, somatization
Use of suicidal gestures and threats to get attention

Narcissistic Personality Disorder

Grandiose view of self
Lacks empathy toward others
Need for admiration
Preoccupation with fantasies of success, brilliance, beauty, ideal love

Box 12-3 Epidemiology of Cluster B Personality Disorders

Antisocial Personality Disorder

Usually diagnosed by age 18 years old.
Individuals have a history of conduct disorders before age 15 years old.
Males are diagnosed more often than females.
Characteristics are evident by early childhood in males and by puberty in females.
High percentage of diagnosed individuals are in substance abuse treatment settings and prisons.
Incidence is more common in the lower socioeconomic classes.
Substance abuse is common.
Impulsive behavior is common.

Borderline Personality Disorder

Diagnosed in 2% of the general population.
10% of this population are in outpatient mental health clinics.
20% are in inpatient psychiatric settings.
75% of diagnosed individuals are female.
60% of the diagnosed disorder population have borderline personality disorder.
Diagnosed individuals have a history of physical and sexual abuse, neglect, hostile conflict, and early parental losses or separation.

Histrionic Personality Disorder

Females are diagnosed more often than males.
Diagnosed in 2% to 3% of the general population.
10% to 15% of the individuals who seek treatment have this disorder.

Narcissistic Personality Disorder

Diagnosed in less than 1% of the general population.
Diagnosed in 2% to 16% of the clinical population.
50% to 75% of those diagnosed are male.

an individual whose personality pattern meets the general criteria for a personality disorder, but the person is considered to have a personality disorder that is not included in the current classification such as passive-aggressive personality disorder.

PROGNOSIS

When providing nursing care to clients with personality disorders, it is important to consider the prognosis for improvement. This is especially important during the planning and evaluating portions of the nursing care plan. By definition, individuals with personality disorders have demonstrated pervasive and inflexible behaviors and thoughts that deviate from their cultural expectations (APA, 2000). These patterns first begin in adolescence or early adulthood and are stable over time. The symptoms lead to distress and functional and relationship impairment in the individual. With this definition in mind, the prognosis for individuals with personality disorders is guarded.

An example of how the manifestations of a personality disorder can be demonstrated in adolescence is made by examining the symptoms of conduct disorder in adolescence and the development of antisocial disorder in adulthood. Pajer (1998) studied the literature to determine if girls who displayed symptoms of conduct disorder continued the symptoms to demonstrate antisocial personality disorder as adults. The conclusion of this research was that the adults had higher mortality rates; a 10-fold to 40-fold increase in criminal behavior; many psychiatric comorbid symptoms, such as suicidal behavior; disturbed and sometimes violent significant relationships, with a high rate of divorce and ex-

CLINICAL SYMPTOMS

Cluster C Personality Disorders

Avoidant Personality Disorder
Fearful of criticism, disapproval, or rejection
Avoids social interactions
Withholds thoughts or feelings
Negative sense of self, low self-esteem

Dependent Personality Disorder
Submissive, clinging
Unable to make decisions independently
Cannot express negative emotions
Difficulty following through on tasks

Obsessive-Compulsive Personality Disorder
Preoccupation with perfection, organization, structure, control
Procrastination
Abandonment of projects due to dissatisfaction
Excessive devotion to work
Difficulty relaxing
Rule-conscious behavior
Self-criticism and inability to forgive own errors
Reluctance to delegate
Inability to discard anything
Insistence on others' conforming to own methods
Rejection of praise
Reluctance to spend money
Background of stiff and formal relationships
Preoccupation with logic and intellect

Box 12-4   Epidemiology of Cluster C Personality Disorders

Avoidant Personality Disorder
Diagnosis is equal for males and females.
Diagnosed in 0.5% to 1% of the general population.
10% are diagnosed in outpatient settings.

Dependent Personality Disorder
Most frequently diagnosed personality disorder.
More females are diagnosed than males.
Symptoms are demonstrated early in life.
Children or adolescents with chronic physical illness or separation anxiety disorder may be predisposed.

Obsessive-Compulsive Personality Disorder
Diagnosed in 1% of the general population.
Diagnosed in 3% to 10% of the population who seek treatment.
Males are diagnosed twice as often as females.

UNDERSTANDING and APPLYING RESEARCH

Myers et al. studied 137 adolescents who initially received treatment for substance abuse in an inpatient setting. These individuals were followed by the research team for 4 years to determine the correlation between conduct disorder, substance abuse, and the development of antisocial personality disorder. Several tools were used during the study. The Structural Clinical Interview for Adolescents was used to gather data on the subjects' demographic information, as well as academic, social, occupational, family, and health functioning. The Customary Drinking and Drug Use Record was used to determine the substance abuse pattern. The Conduct Disorder/Antisocial Personality Disorder Questionnaire assesses whether an individual has conduct disorder and/or antisocial personality disorder.

The researchers compared the functioning of the subjects in the following domains: schoolwork, interpersonal functioning, emotional well-being, and illegal behavior. Myers and associates found that their results showed a relationship between substance abuse and antisocial behavior. This is reflected in the theoretic models that draw a comparison between adolescents with conduct disorder and substance abuse and those who later develop antisocial personality disorder. The researchers found that individuals with more symptoms of drug and alcohol abuse were more likely to also develop antisocial personality disorder. Adolescents in this study who demonstrated difficulty in functioning in the measured domains of schoolwork, interpersonal functioning, emotional well-being, and illegal behavior also later developed antisocial personality disorder. If there was substance abuse in those individuals who later displayed antisocial personality disorder, there were also more problems in functioning in the domains mentioned above. The researchers concluded that the "prominence of substance use in relation to poorer overall functioning . . . [suggests] that alcohol and drug abuse may be inextricably involved in the progression of antisocial pathology among young people with a history of substance abuse."

This correlation between substance abuse, conduct disorder, and antisocial personality disorder is important in planning treatment. Patients should be carefully assessed for conduct disorder that may occur before, and independent of, substance abuse for treatment considerations. Individuals who have conduct disorder before the substance abuse are at higher risk. These individuals need an intensive treatment program with multisystem therapeutic modalities.

Myers MG, Stewart DG, Brown SA: Progression from conduct disorder to antisocial personality disorder following treatment for adolescent substance abuse, *Am J Psychiatry* 155:479, 1998.

---

tramarital sexual activity; poor educational achievement; less stable work histories; and a high rate of service utilization, such as welfare systems and child protective agencies. Myers, Stewart, and Brown (1998) studied the progression of symptoms from those demonstrated in conduct disorder to antisocial personality disorder, in adolescents who were seeking treatment for substance abuse (see Understanding and Applying Research box). These studies conclude that early, structured therapy may decrease the severity of the personality disorder in adult life.

In another study, Becker et al. (2000) studied the comorbidity of borderline personality disorder with other personality disorders with a group of adolescents who were hospitalized. The researcher compared this finding with adults who were admitted to the same hospital during the same period. They determined that in the adolescent group, schizotypal and passive-aggressive personality disorders occurred concurrently in a significant number of cases.

Realistic expectations for improvement include a commitment by the client to explore and evaluate his or her thoughts and behaviors, especially when under stress. The nurse plays a powerful role by providing support, tools for this exploration, and client teaching. If the client can use the knowledge of his or her dysfunctional patterns to predict how he or she will respond when faced with a stressor, innovative options for problem solving can be planned. In this way, the individual learns new responses and can improve functioning. This process often needs to be repeated over time before behavioral and thought patterns change. Therefore long-term treatment aimed at problem solving and cognitive reframing is indicated for these clients.

Linehan (1993) studied behavioral patterns of individuals with borderline personality disorder, identifying repeating behavioral patterns. She then began to study what interventions could decrease the most destructive behavioral patterns, such as parasuicidal behavior, splitting, and intense emotional reactivity. This research yielded a treatment strategy called dialectical behavioral therapy (DBT). The principal assumption is to use the dialogue to assist the client in reworking destructive ways of dealing with crises. DBT teaches the client that there are choices in working through the crisis that can decrease the suicidal thoughts or emotionally reactive patterns. The therapy focuses on the client's learning new patterns of thoughts and behaviors.

DISCHARGE CRITERIA

Clients with personality disorders are treated in both inpatient and outpatient settings, such as day treatment facilities, partial hospital units, clinics, and private office practices. To determine when to discharge a client from an inpatient hospital setting, it is important to consider the risk factor of safety for the client and others. Some clients with personality disorders have suicidal ideas that are part of their day-to-day thought process. When evaluating clients with this ongoing theme, it is important to ascertain whether the client has a suicidal plan and if he or she intends to implement that plan (see Chapter 24).

Individuals with a personality disorder who are hospitalized often have more than one psychiatric diagnosis. Their lives can be complex and chaotic. Psychiatric follow-up care, whether in a partial hospitalization program, a day treatment center, or with an outpatient psychotherapist, is important to assist the client in working through some of the issues that contributed to the crisis that culminated in the hospital stay. Before discharge from the hospital, it is important for the client to have a plan for outpatient follow-up care and the first posthospital appointment established.

Client teaching is a powerful tool to help the client understand the psychiatric problems that he or she is experiencing, as well as to help prevent a relapse of symptoms. Before discharge from the hospital, each client should receive education in the following areas:

- The need for follow-up care in an outpatient setting
- The psychiatric symptoms that indicate a need for emergent treatment
- An understanding of any medications that the client may be receiving

This client teaching can take place in a group setting or on an individual basis. If one of the milieu activities is a relapse prevention group and/or a medication group, it is helpful for the primary nurse to review the material specific to each client before his or her discharge.

If the client is being treated in an outpatient setting, the following issues must be considered before discharge from treatment:

- The client no longer has active thoughts of wanting to harm self or others.
- The client controls self-destructive impulses such as substance abuse when feeling upset or shoplifting when feeling empty.
- The client has an understanding of the symptoms that precipitated the need for psychotherapy.
- The client understands the types of symptoms that indicate a need for further treatment in the future.
- The client can use community 12-step groups if this is relevant to his or her problems, such as Alcoholics Anonymous, Narcotics Anonymous, Co-Dependents Anonymous, Incest Survivors Anonymous, and Overeaters Anonymous.

THE NURSING PROCESS

ASSESSMENT

The client being assessed for a personality disorder should be interviewed in a comfortable, quiet, private, safe environment. There should be no interruptions during the assessment. Individuals with these disorders may be withdrawn, defensive, guarded, and impulsive, or they may be charming and friendly.

The nurse should not be judgmental or confrontational during the interview. If the client demonstrates an escalation of anger or makes hostile, threatening comments to the assessment questions, a break may help the client regain composure. The client should not be threatened with seclusion or restraints, because this may provoke him or her to impulsively lose control (see Nursing Care in the Community box).

The Nursing Assessment Questions box represents a comprehensive evaluation that can be used with clients who have a personality disorder. The five domains of human behavior examined are the physical, emotional, cognitive, social, and spiritual domains (see Case Study on p. 285).

NURSING CARE IN THE COMMUNITY — Personality Disorders

The community mental health nurse often encounters many challenges when working with clients with Axis II diagnoses. The extent of the client's disorder may not be immediately apparent, as clients with Axis II disorders may appear in control under certain circumstances. Interactions require constant vigilance, as the nurse's suggestions may be distorted by the client as criticism or blame, and professional attention may be perceived as interest in personal involvement. Helpful attempts by the nurse may be negated or rejected by clients with personality disorders, and their distress and complaints will continue, resulting in frustration for both the nurse and the client. The nurse needs to be cautious when clients attempt to pit staff against each other. A client may idealize one staff member while disparaging another in an effort to meet his or her needs inappropriately. Such behaviors are known as "splitting," and need to be addressed by the nurse in a calm, impassive manner. For example, if a client tells a nurse that the nurse is caring and understanding, but that everyone else misunderstands the client, the nurse should remain unimpressed and remind the client of the consistencies in treatment by all staff.

The client may also attempt to influence the nurse by expressing thoughts of suicide or self-mutilation. The client may be at higher risk for self-mutilation and/or a suicidal gesture when feeling intense states of affect, such as anger or abandonment anxiety. The nurse's reaction must always remain calm and thoughtful. An in-depth assessment can determine the client's need for services. Clients need to be encouraged to consider the outcomes of these behaviors and think about other options they could pursue. Control of the interaction and self-awareness are especially important for the mental health nurse in the community. Having knowledge of the local crisis hot line or using the national number 1-800-SUICIDE can provide some assistance to the nurse and client.

Clients with Axis II disorders may often appear charming, engaging, and possessed of insightful humor, although they seem unable to use their intellectual gifts to help themselves break the cycles of substance abuse and/or self-mutilation. A cohesive, team approach is essential, as the demands of this group of clients tend to frustrate and even "burn out" individual case workers. All decisions concerning care of these clients should be made in consensus with the entire health care team.

NURSING ASSESSMENT QUESTIONS
Personality Disorders

Physical Domain

1. Is there evidence of appropriate activities of daily living?
2. Is the client neatly groomed?
3. Is the client dressed appropriately?
4. Does the client appear adequately nourished?
5. Is there evidence of a regular exercise program in his or her life?
6. Is there evidence of any physical illnesses?
7. Does the client concentrate on somatic concerns?
8. Is the client able to maintain eye contact?
9. Is the client experiencing tension?
10. Does the client demonstrate sympathetic stimulation, cardiovascular excitation, superficial vasoconstriction, and/or pupil dilation?
11. Does the client report trouble sleeping?
12. Is the client glancing about?
13. Is the client demonstrating extraneous movements, such as foot shuffling, or hand and arm movements?
14. Does the client show facial tension?
15. Is his or her voice quivering?
16. Does the client report increased wariness?
17. Is the client having an increase in perspiration?
18. Does the client have a history of any of the following physical conditions?
    Temporal lobe epilepsy
    Progressive central nervous system disorder
    Head trauma
    Hormonal imbalance
    Mental retardation
    Abuse of alcohol and/or drugs
19. Is the client dressed inappropriately or in a seductive manner?
20. Does the client have a high incidence of accidents?
21. Is the client overly concerned with physical attractiveness?

Emotional Domain

1. Does the client demonstrate demanding, hostile behavior?
2. Does the client have a history of aggressive actions?
3. Is the client emotionally volatile?
4. Does the client have poor impulse control?
5. Does the client indicate having thoughts of harming self or others?
6. Is the client suspicious of others?
7. Is the client fearful or highly anxious?
8. Does the client express feelings of helplessness?
9. Does the client appear apprehensive?
10. Does the client's thought pattern include feelings of uncertainty?
11. Does the client discuss concerns about unspecified consequences?
12. Does the client have persistent worries?
13. Does the client demonstrate critical behavior toward self and others?
14. Does the client have low self-esteem?
15. Is the client concerned about how others will evaluate him or her?
16. Does the client inflate his or her importance?
17. Does the client describe feelings of guilt or regret?
18. Does the client lack remorse and justify hurting another with excuses?
19. Does the client lack empathy?
20. Is the client vindictive?
21. Does the client demonstrate a low frustration tolerance?
22. Does the client show a lack of motivation?
23. Is the client dependent on others to meet his or her needs?
24. Is the client's behavior passive?
25. Does the client discuss feelings of inadequacy?
26. Does the client deny strong emotions, such as anger and joy?
27. Is the client describing feelings of hopelessness?
28. Does the client demonstrate inappropriate sexually seductive behavior?
29. Does the client manifest a constricted affect?

Continued

NURSING ASSESSMENT QUESTIONS

Personality Disorders—cont'd

Emotional Domain—cont'd

30. Does the client exhibit an inappropriate affect, such as silly or aloof facial expressions?
31. Does the client display lability of his or her mood?

Cognitive Domain

1. Does the client demonstrate inaccurate interpretation of stimuli, both internal and external?
2. Does the client have difficulty understanding abstract ideas?
3. Is the client able to identify problem areas?
4. Is the client able to identify options to solve the problems?
5. Does the client's identification of the problem area involve blaming others or self?
6. Is the client vindictive in his or her problem solving?
7. Does the client lie?
8. Is the client able to identify both good and bad traits in others?
9. Is the client able to distinguish positive and negative options to problem solving?
10. Does the client ruminate over issues of concern?
11. Is the client's thought pattern redundant?
12. Is the client able to tolerate a delay in gratification?
13. Is the client able to identify his or her value system?
14. Does the client have difficulty learning from his or her mistakes?
15. Is the client impulsive?
16. Does the client manifest any deficits in long-term or short-term memory?
17. Is the client preoccupied?
18. Does the client have a lack of consensual validation?
19. Does the client describe any delusions?
20. Does the client experience any hallucinations? What type: auditory, visual, tactile, gustatory, olfactory? What is the content of the hallucinations?
21. Does the client reveal any perceptual experiences?
22. Does the client confirm having any ideas of reference?
23. Does the client discuss any odd beliefs or magical thinking that influence his or her behavior?
24. Is the client's speech impoverished, digressive, vague, or inappropriately abstract?

Social Domain

1. Does the client prefer to be alone?
2. Does the client express a desire to socialize but have concerns that he or she will not be accepted by others?
3. Is the client dependent on others for meeting his or her needs?
4. Does the client participate in family activities?
5. Does the client have any friends?
6. Does the client have unstable relationships that consist of conflict and concerns about abandonment?

7. Is the client able to identify the dynamics of relationship problems?
8. Is the client using manipulative behavior as a means of getting needs met?
9. Does the client show evidence of splitting? Does the client place great value on relating with one person while becoming critical and angry with the other? Does the client devalue and complain about one individual to another person with whom the client has a positive relationship?
10. Does the client identify his or her sense of self by indicating membership in a relationship?
11. Is the client attention seeking, wanting to be the center of attention?
12. Is the client preoccupied with how others view him or her?
13. Is this client extremely sensitive to praise and criticism of others?
14. Is the client reluctant to give time, gifts, and support to his or her friends unless the client can profit?
15. Does the client choose solitary activities?
16. Does the client engage in any social activities?
17. Does the client feel increasingly anxious when in a social situation?
18. Does the client express no desire to have a sexual experience with another person?
19. Does the client have multiple sexual partners?
20. Is this client indifferent to praise and criticism of others?
21. Does the client expect others to exploit him or her?
22. Does the client exploit others to get his or her needs met?
23. Does the client question the loyalty or trustworthiness of friends or associates? Does the client question the fidelity of his or her spouse or sexual partner?
24. Does the client read hidden meanings into benign remarks of others?
25. Does the client bear grudges against others?
26. Is the client reluctant to confide in others?
27. Is the client preoccupied with self to the exclusion of others?
28. Does the client fail to honor financial obligations?
29. Does the client fail to plan ahead, such as traveling without a clear plan or quitting work without plans to begin another job?
30. Does the client provide his or her children with the basic needs for health?
31. Does the client engage in illegal activities?
32. Does the client abuse drugs or alcohol?
33. Does the client demonstrate a belief that he or she is owed a sense of entitlement?

Spiritual Domain

1. Does the client have a belief in a higher power?
2. Is the client able to state a meaning and purpose to his or her life?

CASE STUDY

Brian, a 32-year-old single man, was evaluated by a nurse in an outpatient clinic at the recommendation of his father because of an increase in his isolative behavior. Brian did not want to come in for the interview, as he did not consider "being alone" a problem. He was oriented three times but was not spontaneous with answers to the nurse's assessment questions. His affect was flat, he kept his eyes averted with no eye contact, and his leg was shaking. He was unkempt, with a disheveled appearance and mismatched clothing. He had a vague, wandering, nonspecific way of discussing his problem and his lifestyle.

His mother had been recently hospitalized with pneumonia; however, Brian did not see that as part of his problem. He perceived his boss as "disliking" him, because the boss thought he was "weird." Brian said that he had no friends, found socializing difficult, and tended to withdraw further when forced to interact with others. He was suspicious of the interviewer and of his father's motives for asking him to seek psychiatric intervention.

The problem he identified was that he felt he had to "do more around the house" in his mother's absence. That seemed "unfair and like a burden" to Brian. "She just got sick so she wouldn't have to cook supper or do the laundry," Brian stated. "The doctors put her in the hospital so they can make more money off of her. Dad is in on it; he sent me here so you could make money."

Brian had not visited his mother in the hospital because he was afraid he would get "germs" there. Although he saw no reason for this interview, he consented to return to the clinic to "help" his father.

Critical Thinking

1. What questions should the nurse ask Brian to determine symptoms in the physical domain?
2. How could the nurse assess the emotional domain?
3. How could Brian's problems in the cognitive domain be assessed?
4. What information about Brian helps to determine his functioning in the social domain?
5. What questions could the nurse ask Brian to assess how he functions in the spiritual domain?

NURSING DIAGNOSIS

The nursing diagnosis is developed based on the in-depth assessment of the client's health status. The nursing diagnosis is a statement that defines the problem and its characteristics and contributing factors and guides the development of the nursing care plan (see Nursing Assessment Questions box). The following are the nursing diagnoses that are most common when caring for clients with a personality disorder.

Nursing Diagnoses for Paranoid, Schizoid, and Schizotypal Personality Disorders (Cluster A)

- Anxiety
- Ineffective coping
- Social isolation
- Disturbed thought processes

Nursing Diagnoses for Antisocial, Borderline, Histrionic, and Narcissistic Personality Disorders (Cluster B)

- Ineffective coping
- Disturbed personal identity
- Chronic low self-esteem
- Risk for self-mutilation
- Risk for suicide
- Impaired social interaction
- Risk for other-directed violence
- Risk for self-directed violence

NURSING ASSESSMENT QUESTIONS
Personality Disorders

These questions involve *the nurse's observation of the client's appearance, general nutritional status, and level of observable anxiety manifestations:*

1. Does the client appear appropriately dressed? Is eye contact maintained? Does he or she appear properly nourished? Does the client exhibit signs of anxiety, such as pacing, foot tapping, sighing, or facial tension? Does the client appear hypervigilant? Does the client appear withdrawn?

The following questions are suggestions for the nurse to ask the client *to determine if there are disturbances in the client's relationships, thought processes, and behavior:*

2. How would you describe yourself? What do you like about yourself? What would you like to change about yourself?
3. Describe your relationship with your spouse or significant other, your children, your parents, and other family members. Describe your relationship with your friends. What do you talk about? What types of activities do you do together?
4. How do you feel about your job? Do you get along with your boss and co-workers?
5. If you have a personal problem, who do you trust to help you with it?
6. What are your main worries? How often do you think about them? Do you talk to anyone about these worries? Does that help?
7. Do you ever feel like hurting yourself or anyone else? Have you ever been suicidal? Have you ever hurt yourself by cutting your skin or burning yourself? How often does this occur?
8. Have you ever felt hopeless, helpless, worthless, and a burden? Do you feel this now? Are you getting any support from friends or family?
9. Do you ever use alcohol and/or illegal drugs? Have you ever gone to the doctor to get tranquilizers to reduce your nervousness? What did the doctor give you? What are you taking now?
10. What are your religious beliefs and practices?

Nursing Diagnoses for Avoidant, Dependent, and Obsessive-Compulsive Personality Disorders (Cluster C)

- Anxiety
- Ineffective coping
- Chronic low self-esteem
- Impaired social interaction

OUTCOME IDENTIFICATION

An individual with a personality disorder has disturbances in self-image and relationships throughout life. Identifying outcomes includes the client's ability to demonstrate understanding of problem areas and to display healthy and effective adaptive behaviors. The focus is on helping the individual find patterns of maladaptive behavior, thoughts, and emotions that produce distress. The nurse and client can work together to explore options to change these maladaptive patterns to more effective coping strategies.

The outcome criteria are derived from the nursing diagnoses and are the expected client responses or behaviors that occur as a result of the plan of care. Outcomes are written in clear, measurable terms.

Client will:

- Demonstrate absence of active suicidal ideation.
- No longer have any thoughts of harming others.
- Refrain from self-mutilation.
- Reach and maintain the highest functioning possible, as demonstrated by the ability to function at home, work, and in the community.
- Identify two impulsive behavior patterns that take place during times of stress.
- Recognize when he or she is experiencing cognitive distortions during a stressful period of time.
- Identify a cognitive distortion used most often during times of stress.
- Identify one new method of problem solving.
- Reward self, both with an item (such as some flowers) and a positive thought when able to successfully identify and change a cognitive distortion.
- Identify some patterns of isolative behavior.
- Tolerate short interactive periods with the nurse, family members, and peers (see Case Study).
- Identify with positive role models.
- Contribute one statement in a group setting directed toward facilitating increased socialization.

PLANNING

When planning interventions with a client with a personality disorder, it is important for the nurse to recognize that changes in behavior or thoughts often occur slowly. These changes are a result of the client's perception of the need for that change. Individuals with a personality disorder have disturbed interpersonal relationships and values that do not reflect the views held by the general population. Because of these disturbances, the nurse must collaborate with the client

CASE STUDY

Marie has been working with a nurse for the last 3 years in outpatient psychotherapy. She was recently arrested for stealing some candy and lipstick at a local department store after an argument with her boyfriend. During the session after the arrest, the nurse suggested that Marie explore the dynamics of the incident and how this was related to the argument with her boyfriend. Marie became angry, then scared, expressing concern that she might lose the respect and the therapeutic relationship with the nurse. She ran out of the room, yelling that the nurse did not understand her pain, and slammed the door. Several minutes later, Marie returned, apologized, and asked the nurse to forgive her.

Critical Thinking

1. What responses by Marie would indicate to the nurse that she had some insight into the dynamics of her impulsive stealing behaviors?
2. What changes in behavior are anticipated as a result of Marie's gaining understanding about her impulsive behavior?
3. What two outcomes would be realistic for Marie?

on the goals identified during treatment (see Collaborative Diagnoses table).

IMPLEMENTATION

Implementation of the plan of care for clients with personality disorders includes interventions focused toward modifying lifelong disruptive and dysfunctional behaviors and thoughts, with the promotion of safety (see Nursing Care Plans on pp. 289 and 291).

Nursing Interventions

1. Assess the client for suicidal ideation and determine the level of lethality *to prevent harm or injury.*
2. If warranted, place the client on suicidal precaution, depending on his or her level of lethality (e.g., client who has verbalized plans to hang himself or herself while on the unit should be placed on close individual observation as long as those plans are still viable, with no means or provisions to carry out the intent) *to prevent suicide.*
3. Establish a contract for safety with the client by asking the client to write a statement indicating that he or she will not harm himself or herself. If the suicidal impulse becomes too strong, encourage the client to seek out a staff member to discuss the increase in intensity of suicidal ideation *to protect the client from acting on suicidal impulses.*
4. Encourage the client to attend all unit group sessions *to receive support from peers and to provide opportunities for problem solving.*
5. Assess the client for an escalation of anger to rage and possible impulsive actions against others (obtain a history of violence if possible) *to prevent harm or injury to others.*
6. Contract with the client that he or she will no longer threaten staff or peers during hospitalization *to ensure the safety of others.*

COLLABORATIVE DIAGNOSES

DSM-IV-TR Diagnoses*	NANDA Diagnoses†
Cluster A	
Paranoid personality disorder	Anxiety Ineffective coping
Schizoid personality disorder	Social isolation Ineffective coping
Schizotypal personality disorder	Disturbed though processes Ineffective coping
Cluster B	
Antisocial personality disorder	Ineffective coping Risk for other-directed violence
Borderline personality disorder	Risk for self-directed violence Risk for suicide Risk for self-mutilation Disturbed personal identity
Histrionic personality disorder	Impaired social interaction Chronic low self-esteem Ineffective coping
Narcissistic personality disorder	Impaired social interaction Ineffective coping Chronic low self-esteem
Cluster C	
Avoidant personality disorder	Anxiety Impaired social interaction
Dependent personality disorder	Impaired social interaction Chronic low self-esteem
Obsessive-compulsive personality disorder	Anxiety Ineffective coping Chronic low self-esteem Impaired social interaction

*From American Psychiatric Association: *Diagnostic and Statistical Manual of Mental Disorders*, Fourth Edition, Text Revision. Washington, DC, American Psychiatric Association, 2000.

†From NANDA International (2003). NANDA Nursing Diagnoses: Definitions and Classification, 2003-2004, Philadelphia: NANDA.

7. Teach the client other options to manage angry, impulsive feelings and behavior such as leaving the room where the conflict is occurring or using a quiet area (e.g., an unlocked seclusion room) until the impulse to do harm passes. *Removing the client from a stimulating, provocative environment may decrease angry impulses.*

8. Discuss angry feelings in a group setting focused on exploring alternative problem-solving options. *Alternative actions may distract the client from angry feelings and help to focus energy on constructive activities.*

9. Assess the client for evidence of self-mutilation. *Clients who are self-destructive are likely to repeat such acts and may require further intervention.*

10. Obtain a contract from the client that he or she will approach a staff member when the urge to self-mutilate is present *to ensure the safety of the client.*

11. Place the client on an individual, close watch until the urge to harm self passes or until the client is able to identify another way to obtain emotional relief (e.g., wrapping in a sheet or participating in a movement therapy group) *to protect the client from harmful impulses and redirect the impulses toward alternative, constructive methods.*

12. If self-mutilation occurs, attend to the wounds in a matter-of-fact manner *to provide safe care to the client in a nonjudgmental manner.*

13. Encourage the client to keep a journal of thoughts and feelings the client had before experiencing the urge to self-mutilate *to help the client acknowledge feelings and thoughts and help decrease impulsivity.*

14. Medicate the client with an anxiolytic or antipsychotic medication, prn as ordered *to help the client control his or her intense anxiety or rage rather than self-mutilate.*

15. Use a time-out period, seclusion room, and physical restraints if all attempts of least restrictive measures have been unsuccessful *to protect the client.*

16. Assist the client in recognizing thought patterns that contribute to impulsive behavior. This can be done by helping the client understand the role that intense feelings (e.g., abandonment, anger, rage, or anxiety) play in precipitating impulsive behavior or distorted thinking. Using a journal to document such feelings and thoughts and receiving feedback during group sessions are helpful, instructive methods. *Clients can be taught to manage impulsive behavior and distorted beliefs through a variety of methods within the milieu.*

17. Suggest alternative behaviors that can be learned to deal with the intense feelings, such as:

    a. Recognizing the intense emotional state and writing in a journal or thinking about an action that may help to relieve the intensity of the feeling without resorting to impulsive or self-destructive acts.

    b. Talking about the intense feeling while looking into a mirror, telling the mirror what the client would like to express to the object of anger.

    c. Identifying healthy options to deal with the anger, such as discussing the issue with the person who is involved in the interaction.

    d. Role-playing with the nursing staff different ways to approach the problem that precipitated the intense feelings.

    e. Introducing the issue in the problem-solving milieu group meeting to receive feedback from peers.

    f. Rewarding self with something that is pleasant and healthful, such as buying flowers or reading a novel.

Learning alternative ways to cope with intense feelings can reduce anger/anxiety and provide constructive ways of managing life stressors.

18. Help the client explore behavior that relates to the community, such as safe driving and responsibilities for the environment, *to help the client focus on changes that he or she can do to live in a more healthy and responsible way.*

19. Evaluate the client's family system by observing the family dynamics and determining the client's role within the family. *How the client interacts within the family system and the role the client takes (e.g., victim, placater) offer the nurse insight into the client's self-perception* (see Client and Family Teaching Guidelines box).

CLIENT AND FAMILY TEACHING GUIDELINES

SET Method

Clients with personality disorders often have difficulties recognizing problem areas and identifying options that could be solutions. The nurse could incorporate teaching clients and family members to problem solve more effectively as part of the care plan. One area of difficulty is communication. Kreisman and Straus (1989) have suggested using the "SET" method of communication. This was originally developed for clients with borderline personality disorder who were in crisis and were unable to communicate effectively. Kreisman and Straus's "SET" is a three-part system of communication. This is a particularly useful tool when the client is impulsive, is having outbursts of rage, is harmful to self or others, or is making unreasonable demands on others for care giving. In the SET method:

The *S* stands for *support;* the nurse states a personal statement of concern for the client.

The *E* is for *empathy,* in which the nurse acknowledges the individual's chaotic feelings in a neutral way, with the emphasis on the client's painful experience, not the staff member's feelings.

The *T* is a *truth* statement used to highlight the client's responsibility for his or her behavior and life (Kreisman and Straus, 1989).

For example, Robert had become enraged when his wife, Megan, did not go shopping and cook some meals for him before she went away for a business trip. His anger mounted, and he drank to deal with his intense feelings. He came to his partial hospitalization program, reporting a hangover.

His primary nurse led the following discussion about Robert's response to Megan's travel on business:

Nurse: I know it is hard for you when Megan has to go away. *[E]*

Robert: You got that right. It makes me so angry that she can't complete all her work here.

Nurse: Okay, I hear you *[S]*, but in her job, travel is a big part of how business is conducted. *[T]*

Robert: Yeah, I know, and I think she's good at what she does. I just get so lonely, so empty, I then get angry and scared.

Nurse: Can you look at what type of things you can do when she is away that may help your feelings of emptiness? *[T]*

Robert: Like what?

Nurse: Like going to the movies on the night Megan is out of town and seeing something she isn't interested in. Treat yourself to carryout Chinese or fast-food, so that you can have dinner without a lot of fuss. Does that sound like something that may help? *[T]*

Robert: I'll try.

Kreisman JJ, Straus H: *I hate you—don't leave me: understanding the borderline personality,* Los Angeles, 1989, Body Press.

20. Engage the client in frequent short interactions several times during the shift *to illustrate the value of interacting with others.*

21. Use milieu groups such as problem-solving groups and groups that concentrate on self-care and community responsibilities *to help the client understand the value of interacting with others.*

22. Teach the client assertiveness techniques *to improve the client's ability to relate to others.*

23. Provide direct feedback to the client about his or her interaction with others in a nonjudgmental fashion *to facilitate learning new social skills.*

Additional Treatment Modalities

A team approach, involving nursing staff, the psychiatrist, psychologist, advanced practice psychiatric mental health nurse practitioner/clinical specialist, social worker, occupational therapist, art therapist, music therapist, movement therapist, and recreational therapist, provides the most comprehensive interventions for a client with a personality disorder in an inpatient, partial hospitalization, or day treatment setting (see Additional Treatment Modalities box).

CLINICAL ALERT

Clients with personality disorders have difficulty relating to others. A consequence of this is that these individuals have difficulty defining boundaries between self and others. Part of nursing care is to define boundaries within the therapeutic relationship to develop safe, client-centered therapeutic relationships. This is particularly important for the nurse to think about when he or she is feeling vulnerable, perhaps because of other personal or professional stressors. Smith et al. (1997) have highlighted ways to recognize and prevent sexually inappropriate behavior with a client. It is important that nurses assess their feelings toward the clients that are in their care, as well as nurses' own current stressors. Nurses need to ask: Are the stressors interfering with functioning on the job? What are ways to deal with these issues without becoming vulnerable to the clients under the nurses' care? If nurses recognize that they are experiencing special feelings for a particular client, they should discuss these feelings with a colleague and/or obtain clinical supervision/assistance from the employee assistance program.

Additional Treatment Modalities
For Clients With Personality Disorders

Occupational therapy
Art therapy
Music therapy
Movement therapy
Recreational therapy
Medication therapy
Individual therapy
Group therapy
Family therapy
Milieu therapy

NURSING CARE PLAN

Eric was admitted to the psychiatric unit directly from the Emergency Department because he was involved in a fight with another man at a bar. He was under the influence of PCP, as well as alcohol, while at the bar. The emergency department staff assessed him as medically stable but suggested admission because of his potential for violence.

When Eric arrived on the unit, he was angry, loudly stating that he had been treated unfairly in the Emergency Department and that he did not need admission to the psychiatric unit "with all those nuts!" He demanded a TV in his room and a cigarette. When the staff denied his requests, he became louder and threatening. He told the charge nurse that he would get his way, that he had friends on the hospital board, and that there would be an investigation into the hospital treatment of his case if he was not allowed to smoke or to watch TV in private. He reminded the nurse that he was admitted for fighting in a bar, and he "knows how to get his way."

DSM-IV-TR Diagnoses
Axis I: Substance abuse (alcohol and PCP)
Axis II: Antisocial personality disorder
Axis III: Medically stable, related to withdrawal symptoms
Axis IV: Problems related to the social environment
Axis V: GAF = 40 (current)
          GAF = 60 (past year)

NURSING DIAGNOSIS: Risk for other-directed violence. Risk factors: a perception that others are denying him his rights and control over his environment; a history of violence against others; and an increase in verbal demands, a loud voice, and verbally threatening behavior.

CLIENT OUTCOMES	NURSING INTERVENTIONS	EVALUATION
Eric will be able to maintain control of his anger so that he will not threaten or harm others.	Monitor Eric closely for escalation of the anger to rage or impulsive action. *Close monitoring will help predict any increase in impulsivity and prevent injury to self or others.* Contract with Eric, if appropriate, that he will no longer threaten staff or client peers during the hospitalization. *Contracts used appropriately can assist Eric with impulse control.*	Eric was able to discuss his feelings about entering the hospital without threatening or aggressive behavior.
Eric will use the interactions with the nurse, members of the interdisciplinary team, and groups in the milieu to discuss alternative options to deal with situations that provoke angry, potentially violent responses.	Teach Eric other options to manage the angry feelings, such as leaving the area where the conflict is occurring or using a quiet area such as an unoccupied room until the impulse to do harm passes. *This will provide Eric with other appropriate ways to provide other ways to handle angry feelings, rather than violence.* Discuss angry feelings in the group setting, how the anger can escalate out of control, and what to do to control violent impulses. *Group input will provide alternative solutions to deal with angry feelings rather than resorting to violence.*	Eric was able to control angry outbursts and ask for his needs in a calm manner during his hospital stay and shared his feelings with the group.

NURSING DIAGNOSIS: Ineffective coping related to intoxication from alcohol and PCP, as evidenced by the client's loud and threatening behavior.

CLIENT OUTCOMES	NURSING INTERVENTIONS	EVALUATION
Eric will be able to determine his basic needs, make requests in a calm, thoughtful manner, and make some choices about his treatment and care.	The nurse will observe Eric for symptoms of intoxication and withdrawal from alcohol and PCP, which may require medication, and will administer medications as needed. *Symptoms of intoxication and withdrawal of both substances may include irritability and loss of impulse control.* The nurse will assist Eric in becoming adjusted to the unit by providing a tour, giving statements of support, telling Eric how the hospitalization will help him, and providing Eric with choices regarding his care when appropriate. *Eric will feel more in control, with a greater understanding of the environment and expectations, as well as being able to make some decisions regarding his care.*	Eric was able to decrease his loud and threatening behavior after medication was given to him to decrease withdrawal symptoms, and he was able to make some decisions regarding his care.

Continued

NURSING CARE PLAN—cont'd

NURSING DIAGNOSIS: Chronic low self-esteem related to long-term negative feedback and the client's belief that he is unable to deal with problems, as evidenced by self-destructive behavior (drinking and physical fighting in the bar), inability to accept constructive limit setting from the nursing staff, and demeaning others to increase his own feelings of self-worth.

CLIENT OUTCOMES	NURSING INTERVENTIONS	EVALUATION
Eric will be able to discuss, during a one-to-one session with his primary nurse or in a problem-solving milieu group, that his threatening behavior and demeaning behaviors toward others reveal his own feelings of low self-esteem.	Encourage Eric to attend all verbal milieu groups for problem solving, particularly those that discuss behavior and feelings. *Eric will obtain feedback from other group members about his threatening and degrading behavior toward others, thereby hearing the same feedback from several sources.* Discuss with Eric how his threatening behavior and derogatory remarks toward others distance people. *This discussion will help Eric become more aware of how his behavior contributes to others not attending to his needs, which reinforces his low self-esteem.*	Eric identified a need during a process group without threatening anyone in group. He verbalized other options to meet his identified need if the others chose not to assist him or were unable to help meet his need.
Eric will be able to identify a positive attribute of his personality.	Assist Eric in listing his strengths and areas that need adjustment as he views himself. *Eric only identifies negative parts of himself. Listing both strengths and weaknesses helps Eric have a more balanced view of himself.* Provide positive feedback to Eric when he accomplishes something within the unit milieu or in discussion with others. *Positive feedback reinforces functional behavior.*	Eric was able to identify two strengths in his character that he values, and agreed to recognize these strengths in the future.

Occupational Therapy

The occupational therapist assesses a client's abilities and disabilities and helps the client increase functioning and independent living skills in areas such as self-care, work, or leisure activity. The occupational therapist teaches adaptive skills for home, school, or job functioning. Groups such as stress management, enhancing parenting skills, conflict resolution, time management, money management, budgeting, feeling, and self-awareness are often planned and co-led by the occupational therapist.

Art Therapy

The art therapist uses art as a means of helping the client express thoughts and feelings he or she may not be able to verbalize. This intervention helps the client to understand problem areas from a symbolic standpoint. The art therapist also teaches the client an alternative means of expression and self-soothing. For example, a client who is feeling intense rage and has feelings of wanting to self-mutilate may use art to draw these feelings rather than act on them.

Music Therapy

The music therapist uses music to help the client express feelings and thoughts that may not be easily verbalized. Music is used to help the client relax and learn alternative self-soothing strategies.

Movement Therapy

Movement therapy teaches clients how they move their bodies when stressed and helps them learn methods of relaxation. Movement therapy is helpful for clients who become "numb" when feeling intense feelings, such as abandonment or anger, to use methods of self-touching to reestablish a feeling state rather than self-mutilate.

Recreational Therapy

Recreational therapy helps clients with personality disorders explore ways to enjoy themselves without the use of self-destructive behaviors, such as abusing alcohol or drugs. This modality is helpful for clients who have difficulty socializing, because recreation strengthens social skills.

Medication Therapy

Medications can play a major role in helping the client with a personality disorder. Clients who are demonstrating violence against others may require medications to gain emotional and behavioral control over their impulses. The clinical practice guidelines for the treatment of individuals with borderline personality disorder (APA, 2000) suggest that clients who have affect dysregulation show a reduction in symptoms using a selective serotonin reuptake inhibitor (SSRI). If there is an anxiety component along with the affective dysregulation, an SSRI may need to be augmented

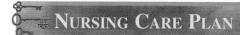

NURSING CARE PLAN

Dawn is a 29-year-old single woman who became suicidal after her boyfriend, Jay, told her their relationship was over. She started to drink and use diazepam (Valium) to calm down after Jay told her they were through. The relationship had become stormy, with frequent threats from Jay that he would stop seeing her. Dawn became vengeful, went to Jay's parent's house where he was staying, and threw a rock into their living room window, shouting that she loved Jay and could not live without him. She shouted, "I don't want to hurt anyone. I just want to die!" and ran into the street in front of an oncoming car. The driver slammed on the brakes and hit Dawn hard enough to knock her down and cause a pelvic fracture. She was admitted to the local hospital, still vowing to harm herself if Jay did not return to her.

DSM-IV-TR Diagnoses

Axis I:	Substance abuse (alcohol and diazepam [Valium])
Axis II:	Borderline personality disorder
Axis III:	Pelvic fracture
Axis IV:	Problems with primary support groups
Axis V:	GAF = 30 (current)
	GAF = 60 (past year)

NURSING DIAGNOSIS: Risk for suicide. Risk factors: intense feelings of abandonment, increased anxiety level, and a history of suicidal attempts.

CLIENT OUTCOMES	NURSING INTERVENTIONS	EVALUATION
Dawn will not act on her suicidal thoughts.	Place Dawn on suicide observations and assess her level of depressed thoughts. *Suicide observations will help prevent any further suicide attempts through early intervention.*	Dawn decreased her suicidal ideation within 2 days of hospitalization.
Dawn will honor the terms of her contract for safety.*	Assist Dawn in writing contract for safety that states she will inform the staff if her suicidal ideation increases. *Contracts can result in early preventive measures that can be taken to prevent a suicidal gesture.*	Dawn was able to use the contract for safety to assist with her impulse control.
Dawn will seek out the staff whenever she experiences suicidal thoughts.	Teach Dawn to inform the staff if there is an increase in her suicidal ideation. *This will enable Dawn to become an active participant in her suicide prevention and be more aware of how her thoughts and feelings influence her behavior.*	Dawn contacted staff when she had suicidal thoughts, feelings of abandonment, and other troubling feelings.

NURSING DIAGNOSIS: Ineffective coping related to ending a significant relationship, as evidenced by the client's vengeful behavior, her impulsive behavior to do self-harm, and her use of drugs and alcohol.

CLIENT OUTCOMES	NURSING INTERVENTIONS	EVALUATION
Dawn will identify her impulsive behavior patterns that occur during times of stress, record these feelings in a journal, and share them in appropriate groups.	Teach Dawn to link her feelings and behavior to how she responds to the events in her relationship by writing her thoughts and feelings in a journal, having one-to-one discussions with her assigned nurse, and listening to the input of the groups in the inpatient milieu. *A journal will help Dawn acknowledge her feelings and thoughts, determine her impulsive behavioral patterns, and decrease her reaction to those thoughts and feelings.*	Dawn was able to talk with her assigned nurse and in the unit process groups about her intense feelings of loss and emptiness. She was able to use her journal as a coping mechanism when her emotions became overwhelming.
Dawn will be able to identify at least one new method of problem solving to manage negative thoughts and impulses.	Teach Dawn healthy ways to manage intense feelings of anger and sadness, such as expressing her feelings to supportive friends and family members. Teach her to use a coping behavior to help calm her intense emotions, such as listening to music, taking a hot bath, going to an exercise class, buying flowers, or writing in the journal. *These activities will help Dawn to learn new coping patterns to deal with intense, painful emotions.*	Dawn was able to use her journal by writing poetry to problem solve and calm herself when feelings became intense during the hospitalization.

---

*Use of contracts for client safety depends on nursing and physician assessment and should not replace observations by a vigilant staff.

Continued

NURSING CARE PLAN—cont'd

NURSING DIAGNOSIS: Dysfunctional grieving related to ending a significant relationship, as evidenced by the client's use of drugs and alcohol, vengeful behavior, suicidal ideation, and impulsive behavior to do self-harm.

CLIENT OUTCOMES	NURSING INTERVENTIONS	EVALUATION
Dawn will identify feelings generated by the ending of her relationship with Jay, such as anger, fear of being alone, and sadness.	Discuss with Dawn her feelings about the end of her relationship with Jay in an open manner. *An open discussion with a trusted nurse will encourage Dawn to share her hurt feelings, fear of loneliness, and abandonment issues, which will facilitate healthy mourning of the loss of the relationship.*	At the end of the hospitalization, Dawn was able to talk about the end of her relationship with Jay without suicidal thoughts or cravings for alcohol or diazepam (Valium).
Dawn will share her loss with group members who also experienced losses.	Encourage Dawn to attend group problem-solving sessions on the unit to discuss her loss with other peers. *Sharing feelings in a safe setting will give Dawn a better perspective on how others have dealt with losses.*	Dawn shared her loss with appropriate group members.
Dawn will use healthy methods to deal with her loss and not use alcohol or diazepam to mask her feelings.	Encourage Dawn to write her thoughts and feelings about the end of the relationship in her journal. *Writing will help Dawn to recognize her thoughts and feelings about the loss of the relationship, which may help her come to terms with the unresolved issues associated with the loss.*	Dawn developed journal writing as a healthy method of dealing with her loss and working through painful issues.

with a benzodiazepine, such as clonazepam (Klonopin). Mood stabilizers such as lithium carbonate, carbamazepine (Tegretol), and valproate (Depakote) have been used with success as an adjunctive treatment for affective dysregulation. For individuals who are demonstrating anger and impulsivity, an SSRI is the treatment of choice. The clinical practice guideline recommends using fluoxetine (Prozac) as the first line of treatment for this symptom. Clients who are very agitated or psychotic may respond to the use of a low-dose neuroleptic or antipsychotic class medication. Clients with extreme violence who are unable to control this impulse may be given intravenous or intermuscular sedative-hypnotics such as barbiturates, benzodiazepines such as diazepam (Valium), or antipsychotics such as haloperidol (Haldol) (Keltner and Folks, 1993). Monitoring side effects is an important nursing function.

Individual Therapy

Individual therapy helps the client explore problem areas, define new options, and discuss how the new behavior may help solve the original problem. With the emphasis in the health care system on short-term therapy, individual therapy is now problem-solving oriented as opposed to explorative based on early trauma. The use of Linehan's Dialectical Behavioral Therapy (DBT) has an excellent rate of symptom reduction with the borderline individual (Swarles, Heard, and Williams, 2000).

Nurses are in a position to encourage and participate in research. The Borderline Personality Disorder Research Foundation is available to assist with a clearer understanding of this complex personality disorder. The more information the client and their family have, the more the choices about the use of treatment services and medication adherence makes sense. Research will assist in more comprehensive care and will aid in answering questions that will drive clinical practice. The website for the Borderline Personality Disorder Research Foundation is www.borderlineresearch.org.

Group Therapy

Group therapy is also problem-solving oriented. The work in group therapy is based on the repeated dynamics of the individuals in the group. This is especially beneficial for clients with a Cluster B personality disorder, who are dramatic and require a lot of attention. The group members will help the client to understand the effect his or her behavior has on each of them so that the client can use this information when relating to significant people in his or her everyday life.

Family Therapy

Family therapy is helpful for clients with a personality disorder because the dynamics of the family system are often repeated in other relationships in the client's life, such as with his or her boss or spouse. The family sessions consist of an assessment of the family system and an exploration of how the family dynamics are affected by the current problems that caused the client to seek care. Because of the current philosophy of short-term therapy, exploration of earlier dynamics and/or trauma is focused on the current issue.

Milieu Therapy

When a client is hospitalized in an inpatient psychiatric setting or participates in a partial hospitalization program or a day treatment facility, the client becomes part of that milieu (environment). The purpose of **milieu therapy** is to recreate a community setting on these units so that the client can interact with other client peers to identify and problem solve issues that occur while relating to others. Such relationship issues may be discussed in community meetings or other problem-solving groups, such as a coping skills group.

The community meetings may be used to delegate tasks of the unit, such as cleaning off the tables at the end of the meal. This meeting can be used to ask each member to think through a daily goal for therapy and discuss how he or she plans to meet that goal. If something happens on the unit (e.g., if someone becomes aggressive or brings drugs or alcohol on the unit), these concerns are discussed in the community meeting.

Problem-solving groups, such as coping skills groups, may pick a common area of concern; the group works together to explore the issues and options necessary to solve the dilemma.

As in any other community, socializing is an important part of the interaction. In an inpatient, partial hospitalization program or day treatment milieu, socialization groups discuss problems with socializing. The socialization group may use a discussion of a movie the group has just seen or current events read from a magazine or a newspaper as a means of enriching the discussion.

EVALUATION

The evaluation stage of the nursing process is ongoing and takes place to ensure accountable nursing practice. There are two steps to the evaluation stage:

1. The nurse compares the client's current functioning with the outcome criteria.
2. The nurse asks questions to determine possible reasons if the outcome criteria were not met (Fortinash and Holoday Worret, 2003).

CHAPTER SUMMARY

- A personality disorder is a long-standing, pervasive, maladaptive pattern of behavior and relating to others that is not caused by an Axis I disorder.
- There are several theories for the development of a personality disorder.
- In psychodynamic theory there is a belief that an individual who develops a personality disorder has deficits in his or her psychosexual development or a failure to achieve object constancy.
- Research has hypothesized biologic considerations as possible causal factors for individuals developing personality disorders.
- The DSM-IV-TR Axis II is set up in a three-cluster format.

- Clients with personality disorders have difficulty relating to others at home, at work, and in the community.
- When working with individuals with personality disorders, it is important to assess each client for the risk of violence toward self and/or others.
- Clients with personality disorders often exhibit self-destructive behaviors such as self-mutilation, eating disorders, alcohol or substance abuse, and shoplifting.
- Realistic expectations for improvement include a commitment by the client to explore and evaluate his or her thoughts, relationships, and behaviors, especially when under stress.

REVIEW QUESTIONS

1. A 50-year-old male client frequently interrupts the members of the group in the partial hospitalization program. He states that he needs to talk about his problems because they are more important. Despite a woman who is crying while discussing the grief she feels after her son passed away 2 years ago, he interrupts her and directs the group to his issues. The nurse assesses that the client must be diagnosed with:
   a. Borderline personality disorder
   b. Narcissistic personality disorder
   c. Antisocial personality disorder
   d. Histrionic personality disorder

2. Which of the following client behaviors indicates that the client diagnosed with borderline personality disorder is improving?
   a. The client cries when her roommate refuses to go to the dining room with her.
   b. She yells at the group facilitator when he points out that she is monopolizing the group.
   c. The client informs staff that she feels unsafe and is having thoughts of harming herself.
   d. The client reported to the evening shift staff that day shift staff excused her from group to have a cigarette break because she was upset.

3. A 26-year-old client is admitted to the partial hospitalization program. She is diagnosed with histrionic personality disorder. An appropriate short-term nursing outcome would be:
   a. The client will not engage in sexually inappropriate behavior.
   b. The client will allow other members of the group to share first.
   c. The client will deny having any thoughts of harming herself.
   d. The client will respond to staff redirection when exhibiting poor boundaries.

4. What Axis I diagnosis would you expect with a client diagnosed with antisocial personality in Axis II?
   a. Major depression
   b. Schizophrenia
   c. Bipolar disorder
   d. Substance abuse

5. A 43-year-old female client arrives to her therapist's office agitated and restless. She is diagnosed with obsessive-compulsive personality disorder. She describes how angry she is after she had to work 16 hours the past week because her staff wouldn't do their jobs. She had to start the project over because they didn't do it the way she directed them. The nurse's best response would be:
   a. "I bet you could use a vacation after this week."
   b. "I understand how frustrating that must be. Part of your responsibilities of being a manager is being able to support your staff to learn and to reach their potential."
   c. "You need to calm down. Why do you feel like you have to do everything yourself?"
   d. "Maybe you should think about changing jobs."

REFERENCES

American Psychiatric Association: *Diagnostic and Statistical Manual of Mental Disorders,* Fourth Edition, Text Revision. Washington, DC, American Psychiatric Association, 2000.

Becker DF et al: Comorbidity of borderline personality disorder with other personality disorders in hospitalized adolescents and adults, *Am J Psychiatry* 157:2011-2018, 2000.

Brown GL et al: Aggression, suicide and serotonin relationships to CSF amine metabolites, *Am J Psychiatry* 139:741, 1982.

Brown GL, Linnoila MI: CSF serotonin metabolite (5-HIAA) studies in depression, impulsivity, and violence, *J Clin Psychiatry* 51(suppl):31, 1990.

Coryell WH, Zimmerman MBA: Personality disorder in the families of depressed, schizophrenia, and never-ill probands, *Am J Psychiatry* 146:496, 1989.

Fortinash KM, Holoday Worret PA: *Psychiatric nursing care plans,* ed 3, St Louis, 2003, Mosby.

Freud S: Three essays on the theory of sexuality, *Standard Edition* 7:125, 1905.

Kavoussi RJ, Siever LJ: Biologic validators of personality disorders. In Oldham JM, editor: *Personality disorders: new perspectives on diagnostic validity,* Washington, DC, 1991, American Psychiatric Press.

Keltner NL, Folks DG: *Psychotropic drugs,* St Louis, 1993, Mosby.

Kernberg OF: *Severe personality disorders: psychotherapeutic strategies,* New Haven, Conn, 1984, Yale University Press.

Kreisman JJ, Straus H: *I hate you—don't leave me: understanding the borderline personality,* Los Angeles, 1989, Body Press.

Linehan MM: *Cognitive-behavioral treatment of borderline personality disorder,* New York, 1993, Guilford Press.

Mahler MS: Thoughts about development and individuation, *Psychoanal Study Child* 18:307, 1963.

Mahler MS: On the first three subphases of the separation-individuation process, *Int J Psychoanal* 53:333, 1972.

Manfield P: *Split self split object: understanding and treating borderline, narcissistic, and schizoid disorders,* Northvale, NJ, 1992, Jason Aronson.

Mann JJ et al: Increased serotonin-2 and beta-adrenergic receptor binding in the frontal cortices of suicide victims, *Arch Gen Psychiatry* 43:954, 1986.

Marin D et al: Biological models and treatments for personality disorders, *Psychiatr Ann* 19:143, 1989.

Masterson JF: *Psychotherapy of the borderline adult: a developmental approach,* New York, 1976, Brunner/Mazel.

Myers MG, Stewart DG, Brown SA: Progression from conduct disorder to antisocial personality disorder following treatment for adolescent substance abuse, *Am J Psychiatry* 155:479, 1998.

NANDA International (2003). NANDA Nursing Diagnoses: Definitions and Classification, 2003-2004. Philadelphia: NANDA.

Oldham JM, Skodol AE: Personality disorders and mood disorders. In Tasman A, Riba MB, editors: *American Psychiatric Press review of psychiatry,* vol 11, Washington, DC, 1992, American Psychiatric Press.

Pajer KA: What happens to "bad" girls? A review of the adult outcomes of antisocial adolescent girls, *Am J Psychiatry* 155:862, 1998.

Roitman SE et al: Attentional functioning in schizoptypal personality disorder, *Am J Psychiatry* 154:655, 1997.

Siever LJ: Biologic markers in schizotypal personality disorder, *Schizophr Bull* 11:564, 1985.

Siever LJ: Schizophrenia spectrum personality disorders. In Tasman A, Riba MB, editors: *American Psychiatric Press review of psychiatry,* vol 11, Washington, DC, 1992, American Psychiatric Press.

Siever LJ, Davis KL: A psychobiological perspective on the personality disorders, *Am J Psychiatry* 148(12):1647, 1991.

Smith LL et al: Nurse-patient boundaries crossing the line: how to recognize signs of professional sexual misconduct and intervene effectively, *Am J Nurs* 97:26, 1997.

Stanley M, Stanley B: Postmortem evidence for serotonin's role in suicide, *J Clin Psychiatry* 51(suppl):22, April 1990.

Swarles M, Heard HL, Williams JMG: Linehan's dialectical behavior therapy (DBT) for borderline personality disorder. Overview and adaptation, *J Ment Health* 9:7-23, 2000.

Tyson P, Tyson R: *Psychoanalytic theories of development and integration,* New Haven, Conn, 1990, Yale University Press.

Widiger TA, Rogers JH: Prevalence and comorbidity of personality disorders, *Psychiatr Ann* 19:132, 1989.

SUGGESTED READINGS

Akhtar S: *Broken structures: severe personality disorders and their treatments,* Northvale, NJ, 1992, Jason Aronson.

Alger I: The dialectical approach to understanding and treating borderline personality disorder, *Psychiatr Serv* 47:927, 1996.

Anonymous, Practice guideline for the treatment of patients with borderline personality disorder, *Am J Psychiatry* 158:2-52, 2001.

Erikson EH: *Childhood and society,* New York, 1950, WW Norton.

Freud S: The development of the libido and the sexual organizations, *Standard Edition* 16:320, 1917.

Freud S: The ego and the id, *Standard Edition* 19:3, 1923.

Freud S: The dissolution of the Oedipus complex, *Standard Edition* 19:72, 1924.

Gunderson JG: *Borderline personality disorder,* Washington, DC, 1984, American Psychiatric Press.

Horner AJ: *The primacy of structure: psychotherapy of underlying character pathology,* Northvale, NJ, 1990, Jason Arnson.

Houseman C: The paranoid person: a biopsychosocial perspective, *Arch Psychiatr Nurs* 5(6):176, 1990.

Kernberg OF: *Borderline conditions and pathological narcissism,* Northvale, NJ, 1985, Jason Aronson.

Layton, M et al: Brain regional alpha-[11C] methyl-L-tryptophan trapping in impulsive subjects with borderline personality disorder, *Am J Psychiatry* 158: 775-782, 2001.

Lencz T et al: Impaired eye tracking in undergraduates with schizotypal personality disorder, *Am J Psychiatry* 150(1):152, 1993.

Mahler MS: A study of the separation-individuation process and its possible application to borderline phenomena in the psychoanalytic situation, *Psychoanal Study Child* 26:403, 1971.

Mahler MS: Rapprochement subphase of the separation-individuation process, *Psychoanal Q* 41:487, 1972.

Valente SM: Deliberate self-injury management in a psychiatric setting, *J Psychosoc Nurs* 29:19, 1991.

Widiger TA, Corbitt EM, Millon T: Antisocial personality disorder. In Tasman A, Riba M, editors: *American Psychiatric Press review of psychiatry,* vol 11, Washington, DC, 1992, American Psychiatric Press.

13

Substance-Related Disorders

Sandra S. Goldsmith

OBJECTIVES

- Trace the historical evolution of substance use and abuse.
- Identify major theories and research findings related to substance abuse and dependence.
- Compare and contrast the etiologic factors related to substance abuse and dependence.
- Describe the effects of alcohol and other drugs on biologic, psychosocial, cultural, cognitive, and spiritual dimensions of clients across the life span.
- Discuss disease concepts specific to substance abuse and addiction (substance dependence).
- Apply the nursing process for clients with substance-related disorders.
- Identify community resources used in rehabilitating clients with substance-related disorders.
- Describe the current treatment modalities in managing the care of clients with substance-related disorders.

A client had been treated for a week in an outpatient clinic for chronic knee joint pain before it was discovered that he had been injecting contaminated material into his knee so he could receive prescription pain medication to support his **addiction (substance dependence).**

Across town, in a psychiatric hospital unit, a homeless person with chronic alcoholism and schizophrenia was experiencing withdrawal and was agitated, cursing, threatening staff, and demanding to be released.

In an Emergency Department, an 18-year-old male was growling like a dog and screaming that the devil was after him. He had been abusing illicit drugs.

The preceding examples are actual cases that demonstrate why individuals with substance abuse disorders can be among the most challenging to assess and treat.

Nurses and other health care clinicians need to develop finely tuned skills of assessment and evaluation. These skills are necessary when working with individuals with substance abuse disorders because, within the context of treatment, there are many opportunities for deception and denial, as well as opportunities to help. Clients may deceive clinicians by denying the use of alcohol or illegal or prescription drugs. They may alter tests designed to identify substances used. They may create symptoms to get the drugs they need, particularly in Emergency Departments. In the legal system, mental illness or substance abuse symptoms may assist in getting a lighter sentence. In a treatment setting, symptoms of mental illness falsely presented may result in prescription medication abuse. Clients with antisocial traits or borderline personality disorders may test the most skillful and experienced health care professional (Withers, 2001). Families and those who care about the addicted individual may also be deceptive or in denial and reflect this in a process called **enabling**.

Millions of individuals genuinely want help after suffering the devastating effects of addiction and may seek it at any point in the disease progression. After accurate assessment and diagnosis are completed, all individuals who care for an addicted person may cooperate to make treatment programs more effective.

Health care professionals, including nurses, can be instrumental in providing hope, encouragement, and effective treatment for those who *are ready* to change their lives. Although nurses must be knowledgeable about the possibilities for deception and denial in those with addiction or abuse disorders, they must also remember that the goal is treatment, remission, and healing for those so affected (Withers, 2001). The nurse's role is to be actively involved in both prevention and treatment aspects of substance abuse, making referrals for intense rehabilitation and recovery programs, treating symptoms of physical illness and addiction, or addressing end-of-life issues. Communities need nurses to be proactive and vigilant regarding the devastating effects of substance use.

HISTORICAL AND THEORETIC PERSPECTIVES

Since the beginning of recorded history, drug use to alter the mind and affect the mood has been documented. Even the earliest of tribes extracted substances derived from plants and roots to use in ritualistic, ceremonial, or medicinal ways to affect their lives. Some substances possessed extraordinary capabilities to alter consciousness. One of the earliest plants used was the glyagaric mushroom, thought to have been documented as *soma,* in a 3500-year-old Sanskrit text (Sadock and Sadock, 2000). In early Greek and Roman societies, alcohol was used as a part of meals, celebrations, and other ceremonies. Before 1800 in America, alcohol and opium were used in combination for calming and sedating effects. Patent medicines contained cocaine, opium, morphine, or (after 1898) heroin, which led to addiction, accidental deaths, or poisonings of both adults and children. The medical profession, as well as so-called "healers," used these drugs to treat illnesses in a world of then mysterious mortal diseases and infections. Sometimes the illness could not be cured but people could be helped to "feel" better.

The development of synthetic or manufactured drugs in the nineteenth century resulted in plentiful supplies of powerful habit-forming drugs. The hypodermic needle permitted direct injection into the body of a powerful, purified substance such as morphine. By 1900 the United States had developed an addicted population of at least 250,000 people, along with a fear of addiction and addicting drugs. This fear led to state and federal antinarcotics laws to regulate the sale and prescription use of narcotics, the most important of which was the Harrison Narcotic Act of 1914 (Sadock and Sadock, 2000).

These regulations and others that are in place today have not eliminated the problems resulting from illegal or legal use of substances. The memory of our nation's past history of drug **abuse** and addiction is essential because today the search continues for more powerful substances, with even greater mood or mind-altering effects, often with tragic results. As one substance is determined to be harmful and a public outcry addresses the problem, its use decreases. Another substance then gains momentum, and efforts are initiated to address that problem. The cycle continues, resulting in social dysfunction, addiction, or even loss of life.

ETIOLOGY

No single theory has adequately explained the etiology of substance abuse. Historically, abuse of addictive substances and alcohol was viewed from a moralistic perspective, with a focus on weakness of personality and lack of will power. More recently, biologic, psychologic, and sociologic theories have contributed to explanations for causes of drug and alcohol use and abuse.

Biologic Theories

Dr. E.M. Jellinek was the premier researcher in the field of alcoholism and was a strong believer of alcoholism as a disease. He proposed that the addictive process might have a biochemical basis. He noted that people with **alcoholism** progress through four stages, with the two more severe stages resulting in dependence. The stages were the *prealcoholic symptomatic phase*, the *prodromal phase*, the *cru-*

cial phase, and the *chronic phase*. His research led to the acceptance of Alcoholics Anonymous (AA) as a respectable treatment modality. Almost every AA-based recovery center teaches the "Jellinek curve," which describes the progression of the disease.

Research highly supports genetic theories of alcoholism. Some studies identify the following genetic influences in the development of alcoholism. There is a threefold to fourfold risk of severe alcoholism in close family members of the person who is alcohol dependent. The rate of problems with alcohol increases with the number of relatives with alcoholism, the severity of the disease, and the closeness of the genetic relationship to the person at risk.

Studies of sons and daughters of parents with alcoholism have led to predictions about who will develop alcoholism based on a lower level of response to alcohol. The lower level of response refers to tests showing that some individuals are more sensitive to the effects of alcohol than others (Schuckit, 2000). It is unlikely that anyone is predestined to be an alcoholic. It is likely that certain genes, traits, and social and cultural factors interact in such a way as to place a person at high risk of developing the disease. There is hope that as the relationship between these factors is further defined, preventive measures can be implemented to avert the development of this disease (Sadock and Sadock, 2000).

Research studies have also demonstrated a strong neurobiologic correlation between stress and drug use, especially in relation to **relapse**. Smokers experiencing stress, for example, may relapse even after long periods of abstinence. Prolonged or chronic stress can also foster the continuation of addiction behaviors. People with mental disorders often resort to drug and alcohol use to alleviate distressful symptoms.

Posttraumatic stress disorder (PTSD) creates a risk for substance use or relapse. Some individuals begin to abuse substances after exposure to trauma. A total of 30% to 60% of persons with substance use disorders meet the criteria for comorbid PTSD. Children who are exposed to severe stress early in life, such as child abuse or loss of a parent, may be at increased risk for substance abuse in adulthood as well as for other mental disorders such as depression and anxiety.

Stress increases the hormone production of corticotropin-releasing factor (CRF), which in turn initiates the body's biologic response to stressors. After exposure to stress, CRF is found in areas of the brain in increased amounts. Almost all drugs of abuse also increase CRF levels, which may indicate a neurobiologic connection between stress and substance abuse (NIDA, Community Drug Alert Bulletin, 2002).

Recently, researchers reported the results of the first "genome scan" for drug abuse. The study provided evidence that specific regions of the human genome differ between abusers of illegal drugs and nonabusers. This study was an important step in identification of individuals who may be at high risk for addiction. This knowledge may make it possible to direct appropriate preventive efforts and treatments to those individuals (NIDA, NewsScan 2002).

Psychologic Theories

Various psychologic theories have been advanced to explain substance use disorders. Some theories identify alcohol or other drugs as helping to decrease tension or feelings of psychologic pain. This hypothesis has not been supported in data collected during real-life situations when heavy drinking or falling blood levels resulted in increased feelings of nervousness and tension.

From a psychodynamic perspective, the earliest theories focused on the use of alcohol to help people cope with self-punitive, harsh superegos as a method of reducing unconscious stress levels. Classic psychoanalytic theory hypothesized that some persons become fixated at the oral stage of development and use substances by mouth to relieve frustrations and attain need satisfaction. Although addictive personality attributes have been studied carefully, no one unique personality profile has been identified that is more prone to addiction than another, with the exception of antisocial personality disorders and conduct disorders (Sadock and Sadock, 2000). Interpersonal theories have focused on the person with a dependent or inadequate personality disorder who uses substances to fulfill gratification needs or to gain a sense of greater competence. Theories of psychologic causation are less well accepted at the present time and are considered to be insufficient to adequately explain the need for excessive substance use.

Family Theories

Family systems theory is useful as a conceptual model to help promote understanding of emotional family functioning. Bowen's use of interrelated and interdependent concepts characterizes what happens in families when a member abuses substances (Bowen, 1978). Children from these families tend to become **enmeshed** in the family system. Their boundaries become blurred within the family and they live solely for each other. Family secrets and myths are used as survival measures by family members. They tend to cut off communication with those outside the family structure. The "multigenerational transmission process" can be used to trace the recurrence of the disease in the family in subsequent generations.

Research about family influence in substance abuse has led to interventions addressed to strengthen the family unit. Social ecology model data suggest that parents have an early influence on development of drug use patterns of their children (Kumpfer and Turner, 1990/1991). Crespi and Sabatelli (1997) identified a connection between the developmental implications of parental alcoholism and the individuation process. Dysfunctional families tend to restrict the individuation process.

Parental support is a strong predictor of decreased drug use in minority youth. Miller (1997) and others have looked at family dynamics related to problem behaviors (e.g., academic failure, antisocial behavior, high-risk sex, and substance abuse). Treatment measures have been designed to improve family involvement, parenting skills, and parental monitoring with the goal of reducing adolescent drug use and associated behaviors.

Learning Theories

Learning theory based on operant conditioning provides other explanations for substance use. In operant conditioning theory, drug use develops and is reinforced through the positive physical and emotional effects of mood alterations that occur as a result of drug use. Initially, the individual experiences increased feelings of self-confidence; reduced feelings of tension, anxiety, and fear; and an overall feeling of well-being. Intermittent reinforcement of the effects of drugs also occurs at several levels. Even though negative consequences occur as a result of excessive use, the initial learned or conditioned response remains. The negative experiences are often insufficient to stop the use of the drug(s).

Peer group pressures and the need to belong to the group have positive reinforcing powers for youth (Newcomb, 1992; Oetting, 1992). Modeling theory suggests that adolescents reared in homes where substances are readily available often repeat the behavior of adults and other role models who use substances to feel good.

EPIDEMIOLOGY

Substance-related disorders constitute a significant health problem and are an onerous financial burden. They may constitute a threat to our national security. The National Household Survey on Drug Abuse (NHSDA) is a major tool that helps track the use of various substances in the United States (*SAMHSA News*, 2002). According to data released for the year 2000, an estimated 14 million Americans were currently using illicit drugs. Approximately 104 million Americans, age 12 years and older, acknowledged current consumption of alcohol. About 66 million Americans reported current use of tobacco in 2000. The total economic cost of alcohol, tobacco, and other drugs has been studied by the White House Office of National Drug Control Policy (ONDCP) since 1985. According to estimates based on 1998 data, the economic cost of substance abuse each year is *more than $414 billion*. This estimate includes premature deaths, treatment and prevention costs, crime, social welfare programs, destruction of property, and costs associated with loss of jobs and earnings (Substance Abuse and Mental Health Service Administration News [SAMHSA], 2001).

Demographic Variables

The use and abuse of legal and illicit substances remain a major problem in the United States. Drug categories include alcohol, marijuana, cocaine, heroin, hallucinogens, inhalants, and some psychotherapeutic or prescription drugs such as tranquilizers, stimulants, sedatives, and opioids. Nondependence-producing substances (such as antidepressants, analgesics, antacids, vitamins, steroids, and hormones) have also been identified as a category of abuse by the International Classification of Diseases (ICD-10). Age, ethnicity, race, gender, and level of education are some of the variables that highlight patterns of substance use by different populations. Preliminary results of the year 2000 NHSDA study yielded the following information about rates of use and types of substances used.

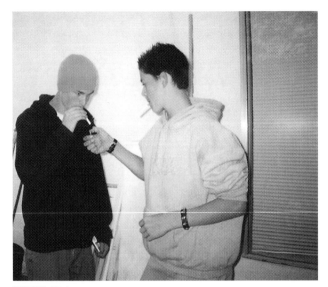

FIGURE 13-1. Cigarettes and alcohol are considered "gateway drugs" because they usually lead to the use of other drugs.

Age

Rates of illicit drug use increased for youth from 12 years up to 18 to 20 years (Figure 13-1). Peak rates of illicit drug use occurred for youth between ages 18 and 20 years. Age 21 years is the age when alcohol use, including binge and heavy drinking, is at its peak for current use by young adults. Alcohol use remained steady for older age groups. Cigarette smoking rates increased steadily in 2000 from a rate of 1.8% at age 12 years to a rate of 41.4% at age 20 years. Rates of smoking then decline slightly from that point on, reaching a rate of 9.8% for those age 65 years or older. A National Institute of Drug Abuse (NIDA)-funded study recently found that adolescent depression, combined with high receptivity to tobacco advertising, plays a powerful role in decisions teenagers make about smoking cigarettes.

Gender Differences

Men had a higher rate of use of illicit drug use than women (7.7% vs. 5%) in the year 2000. However, the rates of prescription nonmedical drug use were similar for men and women (1.8% to 1.7%, respectively). Youth of both sexes had a similar rate of illicit drug use between the ages of 12 and 17 years in 2000 (boys 9.8% and girls 9.5%). Alcohol rates of use between the sexes reflected higher percentages of use for males ages 12 years and older, 53.6%, versus 40.2% for females. Males were more likely to use tobacco products than females in the age bracket 12 years and older (35.2% vs. 23.9%). More young women smoked cigarettes than young men in the age group of 12 to 17 years (14.1% vs. 12.8%).

Race/Ethnicity

The rates of current illicit drug use reported in 2000 showed that no major ethnic group was immune. The rates were 6.4% for Caucasians, 5.3% for Hispanics, and 6.4% for African-Americans. The rates were highest among the

American Indian/Alaska Native people (12.6%) and among people reporting more than one race (14.8%). Asians showed the lowest rate 2.7%, although there were variations in Asian subgroupings. Alcohol rates of current use were highest among Caucasians (50.7%), as compared to people of more than one race (41.6%) and Hispanics (39.8%). African-Americans had a rate of 33.7% and American Indians/Alaska Natives of 35.1%. Current smoking rates by race/ethnicity in 2000 were reflective of rates of illicit drug use. The highest rate was among American Indians/Alaska Natives (42.4%), followed by people of combined races (32.3%), then Caucasians (25.9%), African-Americans (23.3%), Hispanics (20.7%), and Asians (16.5%).

Education

College graduates had a lower rate of illicit drug use (4.2%) compared with those who had not completed high school (6.3%). These rates contrasted with those for alcohol use, which showed increased current drinking patterns with higher levels of education (33.9% for adults with less than a high school education and 63.2% for college graduates). With tobacco use, the more education, the lower the rate of cigarette smoking (13.9% for college graduates, as compared to 32.4% for adults not graduating from high school).

Employment

A much higher rate of illicit drug use was found for those adults who were unemployed (15.4%) than for those who were involved in full-time work (6.3%). Likewise, the rate of current cigarette smokers was higher for unemployed adults (44.2%) compared with those working full-time (28.8%). Alcohol use rates, in contrast, were higher in full-time employed adults (57.3%) than in their unemployed peers (49.1%).

Discussion

The value of research such as the National Household Survey on Drug Abuse, the Monitoring of the Future (MTF) Survey, and the Arrestee Drug Abuse Monitoring System survey cannot be overestimated. Resources developed by the Drug Abuse Warning Network, the Community Epidemiology Work Group, Drug Enforcement Agency, and multiple other agencies can provide nurses and other health care providers with a database and trends that influence the direction of education, prevention, and treatment.

The emerging club drug scene is one example of a trend that is growing across the nation. Methylenedioxymethamphetamine, MDMA (also known as ecstasy) and related synthetic drug use has increased in nearly every city (SAMHSA, 2001). Studies indicate that club drug activity may be moving from nightclubs and raves to high schools, streets, and other open areas. In addition, emergency rooms are seeing youth and adults who have combined the club drugs with other illicit drugs and alcohol, causing violence, increase in crime rates, murders, and deaths (PULSE CHECK Trends in Drug Abuse Mid-Year, 2001).

Box 13-1	Internet Websites

Al-Anon/Al-a-Teen: www.al-anon.alateen.org
Alcoholics Anonymous: www.aa.org
Alcohol-Related Injury and Violence Literature Database: www.andornot.com/trauma
Anti-Drug National Youth Campaign (Freevibe): www.freevibe.com
Centers for Disease Control and Prevention: www.cdc.gov
Center for Substance Abuse Research (CESAR), University of Maryland: www.cesar.umd.edu
Club Drugs: www.clubdrugs.org
International Nurses Society on Addictions, www.intnsa.org
Join Together Foundation: www.jointogether.org
Marijuana Anonymous: www.marijuana-anonymous.org
Monitoring the Future Study, University of Michigan: www.monitoringthefuture.org
Mothers Against Drunk Driving (MADD): www.madd.org
National Asian Pacific American Families Against Substance Abuse: www.napafasa.org
National Association for Children of Alcoholics: www.nacoa.org
National Center on Addiction and Substance Abuse at Columbia University (CASA): www.casacolumbia.org
National Clearinghouse for Alcohol and Drug Information: www.health.org
National Institute on Alcohol Abuse and Alcoholism (NIAAA): www.niaaa.nih.gov
National Institute on Drug Abuse: www.nida.nih.gov or www.drugabuse.gov
National Institute on Drug Abuse: Steroid Abuse: www.steroidabuse.org/
Office of National Drug Control Policy (ONDCP): www.whitehousedrugpolicy.gov
Partnership for a Drug-Free America (PDFA): www.drugfreeamerica.org
Research Institute on Addictions: www.ria.org
Smoke-Free Families: www.smokefreefamilies.org
Substance Abuse and Mental Health Services Administration: www.samhsa.gov
Substance Abuse Librarians and Information Specialists (SALIS): www.salis.org
The Smoker's Quitline: www.quitnet.org

Oxycodone (OxyContin) is another example of a drug whose use increased significantly from 1994 to 2000. Use increased 166% (SAMHSA, 2001). Pharmaceutical companies are taking note of trends like this and are working to develop combinations of medications (such as naltrexone or Antabuse with OxyContin) to preserve the use of this medication for pain relief while countering the drug high sought by those abusing it.

Regardless of the chosen practice area, nurses have a responsibility to stay informed about drug use trends by using resources readily available on the Internet (Box 13-1).

SUBSTANCE ABUSE IN SPECIAL POPULATIONS
Perinatal Concerns

No drug can be considered safe when used by a woman during pregnancy. Research through the years has shown that substances affect the mother and fetus in different ways when used during pregnancy. Many of the substances used by pregnant women are **teratogens** to the offspring, causing developmental malformations in the fetus. Because many women abuse more than one drug, it is difficult to predict the damage to their babies. The effects of specific substances on fetuses is dependent on a number of factors including the type of drugs, amounts, patterns of maternal consumption, and the timing of exposure.

There is no strong evidence of teratogenicity for most of the currently used depressants, but pregnant women should still avoid these substances. Examples of depressants causing changes in infants are thalidomide, phenobarbital, and benzodiazepines (in animals). The belief that caffeine is relatively safe in pregnancy has also been challenged because it readily crosses the placenta to the fetus (Schuckit, 2000).

Smoking in pregnancy accounts for an estimated 20% to 30% of low-birth weight babies, up to 14% of preterm deliveries, and 10% of all infant deaths. Infants also have an increased risk of congenital abnormalities. Even healthy, full-term babies of mothers who smoke have been found to be born with narrowed airways and curtailed lung function. Children of mothers who smoke during pregnancy may also exhibit hyperactivity and have an increased risk of cancer later in life (Schuckit, 2000).

Scientific studies have shown that babies born to marijuana users were shorter, weighed less, and had smaller head sizes than those born to mothers who did not use the drug. In addition, research shows that children born to mothers who used marijuana also have difficulty concentrating when they are older (NIDA, Frequently asked questions, 2002).

Opioids present special problems in pregnant women and their offspring. Fetal damage may be a result of genetic changes caused by the drug. Other medical problems include elevated rates of intrauterine death, low birth weight in infants, premature delivery, and a 2% to 5% risk of infant death (Schuckit, 2000). Newborns of opioid-dependent mothers may exhibit withdrawal symptoms. At birth, children exposed to cocaine prenatally showed more abnormal reflexes, less motor maturity, and poorer ability to regulate their state of attentiveness than did unexposed children (Zickler, 2002).

Prenatal alcohol consumption continues to be a major concern. Drinking during pregnancy is the leading known cause of preventable birth defects and learning difficulties (Figure 13-2). These difficulties and defects are 100% preventable. Some general cognitive deficits were reported after an average of as little as three drinks per day during pregnancy (Schuckit, 2000). The NHSDA Survey looked at pregnant women between the ages of 15 and 44 years for the combined years of 1999 and 2000 and found that 12.4% used alcohol and 3.9% were binge drinkers. These rates, although substantially lower than the rates for nonpregnant women of that age (48.7% and 19.9%, respectively), highlight a major concern because of the effects of alcohol on the fetus. The most severe effects of alcohol on the fetus have

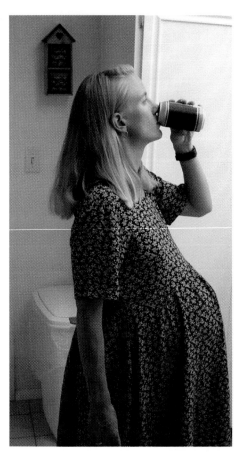

FIGURE 13-2. Alcohol and drug use during pregnancy interfere with normal fetal development.

been categorized into what is called **fetal alcohol syndrome (FAS)** (Figure 13-3). The diagnosis of FAS is determined by the presence of three criteria: (1) growth retardation, (2) central nervous system involvement resulting in mental retardation, and (3) facial abnormalities (Bowden and Rust, 2000). FAS is thought to occur in 1 to 3 per 1000 live births. Surviving infants can exhibit any mixture of the syndrome, which can include a small head, small physical stature, mild to severe mental retardation, facial abnormalities including a flat bridge of the nose, an absent philtrum (medium groove between the upper lip and nose), an epicanthal eye fold (vertical skinfold over the angle of the inner canthus of the eye), an atrial or ventricular septal heart defect, syndactyly (malformations of the hands and feet with fusion of fingers or toes), disorders of the temporomandibular joint, and learning difficulties.

Other signs of FAS include hearing loss or a developmental delay. As children reach school age, they may have problems in reading, spelling, and arithmetic. As they grow older, they have an increased risk for developing alcohol abuse and dependence and may develop antisocial personality disorders and other psychiatric conditions (Schuckit, 2000).

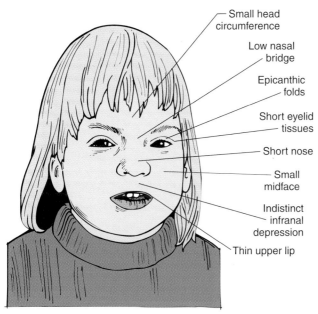

Small head circumference
Low nasal bridge
Epicanthic folds
Short eyelid tissues
Short nose
Small midface
Indistinct infranal depression
Thin upper lip

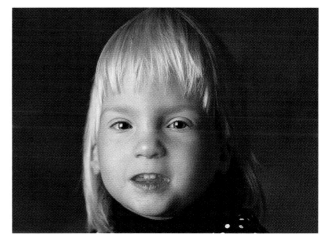

FIGURE 13-3. Fetal alcohol syndrome (FAS). Milder forms of alcohol-induced effects on the fetus and the infant are known as fetal alcohol effects.

Adolescent Substance Abuse

Diagnosis and treatment of adolescent substance abuse are controversial. There are those who believe that this age group should be treated as adults with diagnosed substance-related disorders such as substance abuse, intoxication, withdrawal or dependence. For the most part, the DSM-IV-TR categories focus on *recurrent patterns* of use that result in significant patterns of maladaptive behavior or distress. For some adolescents, it is more relevant to use the term *problematic use*, because this age group experiments or uses drugs in response to specific events such as parties, developmental or emotional crises, and peer group influences and pressures. Teens may not fit in the usual criteria used in the DSM-IV-TR for symptoms of **psychologic dependence** or **physical dependence** because they have not used alcohol or other drugs for sufficient periods of time to develop patterns of use. Some adolescents go on to develop pervasive, recurrent patterns of use, which then result in serious consequences and diagnosable substance-related disorders.

Research conducted over the last 30 years has produced a convincing body of evidence that the use of cigarettes, alcohol, and marijuana by children and adolescents is especially dangerous. These drugs impede social and intellectual development, cause disease or brain damage, and ruin or destroy lives. They often lead to dangerous activities such as driving under the influence, premature or unprotected sex, and violence.

Data on substance use by youth are collected using three major surveys and systems. The MTF tracks more than 44,000 teenagers across the nation in grades 8, 10, and 12 regarding the use of drugs, alcohol, cigarettes, and smoke-less tobacco. The second is the National Household Survey on Drug Abuse (NHSDA), and the third is the Youth Risk Behavior Surveillance System (YRBSS), which monitors six categories of priority health risk behaviors among youth and young adults in grades 9 to 12 throughout the United States.

Of particular note are statistics concerning rave drugs. Both the MTF study and the NHSDA found an increase from 1999 to 2000 in lifetime use of MDMA (ecstasy) among persons ages 12 to 17 years. The increased adolescent consumption of ecstasy is cause for alarm. Since 1999, teen use of ecstasy has increased by 71%. According to Stephen. J. Paserb, President of the Partnership for a Drug-Free America (PDFA), the adolescent experimentation with ecstasy is now equal or greater than teen consumption of all other illicit drugs. "Ecstasy has become the rave generation's cocaine" (PDFA, 2001). The use of other club drugs such as γ-hydroxybutyrate (GHB), flunitrazepam (Rohypnol), ketamine (Ketalar, Ketaject, and Ketavet), methamphetamine, and lysergic acid diethylamide (LSD) is also on the rise.

The Center on Addiction and Substance Abuse (CASA) at Columbia University, analyzed the use of alcohol, cigarettes, and marijuana as entry or gateway drugs that lead to subsequent use of other illicit drugs, regardless of the age, ethnicity, or race of those involved. The highlights of their report emphasize the dangers that gateway drugs present to youth. They found that age at first use, frequency of use, and number of drugs used increase the probability of a youth becoming a regular drug user and addict. The implications of this comprehensive report are clear. If a child/adolescent can make it through the teenage years

CLIENT AND FAMILY TEACHING GUIDELINES

Signs of Adolescent Drug Use/Abuse

Bloodshot, red eyes, droopy eyelids
Wearing sunglasses at inappropriate times
Changes in sleep patterns (e.g., napping, insomnia)
Unexplained periods of moodiness, depression, anxiety, or irritability
Decreased interaction and communication with family
Loss of interest in previous hobbies, sports, etc.
Change in friends; won't introduce new friends
Decline in academic performance, drop in grades
Loss of motivation and interest in school activities
Change in peer group
Disappearance of money or items of value
Use of eye drops/mouthwash
Unfamiliar containers or locked boxes
Money missing from the house

Prevention of Adolescent Substance Use/Abuse

Ensure positive role modeling by parents and adults in the adolescent's world.
Reinforce the dangers of substance use and teach positive behaviors.
Provide support in coping with the social pressure exerted by peers.
Establish limits, structure, and house rules for the adolescent's behavior.
Assist the adolescent to anticipate pressures, and reinforce positive coping behaviors.
Engage the adolescent in life skills training programs where the emphasis is on positive skills training, resistance training, and group support.
Monitor the adolescent's use of television, computer, movies, and video games, as media may portray legal and illegal substances as a part of daily life.

From The Clean Foundation, P.O. Box 28148, San Diego CA, 92198-0148.

without smoking cigarettes, without repeatedly drinking beer or other types of alcohol, the odds are overwhelming that the child will never smoke marijuana. The Client and Family Teaching Guidelines box lists signs of substance abuse in children or adolescents and strategies to prevent substance abuse.

Impaired Professionals

Health care professionals are thought to have the same prevalence of alcoholism and illicit drug use as that seen in the general population. It is difficult to document exact numbers involved because studies are limited and underreporting is common. It is estimated that approximately 9% of physicians are using drugs and/or alcohol (Weir, 2000). About 10% to 20% of nurses are identified as having substance abuse problems, and 6% to 8% of registered nurses are impaired as a result of their abuse of alcohol and drugs (Griffith, 1999). High stress jobs, frequent contact with illness and death, and accessibility to prescription and controlled medications result in susceptibility to use or abuse by some people in the health care field. The medical and legal implications of impaired professionals engaged in the practice of caring for others are profound.

DUAL DIAGNOSIS

Dual diagnosis, comorbidity, and co-occurring disorders are terms used to describe mental illness and drug abuse or alcoholism in various combinations. **Dual diagnosis** is the occurrence of both a substance-related disorder and another serious psychiatric disorder in an individual. These disorders may occur at the same time, or one may follow the other. Even though the diseases of mental illness and drug abuse are comorbid, causality is not implied. Either condition may precede the other. The symptoms of one condition may mask or conceal the symptoms of the other. Either condition may assume priority at any given time. Even though *dual* is common terminology, it is important to recognize that many individuals may suffer from two *or more* disorders concurrently. An individual, for example, may exhibit signs of severe psychosis, depression, and cocaine dependence. It is known that 29% of individuals who are diagnosed as mentally ill abuse drugs or alcohol; 37% of alcohol abusers and 53% of drug abusers also have at least one mental illness (Substance abuse, dual diagnosis, NMHA, 2002). The most prevalent psychiatric disorders among those with a history of substance abuse are antisocial personality disorder, bipolar disorder, and schizophrenia. The drug most often abused is alcohol, followed by marijuana and cocaine. Studies have shown that individuals use different substances to regulate or affect their moods, depending on the psychiatric illnesses involved (Daley, Moss, and Campbell, 1993).

Substance abuse complicates almost every aspect of life for those who are mentally ill. These individuals are difficult to diagnose and to engage in treatment, have often lost their support systems, and may suffer from repeated relapses, hospitalizations, and involvement in the criminal justice system. Violence is more prevalent in this group. The National Institute of Mental Health Epidemiological Catchment Areas study estimated that 90% of inmates in surveyed correctional facilities had dual diagnoses (Hatfield, 1993).

Persons With HIV Disease and/or Hepatitis

The practice of sharing and reusing needles, syringes, and other types of drug injection equipment exposes individuals to risk of multiple infectious processes. Contact with injecting drug users may result in the transmission of human immunodeficiency virus (HIV), hepatitis B virus (HBV), and hepatitis C virus (HCV). Boundaries have blurred between major risk groups who engage in multiple types of drug abuse, unsafe sex practices, and contaminated equipment use. The increase of heterosexual HIV transmission among young women, especially young African-American women, has been linked to the high rate of other sexually transmitted diseases in this group, as well as to the mixing of drugs, alcohol, and unprotected sex. Injecting drug users have one of the highest HBV rates among all risk groups and account for at least half of all new HCV cases. Prevalence rates have been reported as high as 50% for HBV and 65% for HCV among people who have injected drugs for less than a year.

Co-infections of HBV, HCV, and HIV have been identified as clustering in injecting drug users (CDC, 1999).

CLINICAL DESCRIPTION

Most Americans have tried or used at least one substance that could have resulted in further use, abuse, or eventual addiction during their lifetime. Caffeine, tobacco products, and alcohol are the three most frequently used substances. Many, however, learn from negative experiences and do not continue to use the substance. Others perceive only the pleasure from the substances and may go on to develop disorders that require treatment. The substance-related disorders as described in DSM-IV-TR include disorders that are related to use of drugs of abuse, medications, and toxin exposures that may be accidental or intentional. Substances are grouped into 11 different classes (Box 13-2). The DSM-IV-TR also addresses polysubstance dependence and other or unknown substance-related disorders. Many prescription and over-the-counter medications can cause substance-related disorders, particularly when high doses of medication are used.

The DSM-IV-TR divides substance-related disorders into two groups. One group contains the substance use disorders and the other contains the substance-induced disorders. Each of these groups contains criteria for substance dependence, abuse, intoxication, and withdrawal that apply to the different classifications. The criteria for substance abuse and substance dependence are found in the DSM-IV-TR Criteria box.

Alcohol Abuse

Alcohol is the most widely used and most destructive drug in our civilization. When used in a limited consumption by those in good health, any changes in body function that occur are usually reversible. Likewise, some data reveal that alcohol under certain circumstances may have some beneficial effects. In limited amounts, alcohol may increase socialization, stimulate the appetite, and decrease the risk for macular degeneration and gallstones. It is also thought to decrease the risk of cardiovascular disease by increasing HDLs and decreasing platelet adhesion (Schuckit, 2000). When

---

Box 13-2	Classes of Substance Abuse

Alcohol
Amphetamines or similar acting drugs
Caffeine
Cannabis
Cocaine
Hallucinogens
Inhalants
Nicotine
Opioids
Phencyclidine (PCP) or similar-acting substances
Sedatives, hypnotics, anxiolytics

From American Psychiatric Association: *Diagnostic and Statistical Manual of Mental Disorders*, Fourth Edition, Text Revision. Washington, DC, American Psychiatric Association, 2000.

DSM-IV-TR CRITERIA
Substance Abuse and Substance Dependence

Substance Abuse

A. A maladaptive pattern of substance use leading to clinically significant impairment or distress, as manifested by one (or more) of the following, occurring within a 12-month period:
   1. Recurrent substance use resulting in a failure to fulfill major role obligations at work, school, or home (e.g., repeated absences or poor work performance related to substance use; substance-related absences, suspensions, or expulsions from school; neglect of children or household)
   2. Recurrent substance use in situations in which it is physically hazardous (e.g., driving an automobile or operating a machine when impaired by substance use)
   3. Recurrent substance-related legal problems (e.g., arrests for substance-related disorderly conduct)
   4. Continued substance use despite having persistent or recurrent social or interpersonal problems caused or exacerbated by the effects of the substance (e.g., arguments with spouse about consequences of intoxication; physical fights)
B. The symptoms have never met the criteria for Substance Dependence for this class of substance.

Substance Dependence

A maladaptive pattern of substance use, leading to clinically significant impairment or distress, as manifested by three (or more) of the following, occurring at any time in the same 12-month period:
1. Tolerance, as defined by either of the following:
   a. Need for markedly increased amounts of the substance to achieve intoxication or desired effect
   b. Markedly diminished effect with continued use of the same amount of the substance
2. Withdrawal, as manifested by either of the following:
   a. The characteristic withdrawal syndrome for the substance
   b. The same (or a closely related) substance is taken to relieve or avoid withdrawal symptoms
3. The substance is often taken in larger amounts or over a longer period than was intended
4. There is a persistent desire or unsuccessful efforts to cut down or control substance use
5. A great deal of time is spent in activities necessary to obtain the substance (e.g., visiting multiple doctors or driving long distances), use the substance (e.g., chain-smoking), or recover from its effects
6. Important social, occupational, or recreational activities are given up or reduced because of substance use
7. The substance use is continued despite knowledge of having a persistent or recurrent physical or psychologic problem that is likely to have been caused or exacerbated by the substance (e.g., current cocaine use despite recognition of cocaine-induced depression, or continued drinking despite recognition that an ulcer was made worse by alcohol consumption)

Specify if:
   With Physiologic Dependence: evidence of tolerance or withdrawal (i.e., either Item 1 or 2 is present)
   Without Physiologic Dependence: no evidence of tolerance or withdrawal (i.e., neither Item 1 nor 2 is present)

From American Psychiatric Association: *Diagnostic and Statistical Manual of Mental Disorders*, Fourth Edition, Text Revision. Washington, DC, American Psychiatric Association, 2000.

drinking of alcohol increases to more than two drinks daily, or when those in poor physical health drink, however, damage to body systems may be more rapid and pervasive. Any amount of alcohol is considered harmful to a developing fetus, to recovering alcoholics, to people taking medications that interact adversely with alcohol, and for those with certain medical conditions or psychiatric disorders.

Numerous studies have documented the relationship between violence and drugs. Those in treatment for domestic violence, as well as violent criminal offenders, have high rates of substance abuse problems. The severity of violence exhibited escalated when associated with higher drinking levels and use with another drug, cocaine (Chermack and Blow, 2002).

Alcohol Intoxication

Alcohol intoxication, as defined according to DSM-IV-TR criteria, is based on evidence of clinically significant psychologic or maladaptive changes that occur during or shortly after the ingestion of alcohol. These changes include such behaviors as inappropriate sexual or aggressive actions, lability of mood, impaired judgment, and impaired social or work-related functioning. Associated signs related to these changes include slurred speech, incoordination, unsteady gait, nystagmus, impaired attention, memory, and coma or stupor. The breath may smell of alcohol, and toxicology analyses are positive. Other medical or mental disorders must be ruled out.

Effects on the Neurologic System

Cellular damage and loss of brain tissue have been documented as a result of alcohol use. Symptoms such as intense anxiety, psychoses, depressed mood, auditory hallucinations, and/or paranoia may be experienced with intoxication. Most individuals show a clearing of clouded consciousness within a few hours. Those with a previous history of brain damage or trauma, however, may remain confused for days or weeks. Older individuals may be similarly affected. Severe disorders associated with amnesias or dementias may also occur. Alcohol must be considered in all cases of rapidly developing confusion.

Temporary or permanent signs of confusion may also be associated with the direct effects of alcohol and with specific vitamin deficiencies. Wernicke-Korsakoff syndrome occurs as a consequence of a thiamine deficiency in predisposed persons after many years of excessive alcohol consumption. The Wernicke symptoms related to this condition involve neurologic abnormalities including inflammatory hemorrhagic degeneration of the brain. The Korsakoff part of the syndrome is a form of amnesia that is much greater than that seen in a general level of dementia. The person also exhibits an inability to learn new skills. Wernicke-Korsakoff syndrome has a mortality rate of more than 15% (Schuckit, 2000).

Blackouts occur in individuals who have consumed sufficient alcohol, quickly enough, so that the substance interferes with the acquisition and storage of new memories in the brain. The information becomes lost from memory within minutes of its occurrence. About one third of drinkers report at least one alcoholic blackout. Approximately 40% of teenage and young adult males have blackouts (Sadock and Sadock, 2000). The history of a blackout experience indicates at least one episode of a rapidly consumed excessive amount of alcohol. If there are no other symptoms of alcohol-related problems, a blackout may not be indicative of alcohol dependence.

Peripheral nerve deterioration in both hands and feet may result from chronic alcohol intake. This is called peripheral neuropathy and is seen in about 10% of alcoholics after years of heavy drinking. Symptoms include numbness of hands and feet, often bilateral and often accompanied with tingling and paresthesias. Damage may or may not improve with abstinence.

Effects on the Liver

The liver is particularly susceptible to damage by excessive use of alcohol. Alcohol is processed by the liver, and increased alcohol use results in the accumulation of fats and proteins in the cells, producing a reversible swelling called fatty liver. Inflammation of liver cells along with an elevation of some liver function tests and other signs of alcoholic hepatitis such as fever, chills, nausea, abdominal pain, and jaundice can result in excess deposits of hyaline and collagen near blood vessels, early signs of cirrhosis. As damage progresses, normal blood flow through the liver is decreased, dilated veins or varices develop, and fluid seeps from the liver and accumulates in the abdomen as ascites. As liver failure progresses, cognitive impairment can also develop as a result of hepatic encephalopathy (Sadock and Sadock, 2000).

Effects on the Gastrointestinal Tract

Alcohol is associated with ulcers and gastritis or inflammation of the stomach. Esophageal varices may occur in cases of severe alcoholism. Alcohol stimulates gastric secretions and promotes colonization of a bacterium identified in the development of ulcers. Inflammation of the pancreas may occur as a result of blockage of pancreatic ducts along with simultaneous stimulation of the production of digestive enzymes. The result may be either acute or chronic pancreatitis (Schuckit, 2000).

Effects on the Cardiovascular System

Heavy consumption of alcohol increases blood pressure and elevates both low-density lipoprotein cholesterol and triglycerides. These changes in turn increase the risk for myocardial infarction and thrombosis. Alcohol at high doses also produces what may be a reversible deterioration of the heart muscle. Wasting of the heart muscle results in cardiac arrhythmias and congestive heart failure or alcoholic cardiomyopathy (Sadock and Sadock, 2000). Higher levels of alcohol consumption are related to an increased risk for hemorrhagic stroke (Schuckit, 2000).

Other Effects

Blood Cells/Immune System. Alcohol intake of between 4 and 8 drinks a day decreases the production of white blood cells and interferes with the ability of these cells to get to sites of infection. This much alcohol may also interfere with red blood cell production, significantly increase the average size of red cells (the mean corpuscular volume [MCV]), and impair the production and efficiency of clotting factors and platelets (Sadock and Sadock, 2000). A less effective immune system may contribute to increased risks for contracting HIV, tuberculosis, and other infectious or noninfectious disease processes.

Cancer. People with alcoholism have significantly increased risks of cancers of the digestive tract including the esophagus, stomach, head, neck, and lungs. Breast cancer data indicate that as little as one or two drinks a day might be associated with a moderately increased risk of developing the disease (Schuckit, 2000).

Sleep. Alcohol intoxication can interfere with sleep. Persons under the influence may fall asleep more quickly, but have depressed levels of rapid eye movement and less stage 4 sleep. Interruptions between sleep stages, called sleep fragmentation, may occur (Sadock and Sadock, 2000).

Muscles/Bones. Alcohol can cause muscle inflammation or muscle wasting, especially in the shoulders and hips of alcoholics. Data also suggest significant changes in bone strength or density of alcoholics, and the weakened bones are more likely to fracture (Schuckit, 2000).

Hormones. Hormonal changes may occur as a result of alcohol consumption. Acute intoxication may result in transitory alterations of prolactin, growth hormone, adrenocorticotropic hormone (ACTH), and cortisol. It can also produce a reduction in parathyroid hormone associated with lowered levels of blood calcium and magnesium. Some of these changes result in symptoms of menstrual irregularity, decreased sperm production/motility, decreased ejaculate volume, decreased production of testosterone, and impotence.

Nutrition. Alcohol has a profound effect on an individual's metabolism of carbohydrates because it impairs the function of the liver and pancreas to respond normally to insulin. This impairment may result in very high or low levels of insulin in the blood and can have a marked adverse effect on the control of blood sugar in diabetics. Alcohol also interferes with the absorption, storage, and distribution of vitamins such as B_1, B_6, D, and E. Vitamins B_2, A, and K have been found to be deficient in alcoholics (Schuckit, 2000).

Accidents. Accident rates resulting from alcohol consumption dramatically influence mortality and morbidity rates in the United States. In the year 2000, more than 1 in 10 Americans ages 12 years and older (22.3 million persons)

Table 13-1	Alcohol Intoxication
Blood Alcohol Level (BAL)	**Consequences**
20-50 mg/dl blood (0.02-0.05)	No legal consequences; some impaired coordination; potential changes in behavior
80-100 mg alcohol/dl blood (0.08-0.1)	Legal intoxication; impaired ability to drive; slurred speech; staggered gait; impaired sensory function
100-150 mg alcohol/dl blood (0.1-0.15)	Markedly uncoordinated balance; gross cognition and judgment distortions
Levels above 200 mg/dl blood (0.2-0.3)	Notable impairment in all sensory and motor functions
Levels above 300 mg/dl blood (0.3 and above)	Potential for cardiovascular and respiratory collapse; coma and death can occur if lifesaving measures are not initiated

Data from Schuckit MA: *Drug and alcohol abuse: a clinical guide to diagnosis and treatment*, ed 5, New York, 2000, Kluwer Academic/Plenum Publishers.
NOTE: States may differ in defining blood levels for legal intoxication and traffic violations. For example, Colorado has defined a blood alcohol level of 0.02-0.05 as a traffic violation if the driver is under 21 years of age (2000).

stated that they drove under the influence of alcohol at least once in the last 12 months (NHSDA, 2000). Among young adults, ages 18 to 25 years, about 20% drove under the influence of alcohol in the year 2000. There is evidence that a blood alcohol level (BAL) as low as 15 mg/dl (0.01), or about one drink, can significantly impair a person's ability to drive an automobile. Alcohol also significantly contributes to bicycle and pilot errors, and to accidents in the home and workplace (Schuckit, 2000). Table 13-1 describes alcohol intoxication with BALs and their corresponding consequences.

Abuse of Other Drugs
Prescription Drug Abuse

Prescription medications that produce mind- or mood-altering effects are used legally as prescribed or illicitly. Prescribed and taken correctly, prescription medications have the potential to improve the quality of life, stabilize medical or mental health problems, and prevent or reduce pain and suffering. Taken for nonmedical reasons, these medications can cause addiction, overdose, and death. Four categories of prescription drugs were included in the year 2000 NHSDA. These included pain relievers, tranquilizers, stimulants, and sedatives. In the latest survey, 3.8 million people reported using prescription drugs for nonmedical reasons. This represents 1.7% of the population 12 years or older. Prescription drug use is designated as follows: pain relievers (2.8 million users), tranquilizers (1 million users), stimulants (0.8 million users), and sedatives (0.2 million users).

Some trends of concern are seen among older adults, women, and adolescents. Misuse of prescription medications may be the most common form of drug abuse in older adults. This population is especially vulnerable because of the multiple drugs that are often prescribed for medical conditions. Older adults use prescription medications about three times as frequently as the general population, and they have the poorest rates of compliance with directions for taking medications prescribed. Cognitive impairment and physical instability may result in increased risk for automobile accidents and falls. Risks are amplified because older adults have a decreased capability of metabolizing many medications.

Studies suggest that women are more likely than men to be prescribed drugs that can be abused such as opioids and antianxiety medications. NIDA data show that, among men and women who use sedatives, antianxiety drugs, or hypnotics, women are almost two times more likely to become addicted.

Use of psychotherapeutics for nonmedical reasons increased among youths ages 16 and 17 years between 1999 and 2000, from 3.4% to 4.3%. More female adolescents than males had used prescription drugs illicitly in the past month in the 12- to 17-year-old age group (3.3% vs. 2.7%).

Sedative-, Hypnotic-, or Anxiolytic-Related Drugs

Although classes of central nervous system (CNS) depressants work in different ways, they all produce drowsy or calming effects in those using them to help with sleep disorders or anxiety. If they are used over a long period, the body will develop tolerance. Continued use can lead to marked degrees of physiologic dependence and withdrawal if use is reduced or stopped. High doses can be deadly. These medications can produce similar substance-induced and substance use disorders. They can be obtained either by prescription or through other sources "on the street." The medications that are shorter acting with rapid onset are more likely to be abused. When used as drugs of abuse, they are often taken to reduce unpleasant effects of other drugs such as alcohol, cannabis, heroin, methadone, cocaine, and amphetamines. They may be used to "come down" from cocaine.

Medications in the *hypnotic* class include the carbamates, the barbiturates, the barbiturate-like hypnotics, all prescription sleeping medications, and almost all prescription antianxiety medications with the exception of a nonbenzodiazepine antianxiety agent like buspirone (BuSpar). Some medications in this class are also used as anticonvulsants (see Chapter 20). Carbamates include medications such as meprobamate (Miltown, Equanil) and tybamate (Salacen, Tybatran). They can be lethal when taken in overdose amounts. The carbamates also seem to have a higher potential for dependence.

Barbiturates all end in -al in the United States. Examples include phenobarbital (Luminal) and secobarbital (Seconal). Barbiturate-like hypnotics include medications such as methaqualone (Quaalude), etchchlorvynol (Placidyl), and glutethimide (Doriden). Methaqualone has been taken off the market because of its history of abuse. The class of hyp-

notics also includes chloral hydrate (Noctec). Benzodiazepines used as hypnotics include flurazepam (Dalmane), temazepam (Restoril), and triazolam (Halcion). Zolpidem (Ambien), although not specifically a benzodiazepine, has some similarities to those medications.

GHB is a CNS depressant that can relax or sedate the user. It is often used in combination with alcohol. It has been involved in poisonings, overdoses, date rapes, and deaths. GHB is abused either for its intoxicating/sedative/euphoria producing properties or for its growth hormone-releasing effects, which build muscles. The effects last up to 4 hours, depending on the dose. In high doses, it can depress respirations and heart rates until death occurs. Overdose can occur quickly with nausea, vomiting, headache, loss of consciousness, and reflexes. It clears from the body relatively rapidly, so it is difficult to detect in emergency rooms.

Antianxiety medications such as benzodiazepines include chlordiazepoxide (Librium), diazepam (Valium), and alprazolam (Xanax). Valium has been most frequently prescribed for acute anxiety. Benzodiazepines are relatively safe as far as overdose compared with most other types of sedatives and hypnotics. Used in high doses, benzodiazepines disturb sleep pattern and cause changes in affect (Schuckit, 2000).

Rohypnol is a benzodiazepine. It is not approved for prescription use in the United States, although it is used in Europe, Mexico, and more than 60 other countries for treatment of insomnia, sedation, and as a preoperative anesthetic. It is tasteless and odorless and dissolves easily in carbonated beverages. When used as a drug of abuse, its toxic and sedative effects are accelerated by alcohol. Rohypnol can cause anterograde amnesia or blackouts. When used to victimize others, such as in cases of sexual assault or date rape, as little as 1 mg can impair a person for 8 to 12 hours. For this reason it is often called the "forget-me pill."

Stimulants

This category of substances includes caffeine, ephedrine, propanolamine, amphetamines, and amphetamine-like substances. It also includes substances similar in action, but with a different chemical structure such as diet pills. Stimulants are popular drugs of abuse because of their effects on the brain. People become addicted to the sense of high energy, alertness, and well-being that these drugs produce. The effect is similar to a "bipolar high" of a manic state.

These substances are usually ingested orally or intravenously. Methamphetamine, "speed," is also snorted. "Ice" is a very pure form of methamphetamine. It can also be smoked to produce an immediate and strong stimulant effect. Abusers of this stimulant were found to recover from the damage to dopamine receptors substantially after 9 months of abstinence, but not from impairments in motor skills and memory (Mathias and Zickler, 2001).

Stimulants such as methylphenidine (Ritalin) and dextroamphetamine (Dexadrine) are often prescribed for treatment of medical disorders such as narcolepsy, attention deficit disorder/hyperactivity disorder, and obesity. The effects of the stimulants are similar to cocaine, but they do not cause local anesthetic effects. Their effects tend to last longer than cocaine, and they are usually used by someone fewer times a day. In some instances, they are taken on a regular schedule, even when abused, similar to other medications. Users may "binge" and have brief drug-free times. These drugs also may raise blood pressure and body temperature to dangerous levels, and elevate heart rate and respirations. Aggressive or violent behavior occurs with high-dose use. Anxiety, paranoia, and psychotic episodes may occur with abuse and dependence.

Caffeine-related disorders are included in the DSM-IV-TR. Caffeine is the most widely consumed psychoactive stimulant in the world. It is a methylxanthine, as are theobromine (in chocolate) and theophylline (Theo-Dur). It is estimated that more than 80% of adults in the United States consume this substance regularly. That produces a wide variety of symptoms, depending on the individual and levels of consumption. Tolerance may develop. Caffeine is found in beverages, the most well-known of which are coffee, tea, chocolate, sodas, and some medications; and it is added to some brands of bottled water. It is metabolized by the liver, and metabolism is increased in those who smoke tobacco. A person ingesting large doses of caffeine may develop delirium, and rare cases of suicide have been noted in conjunction with high caffeine consumption.

Opioids

Opioids have been used for at least 3500 years. Opioids include natural substances such as morphine, synthetics with morphinelike action, and semisynthetic drugs such as heroin. Codeine and related medications such as oxycodone (OxyContin), hydrocodone (Vicodin), and hydromorphone (Dilaudid) are synthetics with morphinelike action. Fentanyl is a synthetic medication that is injected, and other opioids are either injected or taken orally. Other manufactured, synthetic opioids include meperidine (Demerol), methadone, and propoxyphene (Darvon). Opioids are used as anesthetic agents, antidiarrheal agents, cough suppressants, and pain relievers. Heroin is the most widely abused opiate alkaloid. It used to be prescribed in the United States to treat pain until its abuse potential was realized, but is still used in other countries for pain control. It can be injected, smoked, or snorted when very pure heroin is available.

Opioid dependence can result from prolonged, compulsive self-administration of these substances for the effects alone without a medical need, or for a medical condition in which doses far exceed what is needed. Opioid-dependent people plan daily activities around acquisition and compulsive use of the drugs. Morphine- and heroin-dependent individuals can consume huge amounts (as much as 5000 mg) of the drug. Those addicted to opioids are more likely to overdose on these drugs, with sometimes fatal results. Signs of opioid intoxication include maladaptive behavioral or psychologic changes that develop during or shortly after use. Euphoria may be followed by apathy, dysphoria, psychomo-

tor retardation or agitation, and impaired judgment or functioning. Cognitive changes may occur along with physical symptoms such as pupillary constriction (unless the person has overdosed), drowsiness or coma, and slurred speech.

Nondependence-Producing Drugs of Abuse

The ICD-10 has a category for these medications that may have been recommended initially by physicians. For some persons, individual use continues when it is unnecessary medically, and excessive dosage ranges may occur. Medications in this category include antidepressants, analgesics, antacids, vitamins, steroids, hormones, laxatives, specific herbal or folk remedies, and diuretics. Usually the client has a strong motivation to take these drugs or to continue taking them, but no dependence or withdrawal symptoms develop. In 2002, the Food and Drug Administration announced plans to aggressively pursue the illegal marketing of nonherbal synthetic ephedrine alkaloid products. Herbal ephedrine alkaloids, known as ephedra, are sold in the United States as weight loss, energy, and sports supplements. Adverse reactions to this drug include irregular or rapid heartbeat, chest pain, severe headache, shortness of breath, dizziness, loss of consciousness, sleeplessness, and nausea (Join Together Online, 2002).

Anabolic-Androgenic Steroids

These steroids are manufactured substances related to male sex hormones. *Anabolic* refers to muscle building, and *androgenic* refers to increased masculine characteristics. Since the 1950s, athletes have used these steroids to boost their athletic performance. Anabolic steroids may be taken orally or injected, usually in cycles of weeks or months rather than continuously. This type of schedule, called *cycling,* involves taking multiple doses of anabolic steroids over a specific period of time, stopping for a time, then starting again. Users also combine several types of steroids to maximize effectiveness while minimizing negative effects (called *stacking*). In *pyramiding* a person starts with low doses of stacked drugs, then gradually increases the doses for 6 to 12 weeks. In the second half of the cycle, the doses are gradually reduced to zero.

Over time, anabolic steroids exact a heavy price on health. Abuse is associated with higher risks for heart attacks and strokes, and increased risk of liver problems for those ingesting oral doses. Physical changes include breast development and genital shrinking in men plus increased risk of prostate cancer, infertility, and reduced sperm count. Women experience masculinization of their bodies with growth of facial hair and male-pattern baldness, changes in the menstrual cycle, enlargement of the clitoris, and a deepened voice. Adolescents risk remaining short for the rest of their lives because of changes resulting in cessation of growth. For all individuals, extreme mood swings can occur, with maniclike symptoms leading to violence. Depression, paranoid jealousy, delusions, and impaired judgment may all occur as a result of anabolic steroid use (NIDA Community Drug Alert Bulletin, 2002).

Cocaine

Cocaine is a highly addictive alkaloid stimulant that is similar in clinical pattern, intoxication, and treatment approaches to that of other stimulants such as the amphetamines. The DSM-IV-TR uses almost identical criteria for the clinical conditions of amphetamines and cocaine.

Cocaine is sold on the street as an impure powder that is usually cut with glucose, mannitol, and lactose. The powder is usually injected intravenously or snorted through the nasal passages. Freebase cocaine (which has a lower melting point) is often sprinkled over tobacco or smoked in pipes designed for that purpose. The crystallized form of cocaine, crack, has a relatively low melting point and is readily soluble in water. Freebase or crack cocaine is usually 40% or higher pure cocaine, whereas powdered cocaine is less pure. A single dose of cocaine, especially crack, may cause psychologic dependence. Intranasal use has an onset of about 3 to 5 minutes, with peak effects in 10 to 20 minutes. The high begins to fade in 45 minutes or less. Intravenous use gives a high that lasts 10 to 20 minutes or less. Peak blood levels usually develop quickly, within 5 to 30 minutes. The cocaine effects disappear relatively quickly over 2 hours, although some effect will remain for about 4 hours. Traces of cocaine are found in the urine for at least 3 days, and may be found up to 14 days if high doses were used.

Users who inhale while they smoke cocaine may experience swelling and inflammation of the nasal passages and ulceration of the nose. Those who are sensitive to crack may experience sudden cardiac arrest. Tolerance develops rapidly with cocaine use. The range of tolerance may become very high, with individuals using up to 3 to 10 grams of cocaine daily. For some individuals, however, sensitization develops and users show an increasing effect with repeated doses.

Cocaine intoxication is characterized by changes such as euphoria or affective blunting, hypervigilance, agitation or anger, impaired judgment and social functioning, and anxiety. Depressant effects such as sadness, decreased blood pressure, and psychomotor retardation may be seen with long-term, high-dose use. The course of intoxication is usually self-limiting to approximately 24 hours, after which withdrawal symptoms occur. These withdrawal symptoms are often referred to as the "crash" when the person is depressed.

Hallucinogens

These drugs, classified as intoxicants, alter perception, cognition, and mood. The user typically has insight into the connection between use of the drug and the sensation that follows. LSD was discovered in 1943 by Albert Hofmann. This semisynthetic drug led to the widespread use and abuse of hallucinogenic drugs that could be made more cheaply and distributed more easily than the botanical versions such as psilocybin mushrooms and mescaline (peyote cacti). LSD is marketed illegally as single crystals, drops on blotter paper, or in sugar cubes. Because LSD is difficult to detect, blotter paper often is marked with cartoon figures or other designs.

Other drugs in this class include methylenedioxyamphetamine (MDA) and MDMA. These are referred to in today's society as club drugs or **designer drugs** and are neurotoxic. MDA and 3-4 methylenedioxy-N-ethylamphetamine (MDEA, "Eve") are drugs similar to MDMA.

MDA and MDMA are taken in multiple ways, including orally, snorting, as suppositories, or injected IV or subcutaneously ("skin-popping"). Its effects last between 3 and 6 hours, although confusion, depression, sleep problems, and paranoia may last weeks longer. MDA and MDMA use have resulted in deaths resulting from seroneurotoxicity. Symptoms include drug-induced anxiety or panic, compulsive dancing, hyponatremia, and hyperthermia (temperatures of more than 103° F orally). Autopsies have shown signs of rapid muscle destruction with massive hepatic necrosis, kidney failure, and heat stroke.

Clinical symptoms of hallucinogen use may include panic attacks, flashbacks (unwanted recurrence of drug effects), psychosis, delirium, and mood- and anxiety-related disorders. Tolerance and dependence may occur. Hallucinogens are different from other drugs of abuse because cessation of use after long-term use does not result in a distinct withdrawal syndrome. Hallucinogens may also place a person at higher risk of suicide. A "bad trip" or the negative effects of this drug may end about 6 to 12 hours after the use of a hallucinogen. Psychiatric related disorders may result from as little as one dose of a hallucinogen (Sadock and Sadock, 2000).

Phencyclidine and Ketamine

Phencyclidine (PCP) is abused as a hallucinogen, but has its own set of CNS actions and problems. PCP interacts with a unique high-affinity brain binding site. It is stored in fatty tissues, which causes long-acting effects in some people. It was initially developed as an anesthetic, but its use was discontinued because of severe adverse reactions. It has a long duration of action and, because of its potency, carries a high risk of toxicity. It is usually snorted or smoked, although other routes of administration have been used. PCP is often used as an adulterant with other substances such as tetrahydrocannabinol (THC), cocaine, methamphetamine, or LSD. Clinical indications of significant neuronal hyperexcitability, hypertension, and hyperthermia are regarded as a potential medical emergency. As concentrations of PCP fluctuate, mixtures of features of intoxication, delirium, and psychosis may occur. Confusion, paranoia, hallucinations, and violent outbursts may occur (Schuckit, 2000).

Ketamine, also known as "special K," is an anesthetic that was initially used illegally instead of PCP because it is less potent and has a shorter duration of action. About 90% of ketamine sold today is intended for veterinary use. It is often illegally snorted or smoked with marijuana or tobacco products for its effects of dreamlike states and hallucinations. In some cities, it is being injected intramuscularly. At low doses, it can cause impaired attention, learning ability, and memory. In high doses, it causes delirium, amnesia, impaired motor function, elevated blood pressure, depression, and potentially fatal respiratory problems (Community Alert Bulletin, Club Drugs, 2002).

Nicotine

Nicotine dependence is the most deadly and costly dependence of the substance dependencies. Although nicotine use in the United States has declined in recent years, it remains a major contributor to disease and deaths. Approximately 50% of smokers die of smoking-related illnesses. An estimated 65.5 million Americans reported current use of a tobacco product in 2000. More than 6000 children die each year because of parental smoking, primarily as a result of sudden infant death syndrome (SIDS) and respiratory infections linked to parental smoking and to low birth weights associated with smoking during pregnancy. The types of tobacco products smoked included cigarettes (55.5 million people or 24.9%), cigars (10.7 million people or 4.8%), smokeless tobacco (7.6 million people or 3.4%), and pipes (2.1 million people or 1%). One trend noted in recent years is the increased recognition of the need for treatment of tobacco dependence. Individuals with other substance-abuse problems, especially alcohol abuse, are also typically heavy smokers, as are those with psychiatric illnesses or dual diagnoses.

Dependence on nicotine occurs in a relatively short time period. Reinforcement of smoking may be a result of increases of norepinephrine, epinephrine, and serotonin caused by nicotine. Nicotine is rapidly absorbed into the circulation and reaches the CNS is less than 15 seconds. It has multiple effects on a person that tend to also reinforce continuation of the habit. Nicotine acts psychologically as a motivator for desired personal or professional goals. It improves performance, stabilizes mood, and lessens anger. It decreases appetite and food intake and increases metabolic rate. It is also socially reinforcing for some individuals, particularly youth.

Cannabis

This category includes marijuana and hashish. Both substances are derived from the Indian hemp plant. Marijuana typically refers to the upper leaves, flowering tops, and stems of the plant. Hashish comes from the dried resinous exudates from the tops and back side of the leaves of some plants. Cannabis, the bioactive substances extracted from the plant, remains the world's most commonly used illicit drug. It ranks fourth in the world after caffeine, nicotine, and alcohol. The active ingredient in these substances is tetrahydrocannabinol (THC). This substance produces most of the effects that lead to use. Hashish contains about 10% THC. Most marijuana purchased on the street contains from 1% to 5% THC. Some forms available today, however, may contain up to 40% THC (Bennett and Bennett, 2002).

Cannabis is usually smoked in cigarettes (joints), although it can be ingested in food. It is often adulterated with other drugs such as opium, cocaine, or PCP. Signs of intoxication include a "high" feeling with euphoria accompanied by inappropriate laughter and grandiosity, sedation, lethargy, impairment in cognition, distorted sensory perceptions, impaired motor skills and performance, and a sensation of prolonged time sequences. The psychoactive effects are followed by other signs within 2 hours of use such as conjunctival injection (bloodshot eye appearance), increased appetite, tachycardia, and dry mouth. If cannabis is smoked, the effects develop within minutes and usually last 3 to 4 hours. The severity of symptoms is related to several factors such as dose, method of ingestion, and the individual characteristics of the user. Cannabis is fat soluble, and high-dose effects may persist for 12 to 24 hours longer as it is released from the tissues. Dependence and tolerance develop over time. Data from one research study showed that those who had used marijuana over many years had markedly lower income and education levels than those who did not, regardless of whether they were still using the drug (Zickler, 2002). Another study showed that long-term users performed poorly on most memory, attention, time judgment, and information processing tests (SAMHSA News, 2002).

Inhalants

This classification of substances includes products that are breathable chemical vapors that produce psychoactive effects. More than a million people used inhalants to get high in the year 2000. For young people especially, these substances are cheap and easily accessible. Inhalants fall into three categories:

1. Solvents (paint thinners, degreasers, gasoline, and glues)
2. Gases (butane from lighters; propane; whipping cream aerosols or dispensers [whippets] and refrigerant gases; other types of aerosols such as spray paints, hair or deodorant sprays, and fabric protectors; ether; chloroform; and nitrous oxide [sold as poppers])
3. Nitrites (aliphatic nitrites including cyclohexyl nitrite, amyl nitrite, and butyl nitrite [now illegal])

Inhalants cause effects similar to anesthesia and slow the body functions. Depending on dose, users can experience slight stimulation, decreased inhibition, or loss of consciousness. Sniffing high concentrations can induce heart failure, suffocation, and death. Other irreversible effects include hearing loss, peripheral neuropathies or limb spasms, CNS damage, or bone marrow damage. Reversible effects may include liver and kidney damage and blood oxygen depletion. Amyl and butyl nitrites have been associated with Kaposi's sarcoma.

Club Drugs

As described earlier in the chapter, club drugs or designer drugs are being used by young adults at all-night parties called **raves**, or trances. MDMA (ecstasy), GHB, Rohypnol, ketamine, methamphetamine, and LSD are some of the drugs ingested at these events. All club drugs are potentially deadly or produce long-lasting or permanent damage to the human body. Because they are often colorless, tasteless, and odorless, club drugs can easily be added to drinks by those who want to see the effects on others. Uncertainties about drug sources, chemicals used, and possible contaminants make it difficult, if not impossible, to determine toxicity, consequences, and symptoms of use of these club drugs in any given community.

Multidrug Abuse and Dependence

Although many who abuse drugs try a variety of substances and settle on a "drug of choice," use of multiple substances by those who abuse drugs is also common. Multiple drug use or abuse, sometimes referred to as *polysubstance use,* is also likely to occur in individuals who progress through use or dependence on a variety of drugs over time. For example, some people start use/abuse with nicotine, caffeine, or alcohol. If they then continue on to use other drugs, they may try cannabis, followed by stimulants, hallucinogens, or other CNS depressants. This differs from what is seen in young people who may consume any drug readily available at a party. The ingestion of multiple substances at the same time creates additional risks because of the potential for drug interactions.

Although individuals may mix any combination of substances, some drug mixtures have been identified as more likely to occur. Those individuals with alcohol dependence are more likely to use or develop nicotine dependence. Those who are cocaine dependent are more apt to become dependent on alcohol. Many people with opioid dependence combine heroin and cocaine in a mixture called a *speedball.* The combination both enhances the effects and decreases the side effects. Other combinations of multiple drug ingestion include benzodiazepine use with heroin or methadone, alcohol and methadone, PCP and marijuana combinations found in street drugs, antihistamines, and pentazocine (Talwin), as well as codeine mixed with glutethimide (Doriden) (Schuckit, 2000).

Prognosis

Perhaps the most important factor in determining prognosis or outcome of substance use is the client's ability to recognize that substance use has caused or influenced life's problems and difficulties in functioning. Treatment programs refer to this as "hitting bottom," which means the individual is no longer willing to tolerate his or her own lifestyle because of adverse consequences. The individual must then be motivated to engage in steps to reverse or change the course and pattern of substance use. The steps individuals take may differ, but ultimately the goal is to change patterns of functioning to maintain sobriety. **Sobriety** is the goal for complete recovery from substance abuse or dependence. The client must also learn how to prevent or minimize relapses so that he or she can get back on course toward achievement of abstinence. Most people who seek recovery from substance use disorders do well, especially those who are motivated and capable of functioning at a high level (Schuckit, 2000).

Many clients relapse several times before achieving sobriety or remaining "clean."

The course of substance dependence, abuse, intoxication, and withdrawal varies with the class of substance, route of administration, and other factors as discussed under the specific substances. Nevertheless, some generalizations about prognosis and recovery can be made. **Intoxication** usually develops rapidly after use and continues as long as the substance is used. When use declines or stops, *withdrawal* develops and continues for varying lengths of time, depending on the **half-life** of the substance and related factors. Typically a diagnosis of *substance abuse* is established in persons whose use of substances is recent. For many, substance abuse with particular substances can progress into *substance dependence* for the same substances, especially for drugs that have a high potential for development of **tolerance**, withdrawal, and patterns of compulsive use such as cocaine and heroin. For those drugs with a low potential for repeated use, substance abuse may not progress into dependence.

The course of substance dependence varies. It is usually chronic, with periods of heavy intake that are sometimes stress related and partial or full remission. Substance dependence is at times associated with spontaneous, long-lasting remissions. During the first year after remission begins, one is particularly vulnerable to relapse. Individuals with a history of earlier onset use, higher levels of substance intake and greater numbers of substance-related problems who also exhibit a past history of tolerance or withdrawal may have a worse prognosis. In a similar way, persons who exhibit comorbid serious mental disorders such as conduct disorders, antisocial personality disorder, untreated major depression, or bipolar disorder are more likely to experience ongoing impairments and ultimately, a poorer outcome.

Discharge Criteria

Client will:

- Maintain abstinence or reduce harm (more applicable to some substances than others) from substance use.
- Admit to potential or actual lifelong dependence on psychoactive substances.
- Express knowledge of the continual process of recovery ("one day at a time").
- Verbalize realistic goals.
- Maintain attendance in a support group (Alcoholics Anonymous, Narcotics Anonymous, or others).
- Express increased self-esteem.
- Demonstrate new, constructive coping mechanisms and strategies to manage anxiety, stress, frustration, and anger.
- Engage in use of substitutes to replace drug-seeking, drug-taking behaviors such as hobbies, school, employment, spiritual support, volunteer work, social relationships.
- Express the feeling of being in control of one's life.
- Express hope for the future.
- Abandon people and situations that influence and contribute to drug-taking behaviors.

- State consequences of psychoactive substance use on biopsychosocial/cultural/spiritual well-being.
- State names and phone numbers of resources to contact when unable to cope, or when experiencing a need to revert to substance-taking behaviors.
- Investigate substance abuse assistance programs in the workplace, such as the Employee Assistance Program (EAP).
- Ask family and/or significant others to attend Alanon/Alateen support groups.

THE NURSING PROCESS

ASSESSMENT

If the nurse strives to accurately assess an individual's use, abuse, or dependence on substances, the development of a trust relationship must be a first priority. It is imperative that the nurse convey a nonjudgmental attitude toward the client and/or significant others. Despite these efforts, the nurse may find the tasks of assessment difficult because the signs and symptoms of substance abuse are often concealed, denied, or minimized by the person who is, at the same time, desperately in need of treatment.

The difficulty in assessment is often compounded because the identification of substance-related symptoms is often based on self-report. The nurse may have to serve in the role of detective by being alert and aware of what is *not* said, as well as what is stated by the client. The nurse must make decisions about not only when to ask questions but what to ask, and when to seek more information from those who know the client (see Case Study). In many instances, such as when the client is a poor historian because of the effects of drug use/abuse, history must be corroborated with family members, significant others, and previous treatment facilities. One must also assess the client's readiness for change because motivation is such a key component in the success or failure of treatment efforts. The nurse can maintain hope of obtaining critical assessment data, even when client disclosure is limited, by remembering that assessment is an ongoing process.

In gathering information about drug use, the nurse uses a systematic approach by integrating questions into the general history regarding legal and illicit substances. Age, ethnicity, and demographic factors related to drug use must also be assessed at this time. In addition, information should be obtained about use in other drug categories listed in Box 13-3. A client's positive response regarding any drugs should alert the interviewer to obtain further information about the specific drug or drugs used. The nurse can focus on the age of first use, the period of heaviest lifetime use, patterns of use, the presence or absence of binges, and any occurrence of blackouts. Use during the immediate past must be assessed to determine the possibility of withdrawal symptoms and/or toxicity. If the client is taking methadone, the nurse must ask when the last dose was administered or taken. The other components of a complete health history include a psychosocial history, family history, risk for suicide or violence (toward self or others), and a mental status examination. See the Understanding and Applying Research box on p. 312 for a discussion of recommendations for assessment of older clients with substance use disorders.

Collaboration among the nurse, client, family, and treatment team is essential in the assessment, planning, and implementation of the plan of care. For the client who abuses or is dependent on substances, the road to treatment and re-

CASE STUDY

Donna M. is an 18-year-old Caucasian female who was admitted to the Emergency Department in a local hospital at 0200 hours, after her high school prom. Her boyfriend, who had been drinking, was killed in the accident preceding her admission. She presented with facial lacerations and possible other blunt trauma injuries. She was incoherent and confused. On taking vital signs, the nurse noted that her temperature was 103° F, blood pressure was 140/100 mm Hg, and respirations were 28.

Critical Thinking

1. What is Donna's most immediate problem?
2. Is Donna a danger to herself or others? Why or why not?
3. What symptoms exhibited by Donna are typical of an adolescent with suspected use of a club drug?
4. Given Donna's behavior, what drug screen tests would be appropriate, if any?
5. What nursing diagnoses would be relevant at this time?
6. What complications does the possible drug presence pose to the anticipated use of medical/surgical procedures?

Box 13-3	Drug Categories Considered in an Assessment

Nicotine: cigarettes, chewing tobacco, pipe smoking, snuff, etc.
Alcohol: beer, wine, whiskey, gin, etc.
Cannabis: marijuana, pot, hashish
Cocaine: crack, freebase
Central nervous system depressants: sedatives, hypnotics, and anxiolytic-related drugs
Central nervous system stimulants: caffeine, ephedra, amphetamines, diet pills, benzedrine inhalers
Opioids: heroin, codeine, methadone, oxycodone (OxyContin), hyrocodone (Vicodin), morphine
Hallucinogens: lysergic acid diethylamide (LSD), mescaline, phencyclidine (PCP), mushrooms, peyote
Inhalants: solvents (glue, paint, gasolines), aromatic hydrocarbons (aerosols, gases, hair spray), nitrites
Anabolic-androgenic steroids
Synthetics: meperidine hydrochloride (Demerol), propoxyphene hydrochloride (Darvon)
Over-the-counter (OTC) drugs: antihistamines, cough syrups, sleeping pills, hormones, laxatives, herbal products
Designer/club drugs: ecstasy, MDMA, MDEA, MDA, GHB, Rohypnol, ketamine

UNDERSTANDING and APPLYING RESEARCH

Many senior adults develop alcohol problems related to normal or pathologic changes that occur in the aging process. Researchers also believe that the number of seniors who abuse illicit drugs is much higher than suspected. However, the most common drug dependency problems result from the misuse of prescription drugs. Treatment guidelines suggest that older clients with substance use disorders should receive regular outpatient mental health care after being discharged from the hospital. A longitudinal prospective follow-up study was conducted for older Medicare clients with substance use disorders. Data from Medicare records were used to identify 4961 older inpatients with substance use disorders and to determine their outpatient mental health care for 4 years after hospital discharge. Only 12% to 17% of surviving older clients received outpatient care in each of the 4 years after discharge. Over the 4-year period, about 18% of these clients obtained diagnostic/evaluative mental health services, 22% obtained psychotherapy, and 9% obtained medication management. The study concluded that because of health and economic barriers, this population did not receive the services they needed.

Regardless of setting, nurses have an opportunity to address the needs of the older clients with whom they come in contact. A comprehensive functional assessment of the client will assist the nurse to identify symptoms and/or patterns of change related to substance use as well as normal or pathologic changes resulting from aging. Interventions that will address the needs of this age group include establishing a supportive, caring ongoing relationship; building on identified client strengths; teaching about possible outcomes of medication therapy such as adverse drug reactions, minor side effects, and possible drug-drug interactions; involving family members/significant others in prevention and supportive efforts; providing medication information that is readily available, which addresses sensory deficits and is user friendly such as larger print, verbal, and/or bright visual materials with everyday terminology and primary language of the client; applying principles of teaching-learning and skills training that include repetition, feedback, and practice opportunities; providing compliance aids such as day/hour pill containers; assisting the client with transportation and scheduling of appointments; and identifying helpful resources such as faith-based organizations, physicians, pharmacists, outpatient clinics, self-help groups, and housing options that specialize in the needs of older adults.

Brennan PL et al: Predictors and outcomes of outpatient mental health care: a 4-year prospective study of elderly Medicare clients with substance use disorders, *Medical Care* 39(1): 39-49, 2001.

Box 13-4   CAGE Screening Test for Alcoholism

1. Have you ever felt you ought to **C**ut down on your drinking?
2. Have people **A**nnoyed you by criticizing your drinking?
3. Have you ever felt **G**uilty about your drinking?
4. Have you ever had a drink first thing in the morning to steady your nerves or get rid of a hangover (**E**ye-opener)?

From Ewing JA: Detecting alcoholism: the CAGE questionnaire, *JAMA* 252:1905, 1984.

---

covery requires hope, realistic outcome criteria, and a comprehensive plan of care.

Physical Examination

On examination, identification of specific physical health findings associated with alcohol or drug dependence may suggest the possibility of a substance abuse problem. For alcohol abuse, signs and symptoms include jaundice, arcus senilis (an opaque ring, gray to white in color that surrounds the periphery of the cornea), acnea rosacea (red nose), palmar erythema, enlarged liver, cigarette burns and stains on fingers, upper abdominal pain resulting from inflammation of the pancreas, decreased sensation in the feet or hands resulting from peripheral neuropathy, positive stool guaiac (gastrointestinal bleeding), hypertension, tremor, and tachycardia. For drug abuse, signs and symptoms may include cardiac arrhythmias, needle tracks, cellulitis, conjunctivitis, poor dentition, rapid weight loss, and changes in pupil size. In addition, signs of withdrawal or intoxication specific to each drug class may be present. During the assessment process the nurse observes for and questions the client regarding the incidence of accidents and injuries that might be related to substance use.

Screening Instruments

A wide variety of instruments are available to help in the identification of substance-related or induced disorders. The CAGE questionnaire is a well-validated, brief screening instrument that is readily memorized and useful (Box 13-4). A positive response to two of the four items of the CAGE indicates a potential problem for alcoholism. The Drug Abuse Screening Test (DAST) contains 28 self-reported items and is easily answered. The Alcohol Use Disorders Identification Test (AUDIT) is useful in screening both drug and alcohol abuse disorders. If screening test scoring shows that problems may exist, the nurse should follow up with questions about withdrawal symptoms, tolerance, legal and social complications, and work history. The diagnostic criteria for substance abuse and substance dependence are listed in the DSM-IV-TR Criteria box on p. 303.

Laboratory Tests

In addition to the history and physical examination, part of the assessment process includes laboratory testing for drug use. Ethical issues continue to be a concern with drug testing, such as potential infringement of civil rights and the issue of obtaining the client's informed consent (see Chapter 4). The use of laboratory tests for diagnosing substance abuse continues to become more complex and sophisticated. A large number of variables may affect the results, including the uniqueness of the drug, dosage taken, frequency of use, type of body fluid tested (urine, blood, stool), differences in drug metabolism, half-life of the drug, sample collection time and relationship to the time of use, and the sensitivity of the test itself.

Laboratory tests will not detect alcohol and/or substance dependence if clients are asymptomatic or if the drug used cannot be measured or detected. Relying solely on the results of laboratory tests could therefore be misleading. Despite these limitations, abnormal laboratory test results may suggest substance abuse or dependence problems. They can also be useful in tracking relapse or compliance successes of individuals in treatment or recovery. Blood toxicology tests can be expensive, but can be clinically useful in determining light or heavy alcohol or drug use. These are quantitative measures because they measure serum levels of intoxication. The disadvantages of blood testing include increased expense, the use of an invasive procedure, a narrow window of time for detection of drugs, and lack of usable veins in intravenous drug users. One of the most commonly used laboratory tests is the BAL. In most states, the BAL is used to determine legal intoxication. Table 13-1 provides information on blood alcohol levels and extent of impairment.

Other laboratory test results used as markers include elevated liver enzymes and macrocytic anemia. Elevation of the liver enzyme, GGT, is the most sensitive marker; an increase in the level indicates recent alcohol use. However, GGT is rarely elevated in persons younger than 30 years old. It is also a less sensitive marker in women than in men. More than half of alcoholic clients tracked have elevated GGT, MCV (red blood cell mean corpuscular volume), uric acid, triglycerides, aspartate aminotransferase (AST), and urea. Another indicator of recent heavy drinking (5 or more drinks) is an elevated carbohydrate deficient transferring. The presence of hepatitis C antibody can raise questions regarding substance abuse.

Urine drug screens can provide help in detecting the presence of drug/alcohol consumption within a specified time frame. Urine testing typically is qualitative and notes the presence or absence of the substance. A significant number of false-positive and false-negative findings are reported, so it is important to be familiar with the values reported by a specific laboratory. Urine specimen tests vary, but most are low cost and have well accepted and monitored standards, and the samples can be retested or saved, if necessary. Typical urine drug screens that may be performed in an Emergency Department include morphine, codeine, amphetamine, methamphetamine, cocaine metabolite (benzoylecgonine), THC metabolite, benzodiazepines, barbiturates, and alcohol. Many of these tests are also available for job testing or for home or private use. Shortcomings of urine samples include privacy issues surrounding the sample collection and possibilities of sample dilution/substitution or alteration by deceptive clients. Some of the newer designer drugs cannot be detected in the urine.

To determine heroin or cocaine abuse, a urinalysis collection frequency of three times weekly has been recommended. However, random, intermittent, interval screening may also work and is less expensive. Table 13-2 gives a guideline for the length of time a substance remains detectable in urine. However, rates of excretion are dependent of multiple variables, so figures may vary from those in the table.

Table 13-2 Substance Detection in Urine	
Substance	Days After Last Use
Alcohol	0.5
Amphetamine	1-2
Barbiturates (short acting)	3-5
Barbiturates (long acting)	10-14
Benzodiazepines (Diazepam)	2-4
Cocaine	0.3
Opioids (codeine/morphine)	1-2
Opiates (heroin)	2-3
Phencyclidine (PCP)	2-8
Cannabis (THC)	2-8 (acute)
	14-22 (chronic)

Data from Withers NW: Deceptions in addiction psychiatry, *Am J Forensic Psychiatry* 22(4):7-28, 2001.

NURSING DIAGNOSIS

Nursing diagnoses are identified using the information obtained during the assessment phase of the nursing process. The accuracy of diagnoses depends on a careful, in-depth assessment. Input from the client, family/significant others, and treatment team members is helpful in determining which nursing diagnoses are most relevant in treatment planning. The most frequently used nursing diagnoses when caring for clients with substance-related disorders follow.

Nursing Diagnoses for Substance-Related Disorders

- Anxiety
- Acute confusion
- Chronic confusion
- Ineffective coping
- Ineffective denial
- Interrupted family processes
- Dysfunctional family processes: alcoholism
- Ineffective health maintenance
- Hopelessness
- Hyperthermia
- Risk for injury
- Impaired memory
- Imbalanced nutrition: less than body requirements
- Imbalanced nutrition: more than body requirements
- Risk for poisoning
- Risk for post-trauma syndrome
- Disturbed sensory perception
- Sexual dysfunction
- Disturbed sleep pattern
- Impaired social interaction
- Readiness for enhanced spiritual well-being
- Risk for suicide
- Disturbed thought processes
- Risk for trauma
- Risk for other-directed violence
- Risk for self-directed violence
  See also Collaborative Diagnoses table.

COLLABORATIVE DIAGNOSES

DSM-IV-TR Diagnoses*

Alcohol-related disorders
Alcohol use disorders
Alcohol-induced disorders
Amphetamine (or amphetamine-like)-
 related disorders
Amphetamine use disorders
Amphetamine-induced disorders
Caffeine-related disorders
Caffeine-induced disorders
Cannabis-related disorders
Cannabis use disorders
Cannabis-induced disorders
Cocaine-related disorders
Cocaine use disorders
Cocaine-induced disorders
Hallucinogen-related disorders
Hallucinogen use disorders
Hallucinogen-induced disorders
Inhalant-related disorders
Inhalant use disorders
Inhalant-induced disorders
Nicotine-related disorders
Nicotine use disorders
Nicotine-induced disorders
Opioid-related disorders
Opioid use disorders
Opioid-induced disorders
Phencyclidine (or Phencyclidine-like)-
 related disorders
Phencyclidine use disorders
Phencyclidine-induced disorders
Sedative-, hypnotic-, or anxiolytic-
 related disorders
Sedative-, hypnotic-, or anxiolytic-
 use disorders
Sedative-, hypnotic-, or anxiolytic-
 induced disorders
Polysubstance-related disorder
Other (or unknown) substance-related
 disorders
Other (or unknown) substance use
 disorders
Other (or unknown) substance-induced
 disorders

NANDA Diagnoses†

Impaired adjustment
Ineffective airway clearance
Anxiety
Death anxiety
Risk for aspiration
Risk for impaired
 parent/infant/child attachment
Disturbed body image
Risk for imbalanced body
 temperature
Ineffective breathing pattern
Decreased cardiac output
Impaired comfort
Impaired verbal communication
Decisional conflict
Parental role conflict
Acute confusion
Chronic confusion
Constipation
Ineffective coping
Defensive coping
Compromised family coping
Ineffective denial
Diarrhea
Risk for falls
Dysfunctional family processes:
 alcoholism
Interrupted family processes
Fatigue
Fear
Deficient fluid volume
Excess fluid volume
Risk for deficient fluid volume
Risk for imbalanced fluid volume
Impaired gas exchange

Grieving
Ineffective health maintenance
Hopelessness
Hyperthermia
Risk for infection
Risk for injury
Impaired memory
Nausea
Noncompliance
Imbalanced nutrition: less than
 body requirements
Imbalanced nutrition: more than
 body requirements
Acute pain
Chronic pain
Impaired parenting
Risk for poisoning
Post-trauma syndrome
Powerlessness
Ineffective role performance
Chronic low self-esteem
Disturbed sensory perception
Sexual dysfunction
Impaired skin integrity
Disturbed sleep pattern
Impaired social interaction
Social isolation
Readiness for enhanced spiritual
 well-being
Risk for suicide
Disturbed thought processes
Risk for trauma
Risk for other-directed violence
Risk for self-directed violence

*From American Psychiatric Association: *Diagnostic and Statistical Manual of Mental Disorders*, Fourth Edition, Text Revision. Washington, DC, American Psychiatric Association, 2000.
†From NANDA International (2003). NANDA Nursing Diagnoses, Definitions and Classification 2003-2004. Philadelphia: NANDA.

OUTCOME IDENTIFICATION

Outcome criteria for clients with substance-related disorders are derived from nursing diagnoses and are the expected client responses to be achieved. They may be directed toward short- or long-term changes in behaviors and lifestyle. Different outcomes may be selected, depending on the particular characteristics of the substance(s) abused, the degree of dependence, and the age and other relevant demographic characteristics of the user. Outcomes provide the nurse and client with definitive, measurable steps to achieve before attaining desired discharge criteria.

Client will:

- Maintain vital signs within normal range.
- Verbalize a reduction in delusional thinking, absence of hallucinations or illusions, absence of suicidal or homicidal ideation.
- Maintain normal fluid hydration.
- Remain free of seizure activity.
- Verbalize, "I feel safe in my environment."
- Verbalize a desire to stop drinking or using drugs, or in some instances to decrease/limit use.
- State that there is a reduction in symptoms of withdrawal (which may occur weeks or months after last use).
- Participate in the therapeutic activities of the treatment plan (individual/group/family).
- Ingest a well-balanced diet of sufficient calories to meet prescribed nutritional needs.
- Express a need to contact family members/significant others regarding support.
- Explore factors that may interfere with the treatment plan (e.g., lack of social or family support, lack of financial resources, seeking old "drinking buddies" or drug-using peers).
- Identify realistic goals for rehabilitation (e.g., continue with the 12-step program, random urine drug screens).
- Verbalize that recovery is a lifelong process that occurs one day at a time.
- Verbalize the ability to sleep without sedation.
- Express the desire to establish relationships with non-drinking or nondrugging friends, and avoid situations that previously invoked alcohol or drug use.
- Use community resources to establish and maintain recovery.
- Reestablish structure in lifestyle that limits opportunities for drug or alcohol use (e.g., work, school, or family activities).
- Use healthy coping mechanisms.

PLANNING

The client frequently has a long history of alcohol and/or other drug abuse. Relapse is common, and the nurse and client must develop a plan of care that meets the individual's ongoing needs, whatever they might be in a given period of time. Client care must be based not only on the data gathered during the assessment process but also on a revision of that data as new information becomes available. The immediate needs, often of an emergent nature, as well as the long-range goals of treatment and aftercare must be considered. Collaboration with the client and others who care for or about him or her is essential in developing, revising, and evaluating the plan of care. For the client who abuses substances, the road to abstinence and recovery requires realistic outcome criteria and a consistent plan of care.

IMPLEMENTATION

The nurse working with a client who abuses alcohol and drugs develops a prioritized plan of care for each stage of the recovery process. *Client safety and health are always the first priority,* so the nurse focuses on treating and supporting the client through the drug withdrawal process called detoxification. Nutritional support and supplementation with vitamin B occur in this first stage. If violence or threats toward self or others are a problem, the nurse and staff intervene to provide safety for clients and the environment.

In subsequent stages of recovery the nurse and health team members focus on education concerning the drug abuse/dependence process; physical, psychologic, and psychosocial ramifications of continuing to use drugs; relationship skills training; anger management; and self-esteem building. The client is assisted to identify and reintegrate with healthy supports and to develop a new support system that does not include drug-taking activities or friends. Long- and short-term goals are made and vocational rehabilitation is addressed. It is essential to provide postdischarge contact with the client to monitor progress and provide ongoing support.

Withdrawal/Detoxification Treatment

Sudden withdrawal or rapid decreases in amounts of certain substances in an individual who is physically dependent may require immediate medical intervention. Withdrawal states related to stimulants, depressants, or opioids are the most likely to lead to emergency treatment situations. As in other types of emergencies, initiation of life-support measures is a first priority. These measures include maintenance of respirations and cardiac function and discontinuation of hemorrhage or seizures. A client who is debilitated before going through withdrawal is obviously more at risk of dying. Calmness, along with a reassuring and consistent approach, will benefit the client and his or her loved ones.

Medications are usually avoided because of the potential for drug-drug related interactions. If medications are needed, experts recommend adequate doses to produce the effects desired. If a client who is dependent on CNS depressants has severe withdrawal symptoms, the client undergoes **detoxification**. Enough of the drug (or one to which the person has **cross-tolerance**) is given to relieve the symptoms. The drug used is then decreased gradually over a period of days (Schuckit, 2000).

After stabilization has occurred, accurate history taking, physical evaluation, and laboratory testing will help to iden-

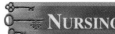
NURSING CARE PLAN

Mr. James H. is a 45-year-old African-American male who is separated from his wife and three adolescent children. He was admitted to a psychiatric acute care unit with initial diagnoses of major depression and multidrug use that includes heavy use of alcohol, cocaine, and pain medication, usually hydrocodone (Vicodin). He had back pain for some time and states he has taken his pain medication regularly, but it is no longer working. He had to supplement his prescription with purchases on the street. He is requesting more pain medication. Since admission to the unit, Mr. H. reports insomnia, nervousness, and loss of appetite. He appears malnourished. He recently was fired from his job as an assistant manager in a bank because of high absenteeism and performance problems. This is his third hospital admission in the past year. He states he drank heavily, about a pint of vodka a day for the past year, but when this didn't seem to alleviate his symptoms of depression and anxiety, he increased his use to a fifth of vodka a day. Money to support his habits dwindled after he lost his job earlier. He states he would like to return home if he can work it out with his wife, but at this time he is unsure of the future. His wife has a part-time job to help pay the bills. The children stay with their grandmother when Mrs. H. is working. She has not yet come to see her husband.

DSM-IV-TR Diagnoses
Axis I   Major depression, alcohol dependence, cocaine dependence, opioid dependence (with physiologic dependence)
Axis II   None
Axis III   Medical diagnoses: malnourished, sleep disturbance, back pain
Axis IV   Severity of psychosocial stressors (Extreme = 4) inadequate finances, fired from job, no health insurance
Axis V   Global assessment of functioning: current
           GAF = 15 (current)
           GAF = 45 (past year)

NURSING DIAGNOSIS: Risk for injury. Risk factors: effects of alcohol, cocaine, and pain medication, and risk for injury secondary to substance withdrawal.

CLIENT OUTCOMES	NURSING INTERVENTIONS	EVALUATION
Mr. H. will verbalize symptoms of withdrawal and comply with the prescribed medication protocol to manage these symptoms. Mr. H. will exhibit no episodes of life-threatening symptoms related to substance withdrawal.	Assess Mr. H.'s physical and mental health status on admission and administer medication as ordered *to relieve initial signs of withdrawal, and to prevent or limit the development of life-threatening withdrawal symptoms.* Reassure Mr. H. about his safety *to develop trust and decrease feelings of anxiety by explaining that he will be monitored continually and that his symptoms can be controlled by use of the appropriate treatment interventions.*	Mr. H. verbalizes that he will do anything to stop feeling so sad and hopeless, and that he is willing to go through withdrawal, no matter what happens to him. Mr. H. states he is able to manage his cravings for alcohol and cocaine and his nervousness, with support.

NURSING DIAGNOSIS: Chronic pain related to history of a lower back injury 2 years ago in an automobile accident, as evidenced by previous documentation in client's medical record, pain level of 5 (on a scale of 1-10) on admission, and difficulty sitting in one position for any period of time.

CLIENT OUTCOMES	NURSING INTERVENTIONS	EVALUATION
Mr. H. will state his pain level is tolerable without use of narcotic medication.	Assess pain level of intensity along with location, duration, and characteristics each time vitals are taken; administer nonnarcotic pain medications as prescribed; evaluate effectiveness and observe for side effects or adverse reactions to medications *because the presence of uncontrolled pain may interfere with his drug withdrawal, and related discomfort will use energy that can be directed toward recovery.*	Mr. H. states that his level of pain is at a level of 2 or 3, and that he can participate in activities related to his recovery.

NURSING DIAGNOSIS: Ineffective coping related to stress, depressed state, and inadequate use of coping methods, as evidenced by dependence on alcohol and cocaine, and loss of job.

CLIENT OUTCOMES	NURSING INTERVENTIONS	EVALUATION
Mr. H. will verbalize that he has a problem with drug use and wants to make changes in his life.	Support Mr. H.'s statement that he is dependent on drugs, and offer hope that he can withdraw safely while his symptoms are managed. *Additional support by the nurse can help him to achieve the first step toward abstinence. Assessing Mr. H. for the presence of suicidal thoughts or plan is an essential intervention in the management of depression.*	Mr. H. verbalizes that he is frightened and depressed, but says he wants to turn his life around. He admits drugs have caused problems.
Mr. H. will practice positive coping skills that were previously effective during difficult times and learn new skills to manage problems related to substance abuse.	Assess Mr. H.'s usual coping style using interview/counseling techniques. Help him explore strengths and areas for growth *because to build new coping skills, previously effective and ineffective coping methods must be explored and new positive ones added.*	Mr. H. is effectively integrating existing coping skills with newly acquired coping methods at the time of discharge.

NURSING CARE PLAN—cont'd

NURSING DIAGNOSIS: Interrupted family processes related to the effects of chronic use of alcohol, cocaine, and pain medication, as evidenced by separation from wife and children.

CLIENT OUTCOMES	NURSING INTERVENTIONS	EVALUATION
Mr. H. will initiate contact with family through phone call and request that family visit.	Encourage Mr. H. to initiate contact with wife and children *to provide a solid family support system to help reintegrate him back into the family and stop substance use/abuse.*	Mr. H. and wife plan to have him return home with his family at the time of discharge.
Mr. H. will attend family counseling sessions with his family.	Teach Mr. and Mrs. H. and children about the benefits of family therapy *because all family members need support with resolution of disabling effects of substance-abuse problems.*	Mr. H. and family are attending family therapy sessions at discharge.
Mrs. H. will attend weekly Al-Anon meetings; children will attend Al-a-teen sessions.	Support family members in their decision to attend Al-Anon and AlAteen meetings *to help them learn new ways to effectively interact with Mr. H. and one another.*	All members are attending meetings at the time of Mr. H.'s discharge.

NURSING DIAGNOSIS: Imbalanced nutrition: less than body requirements related to lack of interest in food and/or substitution of alcohol or drugs for nutrients, as evidenced by malnourishment and vitamin and mineral deficiencies.

CLIENT OUTCOMES	NURSING INTERVENTIONS	EVALUATION
Mr. H. will eat a minimum of 50% of provided nutrients at each meal.	Provide preferred foods high in proteins, carbohydrates, and vitamins, especially the B vitamins, *so Mr. H. will become better nourished in accordance with metabolic needs.*	Mr. H. ate 100% of well-balanced meals at the time of discharge.
Mr. H. will select a diet including "desired" foods.	Assist with dietary choices until Mr. H. feels secure *to support him until he is able to make appropriate choices for himself.*	Mr. H. selected a balanced diet based on the food pyramid at the time of discharge.

NURSING DIAGNOSIS: Disturbed sleep pattern related to the effects of psychologic and physiologic stress and substance withdrawal, as evidenced by irritability, restlessness, depression, and the inability to fall asleep and stay asleep during the night.

CLIENT OUTCOMES	NURSING INTERVENTIONS	EVALUATION
Mr. H. will sleep soundly for at least 5 hours after 1 week.	Provide information regarding supportive measures to induce sleep, such as the use of a darkened room, white noise, and a soothing back rub and soft music *to help him relax and use these techniques as a substitute for drug use.*	Mr. H. was sleeping a minimum of 5 hours at the time of discharge and stated he knew it might take several weeks or months longer before he resumed a normal sleep pattern.

tify additional priorities for care. If an individual is withdrawing from multiple substances, potentiation of symptoms may result in morbidity or death.

CNS Depressants

Early symptoms of withdrawal are usually the opposite of the acute effects of that drug. The length of the withdrawal period can be predicted by the half-life of the drug abused. Withdrawal symptoms from CNS depressants include insomnia; high levels of anxiety; elevated body temperature, pulse, and respiratory rates; fine tremors; gastrointestinal upset; muscle aches; diaphoresis; and labile blood pressure. There is a strong craving to obtain the drug. Confusion and other cognitive changes, delirium, hallucinations, or delusions may be observed in some clinical cases of depressant

drug withdrawal. With the barbiturates especially, grand mal seizures may develop. Withdrawal from depressants lasts from 3 to 7 days for short-acting drugs and up to 3 to 6 months for longer acting drugs. Withdrawal from benzodiazepines results in characteristic symptoms similar to those that occur with alcoholic withdrawal.

Alcohol

For 95% of those experiencing withdrawal from alcohol, symptoms are of mild to moderate severity and include those similar to depressant withdrawal. Withdrawal symptoms include two or more of the following: autonomic hyperactivity (pulse rate greater than 100 or sweating); increased hand tremor; insomnia; psychomotor agitation; anxiety; nausea or emesis; and occasionally grand mal seizures or transient visual, auditory, tactile hallucinations, or illusions. Alcohol withdrawal begins within 12 hours of stopped or decreased alcohol consumption, peaks in 48 to 72 hours, and is usually greatly reduced by 4 to 5 days. Some symptoms may last several weeks or months longer. They cause clinically significant impairment or distress in areas of the individual's life that are important to usual functioning. For those experiencing alcohol withdrawal, the mortality rate is typically low (Schuckit, 2000). As with intoxication, other disorders must be ruled out. Alcohol withdrawal delirium (delirium tremens [DTs]) occurs in less than 10% of those who experience the alcohol withdrawal syndrome. Adequate and rapid medical intervention in clients who are withdrawing from alcohol should eliminate these more severe symptoms. Clients experiencing severe withdrawal symptoms from alcohol usually require B vitamins, including thiamine (vitamin B_1), folic acid, and vitamin B_{12}, as a result of inadequate dietary intake and malabsorption. If alcohol withdrawal delirium is diagnosed, other general medical conditions such as liver failure, pneumonia, or recent head trauma may also exist.

Pharmacologic intervention is not necessary for all cases of alcohol withdrawal. In some instances, general support measures will lead to improvement of comfort. Although any depressant medication can work, most often the benzodiazepines are used because they are less likely to cause neurotoxicity and decreases in vital signs, and are consistently effective. Short-acting benzodiazepines such as oxazepam (Serax) or lorazepam (Ativan) are typically used for clients with severe liver failure or those with severely impaired cognition. Longer acting drugs such as diazepam (Valium) or chlordiazepoxide (Librium) are used for most others undergoing severe withdrawal from alcohol (Schuckit, 2000).

Opioids

Detoxification from opioids requires similar precautions to those mentioned previously. For opioids, beginning withdrawal from the last dose ranges from 4 to 12 hours for heroin, and up to 1 to 3 days for methadone. Peak intensity occurs within 48 to 72 hours. Acute withdrawal symptoms from heroin last about 5 days, and for methadone, several weeks. Withdrawal symptoms may be protracted and decrease over several months. Symptoms of morphine and heroin withdrawal include craving and irritability, lacrimation (tearing of the eyes), rhinorrhea (runny nose), diaphoresis, and yawning. As withdrawal progresses, a restless sleep, involuntary leg movements, restlessness, hypertension, tachycardia and temperature irregularities, dilated pupils, loss of appetite, gooseflesh, back and other muscle or bone pain, and tremor occur. Finally, insomnia, yawning, and a flulike syndrome may occur. Clonidine (Catapres) is the most commonly used nonopioid medication used to treat withdrawal symptoms from opioid use. Side effects from clonidine include sedation and hypotension, so blood pressure must be carefully monitored. Methadone treatment has been the treatment of choice for morphine and heroin ad-

dicts, although new technologies are emerging (see NIDA Web site). L-Alpha-acetyl methadol (LAAM) is another drug used in withdrawal. It is longer acting and is useful in communities not close to methadone clinics. Methadone and LAAM are synthetic opioids given to addicts to suppress withdrawal symptoms. Methadone or LAAM maintenance is continued until the person can be withdrawn from these substitute drugs. Methadone and LAAM are addicting, but individuals can be withdrawn by gradually decreasing the total daily dose until they are methadone or LAAM free. Sometimes addicts have no intention of quitting, but continue to use methadone or LAAM until they obtain the money to buy their drug of choice.

Careful monitoring of methadone or LAAM levels is needed in addition to vital signs. Overdose of these substances may lead to cardiovascular collapse and death.

Stimulants

For cocaine, amphetamines, and other CNS stimulants, the physical signs of withdrawal are limited. Because of tolerance, withdrawal can develop while the person is still taking the drug and may include nonspecific aches and pains. The clinical syndrome includes intense craving and drug-seeking behaviors, agitation, temporary intense depression, and a loss of appetite that gives way over time to fatigue with associated insomnia, continued depression, and a decrease in craving. Cravings for cocaine may be triggered by cocaine-related stimuli such as seeing a white powder substance. These conditioned responses probably contribute to relapse and are difficult to eliminate. Symptoms related to the final phase of withdrawal from stimulants include exhaustion, a rebound in appetite, and a need to sleep. These symptoms, which occur during the first 9 hours to 14 days, are followed by normalization of sleep patterns, decrease in craving, and a more normal mood. Withdrawal then progresses to recurrence of fatigue, anhedonia, and anxiety. Treatment focuses on treating the symptoms and use of medications is generally avoided. An inherent danger is that clients will seek other mood-altering substances, including alcohol and benzodiazepines, to fill the void they experience from giving up stimulants.

Caffeine

Withdrawal from caffeine-related disorders can occur with relatively low doses of caffeine in both adults and children. Caffeine withdrawal occurs around 12 to 24 hours after consumption ends and usually resolves in 2 to 7 days. Symptoms may include headache, fatigue, yawning, nausea, or more disturbing symptoms such as muscle tension, irritability, anxiety, and cognitive changes. Because the symptoms of caffeine withdrawal can overlap with other medical conditions, psychiatric disorders, and drug withdrawal states, a careful assessment of recent caffeine use is an important consideration. If a client consumes caffeine and symptoms are relieved, the diagnosis may be clarified (Sadock and Sadock, 2000). Clients generally respond to comfort measures.

There is no clinically significant withdrawal syndrome for hallucinogens or inhalants. Treatment facilities for inhalant users are difficult to find. Research suggests that chronic users are the most difficult to treat and may exhibit numerous social and psychologic problems. Users may suffer withdrawal symptoms such as hallucinations, nausea, excess sweating, hand tremors, muscle cramps, headaches, chills, and delirium tremens. Relapse is common.

Other categories of illicit or legal drugs are generally associated with mild to moderate withdrawal symptoms. Symptoms of cannabis withdrawal such as irritability, tremor, perspiration, nausea, appetite change, and sleep disturbances have been documented with high doses, but the clinical significance is uncertain. Withdrawal therefore is not a criterion in the DSM-IV-TR (Sadock and Sadock, 2000). Treatment is supportive.

Nicotine

Nicotine withdrawal has characteristic features of dysphoric or depressed mood, insomnia, irritability, frustration or anger, anxiety, difficulty concentrating, restlessness or impatience, decreased heart rate, and increased appetite or weight gain. Craving is a common occurrence after quitting. Most withdrawal symptoms peak in 1 to 3 days, but withdrawal symptoms may last 4 to 6 weeks or more. Craving and weight gain may continue even longer. Symptoms are most acute among those who smoke cigarettes. Nicotine replacement therapies, including gum, patches, sprays, and inhalers, help lessen the impact of withdrawal symptoms and double the cessation rates of tobacco use. Nonnicotine medications such as bupropion (Zyban or Wellbutrin) and clonidine (Catapres) have also been used to treat withdrawal symptoms (Sadock and Sadock, 2000). Without medical assistance, 80% of smokers who quit will relapse within the first 2 years.

Nursing Interventions

1. Maintain a patent airway in the client, monitor vital signs, and intervene in situations involving client hemorrhage, seizures or cardiac arrest *to address the client's life-threatening problems.*
2. Maintain the safety of the client and others (chemical or mechanical restraint may be necessary) *because the client may exhibit unanticipated, out of control, violent, or assaultive behaviors.*
3. Observe for additional signs and symptoms of substance overdose, withdrawal, and drug-to-drug interactions *to establish baseline information about the client's condition.*
4. Assess the physiologic and psychologic symptoms of withdrawal and the effects of medications prescribed during the withdrawal process *to provide safe, effective treatment during withdrawal.*
5. Initiate therapeutic interventions to treat withdrawal symptoms, including anxiety and other complications, *to help the client safely withdraw from the addictive substance.*
6. Provide emotional support to the client/family/significant others *to establish trust and include those important to the client in the treatment process.*
7. Support the client in meeting nutritional/metabolic needs either orally or intravenously, depending on the client's ability to take and retain fluids, *to provide adequate hydration as needed.*
8. Refer to a nutritionist as needed or engage the family in identifying and meeting the client's personal, cultural, or spiritual preferences *to offer holistic and interdisciplinary care.*
9. Increase carbohydrate intake and offer straws or other edible or nonedible but safe objects/foods to chew on (e.g., sugar-free hard candies, trail mix, toothpicks, straws, and gum) *to decrease some of the client's cravings for illicit substances and satisfy the client's oral needs.*
10. Initiate vitamin and mineral replacement therapeutic regimen as prescribed *because low levels of vitamin B and other vitamins and minerals such A, C, D, E, and K, iron, magnesium, and zinc may also be affected with chronic alcohol ingestion.*
11. Provide support to the client/family in acknowledging deception and denial. *A variety of psychotherapeutic techniques may be used with the client/family because interventions involving support and empathy, while not enabling the client, assist the individual/family to work through the denial process and develop awareness that many life problems are related to substance-abuse* (see Chapter 19).
12. Intervene with secondary medical complications or residual effects of substance use exhibited by the client *because the prolonged use/abuse of alcohol and/or other drugs may cause a variety of complications and temporary or permanent damage to major body systems.*
13. Establish a trusting, caring, empathic yet firm therapeutic relationship with the individual *to help the client improve self-esteem and deal with thoughts of guilt and remorse.*
14. Encourage the client's efforts to establish/reestablish/strengthen family/significant other supports through a variety of measures such as role-playing and providing a quiet and private environment for the client to meet with or telephone family *because clients who abuse substances frequently have lost meaningful contact with their family/significant others.*
15. Teach the client, family, and significant others about substance abuse, symptoms, management, treatment, and prevention, individually and as group members. Assess the style of learning that works best for the client to meet learning needs (i.e., verbal, visual, or written communication). Use materials in the language the client is most comfortable with, if possible. Provide factual information about prevention measures that work. *The nurse acts as an advocate and as a re-*

source person regarding successful treatment and prevention efforts and the need for a healthy lifestyle for clients and their families/significant others.

16. Support the client and family in maintaining active involvement with twelve-step or alternative support groups, such as AA, Al-Anon, Al-a-Teen, ACoA, NA, and CA, or Rational Recovery. *Past experience in working with substance abuse clients indicates that lifelong membership in a twelve-step or alternative recovery program is, for many individuals, the key to remaining drug free. Families also benefit from groups that help them to change previous patterns of relating to the client and others.*

17. Encourage the family to be flexible and supportive regarding the client's participation in support groups *because establishing a new lifestyle, such as engaging in a support group network, takes time, effort, and motivation.*

18. Assist the client in establishing a new or different social support system by putting him or her in touch with community organizations where the client may find alternative housing, make new friends, and experience opportunities to build inner strength and develop drug-free coping measures. *The client is faced with the enormous task of establishing a new social network that is drug free; knowledge and guidance regarding resources and recovery programs will provide invaluable assistance in making his or her efforts successful.*

Additional Treatment Modalities

Rehabilitation for substance disorders is a vital part of the treatment process. Now, more than ever before, researchers are evaluating treatment outcomes through funded studies. In 2002, SAMHSA launched a new program called "Changing the Conversation: The National Treatment Plan Initiative to Improve Substance Abuse Treatment." The goal of this program was to ensure that quality treatment services and programs were available to all that needed them. In this initiative, five key guidelines were identified:

1. There is "no wrong door" to treatment (i.e., anyone needing treatment is identified and receives it).
2. Invest for results (i.e., use treatment and services wisely to produce desired results).
3. Commit to quality (i.e., continually strive to improve treatment).
4. Change attitudes (i.e., challenge stigma and misinformation regarding addiction treatment and the nature of the recovery process).
5. Build partnerships (i.e., work together to make needed changes).

Treatment programs offer a wide variety of services and goals. Likewise, clients have different motivations and reasons for seeking treatment. It is important to recognize that there will be no perfect match of client and program. Instead, it is the staff and the approaches used that will help the client to achieve recovery. Collaborative team interventions can enhance successful treatment and rehabilitation outcomes. All available resources should be used. Ulti-

mately, it will be the client's decision and responsibility to achieve and maintain a life of sobriety and recovery.

Psychotherapy

Individual Therapy. Individual psychotherapy is indicated for clients who have a high level of anxiety, inadequate coping mechanisms, and low tolerance for frustration. The primary focus is on the "here and now" of the client's life, as he or she learns to relate to others and adjust to a life without reliance on drugs. Some clients do better in communicating in a one-on-one relationship versus a group setting.

Clients may have strong patterns of denial and deception that must be addressed during the course of therapy. They often continue to test the therapeutic bond between client and therapist. Therapists must often address issues such as relapse, onset of depression, and resistance to continuation of therapy.

Group Therapy. Group therapy is typically more cost effective and can reach greater numbers of people. Group therapy has certain advantages for clients with substance-related disorders that are difficult to achieve in individual therapy. In a group setting, clients with similar experiences and problems can confront and/or support each other in a relatively safe environment. The therapist's role is to facilitate group members' participation and to assist in clarifying interpersonal interactions within the group. In addition to discussions, didactic or educational information regarding substance use and recovery can be shared in the group. Clients in recovery who have maintained sobriety can share experiences and serve as role models for newly admitted clients.

Family Therapy. In recent years family therapy has gained credibility in treatment programs designed for both adults and adolescents. Family therapy is based on family systems theory. The genogram (Bowen, 1978) is a useful instrument to trace intergenerational use of substances. Researchers are scanning genomes to identify which members in a family are more apt to use illicit drugs. Other genetic and environmental research studies are underway that may link family members with specific types of substance use.

Recognition and acceptance of alcoholism as an illness that affects all members of the family support a need for family therapy (Figure 13-4). When the family member who abuses alcohol suddenly attains sobriety, the dynamics of the entire family change. Some clients experience relapse because the family does not know how to relate to the person when he or she is sober. Family members in alcoholic families have a tendency to lack trust for one another, feel unloved and unwanted, and carry a heavy burden of guilt.

Behavioral Therapy. Some programs use behavioral approaches such as relaxation therapy or biofeedback to teach clients how to handle everyday stressors or insomnia. Usually behavioral modification approaches are used in addition to other forms of education and counseling. Approaches may include assertiveness training or aversive conditioning.

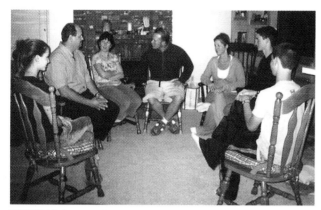

FIGURE 13-4. Family therapy is an important factor when one member is in recovery for substance abuse.

CLINICAL ALERT

All clients taking disulfiram (Antabuse) should carry a card similar to that carried by clients with diabetes or wear a metal bracelet stating that they are taking Antabuse and should be taken to an emergency department if found in a debilitated state, which may include nausea, vomiting, headache, difficulty breathing, and a rapid or irregular heartbeat.

Aversive conditioning is used with nicotine-dependent clients to develop learned negative associations with cigarettes. Aversive conditioning with disulfiram (Antabuse) is the most frequently used technique of behavior therapy for alcoholics. The client is conditioned by pairing the sight, smell, and taste of alcohol with an emetic. Induced nausea and vomiting act as aversions to alcohol. After the conditioning experience, the client is given disulfiram, which inhibits the enzyme aldehyde dehydrogenase; even a small amount of alcohol can cause a toxic reaction because of acetaldehyde accumulation in the blood.

Clients for aversive conditioning must be in good health, highly motivated, and cooperative. They are warned about the consequences of using the drug disulfiram if and when even small amounts of alcohol are ingested. If ingestion occurs, clients experience flushing and feelings of heat in the face, chest, and upper limbs. Other symptoms include pallor, hypotension, nausea, general malaise, dizziness, blurred vision, palpitations, air hunger, and numbness of the upper extremities.

Naltrexone Antagonist Pharmacotherapy

Naltrexone, which is a derivative of naloxone, has been used in recent years in general anesthesia or heavy sedation procedures to shorten weeks of painful withdrawal symptoms into approximately 4 to 6 hours or less. The anesthesia detoxification method has been used in the United States since 1995. Its success in Europe has been documented since the late 1980s. While asleep, the client is given naltrexone, sometimes in combination with midazolam. Naltrexone supplants the narcotics from the receptor sites in the brain and nervous system, thereby ending the addiction.

Clients typically awaken physiologically drug free and remain under the supervision of qualified medical staff until hospital discharge. Naltrexone has few side effects and is the treatment of choice for highly motivated clients such as addicted professionals or individuals in the criminal justice system. Some clinical research trials have shown poor compliance for oral naltrexone use, because its lack of agonist activity does not provide any drug reinforcement when taken, and it produces no negative consequences such as withdrawal symptoms when use is stopped. Methods to enhance naltrexone therapy effectiveness continue to be clinically tested (Schuckit, 2000).

Relapse Prevention

The principles of **relapse prevention** are used throughout the rehabilitation process to help clients avoid or take control of situations in which relapse is possible. The client practices steps to take if relapse occurs and develops a comprehensive plan to follow. The individual identifies situations in which he or she is most apt to relapse or use and makes lifestyle changes including living areas, shopping, and selection of friends and family who will be supportive to a life of abstinence.

Harm Reduction

Harm reduction techniques help an individual to change patterns of use to decrease the risk of harm. This approach, although controversial, has helped some people to adapt healthier lifestyles. Examples include designated driver programs, smoking cigarettes with lower levels of tar and nicotine, needle exchange programs, methadone or LAAM maintenance and hepatitis B vaccination programs for injecting drug users (Heather et al., 1993).

Twelve-Step Support Groups

For decades, Alcoholics Anonymous (AA) and affiliated groups were the only widely available treatment programs. These groups still provide support and reinforcement in recovery for a large number of individuals. More recently, other programs and treatments have become available based on other principles and research (Szalavitz, 2002). For those who benefit from groups, there are options available to meet a wide variety of needs. Individuals who have been active in the groups serve as role models for those who are in different stages of recovery or who are involved with someone in recovery. Help is available 24 hours a day and every day of the week. Generally speaking, the greater the level of participation in the groups and the greater the intensity of exposure, the better the outcomes. Participants in these programs often see recovery as a lifetime effort.

AA is the original self-help group for recovering alcoholics. AA was founded in 1935 and was built on the premise that support and encouragement from others with alcoholism can aid persons on the road to recovery. New members are assigned a sponsor (a recovering alcoholic) who provides 24-hour assistance as needed. The 12 steps of AA are listed in Box 13-5.

Box 13-5	The Twelve Steps of Alcoholics Anonymous

1. We admitted we were powerless over alcohol, that our lives had become unmanageable.
2. Came to believe that a Power greater than ourselves could restore us to sanity.
3. Made a decision to turn our will and our lives over to the care of God as we understood Him.
4. Made a searching and fearless moral inventory of ourselves.
5. Admitted to God, to ourselves, and to another human being the exact nature of our wrongs.
6. Were entirely ready to have God remove all these defects of character.
7. Humbly asked Him to remove our shortcomings.
8. Made a list of all persons we had harmed, and became willing to make amends to them all.
9. Made direct amends to such people wherever possible, except when to do so would injure them or others.
10. Continued to take personal inventory, and when we were wrong promptly admitted it.
11. Sought through prayer and meditation to improve our conscious contact with God as we understood Him, praying only for knowledge of His will for us and the power to carry that out.
12. Having had a spiritual awakening as the result of these steps, we tried to carry this message to alcoholics and to practice these principles in all our affairs.

The Twelve Steps are reprinted with permission of Alcoholics Anonymous World Services, Inc. Permission to reprint this material does not mean that AA has reviewed or approved the contents of this publication. AA is a program of recovery from alcoholism *only*—use of the Twelve Steps in connection with programs and activities that are patterned after AA, but which address other problems, does not imply otherwise.

AA groups are available in each community. Meetings may be open or closed. During open meetings, anyone with an interest, including spouses, friends, and significant others, are invited to attend. Closed meetings are restricted to individuals in the recovery process. Groups are available for specific populations such as women, nonsmokers, business people, and professionals. Groups are conducted in American Sign Language, and many provide access for the handicapped. Many AA groups now accept the need for those with dual diagnoses to take prescribed psychotropic medications to keep their illnesses stabilized.

Narcotics Anonymous (NA) embraces a similar philosophy to AA. It is a support group for individuals addicted to narcotics, especially opiates. Because many individuals are polysubstance abusers or multiple drug dependent, attendees may have problems with one or more substances.

Al-Anon and *Al-a-Teen* self-help groups operate independently from AA groups. Al-Anon is a support group for spouses and friends of individuals with alcoholism. Opportunities are provided to learn about alcohol as a disease and to share common problems and solutions with other spouses. Behaviors and issues common to the disease process are dealt with, such as avoidance, enabling, self-inflicted guilt, and shame. Al-a-Teen is a nationwide support group

for teens (children more than 10 years old) who have alcoholic parents. Similar to Al-Anon, the group helps remove self-guilt as the cause of the parent's drinking and restores feelings of self-worth.

Adult Children of Alcoholics (ACoA) is a support group for adults who were reared in alcoholic homes. Adult children of alcoholics may manifest **codependence,** with issues of control, enabling, making excuses for others' behaviors (especially the behavior of alcoholic individuals), inability to trust self, and feelings of inadequacy and insecurity. Codependent individuals have a constant need to assume responsibility and take care of others' needs. The support groups provide opportunities to discuss problems and feel acceptance from others with similar experiences.

Alternative groups to AA include Rational Recovery, which uses more behavioral approaches, Secular Organization for Sobriety (SOS), and Women for Sobriety (WFS).

Inpatient Care

Generally inpatient care is used to provide a structured treatment program for those who are severely impaired or debilitated, those who fail in outpatient treatment effort, and those who have serious medical or psychiatric problems and/or are in an acute state of crisis. It is typically short term, about 2 to 4 weeks, and is followed by extended aftercare for 6 to 12 months.

Outpatient Care

Outpatient treatment centers teach the client to change and adjust to life without drugs while living in a real life situation. It is less expensive than inpatient hospitalization and just as effective. Outpatient care generally continues until the client is ready for a less intensive level of care.

Halfway Houses

Halfway houses provide shelter as well as support, group therapy, and direct access to AA meetings. These living situations provide opportunities for gradual reentrance into the family and progressive reentry into the work environment and society. Halfway house placement is highly recommended for clients who have been alienated from their families or are homeless.

Day or Night Hospitalization

Partial hospitalization is recommended for clients who need additional professional support. Some clients resume employment and spend the night in the hospital, whereas others spend the day at the treatment center and go home at night. As with the halfway house, partial hospitalization provides additional therapeutic support during early or difficult phases of rehabilitation.

Previous research has shown that a minimum of 90 days of treatment for residential and 21 days for short-term inpatient programs is predictive of positive treatment outcomes for adults. Unfortunately, many long-term treatment programs have been cut or eliminated with the advent of managed care. In the first large-scale study designed to focus on drug abuse treatment outcomes for 1167 adolescents, researchers found that longer stays in treatment programs could effectively reduce substance abuse, symptoms of mental illness, and criminal activity (Hser et al., 2001).

Medications

The use of medications in recovery from alcoholism and other drugs is difficult to evaluate, as studies are limited. No one drug has been shown to guarantee recovery. Typically therefore medications may be used as an adjunct to other therapies. Some being used or investigated for use include acamprosate (Campral), a promising medication used in Europe to calm the withdrawal effects of alcohol and produce an effect of lessening the preference for alcohol, and naltrexone (ReVia or Trexan), a medication whose clinical usefulness has not yet been determined.

Methadone and LAAM Treatment Programs

Methadone is a long-acting opioid similar to heroin in its properties. LAAM is an analog of methadone that has a 72- to 96-hour half-life. These drugs are given for similar reasons: to serve as substitutes for other opioids such as heroin, to reduce criminal activity, and to decrease drug craving.

Methadone and LAAM maintenance for opioid dependence can only be given in facilities that are licensed, that offer counseling services including outreach, and that have security measures in place to minimize illegal use of opioids. The client must have been opioid dependent for a year or more and must not have benefited from drug-free treatment approaches. Some clients stay on these substitutes for 10 years or longer.

Opiate antagonists such as naloxone (Narcan) and naltrexone (Trexan or ReVia) are used to block the effects of heroin and other opioids in rehabilitation and overdose. Most clients are then tested periodically for the resumption of opioid use. Treatment occurs in conjunction with other approaches and has varying degrees of success (Schuckit, 2000).

Community-Based Organizations and Faith and Spiritual Communities

These organizations are often interested in addressing the needs of families and have a positive impact on the problem of substance abuse. Social support from outside influences can moderate or influence the effects of a family history of drug and alcohol problems. Many communities have developed after school programs, mentoring activities, sports and educational programs, and other funded or nonfunded programs to provide opportunities for healthy relationships and activities.

Spirituality is an important part of recovery for many individuals. For 6 out of 10 Americans, religious faith is the most important influence in their lives, and for 8 out of 10, religious beliefs provide comfort and support (*Alcohol, tobacco and other drugs*, 1995). Teens who never attend religious services are at above average risk for drug and alcohol problems, whereas those who attend at least weekly have a lower than average risk (*National survey of American attitudes*, 2001). Factors that have been cited as fostering teen abilities to resist drugs include positive peer affiliations, bonding in school activities, relationships with caring adults, opportunities for school success and responsible behavior, and the availability of drug-free activities.

EVALUATION

The purpose of evaluation in the nursing process is to ascertain changes that occur as a result of nursing and other interdisciplinary interventions. The nurse observes for changes in the client's behaviors and responses to treatment and interventions using the outcome criteria. It is important to recognize that resolution of the acute phase is merely the first step in treatment. Success for the recovery process and rehabilitation depends on many factors including access to treatment programs, twelve-step or other support groups, continuing health care, support of family/significant others, vocational rehabilitation, and community support (see Nursing Care in the Community box).

NURSING CARE IN THE COMMUNITY   Substance-Related Disorders

The nurse in the community who is working with clients who have substance-related disorders may experience judgmental reactions about relapse possibilities. Resumption of substance use is a common occurrence that causes frustration for both the client and the nurse. Both may feel hopeless in the face of this self-destructive behavior. Allowance must be made for impaired thought processes as a result of chronic alcohol or drug use. It is crucial to understand that in some cases relapse is a part of the process. Continual reinforcement of goal-directed recovery, and use of healthy coping skills will ultimately make a difference in the client's behavior.

Resilience is perhaps the most essential quality the nurse can exhibit when treating this client population. Offering help and support when nothing seems to be working requires tenacity and endurance. Knowledge of the predictable stages experienced by clients throughout treatment can help the nurse accept clients while encouraging positive behavioral changes. It is im-

portant to evaluate the client's acceptance of dependence on alcohol/drugs and the harmful impact this dependence has had on the quality of life. The client who is denying the existence of a problem is in need of a strong reality check before making referrals to community programs.

The nurse has opportunities to recommend contact with Alcoholics Anonymous or other support groups, provide encouragement and counseling resources to family members, and enlist the help of other health care professionals, as well as those in recovery. There will also be opportunities to support the client to become involved in a community service group that will increase feelings of self-worth. Interaction between the nurse and the client in the community setting is usually based on choice; thus the development of a trusting relationship is essential. The relationship requires a rigorous and nonaccusatory, nondeceitful honesty, suggesting that both parties aspire to high standards of behavior and responsibility.

Many clients relapse during the rehabilitation process. For this reason it is difficult to predict the time when clients will be motivated sufficiently to change their lifestyle and accept their illness. Evaluation must be an ongoing process. As people attain sobriety, they internalize a commitment to change their lifestyle, which often affects their relationships with family, significant others, and co-workers. Many clients develop a lifetime commitment to their twelve-step program or another program that best meets their needs.

CHAPTER SUMMARY

- Substance abuse causes more deaths, illnesses, and disabilities than any other preventable health condition, and it affects Americans from all walks of life.
- The use of alcohol, tobacco, and illicit drugs has fluctuated in response to shifts in public tolerance and with various political, economic, and social events.
- Assessment for substance abuse and dependence should be a part of every client history and physical examination.
- Alcohol is the number one drug of choice in American society today among both adolescents and adults and is the most widely available drug.
- Nicotine use is a major health problem and, along with alcohol and marijuana, serves as a "gateway" to illicit drug use.
- Fetal alcohol syndrome is 100% preventable if the pregnant woman abstains from alcohol use.
- The incidence of substance abuse varies with cultural groups.
- Dual diagnosis/comorbidity requires in-depth assessment followed by treatment of both the substance abuse and the psychiatric diagnoses.
- Current DSM-IV-TR diagnoses of abuse and dependency do not adequately describe substance use in the adolescent population. It is preferable to use terms such as *problematic* drinking or excessive substance use.
- Secondary complications of drug use may be causative factors for physical illness/health concerns.
- Commitment to long-term treatment and rehabilitation programs strongly improves recovery outcomes.

REVIEW QUESTIONS

1. A 4-year-old client walks into the doctor's office. She is restless, not responding to her mother's directions, and touching everything she sees. You notice that her eyes are small and her nose is short. Based on the nurse's observations, you may conclude that the client may have:
   a. Attention deficit-hyperactivity disorder
   b. Conduct disorder
   c. Fetal alcohol syndrome
   d. Autism

2. A 16-year-old client comes to the therapist's office for the first time. The client's mother reports that her son has been angry, hostile, truant, and disobeying the house rules such as curfew. He has lost weight and sleeps long hours at times. The nurse's first impression is that the client:
   a. Is enmeshed with his mother
   b. Is exerting his independence
   c. Has suffered a traumatic event at school
   d. Is using alcohol and/or drugs

3. A critical care nurse was admitted to the chemical dependency unit after her supervisor discovered that she was abusing Demerol. Which statement by the client demonstrates that the client is ready for discharge:
   a. "I know that Demerol is addictive and the effects it has on the body."
   b. "I don't need to use anymore. I have my friends to help me cope with my stress."
   c. "I think I'm going to have to consider a less stressful job. Critical care nursing is too stressful and dangerous for my recovery."
   d. "I promised my husband that I wouldn't use and I intend to keep my promise."

4. A 53-year-old client was admitted into the hospital for detoxification from alcohol. The client admitted to drinking 12 beers a day for the past 30 years. The case manager suggested that the client transfer to a rehab program. The client refused despite the physician informing him that he has hypertension and his liver function tests were abnormal. The physician informed him that he needed to stop drinking. The client reported to the case manager that he's not an alcoholic because he doesn't get drunk and his father drinks a scotch and smokes a cigar every day and is now 83 years old. The highest priority nursing diagnosis would be:
   a. Ineffective denial
   b. Impaired adjustment
   c. Ineffective coping
   d. Interrupted family processes

5. Which symptoms of detoxification would you be most concerned about?
   a. Tremors
   b. Diaphoresis
   c. Increased heart rate
   d. Hallucinations and delusions

REFERENCES

Alcohol, tobacco and other drug abuse: challenges and responses for faith leaders, DHHS Publication No. (SMA) 95-3074, Washington, DC, 1995, ES Inc. for the U.S. Department of Health and Human Services, Substance Abuse and Mental Health Services Administration, Center for Substance Abuse Treatment (Contract No. 270-91-0016).

American Psychiatric Association: *Diagnostic and Statistical Manual of Mental Disorders*, Fourth Edition, Text Revision. Washington, DC, American Psychiatric Association, 2002.

Bennett SS, Bennett WM: Potency matters, *Drug Watch World News* VII(2):3, 2002.

Bowden R, Rust D: A review of fetal alcohol syndrome for health educators, *J Health Educ* 31(4):231-237, 2000.

Bowen M: *Family therapy in clinical practice,* New York, 1978, Jason Aronson.

Brennan PL et al: Predictors and outcomes of outpatient mental health care: a 4-year prospective study of elderly Medicare patients with substance use disorders, *Medical Care* 39(1):39-49, 2001.

Chermack ST, Blow FC: Violence among individuals in substance abuse treatment: the role of alcohol and cocaine consumption, *Drug Alcohol Dependence* 66:29-37, 2002, retrieved March 2, 2002 from website: www.elsevier.com/locate/drugalcdep.

Crespi TM, Sabatelli RM: Children of alcoholics and adolescence: individuation development and family systems, *Adolescence* 32:407, 1997.

Daly D, Moss H, Campbell F: *Dual disorders: counseling clients with chemical dependency and mental illness,* ed 2, Center City, MN, 1993, Hazelden Foundation.

Ewing JA: Detecting alcoholism: the CAGE questionnaire, *JAMA* 252:1905, 1984.

Griffith J: Substance abuse disorders in nurses, *Nurs Forum* 34:4, 1999.

Hatfield AB: Dual diagnosis: substance abuse and mental illness, 1993, National Alliance for the Mentally Ill, retrieved July 7, 2002 from website: www.schizophrenia.com.

Heather N et al, editors: *Psychoactive drugs and harm reduction: from faith to science,* London, 1993, Whurr Publishers.

Hser Y-I et al: An evaluation of drug treatment for adolescents in four US cities, *Arch Gen Psychiatry* 58(7):689-695, 2001.

Join Together Online, Substance Abuse News Summaries, FDA steps up regulation of ephedrine products. Retrieved June 17, 2002 from website: www.jointogether.org/home/.

Long-term marijuana use affects memory and attention, *Substance Abuse and Mental Health Services Administration (SAMHSA) News* X(2):20, 2002.

Mathias R, Zickler P: NIDA conference highlights scientific findings on MDMA/Ecstasy, *Nida Notes* 16(5):1,5, 6-8,12, 2001.

Miller P: Family structure, personality, drinking, smoking and illicit drug use: a study of UK teenagers, *Drug Alcohol Depend* 45:121, 1997.

NANDA International (2003). NANDA Nursing Diagnoses: Definitions and Classification 2003-2004. Philadelphia: NANDA.

National Institute of Drug Abuse: *Anabolic Steroids. Community Drug Alert Bulletin* (1-3), Retrieved May 27, 2002 from website: www.drugabuse.gov/.

National Institute on Drug Abuse: Club Drugs. Community Drug Alert Bulletin (1-5) Retrieved May 27, 2002 from website: www.drugabuse.gov/.

National Institute on Drug Abuse: Dopamine may play role in cue-induced craving distinct from its role regulating reward effects (2002, May 28). *News Scan* (1-4), retrieved June 22, 2002 from website: www.drugabuse.gov/.

National Institute on Drug Abuse: Frequently asked questions, Retrieved July 4, 2002 from website: www.drugabuse.gov/.

National Mental Health Association: Substance abuse dual diagnosis (n.d.), Retrieved July 7, 2002 from website: www.nmha.org.

National survey of American attitudes on substance abuse VI: teens, New York, 2001, National Center on Addiction and Substance Abuse, Columbia University.

Newcomb MD: Understanding the multidimensional nature of drug use and abuse: the role of consumption, risk factors, and protective factors. In Glantz MD, Pickens R, editors: *Vulnerability to drug abuse,* Washington, DC, 1992, American Psychological Association.

Oetting ER: Planning programs for prevention of deviant behavior: a psychosocial model. In Trimble JE, Boler CE, Niemcryk SJ, editors: *Ethnic and multicultural drug use: perspectives on current research,* New York, 1992, Haworth Press.

Partnership for a Drug-Free America (2001, February) National survey: Ecstasy use continues rising among teens, retrieved April 3, 2002 from website: www.drugfreeamerica.org/.

PULSE CHECK Trends in Drug Abuse Mid-Year 2000, Executive Office of the President, Office of National Drug Control Policy, Washington, DC 20503, NCJ 186747, March 2001.

Sadock BJ, Sadock VA: *Kaplan and Sadock's comprehensive textbook of psychiatry,* ed 7, Philadelphia, 2000, Lippincott Williams & Wilkins.

Schuckit MA: *Drug and alcohol abuse: a clinical guide to diagnosis and treatment,* ed 5, New York, 2000, Kluwer Academic/Plenum Publishers.

Substance Abuse and Mental Health Services Administration, Office of Applied Studies: *Emergency Department Trends from the Drug Abuse Warning Network, Preliminary Estimates January-June 2001 with Revised Estimates 1994 to 2000,* DAWN Series D-20, DHHS Publication No. (SMA) 02-3634, Rockville, Md, 2002.

Substance Abuse: The Nation's Number One Health Problem: Key Indicators for Policy Update (2001, February) Prepared by the Schneider Institute for Health Policy, Brandeis University for The Robert Wood Johnson Foundation, Princeton, NJ, 2001.

Szalavitz M: Breaking out of the 12-step lockstep: commentary, Retrieved June 17, 2002, from website: www.jointogether.org/home/.

Weir E: Substance abuse among physicians, *CMAJ* 162(12):1730, 2000.

Withers NW: Deceptions in addiction psychiatry, *Am J Forensic Psychiatry* 22(4):7-28, 2001.

Zickler P: NIDA studies clarify developmental effects of prenatal cocaine exposure, *Nida Notes,* vol 13, no 3, retrieved July 4, 2002 from website: www.drugabuse.gov/.

Zickler P: Methamphetamine abuse linked to impaired cognitive and motor skills despite recovery of dopamine transporters, *Nida Notes* vol 17, no 1, April 2002.

SUGGESTED READINGS

Beare PG, Myers JL: *Adult health nursing,* ed 3, St Louis, 1998, Mosby.

Grady M: Cognitive deficits associated with heavy marijuana use appear to be reversible, *Nida Notes* 17(1):8, 9, 2002.

Jellinek EM: Phases of alcohol addiction, *Q J Stud Alcohol* 38:114, 1977.

Kavanagh DJ et al: Substance misuse in patients with schizophrenia, *Drugs* 62(5):743-753, 2002.

Kourtis AP et al: Understanding the timing of HIV transmission from mother to infant, *JAMA* 285(6):709-711, 2001.

Martin K: Adolescent treatment programs reduce drug abuse, produce other improvements, *Nida Notes* 17(1):11-12, 2002.

Mathias R: High-risk sex is main factor in HIV infection for men and women who inject drugs, *Nida Notes* 17(2):1, 5-6, 2002.

Mennella J: Alcohol's effect on lactation, *Alcohol Res Health* 25(3):230-234, 2001. NIDA INFOMAX.

Mortality data from the drug abuse warning network 2000, Substance Abuse and Mental Health Services Association, Office of Applied Studies, DHHS Publication No. (SMA) 02-3633. Rockville, MD, 2002.

Musto DF: *The American disease: origins of narcotic control,* New York, 1987, Oxford University Press.

Werner EE, Johnson JL: The role of caring adults in the lives of children of alcoholics, *Children of Alcoholics: Selected Readings* vol 2, 2000.

Williams JS: Cocaine's effects on cerebral blood flow differ between men and women, *Nida Notes* 17(2):1, 6, 2002.

Woll P: *Healing the stigma of addiction: a guide for treatment professionals,* Chicago, 2001, Great Lakes ATTC, Recovery Communities United, Inc., Southeast AATTC.

14 Delirium, Dementia, and Amnestic and Other Cognitive Disorders

Kathleen Pace Murphy

KEY TERMS

OBJECTIVES

- Analyze the various theories of the nature and development of Alzheimer's disease and discuss rationale of the most currently accepted theories.

- Describe the pathophysiologic changes in the brain related to Alzheimer's disease.

- Classify the progressive symptoms of Alzheimer's disease into three stages (mild, moderate, severe).

- Differentiate between the different types of dementia (reversible/irreversible).

- Apply the nursing process in managing clients with cognitive disorders.

- Explain and plan therapeutic activities for clients experiencing dementia.

Dementia is a global impairment of intellectual (cognitive) functions that is usually progressive and of sufficient severity to interfere with a person's normal social and occupational functioning. Many diseases and pathologic processes are categorized under this medical syndrome, of which Alzheimer's disease is the most prevalent.

Alzheimer's disease is a progressive and degenerative disorder of the central nervous system. Alzheimer's disease can be categorized into familial Alzheimer's disease (inherited form) or sporadic Alzheimer's disease (no inheritance pattern seen) (Marin, Sewell, and Schlechter, 2002). It is also defined by onset. Early-onset Alzheimer's disease occurs in clients 64 years and younger, and late-onset Alzheimer's disease occurs in clients more than 65 years old. Alzheimer's disease affects short-term memory first and then progresses to other intellectual abilities such as speech, reading, writing, and comprehension. Clients grow confused and unaware of their surroundings and later become progressively incapable of caring for their basic activities of daily living (ADLs) such as feeding, grooming, and toileting (Figure 14-1).

HISTORICAL AND THEORETIC PERSPECTIVES

Alois Alzheimer (1864-1915), a German-trained neurologist, was inspired by neurologist Franz Nissl (1860-1919) to study neuropathology. In 1895 Nissl moved to Germany to work with the psychiatrist Emil Kraepelin (1856-1926) on the structural basis of psychiatric disease. Kraepelin transferred his operations to Munich in 1903, taking Nissl and Alzheimer with him. At about the same time, a revolution in histologic techniques was taking place in both microscope technology and the advent of metallic stains for nervous tissue. In 1899 Ramón y Cajal demonstrated the usefulness of this new staining technique in studying the structure and form of nervous tissue. Nissl produced his stain for neuronal cell bodies in 1892, and in 1902 Max Bielschowsky, a German neuropathologist (1869-1940), produced the silver-based stain that allowed Alzheimer to demonstrate the now-

familiar neuritic (senile) plaques and neurofibrillary tangles in the brain. In 1906 Alzheimer announced his findings of these lesions in the brain of a 51-year-old woman suffering from dementia and paranoia, and he published these findings in 1907.

In 1910 Kraepelin referred to cases similar to that of Dr. Alois Alzheimer's as Alzheimer's disease or "presenile" dementia (now called *dementia of the Alzheimer's type, with early onset [age 65 years or under]* in the DSM-IV-TR classification), the frequency of which we now know to be much less than that of "senile" dementia (or *dementia of the Alzheimer's type, with late onset [after age 65 years]* in the DSM-IV-TR classification). The incorporation of Alzheimer's disease in Kraepelin's classic text categorized Alzheimer's disease as a psychiatric process rather than a neurologic one, and thus for many decades designated it as the responsibility of specialists in psychiatry.

Early descriptions of Alzheimer's lesions affecting individuals with Down syndrome over the age of 40 years were described initially by Jervis in 1948 and tended to relate Alzheimer's disease to an accelerated aging process (which at that time Down syndrome was thought to be). It was not until the publication in 1968 to 1970 of an important series of articles by the team of British clinical pathologists, Tomlinson, Blessed, and Roth, that Alzheimer's disease moved into its modern era. These authors compared the brains of individuals over age 65 years without dementia to an age-matched group with dementia. Much to their surprise, they found that 62% of cases with dementia had the tangles and plaques described by Alzheimer. Using a neuropsychologic test, they showed that the severity of dementia correlated with the number of cerebral plaques. Only 22% of these cases had evidence of arteriosclerosis and brain softening, indicative of cerebrovascular disease.

ETIOLOGY

Alzheimer's disease is the most common form of dementia. There are, however, many other types of dementia, and some are reversible. A simple way to approach the problem of memory loss is to think of two types of disorders: (1) those that are reversible and (2) those that are irreversible. Table 14-1 lists several types of irreversible de-

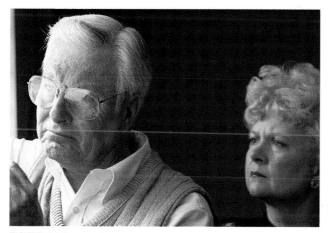

FIGURE 14-1. A wife feels sorrow over her husband's loss of faculties resulting from Alzheimer's disease. (Copyright Cathy Lander-Goldberg, Lander Photographics.)

Table 14-1	Etiologic Factors in Primary Dementia (Irreversible Dementia)	
Diseases That Cause Primary Dementia	**Incidence at Autopsy (%)**
Alzheimer's disease	62.6
Vascular dementia	21.4
Mixed Alzheimer's disease/vascular dementia	6.3
Parkinson's disease	5.7
Pick's disease	3.0
Creutzfeldt-Jakob disease	0.5
Other dementias	0.5

From Glenner GG: Alzheimer's disease, *Encyclopedia of Human Biology* 1:103, 1994.

Table 14-2   Etiologic Factors in Secondary Dementia (Reversible Dementia)

Toxic Causes	Other Electrolyte Disturbances	Infective Causes	Cerebral Disease
Barbiturate intoxication	Hepatic disease	Chronic respiratory infection with cardiac decompensation	Slow-growing cerebral tumor (e.g., frontal meningioma)
Alcoholism	Porphyria	Pulmonary tuberculosis	Multiple cerebral emboli
Polypharmacy	Nutritional	Bacterial endocarditis	Normal-pressure hydrocephalus*
Metabolic disorders	Undernutrition by prolonged neglect or self-isolation	Endocrine disease	
Potassium loss from self-purgation	Chronic malabsorption syndrome	Myxedema	
	Vitamin B$_{12}$ deficiency	Pituitary insufficiency	
	Nicotinic acid encephalopathy	Addison's disease	

*Normal-pressure hydrocephalus is a disorder characterized by dementia, gait disorder, and urinary incontinence. Dilation of the ventricles in the absence of increased cerebrospinal fluid is a prominent manifestation. A shunt is usually effective treatment.

DSM-IV-TR CRITERIA
Dementia of the Alzheimer's Type

A. The development of multiple cognitive deficits manifested by both
   1. Memory impairment (inability to learn new information and to recall previously learned information)
   2. One (or more) of the following cognitive disturbances:
      a. Aphasia (language disturbance)
      b. Apraxia (inability to carry out motor activities despite intact motor function)
      c. Agnosia (failure to recognize or identify objects despite intact sensory function)
      d. Disturbance in executive functioning (e.g., planning, organizing, sequencing, abstracting)
B. The cognitive deficits in criteria A1 and A2 each cause significant impairment in social or occupational functioning and represent a significant decline from a previous level of functioning.
C. The course is characterized by gradual onset and continuing cognitive decline.
D. The cognitive deficits in criteria A1 and A2 are not due to any of the following:
   1. Other central nervous system conditions that cause progressive deficits in memory and cognition (e.g., cerebrovascular disease, Parkinson's disease, Huntington's disease, subdural hematoma, normal pressure hydrocephalus, brain tumor)
   2. Systemic conditions that are known to cause dementia (e.g., hypothyroidism, vitamin B$_{12}$ or folic acid deficiency, niacin deficiency, hypercalcemia, neurosyphilis, HIV infection)
   3. Substance-induced conditions
E. The deficits do not occur exclusively during the course of delirium.
F. The deficits are not better accounted for by another Axis I disorder (e.g., major depressive disorder, schizophrenia).

From American Psychiatric Association: *Diagnostic and Statistical Manual of Mental Disorders*, Fourth Edition, Text Revision. Washington, DC, American Psychiatric Association, 2000.

mentias. Table 14-2 lists the reversible dementias. Approximately 10% of clients with dementia have reversible disease that can be improved and, in a small percentage of cases, cured with proper treatment (see DSM-IV-TR Criteria box).

The Irreversible Dementias

Alzheimer's disease has been called the disease of the century. It is an insidious, irreversible, progressive disease that ultimately leads to death. Several theories are currently being investigated. Among these are:

- Angiopathy and blood-brain barrier incompetence
- Neurotransmitter and receptor deficiencies
- Abnormal proteins and their products
- Genetic defects

Angiopathy and Blood-Brain Barrier Incompetence

Physical alterations of capillary walls have been noted in studies of the brains of persons with Alzheimer's disease. These changes include lumpy thickening and nodular vessels and loss of the fine network of nerve fibers normally investing the blood-contacting surfaces. It has been suggested that these lesions and the resulting devastation of nerves destroy the barrier that prevents many blood serum components from entering the brain (the blood-brain barrier). Amyloid deposition in the walls of blood vessels and in capillaries in the cerebral cortex almost always accompanies Alzheimer's disease, reaffirming that these vascular lesions result in blood-brain barrier incompetence (Scheibel et al., 1987). Thus serum proteins leak into the gray matter (cortex) of the brain. Evidence that a serum protein, sphingolipid activator protein (SAP), can be identified and isolated from the amyloid core of neuritic plaques (Scheibel et al., 1987) strongly suggests that blood-brain barrier incompetence exists in Alzheimer's disease.

Neurotransmitter Deficiencies

Neuronal pathways are altered or destroyed during the course of Alzheimer's disease. The nucleus basalis of Mynert contains many cholinergic pathways. This area is responsible for the integration of complex thought with innervations to the frontal cortex (memory and cognition) and hippocampus (memory and cognition). Choline acetyl transferase is an enzyme responsible for the production of acetylcholine. Acetylcholine is a neurotransmitter whose role is to conduct impulses between neurons. Research findings have demonstrated diminished activity of choline acetyl transferase in the brains of Alzheimer's disease clients. This decrease in available acetylcholine and cholinergic cell loss is directly associated with memory and cognitive impairment. Corticotropin-releasing factor, norepinephrine, and glutamate are also involved in cognition and Alzheimer's disease (Marin, Sewell, and Schlechter, 2002). These neurotransmitters are currently under investigation.

Abnormal Proteins and Their Products

Two proteins have been identified as playing a role in Alzheimer's disease: β-amyloid and τ-proteins interact within the hippocampal and cerebral cortex of the brain. It is believed that they act as part of a communication system that is responsible for memory, cognition, and behavior. The discovery of the major protein that makes up the amyloid fibrillar deposits, the β-amyloid protein, in both Alzheimer's disease and Down syndrome, has initiated biochemical and molecular biologic studies. Based on the presence of β-amyloid protein as amyloid fibrils in 100% of individuals with Down syndrome, it was suggested that the protein was a chemical marker for Down syndrome and that the gene encoding for its precursor would be found on chromosome 21, the abnormally tripled chromosome found in Down syndrome (Barton, 2002).

Genetic Defects

Early onset Alzheimer's disease has been frequently associated with mutations in one of three genes: amyloid-precursor protein (gene 21), presenlin-1 (gene 14), and presenlin-2 (gene 1) (Selkoe, 2001). Chromosome 19, which codes for apolipoprotein E (apo E), may be associated with late-onset Alzheimer's disease. There are three variants of this gene. The E_4 variant, apo E_4, is the one that imparts the increased risk.

Nature of Alzheimer's Disease

Alzheimer's disease is a neurodegenerative disorder in which, predominantly, the cortex of the brain containing nerve cells involved in memory and cognition is destroyed. The loss of gray matter (brain tissue atrophy) causes a separation of the brain from the skull, widening of crevices that produce its convoluted appearance (sulci), and dilation of the cisterns that collect waste fluid and substances from the brain (ventricles). The degradation of the gray matter is caused by the accumulation of destructive lesions, which are the hallmarks of the disease. These are the **neuritic plaques,** which are composed of β-amyloid fibers; **neurofibrillary tangles,** which are composed of paired helical filaments that destroy nerve cells and amyloid deposits in the walls of cerebral blood vessels; and neuronal degeneration. Degeneration in the forebrain diminishes acetylcholine and the activities of choline acetyl transferase (Price et al., 1998).

Vascular Dementia (Multiinfarct Dementia)

Vascular dementia, formerly called multiinfarct dementia, is due to the effects of one or more strokes on cognitive function. Vascular dementia results from the occlusion or obstruction of small arteries or arterioles in the cortex of the brain, preventing nutrients from nourishing the brain (see DSM-IV-TR Criteria box).

DSM-IV-TR CRITERIA
Vascular Dementia

A. The development of multiple cognitive deficits manifested by both:
1. Memory impairment (impaired ability to learn new information or to recall previously learned information)
2. One (or more) of the following cognitive disturbances:
   a. Aphasia (language disturbance)
   b. Apraxia (impaired ability to carry out motor activities despite intact motor function)
   c. Agnosia (failure to recognize or identify objects despite intact sensory function)
   d. Disturbance in executive functioning (i.e., planning, organizing, sequencing, abstracting)
B. The cognitive deficits in criteria A1 and A2 each cause significant impairment in social or occupational functioning and represent a significant decline from a previous level of functioning.
C. Focal neurologic signs and symptoms (e.g., exaggeration of deep tendon reflexes, extensor plantar response, pseudobulbar palsy, gait abnormalities, weakness of an extremity) or laboratory evidence indicative of cerebrovascular disease (e.g., multiple infarctions involving cortex and underlying white matter) that is judged to be etiologically related to the disturbance.
D. The deficits do not occur exclusively during the course of a delirium.

From American Psychiatric Association: *Diagnostic and Statistical Manual of Mental Disorders,* Fourth Edition, Text Revision. Washington, DC, American Psychiatric Association, 2000.

Parkinson's Dementia

Parkinson's disease is a neurologic disorder that causes tremor, rigidity, bradykinesia, and abnormalities of posture and gait (shuffling). Dementia accompanies the disease later in the disease course in approximately 20% to 60% of clients. Nerve cells in the substantia nigra (brainstem), where dopamine is produced, develop pigmented lesions within them that are a sign of the disease. These were first described by Lewy in 1913 and are called Lewy bodies. In about 30% of cases of Parkinson's disease the amyloid lesions of Alzheimer's disease can be seen, whereas, conversely, about 50% of clients with Alzheimer's disease demonstrate typical symptoms of Parkinson's disease.

Pick's Disease

Pick's disease is a degenerative process of nerve cells, usually localized to the frontal and temporal lobe of the brain. It is distinguished clinically by changes in personality early in the course of the disease, deterioration of social skills, emotional blunting, behavioral disinhibition, and prominent language abnormalities.

Creutzfeldt-Jakob Disease

Creutzfeldt-Jakob disease is an infectious (but not contagious) process that can be transmitted by corneal grafts, infected electrodes, and injected crude growth hormone derived from human pituitaries. An infectious agent, called a prion, produces a spongy appearance to the brain (spongiform encephalopathy) with vacuolization of nerve cells (the creation of a clear space in cell protoplasm filled with fluid or air). Its course is more rapid than that of Alzheimer's disease. Creutzfeldt-Jakob disease begins with the insidious onset of confusion, depression, and altered sensation, progressing in weeks or months to dementia, ataxia, palsy, and sometimes cortical blindness. Creutzfeldt-Jakob disease constitutes only 0.5% of primary dementia cases.

Diffuse Lewy Body Disease

Diffuse Lewy body disease is a late-life primary degenerative dementia noted predominantly in men in which Lewy bodies, as seen in Parkinson's disease, are present in neurons in the gray matter. Early ataxic gait and psychiatric symptoms (visual hallucinations, delusions, and violent or aggressive behavior) are not uncommon. Lewy body disease is associated with both Alzheimer's disease and Parkinson's disease lesions.

Progressive Supranuclear Palsy

Progressive supranuclear palsy is a degenerative disease that particularly affects the nucleus of the neuron and presents clinically with dementia, progressive paralysis of downward (vertical) gaze, difficulty in articulation of joints **(dysarthria),** muscular rigidity (most marked in the neck), and ataxic gait. Males are affected more than twice as often as females.

Down Syndrome Dementia

Down syndrome dementia is difficult to diagnose, despite the extensive Alzheimer's disease-type lesions seen in the cortex of the brain on autopsy. Persons with Down syndrome have three copies of chromosome 21 (trisomy 21) and often develop amyloid plaques and Alzheimer's disease at an early age. Only about 50% of individuals with Down syndrome over age 40 years can be determined as having dementia, which is usually first manifested as memory loss. This low percentage is probably due to the difficulty in ascertaining dementia in the face of mental deficiency.

Cerebrovascular Accidents

Cerebrovascular accidents are strokelike episodes that occur in approximately 20% of clients with Alzheimer's disease and are due to the effects of cerebrovascular amyloid deposits either blocking the vessel or causing it to rupture to produce a cerebral hemorrhage. This lesion occurs predominantly in the gray matter and therefore does not result in paralysis. If the vessel ruptures in the leptomeninges (i.e., on the brain surface), however, severe hemorrhage can result in paralysis and death.

The Reversible Dementias

Reversible dementias are a group of processes that represent about 10% of dementia cases. The vast majority of these are treatable. For example, metabolic disease, vitamin B_{12} deficiency, mimics most of the symptoms of Alzheimer's disease. When the client is treated by a physician with injections of vitamin B_{12} before irreversible damage occurs, the dementia symptoms can be eliminated and the well-being of the client readily restored. This is the case with certain superficial benign tumors (meningiomas), which, when completely removed by

the surgeon, eliminate the dementia symptoms. Etiologic factors in secondary dementia are discussed in Table 14-2.

Depression is a common reversible dementia seen in older adults. Older clients may not have the usual signs and symptoms of depression and may present only with memory loss. Depression is easily treated with the newer antidepressant medications. Depression can co-exist with dementia. Lyketsos (1997) demonstrated a 49% clinically significant depression diagnosis in outpatient older adults with Alzheimer's disease.

Disorders Often Confused With Dementia

It is easy to mistake disorders such as delirium or amnestic disorder with dementia, as clients may have some of the same symptoms. Treatment for each of these disorders varies widely, making recognition and diagnosis important.

Delirium

Delirium is a disturbance of consciousness and change in cognition that develops over a short period and tends to fluctuate during the course of a day. The prevalence of delirium in the elderly population ranges from 4% to 53% in hospitalized older adults (APA, 2000). Advancing age, preexisting cognitive impairment (Alzheimer's disease, vascular dementia), certain medications and acute medical conditions are all risk factors for delirium (Richardson, 2003). Delirium is characterized by disorientation to time and place, inability to focus or shift attention, incoherent speech, and continual, aimless physical activity.

The client may or may not be agitated or sleepy and may or may not display hallucinations. There may be periods of lucidity or a change in cognition such as memory deficit, language disturbance, or perceptual impairment. Clients may appear depressed. Delirium always has an organic basis that needs to be carefully assessed.

Delirium is usually seen in clients with Alzheimer's disease when a severe infection or other medical condition is superimposed on the preexisting conditions. Delirium can also be the first or only indicator of illnesses ranging from pneumonia to myocardial infarction to drug toxicity. Failure to recognize delirium can lead to significant morbidity and mortality, both from the underlying illness and from inadvertently self-inflicted injuries. When delirium overlies dementia of the Alzheimer's type, differentiating becomes more difficult yet more vital to positive client outcomes. Criteria for delirium caused by multiple etiologies are listed in the DSM-IV-TR Criteria box. A comparison of delirium, depression, and dementia is found in Table 14-3.

Amnestic Disorders

Amnestic disorders are characterized by a disturbance in memory that is due to either the direct physiologic effects of a general medical condition or the persisting effects of a substance use/abuse or toxin exposure. The main focus is memory disturbance and can be specified as transient (duration of hours or days but less than 1 month) or chronic (duration of more than 1 month) (see DSM-IV-TR Criteria box).

Table 14-3	Delirium, Depression, and Dementia Comparison		
	Delirium	**Depression**	**Dementia**
Onset	Rapid (hours to days)	Rapid (weeks to months)	Gradual (years)
Course	Wide fluctuations; may continue for weeks if cause not found	May be self-limited or may become chronic without treatment	Chronic; slow but continuous decline
Level of consciousness	Fluctuates from hyperalert to difficult to arouse	Normal	Normal
Orientation	Client is disoriented, confused	Client may seem disoriented	Client is disoriented, confused
Affect	Fluctuating	Sad, depressed, worried, guilty	Labile; apathy in later stages
Attention	Always impaired	Difficulty concentrating; client may check and recheck all actions	May be intact; client may focus on one thing for long periods
Sleep	Always disturbed	Disturbed; excess sleeping or insomnia, especially early-morning waking	Usually normal
Behavior	Agitated, restless	Client may be fatigued, apathetic; may occasionally be agitated	Client may be agitated or apathetic; may wander
Speech	Sparse or rapid; client may be incoherent	Flat, sparse, may have outbursts; understandable	Sparse or rapid; repetitive; client may be incoherent
Memory	Impaired, especially for recent events	Varies from day to day; slow recall; often short-term deficit	Impaired, especially for recent events
Cognition	Disordered reasoning	May seem impaired	Disordered reasoning and calculation
Thought content	Incoherent, confused, delusions, stereotyped	Negative, hypochondriac, thoughts of death, paranoid	Disorganized, rich content, delusional, paranoid
Perception	Misinterpretations, illusions, hallucinations	Distorted; client may have auditory hallucinations; negative interpretation of people and events	No change
Judgment	Poor	Poor	Poor; socially inappropriate behavior
Insight	May be present in lucid moments	May be impaired	Absent
Performance on mental status examinations	Poor but variable; improves during lucid moments and with recovery	Memory impaired; calculation, drawing, following directions usually not impaired; frequent "I don't know" answers	Consistently poor; progressively worsens; client attempts to answer all questions

From Holt J: How to help confused patients, *Am J Nurs* 93:32-36, 1993; and Hoffman SB, Platt CA: *Comforting the confused: strategies for managing dementia,* ed 2, New York, 2000, Springer.

DSM-IV-TR CRITERIA
Delirium Due to Multiple Etiologies

A. There are disturbances of consciousness (i.e., reduced clarity of awareness of the environment) with reduced ability to focus, sustain, or shift attention.
B. There is a change in cognition (such as memory deficit, disorientation, language disturbance, perceptual disturbance) that is not better accounted for by a preexisting, established, or evolving dementia.
C. The disturbance develops over a short period (usually hours to days) and tends to fluctuate during the course of the day.
D. There is evidence from the history, physical examination, or laboratory findings that the delirium has more than one etiology (e.g., more than one etiologic general medical condition: a general medical condition plus substance intoxication or medication side effect.)

From American Psychiatric Association: *Diagnostic and Statistical Manual of Mental Disorders,* Fourth Edition, Text Revision. Washington, DC, American Psychiatric Association, 2000.

DSM-IV-TR CRITERIA
Amnestic Disorder

1. The development of memory impairment as manifested by impairment in the ability to learn new information or the inability to recall previously learned information.
2. The memory disturbance causes significant impairment in social or occupational functioning and represents a significant decline from a previous level of functioning.
3. The memory disturbance does not occur exclusively during the course of a delirium or a dementia.
4. There is evidence from the history, physical examination, or laboratory findings that the disturbance is the direct physiologic consequence of a general medical condition (including physical trauma).
Specify if:
Transient: if memory impairment lasts for 1 month or less
Chronic: if memory impairment lasts for more than 1 month

From American Psychiatric Association: *Diagnostic and Statistical Manual of Mental Disorders,* Fourth Edition, Text Revision. Washington, DC, American Psychiatric Association, 2000.

EPIDEMIOLOGY

The prevalence of dementia is approximately 6% in people over 65 years old and 30% in people age 90 years or older (Barton, 2002). It has been estimated that 1 in 45 older Americans will be affected by Alzheimer's disease by 2050 (Alzheimer's disease, 1998). The role of ethnicity is unclear. Prevalence of Alzheimer's disease appears to vary widely in various ethnic groups (Evans et al., 2000). A total of 1 out of 3 families with a member age 65 years or older includes a person with Alzheimer's disease. More than 50% of nursing home clients have been diagnosed with probable or possible Alzheimer's disease (Box 14-1).

CLINICAL DESCRIPTION
Alzheimer's Disease

Alzheimer's disease is an insidious, progressive, and slow disease. Two characteristics make diagnosis difficult in its earliest stage. Initially the hippocampus is attacked by neurofibrillary tangles, producing recent memory loss. This symptom is usually followed by nonsymmetric deterioration of the temporoparietal regions, producing cognitive deficits in learning, attention, judgment, orientation, and/or speech and language use. To further complicate matters, occasionally other regions of the brain may be affected. Thus a constellation of symptoms results. The situation is compounded by the insidious onset of the disease, which to the untrained observer may be perceived as inattention, restlessness, mild forgetfulness, and depression.

Clients with Alzheimer's disease do not present a uniform or coherent history, nor can the time of onset be clearly defined. This can present a serious problem in differential diagnosis. Frequently, family members who have not seen the person for a while fail to notice the subtle changes that have occurred. Rash judgments based on a short visit often lead to conflict between the family caregiver and relatives of the client, particularly when institutionalization comes into question. The loss of a job or a serious auto accident may, unfortunately, be the most convincing evidence of serious cognitive loss and usually motivates the family members to act on behalf of their loved one.

Caregivers may seek medical care for a loved one when specific behavioral difficulties have been observed, such as:

- Difficulty with shopping, which requires performing tasks sequentially, correlating lists, planning, remembering, and calculating money
- Problems in the areas of driving, involving accidents or episodes of getting lost
- Missing social engagements and appointments
- Difficulty with financial tasks, particularly balancing a checkbook, paying bills, or comprehending financial statements
- Aimless pacing or wandering away from home
- Inability to recognize people they should know or misidentifying friends and family members
- Inability to do common household tasks (e.g., cooking and cleaning)

Box 14-1	Dementia Mortality in the United States

374 deaths per 100,000 men
302 deaths per 100,000 women
Death certificates underestimate mortality
35% of persons with dementia spend time in a long-term care facility during the last year of life

Data from Rogers S L et al: A 24-week, double-blind placebo-controlled trial of donezepil in patients with Alzheimer's disease: Donezepil Study Group, *Neurology* 50(1): 136-145, 1998.

Although clients themselves may notice early signs of cognitive impairment, many will use one or more of the defense mechanisms of denial, repression, projection, aggression, regression, or rationalization. Some will succeed in deceiving family, friends, and employers for a time. Distinguishing these behaviors from cognitive deficits further complicates the diagnostic process.

A careful history may reveal many or all of the following symptoms:

- Altered thought processes (**paranoia**)
- Confused or disoriented state
- Impaired intellect and memory (especially short-term memory in the early stage)
- Sensory/perceptual alterations (hallucinations)
- Decreased sensorium
- Loss of body functions
- Self-care deficit
- Fear, anxiety, depression
- Catastrophic reactions
- Self-concept disturbance/powerlessness
- Compromised physical ability
- Social isolation, apathy
- Impaired verbal communication
- Emotional liability
- Sleep disturbances

Stages of Alzheimer's Disease

People with Alzheimer's disease experience cognitive, functional, and behavioral changes. Onset of the disease is usually insidious, and as a result symptoms emerge slowly and often go unrecognized. Progression of Alzheimer's disease is staged according to the level of functional and cognitive impairment. Three stages are detailed next and summarized in Table 14-4. Each stage brings with it additional physical and psychoemotive losses, as well as increasing dependency needs.

Stage 1: Mild. The most distinguishing characteristic of stage 1 is memory loss. Mild cognitive impairment (MCI) refers to elderly patients with mild memory impairment and intact daily functional abilities (Cotter, Clark, and Karlawish, 2003; Peterson, 1999). Often memory impairment is so mild that the client, family, and caregivers attribute it to "normal aging." As this insidious disease progresses, how-

Table 14-4 Stages of Alzheimer's Disease		
Stage 1: Mild	**Stage 2: Moderate**	**Stage 3: Severe**

Recent memory loss
Cognitive loss in:
  Communicating
  Calculating
  Recognition
Anxiety and confusion
Mild behavior problems such as the inability to initiate and complete a task
	Stage 1 symptoms increase
	Behavior problems increase, which may include the following:
	  Catastrophic reactions
	  Sundowning
	  Perseveration
	  Aimless pacing
	  Wandering
	Confusion
	Incontinence, mild
	Hypertonia
		Stage 2 symptoms increase
		Incontinence, total
		Choking
		Emaciation
		Total care needed
		Progressive gait disturbances leading to nonambulatory status

ever, the client often recognizes that there is a problem. Recent memories regarding yesterday's events are lost, yet the client may articulate in detail events from long ago. Inability to find words or using inappropriate words when unable to remember is common. **Neologisms** are also common. It is during this time of self-awareness of loss that many clients suffer profound depression. Approximately 41% of clients with Alzheimer's disease experience depression at some point in their illness (Wragg and Jeste, 1994). Sensory and motor functions are not usually affected at this stage.

Stage 2: Moderate. Intellectual decline continues to increase (amnesia, **disorientation**, **apraxia**, **aphasia**, and depression). Memory and cognitive impairment gradually lead to the loss of the ability to care for themselves. Clients have difficulty making decisions as a result of decreased concentration and lack of cognitive skills to make appropriate judgments. Clients may develop delusions that are fixed false beliefs that may be paranoid in nature. As the disease progresses toward the terminal stages, both short- and long-term memory is affected. The client displays **agnosia**, apraxia, and **perseveration**. Sleep disturbances are common and individuals will often wander during the night. It is not uncommon for clients to experience **sundowning** or catastrophic reactions during this time.

Stage 3: Severe. The client becomes totally dependent on caregivers for all needs. There is loss of communication with the client in a meaningful way. Clients with Alzheimer's disease exhibit weight loss and loss of bowel and bladder control, and develop secondary illnesses and contractions. It is during the severe stage that clients with Alzheimer's disease are often hospitalized. Immobility leads to pneumonia, urinary tract infections, and pressure ulcer development. All decisions regarding medical and social needs must be made by the caregiver.

PROGNOSIS

The duration of Alzheimer's disease averages 10 years, with a range from 3 to 20 years (Marin, Sewell, and Schlechter, 2002). There is no known medical treatment that can prevent,

arrest, or modify the course of Alzheimer's disease, but medications to modify and lessen some of its symptoms exist. Positive interventions by the caregiver can result in behavioral modification and reduce anxiety, avoid incontinence, and eliminate sleep disturbances and depression (see Understanding and Applying Research box on p. 334). A planned therapeutic activity program can increase the client's awareness, verbal and physical response, and level of function.

DISCHARGE CRITERIA

Alzheimer's disease and other primary dementias are progressive, chronic diseases that do not fall into categories of final discharge. As the client and caregiver progress through the three stages, adjustments in care are made, and the following indications of success in specific areas should be considered.

Client:
- Is absent from risk of harm to self or others.
- Accomplishes ADLs and instrumental ADLs (IADLs) with minimal possible assistance.
- Is free from catastrophic reactions.
- Participates in a therapeutic activity program tailored to assess needs.

Primary caregiver(s) has:
- Knowledge of Alzheimer's disease or the related disease.
- Used positive behavior interactions during caregiving.
- Instituted plans and developed resources for self-care.
- Appropriate legal and financial plans in place for the client and self.
- Appropriate backup systems in place in case of emergencies (e.g., sudden illness or death of the client or of the caregiver[s]).

Caregivers

The family deserves special attention because, without support, the burdens of caring for someone with Alzheimer's disease can be overwhelming. Placement in a long-term care facility is usually the final step in the family caregiver's commitment. Many years of concern precede this decision for out-of-home care. Emotional stresses as well as financial expenses become significant. Health care and in-home ser-

UNDERSTANDING and APPLYING RESEARCH

Behavioral problems are estimated to occur in at least half of community-dwelling older clients diagnosed with dementia. This study attempted to test effective nursing interventions between caregivers and clients in a home setting. A total of 54 community-dwelling clients diagnosed with cognitive impairment (probable Alzheimer's disease/multiinfarct dementia) and their primary caregivers made up the study group. The clients had moderate to severe dementia (Mini-Mental Status Examination [MMSE] mean score of 8.9 out of a possible 30).

There were two components to the intervention: an educational program intended to enhance caregiver knowledge and comprehension of dementia and related issues and a behavioral intervention program teaching caregivers techniques to calm clients, enhance functional behaviors, and increase the client's independent ADLs.

The teaching was conducted in the home setting, with both one-to-one instruction and a videotape reinforcing the instruction. The behavioral modification program also was one to one but included role modeling, as well as printed information. Common problems such as wandering were addressed, as were ADLs.

The measurements used to assess change included the MMSE, IADLs, Dementia Behavior Disturbance Scale, Alzheimer's Disease Knowledge Test, and Caregiver (Relative) Stress Scale. Before beginning, the client and caregiver were randomized into one of four groups. Group 1 received both Alzheimer's and behavioral education; group 2 received Alzheimer's education only; group 3 received the behavioral education only; and, group 4 served as a control comparison group, receiving no educational intervention. Assessments were conducted at baseline and in 6 months.

Although this study did not achieve statistical significance because of its small sample size, important clinical information was attained. Caregiver scores for knowledge increased for groups 1 and 2. The caregivers rated the following caring tasks and behavioral approaches as effective based on a 5-point Likert scale (5 indicating the highest level of effectiveness):

Bathing

Be careful not to use physical force. Touching in a forceful way may result in agitation (4.22).

Use visual cues, such as hand motions, to show the client what you want him or her to do (4.22).

Dressing

Use touch cautiously. Forcing the client to dress through use of physical touch may increase resistance and agitation (4.56).
Use praise in an adult tone of voice to let the client know he or she is doing well (4.56).

Toileting

Be flexible. Do not use physical force to assist the client to the bathroom. A personal, gentle touch while walking may be helpful (4.43).
If urine leakage occurs, do not scold the client. A negative or tense response may increase frustration (4.43).

Eating

Keep mealtimes pleasant and relaxed. Do not rush the client while eating (4.83).
Remove unsafe objects, such as sharp knives, from open areas or easily accessible drawers (4.60).

Repeated Behaviors

If the client needs to manipulate objects with his or her hands, find a useful activity using the same motion (e.g., folding clothes or newspapers). These activities allow the client a positive outlet for behavior (5.00).

•••

This study suggests that education and behavioral intervention instructions may be helpful to caregivers in the community setting. This study will be replicated with a larger sample size and a few other minor methodology revisions.

Burgener SC et al: Effective caregiving approaches for patients with Alzheimer's disease, *Geriatr Nurs* 19(3):121, 1998.

vices, special equipment and foods, and loss of income for the client and the caregiver are only a few of the cost factors encountered. More than 50% of nursing home care cost is paid from the private funds of clients and their families. Family education and counseling can ease the demands of caring for a client with Alzheimer's disease (see Case Study on p. 335).

THE NURSING PROCESS

ASSESSMENT

Assessment of clients with dementia is difficult and must rely, to a great degree, on information from several sources. This is especially true of clients with Alzheimer's disease, as often the first symptom reported is recent memory loss, and even remote memory may be adversely affected by the concurrent symptoms of disorientation,

depression, delusions, or hallucinations. A comprehensive assessment should include a thorough history, physical assessment, functional assessment, and mental status evaluation.

Assessment Environment

When interviewing the client or administering an assessment test, it is critical to have a positive physical and emotional environment. The room should be free from distractions, quiet, and away from the noise of any activity. Visual and auditory deficits may be present in the client, and the evaluator must establish eye contact, speak directly to the client in a low-frequency range (as high tones are usually less discernible), and enunciate clearly. If hearing aids or glasses are usually worn by the client, they should be in clean, working condition. Any printed material that requires a client response should be presented in large, heavy type that is easily read. If English is a second language, someone who speaks the client's primary language should administer

CASE STUDY

Roger has been brought to the Emergency Department by his wife, Kay, for treatment of a large skin tear on his right forearm, which is bleeding and wrapped in a large gauze roller bandage. While the wound is being treated, the nurse interviews Kay and notes that her appearance is disheveled, grooming is poor, and there are dark circles under her eyes. Roger is 68 and has been retired for 7 years, and Kay is 64 and still trying to work part-time as a clerk to supplement their income. Kay relates that Roger has been "acting crazy," "never sits still," "has accidents in the bathroom," and has kept her up for the last three nights. She states that she is exhausted and says, "If I don't get some sleep, I'm going to hit him or something." Further questioning reveals that Roger lost his job as a clerk because of low production and errors in mathematics. Roger's affect is flat and he states, "I can't remember how I hurt myself." His hygiene and grooming are poor, which is evidenced by his untidy appearance, soiled clothing, and offensive body odor. Kay con-

firms that neither has seen a physician "in a long time," as Roger decided that physicians "are all useless."

Critical Thinking

1. What are the primary immediate and long-term needs of Roger and Kay?
2. What therapeutic approach should the nurse use to gain their confidence?
3. Which assessment tools might be used to determine their special needs and psychosocial status?
4. What questions might elicit information about Kay's knowledge regarding Roger's behavior?
5. What teaching approaches might be successful in getting this couple to seek future help?

NURSING CARE IN THE COMMUNITY — Cognitive Disorders

As the older population increases, both in numbers and in longevity, more community attention should be focused on the support of families whose aging members are behaving in unusual and troubling ways as a result of cognitive disorders or other physical or emotional problems.

The mental health nurse may be asked to evaluate a person who resides at home but is no longer able to provide self-care and is resistant to help from caregivers. The nurse needs to assess the reports of caregivers, observe the behavior of the client, evaluate the client's medication regimen/compliance, and attempt an individual interaction, including a mental status examination. It is essential that this personal contact be deferential and exercised with patience.

The identified behaviors may simply be "acting out" demands in an attempt to meet a basic need that may be rectified by a brief intervention, such as providing a more comfortable environment in terms of temperature or level of stimulation. Pain is a critical factor that may be managed or controlled with medication. Apparent confusion may be a result of a hearing loss that can be treated with a hearing aid or with replacement of a malfunctioning one. The older person may have a urinary tract infection, which can lead to restlessness and agitation. Some prescribed or over-the-counter medications may have paradoxic effects of stimulation or disinhibition rather than sedation, which might induce the untrained caregiver to increase the dosage, thereby compounding the problem. Taking multiple medications or a conventional dose that is too much for the person's age may also have adverse effects and lead to delirium. It is crucial that the agitated client be protected from falls or other accidental self-injury. Although one of the goals of community nursing is to empower clients to maintain themselves in the home as long as possible, if the nurse cannot discover a causative agent, the decision to hospitalize the client must be considered.

After delirium from physiologic problems has been ruled out, the two most common mental health disorders for older clients are dementia and depression. Both dementia and depression have a more gradual onset than delirium, and a thorough mental status examination can often assist the nurse in problem identification and treatment recommendations. Apathy is usually found in both depression and dementia, but the cognitive processes are intact in a depressed individual. The disorders may be combined as well; therefore treating for depression can stabilize a person, so that an underlying cognitive difficulty is more apparent.

Effective medications for the treatment of Alzheimer's dementia have recently become standards of treatment, although they gradually lose their effectiveness over time and only offer a window of improved function. These medications have few side effects and are quite beneficial for containing the early stages of the disease, although they do not appear to have much benefit for clients with later stages of dementia.

The caregiver's need for support should also be carefully appraised, with consideration given to establishing a pattern of respite care that would afford the family needed time for themselves. The community nurse should be aware of facilities in the area that provide day treatment or visiting assistants. If such services are not available in a given community, the nurse may suggest their initiation to city governments and nonprofit agencies.

A relatively recent development has been the proliferation of assisted living facilities. Unlike nursing homes, many of these homelike facilities are staffed by unlicensed, minimally medically trained personnel. Services provided by a visiting mental health nurse can effectively improve the quality of care while providing onsite evaluations of residents' mental status and response to or need for medication.

the test and/or translate for the client and interviewer to yield valid results. Paraphrasing questions is permissible to clarify an item. Sufficient time needs to be allotted, as the client may take longer to process the information and form a correct response. In general, the attitude of the evaluator must be friendly, nonthreatening, and nonjudgmental. Giving positive feedback to the client by saying, "You're doing fine," "That was good," or "This is a really hard one," can help relieve the stress of testing. Avoid indications that a re-

sponse is correct or incorrect (see Nursing Care in the Community box).

Cognitive Assessment Tools

Because of the lack of biologic markers, health care professionals must rely on clinical criteria to make a diagnosis of probable or possible Alzheimer's disease. A variety of tools can lend insight into a person's cognitive status. Administering a test in sections is permissible if the client has become too fatigued, has too short an attention span, or shows signs of anxiety. It is best to test the client alone, without an informant/caregiver, so that responses are entirely the client's own and not colored by hints or responses from someone else.

Interviews with the caregiver also should include the same courtesies as used with the client and should be conducted separately and in private. This will ensure honest responses and avoid the danger of talking about the client in front of him or her.

There are cognitive assessment tools that assess orientation, intellectual functioning, memory, and reading and math skills. Among the most common are the Mini-Mental Status Examination (MMSE), the Dementia Severity Rating Scale (DSRS), and the Geriatric Depression Scale.

Mini-Mental Status Examination

The Folstein MMSE (Folstein, Folstein, and McHugh, 1975) allows health care professionals to measure global cognitive performance, follow the course of the illness, and monitor clients' responses to treatment. It is a series of 30 questions that assess orientation, registration, attention span/calculation, language recall, and perception (Richardson, 2003). It can be administered in as short a time as 5 to 10 minutes and provides standardized methods of data collection, scoring, and interpretation in specific areas of cognitive impairment. Scores of ≤24 indicate cognitive impairment.

Dementia Severity Rating Scale

This assessment tool assesses the elderly patient's ability to function in the home (Clark and Ewbank, 1996). The 11-item scale assesses memory, orientation, judgment, community affairs, home activities, personal care, speech/language, recognition feeding, incontinence, and mobility. This functional assessment is most often used for longitudinal assessment throughout the disease course (Cotter, Clark, and Karlawish, 2003).

Geriatric Depression Scale

This is a 30-item questionnaire that asks simple yes and no questions (Yesavage et al., 1983). When an elderly patient attains a score of 11 or higher, further assessment and diagnostic evaluation is warranted. This assessment may be used in Alzheimer's disease patients as long as they comprehend the questions being asked of them. It has established reliability and validity (Cotter, Clark, and Karlawish, 2003).

Neurologic Deficits

The previously discussed pathologic changes in the brain (neuritic plaques, neurofibrillary tangles, and fibrillar deposits in cerebral vessels) result in neurologic deficits with ensuing behavioral changes. Determining the status of a client with Alzheimer's disease or another related dementia must involve assessment of neurologic deficits such as *p*erception and organization, *a*ttention span, *l*anguage, *m*emory, *e*motional control, and *r*easoning and judgment (Zgola, 1987). (The mnemonic *PALMER* may help you to remember these areas.)

Perception and Organization

How well does the client interpret:
- Sensory cues?
- Relationships between objects and between self and environment?

How well does the client organize:
- Movement such as sitting, standing, and transferring?
- Tasks such as dressing in proper sequence?
- Solutions to simple puzzles?

Attention Span

How well does the client:
- Initiate an activity?
- Sustain an activity (shortened attention span or loss of interest)?
- Terminate an activity when completed or in an established pattern (perseveration)?

Language

How well does the client:
- Express thoughts verbally? (Inability—*expressive aphasia*)
- Comprehend the spoken word? (Inability—*receptive aphasia*)
- Read and comprehend the written word? (Inability—*alexia*)
- Express thoughts in writing? (Inability—**agraphia**)

Memory

How well does the client remember:
- Recent events immediately after their occurrence (immediate recall)?
- Recent events within a matter of minutes (recent memory)?
- Events from past events of months or years ago (remote or long-term memory)?

Emotional Control

Is the client's emotional control:
- Consistent with and appropriate to the situation?
- Sustained for an appropriate length of time?
- Changed from previous behavior?

Reasoning and Judgment

How well has the client:
- Made appropriate decisions based on good advice or facts?
- Conformed to social conventions?
- Reacted appropriately in an emergency situation?

Emotional Status
Mood and State of Mind

Each time a nurse approaches a client, an informal assessment of mood and state of mind is done. The Omnibus Budget Reconciliation Act (OBRA) of 1987 requires a more formal psychiatric assessment of a client before ad-

NURSING ASSESSMENT QUESTIONS
Cognitive Disorders

The following questions may be helpful in attaining a thorough nursing history:

1. Has onset been rapid or insidious?
2. Has the progression of cognitive decline fluctuated (delirium) or been a continuous decline (dementia)?
3. What is the duration of the following symptoms?
   a. Difficulty learning and retaining new information?
   b. Difficulty completing multiple-step tasks (e.g., driving, cooking, financial management)?
   c. Problem-solving difficulties?
   d. Disorientation?
   e. Word-finding problems?
   f. Difficulty participating in conversation?
   g. Changes in baseline behaviors (irritability, passivity, suspicious)?

4. Does the client have a history of the following:
   a. Known psychiatric disorders (depression)
   b. Neurologic disorder (head injury, stroke, Parkinson's disease)
   c. Alcohol or drug use
   d. Endocrine disorder (diabetes mellitus, hypothyroidism)
   e. Renal disorders
   f. Infection (pneumonia, urinary tract infections)
5. Ask the client, family, or caregiver to tell you all of the medications the client is taking (prescribed, over-the-counter, and herbal preparations).
6. Inquire if there is a family history of dementia, Down syndrome, or any familial diseases that may lead to dementia (e.g., Huntington's chorea).

mission to a skilled nursing facility (SNF) and before the administration of any psychotropic medications or physical restraints (see Nursing Assessment Questions box and Case Study on p. 335). Consistent use of the following two guidelines to assess clients' symptoms and behaviors will ensure a reliable data assessment tool: (1) significant quoted statements from the client should be noted to increase the objectivity and usefulness of the report and (2) regular documented mental status examinations further assist the professional staff in communicating information in a systematic way.

Depression

Secondary depression can be a concomitant condition with the client with dementia or Alzheimer's disease, and signs and symptoms should be thoroughly assessed and treatment plans developed (see Chapter 10 and Table 14-3). Foreman et al. (1996) distinguished depression from delirium and dementia by the following signs and symptoms: (1) variable onset that is abrupt and reversible with treatment; (2) clear sensorium; (3) normal attention span, but client is easily distracted; (4) selective memory impairment; and (5) intact thinking, but client displays hopelessness and helplessness. Clients may also display changes in sleep patterns and appetite, as well as increased fatigue. The Geriatric Depression Scale can be used as an assessment tool in the mild stage of Alzheimer's disease while language ability is present, and the client may communicate feelings of sadness, guilt, and suicidal ideation.

Functional Ability

Determination of a client's functional ability is essential as nursing diagnoses are formulated. Excess disability can occur when the caregiver responds verbally or physically with more assistance than is necessary and diminishes the client's speaking or activity skills. Maintaining independence in

ADLs and IADLs is vital if clients with Alzheimer's disease are to retain their self-esteem and engage in worthwhile activities.

Behavior

Behaviors often found in clients with Alzheimer's disease and other cognitive disorders can be grouped in the following manner:

Behaviors that are related to mood:
- Pacing, wandering, and rummaging (may indicate anxiety)
- Decreased or inappropriate socialization (may signify apathy)
- Refusal to eat, bathe, or groom (may mean depression)
- Hoarding or accusations of thievery (may manifest paranoia)

Behaviors that result from perceptual/cognitive deficits:
- Day/night reversal
- Inappropriate eating (eating too rapidly or too much, eating nonfood items)
- Falls/accidents (walking into walls or furniture, not being aware of hazards)
- Delusions, hallucinations, paranoia

Behaviors that result from the destruction of impulse control:
- Inappropriate toilet activities
- Inappropriate sexual behavior (display of penis or breasts, sexually explicit comments or language)
- Disinhibited social behavior (inappropriate jokes, neglecting personal hygiene, exhibiting undue familiarity with strangers)

When any change in behavior from previous observations occurs, the client must be reassessed. The client often cannot communicate to others about distressing signs or symptoms of an illness. Determining how a client feels involves use of honed observation skills, especially in the area of assessing body language.

CLINICAL ALERT

Signs of Silent Aspiration (Choking)
Watering eyes
Reddening of the face
Rhonchi on pulmonary auscultation
Variable rates of respiration
Grimacing
Coughing
Gagging
Throat clearing
Pocketing of food in oral cavity

CLINICAL ALERT

Types of Urinary Incontinence
Stress: Involuntary loss of small amounts of urine associated with coughing, sneezing, laughing, etc
Urge: Loss of larger amounts of urine due to inability to delay voiding after feeling the sensation of a full bladder
Overflow: Loss of small amounts of urine due to stresses on an overly full bladder
Functional: Loss of large amounts of urine resulting from cognitive deficits that lead to not recognizing cues from the bladder, inability to find the bathroom, or increasing apraxia

Physical Manifestations

Alteration in nutritional status can be a multifactorial problem. Related reasons could include functional inability to purchase and prepare the food, lack of financial resources to buy food, medical conditions decreasing the older client's appetite, or cognitive dysfunction preventing the client from remembering to eat. *Weight changes* of 3 to 5 pounds or more should be noted, and an assessment made for treatable problems unrelated to the illness of dementia. If no other clinical signs or symptoms are noted, the client's immediate environment must be examined next. The nurse should observe and correct distracting lighting, seating arrangements (groups should be homogenous and compatible), noise level, and the physical comfort of table and chairs.

The family/caregiver should be instructed to keep a food diary and to monitor food intake, being alert for dehydration. Often, older persons significantly decrease oral intake to prevent incontinence. *Dehydration* and *malnutrition* lead to multiple medical diagnoses, including hypoalbuminuria, hypoproteinemia, anemia, hypoglycemia, and other vitamin and mineral deficits.

Aspiration is a risk during stage 3 of Alzheimer's disease, and the resulting aspiration pneumonia is frequently the immediate cause of death. The caregiver monitoring feeding should watch for a swallow after each bite, indicated by the larynx rising and returning to the resting position. If possible, clients should sit at a 90-degree angle and be encouraged to keep the chin toward the chest when swallowing, rather than hyperextending the chin. Thickened liquids are often easier to swallow. As clients become more dependent, they should be left in a sitting position for 30 minutes after the meal; the oral cavity should be checked for "pocketed" food, and any found should be removed. These nursing activities prevent silent aspiration when the client is placed in a lying position.

Changes in gait are noted and nurses must be alert to other disease processes (vision problems, inner ear disturbances, pain from osteoarthritis or an injury) that the client may not be able to identify, neuropathy resulting from vascular or diabetic problems, and general decrease of the "righting reflex" (the reflexes that enable one to maintain the body in alignment to the head and thus maintain the body upright). Treating underlying problems will usually result in better gait in the client in the early stages of Alzheimer's disease, but as the disease progresses, decrease in sensory interpretation, neurologic deficits, and hypertonia will require increased awareness and interventions by the caregiver to prevent falls.

Clients may complain of *feeling cold,* even on the warmest summer days. The level of activity and the amount of body fat present are among several factors that influence body comfort with regard to heat or cold. The best way to judge a client's response to environmental temperature is to actually feel the skin; if perspiration is present, the amount of clothing should be reduced. Conversely, if the skin feels cold to the touch, the client needs the additional layers of clothing, even though they might appear to be excessive.

Incontinence usually occurs in the later stages of Alzheimer's disease. Because of physical and cognitive changes, the client no longer has the ability to maintain bowel and bladder control. Functional incontinence is associated with cognitive impairment. The loss of urinary control is directly related to physical and cognitive functioning or barriers on the environment. Incontinence may also be a physical sign of a urinary tract infection or benign prostatic hypertrophy in older men. A thorough assessment of premorbid bladder and bowel function is essential, as well as continuous assessment of medications, fluid and food intake, and potential environmental constraints (side rails, poor lighting, wheelchair seat belts).

Physical and Laboratory Examination

Physical examination must be careful and thorough to rule out neoplasia (e.g., brain tumors), metabolic disorders, systemic illnesses (e.g., hypertension, human immunodeficiency virus [HIV] infection), and polypharmacy. Physical examination, mental status assessment, and functional assessment are imperative to begin to develop a differential diagnosis list.

No laboratory test exists to the confirm Alzheimer's disease. Diagnostic evaluation is conducted to rule out causes for cognitive changes. Blood studies include a complete

type of depression, and co-existing symptomatology (Sekula, DeSantis, and Gianetti, 2003). Trazodone (Desyrel) is used in behavioral problems of dementia when sedation at night is needed. Older adults who have depression-like symptoms may also use trazodone or a specific serotonin reuptake inhibitor (SSRI). The most useful medications are those with minimal anticholinergic side effects. Citalopram (Celexa) and sertraline (Zoloft) appear to be effective and have few side effects such as sedation and weight gain. In elderly clients it is strongly recommended to start slow and low, increasing the dosage slowly. Fluoxetine (Prozac) is not recommended in elderly clients (Sekula, DeSantis, and Gianetti, 2003) because of the long half-life and potent inhibitor of liver enzymes (potential to increase serum levels of other medications). Venlafaxine (Effexor) is a serotonin/norepinephrine reuptake inhibitor that has demonstrated efficacy in the treatment of anxiety and depression (Roerig, 1999). In depressed older adults with mild Alzheimer's symptoms, sexual dysfunction may occur with the administration of SSRIs and venlafzine (Hirschfeld, 1999). Nefazodone (Serzone), a serotonin modulator, and mirtazapine (atypical/norepinephrine serotonin modulator) should be considered in these patients (Hirschfeld, 1999; McElroy, Keck, and Frieman, 1995).

For treatment of behavioral disorders (delusions, aggression, anxiety, verbalizations), the atypical antipsychotic agents can be used to control these manifestations. Risperidone (Risperdal), olanzapine (Zyprexa), and quetiapine (Seroquel) diminish the risk of developing extrapyramidal symptoms and tardive dyskinesia as compared to the typical antipsychotic agents (de Deyn and Katz, 2000). Patients with mild-to-moderate anxiety or irritability may be prescribed alprazolam (Xanax) or buspirone (BuSpar). Buspirone lacks cognitive and psychomotor effects and has limited drug-drug interactions; these qualities are desirable for treatment of elderly clients (Sekula, DeSantis, and Gianetti, 2003). Low-dose haloperidol (Haldol) is an effective drug of choice for treating anxiety. However, the clinician must be vigilant to assess for the paradoxic symptomatology, such as increased confusion, disorientation, and possible increase in agitation and anxiety, which can be seen with benzodiazepines. In addition, elderly clients must be monitored closely for adverse events, including orthostatic hypotension, instability of gait, and motor stiffness (Chan and Brennan, 1999; Richardson, 2003; Wright, 2000).

Certain anticonvulsants such as valproic acid (Depakene), divalproex (Depakote), and carbamazepine (Tegretol) are used with clients demonstrating impulsivity, aggression, and assaultive behavior (Mayeux and Sano, 1999). Lithium is used in cases of mania. The therapeutic regimen is individualized and based on presenting behavioral problems. Before pharmacologic management is initiated for behavioral problems, it is important to exhaust all behavioral management techniques, as well as environmental and social strategies. If all of these measures fail, medication should be used to modify behavior. The drugs used to modify behavior and increase function are discussed in detail in Chapter 20.

Experimental Drugs in the Therapy of Alzheimer's Disease. Many pharmaceutic research studies are currently underway to find a drug that will slow or reverse the cognitive decline in persons with Alzheimer's disease. The following agents are being studied: nonsteroidal antiinflammatory drugs, COX–2 inhibitors, cholinergic agonists, estrogen, lecithin, nerve growth factor, calcium channel blockers, modafinil (Provigil), vitamin E, gingko biloba, and metabolic enhancers (acetyl-L-carnitine).

Therapeutic Activity Program

An activity is described as any project a person enjoys and that produces a positive feeling. A *therapeutic activity program* is a total plan of care based on assessment of the client's needs and a history of previous endeavors. It is specifically designed to meet identified needs and to keep the person functioning at the highest possible level (Stehman et al., 1991).

Building on retained strengths (e.g., retained remote memory, use of habitual skills, preserved large and fine motor skills, and intact emotional responses) is the basis of success. It is exceedingly difficult, if not impossible, for the person with Alzheimer's disease to learn new skills. "Use it or lose it!" is a truism, especially when working with clients with dementia. Once a skill is lost, it is virtually gone forever and not able to be relearned.

For persons with dementia a therapeutic program is considered a primary treatment, as often the first neurologic losses result in the inability to plan, initiate, carry out in ordered steps (sequence), or remember activities by themselves. Thus it is the role of the caregiver to assist the client throughout the activity, from beginning to end. Positive reinforcement should be used at each step of the way.

Success of a therapeutic activity program can be measured on some objective terms by addressing the following questions:

- Has the number of times per day or week that the client is actively involved increased or decreased?
- Have incidents of catastrophic reactions or sundowning decreased?
- Have incidents of the client aimlessly pacing or wandering and getting lost decreased?
- Has the level of functioning in ADLs and IADLs remained stable, or is it decreasing at a slower pace than before the program was initiated?
- Are caregivers feeling less stress, which might be indicated by fewer incidents of anger or crying, improved sleep patterns, or enhanced feelings of physical and mental well-being?

EVALUATION

Evaluating the client's progress and the degree to which nurses have achieved satisfactory client and caregiver outcomes are especially challenging when Alzheimer's disease and other dementias are involved. Factors that may influence success vary greatly with each situation and must be carefully considered in this process. Below are some questions

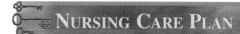

NURSING CARE PLAN

Gina, a 64-year-old female, has been referred to a home health nurse by her primary physician for evaluation for home care. The diagnosis given is probable Alzheimer's disease with a secondary diagnosis of controlled hypertension. After an interview with Sam, Gina's husband, who is 65 years old and still working as a sales representative, the following is determined:

- 2-year history of recent memory loss
- History of being well groomed but now refuses to bathe and change clothes and dresses inappropriately, putting on clothes in the wrong sequence
- Appears to understand spoken language (if thoughts are stated slowly and simply)
- Expressive language lacks correct grammar with evidence of word searching and parroting words used by the interviewer
- Gina's widowed sister, Anna, comes to stay with her during the day and stays overnight if the husband has to be out of town

- Recent episodes of crying, negativity, and angry verbal outbursts have caused the sister concern and fear
- Sam is staying away more often and leaving care to the sister, who is losing weight and dropping out of her personal social activities

DSM-IV-TR Diagnoses

Axis I	Dementia of the Alzheimer's type with perceptual disturbances
	Dementia of the Alzheimer's type with behavioral disturbances
Axis II	Rule out dependent personality disorder
Axis III	Hypertension
Axis IV	Problems with access to health care services
	Other psychosocial problems
Axis V	GAF = 35 (current)
	GAF = 45 (past year)

NURSING DIAGNOSIS: Bathing/hygiene, dressing/grooming self-care deficit related to perceptual and cognitive alterations secondary to neurologic damage in the brain as evidenced by inability to recognize the need for self-care (bathing, changing clothes), inability to dress in the right order, and inability to reason and judge (inappropriate choice of clothing).

CLIENT OUTCOMES

Gina will bathe three times a week.

Gina will be well groomed.

NURSING INTERVENTIONS

Determine habitual time and manner of bathing. *Establishing a pattern based on Gina's previous habits will use her retained remote memory.*
Ensure privacy *to preserve dignity and self-esteem.*
Determine room and water temperature. *Comfort and safety will encourage positive client response.*
Reduce sensory stimulation (e.g., noise from TV, radio, other people) to enable client to attend to the task at hand. Mirrors may need to be covered if the reflection is incorrectly interpreted by the client to be an observer. *Limiting the number of responses required by Gina will facilitate her cooperation and independence.*
Provide a home health aide three times a week for 2 weeks. *Caregivers, Anna and Sam, will increase their knowledge and skills and thus enhance their confidence and ease in assisting Gina. The HHA will teach the caregivers ways in which to maintain skin integrity and general health. The supervising nurse will check on Gina's general health status and hypertension.*

Determine areas of dysfunction in grooming.
Set adequate routines of visual and verbal cues to assist in grooming routines.
Assist directly only as necessary to complete task.
Use positive reinforcement.
Refer for dental prophylaxis and assist the family in preplanning with the dentist and hygienist for a successful visit.
Assist Sam and Anna in formulating follow-up plan for daily oral hygiene.
These interventions will reduce stress for client and caregivers, avoid excess disability, provide a positive environment, and avoid unnecessary physical disabilities.

EVALUATION

Gina was successfully bathed by the home health aide twice in the first week with the help of Anna. During the second week Anna was successful on two occasions with the home health aide (HHA) assisting. Extend HHA assistance for 1 more week and reevaluate.

Anna and Sam were successful on 5 out of 7 successive days in cueing Gina to complete her dental hygiene and in helping with combing her hair. An appointment has been made with the dentist who previously cared for her, and Sam has informed the dentist of the present situation. Evaluate success of visit later.

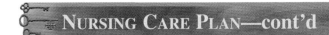

NURSING CARE PLAN—cont'd

CLIENT OUTCOMES	NURSING INTERVENTIONS	EVALUATION
Gina will dress herself appropriately.	Assess clothing supply. Simplify dressing choices for Gina by the following: Remove clothes not currently being worn. Assemble coordinated outfits on one hanger and limit these to six to eight choices. Stack clothes in the order in which they are to be put on. Assess clothes and assist family in choosing those that are appropriate yet easy for Gina to put on (e.g., eliminate buttons, buckles, pantyhose, etc., and replace with elastic waists, snaps, Velcro fasteners, knee- or thigh-high hose). *The client will retain control and independence by making some simple decisions and will be socially acceptable, thus increasing self-esteem and reducing stress for all.*	Family/nurse/HHA see the improvement in Gina's appearance, and Gina is responding with smiles at the compliments about her appearance. Sam is having some adjustment problems in changing her dress style (not putting on hose and heels as she had) and in moving some of his favorite outfits out of the closet. Anna comments favorably on the ease of dressing Gina now and on Gina's increased comfort, evidenced by her willingness to participate in activities and calmer interactions.

NURSING DIAGNOSIS: Disturbed thought processes related to inability to process and synthesize information as evidenced by recent memory loss; decreased ability to analyze, reason, and form judgments; and interruption in logical stream of thought.

CLIENT OUTCOMES	NURSING INTERVENTIONS	EVALUATION
Gina will use her intellect and judgment to the best of her ability.	Develop a stimulating therapeutic activities program. *Cognitive stimulation in deficit areas and positive reinforcement will promote self-esteem and encourage Gina to attain the highest functional level possible.*	Sam and Anna have found that Gina enjoys walks, and they have established routines. Gina has recognized some previously familiar birds and indicated she wanted bird seed to feed them. She also enjoys simple puzzles and assisting Anna in laundry tasks.
Gina will retain some control in her life by exercising her right to choose.	Assess environment and activities and collaborate with all caregivers to: Simplify choices in food, clothes, colors, and activities. Use multiple sensory cues, especially auditory, visual, and tactile senses, to indicate choices. *Choices, even simple ones, give control back to Gina and improve her self-esteem, making her more willing to try to participate in daily activities.*	Gina is responding to the use of multiple cues by increasingly exercising her right to choose. During the first week, Gina made an independent choice five times. During the second week, she made seven choices.
Gina will be oriented to place, time of day, scheduled activities, and family members.	Develop simple calendars with daily routines and easy-to-read clocks. Encourage family members to repeat their names and relationships often in conversations. *These actions will assist in overcoming recent memory loss. Establishing routine decreases the stress of making decisions; verbal cues reinforce recognition and eliminate the need to chat.*	After 2 weeks, Gina knows the time for her walks with Sam and indicates that she wants her supply of bird seed. She is less frequently confused regarding the identification of persons and never fails to recognize Sam and Anna.
Gina will use remote memory.	Formulate daily periods of reminiscence using old photos, specially designed picture books, and rummage boxes. *The use of multiple sensory cues to stimulate remote memory is building on the retained strength of habitual skills to stimulate use of remote memory.*	Gina looked at old photographs with Sam and Anna and indicated her recognition with short phrases or smiles. She independently sought out the box of various colored and textured yarns and handled them with satisfaction, indicating that she remembers knitting when she was well.
Gina will have decreased catastrophic reactions (see Box 14-3).	Analyze with all caregivers what the previous causative factors may have been. Simplify the environment (evaluate furniture and objects, colors, noise level). *Through analyzing and simplifying the environment, the client's safety is maintained and the stressors causing the catastrophic incidents are reduced. Collaborative planning will ensure consistent successful approaches to tasks, and client and caregiver stress will be reduced.*	Gina had two catastrophic reactions during the last 2 weeks. Sam and Anna analyzed each incident and discovered that the underlying causes were (1) increased ambient noise from street repairs in front of the house and (2) being rushed to leave for a dental appointment.

Continued

Nursing Care Plan—cont'd

Nursing Diagnosis: Ineffective community coping related to inadequate understanding of the process of Alzheimer's disease by the caregivers, inability of the spouse to adequately manage the emotional conflicts, role changes, temporary abandonment, weak support systems, and ineffective communication/relationship with the secondary caregiver as evidenced by Sam's being away from home more and Anna's loss of weight and social withdrawal.

FAMILY OUTCOMES	NURSING INTERVENTIONS	EVALUATION
Sam and Anna will verbalize realistic perception of their roles and responsibilities in caring for Gina.	Facilitate meeting with all family members. *Sharing knowledge of status and prognosis will establish the core of a support system based on mutual respect and understanding.* Address knowledge deficits and obtain feedback from participants. *Understanding allays fears and promotes rational planning; each person retains knowledge in unique ways and, common understandings are vital to successful planning and implementation.* Collaborate in developing roles for each caregiver. *Understanding each one's role, including expectations and limitations, will reduce behaviors that might lead to abuse or abandonment and elicit positive care outcomes for the client.*	Anna met with other family members who live in the area, and these family members expressed gratitude for being included and enlightened; they offered assistance with outings and evening care. On two consecutive nursing visits Sam and Anna successfully reviewed information on the pathologic and neurologic deficits of Alzheimer's disease and are coping with Gina's behavior manifestations. Interventions have been successful on four occasions. They have congratulated each other.
Sam and Anna will express their feeling in a mutually supportive manner.	Facilitate sessions directly or provide referrals to appropriate health professionals. *Caregivers need permission to express themselves in a nonjudgmental, supportive environment.*	Sam and Anna join each other for breakfast on most weekdays to plan for the day and critique the previous day's activities. Revisions of plans have been accepted in most cases.
Sam and Anna will demonstrate cooperation of all family/support persons in planning, problem solving, and decision making regarding Gina's care and Sam and Anna's personal needs.	Inform family of support services in the community. Encourage attendance at support groups or individual counseling sessions. *Support services and groups provide external assistance and concern for the caregiver's needs.* Facilitate positive methods (e.g., calendars, defining responsibilities and problem-solving tasks). *Sharing and preplanning will avoid conflict and pursue positive outcomes.*	Sam and Anna attended an Alzheimer's disease support group together while a grandchild stayed with Gina. Sam was late one evening but later apologized to Anna.
Sam and Anna will exhibit effective coping strategies.	Promote healthful methods of caregiver self-care (e.g., socialization, exercise, adequate diet, and time for personal renewal). *Developing positive coping strategies will restore positive physical and mental health and revive a functional family unit.*	Anna has regained only 2 pounds but admits to eating better and feeling more energetic. She attended a sewing class, resuming a previous social activity. Sam is having dinner with an old friend before attending a Lions Club meeting while Anna stays with Gina for the evening.

that need to be clearly answered and understood before specific topics are addressed.

- Is the cognitive impairment reversible or irreversible?
- Is the client experiencing delirium, depression, dementia, or a combination of these?
- What is the setting (i.e., acute care, long-term care, home)?
- What is the caregiving situation?
- What medical and psychiatric problems have been identified in the nursing history?
- What is the current medication profile?
- Is medication compliance a problem?
- What behavioral problems have been identified?
- What is the client's functional status?
- What is the interdisciplinary plan of care?

When the answers to these questions have been agreed on, the nurse and the interdisciplinary team will be better able to determine the degree to which specifics in the outcome identification have been realized.

Chapter Summary

- ▪ The prevalence of dementia increases with age.
- ▪ Alzheimer's disease is the most common form of dementia.
- ▪ The cause of Alzheimer's disease is unclear. Current theories include angiopathy and blood-brain incompetence, neurotransmitter and receptor deficiencies, and abnormal proteins and their products.

- The key pathologic process is abnormal amyloid in the brain, which alters the brain's metabolism.
- The pathologic process of cognitive disorders results in neurologic deficits such as reduced ability to perceive the environment and organize appropriate responses, decreased attention span, language deficits, memory loss, changes in emotional responses, and a decline in the ability to reason and form judgments.
- Alzheimer's disease has three stages: mild, moderate, and severe.
- A variety of cognitive assessment tools can be used to determine medical and nursing diagnoses.
- The nurse should plan and supervise therapeutic activity programs to achieve the highest possible functional status for the client and prevent excess disability.
- Caring for a person with a cognitive disorder is a significant physical and emotional burden for the caregivers.
- All nursing care for clients with cognitive disorders should be done in collaboration with the client's caregivers.
- Care plans should be formulated that are based on assessment of both the client's and caregiver's needs.
- The success of care plans should be based on successful functional status and not on a curative basis.

REVIEW QUESTIONS

1. A 60-year-old female client is admitted to the psychiatric unit. She is confused and disoriented and gets irritable without provocation. The highest priority nursing diagnosis would be:
   a. Risk for other-directed violence
   b. Bathing/hygiene self-care deficit
   c. Chronic confusion
   d. Impaired memory

2. A client with Alzheimer's disease is having difficulty eating. The best nursing intervention to help her eat would be:
   a. Set a time limit because she needs structure
   b. Force the client to eat because nutrition is important
   c. Keep meal times relaxed and do not rush the client
   d. Have the client eat alone in her room for privacy

3. Which statement by a family member of a client who has dementia shows his understanding of dementia?
   a. "When will she recognize me as her son?"
   b. "Can you recommend some resources so that I can have some assistance in caring for my mother?"
   c. "What medication can you give her to make her better?"
   d. "Why does she get so angry with me?"

4. During the third stage of Alzheimer's disease the highest priority to assess for is:
   a. Memory loss
   b. Disorientation
   c. Aphasia
   d. Ability to swallow

5. The best nursing intervention to help orient a client with Alzheimer's disease is to:
   a. Remind the client frequently of upcoming events
   b. Provide a daily routine and easy to read clocks
   c. Do not have the client room with another client with Alzheimer's disease
   d. Post the schedule in the day room

REFERENCES

Alzheimer's disease: estimates of prevalence in the United States (GAO/HEHS –98-16), Washington, DC, 1998, U.S. General Accounting Office.

American Psychiatric Association: *Diagnostic and Statistical Manual of Mental Disorders,* Fourth Edition, Text Revision. Washington, DC, American Psychiatric Association, 2000.

Barton S: Dementia, *Clinical Evidence Concise* 7:165-168, 2002.

Burgener SC et al: Effective caregiving approaches for patients with Alzheimer's disease, *Geriatr Nurs* 19(3):121, 1998.

Chan D, Brennan NJ: Delirium: make the diagnosis, improving the prognosis, *Geriatrics* 54(3):28-41, 1999.

Clark CM, Ewbank DC: Performance of the demential severity rating scale: a caregiver questionnaire for rating severity in Alzheimer disease, *Alzheimer Disease Associated Disorders* 10:173-178, 1996.

Cotter VT, Clark CM, Karlawish JHT: Cognitive function assessment in individuals at risk for Alzheimer's disease, 15(2):79-86, 2003.

de Deyn PP, Katz IR: Control of aggression and agitation in patients with dementia: efficacy and safety of risperidone, *Int J Geriatric Psychiatry* 15(suppl 1):S14-S23, 2000.

Doody RS et al: Practice parameter: management of dementia (an evidence-based review), Report of the Quality Standards Subcommittee of the American Academy of Neurology *Neurology* 56:1154-1166, 2001.

Evans RM et al: Serum cholesterol, APOE genotype and the risk of Alzheimer's disease: a population based study of African Americans, *Neurology* 54(1):240-242, 2000.

Fick E, Foreman M: Consequences of not recognizing delirium superimposed on dementia in the hospitalized elderly individuals, *Gerontol Nurs* 26(1):30-40, 2002.

Folstein MF, Folstein SE, McHugh PR: "Mini-mental state." A practical method for grading the cognitive state of patients for the clinician, *J Psychiatr Res* 12(3):189-198, 1975.

Foreman M et al: Assessing cognitive function, *Geriatr Nurs* 5:228, 1996.

Francis PR et al: The cholinergic hypothesis of Alzheimer's disease: a review of progress, *J Neurol Neurosurgery Psychiatry* 66(2)137-147, 1999.

Glenner GG: Alzheimer's disease, *Encyclopedia of Human Biology* 1:108, 1994.

Henry M: Descending into delirium, *Am J Nurs* 102(3)49-56, 2002.

Hirschfeld RM: Efficacy of SSRIs and newer antidepressants in severe depression: comparison with TCAs, *J Clin Psychiatry* 60(5):326-335, 1999.

Hoffman SB, Platt CA: *Comforting the confused: strategies for managing dementia,* ed 2, New York, 2000, Springer.

Holt J: How to help confused patients, *Am J Nurs* 93:32, 1993.

Jann MW: Rivastigimine, a new generation cholinesterase inhibitor for the treatment of Alzheimer's disease, *Pharmacotherapy* 20(1):1-12, 2000.

Lyketsos CG et al: Randomized, placebo-controlled, double-blind clinical trial of sertraline in the treatment of depression complicating Alzheimer's disease: initial results from the Depression in Alzheimer's Disease Study, *Am J Psychiatry* 157:1686-1689, 2000.

Lyketsos CG et al: Major and minor depression in Alzheimer's disease: prevalence and impact, *J Neuropsychiatry Clin Neurosci* 9(4):445-561, 1997.

Marin DB, Sewell MC, Schlechter A: Alzheimer's disease: accurate and early diagnosis in the primary care setting, *Geriatrics* 57:36-40, 2002.

Mayeux R, Sano M: Treatment of Alzheimer's disease, *N Engl J Med* 341(22):1670-1679, 1999.

McElroy S, Keck PE, Friedman LM: Minimizing and managing antidepressant side effects, *J Clin Psychiatry* 56(S2):49-55, 1995.

NANDA International (2002). NANDA Nursing Diagnoses: Definitions and Classification 2003-2004. Philadelphia: NANDA.

Peterson RC et al: Mild cognitive impairment: clinical characterization and outcome, *Arch Neurol* 56:303-308, 1999.

Price DL et al: Neuropathology of Alzheimer's disease and animal models. In Markesberg WR, editor: *Neuropathology of dementing disorders*, London, 1998, Arnold.

Richardson S: Delirium: assessment and treatment of the elderly patient, *Am J Nurse Pract* 7(1):9-15, 2003.

Roerig JL: Diagnosis and management of generalized anxiety disorder, *J Am Pharmaceutical Assoc* 39(6)811-821, 1999.

Rogers SL et al: A 24-week, double-blind, placebo-controlled trial of donepezil in patients with Alzheimer's disease: Donepezil Study Group, *Neurology* 50(1):136-145, 1998.

Scheibel AB et al: Denervation microangiopathy in senile dementia, Alzheimer type, *Alzheimer Dis Assoc Disord* 1:19, 1987.

Schneider L: Treatment of Alzheimer's disease with cholinesterase inhibitors, *Clin Geriatr Med* 17(2):437-458. 2001.

Scott LJ, Goa KO: Galantamine: a review of its use in Alzheimer's disease, *Drugs* 60(5):1095-1122, 2000.

Sekula LK, DeSantis J, Gianetti V: Considerations in the management of the patient with comorbid depression and anxiety, *J Am Acad Nurse Pract* 15(1):23-33, 2003.

Selkoe DJ: Alzheimer's disease: genes, proteins, and therapy, *Physiol Rev* 81(2):741-746, 2001.

Stehman J et al: *Training manual for Alzheimer's care specialists,* manuscript published in 1991.

Visser PJ et al: Distinction between preclinical Alzheimer's disease and depression, *J Am Geriatrics Soc* 48:479-484, 2000.

Warner JP: Evidence-based psychopharmacology: what is the evidence for treating early Alzheimer's disease with donepezil? *J Psychopharmacol* 13(3):308-312, 1999.

Webster J, Grossberg GT: Strategies for treating dementing disorders, *Nurs Home Med* (6):161, 1996.

Wragg RE, Jeste DV: Cited by Rabins PV. Chapter 26: Noncognitive symptoms. In Latzman R, Bick KO, editors: *Alzheimer disease,* New York, 1994, Raven Press.

Wright S: Delirium in the elderly: recognition and management issues, *Adv Nurse Pract* April 2000, pp 71-74.

Yesavage Ja et al: Development and validation of a geriatric depression screening scale: a preliminary report, *J Psychiatric Res* 17:37-49, 1983.

Zgola J: *Doing things: a guide to programming activities for persons with Alzheimer's disease and related disorders,* Baltimore, 1987, Johns Hopkins University Press.

SUGGESTED READINGS

Agency for Health Care Policy and Research: *Depression in primary care,* vol 1, *Detection and diagnosis,* Rockville, Md, 1996, U.S. Department of Health and Human Services.

Boyd CO, Vernon GM: Primary care of the older adult with end stage Alzheimer's disease, *Nurse Pract* 23(4):63, 1998.

Evans DA et al: Cited by Clinical Practice Guidelines: No. 19. Recognition and initial assessment of Alzheimer's Disease and related dementias. Characteristics, epidemiology and costs. US Department of Health and Human Services. AHCPR Publication 97-0702: 27.

Leon J, Cheng CK, Neumann PJ: Alzheimer's disease: cost and potential savings, *Health Affairs* 17(6):206-216, 1998.

Mangeno M, Middemiss C: Alzheimer's disease: preventing and recognizing misdiagnoses, *Nurse Pract* 22(10):58, 1997.

McNiel C: *Alzheimer's disease: unraveling the mysteries,* Rockville, Md, 1995, National Institutes of Health.

Morris JH: *Alzheimer's disease: the neuropathology of dementia,* Cambridge, England, 1997, Cambridge University Press.

Needham J: Alzheimer's disease: diagnosis and management, *Cont Med Educ Resources,* p. 15, 1998.

Prusiner SB: Molecular biology of prion diseases, *Science* 252:1515, 1991.

Tomlinson BE et al: Observations on the brains of demented old people, *J Neurol Sci* 11:205, 1972.

U.S. Department of Health and Human Services: Quick reference guide for clinicians: early identification of Alzheimer's disease and related dementias, *J Am Acad Nurse Pract* 9(2):85, 1997.

Winblad B et al: Pharmacotherapy of Alzheimer's disease: is there a need to redefine treatment success? *Int J Geriatr Psychiatry* 16:653-666, 2001.

Wong CW et al: Neuritic plaques and cerebrovascular amyloid in Alzheimer's disease are antigenically related, *Proc Nat Acad Sci USA* 82:8729, 1985.

15

Disorders of Childhood and Adolescence

Richard C. Lucas and Chantal M. Flanagan

OBJECTIVES

- Describe child/adolescent developmental disorders such as pervasive developmental disorders, Asperger's disorder, and mental retardation.

- Identify attention deficit/hyperactivity disorders in children and adolescents.

- Distinguish between oppositional defiant disorder and conduct disorder.

- Describe tic disorders, separation anxiety, and elimination disorders.

- Learn the components of a thorough nursing assessment and application of the nursing process for children or adolescents.

Nurses have the opportunity to assess and treat children and adolescents in diverse health care settings. Children and adolescents frequently present for medical problems when in fact the underlying problem may be a mental disorder requiring treatment. The nurse's assessment must be comprehensive to identify those children and adolescents and their families in need of mental health referrals and early intervention. The earlier identification is made the sooner the client and family can receive necessary treatment and community resources.

Children and adolescents are treated within the context of the family system. One cannot be separated from the other. It is important for the nurse to understand the mental health problems and needs that children and adolescents face and the impact these issues have on their growth and development. This chapter discusses the major mental disorders affecting children and adolescents and provides direction for applying the nursing process in the assessment, diagnosis, and treatment of this population.

HISTORICAL AND THEORETIC PERSPECTIVES

History tells of a time when there was a lack of concern for, and little attention paid to, understanding or treating children. Children were seen as miniature adults. There was no understanding of the developmental process. A child's perspective, opinion, or desires traditionally were of little importance for adults. Before the 1900s, children had few rights and were viewed as property owned by their parents. Not until 1889 did children and adolescents get their own juvenile justice system. In 1912, the Federal Children's Bureau was developed to safeguard the welfare of children. Children were finally recognized with their own mental health clinics when William Healy started the Juvenile Psychopathic Institute in Chicago and Ernest Southard was assigned director of an outpatient clinic in Boston in the early 1900s (Hirshberg, 1980). The expansion of child guidance clinics was slow, however, including only those children who were affiliated with the juvenile justice system.

Eventually the services were open to the community, but treatments were not provided in hospitals or taught in medical schools. In the 1930s and 1940s child psychiatry developed into its own specialty with the first child psychiatric textbook and the introduction of amphetamines to treat children.

Reactive theories of psychology maintain that a child's mind starts as a blank slate and that environmental influences promote healthy or pathologic development. Major reactive theories include stimulus-response (eliciting a behavior or a response by conditioning a stimulus [e.g., Pavlov's salivating dogs]), environmental learning (learning is not only biologic or maturational but is also acquired, whereby experience in the environment brings about change in behavior), classical conditioning (learning which events in the environment go with each other, thereby being able to anticipate the events instead of only reacting to them), and operant conditioning (behavioral changes occur because of the positive or negative consequences produced as a result of the behavior [e.g., positive reinforcement will increase the chance that the behavior will recur]). These theories imply that symptoms are learned and that improvement comes through relearning and environmental changes (Hirshberg, 1980).

Structural theories start with the belief that the child has a genetically determined ability for developing behavior and acts on the environment. Major structural theorists include Bowlby (attachment), Freud (psychosexual developmental lines), Erickson (psychosocial development), and Piaget (cognitive development). Treatment according to structural theory involves *reorganization of the child's or adolescent's beliefs* (e.g., resolution of intrapsychic conflicts as occurs when an unwed teenage mother who feels anger towards her infant because of her lost youth becomes overprotective and smothering because she cannot display her anger; *alteration of family patterns of interaction,* for example, if the child is aligned with one parent against the other parent; or *acquiring a new schema*) (Lewis, 1980). Additional detailed information about child and adolescent development is found in Chapter 8.

MENTAL DISORDERS

MENTAL RETARDATION
Etiology and Epidemiology

Despite extensive evaluations, no definitive etiology can be found in 58% to 78% of individuals with mild mental retardation and 23% to 43% of individuals with severe or profound mental retardation. When found, the etiology may be genetic, medical, environmental, or a combination of these (Szymanski, 1999) (Box 15-1).

Box 15-1   Etiology of Mental Retardation

Genetic
Genetic causes result from an abnormality of genes inherited from parents, such as Down syndrome, which is a disorder of chromosome 21 (trisomy 21).

Medical
Any medical condition that can cause brain damage may result in mental retardation such as in utero infections, prematurity, low birth weight, and childhood diseases such as whooping cough, measles, and meningitis. Brain injuries from accidents may also result in mental retardation such as drowning or a blow to the head.

Environmental
The use of alcohol or drugs by the pregnant mother may cause mental retardation. Smoking while pregnant may increase the risk for mental retardation. Other risks include malnutrition, certain environmental contaminants such as lead poisoning, and illnesses of the mother during pregnancy, such as toxoplasmosis, cytomegalovirus, rubella, syphilis, and HIV.

The prevalence of mental retardation is estimated at 1% of the U.S. population (Szymanski, 1999) (see DSM-IV-TR Criteria box).

Clinical Description and Prognosis

Individuals who are diagnosed with mental retardation (subaverage intellectual function) also typically present with problems in adaptive functioning, defined as "how effectively individuals cope with common life demands and how well they meet the standards of personal independence expected of someone in their particular age group, sociocultural background, and community setting" (APA, 2000). Several factors may influence adaptive functioning: education, motivation, personality characteristics, social and vocational opportunities, and other coexisting mental and physical conditions (APA, 2000).

Types of Mental Retardation

Mild. Approximately 85% of individuals with mental retardation have *mild retardation*. These children typically develop social and communication skills during the preschool years, suffer only minimal sensorimotor problems, and often are not identified until a later age. They can generally acquire academic skills up to approximately the sixth grade level. In adulthood they generally achieve social and vocational skills adequate for minimum self-support, and they usually require supervision, guidance, and assistance. However, in most cases they live successfully in the community—some independently and some in supervised settings.

Moderate. About 10% of the population with mental retardation have *moderate retardation*. Most individuals with

moderate mental retardation acquire some communication skills during early childhood and may benefit from vocational training, but they seldom advance academically beyond the second grade level. With moderate supervision, they can usually provide for their own personal care and learn to travel in familiar areas. Peer relationships often deteriorate in adolescence because of problems in recognizing and acquiring socially correct interactions. During adulthood they generally can perform unskilled or semiskilled work and live and function in the community in supervised settings.

Severe. About 3% to 4% of individuals with mental retardation have *severe retardation*. They typically acquire little if any communicative speech during early childhood but may learn to use rudimentary communication and develop elementary self-care skills in the school-age period. They may profit from learning to sight-read some "survival" words. As adults they may be able to perform simple skills in closely supervised settings. They can generally live in the community in group homes or with their families unless some other handicap requires specialized nursing or other care.

Profound. Only 1% to 2% of mentally retarded individuals suffer from *profound retardation*. Most also have an identified neurologic condition such as cerebral palsy, sensory deficits, epilepsy, and other neurologic disorders causing their retardation. They have considerable sensorimotor problems recognized during early childhood, such as poor head control, feeding problems, and the inability to roll over. They require a highly structured setting with constant monitoring and assistance in an individualized relationship for optimal development. Under this sort of care, they may develop enough motor skills, self-care skills, and communication to perform simple tasks in a closely supervised and sheltered setting (APA, 2000).

Associated Features

Individuals with mental retardation demonstrate no consistent or specific personality or behavioral features that are generalized to this population. Individual traits range from passive, placid, and dependent styles to aggressive and impulsive styles. Individuals with more severe retardation and associated communication deficits may demonstrate more aggression and impulsivity resulting from frustration and lack of ability to interact adequately with their environment. Any mental disorder may present in retarded individuals, and no evidence indicates any difference in the nature of the mental disorder. Problems frequently occur in diagnosing mental disorders, however, because of communication skills deficits and other handicaps. The most commonly diagnosed mental disorders in this population include attention deficit/hyperactivity disorder (ADHD), mood disorder, pervasive developmental disorder, stereotypic movement disorder, and mental disorders resulting from a general medical condition (e.g., dementia resulting from head trauma) (APA, 2000). Medical comorbid problems include seizures in 15% to 30% with severe mental retardation, motor problems in 20% to 30% including the inability to walk or talk as a result of little muscle coordination and hearing, and vision problems in 10% to 20%. The prognosis reflects the interaction of biomedical, psychologic, and environmental factors. Studies have shown that those with severe to profound mental retardation have a shortened life expectancy because of medical conditions, such as epilepsy and feeding problems, and because of limitations of self-care and communication that are associated with these degrees of retardation (Szymanski, 1999).

ELIMINATION DISORDERS
Encopresis
Etiology and Epidemiology

Certain conditions such as inadequate, inconsistent toilet training and psychosocial stress (e.g., entering school or the birth of a sibling) may predispose the child to **encopresis** (APA, 2000), which is the repeated passage of feces into inappropriate places, whether involuntary or intentional. However, physiologic variables are the predictive measures of outcome (Mikkelsen, 2001).

Approximately 1% of 5-year-olds have encopresis. It is more common in males than in females (APA, 2000) (see DSM-IV-TR Criteria box).

Clinical Description

Most often the fecal soiling is involuntary. At times it may be intentional when it is the result of a power struggle between the child or adolescent and an authority figure or is a regressive activity resulting from an emotionally charged event such as a birth of a new sibling or starting in a day care center. It is not due to the direct physiologic effects of a substance such as laxatives or a medical condition. Involuntary soiling often involves constipation, impaction, and retention with leakage around the hardened stool. The underlying reason for constipation typically involves a psychologic reason such as anxiety specific to a place or a more general pattern of oppositional or anxious behavior.

Associated Features

Individuals with encopresis often feel ashamed about the condition and attempt to avoid situations that would lead to further embarrassment, such as camp, school, and sleep-

overs. Impairment generally relates to the effects of social ostracism, as well as anger, punishment, and rejection by caregivers, that affect the child's self-esteem. Smearing as an associated feature may be due to an attempt to clean or hide feces or may be more clearly deliberate. When deliberate, the individual often exhibits features of oppositional defiant disorder or conduct disorder (APA, 2000).

Prognosis

Encopresis can persist for years with remissions and exacerbations but rarely becomes chronic (APA, 2000). The best treatment remains a combination of educational, behavioral, dietary, and physiologic approaches (Mikkelsen, 2001).

Enuresis
Etiology and Epidemiology

Enuresis is the repeated voiding of urine into the bed or clothes, whether involuntary or intentional. Some possible predisposing factors include delayed or lax toilet training, psychosocial stress, dysfunction in the ability to concentrate urine, and a lower bladder volume threshold for involuntary voiding (APA, 2000).

At age 5 years, 7% of boys and 3% of girls experience enuresis. At age 10 years, 3% of boys and 2% of girls experience it (APA, 2000) (see DSM-IV-TR Criteria box).

Clinical Description and Associated Features

Diagnostic criteria for enuresis include voiding in inappropriate places during the day or night when control is expected. Impairment usually comes from interference with social activities or the effects of social ostracism and caregiver anger, rejection, and punishment that affect the child's self-esteem. Other disorders sometimes associated with

DSM-IV-TR CRITERIA
Encopresis

A. Repeated passage of feces into inappropriate places (e.g., clothing or floor) whether involuntary or intentional
B. At least one such event a month for at least 3 months
C. Chronologic age at least 4 years (or equivalent developmental level)
D. Behavior not due exclusively to the direct physiologic effects of a substance (e.g., laxatives) or a general medical condition except through a mechanism involving constipation

From American Psychiatric Association: *Diagnostic and Statistical Manual of Mental Disorders*, Fourth Edition, Text Revision. Washington, DC, American Psychiatric Association, 2000.

DSM-IV-TR CRITERIA
Enuresis (Not Due to a General Medical Condition)

A. Repeated voiding of urine into bed or clothes (whether involuntary or intentional)
B. Behavior clinically significant as manifested by either a frequency of twice a week for at least 3 consecutive months or the presence of clinically significant distress or impairment in social, academic (occupational), or other important areas of functioning
C. Chronologic age at least 5 years (or equivalent developmental level)
D. Behavior not due exclusively to the direct physiologic effect of a substance (e.g., a diuretic) or a general medical condition (e.g., diabetes, spina bifida, or a seizure disorder)
Specify type:
Nocturnal only
Diurnal only
Nocturnal and diurnal

From American Psychiatric Association: *Diagnostic and Statistical Manual of Mental Disorders*, Fourth Edition, Text Revision. Washington, DC, American Psychiatric Association, 2000.

enuresis include encopresis, sleepwalking disorder, and sleep terror disorder (APA, 2000).

Prognosis

Enuresis persists at age 18 years in only 1% of boys and less than 1% for girls. Only about 1% of cases continue into adulthood. About 75% of all children with enuresis have a first-degree relative who had the disorder (APA, 2000). The primary treatment approach uses the "bell-and-pad" approach as a behavior modifier. Imipramine and DDAVP are frequently used pharmacologic interventions (Mikkelsen, 2001).

PERVASIVE DEVELOPMENTAL DISORDERS
Autistic Disorder

Pervasive developmental disorders are a collection of neuropsychiatric disorders in which the child experiences deficits in a broad range of developmental areas, including reciprocal communication, social interactions, cognitive skills, and stereotypic behavior. **Autism** is the most common of these disorders (see DSM-IV-TR Criteria box) (Volkmar, 1999).

Epidemiology

Studies suggest that the rate of autistic disorder is as high as 1 in 1000, whereas other sources such as DSM-IV-TR report 5 per 10,000. Rates are three to four times higher in males than in females. Females, however, tend to have more severe mental retardation. Siblings of individuals with the disorder have an increased risk of developing autistic disorder (APA, 2000; Volkmar, 1999).

Clinical Description

Behavioral Manifestations. A variety of behavioral symptoms may present, including any of the following: hyperactivity, short attention span, impulsivity, aggressiveness, self-injurious behaviors, and temper tantrums. Abnormalities of eating (e.g., limiting intake to a few foods or eating nonnutritious objects) or sleeping (e.g., recurrent awakenings with rocking) may be found. Individuals often have restricted, repetitive, and stereotyped patterns of behavior, interest, and activity. They become preoccupied in a way that is abnormal, either in intensity or focus, with an inflexible adherence to specific, nonfunctional routines or rituals; or they use stereotypic and repetitive mannerisms or become persistently preoccupied with parts of objects. For example they may demonstrate an obsessive need to maintain sameness and orderliness by insisting on lining up objects over and over again. They may be unable to tolerate even minor changes in the environment and have catastrophic reactions to minor changes such as a new chair or new seating arrangement at dinner. They may insist on maintaining non-functional and unreasonable adherence to rituals and routines. For example, a child who is used to brushing teeth before getting into pajamas may become very upset if asked to change the order and put on pajamas first and then brush teeth. Self-injurious behavior can include head banging or biting of various body parts.

Autistic children often demonstrate stereotypic motor activities (e.g., clapping hands, spinning, rocking, swaying) and postural peculiarities (e.g., walking on tiptoes, odd postures, or strange hand movements). Play cannot be disrupted from preoccupation with objects such as buttons. They frequently show a fascination with movement of such things as

DSM-IV-TR CRITERIA
Autistic Disorder

A. A total of six (or more) items from 1, 2, and 3, with at least two from 1, and one each from 2 and 3:
   1. Qualitative impairment in social interaction, as manifested by at least two of the following:
      a. Marked impairment in the use of multiple nonverbal behaviors such as eye-to-eye gaze, facial expression, body postures, and gestures to regulate social interaction
      b. Failure to develop peer relationships appropriate to developmental level
      c. A lack of spontaneous seeking to share enjoyment, interests, or achievements with other people (e.g., by a lack of showing, bringing, or pointing out objects of interests)
      d. Lack of social or emotional reciprocity
   2. Qualitative impairments in communication as manifested by at least one of the following:
      a. Delay in, or total lack of, the development of spoken language (not accompanied by an attempt to compensate through alternative modes of communication such as gesture or mime)
      b. In individuals with adequate speech, marked impairment in the ability to initiate or sustain a conversation with others
      c. Stereotyped and repetitive use of language or idiosyncratic language
      d. Lack of varied, spontaneous make-believe play or social imitative play appropriate to developmental level
   3. Restricted repetitive and stereotyped patterns of behavior, interests, and activities, as manifested by at least one of the following:
      a. Encompassing preoccupation with one or more stereotyped and restricted patterns of interest that is abnormal either in intensity or focus
      b. Apparently inflexible adherence to specific, nonfunctional routines or rituals
      c. Stereotyped and repetitive motor mannerisms (e.g., hand or finger flapping or twisting, or complex whole-body movements)
      d. Persistent preoccupation with parts of objects
B. Delays or abnormal functioning in at least one of the following areas, with onset before age 3 years: (1) social interaction, (2) language as used in social communication, or (3) symbolic or imaginative play
C. Disturbance not better accounted for by Rett's disorder or childhood disintegrative disorder

From American Psychiatric Association: *Diagnostic and Statistical Manual of Mental Disorders,* Fourth Edition, Text Revision. Washington, DC, American Psychiatric Association, 2000.

fans, revolving objects, the opening and closing of doors or drawers, or turning the light switch on and off incessantly. They may become highly attached to some unusual inanimate object such as a piece of string or rubber band and ignore typical items such as a blanket or teddy bear.

Emotional Manifestations.

Individuals with autistic disorder typically lack emotional reciprocity (e.g., not actively participating in simple social play or games, instead preferring solitary activities or only attempting to involve others as tools or "mechanical" aids). Mood or affective abnormalities may be present, such as giggling or weeping for no apparent reason. There is a lack of empathy with failure to show emotional reaction when a reaction is expected. There may be an inappropriate response to danger, such as lack of fear to real danger or excessive fear to harmless objects. If the child acquires sufficient cognitive ability during development, the child may be aware of the seriousness of the limitations. This type of insight may result in depression.

Cognitive Manifestations.

Approximately 80% of individuals with autistic disorder have some degree of mental retardation; approximately 50% have severe or profound retardation and 30% have mild retardation (Volkmar, 1999). Other cognitive areas may also be affected, such as insight, reasoning, and judgment. Communication problems usually present so severely in both verbal and nonverbal areas that spoken language may be absent. Individuals who do speak may not be able to begin or sustain a conversation with others, or they use such stereotyped and repetitive or idiosyncratic language that others find it difficult to continue a conversation with them. Speech may often contain abnormalities of pitch, intonation, rate, and rhythm (e.g., monotonous or inappropriate sing-song pitch and rhythm or questionlike raises of tone at the end of declarative sentences). Grammar is often immature, stereotyped, and repetitive (e.g., inappropriate repetition of jingles or commercials, regardless of meaning) or metaphorical so that the individual can be understood only by those familiar with the individual's idiosyncratic use of language. Some individuals may not be able to understand simple questions, directions, or jokes; others may develop excellent long-term memory of insignificant data such as train schedules, baseball statistics, songs, or dates.

Perceptual Manifestations.

Individuals may respond oddly to sensory stimuli (e.g., high pain threshold, oversensitivity to sound or touch, exaggerated response to light or color, fascination with a particular sensory stimulation such as constantly rubbing a hard surface).

Social Manifestations.

Manifestations of autistic disorder depend on the developmental stage and chronologic age, but autism at any age is a severely limiting disorder. Markedly abnormal or impaired development in social interaction and communication and markedly restricted range of activity and interest severely impair the individual's ability to function in society without a significant amount of persistent family and professional intervention.

Peer relationships produce varied difficulties, depending on the severity of the disorder and the affected individual's developmental level. These children often appear oblivious to others, have no concept of others' needs, and do not notice their distress or joy. They often appear to lack the ability to express themselves and have blunted expressions of joy or distress.

The nature of impairments in social interaction may change over time, depending on developmental levels and the capacity to engage with others. Infants may refuse to cuddle, may show an indifference or aversion for affection or physical contact, may fail to demonstrate eye contact or facial responsiveness, or may not smile socially or respond to parents' voices. Young children may treat adults as interchangeable or cling mechanically to one specific person. Even if the child becomes willing to engage in social interactions, the interactions may demonstrate unusual behavior (e.g., expecting others to answer ritualized questions in specific ways, showing little sense of personal space boundaries, and being inappropriate in social interactions) (APA, 2000; Volkmar, 1999).

Prognosis

Language skills and overall intellectual level are the strongest factors related to the ultimate prognosis. Available studies that have followed the course of this disorder suggest that only a small percentage of individuals progress to live and work independently as adults. In about one third of cases, some degree of partial independence is possible. The highest-functioning adults with autistic disorder typically continue to exhibit problems in social interaction and communication, with restricted interests and activities. Evidence shows the importance of early intense educational interventions in fostering the acquisition of basic social, communication, and cognitive skills through highly structured programs (Volkmar, 1999).

Asperger's Disorder

Asperger's disorder contains many features similar to those of autistic disorder: self-injurious and aggressive behavior; severe and sustained impairment in social interaction; and restricted, repetitive patterns of behavior, interests, and activities that produce significant impairment in social, occupational, or other important areas of functioning. In contrast to autistic disorder, however, no clinically significant delays occur in language, cognitive development, age-appropriate self-help skills, adaptive behavior, or curiosity about the environment (APA, 2000). This disorder follows a continuous course, and duration usually is lifelong. There is a better long-term outcome for individuals with Asperger's than autism. Prognosis is best if treatment is started by age 24 to 36 months (Volkmar, 1999; Tanguay, 2000).

Rett's and Childhood Disintegrative Disorders

The defining characteristic of both Rett's and childhood disintegrative disorder (CDD) is a period of normal functioning perinatally and up to age 5 months for Rett's and 2 years for CDD. That period is followed by multiple deficits and problems in development and socialization.

ATTENTION DEFICIT/HYPERACTIVITY DISORDER

Epidemiology

Rates of ADHD in school-age children are estimated at 3% to 7% of the population. As many as two thirds of those diagnosed with ADHD also meet the criteria for another mental disorder, including up to 50% for oppositional defiant disorder or conduct disorder (see DSM-IV-TR Criteria box). Other disorders that frequently occur with ADHD include mood disorders, anxiety disorders, Tourette's and chronic tic disorders, substance abuse, speech and language delays, and learning disorders.

Etiology

The etiology of ADHD is unknown, but studies have suggested an interaction among psychosocial and biologic factors. Genetic factors likely play a role in ADHD. Concordance is 51% in monozygotic twins and 33% in dizygotic twins. Adoption studies also support genetics over environmental etiology (Cantwell, 1996). ADHD has been found more often in the first-degree relatives of children with ADHD (APA, 2000).

Clinical Description

Behavioral Manifestations. Behavioral manifestations usually occur in various or multiple environments in the child's life, such as school, home, church, or recreational activities. The level of problems typically varies from time to time in the same or different settings. Symptoms generally worsen in situations that require sustained attention and lack appeal or variety to the child or adolescent, such as listening to teachers, performing repetitive or tedious tasks, or reading lengthy materials. Symptoms may actually disappear or become minimal when under strict control, such as during a diagnostic interview or when receiving frequent rewards for appropriate behavior. Symptoms tend to worsen in unstructured group situations such as the typical classroom and playground.

Hyperactivity presents in many forms: fidgeting or squirming in a seat, getting up when one is expected to remain seated, excessive running or climbing when it is dangerous or inappropriate, loud and disruptive playing during quiet activities, and demonstrating a driven verbal or motor quality. Even though toddlers are characterized by a lot of activity and inquisitiveness, toddlers with ADHD present qualitatively different; they are always on the go, darting back and forth, running, jumping, and climbing on furniture,

DSM-IV-TR CRITERIA
Attention-Deficit/Hyperactivity Disorder

A. Either 1 or 2:
1. Six (or more) of the following symptoms of inattention have persisted for at least 6 months to a degree that is maladaptive and inconsistent with developmental level:
   Inattention
   a. Often fails to give close attention to details or makes careless mistakes in schoolwork, work, or other activities
   b. Often has difficulty sustaining attention in tasks or play activities
   c. Often does not seem to listen when spoken to directly
   d. Often does not follow through on instructions and fails to finish schoolwork, chores, or duties in the workplace (not due to oppositional behavior or failure to understand instructions)
   e. Often has difficulty organizing tasks and activities
   f. Often avoids, dislikes, or is reluctant to engage in tasks that require sustained mental effort (such as schoolwork or homework)
   g. Often loses things necessary for tasks or activities (e.g., toys, school assignments, pencils, books, or tools)
   h. Is often easily distracted by extraneous stimulus
   i. Often forgetful in daily activities
2. Six (or more) of the following symptoms of hyperactivity-impulsivity have persisted for at least 6 months to a degree that is maladaptive and inconsistent with developmental level:
   Hyperactivity
   a. Often fidgets with hands or feet or squirms in seat
   b. Often leaves seat in classroom or in other situations in which remaining seated is expected
   c. Often runs about or climbs excessively in situations in which it is inappropriate (in adolescents or adults, may be limited to subjective feelings of restlessness)
   d. Often has difficulty playing or engaging in leisure activities quietly
   e. Is often "on the go" or often acts as if "driven by a motor"
   f. Often talks excessively
   Impulsivity
   g. Often blurts out answers before questions have been completed
   h. Often has difficulty awaiting turn
   i. Often interrupts or intrudes on others (e.g., butts into conversations or games)
B. Some hyperactive-impulsive or inattentive symptoms that caused impairment were present before age 7 years.
C. Some impairment from the symptoms is present in two or more settings (e.g., at school [or work] and at home).
D. There must be clear evidence of clinically significant impairment in social, academic, or occupational functioning.
E. The symptoms do not occur exclusively during the course of a pervasive developmental disorder, schizophrenia, or other psychotic disorder and are not better accounted for by another mental disorder (e.g., mood disorder, anxiety disorder, dissociative disorder, or personality disorder).

From American Psychiatric Association: *Diagnostic and Statistical Manual of Mental Disorders*, Fourth Edition, Text Revision. Washington, DC, American Psychiatric Association, 2000.

or unable to remain still for completion of simple tasks such as putting on a coat or listening to a simple story.

School-age children may settle down somewhat but still display excessive overactivity; they demonstrate difficulty remaining seated by hanging onto the edge of their seats, squirming constantly, playing with objects, or tapping their hands and feet. They can stay focused for activities they enjoy such as watching TV or playing video games, but cannot maintain attention or focus for activities they find boring or difficult. At home they frequently do not finish meals or activities that they have begun. They make excessive noise, interrupting others during quiet times and talking constantly, such as giving a running commentary on a television show. Adolescents often express a subjective feeling of restlessness and report a preference to engage in active rather than sedentary activities.

Impulsivity manifests itself in the following ways: impatience, failing to delay responses, blurting out answers before the question has been finished, difficulty waiting for one's turn or problems waiting in line without pushing and shoving, and frequently interrupting others to the point of social, academic, or occupational problems. In addition, they may also make comments out of turn; fail to listen to directions; initiate inappropriate contact with others by interrupting conversations; grab others by their clothing, limbs, or belongings; touch things that are off limits to them; and clown around at times of expected quiet. Accidents may result from their knocking over objects, running into people, grabbing dangerous objects such as a hot pan, or taking dangerous risks without consideration of the consequences, such as riding a bicycle at night without reflective lights. They often exhibit temper outbursts, bossiness, stubbornness, and excessive and frequent insistence that their requests be met.

Emotional Manifestations. Individuals with this disorder may develop a number of other problems as a result of the underlying attention and hyperactive-impulsive problems, including any of the following: low frustration tolerance, mood lability, demoralization, depressed mood, and low self-esteem.

Cognitive Manifestations. Inattention may take place in various settings. Schoolwork or other activities often contain careless errors, showing lack of close attention to details. Work may be messy, with evidence of not thinking through the project or schoolwork or of not persisting to adequate completion. Often it appears that the child is daydreaming and not listening to what is being said or asked. Shifts may occur from one unfinished task to another, with a growing clutter surrounding the child's path. Children with ADHD are often regarded as lazy, unmotivated, and believed to have below average intelligence. Studies have demonstrated that 10% to 20% of children with ADHD also have a learning disorder and are, in fact, of normal intelligence (Nearns, 1997). Although chores or schoolwork often do not get com-

pleted, care must be taken in attributing this symptom to ADHD, because other problems such as oppositional behaviors often occur that may be considered normal during early childhood development. These individuals often have problems with organizational skills, find tasks that require sustained mental effort unpleasant, and become aversive and take short cuts to such tasks (especially homework). Materials needed for specific tasks typically become scattered, lost, or carelessly handled and damaged. Trivial stimuli such as household noises often distract these individuals, who then leave their assigned task to attend to the interrupting stimuli. They often forget and miss appointments, fail to meet schoolwork deadlines, or forget lunch money. As a result, academic achievement is often impaired.

Perceptual Manifestations. Perceptual problems are rarely seen in ADHD.

Social Manifestations. Social problems may occur as a result of losing the train of conversation and changing topics inappropriately, not following expected rules of games or activities, and appearing uninterested in others. Family members frequently develop resentment and antagonism, particularly when the variability of symptoms leads parents to believe that their child's troublesome behavior is willful. Families likely have more stress, feelings of parental incompetence, marital discord, marital disruption, and social isolation (Dulcan et al., 1997). ADHD can cause rejection by peers and conflicts with family and school authorities. Others often interpret inadequate self-application as laziness, irresponsibility, and oppositional behavior (APA, 2000).

Prognosis

ADHD features persist into adolescence in the majority of children diagnosed as hyperactive and generally attenuate during late adolescence and early adulthood. A family history of ADHD, psychosocial adversity, and comorbidity with conduct, mood, and anxiety disorders increase the risk of persistence. Specific predictors of poor outcome include oppositional and aggressive behavior directed at adults, low IQ, poor peer relations, and continuing ADHD symptoms. Comorbid oppositional defiant disorder raises the risk of conduct disorder. Behavioral management has been validated as the best psychosocial intervention. Education of the whole family is of particular importance in treatment as well (Pliszka, 2000).

DEVELOPMENTAL DISORDERS
Etiology

Learning disorders are associated with a number of factors such as genetic predisposition, perinatal injury, family history, cognitive impairments, environmental factors, and various neurologic or medical conditions; however, these conditions do not inevitably predict learning disorders. Certain medical conditions have a strong association with learning disorders: lead poisoning, fetal alcohol syndrome, and fragile X syndrome. A number of factors must be ruled out when evaluating for a learning disorder: normal variations in academic attainment, lack of opportunity, inadequate teaching, cultural factors, and impaired hearing or vision (APA, 2000; Beitchman et al., 1998).

Epidemiology

A growing consensus supports the theory that genetic factors play a significant role in the determination of reading ability and disability. Two distinct reading problems have been linked to chromosome 6 (phonologic awareness) and chromosome 15 (single-word reading) (Beitchman and Yound, 1997).

Learning disorders are found in about 10% to 20% of children, depending on the nature of assessment and the definitions applied. Approximately 5% of public school students have an identified learning disorder. Reading disorder affects an estimated 4% of school-age children in the United States, and approximately 1% of school-age children have mathematics disorder. Approximately 2% to 3% have a language disorder. Disorder of written expression is thought to occur in 2% to 8% of grade school children. Motor coordination disorder may affect as many as 6% of 5- to 11-year-olds. Developmental expressive language disorder occurs in approximately 1% to 13% of children. The developmental type of mixed receptive-expressive language disorder is estimated in up to 3% of school-age children. About 2% to 3% of 6- and 7-year-olds show phonologic disorder, which falls to 0.5% by age 17 years. Stuttering occurs in 1% of prepubertal children and drops to 0.8% in adolescence. Males predominate, with a ratio of 3:1 over females (APA, 2000; Beitchman et al., 1998). Approximately 50% have an associated psychiatric disorder, 26% a behavior disorder, and 20% an emotional disorder (Toppleberg, 2000).

Clinical Description

Learning Disorders. The National Joint Committee on Learning Disabilities defines learning disabilities as a heterogeneous group of disorders manifested by significant difficulties in the acquisition and use of listening, speaking, reading, writing, reasoning, or mathematic abilities. These disorders are intrinsic to the individual, presumed to be due to central nervous system dysfunction, and may occur across the life span. Problems in self-regulatory behaviors, social perception, and social interaction may exist with learning disabilities but do not by themselves constitute a learning disability (Beitchman and Yound, 1997).

Learning disorders encompass problems with reading, writing, math, and a not-otherwise-specified category when there are difficulties with listening, speaking, or reasoning. Disorders are diagnosed through individually administered, standardized tests when performance is substantially below expected levels (generally defined as 1 to 2 standard deviations below the average) and when there is significant interference with academic achievement or activities of daily living (ADLs). Many problems can result from learning

disorders, including demoralization, low self-esteem, and deficits in social skills. Children and adolescents with learning disorders drop out of school at a rate of nearly 40% (approximately 1.5 times the average rate). A total of 10% to 25% of individuals with conduct disorder, oppositional defiant disorder, ADHD, major depression, or dysthymic disorders have learning disorders as well. Language delay may occur in learning disorders, and learning disorders may be associated with a higher rate of developmental coordination disorder. Underlying abnormalities in cognitive abilities may exist (e.g., deficits in visual perception, linguistic processes, attention, memory, or a combination) that often precede or are associated with learning disorders.

Coordination Disorders. Developmental coordination disorder is diagnosed only if motor coordination significantly interferes with academic achievement or ADLs and is not due to a medical condition (e.g., cerebral palsy, muscular dystrophy). Specific activities or tasks that may be impaired or altered include walking, crawling, sitting, tying shoelaces, buttoning shirts, or zipping pants. Communication disorders also may be associated (APA, 2000).

Communication Disorders. Characteristics of *expressive language disorder* vary and may include a limited amount of speech, limited range of vocabulary, difficulty acquiring new words, word-finding or vocabulary errors, shortened sentences, simplified grammar use, omissions of critical parts of a sentence, use of unusual word order, and slow rate of language development. Intelligence measured by performance tests is usually normal. Expressive language disorder may be either acquired as a result of a neurologic or medical condition (e.g., encephalitis, head trauma, irradiation) or developmental (i.e., no known neurologic condition). *Mixed receptive-expressive language disorder* symptoms include receptive difficulties (e.g., markedly limited vocabulary, errors in tense, difficulty recalling words or producing developmentally appropriate sentences, general difficulty expressing ideas) and language development problems (e.g., difficulty understanding words, sentences, or specific types of words). As with expressive language disorder, mixed receptive-expressive language disorder may be developmental or acquired. A child may initially appear confused or inattentive, follow commands incorrectly, and give inappropriate responses to questions. The child may appear quiet or unusually talkative. Other communication disorders include *phonologic disorder* (problems using expected speech sounds) and *stuttering* (a disturbance in normal fluency and time patterns of speech) (APA, 2000).

Prognosis

The prognosis for reading disorder is favorable when there is early identification and intervention, but the disorder may persist into adult life. The degree of impairment usually depends on the overall intelligence level in mathematics disorder. Brighter children may be able to function at or near grade level in early grades, but by the fifth grade the reading disorder almost always becomes apparent. The course of written expression disorder has not been clearly defined. Motor coordination disorder has a variable course and may last into adolescence or adulthood. Approximately one half of children with developmental expressive language disorder outgrow it, whereas the other half has long-lasting difficulties. In the acquired type, recovery depends on the severity and location of the injury, as well as the child's age at the time of occurrence. Recovery may be rapid and complete, or the injury may get progressively worse. The prognosis for mixed receptive-expressive language disorder of the acquired type is worse than for expressive language disorder. The acquired type has a variable prognosis, as occurs with expressive language disorder. The prognosis for phonologic disorder varies according to the cause and severity. In severe cases speech may not be recognizable and the disorder may persist, whereas mild cases may remit spontaneously. Stuttering typically occurs insidiously and, when noticed, has a waxing and waning course. Recovery occurs in up to 80% of cases and spontaneously in 60%. Recovery typically occurs at age 16 years (APA, 2000; Beitchman et al., 1998).

SEPARATION ANXIETY DISORDER
Etiology and Epidemiology

Separation anxiety disorder appears to be more common in first-degree relatives and may be more common in children whose mothers have panic disorder. It may develop after some life stress (e.g., death of a relative or pet, illness in the child or parent, or a change in the environment) (APA, 2000).

This disorder occurs in approximately 4% of children and adolescents and is more common in females. It typically presents before late adolescence (APA, 2000) (see DSM-IV-TR Criteria box).

Clinical Description

Behavioral Manifestations. With an excessive need to know the whereabouts of their parents or others, individuals with separation anxiety often display attempts to stay in touch with frequent telephone calls. Because of significant discomfort in being away from home, they may become resistant to traveling alone and reluctant to attend activities that other peers enjoy and look forward to such as camp, school, and sleepovers at friends' houses. They may not stay in a room alone. Children with separation anxiety disorder may demonstrate clinging behavior. They may attempt to shadow their parents around the home and with increasing frequency and intensity attempt to shadow their parents outside the home. Bedtime can be difficult, with the child or adolescent insisting that the parent remain with him or her until he or she falls asleep. During the night these individuals may attempt to get in bed with the parents or another significant figure; if their way is obstructed, they may sleep outside the parents or other's door.

Physical complaints often appear during actual or anticipated separation and frequently include stomachaches,

---

DSM-IV-TR CRITERIA
Separation Anxiety

A. Developmentally inappropriate and excessive anxiety concerning separation from home or from those to whom the individual is attached, as evidenced by three (or more) of the following:
1. Recurrent excessive distress when separation from home or major attachment figures occurs or is anticipated
2. Persistent and excessive worry about losing, or about possible harm befalling, major attachment figures
3. Persistent and excessive worry that an untoward event will lead to separation from a major attachment figure (e.g., getting lost or being kidnapped)
4. Persistent reluctance or refusal to go to school or elsewhere because of fear of separation
5. Persistently and excessively fearful or reluctant to be alone or without major attachment figures at home or without significant adults in other settings
6. Persistent reluctance or refusal to go to sleep without being near a major attachment figure or to sleep away from home
7. Repeated nightmares with the theme of separation
8. Repeated complaints of physical symptoms (such as headaches, stomachaches, nausea, or vomiting) when separation from major attachment figures occurs or is anticipated
B. The duration of the disturbance is at least 4 weeks.
C. The onset is before age 18 years.
D. The disturbance causes clinically significant distress or impairment in social, academic (occupational), or other important areas of functioning.
E. The disturbance does not occur exclusively during the course of a pervasive developmental disorder, schizophrenia, or other psychotic disorder and, in adolescents and adults, is not better accounted for by panic disorder with agoraphobia.

From American Psychiatric Association: *Diagnostic and Statistical Manual of Mental Disorders*, Fourth Edition, Text Revision. Washington, DC, American Psychiatric Association, 2000.

---

headaches, nausea, and vomiting. Older children and adolescents may experience a racing or pounding heart, dizziness, and faintness. The somatic complaints often lead to numerous trips to physicians and subsequent medical procedures.

School refusal occurs as a specific type of separation anxiety in about 5% of all school-age children. It usually occurs between ages 5 and 6 and 10 and 11 years (King, 2001).

Emotional Manifestations. Individuals with this disorder often experience recurrent, excessive distress when they are away from home or major attachment figures. Some become extremely distraught and miserable away from home and become preoccupied with reunion fantasies. They may become extremely fearful that some imagined harm will happen to the significant other(s). Fears about danger to themselves or their families may present as fear of animals, monsters, the dark, muggers, burglars, kidnappers, accidents, or plane or train travel. Fears may also present as concerns about death and dying. They may show various moods, such as excessive worry that no one loves them and they therefore want to die, or unusual anger when someone tries to separate them from their parent or significant other. The depressed mood may at times justify a diagnosis of depression. As adulthood is reached, some of these individuals may develop panic disorder with agoraphobia.

Cognitive Manifestations. Nightmares often contain elements of the individual's fears, such as family death through fire, murder, or other catastrophe. Academic difficulties may result from refusal to attend school and thus increase the problem with social avoidance.

Perceptual Manifestations. When alone, young children may experience perceptual problems, such as seeing people peering into their room, scary creatures reaching for them, and eyes staring at them, or they may misperceive usual sounds as ominous.

Social Manifestations. With a typically close-knit family, clients with separation anxiety disorder may exhibit social withdrawal, apathy, sadness, or concentration difficulties at work or play when away from parents or significant others. Families frequently experience significant conflict, with parental resentment and frustration. At times, however, these children may also become unusually conscientious, compliant, and eager to please. Parents may describe children with separation anxiety disorder as demanding, intrusive, and in need of constant attention; the children may physically strike out when prevented from fulfilling their goal of being with the significant parent(s) (APA, 2000).

Prognosis

Typically there are periods of severity and reduction of symptoms. Both the anxiety about possible separation and the avoidance of situations involving separation may persist for many years.

TIC DISORDERS
Tourette's Disorder
Etiology and Epidemiology

Vulnerability to Tourette's disorder appears to be genetic and is transmitted within families (APA, 2000). Tourette's disorder occurs in approximately 5 to 30 children per 10,000 and 1 to 2 per 10,000 in adults. It is approximately two times more common in males than in females. Other disorders associated with Tourette's disorder include ADHD, obsessive-compulsive disorder, and learning disorders (APA, 2000) (see DSM-IV-TR Criteria box).

Clinical Description

Behavioral Manifestations. Tics present as a behavioral symptom. A **tic** is defined as a sudden, rapid, recurrent, non-rhythmic, stereotyped motor movement or vocalization. Although experienced as irresistible, it can often be suppressed

---

DSM-IV-TR CRITERIA
Tourette's Disorder

A. Both multiple motor and one or more vocal tics have been present at some time during the illness, although not necessarily concurrently. (A *tic* is a sudden, rapid, recurrent nonrhythmic, stereotyped motor movement or vocalization.)

B. The tics occur many times a day (usually in bouts) nearly every day or intermittently throughout a period of more than 1 year, and during this period there was never a tic-free period of more than 3 consecutive months.

C. The onset is before age 18 years.

D. The disturbance is not due to the direct physiologic effects of a substance (e.g., stimulants) or a general medical condition (e.g., Huntington's disease or postviral encephalitis).

From American Psychiatric Association: *Diagnostic and Statistical Manual of Mental Disorders*, Fourth Edition, Text Revision. Washington, DC, American Psychiatric Association, 2000.

---

for a varying length of time. Stress typically exacerbates tics, and distracting activities such as reading or sewing may reduce them. Sleep markedly decreases tics.

Simple motor tics include eye blinking, neck jerking, shoulder shrugging, facial grimacing, and coughing. Simple vocal tics include throat clearing, grunting, sniffing, snorting, and barking. Complex motor tics include facial gestures, grooming behaviors, jumping, touching, stamping, smelling an object, and echopraxia (imitation of another's movements). Complex vocal tics include repeating words or phrases out of context, coprolalia (repeating socially unacceptable words, typically obscene or swear words), palilalia (repeating one's own sounds or words), and echolalia (repeating the last-heard word, sound, or phrase).

In Tourette's disorder the number, type, frequency, complexity, and severity of the tics vary over time. Most common tics in Tourette's disorder involve the head and parts of the body such as the torso and limbs. Common vocal tics include clicks, grunts, barks, sniffs, snorts, and coughs. Coprolalia occurs in less than 10% of the cases. Complex motor tics reported in Tourette's disorder include touching, squatting, deep knee bends, retracing steps, and twirling during walking. The most frequent initial tic is blinking. Other initial tics reported include tongue protrusion, squatting, sniffing, hopping, skipping, throat clearing, stuttering, uttering sounds or words, and coprolalia. Other relatively common issues include hyperactivity, distractibility, and impulsivity. Obsessions and compulsions are common features seen in a client with Tourette's disorder. Retinal detachment can occur from head banging; orthopedic problems can occur from knee bending, neck jerking, or head turning; and skin problems can result from picking.

Emotional Manifestations. Shame, self-consciousness, and depressed mood may occur as a secondary result of problems stemming from Tourette's disorder.

Cognitive Manifestations. Various learning disabilities such as dyslexia are commonly found with individuals who have Tourette's disorder.

Perceptual Manifestations. Perceptual problems are not a typical problem area in Tourette's disorder.

Social Manifestations. Frequently reported associated symptoms include social discomfort and rejection by others that interfere with social, academic, and occupational functioning. In severe cases tics may interfere with ADLs such as reading or eating or cause medical complications (APA, 2000).

Prognosis
Tourette's disorder may begin as early as age 2 years but typically presents during childhood or early adolescence. Although it is almost always a lifelong disorder, in most cases symptoms diminish during adolescence and adulthood (APA, 2000).

Other Tic Disorders
Chronic Motor or Vocal Tic Disorder
Chronic motor or vocal tic disorder resembles Tourette's disorder, except the tics may be either motor or vocal and need not be multiple (only one motor or tic movement at a time such as snorting instead of snorting with head jerking). It also tends to be less severe (APA, 2000).

Transient Tic Disorder
The diagnosis of transient tic disorder is made if the tics occur every day for at least 4 weeks but no longer than 1 year. Otherwise, the criteria are the same as for Tourette's disorder, but symptoms typically occur with less severity (APA, 2000).

Tic Disorder Not Otherwise Specified
The diagnosis of tic disorder not otherwise specified is used when other, more specific diagnoses cannot be made. Examples include tics lasting less than 4 weeks or tics with an onset after age 18 years (APA, 2000).

DISRUPTIVE BEHAVIOR DISORDERS
Conduct Disorder
Etiology
Conduct disorder represents the most common reason for referral for psychiatric evaluation and represents 30% to 50% of all referrals in some clinics. Prevalence rates are higher for males than females, but the gap is narrowing.

The following factors have been identified as predisposing the child to conduct disorder: parental rejection and neglect, difficult infant temperament, inconsistent child-rearing practices with harsh discipline, physical or sexual abuse, lack of supervision, early institutional living, frequent changes of caregivers, large family size, association with a delinquent peer group, and certain family psychopathology. Conduct disorder occurs more frequently when a biologic or adoptive parent has antisocial personality disorder; a biologic parent has alcohol dependence, a mood disorder, schizophrenia, or a history of ADHD or conduct disorder; or a sibling has conduct disorder.

Although definitive etiology for conduct disorder has not been developed, one possible model proposes a genetic liability triggered by environmental risk and mediated by factors such as poor coping skills (APA, 2000; Steiner et al., 1997).

Comorbid conditions frequently include ADHD, oppositional defiant disorder, mood and anxiety disorders, borderline personality disorder in girls, antisocial personality disorder in boys, mental retardation, and specific developmental disabilities (Steiner et al., 1997; Loeber, 2000).

Epidemiology
According to DSM-IV-TR, rates appear higher in urban than in rural settings and vary depending on the nature of the population sampled and methods of ascertainment used (APA, 2000) (see DSM-IV-TR Criteria box on p. 361). Bauermeister et al. (1994) found the pattern of conduct disorder to be highest in 13- to 16-year-olds, with a sharp decline thereafter. In boys the prevalence reached a high point from age 10 to 13 years, with a gradual decline from ages 13 to 20 years. In girls a gradual increase occurred in late childhood and early adolescence, peaking at age 16 years and followed by a sharp decline.

Clinical Description
Behavioral Manifestations. Conduct disorder presents mainly with a repetitive and persistent pattern of behavior that violates the basic rights of others or major age-appropriate societal norms or rules. The behavior typically presents in a variety of settings, including home, school, and the community. It can be difficult to detect, however, because the child or adolescent tends to minimize the problems, and adults may not have full knowledge because of their inability to adequately supervise the child or adolescent (Loeber, 2000).

Clients with conduct disorder manifest aggressive behavior and react aggressively toward others. They bully, threaten, and intimidate; initiate physical fights; use weapons in ways that could lead to injury; act cruelly to people or animals; steal; and force sexual activity. The severity of these behaviors may involve rape, assault, or (rarely) homicide. Deliberate destruction of property may result in fire damage, vandalism, and destruction of others' property for simple vengeance. In addition to theft or robbery, the child or adolescent may be deceitful, demonstrating frequent lying or breaking promises to obtain goods or favors or to avoid obligations, responsibility, or retribution.

These clients also frequently attempt to avoid consequences by attempting to blame others. Early onset of behavior usually includes sexual activity, drinking, smoking, use of illegal substances, and other high-risk behaviors.

DSM-IV-TR CRITERIA
Conduct Disorder

A. A repetitive and persistent pattern of behavior in which the basic rights of others or major age-appropriate norms or rules are violated, as manifested by the presence of three (or more) of the following criteria in the past 12 months, with at least one criterion present in the past 6 months:

Aggression to people and animals
1. Often bullies, threatens, or intimidates others
2. Often initiates physical fights
3. Has used a weapon that can cause serious physical harm to others (e.g., a bat, brick, broken bottle, knife, gun)
4. Has been physically cruel to people
5. Has been physically cruel to animals
6. Has stolen while confronting a victim (e.g., mugging, purse snatching, extortion, armed robbery)
7. Has forced someone into sexual activity

Destruction of property
8. Has deliberately engaged in fire setting with the intention of causing serious damage
9. Has deliberately destroyed others' property (other than by fire setting)

Deceitfulness or theft
10. Has broken into someone else's house, building, or car
11. Often lies to obtain goods or favors or to avoid obligations (i.e., "cons" others)
12. Has stolen items of nontrivial value without confronting a victim (e.g., shoplifting, but without breaking and entering; forgery)

Serious violations of rules
13. Often stays out at night despite parental prohibitions, beginning before age 13 years
14. Has run away from home overnight at least twice while living in parental or parental surrogate home (or once without returning for a lengthy period)
15. Is often truant from school, beginning before age 13 years

B. The disturbance in behavior causes clinically significant impairment in social, academic, or occupational functioning.

C. If the individual is age 18 years or older, criteria are not met for antisocial personality disorder.

From American Psychiatric Association: *Diagnostic and Statistical Manual of Mental Disorders*, Fourth Edition, Text Revision. Washington, DC, American Psychiatric Association, 2000.

Behaviors usually persist into adulthood. These behaviors frequently lead to school suspensions, unplanned pregnancy, physical injury, sexually transmitted diseases, legal problems, dismissals from work or other activities, and the inability to attend regular schools.

Children or adolescents with conduct disorder generally exhibit callous behavior but may express guilt or remorse because they have learned that it may reduce or prevent punishment. This stated sense of remorse is often insincere and fabricated.

Although they may project an image of "toughness," they often experience low self-esteem with resulting poor frustration tolerance, irritability, temper outbursts, and reckless behavior. Two subtypes have been identified. One consists of overt (confrontational, fighting) aggression and the other of covert (concealing, theft) disruptive behaviors (Loeber, 2000).

Emotional Manifestations. Individuals with conduct disorders usually have little empathy or concern for the feelings, wishes, and well-being of others. Suicide ideation, attempts, and completions occur at a higher rate than the norm (see p. 363 and Chapter 24).

Perceptual Manifestations. Clients with conduct disorder often have misconceptions about the intentions of others, especially in ambiguous situations. They typically perceive others as threatening and hostile and therefore feel justified in responding aggressively.

Cognitive Manifestations. Individuals with conduct disorder may have various learning disorders or impairments in cognitive functioning, such as borderline intelligence, but none appears specific to conduct disorder.

Social Manifestations. Accident rates are higher. Peer relationships often are impaired as a result of the behaviors associated with conduct disorder (APA, 2000; Loeber, 2000).

Prognosis

Less severe symptoms tend to emerge initially. Males dominate in the childhood-onset group and tend to exhibit more fighting, stealing, vandalism, and school discipline problems. Females tend to have symptoms of lying, running away, substance use, and prostitution. Males tend to use more confrontational aggression; females tend to use more nonconfrontational behaviors. An onset of conduct disorder before age 10 years (childhood-onset type) generally indicates a more severe and persistent type that often develops into adult antisocial personality disorder. These individuals typically are male, display more physical aggression, are more likely to have oppositional defiant disorder during childhood, and meet full criteria for conduct disorder before puberty. Individuals in the adolescent-onset group (no symptoms of conduct disorder before age 10 years) display less aggression, are likely to have better peer relationships, and display conduct problems in groups. The most serious outcomes are antisocial personality and psychopathy. Psychopathy consists of the dimensions of egocentricity, callousness, and manipulativeness. Antisocial personality consists of impulsivity, irresponsibility, and antisocial behavior (APA, 2000; Loeber, 2000).

Oppositional Defiant Disorder
Etiology

Oppositional defiant disorder occurs more often in families where childcare has been disrupted by a succession of different caregivers, or where harsh, inconsistent, or neglectful child-rearing practices occur. The disorder occurs more commonly when serious marital problems are present (APA, 2000) (see DSM-IV-TR Criteria box on p. 362).

DSM-IV-TR CRITERIA
Oppositional Defiant Disorder

A. A pattern of negativistic, hostile, and defiant behavior lasting at least 6 months, during which four or more of the following are present:
1. Often loses temper
2. Often argues with adults
3. Often actively defies or refuses to comply with adults' requests or rules
4. Often deliberately annoys people
5. Often blames others for his or her mistakes or misbehavior
6. Is often touchy or easily annoyed by others
7. Is often angry and resentful
8. Is often spiteful or vindictive
   NOTE: Consider a criterion met only if the behavior occurs more frequently than is typically observed in individuals of comparable age and developmental level.
B. The disturbance in behavior causes clinically significant impairment in social, academic, or occupational functioning.
C. The behaviors do not occur exclusively during the course of a psychotic or mood disorder.
D. Criteria are not met for conduct disorder, and, if the individual is age 18 years or older, criteria are not met for antisocial personality disorder.

From American Psychiatric Association: *Diagnostic and Statistical Manual of Mental Disorders*, Fourth Edition, Text Revision. Washington, DC, American Psychiatric Association, 2000.

Epidemiology

Rates vary considerably from 2% to 16%, based on the nature of the population sample and method of assessment. Oppositional defiant disorder occurs more frequently in males before puberty and with approximately equal frequency after puberty. The disorder also occurs more commonly when at least one parent has a history of one of the following: mood disorder, oppositional defiant disorder, conduct disorder, ADHD, antisocial personality disorder, or a substance-related disorder. ADHD, learning disorders, and communication disorders tend to be associated with oppositional defiant disorder (APA, 2000).

Clinical Description

Behavioral Manifestations. The essential features of negativism, defiance, disobedience, and hostility toward authority figures typically present with persistent stubbornness, resistance to directions, and unwillingness to compromise, give in, or negotiate with adults. Evidence of defiance can also present as deliberate or persistent testing of limits, typically by ignoring directions, arguing, and refusing to accept responsibility for misbehavior. Hostility may be directed at adults or peers and includes deliberately annoying others verbally. Symptoms invariably present at home but may be absent or minimal at school and are generally directed toward those the child knows best. Individuals with oppositional defiant disorder do not tend to regard themselves as troublesome but blame others for making unreasonable demands or blame the circumstances.

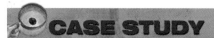
CASE STUDY

Brian, an intelligent 9-year-old boy, is reported by his parents to be argumentative, irritable, and not able to follow through on simple instructions, needing constant reminders. It takes him hours to complete his homework every evening. He becomes easily frustrated and is not able to finish his assignments. At school, his teacher reports that he is restless, talks out of turn, interrupts, and frequently leaves his seat to disturb other students in the classroom. During recess he is constantly fighting with peers and is unable to make friends at school. In his neighborhood, none of the children want him on their team because he is a poor sport and argues about all the rules.

Critical Thinking
1. What is an appropriate level of adult supervision for a 9-year-old? Why?
2. What effect will restrictions have on Brian's school progress?
3. Is Brian's self-esteem positive or negative, based on his peer interactions?
4. Are Brian's frustrations a result of being a disciplined child or being a child in need of therapeutic intervention?

Emotional Manifestations. During school years the following problems may be seen: low self-esteem, mood lability, and low frustration tolerance.

Cognitive and Perceptual Manifestations. Cognitive and perceptual symptoms do not usually present as significant symptoms in oppositional defiant disorder.

Social Manifestations. During early childhood, evidence of difficult temperament (e.g., high reactivity, difficulty in being soothed) or high motor activity has been noted. There may be swearing and precocious use of alcohol, tobacco, or illicit drugs that impact peer relationships and disrupt adult relationships. A negative relationship frequently exists between parent and child that elicits the worst characteristics in each (APA, 2000) (see Case Study).

Prognosis

The onset is typically gradual, usually occurring over months or years. In a significant number of cases, oppositional defiant disorder develops into conduct disorder. This disorder tends to persist over time in approximately half of the cases (Loeber, 2000).

DISCHARGE CRITERIA

Client will:
- Engage in self-care within level of capability.
- Demonstrate emotional control within capacity.
- Attend to tasks, schoolwork, and performance without undue anger or frustration.
- Exhibit healthy self-concept and self-esteem.
- Demonstrate functional eating habits and behaviors appropriate for age and stature.

- Use cognitive, communication, and language skills to make self understood and to get needs met.
- Demonstrate interactive skills appropriate for level of development.
- Verbalize satisfaction with gender identity and sexual preference.
- Interact meaningfully with staff, peers, and family within capability.
- Seek attention and assistance appropriately from significant persons and refrain from undue or unnecessary interactions with strangers.
- Adhere to treatment regimen, including medication as needed.
- Play appropriately with peers.
- Engage in educational and vocational programs within capacity.
- Use adaptive coping techniques and stress-reducing strategies.
- Respond satisfactorily to others' attentions and requests.
- Use community resources to enhance quality of life.
- Engage in ongoing individual and family therapy.

OTHER PROBLEM AREAS

ADOLESCENT SUICIDE

Adolescent suicide does not neatly fall under any diagnostic category. Adolescent suicides have quadrupled since 1950 from 2.5 to 11.2 per 100,000 and currently represent 12% of all deaths in this age group. Approximately 2 million U.S. adolescents attempt suicide, 700,000 receive medical attention, and 2000 die each year. It ranks third as the leading cause of death in adolescents. For every completed suicide it is estimated that there are 20 to 200 attempts. Between 80% and 90% of the attempters have a diagnosable psychiatric disorder. Reported predisposing factors include anxiety, disruptive disorder, bipolar disorder, substance abuse and personality disorders, a family history of mood disorders, a family history of suicidal behavior, exposure to family violence, impulsivity, abuse and molestation, stress events (real or perceived), and availability of methods (Shaffer et al., 2001). Substance abuse/dependence enhances the risk of suicide thoughts becoming suicide attempts (Gould, 1998). Wagner et al. (2000) found that nearly half of the children and adolescents who were hospitalized for suicidal ideation attempted suicide at least once in the past.

Hanging was the most common method in the 10- to 15-year age group, and firearms were the most common method in later adolescence. Fewer warning signs and fewer precipitating events preceded the suicide in children and young adolescents. Intoxication and romantic failure did not appear to constitute a risk in those younger than 15 years, as so often occurs in older adolescents. Significant risk factors for suicide include the following: males with a prior attempt who are older than 16 years with an associated mood or sub-

stance disorder, females with a mood disorder, and prior attempt. Immediate risk is predicted by a diagnosis of major depression and agitation (Shaffer, 2001).

YOUTH VIOLENCE

Youth violence is becoming more prevalent, with younger children committing more aggressive acts than ever before. Early childhood aggression has a relatively high likelihood of persistence over time (Vance et al., 2002). Students bringing guns and knives to school have prompted the school systems to implement stricter "no tolerance" rules and higher security such as metal detectors and on site police officers. The Surgeon General (Report of the Surgeon General, 2001) published a report on youth violence summarizing research studies that discussed possible risk factors, interventions, and preventions for youth violence.

There was an epidemic of violence in the United States between 1983 to 1993 resulting from an increase in gang violence, drug usage, and easier access to guns. A total of 10% to 15% of high school seniors admitted to committing at least one serious violent act the previous year. Approximately 30% to 40% of males and 15% to 30% of females are reported to have committed a serious violent act at some point in their lives. There were more arrests for violent crimes committed by African-Americans and Hispanics, but confidential surveys completed by adolescents demonstrated a more narrow racial disparity (Report of the Surgeon General, 2001).

There are many factors that predict risk for violence (Box 15-2).

| Box 15-2 | Risk Factors for Violence |

Childhood
Low IQ
Attention deficit/hyperactivity disorder
Delinquent behavior
Substance abuse
Poverty
Neglect
Parents with antisocial personality
Single-parent homes

Adolescence
Peer rejection or isolation
Substance use
Gang involvement
Associating with delinquent peers who commit crimes

Both
Male gender
Divorce of parents
Separation
Negative parent-child interaction
Witnessing domestic violence
Physical and sexual abuse

Studies have shown that exposure to violence on TV, the Internet, and video games increases aggressive behavior in children. Continued research is needed to study the long-term effects of exposure to violence (Report of the Surgeon General, 2001; Rae-Grant, 1999). Other research has also documented the relationship between aggressive behavior and exposure to violence; in particular violent interactive entertainment increases several other risk-taking and self-defeating behaviors including use of substances and alcohol, accelerated onset of sexual activity, lower grades in school, less exercise, reading fewer books, being desensitized to violence and the suffering of others, and being more fearful of the world. Children with emotional problems appear especially vulnerable (American Academy of Child and Adolescent Psychiatry, 2000, 2001; APA, 2000; Villani, 2001).

On the more positive side some protective factors have been identified. These include positive and consistent parental discipline, daily structure, positive parent-child relationships, family church involvement, parents having a high school or higher education, belief that parents care, family support, good problem-solving ability, living at home, having an internal locus of control, use of faith as a coping method, competence in daily life, and good interpersonal skills (Vance, 2002).

ADULT DISORDERS IN CHILDREN AND ADOLESCENTS
Substance Abuse
Although a large number of adolescents try drugs or alcohol, the majority do not progress to abuse or dependence. In 1996 the annual Monitoring the Future Study found that nearly one third of high school seniors reported having been drunk in the past month and one fifth reported marijuana use. Nearly 5% reported daily marijuana use (Weinberg et al., 1998). By the end of high school approximately 90% of students have tried alcohol and 40% have tried an illicit drug, typically marijuana (Bukstein et al., 1997).

It is believed that drug use appears to be more a function of social and peer factors, whereas abuse and dependence are more related to biologic and psychologic processes. Risk factors include the following: executive cognitive dysfunction; disorders of behavioral self-regulation; difficulties with planning, attention, abstract reasoning, foresight, judgment, self-monitoring, and motor control; need for sensation seeking; difficulties with affect regulation; drug-abusing parents; maternal depression; and anxiety. Factors that are thought to protect against use include the following: intelligence, problem-solving ability, social facility, positive self-esteem, supportive family relationships, positive role models, and affect regulation (Weinberg et al., 1998).

Depression
Population studies report a prevalence of major depression and dysthymia of approximately 0.4% to 2% in children and 4% to 8% in adolescents, with a lifetime prevalence of major depression in adolescents of 15% to 20% (Birmaher, 1996). Developmentally, symptoms of melancholia, psychosis, suicide attempts, lethality of attempts, and impairment of functioning increase with age. Symptoms of separation anxiety, phobias, **somatic complaints,** auditory hallucinations, temper tantrums, and behavioral problems occur more frequently in children. Psychotic depression manifests in children as auditory hallucinations instead of delusions, as seen in adolescents and adults. Children and adolescents with depression have a comorbid diagnosis in 40% to 70% of cases; those with dysthymic disorder or anxiety have a comorbid diagnosis in 30% to 80% of cases; those with disruptive disorders have comorbidity in 10% to 80% of cases; and those with substance abuse have comorbidity in 20% to 30% of cases (Birmaher et al., 1996).

Bipolar Disorder
Children frequently present with atypical symptoms that are often markedly labile and erratic rather than persistent, and irritable, belligerent, or mixed rather than euphoric. Reckless behavior often leads to school failure, fighting, dangerous play, and inappropriate sexual activity. These symptoms must be differentiated from common childhood phenomena of boasting, imaginary play, overactivity, and youthful indiscretions (McClellan et al., 1997; Beiderman, 1998).

A child may appear amusing and show misleading infectious cheerfulness in the midst of significant problems such as school suspensions and family fights. The thinking of these children frequently defies logic. These children or adolescents often harass teachers about how to teach the class. They may fail intentionally because they believe they are being taught incorrectly.

They may hold a belief that they will achieve in a prominent profession despite failing grades. They may believe that stealing is legal for them. In contrast, conduct-disordered children and adolescents know that stealing is wrong but believe they are above the law.

They often overreact to minor perturbations in the environment, behave inappropriately sexually by propositioning teachers and making overt comments to peers, or calling sex phone (1-900) lines. Individuals may become overly interested in money and purchase items from (1-800) lines with others' credit cards, and take more dangerous dares, believing that they are above the possibility of danger.

Psychosis
Schizophrenia rarely presents before age 13 years, although cases have been documented as young as 3 and 5 years. An onset before age 13 years (very-early-onset schizophrenia) usually has an insidious nature and includes withdrawal, odd behavior, and isolation. Other developmental delays have been noted, including lags in cognitive, motor, sensory, and social functioning.

The presence of psychosis in preschool-age children is an extremely difficult problem. Transient hallucinations under stress, imaginary friends, and fantasy figures are common. By the school-age years, persistent hallucinations are associated with serious disorders. Delusional content and hallucinations usually reflect developmental concerns. Hallucinations often include monsters, pets, or toys, and delusions typically revolve around identity issues and are less complex and systemic. After age 7 years, loose and illogical thinking does not usually occur in normal children (McClellan et al., 1997).

Anxiety Disorders

A pediatric primary care sample revealed a 1-year prevalence of anxiety disorders of 15.4% in 7- to 11-year-olds. Epidemiologic studies in nonreferred 11-year-olds documented the following prevalences: separation anxiety, 3.5%; overanxious disorder, 2.9%; simple phobia, 2.4%; social phobia, 1%. Risk factors for development of anxiety disorders in children include behavioral inhibition, insecure attachment, cognitive factors, developmental events, traumatic events, and access to support systems (Bernstein, Borchardt, and Perwien, 1996).

Developmental differences exist in the symptoms of anxiety. Children ages 5 to 8 years most commonly report unrealistic worry about harm to parents and attachment figures and school refusal. From ages 9 to 12 years, children report excessive distress at times of separation. Adolescents typically report somatic complaints and school refusal. At any age, unrealistic worry about future events is key in overanxious disorder in children and adolescents. School refusal is present in three fourths of those identified with separation anxiety disorder.

In a community sample, more than two fifths of youths met criteria for exposure to at least one major trauma by age 18 years. A total of 6% met the criteria for a lifetime diagnosis of posttraumatic stress disorder. Avoidance symptoms were more common in younger children. They were more likely to have spontaneous intrusive phenomena (e.g., preoccupation with words or symbols that may be related to the trauma). Older children reported more reexperiencing and arousal, particularly with specific reminders. After a natural disaster, separation from parents, ongoing maternal preoccupation with the event, and altered family functioning were greater predictors of symptom development than exposure alone (Cohen et al., 1998). Pilowsky et al. (1999) found that adolescents with panic attacks were three times more likely to verbalize suicidal thoughts and two times more likely to have attempted suicide in the past than adolescents without panic attacks.

Obsessive-compulsive disorder has a 6-month prevalence of 1 in 200 children and adolescents. Children typically demonstrate normal age-dependent obsessive-compulsive behaviors such as wanting things done "just so" and may insist on elaborate bedtime rituals. These behaviors are usually gone by middle childhood and are replaced by collections, hobbies, and focused interest. Frequently observed symptoms in children and adolescents include the following: obsessions (contamination fears); worry about harm to self or others; aggressive themes; sexual ideas; scrupulosity/religiosity; forbidden thoughts; symmetry urges; need to tell, ask, or confess; and compulsions (washing, repeating, checking, touching, counting, ordering/arranging, hoarding, praying).

THE NURSING PROCESS

The nursing process (assessment, nursing diagnosis, outcome identification, planning, implementation, and evaluation) is applicable to children and adolescents in the psychiatric setting. Knowledge of growth and development is essential, as is the ability to do a thorough clinical assessment, including both medical and psychosocial aspects. The child or adolescent must be assessed within the context of the entire family structure and dynamics, including the cultural and socioeconomic situation.

Parents often seek treatment for the child or adolescent after being referred by the school system or after their own multiple attempts to change the child or adolescent have been unsuccessful. Parents may present a medical concern (e.g., a stomachache) as the primary identified problem, when the underlying primary problem is often a psychiatric one. It can be difficult for adults to comprehend that children, especially young children, have mental disorders. As a result, treatment may be delayed for years in the hope that the child will "grow out of it."

Although it is common for a family to present a child or adolescent as the "identified client" (family member with the problem), it is important to remember that children often act out the underlying family dynamics or family psychopathology. In addition, families may deny that the child may have a disorder, such as tic disorders, obsessive-compulsive disorders, mood disorders, or psychosis, that has been identified in other family members.

Families can be skeptical of proposed treatment recommendations and discredit the therapeutic interventions. They may continue to use unhealthy multigenerational parenting techniques. Families may see initial improvement in a child or adolescent who is in treatment and then prematurely discontinue newly adopted interventions. This will inevitably result in the relapse of the child or adolescent's condition and family dysfunction. The child or adolescent may suffer academically and socially because of lack of implementation of treatment. With time and continuing growth of the child or adolescent, months or years of progress and development may be lost if the family does not continue with recommended treatment.

Treatment success and outcome depend on family commitment to learning new skills and consistently applying them. Early assessment and intervention from all caregivers and educators are the most ideal treatment goals.

ASSESSMENT

The nurse takes a thorough history, which reveals the child or adolescent's baseline level of functioning for the past year, as well as the current level of functioning. As the nurse obtains

CLINICAL ALERT

The nurse must be acutely observant of the child or adolescent who has ADHD and taking medications. Children or adolescents taking stimulant medications such as methylphenidate hydrochloride (Ritalin) may demonstrate adverse changes in appetite, sleep, and levels of restlessness. In addition, children or adolescents may develop new tics or have an exacerbation of previously existent mild tics. It is imperative that the nurse holds the medication, document the findings, and notify the provider of the clinical observations. Often changes in dosage or discontinuance of the medication are required.

CLINICAL ALERT

When working with children, the nurse must remember that the child or adolescent is a minor and that the primary caregiver/guardian has legal rights in addition to the child's rights. Children and adolescents can give **assent**, and caregivers/guardians give *informed consent*. This applies to all forms of treatment such as medications and research studied and, in the inpatient setting, to all client rights, including admission to the mental health units, and seclusion and restraint.

Whenever possible, the nurse should obtain the child or adolescent's signature on all assent and consent forms in addition to the caregiver/guardian's signature.

the history, it is important to identify and ask caregivers about the child or adolescent's strengths and positive characteristics. Children and adolescents often do not demonstrate the negative behaviors for several weeks in both inpatient and outpatient settings. Once the child or adolescent begins to act out his or her true behavioral problems, knowing and using the child's strengths can enhance the nurse-client relationship.

Developmental Stage

Each child and adolescent attempts to progress along the course of growth and development in all aspects of his or her life. Some, however, struggle in areas such as social skills; language; cognition; or the moral, psychologic, cultural, or behavioral aspects of development. Because each child and adolescent has unique strengths and weaknesses, the nurse is challenged to assess the client in the context of the family culture and socioeconomic circumstances throughout the phases of normal growth and development. Children and adolescents may experience developmental delays as a result of family traumas, social deprivation, abuse, neglect, or complications from a major mental disorder. Children and adolescents may be advanced in developmental phases in some aspects of their life, such as cognition, but may be retarded at the same time in other aspects, such as social skills.

Physical Assessment

A thorough physical assessment involving all body systems and a history of past physical development and problems are important in providing a comprehensive mental health evaluation. The nurse plays a key role in identifying potential health conditions that may contribute to the overall health and well-being of the child or adolescent. The nurse assesses the child or adolescent's immunization history, nutrition, grooming, and dental hygiene status. In addition, the nurse must assess for other health information, such as neurologic history that includes previous brain injury or seizure disorder, allergies, otitis media, sinusitis, asthma, gastrointestinal and gastrourinary functioning, patterns of food restriction, history of laxative or diuretic use and purging, diabetes, scoliosis, or other preexisting conditions. It is critical to obtain a thorough alcohol and drug history including the amount used, length of use, and the date and time of use. A drug history should consist of questions that cover all

potential methods of drug use such as sniffing paint thinner, glue, or aerosol cans; smoking; drinking; or injecting.

Family Life

The child or adolescent's family life and home environment are crucial aspects of assessment that lead comprehensive understanding of the presenting mental health problems. Many of today's families are blended and diverse, with mixed races, cultures, religions, and beliefs. An increasing number of families are affected by separation and divorce. The traditional family unit is no longer the only model. Our society has families in which children and adolescents are being raised by homosexual parents or parents who elect to live with significant others without marriage. In other families grandparents assume the role of primary caregivers as a result of financial problems, drug abuse, human immunodeficiency virus or AIDS, death, or other situations that make the biologic parents unable to raise the child or adolescent.

The nurse must gain an understanding of the types of interactions within the family relationships and each member's perception of the issues. It is important for the nurse to understand characteristics of the home environment, including cleanliness and the size of the home, where and with whom the child or adolescent sleeps, patterns for meals, pet care, chores, homework, times and frequencies of recreational activities, and bedtime rituals.

Activities of Daily Living

The child or adolescent's ADLs reveal much about the child or adolescent's level of independence or dependence and current level of developmental functioning. Many families struggle with their children or adolescents over ADLs, and a thorough assessment may reveal family dynamics with expectations that are either too high or too low for the child or adolescent. Children and adolescents often act out family power struggles over the expectations of ADLs. These power struggles may occur daily in the morning when getting the child or adolescent up and off to school, on return from school, and at bedtime. Excessive consequences or punishments, and even negative rituals, may develop within the family structure centered on the ADLs. The nurse may have a powerful impact in the role of establishing age-appropriate

COLLABORATIVE DIAGNOSES

DSM-IV-TR Diagnoses*	NANDA Diagnoses†
Autistic disorder	Impaired social interaction
	Self-care deficit
	Risk for self-mutilation
Conduct disorder	Risk for other-directed violence
	Risk for self-directed violence
	Impaired social interaction
Separation anxiety disorder	Anxiety
	Ineffective coping

*From American Psychiatric Association: *Diagnostic and Statistical Manual of Mental Disorders*, Fourth Edition, Text Revision. Washington, DC, American Psychiatric Association, 2000.
†From NANDA International (2003). NANDA Nursing Diagnoses: Definitions and Classification 2003-2004, Philadelphia: NANDA.

expectations and in teaching successful behavioral techniques to the child or adolescent and the caregivers.

NURSING DIAGNOSIS

All currently used NANDA nursing diagnoses are applicable to children and adolescents. Because of the tendency for children and adolescents to act out the many issues with which they struggle, however, some diagnoses may be more important than others. Safety issues are a first priority with any client in the mental health setting. It is even more crucial for children and adolescents, because even children who are developing normally may have little impulse control. Thus diagnoses such as risk for self-directed violence, risk for other-directed violence, and risk for injury are important for the nurse to consider. This is especially true in some of the pervasive developmental disorders in which autistic behaviors can lead to self-mutilating activities and, in the case of ADHD, where extreme impulsivity and hyperactive behavior can result in injury (see Collaborative Diagnosis table).

Communication and relationship issues present a challenge for the diagnostic process. Children, especially young children, often do not have adequate verbal skills to effectively communicate their needs and feelings to the nurse. In some developmental disorders this may be even more of a complicating factor. For adolescents, mistrust of authority and power may cause difficulty in the development of the nurse-client relationship and hinder care. Thus diagnoses related to difficulties in communication may be indicated. In addition, the diagnosis of delayed growth and development should be considered when there is a series of deficits that affect nursing care and discharge planning.

Finally, family issues may be more pertinent for the nurse to consider than other client needs or problems. Ineffective role performance, impaired parenting, and interrupted family processes are all important diagnoses for the nurse to

consider. The needs of the family must always be considered in the process of assigning nursing diagnoses.

OUTCOME IDENTIFICATION

Outcome criteria flow from the nursing diagnosis in the nursing process and are stated in simple terms. Outcome criteria for children and adolescents focus on promotion of normal growth and development in an effort to improve areas of current developmental deficits in addition to improving any dysfunction that is identified. Outcome criteria integrate treatment goals of the interdisciplinary team, caregivers, and the child or adolescent. Children and adolescents are more motivated to actively participate in the treatment process when they are included in decisions.

Examples of outcome criteria are:
Client will:
- Demonstrate age-appropriate relationships with adults.
- Demonstrate age-appropriate relationships with peers.
- Demonstrate a decrease or elimination of aggressive behaviors toward self and others.
- Use age-appropriate play and recreational activities to express self.
- Identify triggers that may provoke negative behavioral responses.
- Seek assistance and support from adults before losing self-control.

PLANNING

In the beginning phases of the nursing process, the nurse sets realistic expectations based on the child or adolescent's developmental level of ability and function. The nurse is aware that negative behavioral patterns may have been an integral part of the family dynamics and often have been established for long periods. Children and adolescents want the world to be fair, and they resist treatment plans that are set too high and too suddenly. They also resist insincerity from adult authority figures. Ideally the nurse plans for small, incremental changes in behavior, with obtainable goals. The nurse's effort for mutual goal setting will demonstrate respect and trust with the child or adolescent. The nurse may explain the plan to the child or adolescent in simple terms, requesting their active participation and best effort, with the understanding that the nurse will work in a cooperative effort with the patient to obtain these treatment goals.

IMPLEMENTATION

As the nursing plan is implemented, the nurse's role is to support the child or adolescent and the family through the behavioral change process. The child or adolescent will be tempted to continue to use previously established behaviors, many of which may be negative. The nurse can demonstrate clear, consistent, and realistic expectations using role-modeling and communication skills. The nurse needs to set consistent boundaries and limits as the child or adolescent questions authority and struggles to learn adaptive developmental functioning.

NURSING CARE PLAN

Michael, a 9-year-old boy, was admitted to the children's unit after he attempted to stab his teacher with a pencil. He has a history of poor peer and sibling relationships, frequently being placed on detention at school for fighting with peers during recess. He has taken Ritalin for the past year after he was diagnosed with attention deficit hyperactivity disorder. His mother complains that Michael continues to have a low frustration tolerance, often displaying temper outbursts when he does not get his way or when he is asked to do his homework or chores. He physically assaulted his 6-year-old sister when she was playing with his toy and then proceeded to break her toys. The family history includes marital discord between Michael's parents related to his father's excessive drinking. Michael's mother acknowledges that she has difficulty being consistent and firm with Michael. She thinks that her husband is too strict and she tries to compensate by being more flexible. The mother related that she has suffered from depression for the last 2 years and has been taking Paxil. The family has recently started family therapy.

DSM-IV-TR Diagnoses

Axis I:	Attention deficit/hyperactivity disorder: rule out intermittent explosive disorder
Axis II:	None
Axis III:	Asthma
Axis IV:	Severity of stressors = 3 (moderate): school detentions; alcoholism of biologic father; mother's depression
Axis V:	GAF = 45 (current)
	GAF = 55 (past year)

NURSING DIAGNOSIS: Risk for other-directed violence. Risk factors: a positive history of aggression toward peers, sibling and teacher (e.g., attempted to stab his teacher with a pencil, detentions at school).

CLIENT OUTCOMES	NURSING INTERVENTIONS	EVALUATION
Michael will demonstrate safe behaviors.	Provide close observations as indicated *to ensure the client's safety and to maintain a safe milieu.* Set firm limits and consequences for aggressive behaviors. *Structure and clear expectations clarify boundaries for improved self-control.* Identify situations that precipitate Michael's aggressive outbursts *to assist the client to identify sources of frustration.*	Michael continues to push peers and throw objects when he is angry, which results in "time out."
Michael will demonstrate alternative behaviors to violent outbursts.	Assist Michael to identify three alternative behaviors that he can use when he becomes frustrated or angry. *A specific plan precedes successful action.* Give Michael stickers for the star program every time he uses alternative behaviors *to reinforce appropriate behaviors and build self-esteem.* Encourage Michael to play with harmless foam basketball when he is frustrated or angry *to promote socially acceptable and safe ventilation of negative feelings.* Encourage Michael to draw his feelings on paper *to express his hostile feelings in safe manner.*	Michael seeks staff when he is feeling angry and on the verge of losing control 75% of the time. Michael is currently on the silver and has been able to use his Game Boy and eat in the cafeteria. Michael plays foam basketball 80% of the time when he feels frustrated. Michael draws pictures daily to help identify his feelings.
Michael will identify three situations that precipitate violent outbursts.	Encourage Michael to verbalize feelings in daily one-to-one conversations *to provide a healthy outlet for frustrations.* Discuss possible situations that precipitate Michael's violent outbursts *to connect negative feelings with aggressive actions.*	Michael verbalizes when he feels angry with peers and staff 50% of the time. Michael identifies situations that cause him to get angry (when he does not win at a game, when peers make fun of him, and when he's told he did something wrong).
Michael will follow the unit rules and maintain the silver or gold on the star program.	Provide consistent staffing *to build trusting relationships.* Set firm limits and consequences for breaking the unit rules. *Structure and clear expectations clarify boundaries for improved self-control.*	Michael is beginning to respond positively to his designated staff. Michael continues to provoke peers and require frequent time-outs during the shift. He continues to be on bronze level with no privileges.

NURSING CARE PLAN—cont'd

NURSING DIAGNOSIS: Impaired social interaction related to low self-esteem, lack of positive peer and family relationships, as evidenced by physical altercations with peers and sibling.

CLIENT OUTCOMES	NURSING INTERVENTIONS	EVALUATION
Michael will interact with peers and sibling without exhibiting aggressive behaviors.	Give Michael a sticker every time he verbalizes his anger and frustration appropriately *to reinforce appropriate behaviors and build self-esteem.*	Michael has verbalized to peers when he was angry 90% of the time and is currently on the gold of the star program. He has earned snack privileges and extended bedtime.
Michael will demonstrate good sportsmanship by not crying, yelling, or becoming aggressive when he does not win a game or by not arguing over the rules of the game.	Engage Michael in activities with peers that encourage teamwork and good sportsmanship. Give Michael a sticker every time he demonstrates good sportsmanship. *Consistent reinforcement encourages postiive responses and sets clear parameters of acceptable social interactions.*	Michael was able to accept that his team lost in a game of kickball and received positive recognition from his peers and staff for his response.

The nurse-client relationship is essential in the implementation phase. The child or adolescent looks to the nurse for the trust and respect that was set forth in the planning phase. However, the implementation phase is often the most challenging as the child or adolescent tests limits, acts out, and may become manipulative, deviant, defiant, or aggressive in an effort to revert to preexisting family dynamics and behaviors. Maintaining the safety of the child or adolescent may be a target goal in the implementation phase. It is common for the adolescent to be increasingly aggressive, often resulting in seclusion and restraint. The child or adolescent may fail repeatedly in the initial phases of treatment. The nurse is the catalyst to promote the change process, and the child or adolescent looks for reassurance, encouragement, and support from the nurse. The nurse constantly reassesses the expectations throughout the implementation phase to ensure realistic and obtainable goals for the child or adolescent. It may be necessary to reset expectations if they are either too easy or too difficult to achieve.

Therapeutic Play

For the younger child, nursing interventions take place in activities of **therapeutic play.** Play is the work of children. Children can use recreational and creative play activities in relationships with peers and adults as they work to master new developmental tasks. Because language skills are not fully developed, they may express their thoughts, feelings, frustrations, fears, and hopes through therapeutic play. The astute nurse keenly observes the child in play and interacts to modify distortions and reestablish healthy boundaries and safe parameters as the child redefines behaviors through play.

Group play and recreational activities are other means to assist the child or adolescent in developing positive peer communication and improve interpersonal relationships. Group play can be an excellent opportunity for the nurse to role model and teach new age-appropriate skills, reinforce positive behaviors, and promote nurturing peer relation-

ships. The nurse sets limits in group play to promote a safe environment and to demonstrate showing cooperation and respect to peers. Children and adolescents often have learned to tease and provoke peers in group settings. The nurse can assist them in redefining successful relationships.

The Adolescent

Interventions with adolescents are often more difficult than with children, depending on the clinical presentation. It is normal growth and development behavior for adolescents to question authority and test limits and rules. The nurse must establish rapport and a therapeutic alliance with the adolescent early in the course of treatment. Nursing interventions that promote development of a trusting nurse-client relationship are fundamental to working with adolescents. The nurse sincerely communicates empathy and understanding regarding the difficult developmental issues the adolescent encounters at this stage. Adolescents resist the nurse's efforts to exercise authoritative power over their point of view. The nurse works to integrate the caregiver's perspective with that of the adolescent.

Because adolescents need and search for role models, it is imperative that the nurse maintain appropriate boundaries and not behave as an adolescent or peer friend to gain their acceptance. Adolescents may attempt to be flirtatious with nursing personnel of both genders, and the nurse has the opportunity to demonstrate self-control, respect, and mature modeling of healthy interpersonal relationships. The nurse continues to demonstrate empathy, understanding, sincerity, and caring, while at the same time role modeling consistent adult interactions and boundaries.

Group activities provide an excellent opportunity for the nurse to interact with adolescents during treatment. Group activities enable the adolescent to develop interpersonal skills, give and accept feedback and communicate with peers, attempt to implement more adultlike relationships, and listen and learn successful and appropriate ways to interact with the world.

Behavior Modification Programs

For the child approximately 3 to 11 years old, a behavior modification program is frequently used in treatment plans. **Behavior modification** involves a systematic and structured program that is extremely effective. A behavior modification program establishes developmental and age-appropriate goals that are observable and measurable within an established time frame. The goals are often geared toward ADLs, impulse control, and peer and sibling relationships. The child is rewarded for the accomplishment of each goal. There often is a chart that correlates with each goal, and the child is rewarded with stars, stickers, or colors to signify progress. Many school systems use colored charts, and a behavior program can be implemented in the home to correlate with the school program. This provides the necessary consistency and a stable, structured program for the child and the family to use.

Preadolescents and adolescents are less likely to use a structured behavior modification program with a chart that uses rewards such as stars and stickers. They may perceive this program as insulting as they strive for independence and autonomy. Preadolescents and adolescents often use behavioral contracts. These contracts may emphasize one to three goals that are more psychodynamic in nature (e.g., will speak to others with respect; will actively participate in group activities). Instead of giving such things as stars and stickers when the preadolescent or adolescent accomplishes goals, a checkmark can be placed after each goal to signify that the adolescent has accomplished that goal. Rewards in the form of increased privileges may be one outcome of maintaining the contract.

Nursing Interventions

1. The most critical intervention is to maintain a safe environment at all times. Assess for potential dangers, **contraband,** the presence of suicidal ideation, and plans or access to a method (pills, weapons, etc.) and always ensure safety.
2. Monitor and continually assess for behavioral changes and signals that may indicate increasing irritation, frustration, anger, hostility, or distorted thinking that may result in assaultive behaviors *to prevent violence.*
3. Communicate respect and trust, both verbally and nonverbally, *to promote a therapeutic alliance with the child or adolescent.*
4. Maintain a therapeutic environment by setting simple, fair, and consistent limits *to promote healthy boundaries and expectations.*
5. Use positive reinforcement and praise with genuine sincerity *to promote and increase self-esteem and confidence.*
6. Communicate effectively with the family and child or adolescent *to reinforce treatment gains and application of new skills in the home.*

Additional Treatment Modalities

A variety of collaborative interventions are used with children and adolescents in the mental health setting. Medications have been used for decades, often with great success. The classifications and doses are changing rapidly, with the emphasis on biologic psychiatry in the twenty-first century. Many medications used with adults can be used with children and adolescents. The predominant classifications remain stimulants, antidepressants, antianxiety agents, anticonvulsants, and antipsychotics. The nurse plays a crucial role in administering medication, monitoring for clinical effectiveness and adverse reactions, assessing for titration of dose and times of medication administration, and promoting optimal health functioning. The nurse plays a key role in the communication of these findings to the multidisciplinary treatment team and to the primary care provider. The nurse must continually be educated regarding current and newly developed medications and their clinical impact on this population.

Recreational, occupational, music, and art therapies, as well as school, group, family, and individual therapies, are treatment modalities that also play a significant role in this population to promote overall health and well-being for the child and adolescent. Close coordination and communication by the entire multidisciplinary team enhance developmental gains and reinforce newly established therapeutic skills. The nurse involved in these modalities can assess the patient in various settings while at the same time promoting development of growth and fine motor skills and interpersonal development.

The nurse remains realistic during the intervention phase of treatment while maintaining a hopeful outlook. Most individuals with moderate mental retardation acquire some communication skills during early childhood and may benefit from vocational training, but they seldom advance academically beyond the second grade level. They can generally live in the community in group homes or with their families unless some other physical or mental challenge requires specialized care.

EVALUATION

The evaluation phase of the nursing process documents the treatment progress as evidenced by actual outcomes. The observant nurse objectively reviews the evaluation phase to determine the effectiveness of the treatment plan. In addition to outcomes, the nurse examines other factors. For instance, were the treatment goals cognitively and developmentally appropriate for the child or adolescent? Are there other stressors within the family or social support system that may be compounding the presenting problems, thus contributing to unrealistic expectations of the child or adolescent (e.g., health, financial, or placement problems)?

It is possible to have the correct treatment goals but overestimate or underestimate the potential for the child. This may be easily corrected by modifying the measurable component. For example, if the nurse stated that Johnny would decrease negative peer interactions by 90% in 1 week and at the end of 1 week Johnny has made no progress whatsoever, it would be unrealistic to continue to expect a 90% decrease. Modification of the percentage (e.g., decreased to 60%) and/or the time frame (e.g., increased to 3 weeks) would result in a more realistic expected outcome for the child to accomplish.

It is wise to use the expertise of the multidisciplinary team to coordinate care plan modifications in an effort to maintain implementation cohesiveness. It is also important to continually communicate the treatment evaluation with the caregivers. This helps to reinforce treatment gains, reinforce new methods of parental interventions, and assist the caregivers in monitoring and reestablishing new and realistic expectations. As stated earlier, many of the behavior problems have been longstanding, so it will take an increased amount of time to see marked change.

Inpatient hospitalization time has been severely shortened as a result of pressures from the insurance and health care industries. Therefore it is critical for the nurse to assist the caregivers in comprehending the treatment goals and teach them to implement and evaluate the care plan in the home setting. It is recommended that the nurse begin early in the course of treatment with the family to prepare them for the potential and pending discharge. Work initially begun in an inpatient setting is transitioned to home or other placement such as day treatment, residential care, or a group home. In more severe and chronic cases, state hospitals for the mentally ill may be a placement setting for the discharged child or adolescent. These placements are becoming severely limited as states and counties throughout the country privatize mental health services. More and more often, children with severe and chronic mental disorders are returning to the home setting, with the responsibility and burden of care falling on the family.

When working with children and adolescents, the nurse is aware of the significance of the nurse-client relationship and permits appropriate time for healthy termination. Children and adolescents frequently act out with increasing negativity at the time of termination. It can be a challenge for the nurse to continue to be nurturing and therapeutic while role modeling the termination process in a manner that maintains the integrity, respect, and trust established in the treatment process. This role modeling may set a lifelong impression for healthy termination, and its significance to the child and adolescent in the mental health setting must not be underestimated.

In the evaluation phase, the nurse encourages the child or adolescent and the family to make healthy transitions to the ongoing therapeutic relationship that will be maintained with the next primary mental health provider (i.e., nurse specialist, social worker, psychologist, or psychiatrist). The nurse's role is fundamental for the child or adolescent during the therapeutic treatment process, even if much work lies ahead in the future treatment of the client and family.

CHAPTER SUMMARY

- Encopresis often is the result of a major power struggle between the child/adolescent and an authority figure.
- Of mentally retarded individuals, 85% are mildly retarded, 10% are moderately retarded, 3% to 4% are severely retarded, and 1% to 2% are profoundly retarded.

- Children with autistic disorder present with repetitive movements, no emotional reciprocity, impaired communication (both verbal and nonverbal), and an indifference to affection; 75% have some degree of mental retardation.
- The most commonly diagnosed mental disorders are attention deficit/hyperactivity disorder (ADHD), mood disorder, pervasive development disorder, stereotype movement disorder, and mental disorders resulting from a general medical condition.
- Children with ADHD may have the following histories: child abuse or neglect, multiple foster placements, neurotoxin exposure, infections, drug exposure in utero, low birth weight, and mental retardation.
- ADHD causes problems in academics, social relationships, self-esteem, and occupation because of its manifestations of demanding personality, impulsivity, and seeming laziness.
- Separation anxiety is a disruptive disorder that prevents children from engaging in normal activities because of incessant fear that their loved ones will be harmed in their absence.
- Like autistic disorder, Tourette's disorder involves repetitive movements, sounds, and actions; however, unlike autistic disorder, these symptoms diminish during adolescence and adulthood.
- One of the main characteristics of conduct disorder is the client's violent and/or aggressive behavior with little concern for those who are affected by his or her actions.
- Behavior modification programs are systematic structured plans with specific goals and time frames. The client is rewarded for goal attainment.
- Early identification and treatment of the child and adolescent may assist the client in the home, school, and social setting for both the long and short term.
- Nursing interventions with children and adolescents are intense and challenging. The nurse must work closely with the family and the multidisciplinary team.

REVIEW QUESTIONS

1. Which statement by the parent of a 4-year-old who was diagnosed with moderate mental retardation show his understanding of mental retardation?
   a. "If I have tutors to assist with my daughter's education, can she still go to college?"
   b. "I will give my daughter all the support necessary so that she can develop skills to help support herself when she is an adult."
   c. "She will never be able to talk to me and tell me how she feels."
   d. "I told my wife to stop drinking caffeine when she was pregnant."

2. A father brings his 3-year-old child to be assessed. The father states that his son doesn't play with other kids, doesn't enjoy playing with his toys, hasn't spoken his first word yet, and spins the tire of his toy constantly. The nurse determines that the client may have:
   a. Mental retardation
   b. Tourette's disorder
   c. Autism
   d. Attention deficit/hyperactivity disorder

3. Which statement demonstrates that the mother understands the diagnosis of attention deficit/hyperactivity disorder?
   a. "My son will never go to college."
   b. "My son's performance will improve in a structured setting that provides rewards for appropriate behavior."
   c. "My son doesn't have anything wrong with him. He just had bad teachers."
   d. "He's just going through a stage."

4. Which nursing intervention would be the most effective for a 9-year-old client diagnosed with ADHD?
   a. Play therapy
   b. Milieu therapy
   c. Family therapy
   d. Behavior modification

5. A 16-year-old client hospitalized for out of control behavior and diagnosed with oppositional defiant disorder is preparing for discharge. Which discharge criterion must be met before discharge?
   a. The client agrees to develop a behavior contract with rules and rewards and consequences.
   b. The client has an absence of anger or frustration for 1 week.
   c. Nurse arranges for discharge placement with someone other than the client's parents until they can develop better communication skills.
   d. Physician arranges for the client to enter a military academy for structure and discipline.

REFERENCES

American Academy of Child and Adolescent Psychiatry: Children and Watching TV, *Facts for Families No 54* 2001.

American Academy of Child and Adolescent Psychiatry: AACAP Joint Health Organizations' Consensus on Entertainment Violence Danger, *News Release* 2000.

American Psychological Association: Family and Relationships: Children and Television Violence, website: helping.apa.org/family/kidtvviol.html.

American Psychiatric Association: *Diagnostic and Statistical Manual of Mental Disorders*, Fourth Edition, Text Revision. Washington, DC, American Psychiatric Association, 2000.

Bauermeister J et al: Epidemiology of disruptive behavior disorders, *Child Adolesc Psychiatry Clin North Am* vol 3, no 2, 1994.

Beiderman J: Resolved: mania is mistaken for ADHD in prepubertal children: affirmative, *J Am Acad Child Adolesc Psychiatry* 37:1091-1093, 1998.

Beitchman J et al: Practice parameters for the assessment and treatment of children and adolescents with language and learning disorders, *J Am Acad Child Adolesc Psychiatry* 37(suppl 10):46S-62S, 1998.

Beitchman J, Yound A: Learning disorders with emphasis on reading disorders: a review of the past 10 years, *J Am Acad Child Adolesc Psychiatry* 36:8, 1997.

Bernstein GA, Borchardt CM, Perwien AR: Anxiety disorder in children and adolescents: a review of the past 10 years, *J Am Acad Child Adolesc Psychiatry* 35:9, 1996.

Birmaher B et al: Childhood and adolescent depression: a review of the past 10 years, part I, *J Am Acad Child Adolesc Psychiatry* 35:11, 1996.

Bukstein O et al: Practice parameters for the assessment and treatment of children and adolescents with substance use disorders, *J Am Acad Child Adolesc Psychiatry* 36:10, 1997.

Cantwell DP: Attention deficit disorder: a review of the past 10 years, *J Am Acad Child Adolesc Psychiatry* 35:8, 1996.

Cohen J et al: Summary of the practice parameters for the assessment and treatment of children and adolescents with posttraumatic stress disorder, *J Am Acad Child Adolesc Psychiatry* 37:9 1998.

Dulcan M et al: Practice parameters for the assessment and treatment of children, adolescents, and adults with attention-deficit/hyperactivity disorder, *J Am Acad Child Adolesc Psychiatry* 36(suppl 10):85S-121S, 1997.

Gould MS et al: Psychopathology associated with suicide ideation and attempts among children and adolescents, *J Am Acad Child Adolesc Psychiatry* 37(9):915-923, 1998.

Hirshberg JC: Child psychiatry: introduction. In Kaplan H et al, editors: *Comprehensive textbook of psychiatry/III*, ed 3, vol 3, Baltimore, 1980, Williams & Wilkins.

King NJ: School refusal in children and adolescents: a review of the past 10 years, *J Am Acad Child Adolesc Psychiatry* 40:2, 2001.

Lewis M: A structural overview of psychopathology in childhood and adolescence. In Kaplan H et al, editors: *Comprehensive textbook of psychiatry/III*, ed 3, vol 3, Baltimore, 1980, Williams & Wilkins.

Loeber R: Oppositional defiant disorder and conduct disorder: a review of the past 10 years. Part I, *J Am Acad Child Adolesc Psychiatry* 39:12, 2000.

McClellan J et al: Practice parameters for the assessment and treatment of children and adolescents with bipolar disorder, *J Am Acad Child Adolesc Psychiatry* 36(suppl 10):157S-176S, 1997.

Mikkelsen E: Enuresis and encopresis: ten years of progress, *J Am Acad Child Adolesc Psychiatry* 40:10, 2001.

NANDA International (2003). NANDA Nursing Diagnoses: Definitions and Classification 2003-2004, Philadelphia: NANDA.

Nearns J: Attention deficit/hyperactivity disorder, *CME Resource* 1-28, 1997.

Pilowsky E et al: Panic attacks and suicide attempts in mid-adolescence, *Am J Psychiatry* 156:1545-1549, 1999.

Pliszka S: The Texas Children's Medication Algorithm Project: Report of the Texas Consensus Conference Panel on Medication Treatment of Childhood Attention Deficit/Hyperactivity Disorder: Part II Tactics, *J Am Acad Child Adolesc Psychiatry* 39:7, 2000.

Rae-Grant N: Violent behavior in children and youth: preventive intervention from a psychiatric perspective, *J Am Acad Child Adolesc Psychiatry* 38:3, 1999.

Shaffer D et al: Practice parameters for the assessment and treatment of children and adolescents with suicidal behavior, *J Am Acad Child Adolesc Psychiatry* 40:7, 2001.

Steiner H et al: Practice parameters for assessment and treatment of children and adolescents with conduct disorder, *J Am Acad Child Adolesc Psychiatry* 36(suppl 10):122S-139S, 1997.

Szymanski L et al: Practice parameters for the assessment and treatment of children, adolescents and adults with mental retardation and comorbid mental disorders, *J Am Acad Child Adolesc Psychiatry* 38:12, 1999.

Tanguay PE: Pervasive developmental disorders: a 10-year review, *J Am Acad Child Adolesc Psychiatry* 39:9, 2000.

Toppleberg CO: Language disorders: a 10-year research update review, *J Am Acad Child Adolesc Psychiatry* 39:2, 2000.

Vance JE et al: Risk and protective factors as predictors of outcome in adolescents with psychiatric disorder and aggression, *J Am Acad Child Adolesc Psychiatry* 41:1, 2002.

Villani S: Impact of media on children and adolescents: a 10-year review of the research, *J Am Acad Child Adolesc Psychiatry* 40:4, 2001.

Volkmar FR: Practice parameters for the assessment and treatment of children, adolescents, and adults with autism and other pervasive developmental disorders, *J Am Acad Child Adolesc Psychiatry* 38:55S-76S, 1999.

Wagner K et al: Cognitive factors related to suicidal ideation and resolution in psychiatrically hospitalized children and adolescents, *Am J Psychiatry* 157:2017-2021, 2000.

Weinberg NZ et al: Adolescent substance abuse: a review of the past 10 years, *J Am Acad Child Adolesc Psychiatry* 37:3, 1998.

Youth Violence: *A report of the Surgeon General*, Washington, DC, January 2001, USPHS, Office of the Surgeon General.

ONLINE RESOURCES
Publications/Journals

American Psychiatric Publishing, Inc: www.appi.org

Journal of the American Academy of Child and Adolescent Psychiatry: www.jaacap.com

Youth Violence: Report of the Surgeon General: www.surgeongeneral.gov./library/youthviolence/

Associations

American Psychiatric Association: www.psych.org

American Psychiatric Nurses Association: www.apna.org

American Academy of Child and Adolescent Psychiatry: www.aacap.org

Association of Child and Adolescent Psychiatry Nursing: www.ispn-psych.org/html/acapn.html

National Alliance for the Mentally Ill: website: www.nami.org

National Joint Committee on Learning Disabilities: www.ldonline.org/njcld

National Association for Prevention of Child Abuse and Neglect: www.napcan.org.au/

National Youth Violence Prevention Resource Center: www.safeyouth.org/home.htm

16 Eating Disorders

Anne Clarkin-Watts

OBJECTIVES

- Identify the behavioral and psychologic symptoms of anorexia nervosa and bulimia nervosa.

- Compare and contrast the medical complications of anorexic and bulimic behavior.

- Analyze the complex interplay of biologic, sociocultural, familial, and psychologic factors that contribute to the etiology of eating disorders.

- Explain the "vicious cycle" of eating disorder behavior.

- Discuss the psychologic issues that underlie eating disorder behavior.

- Describe the type of therapeutic relationship that is most effective with clients with eating disorders, including the approach and attitude the nurse should demonstrate to achieve this relationship.

- Apply the nursing process for clients with eating disorders.

Eating disorders have many facets and many causes. Although they have become quite common and are seen in a variety of clinical settings, eating disorders are considered to be a relatively new phenomenon. Self-starvation, bingeing, and purging have existed for centuries, but historically have been rare and poorly understood conditions. The incidence of **anorexia nervosa,** characterized primarily by self-starvation and distorted body image, and **bulimia nervosa,** characterized primarily by binge eating and purging behavior, has increased dramatically in the last quarter-century. With this increase has come a rapidly growing body of literature, including medical research, psychiatric research, psychologic literature, and popular press, as well as enormous media attention. This information has helped to educate us about eating disorders, but many controversies and conflicts have ensued.

Throughout history it appears that women have used food as a symbol to express a variety of issues in a variety of contexts. Because food has always been a compelling cultural symbol (of wealth, nurturing, and survival), the rejection of food and denial of appetite are always attention-getters. Although most individuals with eating disorders are female, some males also suffer from anorexia nervosa and bulimia nervosa.

The increase in eating disorders in the late twentieth century has coincided with three major cultural trends: the fashion industry, the diet and fitness industry, and the women's movement. A trend toward thinness in fashion, the creation of the diet and fitness industry, and changes in the women's movement have all contributed to the current epidemic of eating disorders. Box 16-1 summarizes these cultural trends.

HISTORICAL AND THEORETIC PERSPECTIVES

Eating disorders are not just a late twentieth-century fad of young, fashion-conscious American women; they have existed in various forms for hundreds of years. The explosion of written material on eating disorders includes some careful and thorough research into the history of both anorexia nervosa and bulimia nervosa (Bell, 1987; Brumberg, 1989).

Incidence in History

Brumberg, in *Fasting Girls* (1989), and Bell, in *Holy Anorexia* (1987), note that medieval women commonly starved themselves in devotion to Christ. Both authors detail the case of Saint Catherine of Siena, Italy (1347-1380), who kept an extensive diary of her fasting and self-induced vomiting. Her piety also included self-flagellation and other self-punishing behavior, not very different from the self-destructive behavior common today among clients with anorexia and bulimia. This demonstrates the intertwining of anorexic and bulimic behaviors from the beginning of their known existence.

Few clinical accounts of normal-weight bulimia nervosa existed until the twentieth century, when case histories began to appear in psychoanalytic literature. In "The Case of Ellen West," American psychoanalyst Binswanger (1958) described a woman he treated in 1915. She dieted from 165

Box 16-1   Cultural Trends and Eating Disorders

Fashion Industry

Cultural ideals of beauty have always been reflected in the fashion of the day. The trend in fashion since the 1960s has been more and more toward thinness. By the late twentieth century, fashion had become a huge industry, fueled by advertising dollars and exerting great influence on women. With the media as the vehicle, women are bombarded with images of the thin, fit, "perfect" woman, an ideal that is unattainable for most women. Epidemiologic studies show that 0.1% of women have a natural body type that matches the ideal, leading most to believe that their normal, healthy shape is too fat. The pervasiveness of this trend is reflected in the dieting behavior and body dissatisfaction among high school, elementary school, and middle school children.

Diet and Fitness Industry

The second trend is the birth of the diet and fitness industry. Since the 1950s, weight management has moved out of the doctor's office, into multibillion-dollar businesses run by opportunistic entrepreneurs who are not part of the health professions. Women are deluged by the media with an array of products such as pills, powders, packaged food, diet books, videos, and a variety of health club and diet program memberships designed to help them attain the "perfect body."

Women's Movement

A third trend is the ongoing women's movement. Although women's struggles for equality are not new, women's roles have changed dramatically during the last 20 to 25 years. Pressure to be "superwoman"—to balance motherhood, marriage, and career—is new, and has influenced women of all generations. The need for women to achieve success both academically and professionally, while still fulfilling their traditional female roles, creates conflicts, even as it affords women greater societal rights and freedom.

Professional women need to be assertive and even aggressive to successfully compete in the business world, yet women are still socialized to be passive and accommodating. Some feminist writers, such as Susie Orbach and Susan Wooley, view the drive for thinness as possibly symbolizing a woman's attempt to destroy her femininity to compete in a man's world, or as male society's backlash against the women's movement. Pressuring women to strive for an impossible ideal of thinness may promote feelings of inadequacy that drive women to constantly diet and exercise to please men (Orbach, 1978; Wooley and Wooley, 1985).

---

to 92 pounds; she binged and purged with self-induced vomiting, excessive exercise, and laxative abuse. Obsessed with food and clinically depressed, she committed suicide 13 years later. In *The Fifty Minute Hour,* psychiatrist Robert Lindner (1955) describes the case of "Laura," a client with bulimia nervosa.

Given that these are psychoanalytic case studies, they do not include any discussion of sociocultural or biologic influences, but instead focus on the bulimic symptom complex as a manifestation of oral impregnation fears, oral eroticism, rejection of femininity, and unconscious hatred of the mother. A few less well-known case studies noted bulimic behavior among young girls in boarding schools and refugee children (Johnson and Connors, 1987). These cases were clearly related to separation issues, a primary factor in the development of bulimia nervosa among college women today.

In the 1950s binge eating among the overweight and obese population was described as another form of eating disorder (Hamburger, 1951; Stunkard, 1959). This common condition was compared with alcoholism, with its similar cravings and secret binges, followed by shame and guilt. The term *compulsive overeating* was used to describe this disorder until *binge eating disorder (BED)* was proposed as a diagnosis.

In the mid-1970s psychologist Marlene Boskind-Lodahl described a group of normal- and low-normal-weight women she saw at Cornell University's mental health clinic, who shared the anorectic individual's fear of fat and drive for thinness and who regularly binged and purged, but were not emaciated. In her 1983 book, the author described her extensive clinical experience and groundbreaking research with this group, who represented the first wave of the current outbreak of eating disorders (Boskind-Lodahl and White, 1983). The term *bulimia nervosa* was coined by Russell (1979), linking bulimia to anorexia nervosa.

ETIOLOGY

A variety of etiologic theories regarding eating disorders have been explored. Except for a few extremists, there has been a convergence among many disparate etiologic views from biology, sociology, psychoanalysis, and other models, to form a model of eating disorders as multifaceted, multi-determined syndromes. Most of the current literature describes eating disorders as complex, with biologic, sociocultural, and psychodynamic variables (Box 16-2).

Box 16-2 Etiologic Factors Related to Eating Disorders

Biologic Factors
Family history of depression
Tendency to be overweight

Sociocultural Factors
Diet and fitness industry
Fashion industry
Women's movement
Developmental peer pressure

Psychologic Factors
Low self-esteem
Perfectionism
Affective instability
Interoceptive deficits
Ineffectiveness
Compliance—a "people pleaser"

Familial Factors
Enmeshment
Poor conflict resolution
Separation/individuation issues
Some incidence of alcoholism or physical or sexual abuse

Biologic Factors

The many physiologic abnormalities found in anorexia nervosa and bulimia nervosa suggest a biologic basis for eating disorders. Although a great deal of research has examined abnormal hormone functioning, hypothalamic dysfunction, and neurologic aberrations, it is difficult to determine whether the abnormalities are causes of eating disorders or effects of the extreme behaviors of starving, bingeing, and purging, especially because most of these neuroendocrine changes reverse with weight gain and proper nutrition. Further complicating the picture is the fact that many of the biologic effects of eating disorder behavior sustain and perpetuate them. For example, starving can decrease appetite and the sense of smell, resulting in less desire to eat (Polivy and Herman, 2002).

Twin and family studies suggest a genetic link in that eating disorders definitely run in families (Fairburn et al., 1999). New research has located preliminary evidence that a gene on chromosome 1 may render some individuals susceptible to anorexia nervosa and that genes that control ovarian hormones may be related to eating disorders (Grice et al., 2002; Klump, Kaye, and Strober, 2001).

The high comorbidity of depression and eating disorders has been carefully studied for a biologic link. Serotonergic abnormalities have been noted in both anorexia nervosa and bulimia nervosa, even among recovered bulimics (Kaye et al., 2001b). Bulimia nervosa responds favorably to selective serotonin reuptake inhibitors (SSRIs), particularly fluoxetine (Prozac) (Romano et al., 2002).

Sociocultural Factors

By adolescence the preanorexic or prebulimic woman has been exposed to countless advertisements, fueled by the diet and fashion industries, that encourage her to eat, dress, and exercise to look beautiful. She has learned from an early age to idealize an unrealistically thin shape and thus likely be dissatisfied with her own body (Groesz et al., 2002). She has likely equated food with pleasure, comfort, and love and may have been nurtured, punished, or rewarded with food within her family.

Frequently the person with anorexia nervosa or bulimia nervosa has been observing her mother's struggles to balance all of society's expectations. She may have watched her mother try to maintain a feminine image while striving to achieve the superwoman role. Such conflicting dynamics influence the woman's eating patterns.

Psychologic Factors

Although the same sociocultural pressures challenge all adolescents, only a few, approximately 8%, develop eating disorders. Some teens seem to cope more effectively than others based on their personalities and support systems. Personality traits common among those with eating disorders include:

- Low self-esteem
- Perfectionism
- Social insecurity
- **Affective instability** (rapidly fluctuating moods)

- **Interoceptive deficits** (inability to correctly identify and respond to bodily sensations)
- **Alexithymia** (difficulty naming and expressing emotions)
- Immaturity
- Compliance
- A sense of ineffectiveness in dealing with the world
- Interpersonal distrust

These traits increase vulnerability to eating disorders (Garner, 1991). Cognitive therapy literature describes certain distorted thinking patterns as characteristic of eating disorders (Bauer and Anderson, 1989). They include **dichotomous thinking** (individuals view situations as either all good or all bad), erroneous control issues (individuals feel solely responsible for the happiness and failure of others), and personalization (individuals compare themselves endlessly with others and believe everything other people do is a reaction to them).

Familial Factors

Personality characteristics can be influenced by family environment. In 1978 Minuchin, Rosman, and Baker described a stereotypical "eating disorder family" as Caucasian, upper-middle class, intact, enmeshed, rigid, and hostile. Nowadays, eating disorders can be found in all socioeconomic levels, races, and cultures, with a range of interactive styles. However, many family environments of persons with eating disorders are tense, rigid, and enmeshed. **Enmeshed families** have poor boundaries, overinvolvement among members, and a pattern of relating in which individuality is discouraged and conformity is expected. Parents discourage the direct expression of feeling. They tend to demonstrate poor conflict resolution skills, in which disagreement may be displayed as denial of conflicts, conflict avoidance, repetitive and unproductive arguments, or escalation to violence. The result is ongoing tension, fear of conflict, and a belief that conflict is dangerous. An interesting study showed that a significant number of adolescents with eating disorders were overprotected as infants (see Understanding and Applying Research box).

These families often put a great deal of importance on outward appearance, social acceptance, and achievement. Recent research demonstrates the powerful influence of parental encouragement of dieting and preoccupation with body image. Maternal comments about their elementary school-age child being overweight can cause body dissatisfaction and dieting-strong precursors to eating disorders (Smolak, Levine, and Schermer, 1999). Girls who do not identify with their mothers are at higher risk for low self-esteem and eating disorders (Hahn-Smith and Smith, 2001). A poor marital relationship increases the risk of eating disorders in children (Wade, Bulik, and Kendler, 2001). As mentioned previously, many girls with eating disorders have a parent, sibling, or other close relative who practices eating disorder behavior (Strober et al., 2000). If a young woman sees the drive for thinness, dieting, or other extreme behaviors in her role models, she is likely to try dieting as

an attempt to improve self-esteem (Agras, Hammer, and McNicholas, 1999).

In extremely dysfunctional families the damage can be severe. Alcoholism and physical and sexual abuse have devastating effects. Emotional abuse is more subtle but very damaging. The child may not feel encouraged to be independent, to develop self-trust, or to have confidence in the child's own individual abilities. If the child learns to avoid conflict to please others, and to fear adult responsibilities, adolescence is a crisis. The sense of self never fully develops, and the pressures to separate and be an individual in adolescence can be terrifying, not only to the child but also to the parents.

Confronted with this crisis, it is not surprising that a young woman feels overwhelmed. She perceives her life as out of control and desperately wants to feel in control. The myth of thinness as the key to confidence and success portrayed in the diet program advertisement is compelling and perceived as a good way to "get control of my life." The young woman then begins dieting, loses weight, and begins to feel better about herself. Consequently, she continues dieting and losing weight, experiencing a sense of accomplishment and feeling more in control. Unfortunately, this behavior is often reinforced by **secondary gains** such as attention and envy from her peers, and often, her parents. Later, when people tell her she is getting too thin and should eat more, she feels a sense of power and control that she has never felt before. By losing weight, she not only has gotten attention, but also has been able to cause envy and to frustrate those who try to make her eat normally. These secondary gains can be very rewarding, especially to an indi-

UNDERSTANDING and APPLYING RESEARCH

Overprotective parenting has always been implicated as a familial factor in the etiology of eating disorders, but until recently there were no good studies investigating this phenomenon. In 2000 researchers in England published a study comparing 40 girls with anorexia nervosa with 40 control subjects well matched for age, ethnicity, parental marital status, birth history, and birth order. Mothers of the anorexic girls were significantly more anxious; provided near-exclusive child-care, meaning that they rarely let anyone, even the father, care for the child; and reported significant stress at the first regular separation from the child (i.e., preschool). These findings show that overprotective parenting existed before the onset of the anorexia nervosa, not just as a reaction to it. Another interesting finding in this study was that a high number of the families had experienced a miscarriage or infant death before the anorexic daughter's birth. This suggests that the parental overconcern that later contributes to the onset of anorexia nervosa may be related to unresolved grief. Clinical implications include the importance of questioning the parents about previous obstetrical losses and encouraging them to deal with unresolved grief. Verbalizing their grief may help decrease enmeshment and facilitate normal separation/individuation.

Shoebridge P, Gowers S: Parental high concern and adolescent-onset anorexia nervosa: a case-control study to investigate direction of causality, *Br J Psychiatry* 176:132, 2000.

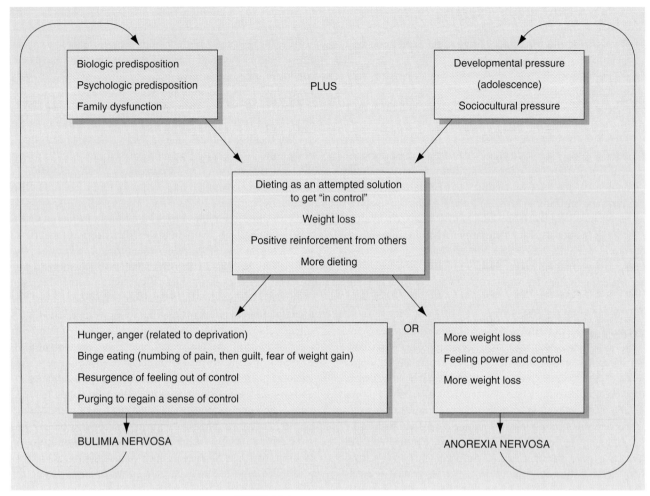

FIGURE 16-1. The cycle of eating disorders.

vidual with low self-esteem. The diet has thus distracted her from her actual conflicts and given her a sense of mastery, albeit false, which she does not want to give up.

Sometimes a young woman in this situation cannot stick to the diet. Bingeing often begins as a reaction to the deprivation of dieting. Binge eating not only relieves hunger, but also numbs pain and distracts from actual conflicts. It may also represent an angry rebellion against the pressure to be thin. The binge is temporary, however, and the problems soon come back. With them, come guilt about eating and panic about loss of control and weight gain. So the young woman purges to undo the binge—and the guilt. Figure 16-1 illustrates the interrelationship of all the etiologic factors in the cycle of eating disorders.

EPIDEMIOLOGY

Studies report wide discrepancies in estimates of the prevalence of bulimia nervosa. Studies using strict DSM-IV-TR criteria estimate that 3% to 10% of adolescent and college-age women and 2% of adolescent males are bulimic. The rate drops to 2% among the general population. However,

disturbed eating patterns, including dieting with occasional use of diet pills, laxatives, or vomiting, occurs in 13% of young women. Binge eating without purging at least once a week occurs in approximately 5% to 20% of all women and slightly fewer men. Anorexia nervosa is consistently reported at a rate of 0.5% to 1% in adolescent and college-age women. Anorexia nervosa is much less common in males. The incidence and prevalence of eating disorders are summarized in Box 16-3.

Sex Ratio

Eating disorders are predominantly female disorders. Some researchers believe eating disorders are underreported in men. Most samples report that 95% to 99% of clients with eating disorders are female.

Age of Onset

The average age of onset of bulimia nervosa is age 18 years, with 80% of cases reported with an onset between ages 15 and 30 years. In anorexia nervosa the peak ages of onset are ages 14 and 18 years. The range of onset ages for both dis-

8 million people suffer from eating disorders in the United States.

Average age of onset is 14 to 18 for anorexia nervosa; 18 for bulimia nervosa.

5%-8% of adolescent and college-age women and 2% of adolescent men have bulimia nervosa.

2% of women and less than 1% of men in the general population have bulimia nervosa.

Less than 1% of the general population has anorexia nervosa.

10% of adolescent and college-age women have subclinical anorexia nervosa; 15% have subclinical bulimia nervosa.

5%-20% of the general population (male and female) binge regularly (but do not purge).

1% of adolescent and college-age women have anorexia nervosa. Anorexia nervosa is much less common in males.

95%-99% of clients with eating disorders are female.

Mortality rates for bulimia nervosa are 0%-19%; for anorexia nervosa, mortality rates are 6%-20%.

Similar incidence and prevalence rates are found among Western countries where food is abundant and dieting is common; eating disorders are not found in developing countries.

Comorbidity

Axis I: Mood disorders; Anxiety disorders; Dissociative disorders; Substance-related disorders

Axis II: Borderline personality disorder; Avoidant personality disorder; Obsessive-compulsive personality disorder

orders is 9 to 50 years. In recent years, more cases of eating disorders, especially anorexia nervosa, are being diagnosed in middle school children.

Cross-Cultural Studies

The incidence and prevalence of eating disorders around the world are similar among European countries, the United States, Canada, Mexico, Japan, Australia, and other westernized countries with plentiful food supplies.

Developing countries do not report a significant incidence of eating disorders. It is generally believed that abundance of food is a necessary sociocultural factor for an outbreak of eating disorders (Gunewardene, Huon, and Zheng, 2001).

In the United States there is no evidence of any significant differences among racial, ethnic, or socioeconomic groups. In past decades, clients with eating disorders were predominantly Caucasian and upper-middle-class women, but this gap has disappeared.

Mortality

The mortality rate in anorexia nervosa is higher than in any other psychiatric diagnosis (Agras, 2001). Lifetime mortality rates are reported from 5% to 20% (Lowe et al., 2001; Emborg, 1999; APA, 2000). Estimates of mortality rates from bulimia nervosa range from 2% to 19%. The lower rates in some studies likely reflect that many deaths from purging are recorded as cardiac arrest or cardiomyopathy and are never connected directly to bulimia nervosa. Suicide is frequently the cause of death in persons with eating disorders.

Comorbidity

Comorbidity is the concurrent existence of two or more disorders. Eating disorders are often accompanied by other Axis I and Axis II disorders. Depression is diagnosed in 40% to 75% of individuals with eating disorders. It is diagnosed more frequently with bulimia nervosa than with anorexia nervosa. Less common than depression, but also frequently seen in clients with bulimia, are generalized anxiety disorders, obsessive-compulsive disorders, panic, dissociative disorders, or substance abuse disorders (von Ranson, Iacono, and McGue, 2002; Lewinsohn, Striegel-Moore, and Seeley, 2000; Lennkh et al., 1998).

In anorexia nervosa, obsessive-compulsive disorder is the most frequent Axis I diagnosis, followed by depression and dysthymic disorders, posttraumatic stress disorder, social phobia, and dissociative disorder (Lewinsohn, Striegel-Moore, and Seeley, 2000; Lennkh et al., 1998; Milos et al., 2002). In anorexia nervosa weight loss and malnutrition tend to exacerbate depressive, anxiety, and obsessive-compulsive symptomatology. These symptoms improve but do not disappear with weight restoration.

Numerous studies have investigated the phenomenon of *comorbid personality disorders*, which is well known to clinicians dealing with eating disorders. Varying rates of prevalence of comorbid personality disorders have been reported, with one third to three fourths of clients with eating disorders having an Axis II diagnosis. Borderline personality disorder is the Axis II diagnosis most commonly associated with eating disorders, with avoidant and obsessive-compulsive personality disorders also prevalent (Rosenvinge, Martinussen, and Ostensen, 2000).

Well-controlled research studies report a high incidence (25% to 30%) of childhood sexual abuse among clients with eating disorders. Those clients with eating disorders who had been sexually abused had a higher incidence of comorbid dissociative disorders and impulsive, self-injurious behavior (Paul et al., 2002; Wonderlich et al., 2001).

CLINICAL DESCRIPTION

Eating disorders are an easily recognizable group of psychiatric diagnoses. Refusal to eat, severe weight loss, and self-induced vomiting are unmistakable indicators of an eating disorder. However, making a precise DSM-IV-TR diagnosis and determining specific nursing diagnoses to reflect a particular client's case can be confusing and complicated tasks.

Anorexia nervosa and bulimia nervosa are the two specific eating disorder diagnoses in the DSM-IV-TR classification. The category of eating disorder not otherwise specified is provided to diagnose individuals with eating disorder symptoms who do not meet the criteria for anorexia nervosa or bulimia nervosa. The DSM-IV-TR Criteria boxes on p. 380 detail the criteria for these three diagnoses. The clinical symptoms of anorexia nervosa and bulimia nervosa are listed in the Clinical Symptoms boxes on pp. 380 and 381.

Obesity is not included as an eating disorder in the DSM-IV-TR classification because it has not been established that

DSM-IV-TR CRITERIA
Anorexia Nervosa

A. Refusal to maintain body weight at or above a minimally normal weight for age and height (e.g., weight loss leading to maintenance of body weight less than 85% of that expected, or failure to make expected weight gain during period of growth leading to body weight less than 85% of that expected)

B. Intense fear of gaining weight or becoming fat even though underweight

C. Disturbance in the way in which one's body weight or shape is experienced, undue influence of body weight or shape on self-evaluation, or denial of the seriousness of the current low body weight

D. In postmenarchal females amenorrhea (i.e., the absence of at least three consecutive menstrual cycles) (A woman is considered to have amenorrhea if her periods occur only after hormone [e.g., estrogen] administration.)

Specify type:

Restricting type: During the current episode of anorexia nervosa, the person has not regularly engaged in binge eating or purging behavior (i.e., self-induced vomiting or the misuse of laxatives, diuretics, or enemas).

Binge-eating/purging type: During the current episode of anorexia nervosa, the person has regularly engaged in binge-eating or purging behavior (i.e., self-induced vomiting or the misuse of laxatives, diuretics, or enemas).

From American Psychiatric Association: *Diagnostic and Statistical Manual of Mental Disorders,* Fourth Edition, Text Revision. Washington, DC, American Psychiatric Association, 2000.

DSM-IV-TR CRITERIA
Bulimia Nervosa

A. Recurrent episodes of binge eating. An episode of binge eating is characterized by both of the following:
  1. Eating, in a discrete period of time (e.g., within any 2-hour period), an amount of food that is definitely larger than most people would eat during a similar period of time and under similar circumstances
  2. A sense of lack of control over eating during the episode (e.g., a feeling that one cannot stop eating or control what or how much one is eating)

B. Recurrent inappropriate compensatory behavior to prevent weight gain, such as self-induced vomiting; misuse of laxatives, diuretics, enemas, or other medications; fasting; or excessive exercise

C. The binge eating and inappropriate compensatory behaviors both occur, on average, at least twice a week for 3 months.

D. Self-evaluation is unduly influenced by body shape and weight.

E. The disturbance does not occur exclusively during episodes of anorexia nervosa.

Specify type:

Purging type: During the current episode of bulimia nervosa, the person has regularly engaged in self-induced vomiting or the misuse of laxatives, diuretics, or enemas.

Nonpurging type: During the current episode of bulimia nervosa, the person has used other inappropriate compensatory behaviors such as fasting or excessive exercise, but has not regularly engaged in self-induced vomiting or the misuse of laxatives, diuretics, or enemas.

From American Psychiatric Association: *Diagnostic and Statistical Manual of Mental Disorders,* Fourth Edition, Text Revision. Washington, DC, American Psychiatric Association, 2000.

DSM-IV-TR CRITERIA
Eating Disorder Not Otherwise Specified

The Eating Disorder Not Otherwise Specified category is for disorders of eating that do not meet the criteria for a specific eating disorder. Examples include:

1. For females, all of the criteria for anorexia nervosa are met except that the individual has regular menses.
2. All of the criteria for anorexia nervosa are met except that, despite significant weight loss, the individual's current weight is in the normal range.
3. All of the criteria for bulimia nervosa are met except that the frequency of binge eating and inappropriate compensatory mechanisms occurs less than twice a week or for less than 3 months.
4. The regular use of inappropriate compensatory behavior by an individual of normal body weight after eating small amounts of food (e.g., self-induced vomiting after the consumption of two cookies).
5. Repeatedly chewing and spitting out, but not swallowing, large amounts of food.
6. Binge-eating disorder: recurrent episodes of binge eating in the absence of the regular use of inappropriate compensatory behaviors characteristic of bulimia nervosa.

From American Psychiatric Association: *Diagnostic and Statistical Manual of Mental Disorders,* Fourth Edition, Text Revision. Washington, DC, American Psychiatric Association, 2000.

CLINICAL SYMPTOMS
Anorexia Nervosa

Behavioral Symptoms
Self-starvation—reported intake restriction and refusal to eat
Rituals or compulsive behaviors regarding food, eating, and/or weight loss
May engage in self-induced vomiting, laxatives, diuretics, or excessive exercise to lose weight
May wear baggy or inappropriate layers of clothing

Physical Symptoms
Weight loss 15% below ideal weight
Amenorrhea—absence of three or more menstrual cycles when expected to occur (primary or secondary)
Slow pulse, decreased body temperature
Cachexia, sunken eyes, protruding bones, dry skin
Growth of lanugo on face
Constipation
Cold sensitivity

Psychologic Symptoms
Denial of the seriousness of current low weight
Body image disturbance (seeing self as unrealistically fat when actually at or near ideal weight, or experiencing parts of the body as unrealistically fat or out of proportion) (Figure 16-2)
Intense and irrational fear of weight gain that does not diminish as weight is lost
Constant striving for "perfect" body
Self-concept unduly influenced by shape and weight
Preoccupation with food, cooking, nutritional information, and feeding others
May exhibit delayed psychosexual development, or may lack age-appropriate interest in sex and relationships

CLINICAL SYMPTOMS

Bulimia Nervosa

Behavioral Symptoms

Recurrent episodes of binge eating (rapid consumption of a large amount of food in a discrete period of time)

Engages in **purging** behavior such as self-induced vomiting, use of laxatives, diuretics, diet pills, ipecac, enemas, excessive exercise, or periods of fasting, to compensate for the binge

Physical Symptoms

May experience fluid and electrolyte imbalances from purging:
  Hypokalemia
  Alkalosis
  Dehydration
  Idiopathic edema
Cardiovascular
  Hypotension
  Cardiac arrhythmia/dysrhythmia
  Cardiomyopathy
Endocrine
  Hypoglycemia
  May experience menstrual dysfunction
Gastrointestinal
  Constipation, diarrhea
  Gastroparesis (delayed gastric emptying)
  Esophageal reflux
  Esophagitis
  Mallory-Weiss syndrome (tears in esophagus)
  Dental
  Enamel erosion
  Parotid gland enlargement

Psychologic Symptoms

Body image disturbance
Persistent overconcern with body weight, shape, and proportions
Mood swings and irritability
Self-concept unduly influenced by body weight and shape

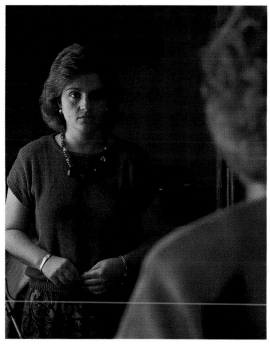

FIGURE 16-2. An individual's appearance influences self-concept. Clients with eating disorders often have a distorted view of their physical appearance, perceiving themselves as unrealistically large. (From Potter PA, Perry AG: *Fundamentals of nursing,* ed 5, St Louis, 2001, Mosby.)

all cases of obesity involve underlying psychiatric illness. Obesity itself is classified in the *International Statistical Classification of Diseases and Related Health Problems* (ICD-10) as a general medical condition (APA, 2000).

Inclusion or exclusion of **binge eating disorder (BED)** in the DSM-IV-TR classification has been a controversial issue. Although it was not included as a separate diagnosis, it is cited as an example of an eating disorder not otherwise specified and is included in the DSM-IV-TR as a proposed diagnosis for further study. BED is described specifically as recurrent episodes of binge eating, in which the individual eats more than most people would eat during a similar period and feels out of control while eating. Other criteria include distress, guilt, and disgust regarding the behavior (APA, 2000).

Anorexia nervosa and bulimia nervosa are classified as distinct diagnoses but have many overlapping features. In clinical practice many low-weight persons with anorexia binge and purge occasionally, and many individuals with bulimia nervosa use fasting and exercise, but not purging, to compensate for binges. The subtypes assist the clinician in making the most precise diagnosis. For example, if an individual meets the criteria for both bulimia nervosa and anorexia nervosa, the diagnosis of anorexia nervosa, binge eating/purging type is made, because it is the only category that includes *all* of the symptoms (neither subtype of bulimia nervosa deals with weight loss).

PROGNOSIS

The course of the illness in eating disorders is variable. A few individuals may recover fully from a single, time-limited episode of anorexia nervosa or bulimia nervosa. Some anorexic teens who recover their normal weight later develop bulimia nervosa. Many individuals with eating disorders follow a chronic course or a pattern of relapses and remissions. Others show slow improvement after several years of treatment.

A number of long-term outcome studies have emerged, showing a more promising prognosis for those clients who seek and continue treatment. More than 50% show improvement after 5 years (Polivy and Herman, 2002; Lowe et al., 2001). A review of the outcome literature indicates that long-term cognitive-behavioral, family therapy, and/or interpersonal therapy, often combined with antidepressant medication, result in the most sustained improvement in symptomatology and psychosocial functioning. Pharmacologic treatment is most effective as an adjunct to psychotherapy in bulimia nervosa and as a relapse prevention tool for weight-restored anorexics (Dare et al., 2001; Keel et al., 2002; Lowe et al., 2001; Mitchell et al., 2001; Peterson and Mitchell, 1999; Romano et al., 2002; Zhu and Walsh, 2002).

DISCHARGE CRITERIA

Client will:

- Be free from self-harm.
- Achieve minimum (within 15%) normal weight as determined by the treatment team.
- Consume adequate calories to maintain a minimum normal weight.
- Demonstrate ability to comply with the treatment regimen recommended for post discharge (i.e., compliance with medication, food plan, control over binge/purge behavior, plan for follow-up care).
- Verbalize awareness and understanding of the psychologic issues related to the eating disorder behavior and the maladaptive use of food and weight control to try to cope with these issues.
- Demonstrate the use of improved coping abilities to respond to stress and to manage emotional issues.
- Exhibit more functional behaviors within the family system.
- Demonstrate decreased enmeshment with family members.
- Attend group therapy sessions that encourage healthy eating patterns and positive self-image and self-concept.
- Interact with peers who assist the client in maintaining healthy coping patterns.
- Keep appointments to monitor behaviors and medications.

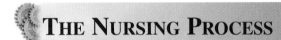

THE NURSING PROCESS

ASSESSMENT

Nursing assessment of clients with eating disorders involves sensitivity, thoroughness, and keen observation skills (Figure 16-3). The first few minutes of the interview are crucial, as first impressions set the tone for the entire treatment experience. Clients with eating disorders are sensitive to others and are quick to judge whether they are trustworthy. If a therapeutic alliance can be forged immediately, much of the power struggles can be avoided (see Case Study and Nursing Assessment Questions box).

Because many clients with eating disorders have one or more coexisting disorders, it is critical for the nurse to assess for the disorders listed in Box 16-4.

NURSING DIAGNOSIS

Nursing diagnoses are made from the information obtained during the assessment phase of the nursing process. The accuracy of diagnosis depends on a careful, in-depth assessment.

Nursing Diagnoses for Anorexia Nervosa

Safety and/or health risks:

- Risk for imbalanced body temperature
- Constipation
- Perceived constipation

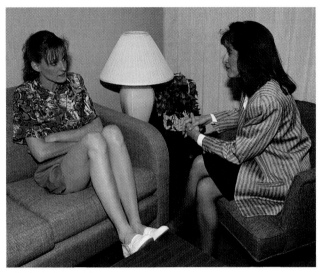

FIGURE 16-3. An initial assessment interview between a nurse and a young woman with an eating disorder.

CASE STUDY

Sarah is a 20-year-old college student who was brought to the Emergency Department by her boyfriend after she fainted in the shower. The boyfriend took the nurse aside and confided that Sarah was bulimic and that he was concerned that her eating disorder was related to the fainting episode. He said that Sarah was very secretive and somewhat defensive about the bulimia. The initial physical examination showed no injuries from the fall, and her vital signs were normal. Her parotid glands appeared enlarged. Her weight appeared within a normal range. Her affect was tense and anxious. She avoided eye contact with the nurse and mumbled that she had recently been up late studying and had not been getting enough sleep.

Critical Thinking

1. How should the nurse approach Sarah? How can the subject of bulimia nervosa be brought up?
2. If Sarah responds defensively or with denial, how should the nurse respond?
3. What further physical assessments should be done?
4. What other information is needed to complete the nursing assessment?

- Deficient fluid volume
- Risk for imbalanced fluid volume
- Delayed growth and development
- Imbalanced nutrition: less than body requirements
- Risk for self-mutilation

Perceptual/cognitive/emotional disturbances:

- Anxiety
- Disturbed body image
- Hopelessness
- Powerlessness
- Chronic low self-esteem

Problems in communicating and relating to others:

- Sexual dysfunction
- Impaired social interaction
- Social isolation

NURSING ASSESSMENT QUESTIONS

1. How do you feel about being here today? *To determine if self-referred or forced into treatment and to assess willingness to engage in treatment*
2. Have you ever talked with anyone before about your eating disorder? *To assess level of self-disclosure and to reduce anxiety and feelings of shame*
3. Have you been in therapy before? *To assess treatment history and get details of previous treatment, including the name of clinician, dates of treatment, outcomes, and client's experience of the treatment*
4. Describe your weight throughout your life. *To determine patterns and perceptions regarding weight*
   Include the following:
   Current weight, including fluctuations during past 6 months
   Desired weight
   Lowest and highest adult weight (excluding pregnancy)
   Lowest and highest adolescent weight
   Perception of childhood weight
   Perception of adolescent weight
   Perception of present weight
   Childhood experiences related to weight
5. How do you feel about the way your body looks? *To assess body dissatisfaction and body image distortion*
6. Assess dieting history:
   When did you first diet?
   What started it?
   What happened?
   Did you lose/gain?
   Has anyone encouraged you to lose weight?
   What dieting behaviors have you used? *To determine use of fasting, structured diet, restriction, diet products/programs*
7. Assess binge eating:
   Do you binge eat?

When was the first time?
Get details about typical binge eating, including when, where, duration, frequency, type and amount of food, any rituals or patterns involved. Ask if secrecy, hiding, stealing, or lying is involved. *To determine use of fasting, structured diet, restriction, diet products/programs*
Assess control (i.e., can client interrupt a binge once it has begun?).
8. Help client identify feeling states associated with the binge: before bingeing, in the planning stages, and during and after the binge.
   Ask client to focus on past binge episodes and answer this question: "Did you feel angry or anxious?" *To determine client's feelings regarding binge behaviors*
9. Assess food cravings (e.g., time of day, weekends, where in menstrual cycle, associated with places [car, work, home, store]. *To determine if client can associate cravings with specific times/situations*
10. Assess purging behavior. Include the following:
    Type (e.g., vomiting, diuretics, laxatives, diet pills, ipecac, thyroid pills, amphetamines, cocaine, exercise [type])
    Frequency (times/week)
    Amount
    Age of first use
    Date of last use
    To identify client's usual methods of purging
11. Assess menstrual history (onset of menses, regularity, premenstrual syndrome, menstrual dysfunction, any hormone therapy). *To determine effect of dysfunctional behaviors on menses*
12. Assess medical side effects of eating disorder. *To identify any concomitant medical problems*
13. Assess comorbidity factors (mood disorders, anxiety, substance abuse). *To determine if these are other factors that may complicate the problem.*

Disruptions in coping abilities:
- Ineffective coping
- Disabled family coping
- Ineffective denial

Client and family teaching needs:
- Deficient knowledge regarding nutrition and medical side effects of anorexic behavior
- Noncompliance with refeeding process

Nursing Diagnoses for Bulimia Nervosa

Safety and/or health risks:
- Constipation
- Perceived constipation
- Risk for imbalanced fluid volume
- Imbalanced nutrition: less than body requirements
- Risk for self-mutilation

Perceptual/cognitive/emotional disturbances:
- Anxiety
- Disturbed body image
- Hopelessness
- Powerlessness
- Chronic low self-esteem

Box 16-4 | Comorbid Disorders Commonly Found in Eating Disorders

Mood Disorders
Dysthymic disorder
Major depressive disorder

Anxiety Disorders
Generalized anxiety disorder
Agoraphobia
Panic disorder
Social phobia
Obsessive-compulsive disorder
Posttraumatic stress disorder

Dissociative Disorders
Dissociative identity disorder

Substance-Related Disorders

Personality Disorders
Borderline Personality Disorder
Obsessive-compulsive personality disorder
Avoidant personality disorder

Problems in communicating and relating to others:
- Sexual dysfunction
- Impaired social interaction
- Social isolation

Disruptions in coping abilities:
- Compromised family coping
- Disabled family coping
- Ineffective coping

Client and family teaching:
- Deficient knowledge regarding nutrition and side effects of bulimic behavior
- Noncompliance with treatment program

The Collaborative Diagnoses table lists DSM-IV-TR and NANDA diagnoses for these disorders.

OUTCOME IDENTIFICATION

Outcome criteria are derived from nursing diagnoses and are the expected client responses to be achieved (see Case Study).

Outcome Identification for Anorexia Nervosa

Client will:
- Participate in therapeutic contact with staff.
- Consume adequate calories for age, height, and metabolic need.
- Achieve minimum normal weight.
- Maintain normal fluid and electrolyte levels.
- Resume normal menstrual cycle.
- Demonstrate improvement in body image with a more realistic view of body shape and size.
- Demonstrate more effective coping skills to deal with conflicts.
- Manage family dysfunction more effectively.
- Verbalize awareness of underlying psychologic issues.
- Achieve ideal body weight for age, height, and metabolic need.

COLLABORATIVE DIAGNOSES

DSM-IV-TR Diagnoses*	NANDA Diagnoses†
Anorexia nervosa	Anxiety
	Disturbed body image
	Imbalanced nutrition: less than body requirements
	Social isolation
Bulimia nervosa	Ineffective coping
	Deficient fluid volume
	Chronic low self-esteem

*From American Psychiatric Association: *Diagnostic and Statistical Manual of Mental Disorders,* Fourth Edition, Text Revision. Washington, DC, American Psychiatric Association, 2000.
†From NANDA International (2003). NANDA Nursing Diagnoses: Definitions and Classification 2003-2004. Philadelphia: NANDA.

- Perceive body weight and shape as normal and acceptable.
- Resume sexual interest and age-appropriate sexual behavior.
- Demonstrate absence of food rituals, preoccupation with food, or fears of food.
- Resolve family issues.

Outcome Identification for Bulimia Nervosa

Client will:
- Participate in therapeutic contact with staff.
- Maintain normal fluid and electrolyte levels.
- Consume adequate calories for age, height, and metabolic need.
- Cease binge/purge episodes while in inpatient setting.
- Demonstrate more effective coping skills to deal with conflicts.
- Manage family dysfunction more effectively.
- Verbalize awareness of underlying psychologic issues.
- Cease binge/purge episodes completely; cease dieting behavior.
- Perceive body shape and weight as normal and acceptable.
- Resolve family and other underlying issues.

PLANNING

The nurse's attitude toward the client with an eating disorder is as critical in the plan of care as any specific therapeutic intervention. Clients with eating disorders appear fragile, and although they are vulnerable, they can also be quite

CASE STUDY

Laura is a 27-year-old married mother of a 3-year-old child. Laura has been hospitalized after a suicide attempt, in which she overdosed on a combination of 100 laxatives and a full bottle of her antidepressant medication. She is currently seeing a psychiatrist for depression and bulimia nervosa. The nursing assessment reveals that Laura currently binges and purges up to three times per day. Purging consists of self-induced vomiting, as well as the use of laxatives (usually 5 or 6 pills every day). She is within normal weight range at 140 pounds and 5 feet 9 inches. Laura is participating in milieu activities willingly, although her affect is depressed. She is eating very little at meals and has agreed not to purge while in the hospital.

Critical Thinking

1. How will the nurse determine Laura's therapeutic involvement with staff and peers?
2. What are realistic expectations of Laura for eating regular meals? What data should be monitored to track her improvement in nutritional status?
3. How will the nurse recognize improvements in eating behavior and cessation of purging?
4. How will Laura demonstrate awareness of the psychologic issues underlying her bulimia?

rigid and frustrating. If a good working alliance is not formed, with the nurse taking a firm, yet compassionate approach, client care quickly turns into a series of power struggles, and the treatment is doomed to fail. Therefore the plan of care includes consistent, collaborative efforts by the client, family, and interdisciplinary staff.

IMPLEMENTATION

For the client with an eating disorder, the nurse needs to implement a balanced plan of action that includes behavioral interventions to interrupt the cycle of eating disorder behavior. Psychologic interventions are used to improve coping skills, communication skills, and insight into underlying issues. Implementation of the plan provides a safe, structured environment to prevent self-harm; promote weight gain and/or nutritional restoration; help the client express in words what the client is acting out with the behavior; teach more effective coping skills; monitor the use of medications; and coordinate the multidisciplinary efforts of the treatment team. Specific issues faced by a community nurse working with a client with eating disorders are discussed in the Nursing Care in the Community box.

Nursing Interventions

1. Provide a safe, nonthreatening environment. *This ensures safety and prevents violence.*
2. Assess any risk of suicide (suicidal ideation, gesture, plan). *This prevents self-harm* (see Chapter 24).
3. Engage the client in a therapeutic alliance. *This encourages expression of a wide range of thoughts and feelings, including any self-destructive urges.*
4. Restore minimum weight and nutritional balance through a behavioral program. *This promotes health and wellness.* (Anorexia includes refeeding with food, food supplements, and tube feedings when necessary. Bulimia includes eating meals prescribed by a dietitian and avoidance of purging by having the nurse remain with the client for at least 1 hour after each meal.)
5. Create a structured, supportive environment with clear, consistent, firm limits. *This helps to establish a predictable routine and promotes an internal locus of control that the client currently lacks.*
6. Construct a behavioral plan that includes weight-gain goals (approximately 3 pounds per week), specific eating goals (eating 90% of all meals), and consequences for compliance (preferably increased privileges for compliance rather than punishment for noncompliance). *Structure helps the client to gain self-control and reduces the anxiety generated by noncompliance and an unpredictable routine.*
7. Encourage the client to express thoughts, feelings, and concerns about body and body image. *Verbalization helps to solidify concerns; helps the client to transform a pervasive sense of shame, guilt, and fear into specific areas of conflict; and clarifies the underlying issues (intimacy, sex, adult responsibility, identity).*
8. Continue to help the client increase understanding of body image distortion. *The goal is for the client to recognize that preoccupation with breasts, hips, stomach, legs, etc. actually symbolizes underlying issues that will not resolve by changing the client's body.*
9. Assist the client in recalling positive eating experiences, such as a time when the client was able to eat a small portion of sweets and stop without bingeing. *This emphasizes the fact that the client is capable of engaging in successful episodes of eating and promotes hope.*

NURSING CARE IN THE COMMUNITY — Eating Disorders

The most overt problem encountered by community mental health nurses in assisting clients with a pattern of eating disorders involves the potential power struggle over participation in a treatment regimen. It is impossible for the community mental health nurse to continually observe the client's eating patterns, including self-starvation and self-induced vomiting. Clients with eating disorders are often evasive about their actual intent or emotions. Clients may say the "right" thing (i.e., what the nurse wants to hear), thereby confusing the nurse's assessment. Only when the client's physical state deteriorates can the counselor obtain a clear picture of what is actually occurring.

The nurse must frequently use the observations of family, friends, and other professionals to validate the client's reports. This may be achieved by offering support groups not only for the clients, but also for their families and significant others. Nurses treating clients with eating disorders must be knowledgeable in the area of reality testing and other cognitive/behavioral therapies. They must also be educated about the signs and symptoms of the disorder, potential problems, and suggestions for positive changes in communication dynamics, including communication among family members. They must be certain to offer support rather than criticism throughout treatment.

The community nurse must plan interventions to empower the client and family to participate effectively in treatment. Written contracts may be engaging tools that offer the client a feeling of involvement and accountability. Clients are encouraged to identify situations that have been problematic for them in the past. They are assured that help is readily available and are encouraged to ask for help in curtailing their habitual dysfunctional patterns. The nurse helps individual clients and groups to use effective coping skills. Bonding techniques are used to extend and expand support groups, especially those clients who are in their teens or early twenties and in need of a comforting peer support group.

The nurse should be aware of community support groups for clients with anorexia and bulimia. Overeaters Anonymous (OA) often has affiliated groups for persons with other eating disorders and can serve as a resource for those experiencing other eating disorders. Clients may also require antidepressant medication, which must be monitored for effectiveness and side effects. As in any prolonged illness, hospitalization must always be an option if the client's behaviors become life threatening.

10. Assume a caring, yet matter-of-fact approach without being overly sympathetic or overly confrontational or authoritarian. *This assists the client in maintaining clear boundaries and avoids power struggles.*

11. Intervene with the client's anxiety by helping the client associate feelings of anxiety with unmet needs and expectations that may represent threats to the self-system. *The client's recognition that anxiety can be a result of unconscious conflicts can, in itself, bring relief and start the process of problem solving.*

12. Offer positive feedback and praise when the client adheres to the treatment plan and strives to maintain the goals of the individual contract. *Praise increases self-esteem, promotes compliance, and encourages repetition of positive behaviors.* Examples: "You have eaten three new foods this week." "You listen attentively in group."

13. Engage the client in therapeutic interactions and groups (e.g., individual therapy, group therapy, family therapy, occupational/recreational therapy). *This will encourage the client to express feelings and conflicts engendered by eating disorder behaviors in a supportive environment and reduce/rechannel anxiety in a more structured and meaningful way.*

14. Assist the client in identifying issues of low self-esteem, identity disturbance, separation, family dysfunction, and fear of maturity. *This will help the client to reveal and process the psychologic conflicts that underlie the eating disorder.*

15. Discuss with the client how obsession with food and weight is a way to avoid more difficult life problems and challenges. *This will help the client increase awareness and gain insight about the dynamics of the eating disorder.*

16. Collaborate with the dietitian to teach the client about adequate nutrition for the client's height and body type. *This will counter the client's erroneous information about ideal weight and size, and provide education regarding cultural pressures to be unrealistically thin.*

17. Collaborate with the social worker, family therapist, physician, and other members of the interdisciplinary team. *This will promote consistency in implementing the treatment plan.*

18. Teach adaptive therapeutic strategies (cognitive, behavioral, assertive). *This will promote realistic thoughts, feelings, and coping behaviors, and help the client realize that it is irrational to believe that losing weight will solve his or her problems* (see Chapter 19).

19. Teach the client, family, and significant others about the eating disorder, symptom management, and prevention. *Knowledge promotes power and control and reduces fear and anxiety.*

20. Educate the family about healthy boundaries and normal separation and individuation versus overprotection and family enmeshment. *Education about these issues will help the family to relinquish unnec-*

CLIENT AND FAMILY TEACHING GUIDELINES

Eating Disorders

TEACH THE CLIENT'S FAMILY MEMBERS:

To not focus exclusively on the client's weight and food intake as indicators of progress. Help them to understand that eating disorder behaviors are symptomatic of underlying psychologic issues. Specify and explain common underlying issues such as low self-esteem, separation/individuation conflicts, interoceptive deficits, fear of maturity, and conflict avoidance.

To encourage the client to share what the client has learned in group and individual therapy regarding the particular psychologic issues underlying the eating disorder.

To encourage the client to verbalize thoughts and feelings about family interactions that the client may previously have been fearful or reluctant to disclose directly.

To relinquish control over the client's behavior; to stop monitoring what, when, and/or how much the client eats and what the client weighs.

To understand how their monitoring and controlling behaviors serve to reinforce the eating disorder behavior by setting up a power struggle in which the client feels controlled and rebels against this indirectly by worsening the behavior.

To decrease enmeshment; to stop behaviors such as preparing separate meals, not setting age-appropriate limits, or not expecting the client to follow family rules.

To understand that their well-intentioned attempts to be supportive backfire by sending the message that their child is helpless and exempt from age-appropriate responsibilities.

TEACH THE CLIENT:

To stop acting out conflicts and feelings with the eating disorder behavior. To stop trying to get needs met indirectly through behaviors, but rather to identify and verbalize conflicts, needs, and feelings.

To express thoughts and feelings verbally in group and one-to-one interactions. To transform diffuse feelings of guilt, anxiety, fear, emptiness, and sadness into concrete concerns. These feelings are expressed as experiences related to the body and about being fat. Ask the client to be very specific about the feeling: "What specifically are you afraid will happen?" or "When you say, 'I'm freaking out,' what thoughts are going through your head?"

essary controls and promote mutually satisfying interpersonal relationships among family members (see Client and Family Teaching Guidelines box).

21. Collaborate with the occupational therapist to teach the client about appropriate exercise. *This will reduce compulsive behavior and encourage the client to exercise in moderation.*

Additional Treatment Modalities
Biologic Modalities

Clients with anorexia who are more than 15% below ideal body weight should be closely monitored medically. After the initial assessment and treatment for effects of starvation, such as amenorrhea, osteopenia and osteoporosis, and vitamin and mineral deficiencies, the client should be closely monitored while refeeding takes place. Refeeding with meals, supplements, and/or nasogastric tube should

CLINICAL ALERT

If the client is compliant with the contract but does not make the expected weight gain, the nurse may suspect that the client is purging and report this to the treatment team, who may recommend that the nurse confront the client with the purging behavior. Increased supervision after meals and during administration of supplements to prevent purging will follow. The nurse remains in the room with the client for an hour after eating or has the client sit at the nursing station for that period. The contract may be amended to include these changes. If weight gain does not occur in a few days, tube feeding may be initiated.

Additional Treatment Modalities
For Clients With an Eating Disorder

Biologic
Pharmacologic
Psychotherapeutic
    Individual psychotherapy
    Behavioral therapy
    Cognitive therapy
    Family therapy
    Group therapy
    Expressive therapies
Adjunctive therapy
    Occupational therapy
    Therapeutic recreation
    Nutrition education and counseling
Social work
    Interdisciplinary treatment team
    Community support groups

begin with approximately 1000 to 1600 kcal/day and slowly increase to 2000 to 4000 kcal/day, depending on the client's ideal weight. A goal of 2 to 3 lb/week is considered safe. The risk of refeeding syndrome, a possibly life-threatening complication, is high in the early phase of treating a severely malnourished client. Edema, congestive heart failure, hypophosphatemia, and other serious electrolyte imbalances can be prevented with slow refeeding and careful monitoring of mineral and electrolyte levels (Treasure and Serpell, 1999; APA Work Group on Eating Disorders, 2000).

Clients with bulimia need to be assessed initially for acute fluid and electrolyte imbalance, particularly serum potassium, and for any of the dangerous side effects related to their individual purging behaviors. Bone mineral density screening for osteopenia and osteoprosis and assessment for amenorrhea should be done as well. If purging is not completely stopped during treatment, electrolytes need to be continually monitored.

There are many other accepted modalities of treatment for eating disorders. These are listed in the Additional Treatment Modalities box and are discussed in the next section.

Pharmacologic Modalities

Data show that SSRI medications, particularly fluoxetine (Prozac), are effective in treating bulimia nervosa. The dose needed to obtain the "antibulimic" effect is usually 60 mg or more. Data on treating anorexia nervosa are more mixed, but fluoxetine (Prozac) can be effective in preventing relapse in weight-restored clients (Kaye et al., 2001a; Mitchell et al., 2001; Peterson and Mitchell, 1999; Zhu and Walsh, 2002). New atypical antipsychotic agents have shown some success in low-weight anorexia nervosa, particularly when accompanied by extreme agitation and/or severe body image distortion (Mitchell et al., 2001).

SSRI medications are used to treat comorbid mood disorders in clients with eating disorders. This indirectly treats the eating disorder by relieving depression and anxiety enough for the client to do the work of psychotherapy. Bupropion (Wellbutrin) is contraindicated because of its tendency to lower the seizure threshold in clients with eating disorders. Antianxiety medications are used sparingly because clients need to learn to tolerate their feelings and cope in more adaptive ways.

Medical side effects of eating disorders require the use of medication. Hypokalemia may be treated with oral or intravenous potassium supplements. Nutritional anemia may be treated with iron supplements. Gastroparesis, or delayed gastric emptying, may be treated with metoclopramide (Reglan). Infected parotid glands may be treated with antibiotics. Laxative dependence is often treated with a combination of stool softeners, bran, fiber, fluids, and decreasing doses of laxatives (if taking very high doses, such as 50 to 100 laxatives at a time, abrupt withdrawal is dangerous and gradual withdrawal is done under close supervision) (see Chapter 20).

Psychotherapeutic Modalities

Individual Psychotherapy. Individual psychotherapy is recommended as the preferred treatment for eating disorders. Psychodynamically oriented therapists recommend long-term, insight-oriented therapy to repair early developmental failures or traumas, which are seen as primary etiologic factors. All but the most conservative psychoanalytic therapists recommend an active therapeutic stance and encourage the use of behavioral techniques for symptom management and cognitive restructuring to alter distorted thinking patterns. Cognitive therapists are likely to recommend structured, short-term therapy with less insight orientation and more focus on thought patterns.

Most therapists, whatever their orientation, use hospitalization as a means to manage acute exacerbations of either the eating disorder symptoms or concomitant affective disorder symptoms.

Behavioral Therapy. Behavioral contracts for weight gain, for regulating eating and exercise behavior, and for diminishing binge/purge behaviors are commonly used tools in inpatient and outpatient treatment. Exposure plus re-

NURSING CARE PLAN

Brittany is an 18-year-old college freshman who is hospitalized for severe cachexia (95 pounds, 5 feet 7 inches) with hypokalemia, nutritional anemia, and cardiac dysrhythmia. She had arrived home after flunking out of her first semester at college, and her parents, who had not seen her in several months, immediately took her to the family physician, who hospitalized her. Brittany's physician reports that she has been dieting and excessively exercising for the past 2 years but that she had always kept her weight within 10% of ideal body weight and that she had been in individual psychotherapy for a year before going to college. Brittany now states that she did not continue with therapy in college, as she had promised. Brittany minimizes her weight loss, complains of feeling fat, is sullen and angry, and wants to be discharged.

DSM-IV-TR Diagnoses

Axis I	Anorexia nervosa, binge eating/purging type
Axis II	Rule out borderline personality disorder
Axis III	Deferred
Axis IV	Moderate—3 (moving away from home to college)
Axis V	GAF = 50 (current)
	GAF = 65 (past year)

NURSING DIAGNOSIS: Imbalanced nutrition: less than body requirements related to self-starvation and possible purging behavior, as evidenced by severe weight loss, hypokalemia, and cardiac dysrhythmia.

CLIENT OUTCOMES	NURSING INTERVENTIONS	EVALUATION
Brittany will consume adequate calories for age, height, and metabolic need (e.g., 75% of each meal will be consumed by the end of the hospital stay).	Initiate refeeding in collaboration with treatment team (Box 16-5). *Starving behavior is out of control, and Brittany cannot begin eating again on her own.* Encourage Brittany to choose her own menu. *Brittany may be more cooperative if she feels she has some control over the refeeding process.*	Brittany ate only 25% of meals on Day 1, but on Day 2, she ate 50% and drank all three dietary supplements. After 7 days, she was eating 75% of all meals and the supplements were discontinued. Brittany selected her own meals on Day 3.
Brittany will achieve minimum normal weight (less than 15% below ideal weight: for 5 feet, 7 inches, approximately 115 pounds).	Weigh daily with the client's back facing the scale. *Brittany's obsession with weight may be reinforced by her knowledge of daily weight changes. Not knowing may help her tolerate weight gain and help her to let go of overcontrol of her body.*	Brittany achieved her goal weight by discharge.
Brittany will gain an average of 4 pounds per week.	Continue to implement the refeeding plan and contract as needed *to maintain the client's expected weight.*	Brittany maintained her expected weight.

NURSING DIAGNOSIS: Disturbed body image related to underlying psychologic conflicts (fear of growing up, fear of sexuality), as evidenced by complaints of body dissatisfaction, fear of weight gain, and minimizing weight loss when more than 15% below minimal normal weight (e.g., 95 pounds, 5 feet 7 inches).

CLIENT OUTCOMES	NURSING INTERVENTIONS	EVALUATION
Brittany will demonstrate realistic perceptions of body shape and size. Brittany will demonstrate increased insight into body image distortion.	Encourage expression of thoughts and feelings regarding body. *Verbalizing specific concerns may help Brittany uncover psychologic issues related to her body image.* Collaborate with dietitian to give fact-based information to counter irrational beliefs about body size and shape (e.g., "You are 20 pounds below minimum healthy weight for your age and height"). *Factual information from more than one professional provides reality orientation of discrepancy between ideal weight and current weight.*	Brittany verbalized awareness that she is underweight and that her dissatisfaction with her body has to do more with psychologic issues than with her weight. Brittany verbalized that she perceives herself as heavier than her actual weight.
Brittany will demonstrate an enhanced self-concept based on positive attributes, rather than based totally on her body shape.	Give Brittany feedback regarding positive qualities that she demonstrates in the milieu. *Brittany's self-concept is overly defined by her body, and she needs to view herself more realistically.*	Brittany verbalized positive qualities about herself that were unrelated to her body.

NURSING CARE PLAN—cont'd

NURSING DIAGNOSIS: Noncompliance with the treatment plan related to underlying psychologic conflicts (control issues or separation issues), as evidenced by anger, refusal to self-disclose to the staff, and requests to be discharged.

CLIENT OUTCOMES	NURSING INTERVENTIONS	EVALUATION
Brittany will participate in therapeutic contacts with staff.	Engage Brittany in therapeutic alliance (e.g., using Brittany's input to develop a collaborative treatment plan). *Including Brittany as a part of the treatment team increases her power base and decreases power struggles, strengthening the therapeutic alliance.*	Brittany participated as part of the treatment team.
Brittany will comply with the interdisciplinary treatment plan.	Use interdisciplinary-designed contracts, with clear expectations and consequences, *to increase client compliance and further reduce power struggles.*	Brittany complied with the expectations of her behavioral contract.
Brittany will acknowledge her condition and the need for treatment.	Use reality orientation to challenge Brittany's minimization of the seriousness of her condition. Give information about laboratory results, medical status, etc. *Brittany's denial will decrease when challenged with concrete information.*	Brittany verbalized awareness of the need for hospitalization and treatment.

Box 16-5   Refeeding Procedure

If Brittany does not eat 75% of her meals on Day 1, she will receive three dietary supplements on Day 2. Supplements will continue daily until she eats 75% of her meals.

If she does not finish her supplements on Day 2, she will be tubefed on Day 3. Tube feeding will continue until she eats 75% of all meals for 1 day.

If she refuses tube feeding, she will be discharged.

---

sponse prevention, in which clients eat "scary" or binge foods and are then prevented from purging, is an effective intervention for bulimia nervosa.

Cognitive Therapy. Most clients with eating disorders demonstrate distorted thoughts and beliefs related to food and weight, as well as to self-concept. Techniques such as reframing, cognitive restructuring, and rational-emotive therapy are commonly used to alter these cognitive distortions.

Family Therapy. Adolescents with eating disorders almost always participate in family therapy. Educating the family about eating disorders is essential, as the eating disorder behavior often becomes the focal point of the family, leading to overinvolvement and power struggles that inadvertently reinforce the behavior. Decreasing secondary gains and uncovering underlying family dysfunction are the initial goals of family therapy. Improving family interaction is the goal for the longer term.

Group Therapy. Clients with anorexia and bulimia often set themselves apart from others with their unusual stance toward food and eating, resulting in secretiveness, feeling misunderstood, and secondary gains related to feeling "special." Being in a group with others with eating disorders allows them a safe place to self-disclose and be accepted/understood while preventing manipulation and secondary gains related to being "different."

Expressive Therapies. Because eating disorder symptoms are an indirect physical expression of emotional pain, many clients have great difficulty translating their pain into the words needed for "talking" therapy. The use of nonverbal techniques in art, music, and dance therapies; journal writing; and poetry may allow for greater self-disclosure and exploration of underlying issues.

Adjunctive Therapy

Occupational Therapy. Many clients with eating disorders need assistance in learning how to plan meals, shop, and cook for themselves, especially if they have not eaten properly for many years. Although the dietitian will do the actual meal planning, occupational therapy can help the client carry out the plan. Education concerning healthy moderate exercise is also necessary to alter compulsive exercise patterns (see Chapter 19).

Nutrition Education and Counseling. Although clients with eating disorders are obsessed with food, most have distorted information about nutrition. Consultation with a registered dietitian includes determining the client's ideal weight range using the basal metabolic index and other types of calculations, planning a refeeding program, and meal planning. The dietitian provides nutritional counseling and assists the client with postdischarge meal planning.

Clients with chronic eating disorders often do not function well in society. Hospital social workers can be helpful in finding community resources such as day treatment services, board-and-care homes, group homes, residential treatment facilities, or vocational rehabilitation. Social workers often provide family therapy.

Interdisciplinary Treatment Team

In both inpatient and outpatient settings, a successful treatment outcome depends on the collaboration of nursing, psychiatry, medical physician, psychology, pharmacy, dietary, social work, occupational therapy, counseling, and spiritual guidance as needed. Interdisciplinary treatment team meetings are the recommended forum for sharing assessment information and developing the multidisciplinary treatment plan. Nurses often coordinate this plan and ensure that it is implemented. Since managed health care has taken over more of the mental health care industry, hospital stays have become shorter, and specialty units such as eating disorder units have all but disappeared. Clients with eating disorders are usually admitted to general psychiatric units or medical units. Nursing is therefore taking more of a leadership role in the coordination of the treatment team.

Community Support Groups

Community-based support and self-help groups are available in some areas. Twelve-step programs for eating disorders (Anorexics Anonymous, Bulimics Anonymous) and national nonprofit organizations, such as Anorexia Nervosa and Associated Disorders (ANAD), provide support groups for people with anorexia nervosa and bulimia nervosa.

EVALUATION

The nurse evaluates the progress of the client with an eating disorder in an organized, timely manner, in accordance with the outcomes delineated in the care plan. For the client with an eating disorder, the evaluation includes physiologic, behavioral, psychologic, social, and cultural spheres. Monitoring laboratory values, vital signs, weight, and food/fluid intake provides the data to evaluate physiologic responses to treatment. Observing and recording the client's affect, level of program participation, specific eating behaviors, peer interactions, and responses to staff provide evaluative data that help the team track behavioral responses to treatment. Listening to and interacting with the client in group therapy, in milieu activities, and during individual interactions regarding specific issues, the treatment plan, or the behavioral contract, provide additional data from which to evaluate the client's psychologic and behavioral responses to treatment (see Case Study).

CASE STUDY

Eileen is a 16-year-old young woman admitted to the hospital for increasingly out-of-control bulimic symptoms, including bingeing and purging up to 10 times a day and abuse of laxatives.

During her first week of hospitalization, the primary focus was to correct Eileen's fluid and electrolyte balance, and monitor her to prevent purging. Eileen slept a great deal her first week. She participated superficially in group sessions, complaining mainly of physical discomfort related to stopping purging and laxatives. During the second week of treatment, the team set goals to help Eileen become "more involved" in the psychologic issues related to her bulimia. The interventions included encouraging Eileen to work on underlying issues of self-esteem and family dysfunction.

Critical Thinking

1. How will the nurse evaluate Eileen's progress in working on underlying issues? What are three specific client outcomes that would indicate such progress?
2. What specific observations should the nurse make during group sessions to evaluate Eileen's progress?
3. What verbalizations, if made by Eileen, would indicate progress in her work on "underlying issues"?

CHAPTER SUMMARY

- Eating disorders are syndromes with physiologic, behavioral, and psychologic features.
- Self-starvation, binge eating, and purging behaviors have existed for many centuries, having various psychologic meanings in different cultural eras. Until recent times, eating disorders were a rare occurrence.
- The recent outbreak of eating disorders is related to current cultural trends in the fashion industry, the diet industry, and the women's movement.
- Eating disorders have a multidetermined etiology, including biologic, possibly genetic, sociocultural, psychologic, and familial factors.
- There is a high incidence of depression among clients with eating disorders and their families.
- Personality traits that are common among individuals with eating disorders include low self-esteem, perfectionism, affective instability, interoceptive deficits, ineffectiveness, and people pleasing.
- Common dynamics in families of origin of persons with eating disorders include enmeshment, poor conflict resolution, and incomplete separation, and may include alcoholism and physical or sexual abuse.
- Most individuals with eating disorders are female (95% to 99%). Bulimia nervosa is more common than anorexia nervosa. Eating disorders are most common among high school and college students, although the incidence is growing among children in middle school.

- Clients with eating disorders often have other psychiatric diagnoses. Common Axis I diagnoses are depressive, anxiety, and dissociative disorders. Common Axis II diagnoses are borderline, avoidant, and obsessive-compulsive personality disorders.
- Anorexia nervosa and bulimia nervosa are distinct diagnoses in the DSM-IV-TR classification, but they have many overlapping features.
- The course of the illness may be chronic or episodic, requiring long-term or repeated episodes of treatment.
- Interdisciplinary treatment is indicated to deal with the multifaceted nature of eating disorders.
- Medical complications from eating disorders can be life threatening. Self-induced vomiting and abuse of laxatives and diuretics can cause serious electrolyte imbalances that may lead to cardiac dysrhythmias and cardiac arrest.
- The nurse must take a firm, professional, yet compassionate approach to avoid the power struggles that commonly undermine treatment of individuals with eating disorders.
- The plan of care must balance behavioral interventions that interrupt the cycle of behavior, with psychologic interventions that deal with underlying issues.
- A safe, structured environment must be provided to prevent self-harm, promote nutritional restoration, help the client understand the meaning of his or her behavior, and learn more effective coping skills.
- Refeeding must be done in a structured manner with clear expectations and consequences. Positive reinforcement is more effective than punishment. Consistency is crucial.
- The client must understand how he or she is using the eating disorder to avoid psychologic issues. The nurse assists the client in refocusing attention from gaining weight to underlying issues and conflicts.
- SSRI antidepressants are used to treat the comorbid depression in clients with eating disorders, and may help decrease binge urges in clients with bulimia.
- Long-term individual psychotherapy of various modalities is recommended for all clients with eating disorders. Group and family psychotherapies are also widely used.

REVIEW QUESTIONS

1. Common family interrelationship characteristics of clients with eating disorders are:
   a. Preoccupation with rituals regarding food
   b. Parental neglect and abandonment
   c. Constant changing of rules and family roles
   d. Poor boundaries, overinvolvement among members, and conflict avoidance

2. An appropriate nursing outcome for a client diagnosed with anorexia the first week of hospitalization is that the client will:
   a. Remain on bed rest
   b. Gain 1 to 2 pounds per week
   c. Verbalize a realistic body image
   d. Demonstrate elevated self-concept

3. A 15-year-old female is brought to the Emergency Department after fainting during gym class. She is grossly underweight, wears baggy clothes, and her skin is dry. She complains of feeling cold despite wearing two sweaters. To further assess for the possibility that the client has anorexia nervosa, the nurse should ask:
   a. "Do you often wear such heavy clothing during warm weather?"
   b. "Do you ever lose lapses of time?"
   c. "When was your last menstrual period?"
   d. "Do you use any drugs or alcohol?"

4. A 23-year-old client was admitted to the partial hospitalization program for bulimia nervosa. The most appropriate nursing intervention would be:
   a. Educate the client regarding dangers of purging
   b. Observe the client 1 hour after meals
   c. Discourage the client from eating sweets
   d. Encourage the client to attend a yoga class

5. A 20-year-old college student goes to the Emergency Department with complaints of fatigue and dizziness. After further assessment the nurse discovers that the enamel on her teeth has eroded. The most important nursing intervention would be to:
   a. Discuss with the physician the need to obtain electrolyte and glucose levels and an electrocardiogram
   b. Have a social worker talk to her
   c. Admit her to the psychiatric unit
   d. Bring her lunch since she probably hasn't eaten

REFERENCES

Agras W: The consequences and costs of the eating disorders, *Psychiatr Clin North Am* 24(2):371, 2001.

Agras S, Hammer L, McNicholas F: A prospective study of the influence of eating-disordered mothers on their children, *Int J Eat Disord* 25(3):253, 1999.

American Psychiatric Association: *Diagnostic and Statistical Manual of Mental Disorders*, Fourth Edition, Text Revision. Washington, DC, American Psychiatric Association, 2000.

American Psychiatric Association Work Group on Eating Disorders: Practice guideline for the treatment of eating disorders (revision), *Am J Psychiatry* 157 (suppl 1):1-39, 2000.

Bauer B, Anderson W: Bulimic beliefs: food for thought, *J Counselling Dev* 67:416, 1989.

Bell R: *Holy anorexia*, Chicago, 1987, University of Chicago Press.

Binswanger L: The case of Ellen West. In May R, Angel E, Ellenburger H, editors: *Existence*, New York, 1958, Basic Books.

Boskind-Lodahl M, White W: *Bulima-rexia: the binge/purge cycle,* New York, 1983, WW Norton.

Brumberg J: *Fasting girls,* New York, 1989, New American Library.

Dare C et al: Psychological therapies for adults with anorexia nervosa: randomized controlled trial of outpatient treatment, *Br J Psychiatry* 178:216, 2001.

Emborg C: Mortality and causes of death in eating disorders in Denmark 1970-1993: a case register study, *Int J Eat Disord* 25(3):243, 1999.

Fairburn C et al: Twin studies and the etiology of eating disorder, *Int J Eat Disord* 26(4):349, 1999.

Garner D: *Eating disorders inventory 2,* Odessa, Fla, 1991, Psychological Assessment Resources.

Grice D et al: Evidence for a susceptibility gene for anorexia nervosa on chromosome 1, *Am J Hum Genet* 70(3):787, 2002.

Groesz L, Levine M, Murnen S: The effect of experimental presentation of thin media images on body satisfaction: a meta analytic review, *Int J Eat Disord* 31(1):1, 2002.

Gunewardene A, Huon G, Zheng R: Exposure to westernization and dieting: a cross cultural study, *Int J Eat Disord* 29(3):289, 2001.

Hahn-Smith A, Smith J: The positive influence of maternal identification on body image, eating attitudes and self esteem of Hispanic and Anglo girls, *Int J Eat Disord* 29(4):428, 2001.

Hamburger W: Emotional aspects of obesity, *Med Clin North Am* 35:483, 1951.

Johnson C, Connors M: *The etiology and treatment of bulimia nervosa,* New York, 1987, Basic Books.

Kaye W et al: Double-blind, placebo controlled administration of fluoxetine in restricting and restricting-purging- type anorexia nervosa, *Biol Psychiatry* 49(7):644, 2001a.

Kaye W et al: Altered serotonin 2A receptor activity in women who have recovered from bulimia nervosa, *Am J Psychiatry* 158(7):1152, 2001b.

Keel P et al: Long-term impact of treatment in women diagnosed with bulimia nervosa, *Int J Eat Disord* 31(2):151, 2002.

Klump K, Kaye W, Strober M: The evolving genetic foundations of eating disorders, *Psychaitr Clin North Am* 24(2):215, 2001.

Lennkh C et al: Comorbidity of obsessive-compulsive disorder in patients with eating disorders, *Eat Weight Disord* 3(1):37, 1998.

Lewinsohn P, Striegel-Moore R, Seeley J: Epidemiology and natural course of eating disorders in young women from adolescence to young adulthood, *J Am Acad Child Adolesc Psychiatry* 31(3):284, 2002.

Lindner R: The case of Laura. In *The fifty minute hour,* New York, 1955, Holt, Rinehart & Winston.

Lowe B et al: Long-term outcome of anorexia nervosa in a prospective 21-year follow-up study, *Psychol Med* 31(5):881-890, 2001.

Minuchin S, Rosman B, Baker L: *Psychosomatic families: anorexia nervosa in context,* Cambridge, Mass, 1978, Harvard University Press.

Milos G et al: Comorbidity of obsessive-compulsive disorders and duration of eating disorders, *Int J Eat Disord* 31(3):284, 2002.

Mitchell J et al: Combining pharmacotherapy and psychotherapy in the treatment of patients with eating disorders, *Psychiatr Clin North Am* 24(2):315, 2001.

NANDA International (2003). NANDA Nursing Diagnoses: Definitions and Classification 2003-2004. Philadelphia: NANDA.

Orbach S: *Fat is a feminist issue,* New York, 1978, Berkeley Books.

Paul T et al: Self-injurious behavior in women with eating disorders, *Am J Psychiatry* 159(3):408, 2002.

Peterson C, Mitchell J: Psychosocial and pharmacological treatment of eating disorders: a review of the research findings, *J Clin Psychol* 55(6):685, 1999.

Polivy J, Herman P: Causes of eating disorders, *Annu Rev Psychol* 53(1):187, 2002.

Romano S et al: A placebo-controlled study of fluoxetine in continued treatment of bulimia nervosa after successful acute fluoxetine treatment, *Am J Psychiatry* 159(1):96, 2002.

Rosenvinge J, Martinussen M, Ostensen E: The comorbidity of eating disorders and personality isorders: meta-analytic review of studies published between 1983 and 1998, *Eat Weight Disord* 5(2):52, 2000.

Russell G: Bulimia nervosa: an ominous variant of anorexia nervosa, *Psychol Med* 9:429, 1979.

Shoebridge P, Gowers S: Parental high concern and adolescent-onset anorexia nervosa, *Br J Psychiatry* 176:132, 2000.

Smolak L, Levine M, Schermer F: Parental input and weight concerns among elementary school children, *Int J Eat Disord* 25(3):263, 1999.

Strober M et al: Controlled family study of anorexia nervosa and bulimia nervosa: evidence of shared liability and transmission of partial syndromes, *Am J Psychiatry* 157(3):393, 2000.

Stunkard A: Eating patterns and obesity, *Psychiatry Q* 33:284, 1959.

Treasure J, Serpell L: Osteoporosis in anorexia nervosa, *Hosp Med* 60(7):477, 1999.

von Ranson K, Iacono W, McGue M: Disordered eating and substance use in an epidemiological sample. I. Associations within individuals, *Int J Eat Disord* 31(4):389, 2002.

Wade T, Bulik C, Kendler K: Investigation of quality of the parental relationship as a risk factor for subclinical bulimia nervosa, *Int J Eat Disord* 30(4):388, 2001.

Wonderlich S et al: Eating disturbance and sexual trauma in childhood and adulthood, *Int J Eat Disord* 30(4):401, 2001.

Wooley S, Wooley O: Intensive outpatient and residential treatment for bulimia. In Garner D, Garfinkel P, editors: *Handbook of psychotherapy for anorexia nervosa and bulimia,* New York, 1985, Guilford Press.

Zhu A, Walsh B: Pharmacologic treatment of eating disorders, *Can J Psychiatry* 47(3):227, 2002.

SUGGESTED READING

Johnson J et al: Eating disorders during adolescence and the risk for physical and mental disorders during early adult hood, *Arch Gen Psychiatry* 59:545, 2002.

17 Sexual Disorders

Kathryn Thomas and Shelly F. Lurie

KEY TERMS

Depo-Provera
  (medroxyprogesterone
  acetate) (p. 409)
ego dystonic pedophile
  (p. 406)
ego syntonic pedophile
  (p. 406)
EROS-CTD system (p. 401)
Lupron Depot (leuprolide)
  (p. 410)
nocturnal penile
  tumescence (p. 400)
oxytocin (p. 401)
paraphilias (p. 403)
penile-brachial index (PBI)
  (p. 400)
phermones (p. 401)
plethysmography (p. 400)
psychoeducation (p. 410)
sensate focus (p. 401)
sexual recidivisim (p. 407)
Spontane (p. 401)
testosterone (p. 401)
triggers (p. 407)
vaginal dilator (p. 402)
victimizer (p. 406)

OBJECTIVES

- Discuss possible etiologies for the origins of sexual dysfunctions.
- Provide rationales for the incidence of sexual dysfunctions.
- Describe the clinical picture of various sexual dysfunctions using the DSM-IV-TR and NANDA diagnoses.
- Analyze the efficacy of various treatment modalities.
- Apply the nursing process in caring for clients with sexual dysfunctions.
- Describe the different diagnoses of the sex offender (paraphilic) population.
- Discuss the focus of treatment for paraphilic disorders.
- Explain at least two types of treatment and effects on illness symptomatology.
- Analyze the relationship between treatment and recidivism.
- Apply the nursing process in caring for clients with sexual (paraphilic) disorders.

This chapter explores two categories of sexual disorders: sexual dysfunctions and paraphilias.

SEXUAL DYSFUNCTIONS

HISTORICAL AND THEORETIC PERSPECTIVES

Historically much of the perspective on sexual dysfunctions can be attributed to Sigmund Freud. Freud promulgated his psychosexual theory of development. Childhood experiences were believed to exert a subconscious influence on sexual behavior in adulthood. Infantile feelings such as the fear of castration and penis envy along with actual and overt experiences combined to create sexual dysfunctions. Freud did a significant amount of clinical observation on women and is responsible for coining the term *hysteria*. He believed that sexuality was a root cause of many of the difficulties people faced (Freud, 1977). As a result of Freud's theories, psychoanalysis, the uncovering of old fears and traumas, was used exclusively in the treatment of sexual dysfunctions for more than 50 years. Other prominent sexologists had influence over the understanding of human sexuality as well. Henry Havelock Ellis, Niles Newton, Magnus Hirschfeld, and Theodoor van der Velde all addressed sexual dysfunction; but as with Freud, their work was more theoretic and based less on scientific data.

In 1966 William Masters and Virginia Johnson changed all of that when they published their classic book, *Human Sexual Response*. They directly observed in the laboratory more than 10,000 male and female volunteers (Masters and Johnson, 1966). From this research, they were able to determine exactly what happens to the body during erotic stimulation, from excitement to plateau to orgasm and, finally, to resolution. In 1970 they published a second text, *Human Sexual Inadequacy*, in which they discussed their work in helping others overcome sexual dysfunction. In this book, Masters and Johnson outlined the probable causes for dysfunction and gave detailed prescriptions for treatment.

Masters and Johnson radically moved the theoretic perspective to the behavioral sphere. They postulated that sex therapy should be a series of specifically directed exercises guided by a therapist. Their original treatment program consisted of couple's therapy in which the clients worked with a male/female treatment team. Couples came to St. Louis and lived in a hotel for 13 days. Treatment consisted of careful assessment, roundtable discussions, and homework assignments. In addition, Masters and Johnson developed many specific techniques such as sensate focus, the quiet vagina, and the squeeze technique (Masters and Johnson, 1970).

Since the late 1960s, much has been learned about sexual dysfunctions and about sexuality in general. Although they have their benefits, structured treatment programs such as Masters and Johnson's have not proved to be panaceas. Sexuality is too complex to be reduced to a sex manual solution. Helen Singer Kaplan (1974) identified the need for behavioral techniques to be reintegrated with psychoanalysis in treatment. Many others have researched other approaches. Hartman and Fithian (1972) outlined a treatment approach based on careful observational research. Others such as Anon (1976), Leiblum and Rosen (1989), and LoPiccolo and Friedman (1988) have developed other strategies and therapeutic perspectives. The latest treatments involve physical/biologic techniques such as oral preparations, injections, prosthesis, handheld devices, and surgical interventions. Modern sex therapists believe that the most effective way to treat sexual dysfunction is through a combination of physical/biologic, cognitive-behavioral, communication, and psychodynamic techniques.

ETIOLOGY

Etiologies for sexual dysfunction cover a wide range of possibilities. Three broad categories emerge: physical/biologic, psychologic/behavioral, and couple oriented (Box 17-1). Several factors may coexist within one person or one couple to impede the ability to have satisfying sex.

Physical/Biologic Factors

Biologic factors that may contribute to sexual dysfunction include vascular, neurologic, and endocrine, as well as a range of problems such as cancer, connective tissue and pain disorders, depression, incontinence, and sexually transmitted diseases (Hillman, 2000). Vascular factors include cardiac disease and disease of the blood vessels. Neurologic factors may be stroke, head injuries, spinal cord disorders, epilepsy, Parkinson's disease, or peripheral nerve disorders. Endocrine factors include diabetes and altered hormonal levels. The effects of medications should be considered. It is well known that antidepressants and antihypertensives, as well as sedatives, tranquilizers, narcotics, and alcohol, can all adversely affect sexual functioning. Serotonin reuptake inhibitors have gained increased notoriety for their role in sexual dysfunction (Bancroft, 2002).

Psychologic/Behavioral Factors

As previously noted, early childhood experiences formed the hallmark of beliefs about causation. Indeed, many still believe that psychosocial factors are more important in the etiology of sexual dysfunctions than other reasons. There is currently much literature and discussion about the impact of childhood sexual trauma on later sexual functioning (Berman et al., 2001). Repressive childhood environments that include religious, familial, or cultural restrictions have also been implicated (Money, 1986b).

Other issues such as anxiety and stress may also contribute to changes in sexual functioning. Masters and Johnson (1970) coined the term *spectatoring*. This psychologic factor refers to the tendency to monitor one's own sexual activity, thus de-

Box 17-1   Etiologic Factors for Sexual Dysfunctions

Physical/Biologic Factors

VASCULAR
Cardiac disease
Diseases of the blood vessels

NEUROLOGIC
Stroke
Head injuries
Spinal cord disorders
Epilepsy
Parkinson's disease
Peripheral nerve disorders

ENDOCRINE
Diabetes
Altered hormonal levels, especially testosterone

PHARMACOLOGIC
Antidepressants
Antihypertensives
Mind and mood altering substances
Alcohol

OTHER CAUSES
Cancer
Connective tissue disorders
Pain disorders
Depression
Incontinence
Sexually transmitted diseases

Psychologic/Behavioral Factors

Childhood experiences
Body image
Anxiety and stress
Misinformation and lack of sex education
Learned pattern of response

Couple-Oriented Factors

Differences in sexual desire or interests
Lack of attraction
Lack of communication
Lack of trust

tracting from the actual experience. Stress from any source has been noted to lower sexual drive and to decrease both testosterone and luteinizing hormone levels (Bancroft, 2002). Positive and negative perceptions of one's body image are known to impact sexual interest and function.

Misinformation and a lack of sex education may account for some degree of sexual dysfunction (Ellison, 2000). One example is ignorance about the placement and function of the clitoris, which may severely affect obtaining sexual pleasure. Myths such as those that assert that men are always ready for sex and women are never interested have also influenced attitudes toward sex.

Couple-Oriented Factors

Couple-oriented factors involve differences in sexual drives and interests. Money (1986a) used the term *lovemap* to describe one's idealized picture of who and what types of behaviors make up one's sexual arousal pattern. Lovemaps vary from individual to individual. Thus a couple may not be well matched in their attraction to one another or in the sexual activities that interest them. Communication is another couple-oriented factor that may affect sexual functioning. Couples often do not discuss what they do or do not enjoy sexually or share their feelings about the experience. Trust between partners is also a crucial factor.

ON THE HORIZON

In 1992 the National Institutes of Health Consensus Development Conference on Impotence helped determine the research agenda for male sexual dysfunction. As a result, basic and applied research revolved around organic and physical determinants of erectile dysfunction. The first Consensus Development Panel on Female Sexual Dysfunction began meeting in 1998. They have created new definitions and a classification system for sexual dysfunction with the goal to foster more research and research that is better aimed at unique female characteristics (Basson et al., 2001).

EPIDEMIOLOGY

In 1999 Laumann et al. published the National Health and Social Life Survey, which is the largest and best controlled study of human sexual dysfunction to date. They reported that the prevalence of sexual dysfunction is significant at 43% of women and 37% of men. One third of women said they lack sexual interest and one fourth said they do not experience orgasm. Males report sexual desire and orgasmic disorders, but the most significant finding for males was the incidence of premature ejaculation. Masters and Johnson (1970) suggested that 50% of all couples had a sexual dysfunction.

Kaplan (1974) estimated that 50% of all males would experience erectile problems sometime in their lives. She believed that premature ejaculation was the most common of all sexual dysfunctions. It has been noted that low libido seems to increases with age (Laumann et al., 1999; Hillman, 2000). This is partially but not wholly due to diminishing testosterone levels in males and females.

CLINICAL DESCRIPTION

The DSM-IV-TR divides sexual dysfunctions into sexual desire disorders, sexual arousal disorders, orgasmic disorders, sexual pain disorders, sexual dysfunction due to a general medical condition, substance-induced sexual dysfunction, and sexual dysfunction not otherwise specified (see DSM-IV-TR Criteria box). The first three categories are based on Kaplan's (1974) stages of the sexual response cycle.

CLINICAL ALERT

Hypoactive Sexual Desire Disorder

This disorder is more commonly seen in women, but men are affected as well. One third of all women in the National Health and Social Life Survey (Laumann et al., 1999) reported a lack of sexual interest. It is hard to separate hypoactive sexual desire from arousal or orgasmic difficulties. They may go hand in hand, complicating the picture. According to the International Consensus Development Conference on Female Sexual Dysfunction (Basson et al., 2001), hypoactive sexual desire disorder is the "persistent and recurrent deficiency (absence) of sexual fantasies/thoughts and/or a desire for or receptivity to sexual activity which causes personal distress." The causes of this disorder encompass a range of physical, psychologic, cultural, religious, and couple-related factors. The disorder is widespread, but until recently there was little research or clinical interest in it. It is a hard diagnosis to research because of the lack of clear physiologic and psychologic parameters. In large part it is a phenomenon whose major symptom is lack of interest. Current treatments include exercises where conscious attention is given to sexuality education and cognitive exercises to reverse the negative sexual messages one has acquired. Several pharmacologic agents are being used and evaluated. These include dopaminergic agents, sex steroids, phermones, and psychostimulants. This is an area of sexology where we can hope to see some breakthroughs as more attention is placed on it.

PROGNOSIS

To guide and properly educate their clients, nurses must understand how successful therapy can be for the individual or for the couple. Some prognostic data are available for sexual dysfunctions in general; however, these data cannot be used specifically for each dysfunction. For example, sexual desire disorders tend to have a more negative prognosis than do orgasmic disorders. Sexual desire disorders constitute the largest single reported problem in female sexuality. Current interest in this area is beginning to stimulate research and discussion and should eventually lead to better understanding and better treatments. Beck (1995) found that hypoactive sexual desire has consistently been the most difficult dysfunction to treat.

Masters and Johnson (1970) found that primary impotence treatment had a 40.6% failure rate, whereas the failure rate for secondary impotence treatment was 26.2%. Premature ejaculation treatment failed only 2.2% of the time. Concerning intervention rates for orgasmic dysfunction, the failure rate was 19.7% for males and 19.3% for females. When Masters and Johnson did a follow-up study 5 years later, they found that in males and females combined, only 5.1% had relapsed. Masters and Johnson's evaluation techniques have been sharply questioned. In general it is believed that sexual dysfunctions can be difficult to treat. The combination physical/biologic, psychologic, and couples-oriented programs are considered best (Rosen and Leiblum, 1995). Pharmacology clearly has improved the picture.

DSM-IV-TR CRITERIA
Sexual Dysfunctions

Sexual Desire Disorders
HYPOACTIVE SEXUAL DESIRE DISORDER
A deficiency or absence of sexual fantasy or drive for sexual activity

SEXUAL AVERSION DISORDER
Aversion to or avoidance of genital sexual contact with a partner

Sexual Arousal Disorders
FEMALE SEXUAL AROUSAL DISORDER
Inability to attain or maintain an adequate lubrication/swelling response of sexual excitement

MALE ERECTILE DISORDER
Inability to attain or maintain an adequate erection

Orgasmic Disorders
FEMALE ORGASMIC DISORDER
Delay in or absence of orgasm after sexual excitement phase (must be persistent or recurrent)

MALE ORGASMIC DISORDER
Delay in or absence of orgasm following sexual excitement phase (must be persistent or recurrent)

PREMATURE EJACULATION
Onset of orgasm and ejaculation with minimal sexual stimulation (must be persistent or recurrent)

Sexual Pain Disorders
DYSPAREUNIA
Genital pain associated with sexual intercourse (not resulting from a general medical condition)

VAGINISMUS
Involuntary contractions of the perineal muscles with penetration (not resulting from a general medical condition)

Sexual Dysfunction Due to a General Medication Condition
Use same subtypes as above but indicate which medical condition it is due to

Substance-Induced Sexual Dysfunction
Use same subtypes as above and indicate specific substance

Sexual Dysfunction Not Otherwise Specified
Does not meet criteria for the category of sexual dysfunction

Modified from American Psychiatric Association: *Diagnostic and Statistic Manual of Mental Disorders*, Fourth Edition, Text Revision. Washington, DC, American Psychiatric Association, 2000.

DISCHARGE CRITERIA

Client will:
- Express satisfaction with one's sexuality.
- Develop insight into the disorder, including its etiology and symptoms.

CASE STUDY

Joan and Paul are both 57 years old and have been married for 35 years. They have two adult children. The couple report that they had a good sexual life together until 4 years ago when Paul started having difficulty getting and maintaining erections. After a year he sought treatment and was prescribed Viagra, which helped. Before starting this medication, however, the couple had been drifting apart and went from having sex one to two times per week to less than once a month. Joan says that she found herself less and less interested and she was diagnosed postmenopausal. Two years into the treatment she learned that Paul had an affair. This revelation shook up their lives and they nearly separated. They decided after much work to stay together and are currently seeking help with their sex life. Paul says that, even with Viagra, he can get erections only in the morning, and Joan says that she is not a morning person. They have been having difficulty finding times to be sexual.

Critical Thinking

1. What symptoms of sexual dysfunction do this couple exhibit?
2. What are the precursor/antecedents to the couple's sexual problems?
3. Which nursing diagnoses are appropriate to this couple?
4. How would you help Joan and Paul achieve greater sexual satisfaction in their marriage?

Box 17-2   Principles of Sexual Assessment

1. Before beginning a sexual assessment, examine your own feelings, attitudes, and level of comfort.
2. Ensure a private, quiet space for assessment, ample time, and an unhurried attitude.
3. Questions on sexuality should not be the first asked. Begin with background information and fit the sexual assessment into the context of the overall assessment.
4. Questions asked about sexuality should begin with the least sensitive areas and move to areas of greater sensitivity. For example, begin by asking "Where did you first learn about sex?"
5. Maintain appropriate eye contact and a relaxed, interested manner.
6. Be professional and matter-of-fact about information asked or obtained. Avoid extreme reactions. Maintenance of an open, nonjudgmental attitude is essential.
7. Use language that is professional but understood by the client(s) being interviewed. This can be a good opportunity to teach about the words of sex.
8. Remember, the nurse's tone of voice and manner reflect trust. If clients feel they can trust the nurse, they will be more open.
9. Sex is not something most people are used to talking about and this can make interviewing difficult. If the nurse has the right attitude, however, clients will generally be open, willing, and even eager to talk.

- Use appropriate strategies designed to combat the specific disorder.
- Develop communication strategies with partner by which desires, likes, and dislikes can be expressed.
- Develop coping strategies to deal with frustrations and setbacks.

Sexuality is an essential aspect of every human being. All nurses should have the goal of helping their clients achieve positive sexual expressions. Facilitating this goal is a rewarding but difficult task. It also demands that nurses reflect on their own attitudes, values, comfort, and knowledge of sexuality.

For any given client or couple, it is difficult to predict how long interventions and treatment will last. Some disorders are more difficult to treat (e.g., sexual desire disorders); others are relatively simple (e.g., orgasmic disorders, premature ejaculation). However, the assumption that this will be true in any given case is shortsighted. Individual factors may speed up or complicate the recovery period. The astute nurse is consistently aware of these variables and needs to recognize the importance of flexibility. The overall goal of intervention is achievement of sexual satisfaction. What is meant by sexual satisfaction varies from individual to individual (see Case Study).

THE NURSING PROCESS

ASSESSMENT

For many reasons, sexuality is a sensitive topic for most people. When discussing sexuality with clients, the nurse should consider these sensitivities. Nurses are not immune to the feelings, beliefs, values, and attitudes that affect others. Therefore when the nurse is dealing with client-related sexual dysfunction issues, it may be uncomfortable for both parties. Yet a holistic nursing assessment must consider sexuality as important as other functions. An important step in decreasing discomfort is to have the nurse examine his or her own feelings and comfort level with the topic. The nurse will be better equipped to deal with others in the important area of human sexuality by combining self-understanding, a firm knowledge base, expert use of the nursing process, and a nonjudgmental attitude.

Assessment is a crucial phase in working with clients with sexual dysfunction. A clear understanding of the complexity of the symptoms and what areas of functioning are affected is needed. Sexual dysfunctions may arise throughout various phases of the sexual response cycle. Dysfunctions may reflect individual functioning or may be couple related. Sexual assessment must be seen in the context of overall assessment factors such as background, physical health, religious and cultural beliefs, education, occupation, significant relationships, and social relationships. In addition to the assessment of the specific complaint, the nurse must also consider the individual or couple's perspective of the problem and desire to change. The sexual history is an important aspect of the assessment. It should include early childhood experiences, history of masturbation, teenage experiences, use of erotica and fantasies, contraception history, relationship history, sexual orientation, satisfaction with sexuality, and an opportunity for questions and concerns. Sexual assessment principles are outlined in Box 17-2.

COLLABORATIVE DIAGNOSES

DSM-IV-TR Diagnoses*   NANDA Diagnoses†

Sexual Desire Disorders

Hypoactive sexual desire
- Sexual dysfunction
- Anxiety
- Defensive coping
- Hopelessness
- Ineffective sexuality pattern

Sexual aversion disorder
- Sexual dysfunction
- Anxiety
- Fear
- Ineffective role performance
- Situational low self-esteem

Sexual Arousal Disorders

Female sexual arousal disorder
- Disturbed body image
- Impaired verbal communication
- Ineffective coping

Male erectile disorder
- Impaired verbal communication
- Social isolation
- Situational low self-esteem

Orgasmic Disorders

Female orgasmic disorder
- Deficient knowledge
- Impaired adjustment
- Anxiety

Male orgasmic disorder
- Ineffective coping
- Ineffective role performance

Premature ejaculation
- Anxiety
- Fear
- Ineffective sexuality patterns

Sexual Pain Disorders

Dyspareunia
- Impaired comfort
- Ineffective coping

Vaginismus
- Anxiety
- Fear
- Impaired verbal communication

Sexual Dysfunction Due to a General Medical Condition

Substance-Induced Sexual Dysfunction

Sexual Dysfunction Not Otherwise Specified

*From American Psychiatric Association: *Diagnostic and Statistic Manual of Mental Disorders,* Fourth Edition, Text Revision. Washington, DC, American Psychiatric Association, 2000.
†From NANDA International (2002). NANDA Nursing Diagnoses: Definitions and Classification 2003-2004. Philadelphia: NANDA.

NURSING DIAGNOSIS

After a thorough gathering of assessment data, the nurse is in a position to analyze the findings and arrive at diagnoses. Diagnoses of sexual dysfunctions should be viewed in relation to the psychiatric diagnoses, DSM-IV-TR, as well as nursing diagnoses that reflect the specific problems. A combination of both helps to ensure that adequate plans for intervention are developed (see Collaborative Diagnosis table). Diagnoses are determined on an individual basis and are carefully selected from all that is known.

Nursing Diagnoses for Sexual Dysfunctions

- Impaired adjustment
- Anxiety
- Disturbed body image
- Impaired comfort
- Impaired verbal communication
- Ineffective coping
- Defensive coping
- Fear
- Hopelessness
- Deficient knowledge
- Chronic pain
- Ineffective role performance
- Situational low self-esteem
- Sexual dysfunction
- Ineffective sexuality patterns
- Social isolation

OUTCOME IDENTIFICATION

In this phase the nurse determines clear outcome criteria or expected client outcomes from the nursing diagnosis.
Client will:
- Verbalize specific problem in the sexual area by the time of the second visit with nurse.
- Write a list of feelings associated with the sexual problem by the time of the second visit with nurse.
- Seek a physical examination (if appropriate) by the time of the third visit with nurse.
- Participate in sex therapy sessions (if appropriate) by the time of the fourth visit with nurse.
- Practice recommended strategies learned in sex therapy by the sixth week in therapy.
- Describe two strategies learned to enhance sexual functioning after the sixth week in therapy.
- Incorporate strategies learned in sex therapy into routine sexual activity by the time of discharge.

PLANNING

Planning for client care comes about as the result of thorough assessment and analysis. After formulation of DSM-IV-TR diagnoses and nursing diagnoses that reflect client status, the nurse is ready to begin an individualized plan of care that will address all of the issues. Client care is based on realistic, mutually agreed on goals.

In working with clients and couples with sexual dysfunction, the nurse must carefully consider the long-term goals and what each participant is willing to do to work toward those goals. These may differ in each situation, based on each person's values and attitudes and how each perceives the problem. For example, the client with a primary orgasmic dysfunction may have difficulty with masturbatory exercises that form one basis for treatment because he or she believes that touching one's own genitals is unacceptable and that orgasmic release must come only from partnered sexuality. Obviously such individually held beliefs influence implementation of a care plan.

IMPLEMENTATION

Development of an individualized plan of care is crucial. To do so, one must be aware of the specific nature of the problem and possible etiologies. Implementation includes education, counseling, and assistance in identifying specific strategies, referral, and support (see Client and Family Teaching Guidelines box). The nurse must be aware of various treatment modalities and prognosis of recovery with treatment. The importance of following through on a plan of care, including physical examination and treatments, and on specific sex therapy needs for the individual or the couple must be stressed. The nurse helps the client(s) express concerns about sexual functioning; express feelings about the impact of these concerns; and help enhance client knowledge base, self-esteem, and communication skills. The nurse also recommends a physical examination and/or treatment and sex therapy, monitors client compliance and success in treatment, and helps develop appropriate discharge planning.

CLIENT AND FAMILY TEACHING GUIDELINES

Sexual Dysfunction

TEACH CLIENTS:

Body image exercises, including affirmations and mirror work.

Ways to increase comfort with the body using gradual and progressive touch/caress. This can be done in the shower or bath.

Breathing and relaxation techniques to lower anxiety.

Ways to pleasure themselves using fantasy, erotica, self-stimulation, and toys.

For women: Exercises to increase knowledge and comfort of genitals, using the mirror and touch.

TEACH COUPLES:

Better ways to communicate by telling each other what they like and do not like.

To take turns where one person plans favorite scenario, then both act it out. Switch the next time.

To create a more sexual atmosphere without demand for intercourse through sexual humor, flirtation, touch, enjoyment of one another. Have fun together.

To describe what is sexually unique about them and build on this.

To try something new, for example, full body or specific area massage, sexual play at spontaneous moments or variations in time or location.

Sexuality is a sensitive area of intervention. Having a trusting, open, and comfortable relationship with clients is essential. Without this relationship, many sexual problems go unrecognized and untreated (see Nursing Care in the Community box on p. 400).

The nature of sexuality is partially one of relationships with others. Therefore the nurse must be aware of clients' significant others and how they are affected. Implementation of any plan of care often involves a couple relationship and must be seen in this context. Thus it is often helpful to view the problem as couple oriented instead of placing the blame on either partner. Interventions aimed at the couple, in these instances, are most effective.

Nursing Interventions

1. Help client(s) understand human sexual functioning. Teach them about the human sexual response cycle. Recommend appropriate reading materials, such as Masters and Johnson's *Human Sexual Response* or Helen Singer Kaplan's *The New Sex Therapy. This knowledge forms a foundation for better understanding other sexual functioning issues related to sexual disorders.*

2. Educate client(s) about sexual dysfunctions, including possible etiologies, symptoms, and treatment options. Various methods of assessment should be included such as physical, urologic, gynecologic, and laboratory examinations, as well as a psychosocial sexual assessment. *Education helps to promote client(s) understanding about why changes in sexuality are happening to them and assists them in identifying symptoms that may signal a problem.*

3. Help client(s) enhance communication skills around intimacy/sexuality. Teach and reinforce positive communication skills. *The inability to communicate is often at the root of a sexual dysfunction problem.*

4. Support client(s) in exploring fears/anxieties related to anxiety in a private, trusting, open atmosphere. Encourage client's recall of early learning about sexuality, possibly through journal writing. *An open forum for discussing sexuality helps the client(s) overcome some of the repressions they have felt and be more open to satisfying sexual experiences.*

5. Help client(s) enhance self-esteem related to sexuality. Encourage positive self-talk and body image exercises. Discuss variations of sexual expression techniques. *Lack of self-esteem is often a contributing factor in sexual dysfunction.*

6. Refer client(s) to physical treatment modalities or sex therapy as applicable. *These therapeutic interventions help to maximize client success in dealing with sexual dysfunction.*

Additional Treatment Modalities

After careful assessment to determine the specific diagnosis of sexual dysfunction, a range of treatment modalities can be instituted (see Additional Treatment Modalities box on p. 401).

NURSING CARE IN THE COMMUNITY — Sexual Dysfunctions

Many people find sexual dysfunctions difficult to discuss because of the traditional reticence regarding the subject of sex. The sources of sexual problems may be found in a variety of factors including the natural changes of the aging process, side effects of various medications or disease processes, rape, or a history of abuse. Some clients may have kept their problems a secret for extended periods or may not have been aware of the original precipitant.

Some individuals may experience gender-related conflict or desire for types of sexual experience that are not condoned by society. Any of these dilemmas may be presented to the community mental health nurse with the expectation that nurses have the knowledge and experience to "fix" the problem. The nurse should respond in a nonjudgmental way no matter how different the client's sexual problem seems from the nurse's view or experience. The nurse should not attempt to condone or excuse hurtful behavior related to sexual activity or abuse and should exert patience as the client attempts to express feelings that may never have been shared with anyone else. The nurse also should acknowledge that there are no easy answers to the client's questions and should emphasize readiness to explore individualized options. It is important to remind the client that thoughts are not harmful to others, that he or she is able to make a choice about turning ideas into actions, and that individual or group support is available.

Sexual issues and problems associated with the maturing process are increasingly common because the population that embraced the birth control pill now must cope with the complexities of acquired immunodeficiency syndrome (AIDS), menopause, and "viripause," as some have dubbed the male version of hormonal changes. Women may experience depression and a lack of sexual desire resulting from diminished hormone levels and related painful intercourse. Men may feel trapped in their jobs/careers and/or in their relationships. Sexually active adults who are not in secure monogamous relationships must always have concerns about sexually transmitted diseases (STDs), even though there are protective methods to reduce risk.

Clients in the community may also include those who have already contracted STDs such as gonorrhea, human immunodeficiency virus, genital herpes, or full-blown AIDS. These clients can be helped individually and in support groups to allay their guilt and to evaluate their situations with regard to what sort of relationships are possible for them. They must be encouraged to be scrupulously honest with prospective partners and to explore safer forms of intimacy in their relationships.

The mental health nurse in the community must have up-to-date information about medications, especially antidepressants, which may evoke side effects that affect a client's sexual activity, including impaired desire, delayed orgasm, and impotence. Many persons tolerate these departures from their normal patterns in silence and believe that they are still suffering from depression or that they have developed some other abnormality to add to their problems. They will need assurance that their problems are physiologic and not emotional. At present, there are also recent innovations in drug therapy that support the mechanical bodily response during sexual stimulation. These new medications offer relief from certain types of sexual difficulty and show promise in alleviating the side effects of certain therapies and debilitating diseases.

The difference that the mental health nurse notes between working in the community versus a hospital setting is that relationships with clients are more sustained, holistic, and balanced. A partnership is easier to establish with the client in the community, and there may be more interactions and fewer power struggles between nurse and client than there are in the hospital. For sensitive topics such as sexual disorders, this collaboration can lead to very effective consensual treatment strategies.

Psychophysiologic

Physiologic causation must be ruled out before choosing one or more forms of treatment. Various medical specialties have produced new diagnostic and therapeutic procedures that have quickly changed the practice of sex therapy/clinical sexology.

For men, various psychophysiologic methods are used in both diagnosis and treatment. **Nocturnal penile tumescence** involves the determination of erectile response during the sleep cycle. The client is generally seen in a sleep laboratory where plethysmography is used to monitor erection. **Plethysmography** involves the use of a strain gauge that fits around the penis and detects erection. This information, processed through mechanical and computerized equipment, provides a graphic portrayal of the erectile pattern. This testing is time consuming and relatively expensive, but it clearly detects whether erection is possible without competing psychologic stimuli. Erectile potential can also be determined by daytime evaluation using visual erotic stimuli and the plethysmograph.

Medical testing for males may include endocrine measures, particularly testosterone and prolactin levels. Testosterone is the predominantly male sex hormone produced in the testes that is responsible for the sexual drive. In general, a higher level of testosterone in males is associated with greater sexual desire; a higher level of prolactin is associated with decreased sexual interest (Rowland, 1999). There is currently more understanding and acceptance of male andropause. This phenomenon involves a whole range of symptoms and is due to waning levels of testosterone as men age. The **penile-brachial index,** another useful measure, monitors the difference between penile and brachial blood pressures. There are other invasive and noninvasive tests for evaluation of arterial and venous blood flow to the penis, including pulse-wave assessments, intracorporeal pharmacologic testing, ultrasound (the use of sound waves to evaluate structures and functions within the male genitalia), and cavernosography. Neurologic assessments that carefully evaluate various minute components of neural control of erection are also available.

In women there is a noticeable lack of assessment and treatment in the psychophysiologic realm. Plethysmography is used to determine blood flow to the vagina, which is an indicator of arousal; however, this procedure is inconsistent and invasive. Endocrine studies can be used, but the hormonal control of female sexuality is more complex and is af-

Additional Treatment Modalities
For Clients With Sexual Disorders

Psychophysiologic Modalities

Anxiolytics
Aphrodisiacs
EROS-CTD
Intracavernosal injections
MUSE
Penile prosthesis
Sex steroids (estrogen and testosterone)
Selective serotonin reputake inhibitors (SSRIs)
Viagra
Vibrators
Yohimbine
Possibilities on the horizon:
Adrenocorticotropic hormone (ACTH)
Dopamine compounds
Noradrenergic compounds
Oxytocin
Phermones
Psychostimulants
Spontane

Psychosocial Modalities

Body therapies (massage, chakra balancing, tantric yoga)
Communication techniques
Education
Erotic stimuli training
Gradual dilation of the vagina
Masturbation training
Semans' stop-start technique
Sensate focus

---

fected by the menstrual cycle. Thus the findings may not be useful in diagnosis. The level of estradiol in the bloodstream is sometimes measured, which possibly reflects levels of desire. It is known that the level of testosterone is important in female sexual drive as well. However, the correlation is not well founded or understood (Bancroft, 2002).

At present, practitioners have several methods of treatment. Drug and hormonal therapies often are used as adjuncts. Sildenafil (Viagra) was approved for use in the spring of 1998 and led to immediate worldwide interest. The mechanism of action is to block the enzyme that breaks down cyclic guanosine monophosphate to boost the chemical's relaxing effect on penile muscles. Combined with stimulation, the drug produces erection 1 hour after ingestion. It is currently being tested on women. Early clinical trials suggest that it will increase blood flow to female genitalia, thus increasing arousal. However, consistent prosexual results with Viagra in women have not been demonstrated (Everaerd and Laan, 2000). Apomorphine, which will be marketed under the trade name **Spontane,** will be available soon as a sublingual tablet for the use in male erectile dysfunction (Rowland and Burnett, 2000). A variety of selective serotonin reuptake inhibitors (SSRIs) anti-

depressants have proved useful in the treatment of premature ejaculation.

The use of *yohimbine*, an α_2-adrenoreceptor blocker, is believed to facilitate blood flow to the genitalia (Piletz et al., 1998). Hormonal replacement may also prove useful. This may involve **testosterone** in males (Bancroft, 2002) and estrogen or testosterone replacement in females (Everaerd and Laan, 2000). Anxiolytics have been used successfully in the treatment of vaginismus (Plaut and RachBeisel, 1997).

Intracorporeal injections of vasodilators such as prostaglandins, papaverine, or combinations of these and other drugs are made directly into the corpus cavernosum and produce erection. Intraurethral pharmacotherapy involving the introduction of vasoactive drugs through a system called MUSE is still available. In males, surgery can be done to alter penile arterial blood flow or to implant prosthetic devices. Prosthetic devices come in two different general forms and have been developed over time with more satisfactory results. There is a semirigid rod that can be made of silicone or metal, and there are inflatable pumps of varying degrees of sophistication.

Elaborate physiologic methods of treatment are not available for women but clearly need to be developed. Historically, treatment involved practice sessions and sex therapy techniques that may involve various types of vibrators. However, they are marketed as toys or relaxation devices instead of biomedical instruments and therefore do not have the sanction or the quality of medical instruments. In 2001 the Food and Drug Administration cleared the **EROS-CTD system** for use in treating the symptoms of female sexual dysfunction (see Understanding and Applying Research box on p. 402). This is a device that creates a gentle suction over the clitoris with the goal of bringing increased blood flow to the genitals. The blood flow then puts pressure on the nerves and causes a reaction in the clitoris. An autonomic reflex also results in increased lubrication and an increased ability to achieve orgasm (Women's Sexual Health, 2001).

A variety of prosexual drugs are on the horizon to treat female sexual problems. These include **phermones** or chemical odors that may influence sexual attraction, peptides such as adrenocorticotropic hormone and **oxytocin,** noradrenergic compounds that increase vasocongestion, and dopaminergic agents. Some women find psychostimulants to be helpful in increasing sexual interest (Everaerd and Laan, 2000).

Psychosocial

There are effective sex therapy techniques for both males and females, as well as couples. These techniques were first developed by Masters and Johnson and have become more effective and comprehensive over the years. Masters and Johnson (1970) developed the **sensate focus** technique, which involves focusing on body sensations, especially those in the breasts and genitals, while shutting out other stimuli.

Body therapies have been used in the field for several decades, including hands-on healing, massage, spiritual en-

UNDERSTANDING and APPLYING RESEARCH

This 2001 study involved 32 female patients who agreed to engage in EROS-CTD therapy over six sessions. In all 20 of the participants had complaints of female sexual dysfunction (FSD); 9 of these were premenopausal and 11 were postmenopausal. The remaining 12 study respondents had no sexual function complaints, and of these 10 were premenopausal and 2 were postmenopausal. Participants were screened for a history of depression, sexual abuse, diabetes, dyspareunia, and hypoactive sexual desire disorder. Before beginning therapy they underwent a complete history and physical (including sexual history and serum estradiol and follicle-stimulating hormone levels). Once enrolled, they were given instruction on how to use the EROS-CTD device. They were then told to use the device in the privacy of their home, with or without their partner. For the first three sessions, the participants were asked to adjust the amount of time on the device to their own satisfaction level, but to activate and release the vacuum for 5 to 15 minutes. They were instructed to record changes in sexual pleasure and to complete a Female Intervention Efficacy Index, which ascertains changes in sensation, lubrication, orgasm, and sexual satisfaction. For the last three sessions, study participants were requested to use a stopwatch to determine the amount of time it took before they experienced sexual pleasure or orgasm. Clients kept a diary, had weekly phone conversations with the researchers, and returned for follow-up care.

To analyze the results, researchers divided the groups into those with FSD and those without. Those volunteers without FSD were able to use the vacuum for up to 4 minutes at a maximum vacuum level of 9.8 mm Hg, and none reported any adverse effects. The 20 women participants with FSD were analyzed using the Wilcoxon signed ranks test. A value of $P<0.05$ was considered statistically significant and all paired observations achieved statistical significance. A total of 90% of these women reported increased sensation after using the EROS-CTD system, 80% had increased lubrication, 55% had an increased ability to achieve orgasm, and 80% said they had more sexual satisfaction. Postmenopausal women with FSD reported greater results than the premenopausal women. The authors concluded that the device results in increased vaginal lubrication and clitoral engorgement and is effective in treating the symptoms of FSD. They noted that future research should be directed at long-term restorative use of the device.

Billups K et al: A new nonpharmacological therapy for female sexual dysfunction. *J Sex Marital Ther* 27:435-441, 2001.

ergizing techniques, chakra balancing, and the adaptation of Eastern principles of sexuality such as tantric yoga. Couples massage is often used to enhance pleasure and provide nonverbal communication. Couples are often instructed to give each other weekly hour-long massages that are nondemand; in other words, the partner being massaged must only receive the sensations without feeling the need to reciprocate. Nondemand also implies that there is no demand for sexual arousal or sexual desire completion.

Sex therapy practitioners and clinical sexologists have a wide range of other psychosocial techniques. In general, homework assignments and supportive counseling form the basis of therapy. Sex therapy often involves weekly or bimonthly visits to the therapists during which clients have the opportunity to discuss symptoms, progress, feelings, and observations.

Education provides a first-line technique for sex therapy. Cognitive restructuring, involving replacing negative thoughts about sexuality with positive thoughts, can be helpful as well. Communication training is also beneficial. For desire phase disorders, erotic materials may be used to help train the individual to be more sexually focused. Clients are often asked to include sexual thinking and feelings into their daily schedule. Males and females can undergo masturbation training to help them be more sensitive to sexual stimulation. It may then train males and females to become orgasmic or improve orgasmic potential. Becoming orgasmic may also entail the use of cognitive restructuring of beliefs about sexuality and techniques to reduce the fear of losing control. Hypnotherapy has been used for a variety of sexual dysfunctions. It focuses specifically on the abatement of symptomatology.

For males, the stop-start technique helps overcome premature ejaculation. In this technique, developed in 1956 by Semans, the couple practices foreplay and stimulation until the point of ejaculation. Then direct stimulation is stopped until the feeling subsides. The couple resumes the procedure three times. This technique trains the male to be more aware of the sensation of impending ejaculation and to better control the timing.

After medical etiologies of sexual pain disorders of dyspareunia and vaginismus have been ruled out, appropriate strategies can be used. Insertions of a finger or **vaginal dilator** in the vagina are begun slowly. The gradual introduction of larger inserters, coupled with relaxation techniques, will help the woman overcome her fear and pain and help decrease involuntary spasm. Sets of dilators may be purchased from medical supply firms for this purpose.

The tools and methods of sex therapy have been important developments in the field. But without the sensitivity and attention to other factors in the client's sexual realm, they may not provide satisfactory results. Some other factors include cultural and religious values, other psychologic disorders, poor sexual learning, and body image issues.

Anon (1976) created what is known as the PLISSIT model of sexual intervention. This is an excellent model for the collaborative care of clients with sexual dysfunctions. The P stands for giving *permission,* that is, giving permission for people to be sexual and to have sexual feelings. If the problem persists, go to LI, giving *limited information,* that is, information and education concerning specific sexual problem(s). If the problem persists, go to SS, making *specific suggestions,* that is, calling on the specific treatments for various dysfunctions. If the problem persists, refer the client to a sex therapist/clinical sexologist for IT, *intensive therapy.*

EVALUATION

Evaluation of the effectiveness of intervention is an ongoing process and involves many levels. If the outcome criteria are thorough and carefully defined, evaluation is a relatively simple process of determining whether these outcomes were met. The nursing process is cyclical; if the nurse determines that outcome criteria were not met, he or she must go back to the assessment phase to determine if some key underlying factors were overlooked.

To better understand this cyclic nature in the area of sexual dysfunction, refer to the Nursing Care Plan on pp. 404 to 405. During assessment the nurse learned that Naomi had decreased sexual desire and arousal beginning 6 years ago, although she believed these desires were never very strong. One of the nursing diagnoses identified was sexual dysfunction resulting from a lack of knowledge, beliefs about sexuality, and as a side effect of medication. One of the outcome criteria that the nurse developed with Naomi was that she would acquire and read female erotica on a daily basis. The rationale for this criterion was the theory that consciously putting sex into one's life may help to enhance sexuality and that the practice of reading positive, erotic messages may help to counterbalance some of the previously learned beliefs. If Naomi says she still has not bought the books or has left them on the table unread, what should the nurse do next?

The nurse should go back to assessment. Was something missed? Perhaps something was overlooked in Naomi's history; perhaps she is opposed to erotica as part of her belief structure or is worried she will be embarrassed by reading the stories. Perhaps her reluctance is due to some still unresolved anger at her partner for leaving. Naomi may then be sabotaging her treatment as a way to get back at her partner. If any of these or additional issues are found in assessment, the nurse must revamp the care plan to include them. Nursing diagnosis, outcome criteria, and interventions will then change. If nothing was missed in assessment, perhaps the outcome criteria were unrealistic. The issue of Naomi's anxiety may be complex and deep, and it may be unrealistic to assume that she will be able to relax and read erotic stories by the second session. The need for ongoing evaluation can be seen in this example.

PARAPHILIAS

HISTORICAL AND THEORETIC PERSPECTIVES

The **paraphilias** are a group of behaviors commonly accepted by the clinical description of sexual deviations. Paraphilias present inappropriate sexual fantasies involving deviant sexual acts, inappropriate sexual urges, and acting out of these fantasies and urges.

Once a psychiatric syndrome is described clinically, several steps, including laboratory studies, delimitation from other disorders, follow-up studies, and family studies, are necessary to establish diagnostic validity. It is generally acknowledged that no psychiatric syndrome has yet to be fully validated by the complete series of these steps. However, many syndromes have had a substantial body of data published in most phases of the validation. Little is known, however, about the data in the other areas establishing clinical validity. For instance, although there are some laboratory tests and follow-up studies of sexual deviance, there are few family studies of paraphilias.

LEGAL IMPLICATIONS
Forensic Psychiatry and Paraphilias

Forensic psychiatry is the application of psychiatry for legal purposes. This highly specialized area of psychiatry addresses issues related to criminal responsibility and competency to stand trial for various crimes that have been committed. Formulating a forensic opinion regarding the paraphilias is difficult at best. A person who has committed a sexual crime in response to psychotic processes, such as hallucinations or delusions, may be considered not criminally responsible (insanity plea); however, this individual may not be diagnosed with a paraphilic disorder. A person who commits a sexual crime in response to "recurrent, intense, sexually arousing fantasies, sexual urges or behaviors involving (1) nonhuman objects, (2) the suffering or humiliation of oneself or one's partner, or (3) children or other nonconsenting persons . . ." (APA, 2000) may meet the criteria of a paraphilic disorder and may or may not include forensic issues as previously stated. An important aspect to explore during a forensic evaluation is the client's ability to appreciate the criminality of the behavior (sexual crime) and the ability to conform the behavior to the requirements of the law, which is not intended to address the client's ability to control himself or herself. This is a part of the forensic opinion and depending on the results of this assessment, the outcome may be a prison sentence or a sentence to a maximum security forensic psychiatric facility until such time that the client is assessed as no longer a danger to society.

The Sexually Violent Predator Act

In 1990 the State of Washington's legislature enacted a bill known as the *Community Protection Act*, which provided for the civil commitment of sexually violent predators. After a term of incarceration, a sexually violent predator may be civilly committed against his will to a state psychiatric facility until such time as he is deemed to be safe to return to the community. This was the foundation and model legislation for the development of similar laws referred to as the *Sexually Violent Predator Act*, which has been passed into legislation in 17 states across the United States. This law established a civil commitment procedure for "any person who has been convicted or charges with a sexually violent offense and who suffers from a mental abnormality or personality disorder which makes the person likely to engage in the predatory acts of sexual violence" (Wash. Rev. Code Ann. §71.09.030, 1991). Washington State Law defines a predatory act as "...an act directed toward a stranger or an individual with whom a relationship has been established or promoted for the primary purpose of victimization" (Wash. Rev. Code Ann. §71.09.030, 1991). Therefore it is conceivable that most sexually violent predators are either pedophiles or rapists.

NURSING CARE PLAN

During a routine history and examination, Naomi, a 46-year-old woman, mentions to the nurse that she has some sexual issues to discuss. She tells the nurse that recently her partner of 7 years broke off the relationship because of these sexual problems. Naomi says that she is in generally good health. She was diagnosed with depression 5 years ago and has been taking Paxil, 20 mg q.d. She is on no other medications except for a daily vitamin pill. She tells the nurse that when she and her partner were first dating, sex seemed good in the relationship. They were affectionate to one another and had sex approximately two to three times a week. Shortly after they began living together 6 years ago, sex dropped off to monthly and then became nonexistent. She says her partner tried to initiate sex but gave up after she rebuffed him time after time. Eventually the intimacy and closeness wore away and they fought more often. Without much discussion her partner announced that their relationship was over and promptly moved out. Naomi said she was devastated at first but now believes it is a wake up call to do something about her sexuality.

Naomi explained that she was born in Poland to a conservative Jewish family and that sexuality was never discussed. She had no formal sex education but recalls being interested in sex and sought out books for information. She does not recall any early childhood sexual experiences and says that she has never masturbated. She did not date in high school, partly because of the strictness of her family. During college she had a brief relationship with a man that she considered marrying. However, there was little attraction and she decided to leave Poland to live in the United States. Since arriving in this country she has had several other relationships, none of which was longer than 3 years.

According to the client, she experiences little sexual interest. She reports that she has never put much focus on sex but that in the last 6 years it has gotten less important. She says that she is concerned about this and would like to be "more normal" when it comes to sex. She says she is slow to get aroused and sometimes she and her partner would give up after getting frustrated by the response. She rarely has orgasms. She believes that she has always had these problems to some degree but that they have gotten worse. Now that she is out of the relationship, she is not sure what to do about her sexuality but believes that in future relationships it will again be a factor. She reports being quite stressed about this and says that she has been avoiding social commitments for fear she may meet someone.

Towards the end of the interview, Naomi shyly and reluctantly reveals that she finds sex somewhat "dirty" and that she is a lesbian and has had sexual relationships only with women since she was in college. She says that her family still lives in Poland are unaware of her sexual orientation.

DSM-IV-TR Diagnoses

Axis I	Hypoactive sexual desire disorder
	Major depression
Axis II	None noted
Axis III	None known
Axis IV	Moderate = 3 (primary relationships, socialization, anxiety)
Axis V	GAF = 55 (current)
	GAF = 65 (past year)

NURSING DIAGNOSIS: Sexual dysfunction related to deficient knowledge, beliefs about sexuality, side effects of medication, as evidenced by client's reported lack of sexual interest and arousal and distress about it.

CLIENT OUTCOMES	NURSING INTERVENTIONS	EVALUATION
Naomi will complete one factual book on sexuality by the next session with the nurse.	Suggest that Naomi read *Women's Sexuality* by Ellison by next session. *This can help educate client about human sexuality to overcome some of her deficits.*	Naomi reported that she had read the book and was able to discuss what she read.
	Schedule a follow-up appointment *to ensure continuity.*	
Naomi will read women's erotica on a daily basis.	Suggest that she read female erotica by authors Barbach or Friday for a short time every day. *This can help to enhance her awareness of sexuality and help her overcome some of the previously learned messages.*	Naomi did not buy a book on female erotica until 2 days ago. She has read stories since then.
Naomi will make an appointment with her psychiatrist to discuss her medication by next session with the nurse.	Suggest that Naomi discuss the potentially negative sexual side effects of her Paxil. *The nurse is aware that SSRIs may diminish sexual interest and may affect arousal.*	Naomi reports that after discussing the medication side effects, she and her physician decided to do a trial of Wellbutrin for depression.
Naomi will agree to enter sex therapy with a qualified therapist by next session.	Encourage client to receive treatment for sexual issues. *Sex therapy may be helpful in overcoming sexual difficulty and anxiety.*	Naomi reports that she has an appointment with the sex therapist in 2 weeks.
	Educate her about techniques of sexual therapy. *She will be better informed to make appropriate choices for herself.*	
	Refer client to qualified sex therapist for continued professional help.	

NURSING CARE PLAN—cont'd

NURSING DIAGNOSIS: Anxiety related to stress from recent loss of relationship, fears about sexual functioning, perceived feeling of how others will respond to her orientation, as evidenced by client's statements that she is anxious and unable to relate socially.

CLIENT OUTCOMES	NURSING INTERVENTIONS	EVALUATION
Naomi will be able to discuss her feelings of anxiety with the nurse by follow-up session.	Encourage Naomi to be aware of her anxiety and how it affects her sexually and in other areas of her life. *Knowing more about the nature of the anxiety will help client find better ways to work with it.* Ask Naomi to describe situations that make her anxious. *This will help her prepare better for periods of anxiety and create strategies to overcome them.*	Naomi was able to discuss her fears about entering another relationship and feelings about her sexual orientation with the nurse. Naomi was able to relate that going to all female events in the lesbian community made her anxious and she feared exposure. She decided in the future she would go with a friend.
Naomi will practice breathing and relaxation exercises during her periods of erotic reading and when confronted with social obligations.	Educate Naomi on breathing and relaxation exercises. *This will help Naomi focus on relaxation when she is confronted with sexuality and social contact instead of anxiety.*	Naomi reports that she is able to focus on relaxation during the time she is reading erotic material.

NURSING DIAGNOSIS: Hopelessness related to belief that she will never overcome her sexual problems and be able to have a healthy relationship, as evidenced by her statements concerning this.

CLIENT OUTCOMES	NURSING INTERVENTIONS	EVALUATION
Naomi will be able to verbalize feelings of self-doubt and hopelessness with the nurse during follow-up session.	Encourage Naomi to express her feelings *to provide some relief and to allow her to feel validated.*	Naomi was able to willingly discuss her feelings during the session.
Naomi will report a feeling of hope after she sees her physician and the sex therapist.	Encourage Naomi to follow up with her physician and the sex therapist. Ask her to report progress and ideas she is trying. *To recognize that there are resources to help her with the problems she faces and to provide ongoing support for the work she is doing.*	Naomi reports that with the change in medication and the sex therapy exercises she is using, she believes she is more interested in sex now.

ETIOLOGY

It is unclear as to what may predispose an individual to develop a paraphilic disorder. Several studies have attempted to suggest etiologic factors and the prevalence of sexual deviancies (see Understanding and Applying Research box). Research has not concluded cause-and-effect etiology of the paraphilias.

Biologic Factors

It is important to acknowledge that people do not voluntarily decide what types of sexual arousal patterns they will have. Researchers suggest possible etiologies (Box 17-3). In the biologic domain, two areas are addressed: chromosomal functioning and hormonal levels.

In 1942 Klinefelter and his colleagues described Klinefelter's syndrome as a condition characterized by (1) the development of gynecomastia (enlarged breasts) at the time of puberty, (2) aspermatogenesis (low sperm production), and (3) an increased secretion of follicle stimulating-hormone by the pituitary gland in the brain.

In this particular syndrome, the client presents with 47 chromosomes instead of the normal 46; an extra X chromosome is present. The client may be thought of as a male

UNDERSTANDING and APPLYING RESEARCH

The purpose of this study was to investigate familial patterns of pedophilia. This was done by a double-blind chart review of 33 male clients with paraphilic disorders and 33 male clients with depression as the control group. Information obtained included demographic data, paraphilic diagnoses according to DSM-III criteria, age of onset, and family history for both groups of patients.

The authors identified that the age of risk for developing a paraphilic disorder was between 15 and 40 years. Results were statistically significant in that 18.5% of the families of patients with a paraphilic disorder had family members (mostly males) with a sexual disorder.

This study identified that perhaps pedophilia, as well as other paraphilic disorders, may indeed run in families across generations. Further studies have been done to determine how this transmission occurs.

Gaffney GR, Lurie SF, Berlin FB: Is there familial transmission of pedophilia? *J Nerv Ment Dis* 172(9):546, 1984.

(XY) with an extra X chromosome or as a female (XX) with an extra Y chromosome. Clients with this syndrome look like a male at birth. Hence, parents naturally raise them as males and assign them a male sex role. Money et al. (1957) described an otherwise normal 8-year-old boy with Klinefelter's syndrome who insisted he felt more comfortable dressed in girl's clothing. Klinefelter's clients have very small testes and produce little testosterone and virtually no sperm. They also experience problems with sexual orientation and the nature of their erotic desires.

Some theorists suggest that biologic factors may be etiologic considerations in the development of sexual disorders and that early life experiences may contribute to the development of a paraphilic disorder.

Box 17-3 Etiologic Factors for Paraphilias

Biologic factors
Chromosomal functioning
Hormonal levels

Experiential factors
History of sexual abuse

Environmental factors

Hereditary predisposition

Hereditary/Environmental Factors

Gaffney et al. (1984) found evidence that suggests familial transmission of paraphilic disorders. Groth (1979) identified children who were sexually active with adults during childhood as being environmentally influenced and therefore potentially predisposed for developing a pedophilic disorder. This is an example of victim turned **victimizer,** or sex offender.

EPIDEMIOLOGY

According to the DSM-IV-TR, although paraphilias are not generally diagnosed in clinical facilities, the sizeable commercial market in paraphiliac pornography and paraphernalia suggests that its prevalence in the community is "likely to be higher" (APA, 2000). The paraphilias that most commonly present problems are pedophilia, voyeurism, and exhibitionism. About one half of the clients with paraphilias seen clinically are married (APA, 2000).

CLINICAL DESCRIPTION

The essential diagnostic features of a paraphilia are "recurrent, intense sexually arousing fantasies, sexual urges, or behaviors generally involving (1) nonhuman objects, (2) the suf-

---

DSM-IV-TR CRITERIA
Paraphilias

Exhibitionism
The exposure of one's genitals to an unsuspecting person(s) followed by sexual arousal.

Fetishism
Use of objects (e.g., panties, rubber sheeting) for the purpose of becoming sexually aroused.

Frotteurism
Rubbing up against a nonconsenting person to heighten sexual arousal.

Pedophilia
Fondling and/or other types of sexual activities with a prepubescent child (usually under age 13 years who has not yet developed secondary sex characteristics). Heterosexual pedophiles are sexually attracted to female children under age 13 years. Homosexual pedophiles are sexually attracted to male children under age 13 years. **Ego syntonic pedophiles** do not view this type of behavior as troublesome and will not voluntarily seek treatment for it. **Ego dystonic pedophiles** are concerned and troubled with this type of behavior and might voluntarily seek treatment to deal with it.
Types of pedophiles:
　　Homosexual
　　Heterosexual
　　Bisexual (sexual attraction to both males and females)
　　Limited to incest (sexual attraction to a child in one's immediate family)
　　Exclusive type (sexually attracted to children only)
　　Nonexclusive type (may also be sexually attracted to adults of either sex)

Sexual Masochism
Being the receiver of pain (either physical or emotional), humiliation, or being made to suffer for the purpose of becoming sexually aroused.

Sexual Sadism
The infliction of pain (either physical or emotional) or humiliation onto another person followed by sexual arousal.

Transvestic Fetishism
The act of cross-dressing (heterosexual males wearing female clothing) for the purpose of becoming sexually aroused.

Voyeurism
Observing unsuspecting persons who are naked, in the act of disrobing, or engaging in sexual activity ("peeping Tom") followed by sexual arousal.

Paraphilia Not Otherwise Specified
Disorders that do not meet the criteria for the aforementioned categories:
　Telephone scatologia: Obscene phone calling; "900" sex lines
　Necrophilia: Sexual activity with corpses
　Partialism: Exclusive focus on a particular body part for sexual arousal
　Zoophilia: Sexual activity involving participation with animals (bestiality)
　Coprophilia: Sexual arousal by contact with feces
　Klismaphilia: Sexual arousal generated by use of enemas
　Urophilia: Sexual arousal by contact with urine
　Ephebophilia:* Fondling and/or other types of sexual activities with postpubescent children (usually between the ages of 13 to 18 years) who are developing secondary sex characteristics (e.g., pubic hair, breasts)
　Paraphilic coercive disorder:* Rape; aggressive sexual assault involving an act of sexual intercourse against one's will and without consent

Modified from American Psychiatric Association: *Diagnostic and Statistic Manual of Mental Disorders,* Fourth Edition, Text Revision. Washington, DC, American Psychiatric Association, 2000.
*Not included in DSM-IV-TR.

fering or humiliation of oneself or one's partner, or (3) children or other nonconsenting persons that occur over a period of at least 6 months" (APA, 2000). Another criterion is that "the behavior, sexual urges, or fantasies cause clinically significant distress in social, occupational, or other important areas of functioning" (APA, 2000). The DSM-IV-TR Criteria box summarizes the criteria and description of the paraphilias.

PROGNOSIS

Nurses should be cautioned in attempting to predict **sexual recidivism** (the chronic, repetitive inappropriate acting out of sexual behaviors considered to be unacceptable that have or have not resulted in criminal conviction). Clients currently undergoing treatment for a sexual disorder may have a lower level of sexual recidivism (Berlin et al., 1991). The Berlin et al. (1991) study revealed a higher reoffense rate for those clients who do not receive (or who have never received) treatment than for those engaged in treatment. Treatment compliance is a therapeutic issue that nurses treating this population must address (see Case Study).

It is important for nurses to also acknowledge that treatment efficacy cannot be proven at this time. Further studies are warranted in this area.

DISCHARGE CRITERIA

Client will:
- State nature of specific paraphilic disorder and its impact on self and others (breakdown/absence of cognitive distortions).

CASE STUDY

Martin is a 24-year-old college student who attends the local university and lives at home with his parents and two older sisters. He was referred for treatment after conviction for raping a 22-year-old female. Martin has been an active participant in an eight-member outpatient sex offender group for the last 5 years. The Department of Parole and Probation is about to release him back into the community without any further legal requirements. The nurse group leader is uncomfortable with Martin's desire to be discharged outright from group. Her discomfort is related to the seriousness of the disorder, not to the amount of progress he has made. Martin has been compliant with treatment during the last 5 years. His treatment consisted of weekly group attendance with participation, compliance with medications when prescribed, development and implementation of appropriate relapse prevention strategies, and sound understanding of the nature of his disorder.

Critical Thinking
1. What criteria does the nurse use to effectively evaluate Martin's readiness for discharge from therapy?
2. What concerns might the nurse have regarding Martin's prognosis after discharge?
3. With whom might the nurse consult in rendering her decision regarding Martin's discharge from the therapy group?
4. Would family therapy be indicated on discharge from the group therapy session? What is the rationale for this intervention?
5. How could the nurse be responsible if Martin relapses after discharge from the group?

- Identify **triggers**—stimuli that heighten unacceptable sexual cravings and provoke inappropriate sexual behaviors.
- Develop appropriate relapse prevention strategies.
- Communicate and problem solve effectively.
- Practice appropriate coping strategies.
- Identify support systems.

THE NURSING PROCESS

ASSESSMENT

The client with a sexual disorder may exhibit a variety of behavioral symptoms, depending on the nature of the disorder. Some symptoms are more difficult to assess than others. The client with a pedophilic disorder may exhibit perceptual disturbances. It is not uncommon to hear such a client state, for example, "The child looked older than he was." This may also be perceived as a cognitive distortion (an unconscious defense mechanism).

Cognitive distortions may be present in the client with a sexual disorder. Two cognitive distortions most often present in this client population are denial and rationalization. *Denial* is a defense mechanism used to avoid dealing with problems and responsibilities related to one's behaviors. *Rationalization* is a defense mechanism used to justify upsetting behaviors by creating reasons (rationale) that would allow the individual to believe that the behaviors were warranted or appropriate. These are the most critical issues that the nurse must address early in the therapeutic process. A client making a statement such as, "Well, the child didn't fight me and agreed to have sex with me" is a good indication that such cognitive distortions are present.

Another symptom that requires assessment is a disturbance in feeling. Clients with paraphilic disorders commonly lack remorse for their victims. If they do experience remorse, they may be unable to acknowledge it as a result of cognitive distortions. Occasionally, clients with a pedophilic disorder may claim to experience feelings of "being loved" by the child with whom they have had inappropriate sexual activity.

Clients with a paraphilic disorder should also be assessed for the presence of behavioral and relating disturbances. These are assessed in the client's inability to develop age-appropriate relationships, altered relationships with others, and social withdrawal that may occur secondary to embarrassment or media attention (see Nursing Assessment Questions box on p. 408).

NURSING DIAGNOSIS

After collecting client assessment data, the nurse is ready to begin formulating diagnoses. In doing so, the nurse may find that the client has symptoms indicative of more than one diagnosis, such as a paraphilic disorder, a psychoactive substance disorder, and/or a personality disorder. Multiple diagnoses are not addressed in this chapter.

NURSING ASSESSMENT QUESTIONS
Paraphilias

1. What brings you here for treatment? *To assess client's level of insight*
2. Do you think you have a sexual disorder? *To determine if cognitive distortions are present*
3. Do you think you've caused any physical or emotional harm to your victims? *To determine if there are disturbances of feelings present*
4. How has this problem affected your lifestyle and relationships? *To determine the presence of disturbances in relationships*

COLLABORATIVE DIAGNOSES

DSM-IV-TR Diagnoses*	NANDA Diagnoses†
Exhibitionism	Anxiety
Fetishism	Ineffective coping
Frotteurism	Ineffective denial
Pedophilia	Interrupted family processes
Sexual masochism	Deficient knowledge
Sexual sadism	Disturbed personal identity
Transvestic fetishism	Ineffective role performance
Voyeurism	Risk for situational low self-esteem
	Risk for self-mutilation
	Ineffective sexuality patterns
	Impaired social interaction
	Risk for other-directed violence

NOTE: These nursing diagnoses may be applied to all medical diagnoses for the client with a paraphilic disorder.

*From American Psychiatric Association: *Diagnostic and Statistic Manual of Mental Disorders,* Fourth Edition, Text Revision. Washington, DC, American Psychiatric Association, 2000.

†From NANDA International (2003). NANDA Nursing Diagnoses: Definitions and Classification 2003-2004. Philadelphia: NANDA

However, it is important for the nurse to be aware of this possibility.

When addressing nursing diagnoses for the client with a paraphilic disorder, the nurse has many diagnoses from which to choose and selects those that are specific and appropriate to each individual based on an analysis of comprehensive data collected during assessment (see Collaborative Diagnosis table).

Nursing Diagnoses for Paraphilias

- Ineffective coping
- Ineffective denial
- Interrupted family processes
- Deficient knowledge (of illness and aspects of treatment)
- Noncompliance (with therapeutic regimen)
- Ineffective sexuality patterns
- Impaired social interaction
- Risk for other-directed violence

OUTCOME IDENTIFICATION

Client-centered outcomes should relate to the client's nursing diagnoses and be the opposite of the defining characteristics. Outcomes should be stated in clear, measurable, behavioral terms and include a time frame, when feasible, in which the client is expected to achieve them. Outcomes may be described as expected or anticipated and are viewed as specific goals to be achieved through the implementation of the plan of care. Examples of behavioral terms the nurse may want to use in developing client-centered outcomes include words such as "Client will . . . state, list, perform, and participate."

Client will:

- State two sexually inappropriate behaviors within 3 days of admission.
- Write a list of triggers that provoke inappropriate sexual acting out within the first week of admission.
- Describe two appropriate coping strategies within 1 week of admission.
- List several relapse prevention strategies that are appropriate to his or her disorder within the second week of admission.
- Actively participate in weekly group psychotherapy sessions for clients with sexual disorders.
- Verbalize two appropriate methods to meet sexual needs by the time of discharge.
- Explain the importance of medication compliance and follow-up care with outpatient group psychotherapy by time of discharge.

PLANNING

After diagnoses have been established and client problem identification has occurred, the nurse is ready to begin developing a plan of care specific to the individual client. Client care should be based on mutually agreed on, realistic, client-centered outcomes. The nurse should involve the client in the development of an individualized plan of care, with the expectation that the client will participate in the planning process.

In the population of clients with paraphilic disorders, it is not uncommon to find cognitive distortions. Nurses must be aware of this possibility as they obtain client input into the development of the plan of care. For example, a client who is in denial of a paraphilic disorder may not be able to fully cooperate with the planning of care or view client-centered outcomes as realistic.

CLIENT AND FAMILY TEACHING GUIDELINES

Relapse Prevention Strategies

TEACH THE CLIENT AND SIGNIFICANT OTHER:

How to identify triggers that provoke inappropriate sexual thoughts and desires by listing the precursors to inappropriate sexual acting out (e.g., the client with a pedophilic disorder who claims he must drive by the schoolyard at 3 PM to get home [school yard = trigger]).
Relapse prevention strategies are based on identification of triggers.
To avoid reoffending.

Additional Treatment Modalities
For Clients With Paraphilic Disorders

Antiandrogenic medications
    Depo-Provera
    Lupron Depot
Selective serotonin reuptake inhibitors (SSRIs)
Psychotherapy/psychoeducational groups
    Individual and group
        Insight-oriented
        Goal-directed
Occupational/recreational therapy
Family therapy/couples counseling

IMPLEMENTATION

The nurse should work with the client to develop an individualized plan of care that will help the client identify the presence of cognitive distortions (if appropriate), prevent reoffending by identifying triggers that provoke inappropriate sexual activity, and develop effective relapse prevention strategies (see Client and Family Teaching Guidelines box). The nurse should also explain the significance of treatment on recidivism and stress the importance of medication compliance and follow-up care with outpatient group psychotherapy.

Providing nursing care to such a client may be difficult because of the sensitive nature of this disorder. Nurses must recognize this possibility and be aware of their own comfort level when discussing sexual issues with these clients. Identifying the presence of a paraphilic disorder may have devastating effects on clients and their significant others. It is important for nurses to include significant others in the interventions to the extent that they can participate.

Nursing Interventions

1. Help the client confront cognitive distortions through direct questioning methods that promote reality orientation as to the client's offending behavior. Open confrontation by the nurse may be needed, including an explanation of the impact of these distortions on treatment outcomes. Journaling may assist in the breakdown of cognitive distortions and help the client track inappropriate sexual fantasies. *Client must be aware of the problem and acknowledge it before treatment can begin.*

2. Educate the client and significant others about paraphilic disorders and aspects of treatment, such as identifying triggers that provoke inappropriate sexual activity and methods that help avoid relapse. Encourage active participation in the educational process by compiling lists in a journal for review by the client and the nurse. Copies of these lists should be placed in the client's medical record to inform other team members about the client's progress. *This knowledge forms a foundation for treatment.*

3. Enhance the client's compliance with treatment by openly discussing with him or her the effect of inappropriate sexual behaviors on others. Provide research studies regarding the effects of treatment on recidivism rates and handouts about the scope of treatment and how compliance can assist in regaining control of sexual behaviors. *Compliance with treatment reduces the risk of relapse.*

4. Teach the client appropriate coping strategies, assertiveness skills, and problem-solving techniques *to promote follow-through of the treatment plan and to facilitate appropriate sexual behaviors.*

5. Promote the client's development of appropriate social skills and provide support and encouragement to the client for efforts at control of the disorder. Peer-to-peer mentorship may be appropriate to enhance appropriate social skills and feelings of acceptance. *The client may feel guilty over his or her behavior and become socially isolated. Support and encouragement of the client will signify that there are healthy, functional, acceptable aspects of his or her personality.*

Additional Treatment Modalities

After careful assessment to determine the specific diagnoses of paraphilic disorder, a range of treatment modalities can be instituted (see Additional Treatment Modalities box).

Pharmacologic

The need for medications is based on the collaborative efforts of the multidisciplinary team to assess the intensity and impulsivity of the client's disorder and symptoms.

Depo-Provera (medroxyprogesterone acetate), 500 mg intramuscularly once a week, has been prescribed with some success for clients with a paraphilic disorder (Berlin and Meineke, 1981). This form of external control helps clients develop their own internal controls to avoid relapse. Clients have reported that this medication lowers the frequency and intensity of inappropriate sexual thoughts and fantasies.

The nurse needs to be aware of several side effects. Because this type of medication decreases testosterone levels and sperm production, the client who is receiving Depo-Provera may not be able to father a child. Common side effects include weight gain, increased blood pressure, and fatigue. The nurse may suggest a dietary consultation to help the client maintain weight and decrease the possibility of weight gain. Blood pressures must be taken before each dose. In general, if the diastolic is 100 mm Hg or greater, the medication should be withheld. The nurse must communicate with the physician regarding blood pressure readings and whether to administer the medication.

The medication is viscous and should be given in doses of no more than 500 mg per muscle. The gluteal muscle may also be used in administering Depo-Provera. It is not necessary to administer this medication via Z track because there is no conclusive evidence that this method of injection increases absorption. Clients may complain of pain in the injection sites and need to be reassured that the pain will subside within a day. If given in the deltoid muscle, the nurse may want to instruct the client to engage in range-of-motion exercises (moving the shoulder and arm in a circular motion).

Depo-Provera should not be administered without informed consent and the client's signature on a consent form that explains about the medication and its therapeutic and nontherapeutic effects. The nurse may review this form with the client after a decision has been made by the physician to include this as part of the client's individualized plan of care.

Lupron Depot (leuprolide) is a relatively new form of treatment that is being used more frequently with the paraphilic population. This medication may be a more powerful antiandrogenic drug. It acts similarly to Depo-Provera by lowering testosterone levels in the client with a paraphilic disorder. This medication is usually prescribed as 7.5 mg intramuscularly once a month. It is also available in a nondepo form; the usual prescribed dose is 1 mg/day subcutaneously.

Side effects include a decrease in libido (the desired result), bone pain, osteoporetic changes, gynecomastia, hair growth, weight gain, high blood pressure, dizziness, headaches, mood swings, and phlebitis. The nurse must have the knowledge to assess for the presence of nontherapeutic effects.

In the beginning of treatment with Lupron Depot, clients should be prescribed flutamide (Eulexin), 250 mg PO three times a day, to enhance the testosterone-suppressing aspects of Lupron Depot by blocking testosterone receptors. This should be prescribed secondary to the increase in testosterone production within the first 2 to 4 weeks after having started treatment with Lupron Depot.

Again, it is important for the nurse to monitor the client's blood pressure before administering Lupron Depot. The same criteria should apply to Depo-Provera.

Clients receiving Depo-Provera or Lupron Depot should also be monitored for bone mass density, as these powerful antiandrogenic medications may precipitate osteoporetic changes. Clients may also be prescribed biphosphonate medications, such as Fosamax, to address this potentially dangerous side effect.

Selective Serotonin Reuptake Inhibitors. Current literature contains several case reports regarding the treatment of paraphilic disorders with SSRIs such as Prozac or Zoloft. These medications have fewer side effects than the antiandrogenic medications. Single case reports address the efficacy of paraphilic treatment with SSRIs by increasing serotonin activity, thereby decreasing sexual appetite. It is important to note that further research is warranted because of the absence of double-blind chart studies in this area (Kafka, 1997).

Psychotherapy/Psychoeducation Groups

Nurses may lead or colead psychotherapy/psychoeducation groups with the physician or another member of the treatment team if they have the appropriate group psychotherapy credentials.

The purposes of group psychotherapy/**psychoeducation** are (1) to address cognitive distortions and (2) to provide education to this client population regarding identification of triggers, relapse prevention strategies, importance of treatment compliance, self-esteem issues, appropriate coping strategies, and problem-solving skills.

Recreational and occupational therapy may also be provided to assist the client in time structuring, which may be viewed as a relapse prevention strategy (see Chapter 19 for further information).

Family/couples therapy may also be recommended, depending on the individual client care needs. This form of therapy is usually provided by the social worker but may also be provided by a masters-prepared nurse or physician.

EVALUATION

Nurses must continually evaluate the effectiveness of their interventions on the behavior to successfully treat this population. If identified nursing interventions are not helping the client achieve his or her outcomes, revisions must be made in the nursing care plan. The nurse may want to discuss the plan with the client and obtain his or her assistance in revising it. The areas in which client outcomes have been successfully achieved should be identified as "resolved." If newly identified problems arise, these should also be addressed in the client's plan of care.

In treating the client with a paraphilic disorder, it is not unrealistic to expect the client to acknowledge the presence of the paraphilic disorder, identify triggers, develop relapse prevention strategies, and state the importance of treatment compliance after discharge. If these outcomes are not met by the time of discharge, the client would be at a greater risk for reoffending. The need to protect both the client and society from possible relapse or recidivism is critical.

CLINICAL ALERT

The nurse should be alert for signs of noncompliance with treatment or signs indicative of potential relapse, as evidenced by such things as the client's refusal to take medications and/or attend therapy sessions. Client statements such as "I don't know why I need this; I'm just here because the courts sent me," social withdrawal, presence of cognitive distortions, and lack of candidness may all be viewed as risk factors for noncompliance.

NURSING CARE PLAN

Robert is a 50-year-old vice president of a major corporation who has been diagnosed as having voyeurism. He intermittently acted out by engaging in voyeuristic activities at his country club in the ladies locker room. He would secretly masturbate while "peeping." His wife is currently unaware of his behavior but suspects something is wrong. When she confronted Robert regarding her suspicions, he denied any problems.

Robert voluntarily came for treatment primarily out of concern that his wife would discover his disorder. He also began to recognize that he spends a great deal of time on the job fantasizing and/or engaging in voyeuristic and masturbatory activities. Robert has been lying to his wife about his whereabouts for approximately 10 years.

The treatment team focused on assisting Robert in developing appropriate coping strategies. Treatment also included psychoeducation regarding trigger identification and appropriate relapse prevention strategies. The need for couples counseling to disclose the "secret" of Robert's behavior was also addressed. Robert was given Depo-Provera, 500 mg IM q wk, to help him control his inappropriate sexual acting-out.

DSM-IV-TR Diagnoses

Axis I	Voyeurism
Axis II	Deferred—compulsive traits noted
Axis III	None
Axis IV	Moderate = 3 (marital conflict, job stress, anxiety)
Axis V	GAF = 61 (current)
	GAF = 61 (past year)

NURSING DIAGNOSIS: Ineffective sexuality pattern related to use of cognitive distortions (denial) and sexual behaviors in a socially unacceptable manner, as evidenced by engaging in sexual behavior without regard for others and public masturbation.

CLIENT OUTCOMES	NURSING INTERVENTIONS	EVALUATION
Robert will identify two sexual behaviors that are socially unacceptable within first week of admission.	Assess for presence of cognitive distortions via a thorough sexual history. *If cognitive distortions are present, Robert may not be able to identify socially unacceptable behaviors and further treatment is warranted.* Discuss with Robert what are socially unacceptable sexual behaviors and why *to educate the client about problematic sexual behaviors and their implications on society.* Encourage Robert's participation in a group for clients with sexual disorders. *These clients frequently believe that they are the only ones who experience inappropriate sexual behaviors, which may lead to feelings of hopelessness, embarrassment, and isolation. Group therapy provides confrontation, support, and hope.*	Robert readily identified his voyeuristic and public masturbatory behaviors as inappropriate after 1 week of admission.

NURSING DIAGNOSIS: Ineffective coping related to inability to trust wife with his secret and inadequate problem-solving skills, as evidenced by use of maladaptive coping methods such as lying, ineffective communication with wife (unable to discuss thoughts and feelings regarding disorder), anxiety, and fear of discovery by wife.

CLIENT OUTCOMES	NURSING INTERVENTIONS	EVALUATION
Robert will effectively communicate his thoughts and feelings about his disorder and behaviors with his wife and selected staff within 1 week of admission. Robert will identify concerns he has about disclosing his disorder and behaviors to his wife by the time of discharge. Robert will formulate two relapse prevention strategies by the time of discharge, such as calling his wife before leaving work so that she will expect him at a certain time, to avoid reoffending.	Encourage Robert to verbalize his thoughts and feelings concerning his current coping methods (lying, nondisclosure) *to illustrate to Robert the impact of his present coping strategies on himself and his wife.* Educate Robert and his wife about his disorder, its implications, and treatment. *Educating Robert and his wife about his disorder and aspects of treatment will alleviate their fears and anxiety, develop trust, and establish an effective, supportive relationship.* Help Robert formulate appropriate strategies to use at significant times during his vulnerability *to prevent him from reoffending.*	Robert verbalized many thoughts and feelings about the impact this could have on his marriage. At the time of discharge, Robert was able to share his "secret" with his wife, who was very supportive and eager to learn more about how she could help her husband cope with his disorder. Robert discussed two relapse prevention strategies with the staff. He will call his wife before leaving work, and he will discuss inappropriate thoughts with his wife or therapist.

Continued

Nursing Care Plan—cont'd

NURSING DIAGNOSIS: Deficient knowledge of illness and aspects of treatment related to cognitive distortions, anxiety, and uncertainty, as evidenced by failure to seek prior treatment for his disorder and behaviors.

CLIENT OUTCOMES	NURSING INTERVENTIONS	EVALUATION
Robert will verbalize an understanding of his illness within 1 week of admission.	Assess Robert's current level of knowledge regarding his illness and readiness to learn by asking direct questions. *A client must exhibit readiness to learn for learning to occur.* Create a climate conducive to learning such as a quiet, private, safe environment. *Learning may occur when the nurse has the client's complete attention and distractions are avoided.*	Robert has successfully identified triggers that provoke sexual thoughts/feelings and has developed appropriate relapse prevention strategies at the time of discharge.
Robert will identify triggers, such as unstructured time, that provoke inappropriate thoughts and feelings within 1 week of admission.	Teach the importance of trigger identification and development of relapse prevention strategies as critical steps in treatment *to help Robert gain more effective control of inappropriate behaviors.* Suggest that Robert write a list of triggers that provoke sexually inappropriate activity and review this list with him *to assess Robert's insight into his disorder and symptom occurrence.*	Robert continues to recognize things that trigger his inappropriate sexual thoughts and feelings. Robert is able to write a list of triggers that provoke his inappropriate sexual behaviors.
Robert will formulate two relapse prevention strategies, such as opening lines of communication with his wife, to avoid reoffending by the time of discharge.	Help Robert develop appropriate relapse prevention strategies for his identified triggers *to construct a realistic plan to avoid reoffending.* Encourage Robert's participation in a support group for clients with sexual disorders *to receive feedback from peers regarding realistic qualities of trigger identification and relapse prevention strategies.*	Robert has successfully developed two relapse prevention techniques that will help block triggers and prevent sexually offensive behaviors. Robert agreed to join a support group for clients with sexual disorders.

The minimal expected period for outpatient treatment is 2 years, although actual time for treatment may be considerably longer and is sometimes geared according to the length of the client's probationary sentence. These clients need to be carefully monitored for any changes in their status that could lead to relapse. Monitoring may occur through weekly outpatient group therapy or, if group is not indicated, by periodic visits with the client's therapist.

A client is formally discharged from outpatient treatment based on the level of progress and current status regarding the paraphilic behaviors.

CHAPTER SUMMARY

- The nurse must have an understanding of human sexuality, be aware of his or her feelings and values regarding sexuality, and be committed to incorporating sexuality into client care in a nonjudgmental manner.
- Sexual dysfunctions are the most common of all sexual problems that come to the attention of health care practitioners. Estimates of the prevalence of sexual dysfunctions are as high as 50%.

- The lack of sex education and the high rate of sexual repression may contribute to the high incidence of sexual dysfunctions.
- Establishment of a plan of care should include the significant other. In a couple situation, blame should not be placed on either person.
- Specific, realistic outcome criteria developed by the client (or client and significant other) are necessary for implementing the plan of care.
- Nursing interventions should include client education about human sexual functioning, sexual response, and sexual dysfunctions; helping clients improve their communication; support for the clients' fears and anxieties; support for enhancement of the client's self-esteem; and referral for professional help.
- Many complex diagnostic and treatment modalities have been developed for sexual dysfunctions in the past few decades. These include psychophysiologic and psychosocial methods and involve neurologic, endocrine, and vascular treatments, as well as specific sex therapy techniques. Therapeutic modalities are currently more developed for males than for females.
- Giving permission for sexual feelings and behaviors may be the single most important intervention.

- Paraphilia is defined as sexual deviations/disorders presenting with inappropriate sexual fantasies involving deviant sexual acts, inappropriate sexual urges, and acting out of these fantasies and urges.
- Family history positive for the presence of a paraphilic disorder and/or history of victimization may predispose other family members to developing a similar or different paraphilic disorder.
- Establishing a plan of care should include the client to the extent that he or she is able to participate, and goals should reflect mutual agreement between the nurse and the client.
- Interventions should be based on the client's individual needs. The plan of care should include confrontation of cognitive distortions, exploration of the effects of inappropriate sexual behaviors on others, psychoeducational group therapy to teach the client how to identify triggers that provoke inappropriate sexual thoughts, development of relapse prevention strategies and the effects of treatment on illness symptomatology, the importance of treatment compliance during and after the hospital stay, and development of appropriate coping strategies and problem-solving skills.
- The client with a paraphilic disorder who is compliant with treatment has a decreased risk of sexual recidivism.

REVIEW QUESTIONS

1. Which statement by the client indicates that he feels successful regarding the treatment strategies for his sexual dysfunction:
   a. "I don't believe in masturbation."
   b. "I don't feel like a man because I can't please my wife."
   c. "After 6 months of therapy my wife and I are finally enjoying each other."
   d. "I can't talk about something so personal."

2. A biologic cause for a male client's sexual dysfunction may be:
   a. Agoraphobia.
   b. Altered testosterone levels.
   c. Job-related stress.
   d. Adjustment disorder.

3. A 50-year-old client enters the doctor's office. He avoids eye contact and moves slowly. He looks around the room observing the people in the waiting room. When the receptionist asks the purpose of the visit, he just mumbles. The best nursing intervention at this time would be to:
   a. Wait until the client is in the room, ask some basic medical questions and then ask the purpose of the visit.

   b. Tell him that he must explain the purpose of his visit before he can be seen.
   c. Take his vital signs because he may be having a heart attack.
   d. Suggest that he make another appointment for a different day.

4. A 30-year-old male client is court ordered to attend outpatient therapy after he molested a 12-year-old girl. The client tells the therapist that the girl looked like she was 18 or 19 years old. He is using which defense mechanism:
   a. Denial
   b. Displacement
   c. Rationalization
   d. Identification

5. An appropriate nursing outcome for a client diagnosed with pedophilia for the first week is:
   a. List three relapse prevention strategies.
   b. Identify issues from childhood that may have led to his current situation.
   c. Verbalize two appropriate ways to meet sexual needs.
   d. Identify two sexually inappropriate behaviors.

REFERENCES

American Psychiatric Association: *Diagnostic and Statistic Manual of Mental Disorders,* Fourth Edition, Text Revision. Washington, DC, American Psychiatric Association, 2000.
Anon J: The PLISSIT model, *J Sex Educ Ther* 2(1):1, 1976.
Bancroft J: Biological factors in human sexuality, *J Sex Res* 39(1):15-21, 2002.
Basson R et al: Report of the international consensus development conference on female sexual dysfuntion: definitions and classifications, *J Sex Marital Ther* 27(2):83-94, 2001.
Beck J: Hypoactive sexual desire disorder: an overview, *J Consult Clin Psychol* 63:919-927, 1995.
Berlin FS et al: A five-year plus follow-up survey of criminal recidivism within a treated cohort of 406 pedophiles, 111 exhibitionists and 109 sexual aggressives: issues and outcomes, *Am J Forensic Psychiatry* 12(3):5, 1991.
Berlin FS, Meineke CF: Treatment of sex offenders with antiandrogen medication: conceptualization, review of treatment modalities and preliminary findings, *Am J Psychiatry* 138:601, 1981.
Berman L et al: Pharmacotherapy or psychotherapy? Effective treatment for FSD related to unresolved childhood sexual abuse, *J Sex Marital Ther* 27(5):421-426, 2001.
Billups K et al: A new non-pharmacological therapy for female sexual dysfunction, *J Sex Marital Ther* 27:435-441, 2001.
Ellison C: *Women's sexualities: generations of women share intimate secrets of sexual self-acceptance,* Oakland, Calif, 2000, New Harbinger Press.
Everaerd W, Laan E: Drug treatments for women's sexual disorders, *J Sex Res* 37(3):195-204, 2000.
Freud S: *On sexuality,* New York, 1977, Penguin Press.
Gaffney GS et al: Is there familial transmission of pedophilia? *J Nerv Ment Dis* 172:546, 1984.
Groth AN: *Men who rape,* New York, 1979, Plenum Press.
Hartman W, Fithian M: *Treatment of sexual dysfunction: a bio-psycho-social approach,* Long Beach, Calif, 1972, Center for Marital and Sexual Studies. (classic)

Hillman J: *Issues in the practice of psychology: clinical perspectives on elderly sexuality,* New York, 2000, Kluwer Academic/Plenum Publishers.

Kafka MP: How are drugs used in the treatment of paraphilic disorders? *Harvard Ment Health Letter* 13(9):8, 1997.

Kaplan H: *The new sex therapy,* New York, 1974, Brunner/Mazel.

Klinefelter HF et al: Syndrome characterized by gynecomastia, aspermatogenesis without A-Leydigism, and increased excretion of FSH, *J Clin Endocrinol Metab* 2(2):615, 1942.

Laumann E, Paik A, Rosen R: Sexual dysfunction in the United States: prevalence and predictors, *JAMA* 281:537-544, 1999.

Leiblum S, Rosen R: *Principles and practice of sex therapy,* New York, 1989, Guilford Press.

LoPiccolo J, Friedman J: Broad spectrum treatment of low sexual desire: integration of cognitive, behavioral and systematic therapy. In Leiblum S, Rosen R, editors: *Sexual desire disorders,* New York, 1988, Guilford Press.

Masters W, Johnson V: *Human sexual inadequacy,* Boston, 1970, Little, Brown.

Masters W, Johnson V: *Human sexual response,* Boston, 1966, Little, Brown.

Money J et al: Imprinting and the establishment of gender role, *Arch Neurol Psychiatry* 77:333, 1957.

Money J: *Lovemaps,* Buffalo, NY, 1986a, Prometheus Books.

Money J: *Lovemaps: clinical concepts of sexual/erotic health and pathology, paraphilia, and gender transposition in childhood, adolescence, and maturity,* New York, 1986b, Irvington.

NANDA International (2003). NANDA Nursing Diagnoses: Definitions and Classification 2003-2004. Philadelphia: NANDA.

Piletz J et al: Plasma MHPG response to yohimbine treatment in women with hypoactive sexual desire, *J Sex Marital Ther* 24(1):43, 1998.

Plaut M, RachBeisel J: Use of anxiolytic medication in the treatment of vaginismus and severe aversion to penetration, case report, *J Sex Educ Ther* 22(3):43, 1997.

Rosen R, Lieblum S: Treatment of sexual disorders in the 1990s: an integrated approach, *J Consult Clin Psychol* 63(6):877-890, 1995.

Rowland D: Issues in the laboratory study of human sexual response: a synthesis for the non-technical sexologist, *J Sex Res* 36(1):3-15, 1999.

Rowland D, Burnett A: Pharmacotherapy in the treatment of male sexual dysfunction, *J Sex Res* 37(7):226-243, 2000.

Semans R: Premature ejaculation: a new approach, *South Med J* 49:353, 1956. (classic)

Wilson GD: An ethological approach to sexual deviation. In Wilson GD, editor: *Variant sexuality: research and theory,* Baltimore, 1987, The Johns Hopkins University Press.

Women's Sexual Health: www.womenssexualhealth.com, 2001.

SUGGESTED READINGS

Abel GG et al: Sexually aggressive behavior. In Curran WJ et al, editors: *Forensic psychiatry and psychology,* Philadelphia, 1986, FA Davis.

Abel GG et al: Self-reported sex crimes of nonincarcerated paraphiliacs, *J Interpersonal Violence* 2(1):3, 1987.

Abel GG, Osborn C: Stopping sexual violence, *Psychiatr Ann* 22(6):301, 1992.

Arndt WB Jr: *Gender disorders and the paraphilias,* Madison, Conn, 1991, International Universities Press.

Baker HJ, Stoller J: Can a biological force contribute to gender identity? *Am J Psychiatry* 124(12):1653, 1968.

Beitchman J et al: A review of the long-term effects of child sexual abuse, *Child Abuse Negl* 16:101, 1992.

Bergner RM: Money's "lovemap" account of the paraphilias: a critique and reformulation, *Am J Psychother* 42(2):254, 1988.

Berlin FS: Chemical castration for sex offenders, *N Engl J Med* 336:1030, 2002.

Berlin FS: Special considerations in the psychiatric evaluation of sex offenders against minors. In Rosner R, Schwartz H, editors: *Juvenile psychiatry and the law: critical issues in American psychiatry and the law,* vol 4, New York, 1989, Plenum Press.

Berlin FS: The paraphilias and Depo-Provera: some medical, ethical and legal considerations, *Bull Am Acad Psychiatry Law* 17(3):233, 1989.

Berlin FS, Malin HM: Media distortion of the public's perception of recidivism and psychiatric rehabilitation, *Am J Psychiatry* 148(11):1572, 1991.

Bradford JM, Gratzner TG: A treatment for impulse control disorders and paraphilia, *Can J Psychiatry* 40:4, 1995.

Bradford JM: The treatment approach of sexual deviation using a pharmacological approach, *J Sex Res* 37:248-257, 2000.

Fagan PJ et al: Pedophilia, *JAMA* 228:19, 2002.

Kafka MP: Sertraline pharmacotherapy for paraphilias and paraphilia-related disorders: an open trial, *Ann Clin Psychiatry* 6:189, 1994.

Kansas v. Hendricks, 521 U.S. 346: 1997.

Kaplan HI, Sadock BJ: Paraphilias. In Kaplan HI, Sadock, BJ, editors: *Synopsis of psychiatry, behavioral sciences, clinical psychiatry,* ed 6, Baltimore, 1991, Williams & Wilkins.

Kiersch TA: Treatment of sex offenders with Depo-Provera, *Bull Am Acad Psychiatry Law* 18(2):179, 1990.

Kim MJ et al: *Pocket guide to nursing diagnoses,* ed 5, St Louis, 1993, Mosby.

Laws DR et al: *Remaking relapse prevention with sex offenders, a sourcebook,* Newbury Park, Calif, 2000, Sage Publications.

Leong GB, Silva JA: Sexually violent predator II: the sequel, *J Am Acad Psychiatry Law* 29:340-343, 2001.

Meyer WJ et al: Depo-Provera treatment for sex offending behavior: an evaluation of outcome, *Bull Am Acad Psychiatry Law* 20(3):249, 1992.

Money J: *Venuses penuses: sexology, sexosophy and exigency theory,* Buffalo, NY, 1986c, Prometheus Books.

Money J: Treatment guidelines: antiandrogen and counseling of paraphilic sex offenders, *J Sex Marital Ther* 13(3):219, 1987.

Roesler A, Witztum E: Pharmacotherapy of paraphilias in the next millennium, *Behav Sci Law* 18(1):43-56, 2000.

Simon WT, Schouten PG: Plethysmography in the assessment of sexual deviance: an overview, *Arch Sex Behav* 20(1):75, 1991.

18 Adjustment Disorders

Merry A. Armstrong

OBJECTIVES

- Describe five major criteria for an adjustment disorder.

- Analyze the relationship of life events to adjustment disorders.

- Discuss the implications of the diagnosis of adjustment disorder with depressed mood for the nonpsychiatric hospitalized client.

- Apply the nursing process to clients who exhibit symptoms of adjustment disorders.

- Explain the major therapeutic goals for clients who have a diagnosis of adjustment disorder.

Most people have difficulties managing major, unexpected, or cumulative change events in their lives. **Adjustment disorders** are problematic responses to life events that are considered less serious and often represent transient episodes in the lives of otherwise mentally healthy individuals. Problematic responses are behaviors, feelings, or thoughts that interfere with an individual's functioning or sense of well-being. Some of the symptoms of adjustment disorders are similar to those in other diagnostic groups, such as affective mood disorders or anxiety disorders.

Events such as divorce, relocation, adolescence, or other psychologically challenging events may precipitate problematic responses that meet the criteria for an adjustment disorder. Depending on the intensity of their symptoms, such as anxiety or lack of concentration, and the temporal relation of their symptoms to life events, many of these clients are diagnosed with an adjustment disorder. Individuals seeking outpatient therapy for assistance in dealing with responses to such things as specific problematic life events may also be diagnosed as having an adjustment disorder. After obtaining an appropriate developmental history, completing a mental status assessment, and systematically eliminating other potential diagnoses, the mental health practitioner may decide that the client has an adjustment disorder. The term *mental health practitioner* is used because in some states advanced practice nurses (APN), licensed clinical social workers (LCSW), or other licensed, qualified personnel determine DSM-IV-TR pathology. The diagnosis of adjustment disorder suggests the probability that the client possesses or can rally sufficient resources to resolve his or her problematic response within an appropriate time, in this case by responding to therapeutic intervention as a primary treatment modality.

Like all other clients, the client diagnosed with an adjustment disorder is continually assessed for new or intensifying symptoms that might indicate a developing major depressive disorder or other mental illness. In these situations, the diagnosis implies that the mental health practitioner has reason to believe that the client's problematic symptoms will abate when identified disruptive life events or transitional experiences are resolved and no longer occupy the central focus of the person's life.

HISTORICAL AND THEORETIC PERSPECTIVES

Developmental or incidental changes are an acknowledged part of life. These challenging situations are often briefly disturbing; at other times responses are more problematic. These problematic responses to either developmental or situational stressors have been discussed in psychiatric literature for many years. However, adjustment disorders were first professionally categorized and described in 1968 in the second edition of the *Diagnostic and Statistical Manual of Mental Disorders* (DSM-II) as "transient situational disturbance" (APA, 1968). The newest DSM-IV-TR (APA, 2000) considers adjustment disorders as transient episodes of dysfunction

in response to specific stressors. To be diagnosed as having an adjustment disorder, the client must demonstrate criteria for one of six classifications: adjustment disorder with depressed mood, with anxiety, with mixed anxiety and depressed mood, with disturbance of conduct, with mixed disturbance of emotions and conduct, and unspecified. Adjustment disorders may be acute (symptoms last 6 months or less) or chronic (symptoms persist for more than 6 months) or when the precipitating stressor has long-lasting effects. Examples of these disorders are presented later in the chapter. An important point to remember is that a diagnosis of adjustment disorder suggests that troublesome symptoms may abate with time and therapeutic intervention. Conversely, adjustment disorders may be precursors to more serious mental health problems. In either case, continual reassessment of the client's symptoms, condition, and situation is required. Some debate exists about normal responses that may in some cases be extreme and even expected with severe experiences. In these instances, practitioners debate the appropriateness of labeling a normal response as a disorder (Casey, Dowrick, and Wilkinson, 2001). The same authors note a paucity of research regarding this disorder.

ETIOLOGY

The mental health professional forms a therapeutic relationship with the client and begins to become familiar with the client's patterns of interaction, lifestyle, personality, and environment. The interaction of personality, crisis, stress, developmental factors, and cultural influences must be considered when investigating the formation of adjustment disorders. Often, the convergence of several problematic events results in symptoms of adjustment disorder (see Case Study).

Crisis and Stress Models

Major physical and/or psychologic adjustments occur normally during a person's lifetime. Most people develop a repertoire of skills to manage difficult situations. Because of the intensity, timing, or repetition of the stressor or situation, however, prior methods are sometimes not sufficient to mitigate the problem. Using the model suggested by crisis theory, one might say that an adjustment disorder results from an individual's inability to use existing coping methods or create new methods in response to a situation. Because of this inability, the client feels overwhelmed, confused, and helpless, further depleting his or her ability to rally resources. These feelings may be manifested as depression, anxiety, or other combinations of emotional experience. Problems resulting from stress are classified in the psychiatric literature as posttraumatic stress disorder, grief or bereavement, and adjustment disorders.

Selye's stress-adaptation theory (1956, 1978) suggested a biologic response to stress called the *general adaptation syndrome (GAS)*. Stress was defined as a situation requiring a physiologic response or change. Selye noted that people may respond to the same stressful situation in different

CASE STUDY

Patrick, a 16-year-old high school student, was brought to the counseling center by his parents, who stated that he looked distracted, was not doing well in school, and had developed irregular eating and sleeping patterns. Recent stressors known to his parents included breaking up with his girlfriend of 6 months and being required to lose 15 pounds for the wrestling team. After completion of a thorough medical assessment, the nurse talked with the client about recent events in his life.

Patrick expressed regret about breaking up with his girlfriend but had a positive attitude about this change, feeling that perhaps he was too young for a steady girlfriend. However, Patrick expressed feeling hopeless about losing the 15 pounds and worried that he would fail to make the wrestling team. He confided to the nurse that to lose weight, he had taken pills that another student had given him to ensure weight loss. Patrick found himself unable to sleep or concentrate, so he had started drinking liquor to get to sleep. He had hidden this from his parents and was embarrassed to tell them. He was afraid that if he stopped taking the pills, he would gain weight and not make the team. He felt trapped and also knew that his thinking was affected by his lack of sleep and drug use, and he had occasional, fleeting thoughts that he might be better off dead. He did not know who to talk to and was afraid to talk to his wrestling coach. Although he resisted coming to the clinic, he expressed relief to the nurse that his parents had insisted that he talk to a counselor.

Critical Thinking

1. Patrick is experiencing several problematic life events. What are they?
2. What is Patrick's risk for suicide?
3. What implications does the use of drugs have for suicide and/or mental illness?
4. Do you think Patrick is addicted to drugs and/or alcohol?

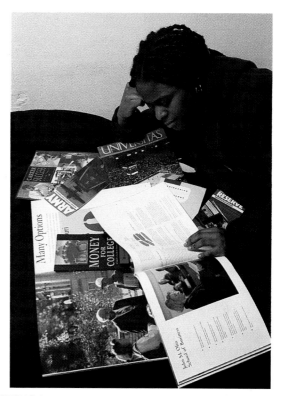

FIGURE 18-1. Adolescents face developmental and situational challenges as they contemplate decisions for their future, such as options for employment or college.

ways. For example, one individual might experience a headache in response to an argument, whereas another might experience physical or psychologic sensations of relief. An experience might be labeled pleasant or unpleasant, but if a biologic adjustment is required, the GAS is activated and the stress response is present. The stress-adaptation and crisis models are similar in that the client feels overwhelmed and without resources to respond to a situation.

Precipitating Factors

Because life is normally a series of changes, there is ordinarily no shortage of events to manage. Life events requiring major adjustments can be developmental, situational, adventitious, or a combination of all three. Adjustment disorders can be triggered by a stressor or series of stressors that may be developmental (adolescence, menopause), situational (job change, divorce, hospitalization), or adventitious (earthquake, war, flood).

For example, serious developmental and situational challenges occur in early adulthood when adolescents graduate from high school and must decide their life direction. Developmental tasks of establishing personal identity and negotiating situational stressors (e.g., decisions after gradua-

tion from high school to explore career, college, surfing, Peace Corps, military) that determine one's life course are complex endeavors (Figure 18-1).

Other stressors challenge the maturing individual. People in their middle and older years have significant developmental challenges that may result in transient situational adjustment problems. For example, retirement is often referred to as a benefit and goal of late adulthood, yet it is sometimes experienced as a loss of identity and purpose. Other life events related to individual physical or psychologic development may include the loss of a significant other or the diagnosis of a major disease. Changes in employment, marital status, childbearing, and other life occurrences may also present individuals with significant challenges. Illness, major family changes, and/or developmental crises are not uncommon and often occur simultaneously.

Recent literature indicates that adjustment disorder is a diagnosis frequently used with difficulties of adolescence and may predict adult problems of depression or other adjustment problems (Aalto-Setala et al., 2002). Adjustment disorders among adult clients who are hospitalized are associated with shorter lengths of stay and with more concurrent substance abuse disorders (Greenberg, Rosenfeld, and Ortega, 1995; Kovacs et al., 1994). Suicidality may also be seen in these clients (Kryzhanovskaya and Canterbury, 2001). Coping with disasters such as floods or other traumatic events increase the likelihood of adjustment disorders and other psychiatric disorders (Ginexi et al., 2000).

Loss

Loss is the psychologic dynamic that often precipitates an adjustment disorder. A key theme underlying life change is that of loss, described by Kubler-Ross (1969) and since explored and refined by others (Levine, 1987; Walsh and McGoldrick, 1991). **Loss** is a process characterized by a series of overlapping stages that include common psychologic and behavioral manifestations of recognition, adjustment, and resolution. Numerous examples of loss have been articulated in this chapter, and all change includes loss. Managing a desired change such as retirement, marriage, or establishing a family requires loss of previous status, freedom, or identity. Walsh and McGoldrick (1991) stated that losses require movement through a process of mourning to get what is needed from the experience or relationship and then continue on with one's life. How persons get what they need from the experience is often contextually determined and influenced by culture and socialization. The nurse plays an instrumental role in educating the client about the loss process and in helping the client mourn the loss.

Grief, mourning, and bereavement are other expressions of loss and are discussed in Chapter 25. According to DSM-IV-TR criteria, persons experiencing severe or prolonged difficulties with grief and bereavement are not diagnosed with an adjustment disorder.

Developmental Influences

Developmental milestones and challenges certainly provide an individual with repeated stress, need for major accommodations, and new situational stressors. A famous and often cited theory by Erikson (1963) proposed that development of the personality is achieved by completing specific tasks at different stages of the life cycle. Erikson postulated that difficulties in adjustment occurred when age-appropriate behaviors or tasks were not completed, resulting in an inability to move forward with developmental tasks. The **adult developmental theory** suggests that individuals continue to evolve as they mature.

A criticism of Erikson's model is that development seemingly ends in adulthood. Colarusso and Nemiroff (1981) contended that individuals continue to refine their sense of identity and self and that adulthood is characterized by normative crises based on adult developmental tasks. According to these authors, themes of adult developmental tasks exist (Box 18-1). As people mature, themes of adult development are continuous and important sources of information for the therapist in the process of identifying the dynamics of the client problem or symptoms.

Using Erickson's model of development, Colarusso and Nemiroff (1981) suggested that adulthood is divided into age groupings: early adulthood (ages 20 to 40), middle adulthood (ages 40 to 60), late adulthood (ages 60 to 80), and late-late adulthood (ages 80 and beyond). These authors

Box 18-1	Themes of Adult Developmental Tasks

Intimacy, love, sex
Body-related issues
Time and death
Relationships with:
    Children
    Parents
    Mentors
    Society
Work
Play
Finances

From Colarusso C, Nemiroff R: *Adult development: a new dimension in psychodynamic theory and practice,* New York, 1981, Plenum Press.

further suggested that adult developmental strands existed on a continuum and were experienced differently, depending on issues that were active in each age category.

Using this model, the strand, or theme, of adult development, "time and death," might likely be applied as an active developmental task for a person in middle adulthood rather than for someone in early adulthood. A person in middle adulthood may concurrently be diagnosed with a chronic health problem, have substantial financial and work responsibilities, be involved in parenting teenagers, and experience the death of a parent. The combination of these influences may result in an adjustment disorder. If adults experience developmental challenges unique to their age and situation, as Colarusso and Nemiroff (1981, 1987) contended, how can mental health professionals help clients to identify, attain, and use new skills?

A common precipitating event that stimulates adult development is the personal experience of an illness, or the illness of a loved one. Clients at risk for, or who have, adjustment disorders are commonly cared for by nurses in general hospitals, long-term care facilities, rehabilitation centers, or in the home. Nurses have unique opportunities for long-term assessment and subsequent intervention regarding clients' emotional and psychologic difficulties. For example, one activity in a mental health assessment is determining the meaning of the situation for the client. Being briefly hospitalized for a hernia repair probably does not have the same meaning for a client of the same age who is hospitalized for stabilization of newly diagnosed diabetes.

Cultural, Social, and Psychologic Influences

The processes of growth and development occur within the context of social and cultural influences. This chapter would not be complete without mentioning the scope and volume of currently debated issues of psychologic and personality development. Beyond historical disputes of nature versus nurture theories, scholars question classification systems of mental illness (Kirk and Kutchins, 1992) and traditional scientific research methods (Blier, 1986). In addition, debate continues in the human sciences regarding differences in development and experience according to one's gender and socialization (Gilligan, 1982; Jordan et al., 1991; Lerner, 1988; Lewis, 1986; Meth and Pasick, 1990; Napier, 1991; Pittman, 1991). Gender, culture, and social factors influence the results of measurements such as the intelligence quotient (IQ). If gender, culture, and social factors partially determine a person's reality, how do we give nursing care using standard nursing diagnoses that may not reflect the reality of our clients?

A nurse who identifies that a client has problems related to the death of a spouse and applies the nursing diagnosis of dysfunctional grieving but does not incorporate the client's sociocultural heritage may not be serving this client well. For example, behaviors that the nurse perceives as problems may be appropriate in the client's culture. In that case, the nurse may be missing identification of important facts. Instead of identifying the client's problems, the nurse might have demonstrated cultural bias in expecting all people to resolve issues in the same way. The nurse must be aware that clients may resolve their grief in a culturally and socially appropriate manner and include assessment activities that reveal this information. This solution sounds simple, but different cultures also refuse to speak to persons outside the family about intimate details. Therefore the nurse must also be aware of communication patterns of the culture and other social customs.

Lowenberg (1989), a nurse researcher, used the framework of an evolving paradigm of health care, **holism,** to explore the practices of consumers and practitioners of American health care. Historically, illness was thought to represent social deviance (Davis, 1972; Parsons, 1951), and stigma and labeling were applied to a variety of problems culturally interpreted as illness. The author observed that emerging concepts of holism and health suggested that people's physical, mental, emotional, spiritual, and social aspects were interrelated and interdependent. The paradigm of holism suggests that illness may be an opportunity for growth and development if the illness promotes an awareness of better health practices. Using this concept, some people have redefined the illness experience from biologic deterioration to a more positive interpretation of illness as a warning sign that adjustments in living are needed.

Contributions of Nursing Research

Nursing research has contributed information leading to a greater understanding of individual experience. Although nursing research has not addressed the diagnosis of adjustment disorders specifically, it has explored meanings of many life events for individual clients and caregivers, using qualitative research techniques (Armstrong, 1992; Beck, 1992; Bergum, 1989; Heifner, 1993; Lowenberg, 1989; Main et al., 1993; Mickley et al., 1992; Murphy, 1993; Tanner

UNDERSTANDING and APPLYING RESEARCH

A case study approach was used in this qualitative retrospective study of the experience of 10 residents who had received psychotherapy for treatment of depression, dysthymic disorder, or adjustment disorder. Six men and four women with an average age of 87.2 (**the old old** are defined as those over age 85 years) who lived semiindependently or in the nursing home facility in the same geriatric center were seen by one of several therapists for individual psychotherapy. Each patient was interviewed for his or her understanding about the content and process of therapy and whether it was thought of as helpful. Interview data were combined with chart information and therapist notes to produce case histories for each patient. Patients had positive recollections of their relationship with the therapist, and the perceived benefit of treatment was related to the positive value of the therapeutic relationship rather than to specific techniques or interventions. The researcher concluded that psychotherapy was a positive experience that provided palliative treatment for these clients. Further research is needed to explore the benefits of psychotherapy for the old old. Little is known about the value of psychotherapy among this age group or with residents of nursing homes in general.

Ruckdeschel H: *Psychotherapy for the old old: ten patients' report on their treatment for depression.* Unpublished doctoral dissertation, 1993, University of Pennsylvania.

et al., 1993). Understanding the process of an illness experience can help nurses and other professionals develop effective assessment techniques, methods for intervention, and models for evaluation of treatment (see Understanding and Applying Research box).

EPIDEMIOLOGY

Popkin (1989) stated that adult adjustment disorders are thought to be common, although data to support this opinion are scarce. A factor contributing to difficulty in gathering statistics regarding adjustment disorder treatment is that the clinical or symptomatic findings in adjustment disorder vary widely, thus making the diagnosis difficult. The DSM-IV-TR (APA, 2000) cites prevalence rates between 5% and 20% in outpatient populations.

Studies were conducted on the findings of psychiatric consultation/liaison personnel who assessed clients in acute care hospitals. Adjustment disorders in medically ill inpatient clients (Popkin, 1990; Razavi et al., 1990; Snyder et al., 1990) were commonly identified. Many clients with terminal diagnoses or severe chronic illness displayed symptoms of either major depression or adjustment disorder.

CLINICAL DESCRIPTION

Six subtypes of adjustment disorder are noted in the DSM-IV-TR (Box 18-2). They are coded on Axis IV according to symptom type and with stressor(s) noted. Because adjustment disorder can present with various combinations of symptomatology, it is difficult to categorize discrete symptoms (see DSM-IV-TR Criteria box on p. 420).

Box 18-2	Types of Adjustment Disorders

Adjustment Disorder With Depressed Mood
Used when the predominant symptomatology are depressed mood, tearfulness, and feelings of hopelessness.

Adjustment Disorder With Anxiety
Used when the predominant symptomatology are nervousness, worry, and jitteriness.

Adjustment Disorder With Mixed Anxiety and Depressed Mood
Used when the predominant manifestation is a combination of depression and anxiety.

Adjustment Disorder With Disturbance of Conduct
Used when the client's conduct violates the rights of others or major age-appropriate societal norms and rules (e.g., vandalism, fighting, defaulting on legal responsibilities).

Adjustment Disorder With Mixed Disturbance of Emotions and Conduct
Used when predominant symptomatology are combinations of emotions (e.g., depression or anxiety) and a disturbance of conduct.

Unspecified
Used for maladaptive reactions (such as physical complaints, social withdrawal, or work or academic inhibition) to psychosocial stressors not classifiable in other specific subtypes.

From American Psychiatric Association: *Diagnostic and Statistical Manual of Mental Disorders,* Fourth Edition, Text Revision. Washington, DC, American Psychiatric Association, 2000.

DSM-IV-TR CRITERIA
Adjustment Disorders

A. The development of emotional or behavioral symptoms in response to an identifiable stressor(s) occurring within 3 months of the onset of the stressor(s).
B. These symptoms or behaviors are clinically significant as evidenced by either of the following:
   1. Marked distress that is in excess of what would be expected from exposure to the stressor
   2. Significant impairment in social or occupational (academic) functioning
C. The stress-related disturbance does not meet criteria for another specific Axis I disorder and is not merely and exacerbation of a preexisting Axis I or Axis II disorder.
D. The symptoms do not represent bereavement.
E. Once the stressor (or its consequences) has terminated, the symptoms do not persist for more than an additional 6 months.
   Specify if:
   Acute: if the disturbance lasts less than 6 months
   Chronic: if the disturbance lasts for 6 months or longer

From American Psychiatric Association: *Diagnostic and Statistical Manual of Mental Disorders,* Fourth Edition, Text Revision. Washington, DC, American Psychiatric Association, 2000.

PROGNOSIS

Most practitioners believe that because the diagnosis of adjustment disorder ordinarily precludes a major psychiatric problem, there is hope that the client can resolve problems by developing coping methods and mobilizing resources. Specific data are not currently available related to specific prognoses for adjustment disorders.

DISCHARGE CRITERIA
Client will:
- Verbalize absence of thoughts of self-harm.
- Identify goals for continuing care after discharge, if indicated.
- Identify and analyze coping resources and plans for using resources.

THE NURSING PROCESS

ASSESSMENT

Clients are not often hospitalized for treatment of adjustment disorder; therefore nurses are more likely to assess clients with an adjustment disorder in an outpatient or home setting (see Nursing Care in the Community box). Outpatient clients may request treatment based on the symptoms of one or more adjustment disorders. Adjustment disorder subtypes with anxious or depressed mood are the most frequently diagnosed types in adult clients (Popkin, 1989).

Nurses need to assess for precipitating stressors that preceded the onset of symptoms of adjustment disorder. Assessment of behavioral symptoms and mood and affect congruity are key to initial nursing assessment (see Nursing Assessment Questions box). Symptoms depend on the type of adjustment disorder and might include:

Sensory-perceptual: Nervousness, worry, and jitteriness; other symptoms congruent with feeling anxious and/or depressed, such as headache, backache, or lethargy

Thought disturbances: Preoccupation with thoughts of death (not suicidal thoughts), inability to attend to tasks, decreased concentration, inattention to external environment, inability to attend to detail, inability to concentrate, and short attention span leading to learning impairment; feelings of ambivalence and inability to make decisions; denial of physical illness and noncompliance with treatment recommendations

Feeling disturbances: Feelings of sadness and sorrow, feelings of emptiness and worthlessness, decreased self-esteem, inability to articulate feelings, excessive worry about life events

Behavioral and relating disturbances: Lack of interest in external events, disruption in relationships, social withdrawal, loss of interest in hobbies, withdrawal from work or academic endeavors, spiritual distress, increased or decreased psychomotor activity, hyperverbal patterns, difficulty continuing conversations, becoming easily distracted,

NURSING CARE IN THE COMMUNITY — Adjustment Disorders

Adjustment disorders are common in the community mental health field. Some are the long-term results of predictable crises of maturation and development, such as the death of a loved one, employment problems, and financial issues. In such cases therapeutic pathways have been fairly well established and the nurse can follow through with standard crisis intervention strategies to reassure the client that the situation should improve with time. Clients can be introduced to support groups focused on similar issues and, if necessary, be prescribed medication to help mitigate the process until the individual has established functional coping patterns. Most clients respond well to education and exposure to peers who have had similar experiences, but prolonged adjustment difficulties may be cause for more intensive interventions. The nurse may consider longer term work with the client, focusing on changes in the client's living situation, and perhaps even lifestyle, to reduce stress, occupy free time, and increase coping abilities.

Unpredictable and sometimes catastrophic crises are much more difficult to manage, requiring active and decisive action on the part of the psychiatric mental health nurse in the community. Assault or other cata-strophic events are examples of such overwhelming trauma, first managed by crisis intervention, but also requiring extremely careful supervision to avoid excessive emotional reactions such as homicidal or suicidal feelings. Nonjudgmental debriefing must be continued to put the situation in perspective and allow the client to both ventilate and distance himself or herself from the trauma.

Prolonged difficulties (e.g., enduring marital problems, adjustment to chronic ill health, or continuing financial problems) require a new level of coping ability. Adjustment should be achieved within 3 to 6 months without attendant anxiety, depression, or changes in typical behavior. The community mental health nurse is in a good position to monitor how well the client has reconciled to the current situation and how positive he or she is about the future.

Finally, if the symptoms of adjustment difficulties continue for more than 6 months, the client's long-term needs are addressed by giving referrals to an appropriate therapist and support group for ongoing treatment. Adjustment disorders often require prolonged psychosocial and practical interventions to promote future safety and functionality.

NURSING ASSESSMENT QUESTIONS
Adjustment Disorders

1. What has happened in your life in the recent past? *To determine if the client can identify a stressor or stressors preceding an adjustment disorder*
2. In the overall picture of your life, how did that event affect you? *To determine the meaning of the event to the person*
3. What have you done in the past when such events occurred? *To determine whether the client has adequate coping skills and potential resources*
4. Tell me about your family and friends and their roles in this event. *To determine current support networks and obtain information about family/significant others*

insomnia, violation of age-appropriate norms or rules, violation of rights of others

NURSING DIAGNOSIS

In adjustment disorders, nursing diagnoses are prioritized based on symptoms. Data gathered in the assessment phase of the nursing process provide information about the client's history, symptoms, and (especially in the case of adjustment disorder) behavior and responses to life stressors. The collaborative and multidisciplinary effort in adjustment disorders is appropriately directed toward helping the client rally resources to achieve a functional level of daily living (see Collaborative Diagnosis table on p. 422).

Nursing Diagnoses for Adjustment Disorders

- Impaired adjustment
- Anxiety
- Ineffective coping
- Dysfunctional grieving
- Chronic low self-esteem
- Situational low self-esteem
- Impaired social interaction
- Spiritual distress
- Risk for other-directed violence
- Risk for self-directed violence

OUTCOME IDENTIFICATION

Based on symptoms related to the specific adjustment disorder, outcome criteria may vary. Regardless of the symptoms, however, client safety is a prime concern. Client outcomes, which are derived from nursing diagnoses, are the expected and anticipated client behaviors or responses to be achieved.

Client will:
- Discuss plans for goal achievement.
- Analyze coping resources and plans for using resources.
- Describe stressors and effective ways of managing stressful situations in the past.
- Evaluate any planned life changes in advance for potential sources of distress.

PLANNING

Clients with adjustment disorder are cared for by a collaborative team. Data from nursing assessment and collaboration with the health care team provide direction for treat-

COLLABORATIVE DIAGNOSES

DSM-IV-TR Diagnoses*	NANDA Diagnoses†
Adjustment disorder with depressed mood	Ineffective coping Ineffective denial Social isolation Spiritual distress
Adjustment disorder with anxiety	Anxiety Ineffective coping Disturbed sleep pattern
Adjustment disorder with disturbance of conduct	Impaired adjustment Anxiety Defensive coping Ineffective coping Ineffective role performance
Adjustment disorder with mixed disturbance of emotions and conduct	Impaired adjustment Anxiety Defensive coping Ineffective coping Ineffective denial Disturbed sleep pattern Social isolation Spiritual distress Risk for other-directed violence Risk for self-directed violence

*From American Psychiatric Association: *Diagnostic and Statistical Manual of Mental Disorders,* Fourth Edition, Text Revision. Washington, DC, American Psychiatric Association, 2000.
†From NANDA International (2003). NANDA Nursing Diagnoses: Definitions and Classification 2003-2004. Philadelphia: NANDA.

ment of clients with adjustment disorder. Because clients have different needs, depending on the symptoms of adjustment disorder, nursing care will be, as always, individualized. Symptoms of adjustment disorder are presumed to be short term, so continuing care may be planned once the client is discharged from an inpatient unit. Continuing care is appropriate if the client's symptoms are active at the time of discharge and provide the opportunity to monitor the client's progress after discharge. The nurse must be alert to detect changes in symptoms or their intensity while caring for the client. For example, a client with adjustment disorder with depressed mood may begin to express thoughts of suicide.

IMPLEMENTATION

For the client diagnosed with an adjustment disorder, nursing interventions are individualized, depending on the symptoms the client exhibits. Any plan of care should include ongoing assessment of symptoms.

CLIENT AND FAMILY TEACHING GUIDELINES

TEACH THE CLIENT, FAMILY, AND/OR SIGNIFICANT OTHER:
To identify the symptoms of adjustment disorders and that:
  Symptoms usually resolve completely.
  Symptoms can be managed using a variety of techniques (e.g., relaxation exercises can be taught to mitigate anxiety).
  Symptoms should be reported to their care provider.
  Thoughts of self-harm or suicide need to be reported immediately to their care provider.
  Their response to a life event is normal because individual people have unique responses to life events.
  They have dealt with difficult life situations in the past using particular coping methods. Reinforce prior successes.
Dosage, frequency, and effects of medication. Include information about common side effects of medication and when to call the physician with questions or concerns regarding medication management.

Nursing Interventions

1. Assess any risk of suicidal ideation, gesture, or plan *to provide for the client's safety and prevent violence to self.*
2. Help the client identify coping strategies *to encourage use of internal resources.*
3. Support activities that increase socialization *to decrease isolation and foster growth of social support networks.*
4. Help the client name thoughts, feelings, and concerns *to help the client identify patterns of thought and provide opportunities for validation of feeling, reflection, and problem solving.*
5. Teach the client, family, and significant others about the disorder including symptom management *to provide control and reduce fear and anxiety* (see Client and Family Teaching Guidelines box).
6. Engage client in a therapeutic alliance *to encourage discussion of thoughts and feelings, particularly noting any suicidal ideation or increase in symptoms of depression.*
7. Support client's progress toward goals *to foster self-esteem and encourage repetition of positive behaviors.*
8. Collaborate with multidisciplinary treatment team *to promote consistency in implementing the treatment plan. Consistency provides structure and communicates involvement of the entire team in the treatment of the client; expectations of the client are agreed on and articulated.*
9. Help the client identify symptoms of anxiety and predisposing situational stressors *to promote problem solving and increased feelings of control.*
10. Help the client recall prior instances of success *to foster self-esteem, support creative problem solving, and instill hope for the future.*

NURSING CARE PLAN

Mr. Brown, a 57-year-old client in a general medical unit, is well known to the nursing staff. He has been hospitalized many times during the past few years for stabilization of diabetes mellitus, which is difficult to control. During his most recent admission, his involvement with plans for his care has not been typical because his interest is minimal. Also, he has eaten foods high in sugar content that belong to his roommate. He denies this behavior, is difficult to engage in client education, and is increasingly withdrawn. He says he tests his blood glucose at home and administers his insulin appropriately.

Mr. Brown has recently retired from his job at a manufacturing plant because of his diabetes, and his retirement benefits are adequate to support his lifestyle. When asked if he feels sad or depressed about his retirement, he denies it in an angry tone of voice. His wife of 10 years died about 8 months ago. He says he has grieved for his wife, acknowledges feeling less sad about her death, and states that he is more at peace with his situation as time goes by. He is able to talk about the good times they had together. At the same time, he acknowledges disappointment at spending his retirement alone and says he feels depressed that his retirement is not as he hoped it would be.

He denies suicidal ideation. Visiting friends told the nurses that he has been reluctant to attend social activities. They say he has told them that he prefers to spend his time alone and just does not feel like being with people. Mr. Brown's inpatient nurse knows that he will be discharged soon and initiates home health follow-up care.

DSM-IV-TR Diagnoses

Axis I   Adjustment disorder with depressed mood
Axis II   None
Axis III Diabetes mellitus
Axis IV   Extreme = 4 (diabetes, death of spouse)
Axis V   GAF = 60 (current)
          GAF = 80 (past year)

NURSING DIAGNOSIS: Risk for self-directed violence. Risk factors: chronic illness, feeling depressed about his retirement, change in marital status (multiple losses).

CLIENT OUTCOMES	NURSING INTERVENTIONS	EVALUATION
Mr. Brown will not harm self while in hospital.	Observe Mr. Brown's behavior frequently during routine client care. *Close observation is necessary to protect client from self-harm.*	Mr. Brown remained safe, unharmed.
Mr. Brown will refrain from verbal suicidal threats or behavioral gestures.	Listen closely for suicidal statements and observe nonverbal indications of suicidal intent, such as giving away possessions. *Such behaviors are critical clues regarding risk for self-harm. Clues regarding potential behavior may be verbal or nonverbal.*	Absence of verbalized or behavioral indications of suicidal intent by Mr. Brown.
Mr. Brown will deny any plans for suicide.	Ask direct questions to determine suicidal intent, plans for suicide, and means to commit suicide. *Suicide risk increases if plans and means exist.*	Mr. Brown denied active suicidal plan.
Mr. Brown will agree to terms of a no-harm contract and will seek staff when feeling suicidal.	Obtain verbal or written agreement from Mr. Brown not to harm self and to seek staff if suicidal feelings and impulses emerge *to confirm that help is available if the client loses control.*	Mr. Brown agreed to terms of contract and sought staff to help maintain control.

NURSING DIAGNOSIS: Ineffective coping related to response to situational crisis (retirement), as evidenced by isolative behavior, changes in mood, and decreased sense of well-being.

CLIENT OUTCOMES	NURSING INTERVENTIONS	EVALUATION
Mr. Brown will identify positive coping strategies, such as structuring leisure time.	Develop trusting relationship with Mr. Brown *to demonstrate caring and encourage Mr. Brown to practice new coping skills in a safe, therapeutic setting.*	Mr. Brown voiced trust in nurse-client relationship.
Mr. Brown will combine past effective coping methods with newly acquired coping strategies.	Praise Mr. Brown for adaptive coping. *Positive feedback encourages repetition of effective coping by Mr. Brown.*	Mr. Brown discussed plans for use of past and newly learned coping methods.
Mr. Brown will cope adaptively by putting anger into words versus actions.	Assist Mr. Brown in expressing anger and exploring angry feelings. *Verbalization of feelings in a nonthreatening relationship may help the client resolve conflicts and provide opportunity to vent feelings.*	Mr. Brown verbalized feelings of anger and loneliness appropriately.
Mr. Brown will verbalize understanding of loss as a process that needs to be worked through over time.	Determine the stage of loss. *Interventions vary with the stage of the loss process. Identification of the stage is necessary for effective interventions.*	Mr. Brown verbalized knowledge that loss is a natural process and will resolve in time.
	Explain to Mr. Brown the feelings and behaviors associated with each stage of loss *to help Mr. Brown understand that feelings such as anger are appropriate and acceptable to resolve loss at this stage.*	Mr. Brown verbalized his understanding of loss stages and identified his own loss process.

Continued

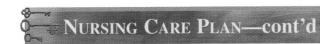

NURSING DIAGNOSIS: Impaired social interaction related to alteration in role (Mr. Brown is now retired), as evidenced by disruption in usual social activities and isolating behaviors.

CLIENT OUTCOMES	NURSING INTERVENTIONS	EVALUATION
Mr. Brown will increase socialization and involvement in activities according to capabilities.	Review Mr. Brown's resources and assist him to identify activities that he enjoys and can resume *to encourage Mr. Brown to focus on positive aspects of himself and his situation.*	Mr. Brown spent more time socializing with client peers than being alone.
Mr. Brown will effectively use social support systems inside and outside the hospital.	Explore Mr. Brown's social support system and his desire to seek help. Identify role changes now that he lives alone. *Opportunity to discuss socialization and preferences for activities helps Mr. Brown identify his own socialization patterns and demonstrates therapeutic alliance.*	Mr. Brown socialized with select client peers and identified aftercare social network and activities.

Additional Treatment Modalities

Inpatient mental health services are designed by a team of caregivers; each member of the team possesses a different expertise. The nurse is an integral part of the multidisciplinary team that identifies key (or target) symptoms or behaviors, designs interventions to address key symptoms, and decides on evaluative methods to measure client movement toward or away from desired outcomes. Before the team meeting, representatives from each discipline should complete their own assessment activities and bring pertinent information to the planning session. In this way, primary functions of the individual disciplines within the team are identified, clarified, and maximized toward resolving the client's problems. Because each discipline has a unique perspective on the treatment issues of each client and focuses collective energy on resolving problems, the resulting team plan is greater than the sum of its parts. For example, the nonverbal client may respond to therapies designed by occupational or art therapists while being relatively nonresponsive to verbal interventional techniques.

Medications

Symptoms of clients with adjustment disorders are expected to resolve after their immediate causes are identified and processed. Therefore medications are used sparingly unless the client meets the criteria for another disorder. Also, because symptoms of adjustment disorder may in some cases progress to include symptoms of major mental disorders, psychiatric mental health nurses may prefer to observe the client without the effects of medication to gather an accurate assessment of client behavior and functioning. Benzodiazepines are often prescribed for brief periods to treat symptoms of anxiety. Antidepressants may be prescribed if symptoms are problematic and interfere with the client's ability to mobilize resources.

Adjunctive Therapies

Typical team care for clients with mental disorders involves collaborative approaches including adjunctive therapies. For example, recreational therapies may be used with the client diagnosed with an adjustment disorder. Discovering the client's preference in leisure activities and providing appropriate resource materials may help the client become more comfortable socially and inspire him or her to become self-directed in pursuing recreational activities. If the client is able to exercise, physical exercise and/or movement can be a constructive outlet for tension and anxiety while enhancing self-esteem.

Supportive Therapies

Many licensed professionals, including clinical nurse specialists, advanced practice registered nurses, physicians, social workers, and psychologists, are prepared to provide therapeutic support for clients diagnosed with an adjustment disorder. Because clients with adjustment disorders are typically treated on an outpatient basis, they have a variety of treatment options and referral sources. Depending on professional preference, assessment of the client's problems, and identification of desired outcomes, therapists may use a variety of interventional methods. Cognitive behavior therapy, interpersonal or psychodynamic psychotherapy, and brief strategic therapeutic techniques may all be used effectively. Family therapy may be indicated when the stressor triggering the adjustment disorder occurs within a family system and the client and family require assistance in resolving the problem. Other therapeutic intervention techniques include biofeedback, relaxation exercises, hypnosis, meditation, journaling, and visual imaging activities.

EVALUATION

Evaluation of outcomes for adjustment disorders depends on the original features of the particular disorder. For the client with depressed or anxious mood, the absence of original problematic symptoms signifies resolution. For most clients, resolution of symptoms signifies a successful outcome to the treatment.

   If the client is hospitalized, the nurse is expected to evaluate the plan of care and the client's response to interventions at least once every 24 hours. Thoughtful discharge planning with attention to follow-up home health care or a visit to the primary physician's office can allay potential problems after the client is discharged. If the client is not completely free of symptoms before discharge, the treatment team should examine options for placement after care in the acute setting is ended.

CHAPTER SUMMARY

- Adjustment disorders are transient episodes of clinically significant emotional or behavioral nonpsychotic symptoms in response to identifiable psychosocial stress or stressors. Symptoms develop within 3 months after the stressful event.
- The diagnosis of adjustment disorder is considered if the client's behaviors or symptoms are different from usual patterns of response and if the symptoms have persisted for less than 6 months (acute), unless symptoms are in response to an ongoing stressor or stressors (chronic).
- The severity of the reaction to the stressor is not predictable from the stressor and is unique to the individual.
- In an adult population the most commonly diagnosed adjustment disorders are adjustment disorder with depressed mood and adjustment disorder with anxious mood.
- Clients with adjustment disorder are often treated as outpatients because the severity of their symptoms or subjective distress does not warrant inpatient hospitalization.
- Supportive psychotherapy is the most frequently used treatment modality with clients with adjustment disorders.
- Clients diagnosed with adjustment disorder may experience a resolution of symptoms or an exacerbation and increase of symptoms, supporting the diagnosis of a major psychiatric disorder such as major depression.
- Research is needed to establish the frequency and incidence of adjustment disorders and to measure outcomes of specific therapeutic interventions.
- Attempting to understand the client's experience from his or her point of view fosters the therapeutic process. Application of clinical models are of little value unless anticipated outcomes of care are meaningful to the client.
- Clients know more than anyone else about their lives and must be considered the resident experts in determining the meaning of life events, mobilizing inner strengths, and determining preferences for care.

REVIEW QUESTIONS

1. A 40-year-old client enters the therapist's office tearful, avoiding eye contact, and pacing the room. She states that her husband of 20 years has left her for another woman, she lost her job a week ago, and she has just discovered a lump in her breast. She complains of insomnia and decreased appetite. The highest priority nursing diagnosis would be:
   a. Disturbed sleep pattern
   b. Imbalanced nutrition: less than body requirements
   c. Powerlessness
   d. Ineffective denial

2. A 50-year-old client suffered a stroke 1 month ago and has not been able to work. He has depended on his wife to help him get dressed and to shower. Which client statement demonstrates that he has adjusted to the changes in his life?
   a. "I'm useless. I'll never be able to do things on my own."
   b. "I'm feeling stronger every day. I know that it will take time before I can become more independent."
   c. "They should have just let met die."
   d. "I don't need medication to control my blood pressure. I feel fine."

3. A 35-year-old client was brought to the psychiatric hospital for assessment. Her 3-year-old son was killed 3 months ago by a drunk driver. Her husband has been unable to cope with the grief, and they are currently talking about a marital separation. The highest priority nursing assessment question would be:
   a. "Do you have any thoughts of killing yourself?"
   b. "How have you coped with your loss?"
   c. "Have you been in therapy?"
   d. "Are you taking any medication?"

4. Which subtype may be found with an adjustment disorder?
   a. Schizophrenia
   b. Bipolar
   c. Depressed mood
   d. Bulimia

5. For a client with adjustment disorder it is important to teach the client and the family:
   a. They will have to cope with this disorder for the rest of the client's life.
   b. The client must keep to himself until the symptoms subside.
   c. The client must develop new coping mechanisms because there are no support systems.
   d. Symptoms can be managed using a variety of techniques (e.g., relaxation techniques, journal writing).

REFERENCES

Aalto-Setala T et al: Depressive symptoms in adolescence as predictors of early adulthood depressive disorders and maladjustment, *Am J Psychiatry* 159(7):1235, 2002.

American Psychiatric Association: *Diagnostic and Statistical Manual of Mental Disorders,* Fourth Edition, Text Revision. Washington, DC, American Psychiatric Association, 2000.

Armstrong M: *Being pregnant and using drugs: a retrospective phenomenological inquiry.* Unpublished doctoral dissertation. San Diego, Calif., 1992, University of San Diego.

Beck C: The lived experience of postpartum depression: a phenomenological study, *Nurs Research* 41(3):166, 1992.

Bergum V: *Woman to mother: a transformation,* Boston, 1989, Bergin & Garvey.

Blier R: *Science and gender,* New York, 1986, Pergamon Press.

Casey P, Dowrick C, and Wilkinson G: Adjustment disorders: fault line in the psychiatric glossary, *Br J Psychiatry* 179:479-481, 2001.

Colarusso C, Nemiroff R: *Adult development: a new dimension in psychodynamic theory and practice,* New York, 1981, Plenum Press.

Colarusso C, Nemiroff R: Clinical implications of adult development, *Am J Psychiatry* 144(10):1263, 1987.

Davis F: Deviance disavowal: the management of strained interaction by the visibly handicapped. In Davis F, editor: *Illness, interaction and the self,* Belmont, Calif, 1972, Wadsworth.

Erikson EH: *Childhood and society,* ed 2, New York, 1963, WW Norton.

Gilligan C: *In a different voice: psychological theory and women's development,* Cambridge, Mass, 1982, Harvard University Press.

Ginexi EM et al: Natural disaster and depression: a prospective investigation of reactions to the 1993 Midwest floods, *Am J Community Psychol* 28(4):495, 2000.

Greenberg W, Rosenfeld D, Ortega E: Adjustment disorder as an admission diagnosis, *Am J Psychiatry* 152(3):459, 1995.

Heifner C: Positive connectedness in the psychiatric nurse-patient relationship, *Arch Psychiatr Nurs* 7(1):11, 1993.

Jordan J et al: *Women's growth in connection: writings from the stone center,* New York, 1991, Guilford Press.

Kirk S, Kutchins H: *The selling of DSM: the rhetoric of science in psychiatry,* New York, 1992, Aldine de Gruyter.

Kovacs M et al: A controlled prospective study of DSM-III adjustment disorder in childhood: short-term prognosis and long-term predictive validity, *Arch Gen Psychiatry* 51(4):535, 1994.

Kryzhanovskaya L, Canterbury R: Suicidal behavior in patients with adjustment disorders, *Crisis* 22(3):125, 2001.

Kubler-Ross E: *On death and dying,* New York, 1969, Macmillan.

Lerner H: *Women in therapy,* Northvale, NJ, 1988, Jason Aronson Press.

Levine S: *Healing into life and death,* New York, 1987, Doubleday.

Lewis H: Is Freud an enemy of women's liberation? Some historical considerations. In Bernay T, Cantor D, editors: *The psychology of today's woman: new psychoanalytic visions,* Cambridge, Mass, 1986, Harvard University Press.

Lowenberg J: *Caring and responsibility: the crossroads between holistic practice and traditional medicine,* Pittsburgh, 1989, University of Pennsylvania Press.

Main M et al: Information sharing concerning schizophrenia in a family member: adult siblings' perspectives, *Arch Psychiatr Nurs* 7(3):147, 1993.

Meth R, Pasick R: *Men in therapy: the challenge of change,* New York, 1990, Guilford Press.

Mickley J et al: Spiritual well-being, religiousness and hope among women with breast cancer, *Image J Nurs Sch* 24(4):267, 1992.

Murphy S: Coping strategies of abstainers from alcohol up to three years post-treatment, *Image J Nurs Sch* 25(1):29, 1993.

Napier A: Heroism, men, and marriage, *J Marital Fam Ther* 17(1):9, 1991.

NANDA International (2003). NANDA Nursing Diagnoses: Definitions and Classification 2003-2004. Philadelphia: NANDA.

North American Nursing Diagnosis Association: *NANDA nursing diagnoses: definitions and classifications, 1999-2000,* Philadelphia, 1999, The Association.

Parsons T: *The social system,* New York, 1951, The Free Press.

Pittman F: The secret passions of men, *J Marital Fam Ther* 17(1):17, 1991.

Popkin M: Adjustment disorder and impulse control. In Kaplan H, Sadock B, editors: *Comprehensive textbook of psychiatry/V,* Baltimore, 1989, Williams & Wilkins.

Popkin M: Adjustment disorders in medically ill inpatients referred for consultation in a university hospital, *Psychosomatics* 31(4):410, 1990.

Razavi D et al: Screening for adjustment disorders and major depressive disorders in cancer inpatients, *Br J Psychiatry* 156:79, 1990.

Ruckdeschel H: *Psychotherapy for the old old: ten patients' report on their treatment for depression.* Unpublished doctoral dissertation, 1993, University of Pennsylvania.

Selye H: *Stress without distress,* New York, 1956, New American Library.

Selye H: *The stress of life,* New York, 1978, McGraw-Hill.

Snyder S, Strain J, Wolf D: Differentiating major depression from adjustment disorder with depressed mood in the medical setting, *Gen Hosp Psychiatry* 12:159, 1990.

Tanner C et al: The phenomenology of knowing the patient, *Image J Nurs Sch* 25(4):273, 1993.

Walsh F, McGoldrick M: *Living beyond loss,* New York, 1991, WW Norton.

SUGGESTED READINGS

American Nurses Association: *Statement on psychiatric-mental health clinical nursing practice and standards of psychiatric-mental health clinical nursing practice,* Washington, DC, 1994, American Nurses Publishing.

Coward D: The lived experience of self-transcendence in women with advanced breast cancer, *Nurs Sci Q* 3(4):162, 1990.

Nemiroff R, Colarusso C: *Psychotherapy and psychoanalysis in the second half of life,* New York, 1985, Plenum Press.

Spector R: *Cultural diversity in health and illness,* ed 3, Norwalk, Conn, 1991, Appleton & Lange.

PART III THERAPEUTIC MODALITIES

19

Interactive, Activity, and Electroconvulsive Therapies

Mary Magenheimer Webster

KEY TERMS

activity therapy (p. 450)
art therapy (p. 451)
attending (p. 430)
boundary (p. 431)
countertransference (p. 429)
electroconvulsive therapy (ECT) (p. 450)
key statement (p. 432)
movement/dance therapy (p. 451)
music therapy (p. 451)
norms (p. 444)
occupational therapy (p. 450)
psychodrama (p. 451)
recreational therapy (p. 450)
safety (p. 431)
social relationship (p. 428)
themes (p. 433)
therapeutic milieu (p. 438)
therapeutic relationship (p. 428)
transference (p. 429)
trust (p. 431)

OBJECTIVES

- Analyze the concepts of boundary, safety, and trust development as they relate to individual, milieu, and group therapy.

- Discuss the foundation that supports the various phases of therapies.

- Identify individual characteristics and attitudes that affect one's ability to function as a psychiatric mental health nurse.

- Describe the appropriate tasks for individual, milieu, and group therapies and how the nurse promotes these tasks.

- Define transference and countertransference and their impact on the therapeutic relationship.

- Distinguish between occupational, recreational, art, music, psychodrama, and movement/dance therapies.

- Identify the goals, objectives, and expected client outcomes for therapeutic activities.

- Describe the effectiveness of the nurse's role for each therapeutic activity.

- Discuss the significance of a multidisciplinary approach to therapeutic activities.

- Describe electroconvulsive therapy (ECT) as a biologic therapy.

- Compare and contrast modern ECT with its early use.

- Discuss the current role of ECT as a treatment for clients with depression and other disorders.

Each human being, family, or group is unique and complex, with a life and style of its own. To work effectively with a client, family, or group, many forms of therapy have been developed. The challenge for the nurse is to develop an awareness of these therapies and the various ways they can be presented in order to select those most beneficial to the specific client, family, or group. This chapter explores three areas of therapy: interactive, activity, and electroconvulsive.

INTERACTIVE THERAPY

Interactive therapy is defined as one individual's therapeutic interaction with another individual, family, or group. This concept is familiar for nurses, as much of nursing's work involves interacting with the client to promote healing. For example, the nurse changes a dressing on one client to assist wound healing or provides antibiotic medication to help another client fight an infection. The nurse also manipulates the many types of equipment required for the client's treatments. All this can be viewed as one individual providing treatment (or therapy) for another; however, this work reveals the nurse doing something very visible for the client. In these instances, most of the nurse's words are used for teaching, assessing the client's status, or exchanging pleasantries.

In contrast, much of the work of psychiatric mental health nursing is initially "invisible." The benefit, as well as the challenge, of psychiatric mental health nursing is that *the nurse uses the self as the therapeutic agent.* The nurse's words and interactions are designed to help the client heal psychically and emotionally. Just as it took time and experience to learn to change dressings, give medications, and manage equipment, it also takes time and skill to use oneself and one's words as tools for healing.

It is essential therefore to examine the nurse-client relationship in psychiatric mental health nursing. This section discusses the role of the nurse with clients in a therapeutic psychiatric environment.

THE THERAPEUTIC RELATIONSHIP

The nurse's goal has always been to promote health. Peplau (1952) defined mental health as: "The forward movement of personality and other ongoing human processes in the direction of creative, constructive, productive, personal, and community living." The psychiatric mental health nurse recognizes that every interaction has the potential to enhance health, and that the use of the therapeutic relationship is an efficient vehicle by which to promote and maintain a client's mental and emotional health.

Social vs. Therapeutic Relationships

The therapeutic relationship is unique in the world of human interactions. It stands apart from other types of relationships in its focus, purpose, and enactment. Beginning nurses and other practitioners tend to act in ways that more closely resemble a social relationship versus a therapeutic one. This is not surprising, as novices in the field may initially be more comfortable using familiar social skills. A **social relationship** exists for the mutual satisfaction of all involved parties, and its duration, focus, and intensity vary according to each participant's wishes. It is a subjective relationship.

In contrast, the **therapeutic relationship** exists to help one of the participants, the client, deal more effectively and maturely with some difficulty. Many theorists have identified the qualities and goals necessary for an effective therapeutic relationship (Peplau, 1969; Travelbee, 1971; Kennedy, 1977). Peplau's theory of interpersonal relations in nursing describes the therapeutic relationship as a personal relationship where "two people come to know each other well enough to face the problem at hand in a cooperative way." Peplau believed that the nursing functions in a therapeutic relationship are (1) to assist the client in identifying emotionally felt difficulties and (2) to apply knowledge of the principles of human relations to the problems or issues that arise at all levels of experiences (Peplau, 1969). This requires nurses to understand themselves and their behavior well enough to be objective and capable of focusing on their clients' needs, and is discussed further in the section on self-development. Travelbee (1971) further illuminated Peplau's work by describing the therapeutic relationship as a transaction between one human being and another, and not simply a nurse-client relationship. She stated that both the nurse and client need to acknowledge each other's uniquely human needs for the therapeutic relationship to be truly effective. Peplau (1991) also believed that education on the part of both nurse and client should occur within the context of a therapeutic relationship and that the nurse needs to view the client as an active participant in reaching the overall goal of the relationship, which is the client's health.

Roles in the Therapeutic Relationship

Roles are the expected social behavior patterns determined by an individual's position or status in a particular group or relationship. The psychiatric mental health nurse enacts several educational and therapeutic roles during various phases of the therapeutic relationship. Peplau (1952) identified four roles: (1) *resource person,* who gives specific information to clients, thus allowing them to understand situations or procedures; (2) *counselor,* who listens to the client's experience and assists in clarifying feelings associated with it; (3) *surrogate,* whom the client casts into roles of past relationships (parent, sibling, spouse, teacher), perhaps needing clarification of feelings; and (4) *technical expert,* who can navigate the complexities of the health care system.

Aspects of the Therapeutic Relationship

The therapeutic relationship is goal directed, client centered, and objective (Fortinash and Holoday Worret, 2003) and involves transference and countertransference.

Goal direction in a relationship implies a purpose for the relationship's existence. The overall goal of any therapeutic relationship is to help the client move toward health by becoming more self-responsible (Kennedy, 1977). Each individual is unique, however, and specific goals need to be defined for each person. The therapeutic relationship is initiated to help the individual deal with offending symptoms in a way that is more conducive to health. It is a highly focused relationship, with both participants agreeing to direct their energies toward achieving the identified goal. This also implies that the relationship has limits: it exists to meet certain defined goals, not to meet all of the client's needs. This concept of boundaries is discussed later in the chapter.

Client centered implies that the relationship is focused on the client; the client's goals, reactions, coping strategies, and growth are at the center of the relationship. The therapeutic relationship requires that the nurse turn attention to another for a while and suspend own preoccupation with life events to experience a client's sense of being (Kennedy, 1977). This does not mean that the nurse's reactions and sense of self are not important; it means that they are not the focus of the relationship. By paying attention to one's own reactions and being able to sort them out, the nurse gains knowledge of the client's interpersonal dynamics. This is some of the most difficult work in psychiatric mental health nursing—to recognize one's own reactions and to use this information in a way that will assist the client in growing toward emotional health. Rogers (1961), in his theory on client-centered therapy, stated that focus and reflection on the client and his needs, regardless of the client's behavior, reflect *unconditional positive regard* for the client's dignity and worth as a human being.

Objectivity is required on the part of the nurse for the therapeutic relationship to be effective. Objectivity implies an analytic approach to the subjective experience (i.e., it requires the nurse to be aware of her feelings and reactions to being with the client, rather than to just responding to the client on a personal level).

Transference refers to the client's feelings toward the nurse and the helping relationship. These feelings actually belong to the significant people in the client's life before the therapeutic relationship with the nurse, and they are transferred and replayed in the therapeutic relationship. Nurses must avoid responding as if the client's feelings are directed at them personally; such feelings are evoked by what the nurse represents to the client. By responding more objectively, nurses can help clients begin to recognize a pattern. For example, instead of responding in anger to anger, nurses can make open-ended comments, opening the door for clients to explore their feelings. By being objective, the nurse allows the client to take a step beyond the act itself and to begin to talk objectively about it rather than continually responding in the same way.

Countertransference is defined as the nurse's feelings toward the client. These feelings may be positive or negative and are a natural part of a therapeutic relationship. Problems arise only when the feeling is discounted because it upsets, surprises, or embarrasses the nurse in some way. Nurses need to recognize, identify, and accept these feelings; otherwise these feelings will influence their responses to clients, whether or not this is apparent (Kennedy, 1977). The success of the relationship depends on the nurse's ability to manage transference and countertransference.

Personal Qualities of Effective Helpers

There is growing recognition that the personal qualities of effective helpers are as important in promoting growth in others as the methods they use (Brammer, 1993). Effective helpers express a positive view of people's abilities to solve their own problems and manage their own lives. Also, they tend to view people as dependable, friendly, and worthy. Effective helpers tend to identify with people rather than things, demonstrate a capacity to cope, and are willing to reveal their thoughts (to the extent that it is therapeutic) rather than conceal them (Brammer, 1993). Helpers care for themselves and others.

PREPARATION FOR INTERACTIVE THERAPY
Self-Awareness

It is clear from the preceding discussion that the psychiatric mental health nurse needs a strong sense of self or at least the willingness to develop one. The term *sense of self* refers to self-awareness or self-knowledge, which is necessary because nurses must be able to separate their own subjective beliefs from the facts. Self-awareness implies recognition of one's thinking, values, conflicts, interaction styles and attitudes, and an awareness of how these can influence interactions with clients. Therefore it is necessary that the psychiatric nurse be committed and open to self-exploration.

There are many ways for the nurse to do this work: support groups, values clarification work, role-playing, and individual supervision. *Self-reflection* is an appropriate first step. Nurses can assess their values, attitudes, and orientation by asking themselves some general questions. Self-assessment increases the nurse's self-awareness and helps develop more effective therapeutic interactive skills.

Areas for Self-Assessment
Need to Be Liked

It is important to assess the need to be liked, accepted, and valued, which can paralyze the nurse in interactions. For example, the nurse is at risk for becoming hurt or angry if the client acts in an angry or hostile manner. Or the nurse may hesitate to comment for fear that the client would be offended in some way and consequently think less of the nurse. With time and experience the nurse learns that the key to an effective approach is simply to be comfortable with the other person. This comfort arises out of a sincere effort to attend to the client's words and listen carefully to the experience. Rapport develops best when nurses focus on their clients and forget their own need to be liked (Kennedy, 1977).

Being Judgmental

Another area to evaluate is being judgmental. Judgments are the quick stereotyping of people to fit them into categories to ease one's own interactive experience and allow one to decide issues of emotional safety quickly. However, judgments can often result in stereotyping, in which individuals lose a personal identity and are clumped into a collective group. Although it is unrealistic to expect anyone to rid themselves of their judgments completely, psychiatric nurses should at least be aware of their judgments and how they affect relationships. "Nursing symbolizes the acceptance of people as they are and assistance in their times of stress" (Peplau, 1952).

Responsibility

Another critical area is assuming responsibility. It is necessary for psychiatric mental health nurses to clarify their own understanding of who is responsible for what in the therapeutic relationship. It is not up to the nurse to define the area, direction, or time frame of the client's growth, but rather to support the client's own work in the therapeutic process. "Real support arises from entering into the experience of other persons, being able to stand there with them as they explore themselves, and not in backing away when the experience threatens to become hard on us" (Kennedy, 1977).

Potential for Human Growth

The psychiatric mental health nurse needs to have some confidence in the client's ability to grow, learn, and make changes. Nurses need to assess their own assumptions about the potential for human growth. One way to achieve this goal is to evaluate their own personal needs for sympathy and protection (Fortinash and Holoday Worret, 2003). If nurses believe that they need to be protected from life experiences, they may also assume that they are not capable of coping with life stressors. Nurses who believe this about themselves may attribute the same qualities to their clients and then try to protect them from the work of psychologic growth rather than help them move through the challenges to achieve growth.

These areas of self-assessment are not meant to be a complete list. Psychiatric mental health nurses will find themselves examining their values and attitudes anew with each client's unique situation.

CONCERNS EXPERIENCED BY THE NURSE

It has been noted that student nurses generally have three concerns: (1) self-consciousness about enacting the role, (2) fears and fantasies about what constitutes professional behavior, and (3) uncertainty about how to proceed technically with clients (Denton, 1987). Novice psychiatric mental

health nurses generally demonstrate these anxieties by worrying about their choice of words. They often fear saying "the wrong thing" or become "awkward" about using words. This heightened self-consciousness is often part of learning to use the self in a therapeutic manner.

This attention to words also extends to the nurse's perception of the client. Students tend to focus solely on what the client says (the content) and often miss the richness of the nonverbal information presented by the client (the intent). They may therefore neglect to follow up on a tone of voice or a special look on the client's face.

Psychiatric mental health nursing is not only about words. It is about therapeutic relationships and focusing on another individual. When nurses are aware of the work occurring at each phase of the relationship, they can consciously use a variety of skills to promote the desired change in the client. When the focus is on the work, words can be used more fluidly as a therapeutic tool.

An important aspect in the development of trust and safety is the nurse's manner or behavior. Nurses must outwardly model or demonstrate their attention to the client. This counseling skill is called **attending** and includes all of the ways in which therapists demonstrate to clients that they are heard; clients are thus encouraged to express feelings and experiences.

The nurse shows this attention nonverbally and verbally. *Nonverbal behaviors* include a relaxed posture (indicating openness and acceptance) with a slightly forward lean (demonstrating interest) (Figure 19-1). The nurse maintains good eye contact, "seeing" the client. It is important not to simply stare or glare at the client, as this is an aggressive behavior, but rather to meet the client's eyes in a relaxed, comfortable manner, occasionally looking away. *Verbal behaviors* associated with attending demonstrate careful listening and include open-ended questions, paraphrasing, reflection of feelings, summarization, and allowing clients to set their own pace (see Chapter 7).

An effective way for nurses to demonstrate attending skills toward clients while earning their trust is to enact the

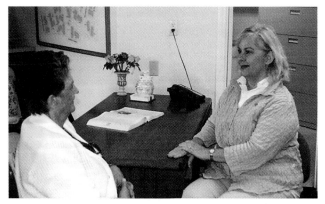

FIGURE 19-1. The nurse therapist's nonverbal behaviors—relaxed posture, attentive expression, and open body position—indicate acceptance and interest in the client and a willingness to listen.

qualities of genuineness, respect, and empathy. *Genuineness* has been defined as verbal and behavioral congruence and authenticity. *Respect* is defined as unconditional positive regard and is conveyed through consistency and active listening. *Empathy* implies seeing the situation from the client's point of view, yet remaining objective. The empathic nurse can intervene to assist clients in their understanding of a situation and suggest appropriate avenues for change (Fortinash and Holoday Worret, 2003).

DEVELOPMENT OF A THERAPEUTIC RELATIONSHIP

Psychiatric clients often misinterpret aspects of reality and relationships. Therefore it is important that the nurse be clear in defining the aspects of the therapeutic relationship to minimize anticipated misinterpretation. Establishing a therapeutic relationship is not magic; it requires hard work and the skillful application of knowledge. Beginners in interactive therapy are often so concerned with the content of the session or the presentation of the client that they overlook the basic concepts at work in every therapeutic relationship. These concepts are boundary development and maintenance, safety development, and trust development. The concepts apply to the individual therapeutic relationship, as well as to the family and group processes, although they are expressed in different ways. These three concepts are tightly interwoven, each affecting the other.

Boundary Development and Maintenance

The term **boundary** refers to the definition of an entity. The boundaries of a country define its shape, size, and location in relationship to other countries. Each country negotiates for itself in various kinds of social interactions. Boundaries separate and define entities at the point where the entity interacts with others.

In psychologic terms, boundaries refer to the definition and separation of the self from others. They define the responsibilities and duties of one's self in relationship to others. This is an extremely important concept in working with psychiatric clients whose sense of self is often unclear in some way. Often, psychiatric clients do not have a sense of what constitutes their own responsibility and ask nurses to do things that are not the nurse's responsibility. Consequently, nurses must have a clear sense of self and of their role to prevent collusion with clients in this way.

Safety Development

Safety is the sense of security within the therapeutic relationship. Well-defined boundaries are essential to developing safety. Safety comes from knowing the expectations of the relationship and the responsibilities of the parties involved (nurse and client). By defining the structure of the therapeutic relationship, clients are safe to experiment within these boundaries while knowing that there are definable limits. All individuals need to feel safe when experimenting with new ways of being; this is especially true of psychiatric clients.

Consequently, part of the nurse's role in a therapeutic relationship is to enhance safety by acting consistently within the defined boundaries. It is confusing and dangerous for clients if a nurse introduces social elements into a therapeutic relationship in an attempt to be "friendly." Nurses should act within the boundaries of their role by assisting the client in focusing on the assigned task and exploring new options for growth, healing, and understanding.

Trust Development

Trust is the reliance on the truthfulness or accuracy of the relationship. As the nurse exercises the concepts of boundary and safety, trust develops within the nurse-client relationship. Congruence between words and actions is essential for trust to grow. If nurses consistently do what they say they will, the client is free to focus on the work and tasks of therapy. For many clients the relationship with the caregivers may be the most trusting one in their lives. As nurses continue to model their responsibilities in maintaining a trusting relationship, clients can begin to trust themselves and their reactions more. Trust is essential to the development of a sense of self.

Acting in a trustworthy manner does not imply that conflicts will not occur. Trust does not imply agreement, only consistency. If the client makes an inappropriate demand, the nurse is not expected to meet it to maintain trust. (In fact, trust could be damaged when a nurse meets a demand that is inappropriate for the relationship.) Trust does not develop from doing everything the client asks; trust develops from doing what one said one would do.

These three concepts of *boundary development and maintenance, safety development,* and *trust development* are the foundations of every therapeutic relationship. The nurse constantly works to develop these in each relationship; it is the "invisible work" of psychiatric nursing. Within these three concepts, the nurse works with the client in a goal-directed, objective, and client-centered way, using a variety of skills such as listening and reflecting.

PHASES OF THE THERAPEUTIC RELATIONSHIP
Orientation Phase

The *orientation phase* is the first phase of the therapeutic relationship. It occurs when clients enter the system and are experiencing the tension and anxiety associated with their own needs, as well as those generated by exposure to a new and uncertain situation. Successful orientation is essential in helping the client to combine these experiences (rather than split them away in some manner—repression or dissociation) so as to be able to participate fully in the therapeutic relationship. Orientation serves to define and clarify the relationship: the formulation of the client's issue or conflict, the purpose or goal of the work, and the relationship between the client and the nurse. The major "invisible work" of the orientation phase is boundary formation. The nurse works to assist clients in clarifying their impression of the problem, thus defining the scope or boundary of the work. In addition, the nurse helps the client to function within the relationship and to have questions answered, needs expressed, and sincerity developed, thus defining the scope or boundaries of the relationship itself (Peplau, 1952).

Boundary development is done in specific ways. Nurses initially approach clients as strangers and must work to define themselves as allies and helpers. In introducing themselves to clients, nurses must state their purposes clearly. For example, if meeting a depressed client on an inpatient unit, the nurse could say, "Hello, I'm Mary, your nurse. I'll be working with you while you're here, to help you get used to the hospital and to look at areas in your life that are troubling you." This introduction clearly establishes the relationship as therapeutic and defines the nurse's role as a helping professional. Vague introductions do not work because they do not address the formation of the boundary. The purpose of the introduction is to begin to define the scope of the work and the relationship.

The next step of the introduction builds on boundary development by defining the time frame when the work can be done. Defining the time boundary includes the approximate number of sessions, the length of time for each session, and the total number of sessions, which is the overall length of the relationship. This may be done formally, as with a contract for scheduled outpatient appointments, or simply as an agreement to meet daily. The specifics vary with different clients and in different settings, and the words vary with the nurse's personality style. These variances are to be expected and encouraged. Whatever the approach, each introduction must define the boundaries for the nurse's role, the scope of the work, and the time frame for doing the work.

Application to Short-Term Psychiatric Hospitalization

With the advent of managed care and concomitant payer systems, many inpatient settings may function as short-term assessment and crisis intervention units, with clients referred to other areas of care, such as day treatment programs, long-term care facilities, or the community. This means that the nurse may have only 1 to 3 days to work with the client and needs to incorporate the important work of boundary development, trust building, and safety development within that limited time frame. Box 19-1 describes some specific skills that may help the nurse fulfill these critical relationship components within the shorter time frame.

Work of the Orientation Phase

The work of the orientation phase is to help the client become a full participant in the therapeutic process by developing safety and trust. To do this, the nurse must follow through on the agreements made in the introduction. As Peplau (1952) has noted, "A relationship that is useful to the

| Box 19-1 | Nursing Skills to Establish a Therapeutic Relationship Within a Limited Time Frame |

During the client's short-term hospitalization, the nurse will:
- Make rounds on clients immediately after the shift report and introduce self. Meet family/significant others as appropriate.
- Explain the roles and responsibilities of the client, nurse, and other disciplines as appropriate.
- Discuss the time frame of the therapeutic relationship and client goals to be achieved within that time.
- Help the client to prioritize achievable goals and list resources for long-term goals that may be met after discharge.
- Inform the client of his or her rights and of the expectations of the nurse and other caregivers.
- Provide the client with a schedule of groups, activities, medications, and other treatments appropriate for the estimated length of stay and plan of care.
- Educate the client/family/significant others about medications and other treatments and provide written literature approved by the treatment team to help the client meet discharge and aftercare needs.
- Discuss discharge plans (with the client/family/significant others) in collaboration with the treatment team.

client is one in which what is expected of him is made clear and adhered to consistently, . . . one in which he is treated with understanding and respect as a person."

This goal is accomplished in specific ways. The nurse demonstrates dependability by being punctual and willing to discuss with the client the length of meetings, location, confidentiality of information; roles of the nurse and the client; and other specifics such as the reason for the hospitalization, the source of the client's problem, or which alternative choices may help the client (Fortinash and Holoday Worret, 1999). The nurse's remarks should be simple and clear to orient the client to the situation.

In addition, the nurse focuses on clients and their concerns to help them identify and formulate goals. Nurses should listen carefully to what clients say about their own lives (the content) and observe how clients present this information (the process). Questions should be asked to further both the nurse's and the client's understanding of the client's experience. For example, a client may be describing the death of a parent and the subsequent breakup of the family (this is the content, i.e., *what* is said). Yet the client may relate all of this information in a matter-of-fact way (this is the process, *how* it is said). The nurse's response should broaden the client's knowledge of the experience. For example, the nurse could comment, "Please tell me more about what this was like for you." Or the nurse may simply reflect back an important **key statement**. Rather than interpreting, nurses should encourage clients to recognize their own feelings (Peplau, 1952). These responses help clients to focus and expand their experiences. Questions are focused on clients' experiences and are open ended to allow clients to expand and clarify their thoughts.

Client Responses to Orientation

Psychiatric clients often have not been able to tell their story. Families may develop their own version around specific issues, and the family myth is difficult to challenge. Friends may tire of the story or respond in a socially conventional way. As a result, clients have no one to tell their story to, and thus the story gets stopped at a certain point and is never allowed to reach a conclusion. Consequently, many of the emotions are also blocked and never worked through to resolution. The nurse's work in orientation is to help the client continue the story.

Although some clients are open to continuing their story, others do not welcome this opportunity or even know how to use it. There is a great deal of anxiety whenever one ventures beyond the known social conventions, and this anxiety may be manifested in several ways. The client may test the nurse in some way, such as being late for meetings, ending them early, or questioning their usefulness. The client may focus on the nurse personally by questioning the nurse's competence, showing sexual interest, or attempting to shock the nurse through profanity, confrontation, or sharing bizarre experiences or behavior (Fortinash and Holoday Worret, 1999).

The nurse needs to observe this behavior sensitively and objectively and consider it as both the client's interactive style and as a level of the client's anxiety. The nurse responds by focusing the client on the therapeutic work based on assessment of the situation.

Assessment

In addition to establishing the relationship, the orientation phase gives the nurse an opportunity to assess the client.

Themes. The nurse listens for themes that run throughout the client's stories. **Themes** are recurring patterns of interactions that the client experiences. The following are examples of themes: every close relationship ending in anger, clients doubting their abilities in every instance, clients blaming others for life situations, and clients portraying themselves as victims. Themes are the underlying dynamics of many encounters. It is important to discern these patterns, and it takes time. The patterns become more evident as the work progresses; the client may or may not be aware of them.

Themes are often linked to the client's problem areas. Clients are usually aware of their problem areas and can assist in identifying them. Generally, clients can give the nurse some idea of what would make the situation "right" for them (i.e., their thoughts about what is unhealthy for them and what would "fix" it). The function of the psychiatric mental health nurse is to accept this understanding and work to safely create opportunities for the client to learn healthy ways of assessing and achieving appropriate parts of the goal. Together, the client and nurse can prioritize the identified problem areas.

Observations. Psychiatric mental health nurses can enhance their effectiveness by making observations about the clients and the relationship. The nurse could make note of the client's affect and demeanor, noticing whether either changes when certain topics are discussed and in what way. The nurse also listens for what is *not* said—in terms of the major players in the client's life who are not part of the story and the omission of feelings, reactions, or thoughts. Nurses need to listen and identify their own feelings evoked in the relationship with the client. These feelings provide valuable information about the client's interactive style. The nurse must assess the client's mood, cognitive functioning, and potential for suicide or homicide.

Strengths. One of the most important aspects of the orientation period is to assess the strengths and positive aspects of the client's personality. These healthy parts of the individual can be used to heal the more problematic areas. If the work of psychiatric mental health nursing is to move the client toward health, then it is critical to know "the allies." Much of the work of psychiatric mental health nursing is to expand and enlarge the healthy aspects of a person's personality while minimizing the dysfunctional aspects.

It is a skill to assist clients in using their own strengths in ways that benefit them. Together, the nurse and client identify these strengths. It is helpful for clients to view themselves as more than the sum of their problems. Such an expanded self-view may be the first step toward altering clients' self-perception and increasing their objectivity; it will assist them as they begin to engage in problem solving.

Nursing Care Plan. Once the assessment is completed, the nurse identifies the client's problems, nursing diagnoses, and outcome criteria; formulates the nursing care plan; implements the plan with nursing interventions; and evaluates the efficacy of the care plan, modifying it as needed (Fortinash and Holoday Worret, 2003).

In summary, the work of the *orientation phase* is to (1) define the boundaries of the therapeutic relationship (i.e., identification of the work to be completed, the relationship between client and nurse, and the time frame; in effect, the "contract" between the nurse and client), (2) begin the development of safety and trust by acting congruently within the defined boundaries, (3) complete the nursing assessment of the client, and (4) formulate the nursing care plan.

Working Phase

There is no clear ending to the orientation phase or beginning to the next phase, known as the *working phase*. The phases of the relationship overlap. As the working phase begins, the boundaries of the relationship have been established and the client acts within these boundaries. Safety and trust have also developed to the point that the client is willing to risk further exploration of issues. The nurse and client have come to know each other well enough to be able to cooperate in dealing with a problem.

The working phase is a problem-solving time and involves both understanding the problem and assisting clients

The Working Phase: Steps in Problem Solving

1. Identify the problem.
2. Clarify understanding of the problem.
   a. Identify triggers to maladaptive behaviors.
   b. Increase specificity (i.e., decrease generalizations).
3. Identify past solutions.
4. Evaluate the effectiveness of past solutions.
5. Generate new solutions (NOTE: This is often done with peers or in group discussions.)
6. Test new solutions.
7. Evaluate effectiveness of new solutions.

in translating this understanding to actions that work to their benefit. Box 19-2 lists the steps in problem solving.

Identifying and Clarifying the Problem

Identifying and clarifying the problem includes facilitating both the nurse's understanding of the client's position and the client's own understanding. This task is commonly known as *problem formulating,* and is the first step of problem solving. To do this, the nurse asks open-ended questions designed to promote the client's recognition and integration of his or her own experiences and perhaps gain a new perspective on them. The function of the nurse as a counselor is to assist the individual's self-directed learning in ways that promote health and integration of experience (Peplau, 1952).

Keen listening and open-ended, nonjudgmental responses are necessary skills for this phase of work. The nurse's response to a client's statement must not obstruct the possibility of identifying feelings or thoughts that help the client to learn about himself (Peplau, 1952). For example, consider a homemaker in crisis. She states, "I just can't do it all anymore." The nurse's goal is to further the client's understanding of her own situation. Evaluate the following conversations to see which statement accomplishes this task.

CONVERSATION 1

Client: It's all too much for me. I can't do it all anymore!
Nurse: We all have our bad days.
Client: I've had too many of them.
Nurse: Then they must be nearly over. Hang in there.
Client: Thanks. I will.

CONVERSATION 2

Client: It's all too much for me. I can't do it anymore!
Nurse: I'm not sure I understand. What do you mean by "It's"?
Client: My life.
Nurse: Your whole life is "all too much" for you?

Client: No, well, yes. There's just so much to be done!
Nurse: You have a lot to do?
Client: I'll say I do! I take care of the kids and the house, and my husband is never around to help out.
Nurse: You're taking care of the kids and the house without much help?
Client: Much help? *No* help! He's never there for me! He's always out doing something while I'm stuck at home with his kids from his first marriage.
Nurse: What's that like for you?
Client: It makes me mad. I'm not his slave.
Nurse: So, you're angry about this?
Client: Sometimes. At other times, I am not so mad because my first marriage was pretty bad.
Nurse: It sounds like you have more than one feeling about this.

In the first example, the nurse blocked any chance for exploration by injecting her own viewpoint as a reassurance. The client could justifiably assume herself to be a self-pitying whiner. Most likely, the client will keep further "failings" from this nurse. In the second example, however, the nurse was open to exploring the client's reality with her. Her questions provided focus for the work of exploring, but did not limit the client's responses, thereby allowing the client to begin to gain perspective on her situation.

To further demonstrate nursing responses that promote the client's understanding of the situation, consider the following example of a suicidal client.

Client: I just want to die.
Nurse: You're thinking about death quite seriously.
Client: Yes. It would take care of everything.
Nurse: You're seeing death as a solution.
Client: Yes.
Nurse: I'm not sure I understand. Tell me more.
Client: About what?
Nurse: About death as a solution.
Client: Well, the insurance money would pay off my debts, and my wife would have money to live on.
Nurse: You're thinking that your wife would benefit financially from your death?
Client: Yes. She would probably be happier, too . . . without me. I'm not worth much these days.
Nurse: You think your wife would be happier if you were to die.
Client: Yes . . . well, not right away, of course. She'd be sad at first . . . but she'd get over it . . . find somebody worthy of her.
Nurse: It sounds as if you think highly of your wife.
Client: Oh, yes! I just don't know why she puts up with me. I've been terrible to be around.
Nurse: You sound puzzled that she could love you even during this difficult time.

In this case the nurse did not argue against the client's solution of suicide but explored the dynamics behind it. The questions/statements also helped to introduce different perspectives to the client (the fact that he is worthy of love even during his depression and the possibility that the depression is time limited).

Further exploration with both these clients clarifies the patterns of thinking and acting that contribute to their anguish. This is crucial information. It is the meaning of the behavior, mood, or thoughts perceived by the client that gives the nurse clues to determine which needs must be met. The nurse obtains this information as purely as possible without contaminating it. To do this, the nurse acts as a neutral sounding board so that clients can voice their views in a relationship that is safely defined and nonjudgmental (Peplau, 1952). Another part of understanding the problem involves the client and nurse determining what sorts of things trigger the maladaptive response. The nurse can help clients determine whether their reactions are a global response to any stressor, or whether certain situations set them off or make them worse. This is important to know because it guides the nurse in assisting the client to develop effective responses.

The nurse continues to help the client explore the problem by asking the client how he has previously dealt with the problem, and having him determine which of these methods, if any, produced an effective solution. The client usually identifies one or two ways that were effective to some extent, but many of the attempted solutions did not bring the expected relief. The work here is to pull out the effective methods and help the client expand on them either through nurse-client discussions or with the input of peers. This will often result in new solutions or effective refinement of solutions that the client has already attempted. For example, the housewife in crisis in the preceding example may have sought relief with alcohol or drugs, long walks, talking to a friend, arguing with her husband, and/or ignoring her children. When asked how effective these methods were in relieving her distress, she would probably note that talking with her friend and taking a long walk helped the most, arguing with her husband had some effect, and the other methods made her feel worse. The nurse would then help her explore, refine, and expand these helpful solutions.

Safety Development

During the working phase of the relationship, the concepts of safety and boundaries become important again. As noted earlier, the client feels safe when he knows what the expectations are in a given situation, as well as his responsibilities in meeting those expectations. Clients are expected to tell their story and explore various aspects of it. This may cause them a good deal of anxiety, but the nurse maintains a climate of safety by setting the pace of the work and maintaining healthy boundaries, which prevent the client from becoming overwhelmed (Peplau, 1952).

Translating Understanding Into Action

The next part of the working phase is to assist the client in translating his expanded understanding of the situation into behavioral changes or actions that promote health. There are many ways to do this, depending on the client's situation and the nurse's theoretic perspective. One aspect common to all client situations is that the behavioral changes are practiced in the here and now. The client actually attempts behavioral change in the clinical situation with nursing support. The formulation of a daily goal is an effective way to help the client try new behaviors. The nurse can interact throughout the day about goal accomplishment and how it is influenced by various events. For example, perhaps the suicidal man described previously has learned that his days are much worse when he does not get out of bed in the morning. Together with the nurse, he has identified a behavioral pattern in which he stays in bed isolated from his wife, reflects on his worthlessness, and becomes more despondent as the day goes on. This pattern has been repeated on the unit. The client and nurse have decided to evaluate whether a change in this pattern would effect a change in his self-perception; they decide to test this by having the client get out of bed promptly in the morning and interact with at least one person at breakfast. (This would be consistent with a cognitive therapy approach.)

The homemaker has discovered an inability to say "no" to requests or to ask for any assistance at all. On the unit she has been helpful to other clients, caring for them and negating her own needs. After learning some assertiveness skills, she and the nurse devise a plan in which she has to say "no" to three requests made of her and to ask for help once. In both cases the nurse continues to help the client to clarify feelings associated with the task and integrate the experience into the client's life (see Chapter 7 for further information on assertiveness).

Working in the here and now is always possible and is especially appropriate for short-term hospitalizations. Beginners will often focus on the situation outside of the therapy as if it were a separate entity. More experienced practitioners know that everything that happens "outside" of the relationship also happens within it. If nurses focus on the problem situation as one occurring outside the client, they can assist clients in dissociating from the situation (Peplau, 1952). However, the nurse's function is to assist the client in seeing that the locus of control is within the self, and that the client can either possess or learn the skills to deal with this and other situations. Clients must experience this first in order to learn it. Once the client has experienced the ability to act in new ways, the nurse can help the client to evaluate the effectiveness of these new solutions and to use them as more typical responses in the future.

The nurse often teaches new skills for the client to explore. The nurse's teaching must be appropriate to each client's plan of care, and generally consists of both instruction and experience. The nurse evaluates the client's current level of knowledge and uses this experience to expand the client's levels of understanding. The nurse may select from such skills as the relaxation response, stress reduction techniques, assertiveness training, and cognitive therapy.

Roles

Much of this learning happens within the client's relationship with the nurse, and it requires a sensitivity to the different roles that clients assign nurses. As noted earlier, clients often respond to nurses *as if* they were someone else from a previous relationship. This unconscious pattern occurs when the client's situation reactivates feelings that were generated in a prior relationship (transference) (Peplau, 1952). By stereotyping the nurse, clients limit their own actions and reactions to those in the original experiences. This repetitive pattern of interacting is limited and can serve to reinforce maladaptive behavior. As nurses gradually reveal their own individuality, they demonstrate the variety of human responses to their clients, who are then free to explore their own various responses.

For example, imagine the homemaker in a creative group setting where she accidentally spills the paint. She seems horrified by this and begins to frantically clean up the spill. The nurse approaches her.

Client:	I'm so sorry! I'm so sorry. I can't believe how clumsy I am! I can't seem to do anything right.
Nurse:	[Recognizing that the client seems to want the nurse to participate in this "critical parent" stance] Are you expecting me to criticize you?
Client:	Well, you should. I've made a mess of everything! Don't you see what I've done?
Nurse:	What I see is that you had an accident and you're cleaning it up. That looks like being responsible to me. Can I help you?
Client:	No, it's almost done. The spill wasn't that huge.
Nurse:	I appreciate your taking care of it.

By being genuine and sharing her viewpoint, the nurse provided the client with an important learning experience. The nurse did not respond in the anticipated critical way, but instead offered her own point of view and acknowledged the client's appropriate response.

From the nurse's viewpoint the client was acting responsibly. The client may have never considered this possibility, as her self-perceptions were locked in a self-critical mode, a pattern she enacted in the here and now in the presence of the nurse. The nurse used the opportunity to reject the critical role the client attempted to assign her and to acknowledge the client's strength instead.

The psychiatric nurse recognizes that *every* interaction provides an opportunity to be therapeutic and promote health.

Trust Development

In the preceding scenario, the nurse promoted trust between herself and the client by congruent words and actions. As noted earlier in this chapter, trust develops when there is

congruence between words and actions. As clients learn to trust the nurse's genuineness and experience the nurse's acceptance, they begin to trust their own genuineness. This is one of the remarkable healing features of an effective therapeutic relationship. As clients experience trust and safety in the relationship, they begin to incorporate these elements into their sense of self. The nurse often has to point out the areas of growth or change in the here and now because there may not be another opportunity. It is especially helpful if these comments are geared toward clients' daily goals so that they can see the work they have done, which they otherwise may not recognize.

The client eventually develops an understanding of the situation, its causes, some skills for dealing with it, and some self-confidence to enact those skills. It is then time to terminate the therapeutic relationship.

Termination Phase

Terminating relationships is not generally done effectively in many Western cultures. There is a tendency to ignore, belittle, or hasten terminations in relationships, whether they are superficial or intimate. *Termination* is often a difficult phase in therapy as well. Because it represents an ending and is consciously or unconsciously associated with death, termination brings out many fears and anxieties in people. Termination forces one to come to terms with the limits of the relationship and therefore acknowledges the limits of life itself. In a more concrete sense, termination is the real loss of the nurse for the client. The relationship ends, and the client must face life without the external support of the nurse. At the same time that endings are being acknowledged, however, accomplishments, growth, and individuality are also being realized. The therapeutic work of the nurse is to help the client accept the closure of the boundaries of the relationship and the transfer of safety and trust to the client.

Before Termination

As noted earlier, termination work begins during the introductory phase when the nurse defines the time frame and eventual end of the relationship. In addition, the work of the relationship, including specific goals, has been clearly defined during the introductory period. Given the current short lengths of stay, it is imperative that the nurse be as clear as possible about client goals, time frame, therapeutic regimen, and termination issues (see Box 19-1).

The nurse must also continue to acknowledge the end of the relationship during the working phase. Comments such as "While we're still working together . . ." or "During the time we have remaining . . ." reinforce the given time boundaries and help the client get used to the idea of termination.

It is also effective to acknowledge the client's growth or accomplishments toward goal achievement or attainment as they occur during the working phase. By noting movement toward goal achievement, the nurse marks the client's progress and reinforces the concept that the relationship exists to accomplish certain things. Such comments also pro-

Box 19-3	Acknowledging Client Goals in the Working Phase

1. The nurse assists the client in acknowledging the work done on the daily goal and the remaining issues. A review of the day is helpful and reinforcing.
2. The nurse offers his or her observations of the client's progress toward goal accomplishment.
3. Preliminary goal setting for the next shift or day is appropriate because it helps the client to recognize progress made toward goal achievement.

Box 19-4	Typical Client Responses to Termination of the Relationship

Denial
Minimizing the relationship
Rejection
Regression
Anger
Suicide attempt
Acceptance

mote trust and safety in clients by encouraging them to trust themselves to be effective in specific areas of their lives and, consequently, feel safer.

As clients begin to do more for themselves, the nurse can transition to the termination phase by spacing contacts further apart to allow clients more time to "stand on their own" according to their capabilities. This gives clients the opportunity to support themselves gradually, which the nurse acknowledges.

During the transition to the termination phase (and during termination itself), new or intense topics should not be introduced. This is a time of solidifying gains and acknowledging the work accomplished. If other issues exist, they may be acknowledged as areas for future work. It is unfair to the client to raise issues that cannot be resolved within the time that remains (Box 19-3).

Client Responses to Termination

As the reality of termination approaches, clients may respond in a variety of ways depending on their personality and coping skills. Some may deny the occurrence or imminence of separation. Clients involved in denial try to make plans to visit the nurse after discharge or ask about making arrangements to "drop by" the hospital some time. By guaranteeing future contact, they can deny the impact of the current separation. Other clients minimize the importance of the relationship and may make comments comparing the nurse with other supportive people in their lives, as if discounting the work done and the importance of the nurse's role. They may even ignore or avoid the nurse. Another common reaction is anger. The client may express anger at the nurse, the institution, or other clients in an attempt to cover the pain of separation. The client may experience the termination as a rejection, which may activate old feelings of inferiority or a negative self-concept. Some clients may attempt to avoid the whole situation through premature discharge or noninvolvement in groups. Others may regress as if to demonstrate their continuing need for the nurse, stemming from their perceived inability to deal with life on their own. A few clients may actually attempt suicide to keep the nurse involved. Finally, some clients accept the termination and demonstrate some perspective on their various reactions (Fortinash and Holoday Worret, 1999). Careful review of these various reactions will remind the reader of the stages of grief (denial, anger, bargaining, and acceptance) (see Chapter 25). This is not surprising when termination is viewed as a loss (Box 19-4).

The Nurse's Role in Termination

As noted earlier, American culture does not deal well with endings. Consequently, few clients have a frame of reference for handling this crucial aspect of life. The nurse has the unique opportunity to assist the client in a successful separation and ending, allowing the client to transfer this knowledge to the next situation. To do this, the nurse must model effective parting for the client. The first step is for the nurse to clearly understand the goal of termination, which is to dissolve the therapeutic relationship while assuring the client of an improved ability to function independently (Fortinash and Holoday Worret, 2003).

The second step is for the nurse to have a clear understanding of the dynamics of loss (see Chapter 25) and how these concepts affect the client and the nurse. Preparing to terminate the therapeutic relationship takes time. As a general rule, one third of the entire length of the therapeutic relationship should be spent on termination issues. Although this may not always be possible given the current system of health care, it does emphasize the importance of this aspect of care.

Although termination is addressed initially and throughout the relationship, it begins formally when the client has accomplished the appropriately defined goals and has improved to a higher level of self-sufficiency.

The nurse acknowledges the upcoming ending of the relationship by engaging the client in open discussions of his or her feelings. The nurse continues to be accepting and nonjudgmental, even if the client expresses anger, apathy, or denial. By accepting the client's response, the nurse acknowledges that such reactions to loss are normal. The nurse's acceptance allows clients to accept and experience their own reactions (instead of defending them) and to view them as part of the whole process.

The nurse helps the client acknowledge the gains made during their work together. It is often useful to review the progress made throughout the relationship, acknowledging the client's initial distress, the significant learning that took place, and the changes in behavior at the end. Although most of this review is done by the client, nurses also share their perceptions of the work. This sharing is incredibly powerful, and nurses need to express themselves positively to continue to promote health. The nurse's emphasis is on summarizing the important learning and the aspects of the client's growth. The nurse also shares what he or she has learned while working with the client. Clients are often surprised that nurses learn something from being with them, and such knowledge reinforces their self-esteem and self-worth.

A realistic and natural part of any discussion of termination is the disappointment about what was not achieved. This will be a major part of the work for some, whereas for others it will be a mere footnote. In either case, the topic of things not achieved should not be avoided, as it provides the opportunity to help the client recognize that growth continues throughout life. Frequently the clients and nurses who are most disappointed at termination are those who set goals that are unrealistic or inappropriate to the time frame.

Nurses, like clients, need to express their own mixed feelings about the separation. For example, "I also feel sad that this relationship is ending, and I am happy about the work we've accomplished" is a statement that helps clients perceive their own reactions to termination as normal.

Even with the best preparation, most clients are anxious at the time of discharge or termination because of fears about their ability to cope on their own. A list of available community resources will help clients know that "the door has not been closed" and that help is available whenever needed.

Because the focus of short-term hospitalization is often on assessment, medication stabilization, and crisis intervention, follow-up care is essential for treatment. Arrangements for follow-up care are best discussed throughout the hospitalization. At discharge, the client should have an established link to care in the community.

THERAPEUTIC MILIEU

The therapeutic milieu is the environment designed to promote health. Since its earliest days, nursing has recognized the importance of the environment, or milieu, to healing. Indeed, Florence Nightingale defined her work as organizing the environment to allow the body to heal. The same principle holds true in psychiatric mental health nursing.

The psychiatric unit is a social system in its own right, with clients at various points of length of stay, each with an agenda, interacting and meeting unique personal and social needs. As such, the milieu can be seen both as a large work group with the definitive task of healing and as a community with all the tasks of communal living. The psychiatric mental health nurse is a constant in this system, interacting with clients and staff in a variety of ways. These interactions are significant and greatly assist in creating the atmosphere or culture of each particular psychiatric unit.

Historical Development

Maxwell Jones developed the concept of the therapeutic community in the 1950s. His goal was to design an entire culture that would promote healthy personalities (Jones,

1953). Jones's goal for clients was improved behavior, and he was one of the first to act on the knowledge that the hospital environment affects the symptoms, behaviors, and progress of clients.

Since the 1950s this work has been expanded and revised, and the language has changed from *therapeutic community* to the French term *therapeutic milieu,* meaning environment or setting. Thus a **therapeutic milieu** is an environment designed to promote health. It is also an environment designed to provide corrective or healing experiences that enhance the client's coping abilities.

It is one of the challenges of psychiatric mental health nursing to use this environment in a conscious manner to promote the healthy functioning of individuals and the group as a whole. The nurse, who is involved in most of the activities on the unit, is key to effective milieu development.

Principles of Milieu Therapy

To be effective, the nurse must understand the underlying assumptions of milieu therapy and promote its principles. The basic underlying assumption of milieu therapy is that *clients are active, not passive, participants in their lives.* This assumption implies that clients own their behavior and environment and consequently need to be involved in the management of both. In the milieu, human beings are seen as independent. Distortions, conflicts, and inappropriate behaviors are dealt with in the here and now and in the context of their impact on others. Peers are assumed to be necessary for the learning that comes from various interactions, as well as the potential healing effect of peer pressure. The principles of milieu therapy are:

- To promote a fundamental respect for individuals (both clients and staff)
- To use opportunities for communication between client and staff for maximum therapeutic benefit
- To encourage clients to act at a level equal to their ability and to enhance their self-esteem
- To promote socialization
- To provide opportunities for clients to be part of unit management (Herz, 1969; Jones, 1953).

The nurse's function is to act in ways that consistently promote these goals.

Boundary, Safety, and Trust Development in a Milieu

The concepts of boundary, safety, and trust assist in formulating this task just as they help formulate the therapeutic relationship discussed earlier. At this level, however, they are expanded to meet the needs of a type of community, which is the psychiatric unit.

Boundary

As mentioned earlier, boundaries define functions and consequently imply responsibility. The nurse must clarify boundaries for clients. It is not easy for anyone to walk into a new culture (such as a psychiatric unit) and make sense of it. It is considerably more difficult if that person is experiencing the cognitive or emotional stress of a psychiatric disorder. By defining functions and tasks of the various groups and activities offered on the unit, the nurse promotes the opportunity for each group or activity to be used efficiently. Appropriate task completion is essential for health.

For example, most units have some type of meeting for staff and client that is designed to orient clients to the staff, activities of the day, and any issues of communal living. This is frequently called the *community* or *contact meeting,* and it provides an excellent opportunity for boundary definition because one of its purposes is the orientation of clients. This meeting roughly correlates with the orientation phase in the development of a therapeutic relationship. Introductions and explanation of purpose and role are needed, but now these introductions address the relationship of the client to the unit and staff, rather than to the individual therapist.

All too often, the community meeting is reduced to superficial introductions of the members (clients and staff) and a cursory schedule of activities. A rich opportunity to help clients structure their time and focus their work is wasted.

Consider the effects of these two examples of community meetings. In this first example, the nurse leader does little to define the structure, or purpose, of the work.

EXAMPLE 1 (NONTHERAPEUTIC)

Leader defines function of the meeting as introductory. Clients follow defined function of introductions.	**Leader:** OK. This is community meeting, and we generally introduce ourselves. I'm Tracy, the nurse. I'll be passing out meds today.
	Client: Cory.
	Client: Mark.
	Client: Patty.
	Client: Lynette.
	Client: Claire.
	Staff: I'm Jana, the O.T. I'll see most of you at my group.
Leader offers minimal assistance in organizing.	**Leader:** OK. The schedule of groups is posted on the board. Who are the contacts?
Leader does not define function of contacts.	***Jana:*** I'll be working with Cory, Patty, and Lynette today.
	Leader: And I'll work with the rest.
Leader uses *stuff,* a vague term that does not focus group to work.	**Leader:** Any questions about unit stuff?
	Lynette: I still don't have any hot water in my room.
Leader does not allow for group problem solving.	**Leader:** I know. Engineering's working on it. Anything else? [Pause] OK? Meeting adjourned.

On the surface, boundaries were addressed in a cursory way. The nurse defined one of her functions (giving medications) and informed the clients that groups would be formed. Clients picked up on this role modeling and responded with cursory information of their own. It is difficult to see how they could understand unit organization in order to function effectively within it. A rich opportunity was missed.

Now, consider the difference in tone and expectations when boundaries and tasks are more clearly defined as in the following example.

EXAMPLE 2 (THERAPEUTIC)

Leader defines purpose of meeting.	**Leader:** Good morning. It's Tuesday, June 14, and this is our community meeting. This is the meeting where we get ourselves organized for the day and take care of any business that comes up just from so many people living together.
Leader provides structure for task.	**Leader:** Let's do first things first and introduce ourselves and what we do here.
Leader defines tasks and explains how clients can use her in this role.	**Leader:** I'm Tracy, and I'm one of the nurses. I'll be passing out the medications today, so if any of you have questions about your medications, please see me. I'll also be leading the process group, and I'll tell you more about that later.
Leader provides structure.	**Leader:** [To each client] Would you please introduce yourself to everybody and say something about yourself?
	Client: Well, I think everybody knows me. I'm Sara. I've been here since Friday. I'll probably go home Wednesday or Thursday.
	Client: I'm Cory. I don't know if I'll every go home.
	Client: I'm Mark. I'm Cory's roommate, and he snores! So loud!
Leader focuses on task.	**Leader:** Please say something about yourself.
	Client: I'm tired. I'm not sleeping well.
	Leader: Thanks.
	Client: I'm Patty. I just came in yesterday, and I've met a few of you. This is a real nice place.
	Client: I'm Lynette. I've got nothing to say.
	Client: I'm Claire, Uh—I don't like to talk in front of people.
Leader models acceptance.	**Leader:** I appreciate your effort.

Staff: I'm Jana. I'm the occupational therapist. I'll be leading the 9 AM and 2 PM groups today in the activity room. I also want to meet with you, Patty, to get to know you and make some plans with you about how you can best use occupational therapy. Could you meet with me after the meeting to set up a time?

Patty: Sure.

Leader: Thanks for your introductions.

Leader: Each one of the staff acts as a contact person for each of you. A contact is the person who is working with you for the day. You can talk to your contact about anything that concerns you. I'll be the contact person for Sara, Mark, and Claire. Jana will be the contact person for Cory, Patty, and Lynette. Any questions so far?

Leader defines role and how to use contact person to promote task accomplishment.

Leader: Let me introduce today's schedule to you. It's posted on the bulletin board if you forget the times. We mostly want to tell you about the activities.

Leader promotes self-responsibility by telling clients how to meet their own needs.

Jana: From 9 to 10 AM is roles group. This group helps you look at the different parts you play in your various relationships. It's a good place to look for patterns that recur in your life. I will be the leader.

Leader defines purpose.

Leader: You have free time until 10:30 AM. From 10:30 to 11:30 AM is process group. This is the group I'll be leading. This is the group where we pay attention to how we communicate with each other. It's a good place to look at any problems you may be having communicating with other people. Lunch is at 11:45 AM, and at 1 PM you have a choice of taking a walk (if you have privilege to do so) or playing a game like Bingo here on the unit. From 2 to 3 PM is the activity group that Jana leads. This is where you can make something. It's a good opportunity to look at how you approach doing a task. At 3:30 PM we go home, and the evening staff will meet with you to go over the evening schedule and staffing. Any questions?

Cory: Do we have to play Bingo? I hate that game.

Leader: No, that was just what came to mind. Actually, as a group you can choose any game you'd like at that time.

Client uses information and responds to cooperative style modeled by leaders.

Leader: Thanks for asking. It helps us to make ourselves clear and share understanding of what happens here on the unit.

Leader supports client initiative, clarifies the situation, and models acceptance of question asking.

Leader: Any other questions about the schedule? [Pause] It's a lot to remember. If any questions come up during the day, check the schedule on the bulletin board or see your contact person.

Leader reiterates ways to be self-responsible.

Leader: I think we can move to the last piece of business for this meeting and that's to deal with any issues that come up whenever so many people live together. Anything you want to bring up?

Leader continues providing structure.

Lynette: I still don't have any hot water.

Leader: I heard about that from night staff again. It's been a while, hasn't it?

Leader promotes interaction.

Lynette: Three days, and nothing has happened yet.

Leader: Well, actually, something is happening. Engineering found that the valve is broken and they're waiting for a replacement.

Leader clarifies information. Group follows up on problem solving (probably based on leader's earlier modeled acceptance and encouragement to be self-responsible).

Lynette: [Sarcastically] Great! They're waiting, and I still don't have any hot water.

Sara: No hot water at all?

Lynette: Well, my shower works, but I don't have any hot water in my sink to wash up. I don't want to take a whole shower just to wash my face.

Mark: Why don't you just wet your washcloth in the shower?

Lynette: That's what I've been doing, but I get soaked and my clothes get soaked.

Sara: Well, I don't mind if you want to use my sink for washing up, as long as you give me notice.

Clients have clarified their action appropriate to their role.

Lynette: Really? Thanks. I'll do that.

Leader clarifies her action appropriate to her role as staff member.

Leader shares information not available to clients and offers solution.

Leader acknowledges contribution.

Leader acknowledges issue and ways to work on it while keeping group focused to accomplish task of this meeting.

Supportive and accepting approach.

Leader continues to focus client on task of meeting to promote goal accomplishment.

Leader models self-acceptance of faults.

Leader provides further clarification on unit structure.

Leader: That worked out . . . I'll see what engineering can do today, Lynette.
Lynette: Thanks.
Leader: Any other issues?
Mark: The radio is broken.
Cory: No, it's not really broken, just out of batteries.
Leader: We keep batteries at the desk. Mark, would you bring the radio to the desk after this meeting and we'll see what new batteries can do.
Mark: Sure.
Leader: Thanks. What else?
Patty: I just don't know what to do about my son. He never listens to me anymore. He used to be such a good kid and now I just worry all the time.
Leader: Patty, this sounds very important to you and something I know you'll want to work on while you're here. Process group or role play, or even a talk with your contact would be good places to talk about that; that's their purpose. In this meeting we try to handle the nuts and bolts of living on this unit.
Patty: I'm sorry. I didn't know.
Leader: It's OK. It takes a bit of time to learn how to use this place and what all the meetings are for. It sounds like you have a good idea of some of the issues you want to work on.
Patty: Oh, yes, that's for sure.
Leader: That's how it starts. Any questions about living here?
Patty: You mentioned that you would be passing out medications? I know I'm on some. Where do I go?
Leader: Thank you. That's an important point, and I forgot to mention it.
Leader: Medications are passed out at the medication cart at 9 AM, right after this meeting, and again at 1 PM. The evening shift will pass them out at 5 and 9 PM. Not everyone gets medications at all these times. If you'd like, I can meet with you after this meeting to see when you get your medicine.

Supportive comment from peer.

Leader continues to focus on task appropriateness.

Leader makes supportive and educational comment.

Leader models reality orientation and acceptance of limits.

Leader keeps group focused on task of problem solving and does not allow group to degenerate into gripe session.

Leader supports client initiative and provides link to other shifts as appropriate for staff member role.

Patty: Thanks. I'd like to do that. There's so much to know.
Sara: Don't worry. You'll get used to it.
Patty: [Smiles at Sara]
Leader: Anything else?
Mark: I don't know if I should bring this up.
Leader: Does it have to do with the business of living together?
Mark: Yes.
Leader: Then this is the place.
Mark: OK then—well, I like Cory, don't get me wrong, but I can't sleep with his snoring and I don't think that's healthy for me.
Cory: I do snore. I've heard that all my life.
Leader: Sleep is important to being able to function. Any solutions?
Mark: Well, I'd like a new room.
Leader: That would be a great solution, but we don't have another room, and with our current mix of males and females we can't do any swaps.
Lynette: Well, it's not fair! He should be able to sleep, for God's sake. This is a hospital.
Leader: I couldn't agree with you more. But a hospital has its limits, too. Apparently right now there is limited bed space. So we have to figure out a solution with what we've got.
Lynette: Isn't this ridiculous! What can we do? Sleep in shifts?
Leader: There's one idea on the table. Any others?
Patty: Maybe he could get a bed on another unit?
Mark: Well, I actually have an idea that might work.
Leader: What is it?
Mark: Well, I was wondering if I could sleep in the quiet room, as long as it wasn't in use.
Leader: What do you all think?
Group: [Murmurs assent]
Leader: That's a very workable solution, Mark. I'll tell the evening and night staff, and you can start tonight.

Leader promotes functional communication by assisting in message completion.

Mark: Thanks! [To Cory] No hard feelings? [No response]
Leader: Any hard feelings, Cory? Mark wants to know.
Carl: No hard feelings. Like I said, this is an old problem.
Leader: OK, anything else? [Pause] It seems like we've taken care of a lot of business. Thanks for your contributions here. If there are no objections, this meeting is adjourned.

What a different meeting and tone! The first meeting had a rather superficial feeling, whereas this second meeting actually facilitated movement toward the stated goals of introductions, orientation, and organization. In addition, the nurse has had the opportunity to assess the general tone of the milieu; for example, Patty seemed somewhat bewildered and Lynette appeared angry. This information will be extremely useful to the rest of the staff as they interact with the clients throughout the course of the day. In effect, the clearly defined boundaries greatly assist the nurse in becoming oriented to the tone of the unit and the status of the clients. This information will help the nurse to organize the day while considering clients' needs.

Boundaries continue to be addressed throughout the day. Groups are introduced, duties of staff and clients are defined, and responsibility for various actions is acknowledged. Just as boundaries provide structure for individual work by defining the work, its limits, and time frame, so do boundaries in the milieu.

Safety

Safety and trust are developed in a similar manner as well. As noted earlier, safety is developed by knowing what one's responsibilities are in a given situation, and trust develops through actions that are consistent with an individual or group's stated intent. It is important that these issues be addressed in terms of the milieu. To feel safe, clients need to know what is expected of them in their role as clients. Do they make their own beds? Are they called to group or expected to arrive at the stated location on time? Do they go to a certain spot to get medications, or are medications delivered? How do they contact a staff member if they want to talk?

The psychiatric staff may not inform clients of their responsibilities, thinking that these expectations are obvious. By addressing these issues in a timely manner, however, the staff is able to ensure that safety is promoted, and work may proceed more quickly.

Development of safety is addressed consistently throughout a client's stay through this clarification of expectations and responsibilities. This clarification of responsibilities is often necessary as it relates to other clients. Often psychiatric clients will attempt to "help" other clients in certain ways.

Such "help" is usually unhelpful because it violates the boundaries of each individual's responsibilities (completing a task, speaking for oneself). Safety is promoted by clarifying what each member's tasks are and are not and assisting all clients in meeting their appropriate responsibilities.

Consider the following scenario that occurs on the same day as the community meeting just outlined.

Patty: I need to find a blanket.
Nurse: We keep them on the linen cart.
Patty: Are the sheets and pillow cases kept there, too?
Nurse: Yes. It sounds like you're making a bed. I thought you had already done that.
Patty: Oh, I have done mine. I just wanted to help Mark out and make up the quiet room for him.
Nurse: How did you decide to do that?
Patty: Oh, it's just my way. I'm always doing things like that for people.
Nurse: How does that work for you?
Patty: Pretty well; people always ask me for help, so I know I'm needed.
Nurse: So, you're always needed.
Patty: Yes, and always tired.
Nurse: It gets tiring doing things for other people.
Patty: Yeah, I don't know any other way, though.
Nurse: So, you're doing the same thing here that you do outside the hospital?
Patty: Yes.
Nurse: I wonder what would happen if you just took care of yourself and your needs here, and let others do the same for themselves. Do you think Mark can make his own bed?
Patty: He's a grown-up so I don't see why not.
Nurse: Do you think you can let him make his own bed and do his own work?
Patty: I suppose I could, but it would be so different.
Nurse: It is a different way for you, to let each person do his or her own work. Are you willing to try it?
Patty: OK.
Nurse: Let me know later on what it's been like for you.

In this scenario the nurse was able to turn a casual question into a therapeutic conversation, using this interaction to reinforce the boundaries of personal responsibility (each does own task), focus Patty on her work (exploring self-defeating patterns), and promote safety by clarifying the expectations of each person's work. The nurse functioned within the role of a nurse in the milieu by (1) performing within the role to use communication for therapeutic benefit, (2) helping the client to function within the limits of self-responsibility, (3) promoting the appropriate self-functioning of each client, and (4) demonstrating respect for both the client and the process.

Trust

Trust in a milieu is nurtured in a similar manner: the promotion of consistency between words and actions. Again, the nurse acts in a consistent manner to achieve defined purposes. For instance, nurses who say that they are medication nurses work to achieve the stated objectives: they pass out the medications on schedule and are available to answer questions about the medications. Nurses who say they orient a new client to the unit follow up by actually doing it.

More subtle, however, is the accomplishment of the overall goal of promoting a functional milieu that fosters self-responsibility, growth, and clear communication patterns. Nurses are involved in creating this type of milieu each time they interact with clients and staff. In the preceding conversation between Patty and the nurse, the nurse used a client's casual question to more clearly define areas of responsibility for both Patty (the client) and her peers. Psychiatric mental health nurses must be aware of the various goals of the therapeutic milieu and their own role in facilitating trust; they must then work in a consistent manner to promote trust as a major goal of milieu work.

Working effectively in a milieu is some of the most challenging work for the psychiatric mental health nurse. Each nursing interaction affects the milieu in some way. The challenge, then, is to make every interaction a therapeutic one. This is accomplished by acting in a manner that promotes achievement of identified therapeutic goals within the milieu.

GROUP THERAPY

Humans spend much of their time in some form of group interaction. We are raised in family groups, participate in work groups at all ages, and socialize in formal or informal group settings. Much of our "humanness" is defined by our interactions with others. Before looking specifically at the use of groups as a form of therapy, it would be helpful to examine some universal characteristics of all groups.

The Group As a Microcosm

Groups offer individuals the opportunity to interact with other individuals in a meaningful way. Groups provide the opportunity for self-definition through human interaction and task accomplishment. All groups have a task or purpose; family groups are for mutual nurturance and support (especially in caring for offspring); work groups are designed to accomplish or produce certain defined tasks; social groups of various types exist to foster interactions. Each group functions as a microcosm, or miniature universe, reflecting its own specific group culture and set of values. People interact within this microcosm to meet their own needs.

Roles

For the group to do its work, specific duties need to be accomplished. These duties are formulated into roles. Individuals enact roles based on their own personal dynamics and group needs. Roles are described as either *ascribed* or *achieved*. Ascribed roles are based on certain intrinsic characteristics that are beyond a person's control, such as age or sex; achieved roles are based on a person's achievements through interests, education, and talents (Sampson and Marthas, 1990). Examples of achieved roles are teacher, nurse, musician, and athlete. Achieved roles are played out in relation to other roles; thus to fulfill the role, a parent needs a child, a teacher needs a student, a nurse needs a client, and so on.

Roles exist in all groups and are related to the group's main issues of (1) accomplishing its defined task and (2) maintaining member relations (Sampson and Marthas, 1990). Special roles develop in the group to deal with these issues. A *task specialist* is someone within a group who works toward accomplishing the group's defined task. A *social specialist* is someone who maintains relative harmony in member relationships throughout the group process (Sampson and Marthas, 1990). Members enact these roles and others based on personal preference and group need. Roles that serve the individual's personal needs rather than the group's needs are referred to as *individual functions;* Box 19-5 summarizes these roles.

Box 19-5 | Individual Functions Within a Group

Roles Involving Task Functions

Initiator: Proposes new ideas, directions, tasks, methods.

Elaborator: Expands on existing suggestions and develops the group's plans further.

Evaluator: Critically evaluates ideas, proposals, and plans, examining the practicality of proposals and the effectiveness of procedures.

Coordinator: Helps to pull together ideas and themes to clarify suggestions that have been made and to help various subgroups work more effectively together toward their common goals.

Roles Involving Group Maintenance Functions

Encourager: Offers praise to and agrees with other members; communicates acceptance of others and their ideas and an openness to differences within the group.

Harmonizer: Mediates conflicts and disagreements that crop up, trying to relieve or reduce tension within the group.

Compromiser: Seeks a position between contending sides; seeks a compromise that all parties can accept.

Roles Involving Primarily Personal, Individualistic Functions

Aggressor: Acts negatively, with hostility toward other members; criticizes others' contributions; attacks the group and its members.

Recognition-seeker: Calls attention to own activities; boasts; redirects things toward self.

Help-seeker or *confessor:* Uses the group as a vehicle either to gain sympathy or to achieve personal insight and self-satisfaction without consideration for others or the group as a whole.

Dominator: Asserts authority and seeks to manipulate others so as to be in control of everything that happens.

Norms

Norms are the group's standards of behavior, attitudes, and perceptions of its members. They represent the shared expectations of appropriateness in behavior (Sampson and Marthas, 1990). Norms serve certain purposes for groups. One major function of norms is to allow a group to act in a fairly coordinated manner to accomplish its goals and tasks. In this way norms fulfill a *task function*. Norms also fulfill a *maintenance function* by regulating maintenance issues around attendance, conflict resolution, and personal relations. Finally, norms serve a *social reality function*. Much of what we know to be true has been socially determined. Overall, group norms provide a framework for the interpretation of data (Sampson and Marthas, 1990).

Norms can be *enabling* (assist the group in accomplishing its work) or *restrictive* (hinder movement toward goal accomplishment).

Universal Tasks

Finally, all groups must deal with the issues of group life: forming, working, and ending. Often this work is unknown to the group, but work in human relations theory implies that it is always being addressed. During the *forming phase*, group members deal with issues of joining a group. They wrestle with questions of how to join a group and issues of pairing with other group members. Acceptance/rejection by group members, issues of sexual attractions, and position within the group are also addressed at some level. During the group's working phase, task accomplishment is emphasized. The group deals with issues of leadership, completion, competence, and trust. At the final or termination phase, the group deals with issues that apply to endings, such as death, loss of the group, grief, separation, loneliness, and limitations.

These issues underlie all group processes and are always being addressed by the group, even if only at an unconscious level.

Types of Groups

Groups in the health care setting vary according to whether they are *content oriented* or *process oriented*. Content refers to the discussion of goals and tasks. Process refers to the discussion of interpersonal relations. Although all groups contain both elements, they vary with the degree of emphasis given (Northouse and Northouse, 1992).

Task groups focus on content issues: defining the tasks and what work is needed to accomplish them. It is rare, however, to find a group that is totally task oriented. There is generally some processing going on among members. Examples of task groups are committees formed to develop clinical or critical pathways or to monitor quality improvement.

Process groups focus on relations among members and their communication styles or patterns. Therapy groups designed to discuss client issues on an inpatient psychiatric unit fall into this category.

Finally, there are the *mid-range* groups that combine both functions of task and process. Many support groups with an emphasis on education and adjustment are in this category (Figure 19-2).

Aspects of Group Therapy

Groups, like milieus, function as social communities, and individuals tend to function in groups as they do in other parts of their lives. Likewise, individuals' behavior in group therapy imitate their behavior in other group settings. A key assumption of group therapy is that psychopathology has its source in disordered relationships (Yalom, 1985). The goal of the therapy group is to help individuals develop more functional and satisfying relationships. Because the individual dysfunction is demonstrated in the group, the task of the group is to assist members in understanding their patterns of interacting within the group so as to be able to generalize to the larger arena of life outside the group. To do this, members must (1) get information on how they present them-

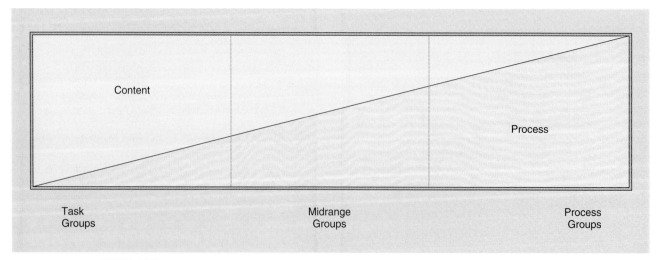

FIGURE 19-2.   The emphasis on content and process in different types of groups. Psychiatric mental health nurses are most involved with process group therapy. (Modified from Loomis M: *Group process for nurses,* St Louis, 1979, Mosby.)

selves to others, (2) assess whether their fixed patterns are realistic to continue in the current situation, (3) discover previously unknown parts of themselves (strengths, skills, abilities, desires), (4) gradually try new behaviors within the safety of the group, and (5) accept ultimate responsibility for the way they live (Yalom, 1985).

Cohesiveness

The extent to which group members work together to accomplish these stated goals is called *cohesion* or *cohesiveness:* the sense of "we-ness" that a group experiences and that acts as a bond between group members. Cohesion has been associated with positive group outcomes: increased interactions, norm conformity and goal-directed behaviors, and member satisfaction (Northouse and Northouse, 1992). Factors that influence group cohesiveness are summarized in Table 19-1.

Therapeutic Factors

Researchers have attempted to define the factors of a group process that have a positive effect on its members. To be effective as a group leader, the nurse must have an appreciation of these therapeutic factors of group therapy and be able to promote them. In his landmark work on groups and group therapy, Yalom identified 11 curative factors, which are listed in Box 19-6.

Inpatient Groups

To effectively lead an inpatient group, the nurse must be aware of the various factors influencing the group so as to develop a style that is responsive to the unpredictable conditions of inpatient group therapy (Box 19-7). The membership of an inpatient group requires leadership that provides orientation and continuity of group norms, defines the structure and limits of the group, promotes safety development, clarifies the relevant group task, and assists in the group's accomplishment of that task.

The careful leader recognizes the need for boundary definition, safety, and trust development as just noted. These concepts must be expanded to create a therapeutic relationship at the group level. Instead of applying these concepts to individuals, the nurse leader must now apply them so that they are useful to the unique requirements of group functioning. This work is accomplished in some specific ways, as are summarized in Table 19-2.

Group Boundaries

Boundaries refer to the definition of structure surrounding tasks, group norms, roles, and time. In working with groups, boundaries between people also must be defined clearly. Guidance ought to be given to help group members understand how to work together to accomplish a specific task.

In expanding the concept of boundary to group work, location must be added: an area must be defined as the specific location for the group to do its work. As noted by Yalom (1985), an externally imposed structure is the first step to the internal structure needed by the frightened, confused, and disorganized inpatient. Therefore the group leader needs to provide clear spatial boundaries for the group. The ideal space is a comfortable room with a door that can be closed when the group session begins and opened when the session ends. This arrangement not only provides privacy for the group but also serves as a visual reminder of structure. Everyone in the group should be able to see each other (a further expansion of the therapeutic relationship); chairs should be arranged in a circle. This structure promotes interaction in the group. If the clients cannot see each other, they will tend to speak only to the nurse (Yalom, 1985). The space should be consistent from session to session. Group size is also a consideration. The ideal number for an inpatient process group is 6 to 10 clients (Yalom, 1985). This number allows for enough interactional material for processing, yet is small enough for all members to interact.

Table 19-1	Factors That Influence Group Cohesiveness
Group goals	Clear goals, based on similar member values and interests, motivate members to seek or maintain group membership.
Similarity among members	Members are frequently attracted to other members who share similar values and beliefs. There are some instances, however, in which people are attracted to those who are dissimilar in values and attitudes.
Type of interdependence among members	Groups that function in a cooperative versus competitive manner tend to have higher cohesion among members.
Leader behavior	For the most part, democratic styles of leadership are associated with higher group cohesiveness than are other styles of leadership (e.g., autocratic).
Communication structures	Decentralized communication structures, characterized by increased member interaction, are associated with higher morale and increased satisfaction among members.
Group activities	Members who are asked to perform group activities they believe are beyond their capabilities will feel less attraction toward the group, whereas members who believe group activities are within their capabilities will feel more attracted toward the group.
Group atmosphere	Members are frequently attracted to groups that help them feel valued and accepted.
Group size	Group size should match the number of members needed to complete the task. Later groups, in which the group size interferes with group goals, can decrease cohesiveness.

From Cartwright D: The nature of group cohesiveness. In Cartwright D, Zander A, editors: *Group dynamics: research and theory,* ed 3, New York, 1968, Harper & Row.

Box 19-6 Yalom's Curative Factors of Group Therapy

1. *Instill hope:* Group members are at various points of the health continuum. Those who are not coping well can gain hope from those who have benefited from the group experience.

2. *Universality:* Members come to learn they are not unique or alone in their discomfort. They learn that others have reactions and thoughts similar to their own.

3. *Imparting information:* Both formal and informal learning occurs in groups. Some groups such as Alcoholics Anonymous (AA) and medication-education or symptom recognition groups are designed specifically to impart information. Through groups designed to assist with interpersonal dynamics, members learn about the effects of their interactions on group dynamics.

4. *Altruism:* By and large, members of groups give credit to the other group members for their support and insight. Members view their improvement as related to the work done by all group members. By learning they can be useful, members experience an improved sense of self-value.

5. *Corrective recapitulation of the family group:* As noted earlier, people act as they were taught to act in their families. As is often the case with psychiatric clients, these patterns are dysfunctional and the client continues to repeat these dysfunctional patterns in all interactions. Group therapy provides the opportunity for these patterns to be identified, evaluated, and changed.

6. *Development of social techniques:* By interacting with others, members can improve their social skills. Members will often give each other feedback on their reactions to each other's interpersonal style. This enriches member recognition of the various effects of their style on others and gives them opportunities to choose and practice styles that are more in keeping with their goals.

7. *Imitative behavior:* Group members are often "caught" or trapped in ways of interacting because they cannot conceive of another way. In a group situation members are able to see how others interact

and can choose to model their behaviors on those of other group members or the therapist. By looking at options, group members get the help they need to dissolve their rigid behavioral styles and become more flexible in their interactions.

8. *Catharsis:* Catharsis is the release of intense emotions. Psychiatric clients are often hesitant to express these emotions for fear that they will be too overwhelming for anyone to handle and that the consequence of expressing them would be grievous. In group therapy, members learn how to express these emotions and experience the immediate relief catharsis can bring. In addition, members learn that they and the group have survived the expression of emotions without calamity.

9. *Existential factors:* All human beings must deal with one basic issue of existence: that we are ultimately alone despite the presence of others. Psychiatric clients (and others) may tend to be unrealistic in their expectations of human relationships, thinking that with the perfect mate, friend, or family all feelings of aloneness would vanish. In group therapy, members learn that feelings of loneliness can be decreased by human companionship but not completely eliminated. By not reaching for what is unattainable, members may be able to enjoy what is attainable.

10. *Cohesiveness:* This is one of the most powerful benefits of an effective group. Many members experience extreme isolation from others in their daily lives and consequently experience a feeling of disconnectedness from others. By being part of a group that is achieving its stated goals, members experience a sense of belonging, a feeling of being part of a whole that is greater than each individual self.

11. *Interpersonal learning:* In groups designed to examine interpersonal relationships, the members learn to identify, clarify, and modify maladaptive behaviors.

From Yalom ID: *The theory and practice of group psychotherapy,* ed 3, New York, 1985, Basic Books.

Box 19-7 Factors Affecting Inpatient Groups

1. *The turnover of clients in today's psychiatric hospitals is rapid.* This means it is probable that group membership will not be constant from one meeting to the next. Thus some members may be in totally different phases of the group process (e.g., orientation, working, termination). This has critical implications for how group routines and dynamics are played out and carried over from one group to the next. Rapid turnover may compromise group cohesion. This greatly affects safety development within the group. Because it is rare for all group members to share a single specific diagnosis, the variety of disorders also affects group safety and cohesiveness.

2. *The clients are inpatients and, by definition, fragile.* They are often frightened, confused, and disorganized. Again, the creation of safety and structure becomes important.

3. *Many clients are unmotivated.* They attend group sessions because they "have to" by unit rules, but it would not be their choice. The nurse leader must find ways to make the group relevant for them and their needs. There is often too little time to prepare clients for the

group experience. Staff may frequently be too busy to effectively orient clients to the group; all too often the orientation must happen within the group.

4. *The therapy group may have varied leadership based on staff scheduling.* This affects the continuity of routine, as well as safety development.

5. Another consideration related to staffing is that *the clients see the group leader in a variety of roles throughout the day.* The nurse may be their contact person, their medication nurse, and part of the treatment team, in addition to leading the group. It would be easy for clients to confuse these various roles. Consequently, leaders have the responsibility to clarify their roles and functions in the group.

6. *There is little time for the more subtle aspects of psychiatric treatment.* Clients are generally preoccupied with seeking relief from their despair and are not interested in subtle nuances. This implies that the work must be direct, effective, and limited in scope to accomplish goals.

Table 19-2	Summary of Inpatient Group Considerations			
Considerations of Inpatient Group Work	**Clients' Requirements**	**Nurse's Technique/ Functions of Nurse**	**Nurse's Style to Promote Function**	**Promote Function**
High severity of distress in group members caused by: Personal distress Secondary anxiety of hospitalization Rapid turnover Little preparation Many roles of therapist	Defined structure to work within	Lessen the ambiguity of therapy situation through clarification of details	Provide boundaries: Room Time frame Orientation Expectations for behavior (therapist's and client's) Sequence of group Norm clarification	Firm, explicit, and active Explain actions Model contradictory feelings and solicit feedback
Brief duration of therapy Provide opportunity to explore (not necessarily resolve) questions of interpersonal relationship	Goals that can be achieved: How am I seen by others? How does my behavior affect others? Finding a safe arena to try new behaviors	Enhance client strengths by: Discouraging self-defeating behavior Acknowledging contributions	Support client by: Modeling feedback Providing positive interpretation Showing relevance of interactions to life outside hospital	Model respect as shown by: Being supportive, constructive, and accepting feedback Using data as learning opportunity Acknowledging client's contributions during summary statement
Group exists as part of a larger whole: Client is member of unit milieu Group session is only one of many groups	Facilitating client-to-client relations	Problem identification	Promote direct communication Client to client Abstract to specific Questions support furthering of relationships: What aspect of behavior gets in way of ideal relationship?	Modeling of openness, selective self-disclosure, risk taking
Fragility of clients	Avoiding and managing stress	Conflict management	Immediate intervention Promoting resolution, objectivity, and learning	

Linked to the concept of spatial boundary is the temporal or time boundary. The group needs a definite time to begin and end its work. The best way for this to occur is for the leader to model promptness. The leader should be in the room, ready to begin work at the appointed time. It is also the leader's responsibility to ensure that the group meets its tasks within the appointed time frame and ends on time. The leader must recognize that the effective life span of the group is one group session long. Because of the rapidly changing membership, it is unlikely that the same group members will ever meet twice; therefore the leader must provide a beginning, middle, and ending structure to every group session.

Perhaps the greatest opportunity for the leader to define group structure and boundaries is in the introductory comments to the group. As in developing a therapeutic relationship with an individual, the introduction serves to clarify:

- The role of the nurse
- The role of the client
- The tasks of the group
- The ways to accomplish these tasks
- The time frame for accomplishing these tasks

An example of such an introduction follows (Yalom, 1985).

Orientation to names Defining spatial and time boundaries Defining a leadership function Task definition Limits of work defined	"Hello, I'm Mary and this is the daily therapy group. We meet in this room every day for 1 hour, from 10 to 11 AM. I'll keep track of the time and make sure we end on time." "The purpose of this group is to help members understand their problems better and to learn more about the way they communicate with others. I know there are many different reasons why people come into the hospital, and you may not want to talk about some of these reasons in a group."
Restating task	"But one thing almost all of the people here have in common is some unhappiness in their relationships with people who are impor-

Tasks definition (and method to accomplish)

tant to them. What groups do better than any other form of therapy is help people understand more about their relationships with others."

"One of the ways we'll work on this task is to look at relationships that may go on between people in this room. We're not very different inside the hospital than we are outside of it, so the better we can understand relationships that happen here, the better we'll understand the important relationships outside the hospital."

Information boundary addressed
Confidentiality issue to promote safety

"You'll be learning a lot about yourself and other people while you're in the group. It's very natural to want to share what you learn with your family and friends, but confidentiality is of utmost importance. We ask you to pass on the valuable information but to keep the names of the people or other identifying information confidential. This information is only for group members and staff."

Consistent explicit sequence (provides for method to accomplish task)

"As I mentioned before, the group lasts 1 hour. We start by going around the group and asking each member to say something about the kinds of problems he or she is having and would like to work on in group. Then we talk about as many of those as possible. We save the last 10 minutes or so to check in on everybody again, about how everybody feels and what kind of work we saw happening, and to finish up any leftover business."

This type of structured and consistent introduction serves many purposes:

- It provides an orientation to new members as to the purpose and sequence of the group, thus relieving some anxiety.
- It facilitates the transfer of norms from one meeting to the next, even in the absence of returning members.
- It defines the work of the group (i.e., relating to others) in relevant terms.
- It sets limits (i.e., not every problem is appropriate for group discussion).
- It defines the role of the nurse implicitly as the one with the sense of group tasks and appropriateness and explicitly as timekeeper and organizer.

The introduction alone, however, does not meet all of the boundary issues. The group leader must actively continue to work to shore up the boundaries and structures of the group

throughout the meeting by using an active, focused style of leadership that promotes task accomplishment. Yalom (1985) suggested that clients are reassured by a leader who is firm, explicit, and decisive, and who also shares the reasons for his or her actions.

Thus the leader of an inpatient group will actively identify group themes, focus discussion on learning from relationships within the group, share his or her ambivalence and thinking about difficult decisions he or she makes within the group, and maintain a consistent order to the group. His or her choice of actions, directions, and words is consistent with the goal of furthering learning about relationships.

Safety and Trust

Safety has been defined in terms of knowing what is expected of oneself in a given situation. As has been mentioned earlier, in group situations this concept must be expanded to knowing what is expected in relationship to others. In this example, it is expected that group members explore their relationships with each other to better understand their outside relationships. Recognizing that psychiatric clients may have tumultuous relationships with others, the group leader strives to maintain a safe and supportive environment in which to do the work. In group work, as in other forms of the therapeutic relationship, safety is developed when the nurse demonstrates a personal acceptance or valuing of each member, treats each member with respect, and empathizes with each one's situation as much as possible within the boundary context. The nurse works to reinforce the client's strengths and encourages higher level behavior (Yalom, 1985). The nurse models these safety-promoting behaviors by acknowledging each client's contributions openly to the group and by taking each client seriously. These tasks are often accomplished by providing a framework for the group to understand the client's behavior, discouraging self-defeating behavior before anger builds in the group, and acknowledging at some point each client's contribution to the group. The nurse must actively intervene if a client is being verbally attacked by another and use the opportunity to promote reflection on relationships appropriate to the group's goal. The leader consistently works to help members meet their responsibilities to each other in a safe and nonthreatening manner.

FAMILY THERAPY

Family therapy is the most intimate form of group therapy. In most cultures, families are given the task of raising children within the expectations of the culture and must also provide nurturing and support for its members. A well-functioning family has a collaborative power structure, an acceptance of individual family members and their special qualities, mutual affection, and the ability to adapt to social change.

Families generally seek therapy when they experience some difficulty in performing one or more of these tasks. These difficulties generally arise during times of crisis or transition, such as births, deaths, marriage, financial changes, illness, divorce, and major growth transitions from childhood to adulthood.

The identified difficulty is generally expressed by one member of the family, who experiences symptoms. Most often it is a child who develops certain symptoms such as failing in school work, drug abuse, acting out behavior, withdrawn or passive behavior, or sexual promiscuity. This behavior is usually of great concern to the parents who initiate therapy. At times, however, the parents may be coerced into treatment by the various social systems with which the child interacts, such as schools, judicial organizations, and social welfare agencies. These institutions often define the behavior as a problem and recommend therapy, even against parental wishes. Thus not everyone willingly comes to family therapy. The child's behavior is generally viewed as the child's problem by the parents who assume that the family will become functional once the child's problems are solved. Therefore the child is seen as the "identified client" (i.e., the one whose behavior is causing the problem). Occasionally, an adult is the identified client. For example, the problem may be seen as the mother's drinking or the father's absenteeism, and the family believes that once this behavior (or person) is "fixed," the family will be fine.

Theoretic Perspective

Family therapists view the behavior of the identified client as merely relaying a message about the overall functioning of the family in general. Instead of seeing the identified client as the cause of the family's distress, the family therapist sees that person more as the "symptom carrier" for the family. The process of family therapy is geared toward the family as a whole rather than toward any individual member.

Family Therapy and Systems Theory

Family therapy is based on systems theory. Systems theory views the family as a system that strives to maintain homeostasis or balance. Consequently, even if the identified client's behavior were to change, systems theory predicts that another symptom would develop in another member of the family in an attempt to maintain the previous balance of a dysfunctional system. A dysfunctional system cannot tolerate health in one member. The entire system must be made functional to restore health.

Goals

The goals of family therapy are to relieve the family's pain and to promote the functional nurturing of its members. Satir (1972), in her landmark work, has identified four areas that may result in family conflict and four goals of family therapy that help to ameliorate it (Box 19-8).

Settings for Family Therapy

Family therapy can take place in a variety of settings. It most often occurs in a nurse's office, in a structured, formal, outpatient setting. Families can also undergo therapy sessions in hospitals, when the identified client is admitted. It is difficult to complete the work of family therapy on an inpatient basis, however, and generally arrangements are made for follow-up family therapy on discharge. The family's home is one of the most valuable settings for family therapy from a nurse's viewpoint, as it provides the nurse with much information about the family's unique interactive style.

Box 19-8   Satir's Sources of Family Conflict and Goals of Family Therapy

Sources of Family Conflict
1. Self-worth or the feelings and ideas a family or member has internalized
2. Communication styles in the family, which can be indirect, vague, and dishonest
3. The rules the family uses to define behavior, as well as the way the rules are negotiated
4. The links to society (the way the family relates to outside institutions)

Goals of Family Therapy
1. To foster a greater self-worth in all family members
2. To promote communication that is direct, clear, specific, and honest
3. To create rules that are flexible, humane, and responsive to varying needs
4. To link with society in ways that are open and hopeful

From Satir V: *Peoplemaking*, Palo Alto, Calif, 1972, Science & Behavior Books.

Box 19-9   Examples of Role Confusion and Task Confusion

Role Confusion
- A parent dies and the oldest sibling takes over the role functions of the deceased parent.
- A child is ill and the family revolves around the child's needs, giving the child the authority role.
- A couple is unhappy with their relationship, and each develops a strong alliance with one of the children, thus displacing the spousal unit's role as the primary unit of the family.

Task Confusion
- The birth of a new child: The family task is to meet the baby's needs as well as the needs of other family members. This can be especially traumatic if the infant is ill, colicky, or premature.
- The transition of a child to a teenager: The family task is to increase separation and individuation, and support the growing adolescent in successfully completing new tasks.
- The move of a family from one geographic location to another: The family task is to connect with the resources of the community (school, work, social, spiritual) for all family members.

Family Role and Task Confusion

Sometimes family members are unable to enact their roles or tasks properly for a variety of reasons. This inability is often likely to occur during times of stress and transition, especially if the family or its members are vulnerable. As with other groups, families also have defined tasks, roles for its members, norms, and communication patterns.

The nurse can help to identify how members enact their roles and meet their tasks to help them recognize the negative effects of role confusion and task confusion on individual members and on the family as a whole. Family therapy promotes the health and functioning of individual members and the family as a system. Box 19-9 lists examples of role confusion and task confusion.

ACTIVITY THERAPIES

Activity therapies, also known as therapeutic activities, expressive therapies, experimental therapies, or adjunct therapies, have been commonly practiced in psychiatric mental health settings since the 1980s. With the onset of managed care and cost containment, the use of these activities have diminished, and in many instances, nurses pair up with recreational therapists to conduct these activities in inpatient, outpatient, and community settings.

Types of therapeutic activities include recreational, occupational, art, music, movement/dance, and psychodrama. These activities provide service to children, adolescents, adults, and older adults of all functional levels and diagnostic categories. The primary intent of these activities is to increase the client's awareness of feelings, behaviors, thoughts, and sensations through the medium of art, music, or dance and to use that medium to minimize pathology and promote mental and emotional health. Activities also allow clients to express themselves on multiple levels, to be creative, and to demonstrate conflicts, strengths, and limitations in a safe, nonthreatening environment, which will help prepare them for life outside the hospital. Activity therapists and nurses generally collaborate to recommend activity therapies to the client's primary physician.

HISTORICAL PERSPECTIVES

Activity therapies date back to 2000 BC when exercise and the arts were found to be healing, especially for melancholia, known today as depression. In the eighteenth and nineteenth centuries the moral treatment of persons with mental illness increased, and nurses were among the first to recognize the therapeutic value of these activities. Two nurses, Florence Nightingale and Susan E. Tracy, contributed greatly to the birth of recreational therapy and occupational therapy. As the activities evolved and became more complex in theory and practice, activity therapy eventually became recognized as its own specialty with professional, ethical, and educational standards.

THE ROLE OF NURSING IN ACTIVITY THERAPIES

The nurse's role in activity therapies is extremely valuable for the following reasons:

- Involvement of nurses provides more availability for client activities.
- The nurse is an additional trained professional observer who represents safety and comfort, which may help reduce the client's anxiety and inhibitions.
- The collaboration of nurse and therapist, along with the physician, allows multiple disciplines to view client problems from different perspectives, which increases the opportunity for more effective outcomes.

Occupational Therapy and the Nurse's Role

Occupational therapy focuses on assessment of task performance, cognitive functioning, psychosocial development, recognizing strengths, ameliorating weaknesses, and adapting to change. The nurse's role in occupational therapy includes daily contact with clients to provide encouragement, support, role modeling, teaching, discussion, and reality testing of prescribed tasks. The nurse's assessment of overall client functioning provides valuable information for occupational therapists. For example, a client who is experiencing cognitive decline based on the nurse's mental status assessment may benefit from the occupational therapist's evaluation and perspective of cognitive functioning. Also, nurses can observe a client's frustration tolerance and problem-solving skills as the client performs activities of daily living or attempts other simple tasks. Nursing and occupational therapy work together and with the physician to provide the best possible outcomes for the client by promoting client strengths based on the specialized roles of each discipline.

Recreational Therapy and the Nurse's Role

Recreational therapy, also known as therapeutic recreation, has been described as the art of work, love, and play. The nurse's role in recreational therapy includes promoting activities and interactions that foster independence, responsibility, problem-solving skills, leisure activities, and interactive skills. The various types of recreational therapy and the nurse's role in each type are described in Table 19-3.

ELECTROCONVULSIVE THERAPY

Many healing methods focus on effecting changes on the physical parts of the body that may result in positive effects on the individual's mental or emotional state. This is one of the premises for nutrition therapy, for example, which suggests that a well-balanced diet, based on all the food groups, tends to promote a healthier physical state, which in turn positively affects one's emotions. Psychiatry has a unique form of biologic treatment known as **electroconvulsive therapy (ECT)**, which stipulates that a brief controlled electrical stimulus applied to the brain can produce a change in brain chemistry that results in an improved mood state, even though the precise mechanism of action is unknown. In this instance, the individual's physical state may also improve once the depression has lifted. Unlike nutritional therapy, ECT was not always favorably viewed, and even today this mainstream biologic-based treatment has its share of skeptics.

HISTORICAL PERSPECTIVE

ECT, sometimes known as electroshock therapy, is not a new discovery. It was first used as a treatment in 1934 to "cure" psychotic disorders by inducing convulsions.

Table 19-3 Recreational Therapy and the Nurse's Role

Therapy	Description	Nurse's Role
Art therapy	The use of art to help resolve conflicts and promote self-awareness through nonverbal media	Observing client's use of art, encouraging verbal responses to artwork, and noting content of artwork and how it relates to client's specific issues. NOTE: The nurse should not comment on the quality of the artwork or the client's artistic talents, as this is not an art contest, but simply each client's self-expression.
Music therapy	The use of music in a defined structure to bring about change and promote self-organization, social connection, and expression	Observing whether the client is active or passive during the experience, and noting any verbal and nonverbal feelings expressed by the client. NOTE: The client's taste in music is not the focus of this activity.
Movement/dance therapy	The use of movement (kinesics) to express emotions, work out tensions, develop improved body image, and achieve body awareness and social interactions through rhythmic exercises and responses to music	Participating in the activity, observing and encouraging all clients to participate, and promoting discussion when possible. NOTE: The client's dancing talents are not the focus of this activity.
Psychodrama	The use of spontaneous expression and dramatic technique to act out emotional problems to promote health through the development of new perceptions, behaviors, and connection with others	Observing the client's reactions and encouraging client to relate these reactions to his own issues. NOTE: A client's acting talent is not the focus of this activity. Psychodrama is not a mainstream activity in most psychiatric mental health facilities. However, it may be used in a simpler form, such as role playing, in which individuals are encouraged to act out conflicts with significant others in a safe setting. Role playing is often used to help children and adolescents reenact conflicts with a trusted nurse or therapist.

Paracelsus, a sixteenth century Swiss physician gave camphor to induce convulsions as a method of treating "lunacy." von Auenbrugger in 1764 used the same intervention to treat symptoms of mania. In 1934 Meduna administered an injection of camphor oil to a patient with schizophrenia who had been in a catatonic stupor for 4 years. After a series of these treatments, the patient made a remarkable recovery. Meduna administered this same treatment to 26 patients, 13 of whom showed significant improvement. Reports of the success of this new form of therapy spread, and others soon explored additional methods to induce convulsions. By 1938 two Italian scientists, Cerletti and Bini, administered 11 separate transcerebral treatments using an electrical stimulus to induce a seizure in a client with schizophrenia. The client fully recovered from his illness and Cerletti and Bini received worldwide acclaim for their efforts (Abrams, 1988). It is doubtful that this client would be diagnosed with schizophrenia by today's standards, but the relative safety and efficacy of this procedure opened up a whole new treatment technique in psychiatry.

STATISTICS

Despite advances in the pharmacologic treatment of major depression, approximately 15% of depressed people do not respond to medications and continue to experience depression. Of this 15%, however, approximately 90% find relief from depression through ECT, making it an effective treatment for clients who are resistant to pharmacotherapy.

MODERN ELECTROCONVULSIVE THERAPY

ECT is a safe and effective treatment for major depression. It involves sending an electrical current through the brain of an anesthetized client to induce a grand mal seizure. The exact mechanism of action is not known. Because of this lack of understanding, as well as issues surrounding patient rights, ECT has gained undeserved notoriety in the public mind based on media portrayal of this treatment. The most appropriate candidates are those experiencing a major mood disorder. Clients with melancholic, delusional, and psychotic depression also tend to respond well to ECT.

Other indications for ECT include previous positive results from ECT, clients who cannot tolerate side effects of antidepressant medications, clients with acute suicidal ruminations and behaviors, and clients in danger of fluid and electrolyte imbalance as a result of inability to eat or drink because of severe depression. ECT has also been used in the treatment of mania, severe catatonia, and in schizophrenia that is unresponsive to antipsychotic medications.

ECT is also considered in the first trimester of pregnancy when pharmacotherapy is contraindicated, and may be an effective treatment for older adult clients who cannot tolerate the effects of pharmacotherapy.

Absolute contraindications of ECT include clients with space-occupying lesions in the brain with increased intracranial pressure. Risk factors to be considered are clients with recent myocardial infarction, aneurysms, acute respiratory infection, cardiac arrhythmias, organic syndromes, thrombophlebitis, and narrow-angle glaucoma.

ECT is not indicated for clients with the following diagnoses: drug dependence, personality disorders, reactive depression, and paranoid schizophrenia. ECT treatments are generally administered three times a week, with an average series of 8 to 12 treatments.

Informed Consent for Electroconvulsive Therapy

Informed consent authorizes the physician to perform ECT. It is given to the client before treatment and obtained only after the client is thoroughly educated about the procedure and prepared for any possible effects (Box 19-10). The nurse is often a witness to informed consent.

Preparation for Electroconvulsive Therapy Procedure

Basic preliminary tests before ECT include a complete blood count, a comprehensive metabolic profile, a urine analysis, an electrocardiogram, and a physical examination. ECT currently may be performed on an inpatient or outpatient basis depending on the physician's assessment of the client's condition and support system. Clients scheduled for ECT must fast overnight and are prepared as if they were undergoing a routine operative procedure (i.e., they empty the bladder and remove any jewelry, dental work, or nail polish).

Approximately 30 minutes before ECT, the client receives an intramuscular injection of atropine, typically 0.5 mg. This drug reduces secretions and protects against vagal bradycardia, which can occur with application of the electrical stimulus.

Electroconvulsive Therapy Procedure

In the ECT treatment room, blood pressure, cardiac, and electroencephalogram monitors are placed to assess the client's vital functions. Emergency equipment such as oxygen, suction, and a cardiac arrest cart (crash cart) are also available. Minimum staff in attendance include the treating psychiatrist, an anesthesiologist, and a nurse.

A short-acting anesthetic and a muscle relaxant are given intravenously, as muscle paralysis prevents increased

Box 19-10   Role of Informed Consent for ECT
States the purpose of the ECT procedure
Stipulates the proposed number of treatments
Lists the risk factors associated with ECT
Authorizes the physician to perform ECT

ECT, Electroconvulsive therapy.

movement, which reduces the risk of fracture or injury. A mouth guard and 100% oxygen are administered. After anesthesia and paralysis are obtained, the ECT electrodes are placed. For bilateral ECT, electrodes are placed on the right and left anterior portion of the client's temples. For unilateral ECT, the electrode is placed on the anterior side of the client's nondominant temple. For example, if the client is right-handed, the electrode is placed on the right temple.

Once the electrodes are placed, a brief electrical stimulus (generally no more than 2 seconds' total duration) is applied. The body does not move because of the paralyzing agent, and the seizure is confirmed by EEG monitoring. The client wakes in a few minutes and oxygen is discontinued accordingly. The client is monitored for any respiratory distress or excess secretions that need to be suctioned.

Post-Electroconvulsive Therapy Procedure

After ECT the client remains in the recovery room for about 1 to 3 hours, until vital signs are stable and the client is alert, oriented, and able to walk without assistance. The client may now eat and resume normal activity. Some clients may feel sleepy and return to bed for awhile. Side effects most associated with ECT are headache and memory loss.

Clients experiencing headache may be given a mild analgesia and instructed to rest. Memory impairment tends to be more pronounced with bilateral ECT. It can be quite severe during the course of treatment but generally improves significantly after completion of a series of treatments.

The Nurse's Role in Electroconvulsive Therapy

Nurses play an integral role in ECT treatment by providing accurate education to the client and family to reduce fear and prevent distortions and myths regarding the use of ECT. Nurses need to fully understand the indications, contraindications, procedures, and side effects of ECT in order to educate, prepare, monitor, and support the client and family.

The nurse also witnesses the informed consent procedure and ensures that patient rights regarding treatment are understood by the client and accurately documented. Before and after the procedure, the nurse allays the client's fears, anxieties, and concerns; administers vital signs; and performs other necessary nursing interventions. The nurse also offers support, comfort, and reassurance to clients experiencing headache or memory loss and recognizes the need for repetitive teaching for clients with memory loss throughout the course of treatment. This can be challenging, as the depression itself may impair memory and concentration. Nurses need to be aware that there is still some controversy about whether mild cognitive deficits remain after ECT (Blazer and Cassel, 1994). Nurses work closely with the client, family, physician, and anesthesiologist to provide a safe, effective ECT procedure and to prepare the client for transition to another unit or discharge home.

CHAPTER SUMMARY

- The nurse in the therapeutic relationship acts as a resource person, counselor, surrogate, and technical expert for the client.
- The nurse continually assesses his or her personal values and attitudes in order to be an effective counselor.
- The basic concepts a nurse strives to develop in each therapeutic relationship are boundaries, safety, and trust.
- The orientation phase of the relationship defines the client's issues/conflicts, the goal of the work, and the nature of the relationship between the nurse and the client.
- During the working phase of the relationship, the nurse demonstrates understanding of the client's problem and assists the client in finding effective coping strategies.
- The termination phase of the relationship involves helping the client acknowledge gains already made, and progress yet to be made.
- The basic purpose of milieu therapy is to help the client become an active rather than a passive participant in life.
- Group therapy allows the client to define himself through human interaction and task accomplishment.
- Family therapy promotes the health and functioning of the entire family system as it helps to define the member's roles and tasks during times of stress and transition.
- The goal of activity therapy is to increase the client's awareness of sensations, feelings, perceptions, thoughts, and behaviors.
- Activity therapy includes occupational, recreational, art, music, movement/dance, and psychodrama.
- Occupational therapy focuses on assessment of task performance, cognitive functioning, and psychosocial development.
- Recreational therapy focuses on assessing the individual's capacity to incorporate the curative elements of play and leisure into his or her lifestyle.
- The nurse's role in therapeutic activities is that of a professional observer and participant who works with the therapist to enhance the client's capabilities and functioning within the parameters of the assigned activity.
- Electroconvulsive therapy (ECT) is a safe, effective treatment for major depression and other select diagnoses despite lingering consumer beliefs.
- Nurses play an integral role in preparing and educating clients and families about ECT.

REVIEW QUESTIONS

1. A nursing supervisor is evaluating a new nurse's group therapy skills. The nurse must demonstrate that the group therapy:
   a. Is client centered
   b. Has flexible rules
   c. Is mutually satisfying
   d. Has flexible boundaries

2. After 8 weeks of group therapy, a client yells, "This group was a complete waste of my time. You don't even know what you're talking about. You certainly don't care about us. You only care about getting paid." The group is in which stage of development?
   a. Orientation
   b. Working
   c. Termination
   d. Processing

3. A family of a 10-year-old client with attention deficit/hyperactivity disorder and school behavioral problems is referred to family therapy. An appropriate goal for family therapy would be:
   a. The client will develop stress reduction techniques.
   b. The parents will provide structure and limit-setting skills.
   c. The client will be compliant with medication.
   d. The client will be free from aggressive behavior.

4. A goal for a client in art therapy would be:
   a. The client will develop artistic skills.
   b. The client will understand the importance of following directions.
   c. The client will verbalize feelings in a safe and therapeutic environment.
   d. The client will learn how to critique others' work.

5. Psychodrama is an intervention that would be beneficial to express emotionally charged issues. What type of client issues would be appropriate for this level of psychodrama?
   a. Delusional thinking
   b. Consistent feelings of paranoia
   c. Racing thoughts
   d. Sexual abuse by a parent

REFERENCES

Abrams R: *Electroconvulsive therapy*, New York, 1988, Oxford University Press.

Blazer DG, Cassel CE: Depression in the elderly, *Hosp Pract* 29:37-41, 1994.

Brammer LM: *The helping relationship: process and skills*, Boston, 1993, Allyn & Bacon.

Denton PL: *Psychiatric occupations therapy: a workbook of practical skills*, New York, 1987, Little, Brown.

Fortinash KM, Holoday Worret PA: *Psychiatric nursing care plans,* ed 3, St Louis, 1999, Mosby.

Fortinash KM, Holoday Worret PA: *Psychiatric nursing care plans,* ed 4, St Louis, 2003, Mosby.

Herz MI: The therapeutic milieu: a necessity, *Int J Psychiatry* 7:209, 1969.

Jones M: *The therapeutic community,* New York, 1953, Basic Books.

Kennedy E: *On becoming a counselor,* New York, 1977, Seabury Press.

Northouse P, Northouse L: *Health communication: strategies for health professionals,* Norwalk, Conn, 1992, Appleton & Lange.

Peplau HE: *Interpersonal relations in nursing,* New York, 1952, GP Putnam's Sons.

Peplau HE: *Basic principles of patient counseling,* ed 2, Philadelphia, 1969, Smith, Kline and French Laboratories.

Peplau HE: *Interpersonal relations in nursing,* New York, 1991, Springer Publishers.

Rogers CP: *Client-centered therapy,* Boston, 1961, Houghton-Mifflin.

Sampson E, Marthas M: *Group process for the health professions,* New York, 1990, Delmar.

Satir V: *Peoplemaking,* Palo Alto, Calif, 1972, Science & Behavior Books.

Travelbee J: *Interpersonal aspects of nursing,* Philadelphia, 1971, FA Davis.

Yalom ID: *The theory and practice of group psychotherapy,* ed 3, New York, 1985, Basic Books.

SUGGESTED READINGS

Cartwright D: The nature of group cohesiveness. In Cartwright D, Zander A, editors: *Group dynamics: research and theory,* ed 3, New York, 1968, Harper & Row.

Corey G: *Becoming a helper,* Pacific Grove, Calif, 1989, Brooks/Cole Publishing.

Corey G: *Case approach to counseling and psychotherapy,* ed 3, Pacific Grove, Calif, 1991, Brooks/Cole.

Corey G: *Theory and practice of group counseling,* ed 3, Pacific Grove, Calif, 1990, Brooks/Cole.

Cosgray E et al: A day in the life of an inpatient: an experiential game to promote empathy for individuals in a psychiatric hospital, *Arch Psychiatr Nurs* 6:6, 1990.

Dunton WR: *Occupational therapy: a manual for nurses,* Philadelphia, 1915, WB Saunders (classic).

Folsum JC, Hildreth NH, Blair DT: Behavioral interventions in the dementias by a multi-therapist team. In Morley JE et al: *Memory function and age related disorders,* New York, 1992, Springer.

Freud SL: *Dreams, new introductory lectures on psychoanalysis,* vol xv, London, 1963, Hogarth Press.

Gaston E: Factors contributing to responses in music. In *Book of proceedings,* Kansas City, 1957, National Association for Music Therapy.

Jung: CG: *Man and his symbols,* New York, 1998, Doubleday.

Kety SS et al: Cerebral blood flow and metabolism in schizophrenia: the effects of barbiturate semi-narcosis, insulin coma and electroshock, 1948, *Am J Psychiatry* 151(suppl 6):203, 1994.

Lepola I, Vanhanen L: The patient's daily activities in acute psychiatric care, *J Psychiatr Mental Health Nurs* 4:29, 1997.

McCaffery G: The use of leisure activities in a therapeutic community, *J Psychiatr Mental Health Nurs* 5:53, 1998.

Moreno J: *Psychodrama,* vol 1, New York, 1964, Beacon House.

O'Toole AE: Review of Hildegard Peplau: psychiatric nurse of the century, by Barbara Callaway, New York, 2002, Springer Publishing, *J Am Psychiatric Nurses Assoc* 8(4):135-140, 2002.

Rosen F: *Dance in psychotherapy,* New York, 1974, Dance Horizons Republication.

Sackheim HA: Continuation therapy following ECT: directions for future research, *Psychopharmacol Bull* 25:501-521, 1995.

Sadock BJ: Group psychotherapy, combined psychotherapy and psychodrama. In Kaplan HL, Sadock BJ, editors: *Comprehensive textbook of psychiatry,* ed 6, Baltimore, 1995, Williams & Wilkins.

Sayre J: Common errors in communication made by students in psychiatric nursing, *Perspect Psychiatr Care* 5:175, 1978.

Ulman E, Dachinger P, editors: *Art therapy in theory and practice,* New York, 1975, Schocken Books.

ONLINE RESOURCES

American Art Therapy Association: www.arttherapy.org

American Dance Therapy Association: www.adta.org

American Music Therapy Association: www.musictherapy.org

American Occupational Therapy Association: www.aota.org

American Society of Group Psychotherapy and Psychodrama: www.asgppp.org

American Therapeutic Recreation Association: www.atra-tr.org

Internet Mental Health: www.mentalhealth.com/

Mental Health InfoSource: www.mhsource.com

PsychPro Online: www.onlinepsych.com.aboutpro.htm

20 Psychopharmacology

Pauline Chan and Jay Sherr

OBJECTIVES

- Describe and discuss the pharmacologic issues related to antipsychotic medication therapy.

- Describe and discuss the pharmacologic issues related to antidepressant therapy.

- Describe and discuss the pharmacologic issues related to mood stabilization therapy.

- Describe and discuss the pharmacologic issues related to anxiolytic and hypnotic medication therapy.

- Describe and discuss the pharmacologic issues related to stimulant medication therapy.

- Explain nonpharmacologic modalities related to the treatment of individuals with mood disorders.

- Explain the nursing issues related to psychopharmacology and nonpharmacologic treatment and modalities.

ccording to the National Institute of Mental Health, an estimated 22.1% of Americans 18 years and older—about 1 in 5 adults—suffer from a diagnosable mental disorder in a given year. When applied to the 1998 U.S. Census residential population estimate, this figure translates to 44.3 million people. In addition, 4 of the 10 leading causes of disability in the United States and other developed countries are caused by mental disorders: major depression, bipolar disorder, schizophrenia, and obsessive-compulsive disorders (OCDs). Many people suffer from more than one mental disorder at a given time, and the cost of mental illness accounts for billions of dollars a year, including treatment costs and loss of wages and income resulting from disability. In fact, psychiatric disease emerges as a significant component of the global burden of disease (Murray and Lopez, 2000) when disability, as well as death, is taken into account (Box 20-1).

Until the discovery of chlorpromazine (Thorazine) and other psychoactive medications, clients with mental illness had few options and often were left untreated. Edward Shorter, in his book *History of Psychiatry,* summarized the discovery of chlorpromazine as analogous to the discovery of penicillin in general medicine. The discovery that chlorpromazine reduces agitation, hallucinations, and psychotic symptoms marked the beginning of the era of psychopharmacology. In subsequent years, additional antipsychotic medications were discovered. Initially these included more phenothiazines, as represented by chlorpromazine and then other structurally different chemical compounds such as the butyrophenone class, as represented by haloperidol (Haldol). In the 1960s these drugs were studied to establish clinical efficacy using the double-blind, placebo-controlled study method, which greatly increased our knowledge of the mechanism of actions of these drugs. These studies also provided evidence that the various antipsychotic drugs are equally effective, although their potency varies.

MODE AND MECHANISM OF DRUG ACTION

The mode of action of a drug describes what it does to the body; the mechanism of action describes how the drug works to affect the symptoms, cure the disease, or cause **side effects**.

Neurotransmitters

To understand the modes of action of **psychotropic** drugs, it is important to have an understanding of the neurotransmitter systems in the brain (Kramer, 2002). The classic neurotransmitters include the following: acetylcholine, histamine, serotonin, dopamine, norepinephrine, epinephrine, aspartic acid, γ-aminobutyric acid (GABA), glutamic acid, glycine, homocysteine, and taurine.

The four neurotransmitters that are *most* important in the study of psychotropic drugs are:
1. Acetylcholine
2. Dopamine
3. Serotonin (also called 5-hydroxytryptamine or 5-HT)
4. Glutamate (blutamic acid)

Box 20-1	Leading Causes of Years Lived with Disability Worldwide in 1990

1. Unipolar major depression
2. Iron deficiency anemia
3. Falls
4. Alcohol use
5. Chronic obstructive pulmonary disease
6. Bipolar disorder
7. Congenital anomalies
8. Osteoarthritis
9. Schizophrenia
10. Obsessive-compulsive disorders

Acetylcholine

Numerous receptors exist for acetylcholine. The major subdivisions are the nicotinic and muscarinic cholinergic receptors. There are numerous muscarinic receptors; the M1 postsynaptic receptor is the most important because of its mediating effect in the memory function linked to cholinergic neurotransmission. It is also related to the side effects of anticholinergic drugs such as dry mouth, blurred vision, urinary retention, and constipation.

Dopamine and acetylcholine have a reciprocal relationship. Dopamine suppresses cholinergic activities in the nigrostriatal dopamine pathway.

Dopamine

Dopamine is produced in dopaminergic neurons from the precursor tyrosine. Receptors for dopamine regulate dopaminergic neurotransmission. There are four dopamine receptor pathways in the brain:
1. *Nigrostriatal dopamine pathway* is thought to control movements.
2. *Mesolimbic dopamine pathway* is thought to be involved in behaviors such as pleasurable sensation, euphoria resulting from drugs of abuse, and delusions and hallucinations resulting from psychosis.
3. *Mesocortical dopamine pathway* is thought to mediate positive and negative psychotic symptoms, as well as cognitive side effects of antipsychotic medications.
4. *Tuberoinfundibular (endocrine) dopamine pathway* controls the release of prolactin.

Serotonin

Serotonin is produced when tryptophan is converted by the enzyme tryptophan hydroxylase, after being transported into the serotonin neuron. It is first converted to 5 hydroxytryptophan (5HTP) and then further converted to 5-HT by the enzyme aromatic amino acid decarboxylase. Serotonin is stored in the vesicles until it is released by a neuronal impulse. It is an inhibitory catecholamine.

Serotonin is destroyed by the enzyme monoamine oxidase type A, forming an inactive **metabolite**.

There are numerous subtypes of serotonin receptors. The key receptor, $5HT_{1D}$, is a presynaptic receptor. Other key postsynaptic receptors are $5HT_{1A}$, $5 HT_{2A}$, $5HT_3$, and $5HT_4$.

There are at least five serotonin pathways in the central nervous system (CNS). Serotonin mediates cognitive effects, emotions including panic, memory, and anxiety; violence and aggression; sexual function; and sleep-wake cycles through the various serotonin pathways.

Serotonin also interacts with many dopamine pathways and has the ability to inhibit dopamine release.

Glutamate

Glutamate, or glutamic acid, is an amino acid that is synthesized in the brain, where it functions as a major excitatory neurotransmitter. Glutamate has been implicated in an increasing number of neurologic and psychologic disorders. The psychoactive drug phencyclidine (PCP) has the ability to block the N-methyl D-aspartate receptor channel. Because glutamate is the neurotransmitter of cortical and hippocampal pyramidal neurons, it has been hypothesized that the effects of PCP may reflect interference with glutamatergic neurotransmission in these brain regions.

PSYCHOTROPIC PHARMACOTHERAPY ASSESSMENT

Before starting pharmacotherapy treatment, a thorough assessment of the client is necessary. Many drugs may cause psychotic symptoms (Drugs, 2002), and it is important to evaluate the client carefully. Treatment is aimed at stabilization of the illness with the goal of achieving remission, defined as complete return to baseline level of functioning and absence of symptoms. After remission, the client enters the maintenance phase. The goal of the maintenance phase is to optimize protection against recurrence of illness. Equally important is consideration of treatment that maximizes client functioning and minimizes subthreshold symptoms and adverse effects of treatment.

Variables Affecting Drug Therapy

Sherr advocates that when assessing clients before or during pharmacotherapy, it is necessary to incorporate information from both drug-related and client-related variables before initiation of therapy. Common drug- and client-related variables are described in Box 20-2.

ANTIPSYCHOTIC MEDICATIONS

Antipsychotic medications, previously known as *major tranquilizers* and **neuroleptics**, have been the mainstay of treatment for schizophrenia since the introduction of chlorpromazine in 1952. These medications are effective and probably responsible for deinstitutionalization of clients diagnosed with schizophrenia during the 1950s and 1960s. Antipsychotic medications can be generally divided into two broad categories, the *conventional* or *typical* antipsychotics and the *atypical* or *unconventional* antipsychotics. The **conventional antipsychotics** are similar in mode of action and efficacy but differ in side effects and potency. The mechanism of action is the ability to block D_2 receptors in

Box 20-2	Variables Affecting Drug Therapy

Drug-Related Variables

Mode/mechanism of action
Available dosage form: oral (solid, liquid, sublingual), parenteral
Bioavailability of various formulations
Onset, peak, and duration of action
Serum half-life
Method of elimination from the body (hepatic or renal)
Side effects/toxicities (both predictable and idiosyncratic)
Cost (drug price, administration, and monitoring costs)

Client-Related Variables

Diagnosis
Other disease states (cardiovascular, liver, renal disease)
Age
Weight
Anticholinergic susceptibility
History of side effects
Previous response
Family history of response
Willingness to comply/insight into illness
Financial and/or health insurance
Support systems

the limbic region of the brain. The **atypical antipsychotics** differ in mode of action, side effects, and potency, and, compared to conventional antipsychotics, generally have lower potential for extrapyramidal effects; greater efficacy in negative symptoms, cognitive symptoms, and **refractory** illness; lower potential to cause prolactin elevations; and greater serotonin/dopamine D_2 effects.

PSYCHOSIS
The Dopamine Hypothesis of Psychosis

Psychosis was thought to be due to overactivity of dopamine neurons. Psychosis is traditionally described as having positive and negative symptoms. Research has concluded that psychosis is not adequately described with merely positive and negative symptoms, but is better described with five symptom dimensions: positive symptoms, negative symptoms, cognitive, aggressive/hostile, and anxious/depressed (Box 20-3).

Positive Symptoms

It is thought that positive symptoms are mediated as a result of the overactivity of the dopamine neurons in the mesolimbic dopamine pathway.

The positive symptoms of psychosis are associated with increased mental activities with clients suffering from delusions, hallucinations, disorganized speech, disorganized behavior, catatonia, and agitation.

Negative Symptoms

It is thought that negative symptoms are mediated as a result of the cortical dopamine deficiency in the mesocortical pathway, and are associated with decreased mental activities.

Box 20-3	Symptoms of Psychosis

Positive Symptoms
Delusions
Hallucinations
Disorganized speech
Disorganized behavior
Catatonia
Agitation

Negative Symptoms
Blunted effect
Passiveness
Social apathy and withdrawal
Alogia (inability to speak)
Avolition (inability to decide)
Anhedonia (lack of pleasure)
Lack of attention or spontaneity

Cognitive Function Impairment
Thought disorder
Incoherence
Loose association
Difficulty processing information

Aggressive Symptoms
Hostility
Verbal abuse
Assault
Sexual acting out
Poor impulse control

Depressive Anxious Symptoms
Worry
Guilt
Irritability
Anxiety
Depression

Clients may display behaviors such as blunted affect, passiveness, social apathy and withdrawal, alogia, avolition, anhedonia, and lack of attention or spontaneity.

Cognitive Function Impairments

Cognitive function impairments may include thought disorder, incoherence, loose association, and difficulty processing information.

Aggressive Symptoms

Aggressive and hostile symptoms may include hostility, verbal abuse, assaultive behavior, sexual acting out, and poor impulse control.

Depressive/Anxious Symptoms

Depressive and anxious symptoms may include excessive worry, guilt, irritability, anxiety, and depression.

Indications

Antipsychotics are indicated for the treatment of psychosis (APA, 2000) including a wide spectrum of illnesses such as schizophrenia, schizoaffective disorders, and delusional disorders. Atypical antipsychotics are used as adjunctive or monotherapy for bipolar disorders (Schatzberg, 2001). Psychosis from secondary causes, such as electrolyte or hormonal imbalances, drug abuse, brain tumors, mania, or depression with psychotic features, may also benefit from short-term antipsychotic medications while the underlying illness is being treated. Table 20-1 lists the various types of antipsychotic medications and their dosages.

Goals of Therapy

Typical (conventional) antipsychotic medications are effective in reducing or alleviating the positive symptoms of psychosis. Atypical antipsychotics are better in alleviating negative symptoms and other symptoms associated with psychosis. It is important to observe clients for signs and symptoms and to assess clients regularly, documenting specific behaviors that have improved. The overall goal is to enable the client to return to normal daily functions and to be able to provide self-care. Another important goal is to minimize side effects using the optimal dose with the least possible side effects, and to help clients manage these side effects so that they will continue to be medication compliant on a long-term basis.

Absorption, Distribution, Metabolism, and Excretion

The absorption of drugs may be influenced by the presence of food, antacids, anticholinergics, and smoking. Cigarette smoking tends to activate hepatic enzymes and the drugs are metabolized faster, thus requiring higher doses. Distribution of the drug depends on the route of administration, with intramuscular injections generally having greater bioavailability than oral preparations. All the drugs are metabolized in the liver and excreted through the kidneys.

Drug Level Monitoring

Because many of these drugs are metabolized to active metabolites, it is difficult to correlate their plasma levels of the drugs to therapeutic response; therefore therapeutic drug level monitoring is not necessary in most clinical settings. In some situations, however, monitoring drug levels can be useful, for example when (1) the client is an older adult or very young, (2) the client is using multiple medications with known potential drug interactions, (3) the client fails to respond with usual doses, and (4) noncompliance is suspected.

Clinical Use and Efficacy

Although they are important and effective medications, antipsychotics are also the most toxic drugs used in psychiatry. The lowest possible effective dose should be used for the shortest amount of time.

Table 20-1 | Antipsychotic Medications Dosage Ranges, Equivalency, and Dosage Forms

Medication	Trade Name	Potency	Dosage Range	Equivalent Dose
Clozapine	Clozaril	—	200-900 mg/day	—
Olanzapine	Zyprexa	—	5-20 mg/day	—
Risperidone	Risperdal	—	2-8 mg/day	—
Quetiapine	Seroquel	—	250-750 mg/day	—
Ziprasidone	Geodon	—	80-160 mg/day	—
Chlorpromazine	Thorazine	Low	200-1600 mg/day	100 mg
Thioridazine	Mellaril	Low	200-800 mg/day	100 mg
Mesoridazine	Serentil	Moderate	100-400 mg/day	50-60 mg
Thiothixene	Navane	High	10-120 mg/day	5 mg
Perphenazine	Trilafon	High	12-64 mg/day	10 mg
Trifluoperazine	Stelazine	High	10-60 mg/day	5 mg
Loxapine	Loxitane	High	40-225 mg/day	15 mg
Molindone	Moban	High	40-250 mg/day	15 mg
Fluphenazine	Prolixin	Very high	2-60 mg/day	2-5 mg
Fluphenazine Decanoate	Prolixin decanoate	Very high	6.25-75 mg/3 weeks	—
Haloperidol	Haldol	Very high	4-40 mg/day	2-5 mg
Haloperidol Decanoate	Haldol decanoate	Very high	100-450 mg/mo	—

Target symptom response varies with time. Positive symptoms are the most responsive. Symptoms such as combativeness, hostility, psychomotor agitation, and irritability are often relieved within hours. Affective symptoms, anxiety, tension, depression, inappropriate affect, reduced attention span, and social withdrawal may take 2 to 4 weeks to respond. Cognitive and perceptive symptoms such as hallucinations, delusions, and thought broadcasting may take 2 to 8 weeks to respond. The most negative symptoms—poor social skills, unrealistic planning, poor judgment and insight—respond the slowest and the least. Many clients have fixed hallucinations and delusions that respond minimally to medications. Given the varied time course of different symptoms, it should be kept in mind that increases in medication dose will not hasten the relief of slow-responding symptoms.

Antipsychotic therapy may be started using divided doses three or four times a day. This regimen is useful in determining a client's ability to tolerate a medication and to minimize the initial impact of side effects. Once an effective total daily dose has been established and the client has had time to develop tolerance to side effects, the medication is often reduced to once or twice a day. Reduced frequency of administration increases the likelihood of compliance with the regimen.

In general, antipsychotics are well absorbed from the gastrointestinal (GI) tract and are extensively metabolized in the liver. The half-life varies highly among individuals but is usually between 20 and 40 hours in adults, with steady state being reached in 4 to 7 days. **Serum level monitoring** (i.e., obtaining blood samples to determine drug concentration) is not routinely useful. Serum level monitoring may be revealing in specific situations, including lack of response to nor-

mal doses after 6 weeks, severe or unusual adverse reactions, with clients taking multiple medications, in the physically ill, in the elderly or young children, and as a check for compliance. The choice of medication is determined largely by the side-effect profile and specific needs of the client.

Treatment Therapy for Acute Episodes

Atypical antipsychotics such as olanzapine (Zyprexa) 10 to 20 mg daily, risperidone (Risperdal) 4 to 6 mg daily, and quetiapine (Seroquel) 300 to 400 mg daily in divided doses are currently first-line treatment for acute episodes. Clozapine (Clozaril) is *not* a first-line treatment and is reserved for refractory illness because of the risk of the serious adverse effect of agranulocytosis.

Adverse Effects of Antipsychotics and Nursing Management

The conventional antipsychotics block the D_2 receptors and the extrapyramidal motor system. Therefore their effectiveness to treat psychosis also induces **extrapyramidal side effects (EPS)** (movement disorders). In addition, these drugs also block noradrenergic, cholinergic, and histamine receptors to varying degrees, resulting in a unique side-effect profile for each drug. Table 20-2 lists side effects associated with receptor blockade.

Drowsiness

Drowsiness is most common during the first days of treatment and usually disappears in 1 to 2 weeks. Sedation is particularly significant with the *low potency conventional* antipsychotics such as chlorpromazine and thioridazine (Mellaril). Clients should avoid alcohol, medications such as

Table 20-2 Side Effects Associated with Receptor Blockade

Dopamine$_2$	Histamine$_1$	Cholinergic	Alpha$_1$	Serotonin$_2$
Extrapyramidal side effects Prolactin	Sedation Weight gain	Dry mouth Blurred vision Sinus tachycardia Constipation Impaired memory/cognition	Orthostatic hypotension Reflex tachycardia	Weight gain Gastrointestinal upset Sexual dysfunction

antihistamines (common in some cough and cold preparations), and sleeping aids. The daily dose may be given at bedtime instead of during the daytime.

Extrapyramidal Side Effects

The use of *high potency conventional* antipsychotic medications poses a higher risk for EPS. *High potency conventional* antipsychotic medications include fluphenazine (Prolixin), perphenazine (Trilafon), trifluoperazine (Stelazine), and haloperidol.

Dystonias. These reactions include spasms of the eye (oculogyric crisis), neck (torticollis), back (retrocollis), tongue (glossospasm), or other muscles, which can be frightening to the client. Fortunately these symptoms can be readily reversed with intramuscular injection of 50 mg of diphenhydramine (Benadryl) or 1 or 2 mg intramuscularly of benztropine (Cogentin), followed by oral agents to prevent recurrence.

Dystonia usually occurs during the early stages of treatment and is common after intramuscular injections of antipsychotics. They seldom occur after 3 months of treatment. Risk factors include administration of high potency agents, large doses, and parenteral injections.

Pseudoparkinsonism. Symptoms include decreased movements (bradykinesia, akinesia), muscle rigidity (cogwheel and lead pipe), resting hand tremor, drooling, masklike face, and shuffling gait. This EPS is often misdiagnosed, untreated, or unrecognized. Some clients have a behavioral form of akinesia, characterized by lack of motivation, blunted affect, decreased speech, and apathy. This can be difficult to distinguish from their illness. Physicians should be on the alert for this symptom complex for proper diagnosis.

Treatments include reduction of the antipsychotic medication dose, change of antipsychotic medications to one with less potential for EPS, and use of an oral anti-Parkinson agent such as benztropine, trihexyphenidyl (Artane), diphenhydramine, or amantadine (Symmetrel). It is not recommended to treat EPS prophylactically. Table 20-3 lists adjunctive medications used to treat EPS.

Akathisia. Symptoms of **akathisia** include restlessness, pacing, rocking or inability to sit still, and anxiousness. These symptoms are often dose related. Akathisia can be confused with anxiety and agitation. To differentiate the diagnoses of akathisia and anxiety/agitation, careful observa-

Table 20-3 Adjunctive Medications Used to Treat Extrapyramidal Side Effects

Generic Name	Trade Name	Equivalent Dose (mg)	Dose Range (mg)	Dosage Forms*
Anticholinergic				
Benztropine	Cogentin	1	1-8	Injectable
Trihexyphenidyl	Artane	2	2-15	Capsule-extended release, elixir
Antihistamine				
Diphenhydramine	Benadryl	50	50-400	Capsules, liquid, injectable
Dopamine Agonist				
Amantadine	Symmetrel	N/A	100-400	Capsule and liquid only

*All available as tablets unless noted.

tion of the client is warranted. Akathisia improves with decreasing antipsychotic dose, whereas anxiety/agitation worsens; akathisia is difficult to control over a period of time, whereas anxiety/agitation can be controlled over time. Propranolol (Inderal) with daily dose of 80-120 mg (divided dose) can be an effective treatment. It is advisable to monitor the client's blood pressure when using this agent. A benzodiazepine such as lorazepam (Ativan) 1 mg orally can be helpful.

Tardive Dyskinesia. **Tardive dyskinesia** manifests as abnormal movements of voluntary muscle groups after a prolonged period of dopamine blockade. These movements may affect any muscle group, but the most commonly affected are those of the face, mouth, tongue, and digits and include grimacing, lip smacking, tongue poking, and writing movements of the fingers and toes. These movements can be severe and disabling. Risk factors include longer lengths of time of antipsychotic use and exposure, high doses, high potency drugs, and use of conventional antipsychotics. There is no effective treatment for tardive dyskinesia; the use of vitamin E has shown some benefit. Atypical antipsychotics have much lesser

CLINICAL ALERT

Tardive dyskinesia (TD) occurs as a result of upregulation of dopamine receptors (i.e., prolonged blockade results in the increase in the number of receptors). Extrapyramidal side effects (EPS), on the other hand, occur as a result of temporary blockade of these same receptors. Therefore, when TD occurs, decreasing the dose temporarily worsens TD but improves EPS; increasing the dose temporarily improves TD but worsens EPS. A long-term solution is to decrease the dose and change to an atypical antipsychotic medication.

Recognition of TD during its early stage is crucial. Clients should be examined using the Abnormal Involuntary Movement Scale (AIMS) or Dyskinesia Identification System: Condensed User Scale (DISCUS).

Box 20-4 Antipsychotics Associated with Weight Gain*

Clozapine
Olanzapine
Low-potency conventional antipsychotics (e.g., chlorpromazine)
Quetiapine
Risperidone
High-potency conventional antipsychotics (e.g., haloperidol)
Ziprasidone and molindone

*From greatest to least potential.

risk of causing tardive dyskinesia (less than 1% with risperidone and olanzapine) and clozapine carries no risk of causing tardive dyskinesia. Conversion to atypical antipsychotics is warranted.

Anticholinergic Side Effects

The use of *low potency conventional* antipsychotics such as chlorpromazine and thioridazine presents a greater risk of anticholinergic side effects. Tolerance may develop over the first 4 to 8 weeks. Side effects are mostly annoying but not serious. Anticholinergic side effects include dry mouth, blurred vision, constipation, urinary retention, nasal congestion, and ejaculatory inhibition. The following interventions may be useful:

- *Dry mouth:* Use of ice chips, lemon swabs, sugarless gums or candies.
- *Blurred vision:* Read in well-lighted areas, read for short periods, and vary the distance of the reading materials.
- *Constipation:* Exercise (including walking) regularly, drink plenty of fluids, eat plenty of fruits and vegetables, and use a stool softener such as docusate sodium (Colace).
- *Urinary retention:* Medical attention is advised. Oxybutynin (Ditropan) may be tried.
- *Nasal congestion:* Nasal decongestants may be useful to relieve symptoms.
- *Ejaculatory inhibition:* This is more prominent in men using thioridazine. The client should be referred to a physician for further interventions.

Cardiovascular Side Effects

Postural Hypotension. Postural hypotension is dizziness associated with sudden changes in position such as lying down and getting up. The use of *low-potency antipsychotics* such as chlorpromazine and thioridazine presents a greater risk for postural hypotension as a result of α-adrenergic receptor blockade.

Clients should be advised to rise from bed slowly and to avoid the risk of falling. This is especially important with older adults.

Arrhythmias, Palpitations (Changes in Heart Rhythm). Arrhythmias or palpitations may be seen with higher doses or in clients with preexisting heart disease, as well as in combination with certain drugs such as thioridazine and ziprasidone (Geodon).

Changes in QT intervals. Baseline electrocardiogram (ECG) and repeat at maximum dose **titration**. Changes in ECG should be carefully monitored and an alternative medication may need to be used (Taylor, 2002).

Weight Gain

Clozapine and olanzapine have higher weight gain potential (Box 20-4). The client should be carefully monitored with blood glucose levels and adult onset diabetes should be carefully screened and monitored. Weight gain is especially significant when the client is taking other drugs, such as lithium, divalproex sodium (Depakote), or mirtazapine (Remeron), that also cause weight gain.

Clients should be counseled on weight gain and obesity at the initiation of antipsychotic therapy. The client's weight should be recorded at baseline and monitored weekly. Excessive weight gain may warrant a change of antipsychotics. Preventive education should include dietary counseling, including calorie counts, portion size, choice of low-fat/low-calorie foods, and exercise.

Neuroleptic Malignant Syndrome

Neuroleptic malignant syndrome (NMS) is a medical emergency (Berkow, 1992). The neuroleptic syndrome is characterized by decreased level of consciousness, greatly increased muscle tone, and autonomic dysfunction including hyperpyrexia, labile hypertension, tachycardia, tachypnea, diaphoresis, and drooling. Muscle necrosis can be so severe as to cause myoglobinuric renal failure, as large amounts of myoglobin are released from the muscle tissue and excreted in the urine causing myoglobinuria.

NMS is potentially fatal; the mortality rate is about 10%. It occurs in approximately 1% of clients taking antipsychotics. Major risk factors identified for the development of NMS include history of NMS, adjunctive and polypsychotropic medications, rapid dose titration, use of high potency antipsychotics at high dose, or use of parenteral antipsychotics. Young male clients are more frequently affected. Most of the time NMS occurs during the early stages of treatment with antipsychotics, but may at times occur even after years of treatment.

Laboratory findings are an important aid with this diagnosis. Typically, laboratory abnormalities include leukocytosis (15,000 to 30,000 cells/mm^3), greatly elevated creatine phosphokinase levels (over 3000 IU/ml), and myoglobinuria (Hermesh et al., 2002).

Treatments include:

- Discontinuation of all antipsychotic medications.
- Hydration of client, including administration of intravenous infusion of fluids.
- For hyperthermia, administration of acetaminophen (Tylenol), along with cooling blankets.
- Consideration of intravenous heparin infusion to reduce the risk of pulmonary emboli.
- Management of arrhythmias.
- Intravenous infusion of dantrolene (Dantrium), a direct muscle relaxant, to reduce muscle rigidity and to treat hyperthermia resulting from breakdown of muscle tissues.
- Consideration of use of dopaminergic drugs such as bromocriptine (Parlodel), amantadine, or anticholinergic drugs.

Most clients recover from NMS. Once the client has recovered, it is advisable to wait for 1 to 2 weeks before restarting the antipsychotic medication. Clients should be carefully evaluated for the need for antipsychotics. Possible alternatives such as lithium, carbamazepine (Tegretol), and divalproex sodium should be considered. If it is determined that the client should continue with an antipsychotic medication, another antipsychotic medication with a different chemical structure should be used, and doses should be titrated slowly. A history of NMS should be noted in the client's medical record, and depot antipsychotic drugs (haloperidol or fluphenazine) should not be used because of their long half-lives.

Recently the atypical antipsychotics clozapine and risperidone have been advocated for clients with a history of NMS. It is important to note that NMS has also occurred with the use of these agents. The most important rule is careful monitoring for recurrence and relapse. Clients should be monitored for signs and symptoms such as psychomotor excitement, refusal of food, anuria, and weight loss.

Photosensitivity

Phenothiazines such as chlorpromazine are known to induce photosensitivity reactions. Haloperidol may cause photosensitivity but is considered rare. The word *photosensitivity* is a general term used to describe either the common phototoxic response or the uncommon photoallergenic reaction. Phototoxic response is nonimmunologic and resembles sunburn; it can occur immediately after exposure to sunlight, usually within hours. Clinical signs and symptoms include erythema, pain, and edema. Photoallergenic reactions are immunologic and require previous exposure to the photosensitizing agent, and are commonly seen as a delayed reaction (i.e., usually in 1 day to 2 weeks after exposure to sunlight). Clinical signs and symptoms include papillovesicular eruption, pruritis, and eczematous dermatitis. Treatment of sunburn includes topical burn cream and antihistamines. Steroids may be indicated for photoallergenic reactions. Clients should be advised to wear protective clothing and to use a good sunscreen during outdoor activities. Titanium dioxide is the least likely sunscreen product to cause photosensitivity disorders (Reid, 1996). Skin coloration such as gray-blue skin is associated with antipsychotic use. Low-potency conventional antipsychotics such as chlorpromazine and thioridazine are associated with skin pigmentation. Management of these side effects may require switching to another antipsychotic.

Poikilothermia

The loss of ability to regulate internal body temperature with environment temperature change can occur and can be problematic with older adults. Older clients on antipsychotics should not be left unmonitored in the outdoors during hot weather.

Galactorrhea and Gynecomastia

These conditions are due to dopamine blockade, which results in hyperprolactinemia. Management of these side effects includes client counseling.

DEPOT ANTIPSYCHOTICS

Two depot antipsychotic medications are marketed in the United States: haloperidol decanoate and fluphenazine decanoate. Fluphenazine enanthate has been discontinued by the manufacturer.

Clinical Use and Dosage Regimen

In general, antipsychotics should be administered initially in divided doses to minimize side effects and to determine the client's ability to tolerate the medication. Once an effective dose has been established, the dosage regimen should be simplified to once-a-day dosing. Studies have shown that client medication compliance improves with daily dosing or less frequent dosing.

In general, antipsychotic medications are well absorbed in the GI tract. To improve compliance, liquid doses are available, and olanzapine is available in an orally disintegrating tablet form, which readily dissolves on the tongue. It is generally not necessary to obtain serum blood samples to determine the drug concentration in the blood. Serum levels are indicated in specific situations such as lack of response to normal dose after an adequate trial period (6 weeks), severe or abrupt adverse drug reactions, or when a client is seriously ill.

Fluphenazine Decanoate Injection

Once it is determined that a depot injection is indicated and the client is able to tolerate the adverse effects, an initial dose of 12.5 to 25 mg (0.5 to 1 ml) may be given. Fluphenazine decanoate may be given intramuscularly or subcutaneously. The onset of action is about 24 to 72 hours. Effects of the drug can be seen within 48 to 96 hours. Subsequent dosage intervals are given in accordance to the client's response. For maintenance therapy, effects of the drug can be seen in 4 weeks.

Dosage Conversion

A controlled multicenter study showed that fluphenazine hydrochloride 20 mg daily (orally) is equivalent to 25 mg of fluphenazine decanoate every 3 weeks. This represents a conversion of every 10 mg daily dose to be equivalent of 12.5 mg (0.5 ml) of fluphenazine decanoate every 3 weeks.

Haloperidol Decanoate Injection

Haloperidol decanoate can be given only as a deep intramuscular injection. The maximum dose should not exceed 100 mg. If an additional dose is required, the initial injection should not exceed 100 mg, with the balance of the dose given in 3 to 7 days as a separate injection. Haloperidol decanoate is usually given every 4 weeks or monthly.

Dosage Conversion

The initial conversion of an oral haloperidol daily dose to decanoate injection can be achieved by administering 10 to 20 times the daily oral dose; for older clients, a conversion factor of 10 to 15 should be used. In clients previously maintained on higher doses of antipsychotics for whom a low-dose approach risks recurrence of psychiatric decompensation, and in clients whose long-term use of haloperidol has resulted in a tolerance to the drug, 20 times the previous daily dose in oral haloperidol equivalents should be considered for initial titration, with downward titration on succeeding injections.

Maintenance dosage should be 10 to 15 times the previous daily oral dose. Table 20-4 compares haloperidol decanoate and fluphenazine decanoate in onset, peak time, half-life, and therapeutic range.

The pharmacokinetic response after intramuscular injections may be variable among clients.

Table 20-4	Pharmacokinetics Comparison of Depot Antipsychotics	
	Haloperidol Decanoate	Fluphenazine Decanoate
Onset	Slow onset	1-3 days
Time to peak	6 days	2-4 days
Half-life	21 days (3 weeks)	14-26 days (2-3 weeks)
Therapeutic range	100-450 mg/month	12.5-75 mg/3 weeks

Administration of Depot Injections

According to the manufacturers' instructions, the following procedures should be followed when administering depot injections:

- Parenteral products should be inspected visually for particulate matter and discoloration.
- A dry syringe and 21-gauge needle should be used. Using a wet syringe will cloud the solution.
- Maximum volume per site per injection should not exceed 3 ml.
- Before administering a depot injection, it is always advisable to start with a short-acting dosage form (e.g., oral) so that the client can be assessed with potential side effects.

ATYPICAL ANTIPSYCHOTICS

Clozapine is the first atypical antipsychotic that demonstrated efficacy in the treatment of negative symptoms in schizophrenia. Subsequently, risperidone, olanzapine, quetiapine, and ziprasidone were approved for use in the United States. In general, the atypical antipsychotics are superior in efficacy over the typical antipsychotics in the treatment of negative symptoms. EPS occur much less frequently, and there is much less risk for developing tardive dyskinesia. These drugs also may improve the cognitive function of clients with schizophreinia. Olanzapine, risperidone, and quetiapine are first-line treatment of schizophrenia because of their effectiveness and favorable side-effect profiles. Ziprasidone is also considered first-line treatment, but it has greater capacity to prolong the QT/QTc interval compared to other antipsychotics, and should be used with caution. Clozapine is not a first-line therapy because of the risk of agranulocytosis. It is reserved for refractory illness.

Clozapine

Clozapine is a dibenzodiazepine. It was the first atypical antipsychotic introduced for use in the United States.

Mechanism of Action

Clozapine has high receptor affinity for the D_4, 5-HT_2, α-1 adrenergic, muscarinic, and histamine H_1 receptors, and relatively weak receptor affinity for the D_1, D_2, and D_3 receptors. The high-receptor affinity for D_4 and 5 HT_2 is thought to be responsible for the many advantages of clozapine over the typical antipsychotics.

The difference between the atypical antipsychotic clozapine and the conventional antipsychotic haloperidol can be dramatically demonstrated using positron emission tomography scan techniques (Figure 20-1).

Clinical Use

Clozapine is not a first-line antipsychotic and is reserved for refractory illness. The dose should be titrated slowly to avoid side effects such as sedation and orthostatic hypotension. The initial dose is 12.5 mg daily on the first day, which is then quickly titrated to 12.5 mg twice a day. The

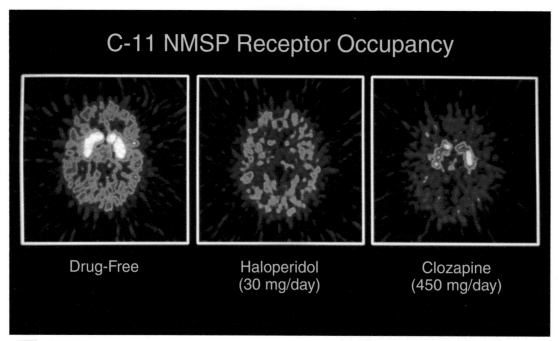

FIGURE 20-1. A transaxial positron emission tomography (PET) scan image at the level of the basal ganglia. Carbon-11 *N*-methylspiperone (NMSP) is a radioactive tag that binds and thus highlights dopamine type 2 (D₂) receptors. The three panels are from the same 36-year-old man with schizophrenia. In the first panel the man is drug free, and the D₂-rich basal ganglia are highlighted by the NMSP. Note the absence of NMSP in the next panel, 6 weeks later, when the client was taking haloperidol, 30 mg/day, with 85% of his basal ganglia D₂-receptors occupied with haloperidol. Finally, with the man taking clozapine, 450 mg/day, only 37% of the D₂-receptors are occupied by drug. Although the psychosis was responsive to both medications, motor side effects were considerable with haloperidol and absent with clozapine. (Data from Tamminga CA et al., Maryland Psychiatric Research Center, University of Maryland at Baltimore, unpublished research.)

dose could be increased in 25-mg increments every other day until reaching an optimal dosage of 300 to 500 mg/day. To avoid oversedation, the larger dose is given in the evening. Serum therapeutic level monitoring is not required, but a serum level of 350 ng/ml or greater is necessary for optimal response. The typical trial period of clozapine is 6 months, and if the client does not respond, a higher dose may be considered.

Risks

Agranulocytosis. **Agranulocytosis** occurs in 1% to 3% of clients. In the United States clients on clozapine are required to be registered with the Clozaril National Registry. The physician is required to register the client by filling out a Clozaril Client Safety Assurance Form at the initiation of therapy, and also to apply for a rechallenge clearance authorization from the national registry. To limit "rechallenge" of clients at risk, weekly white blood cell (WBC) counts and evaluation (normal and abnormal) must be submitted to the pharmacy that is dispensing the medication for submission to the National Registry within 7 days of collection. The physician must also agree to notify the National Registry promptly of all clients who have discontinued therapy and submit to the National Registry the results of the four required weekly blood tests after discontinuation of therapy.

A weekly WBC is drawn for the first 6 months of therapy and every other week thereafter. If the weekly WBC count is between 3000 and 3500/mm³, these counts may need to be obtained more frequently, such as twice a week. If total WBC falls between 2000 and 3000/mm³, and the absolute neutrophil count is between 1000 and 1500/mm³, the client should be carefully monitored, and WBC with differentials should be checked daily. Clozapine should be discontinued permanently if the total WBC count falls below 2000/mm³, or absolute neutrophil count falls below 1000 mm³. The client should never be restarted on clozapine. Allergy history must be updated to include clozapine to prevent readministration. If no WBC is available from the client, therapy should be discontinued. Granulocyte colony-stimulating factor may need to be administered to reduce the risk of prolonged agranulocytosis and infection.

Clients who are at risk of agranulocytosis, such as immunocompromised clients (e.g., clients with AIDS or active tuberculosis), are not good candidates for clozapine therapy. Also the client should not receive other medications, such as carbamazepine, that carry the risk of agranulocytosis.

Side Effects

Sedation. Sedation is the most common side effect of clozapine, especially during initiation of therapy. Dose reduction may be warranted in some situations. Giving a larger dose at bedtime and a smaller dose during the day can be helpful.

Anticholinergic Side Effects. Dry month, blurred vision, GI upset, urinary retention, and constipation are common.

Extrapyramidal Side Effects. EPS are uncommon with clozapine, even with higher doses. However, akathisia may be common.

Neuroleptic Malignant Syndrome. Clozapine is not risk free with NMS.

Cardiovascular Effects. Tachycardia may occur. Orthostatic hypotension can be significant. Clients should be advised to rise slowly to prevent falls.

Weight Gain. Weight gain can be significant. Clients should receive nutritional counseling before initiation of therapy. Clients may be at higher risk for diabetes mellitus (Wang et al., 2002).

Hypersalivation. Hypersalivation is common and symptoms may be alleviated with an anticholinergic medication.

Fever. Transient rise of temperature is seen in clients treated with clozapine, especially during initiation of therapy. Clients with fever should be monitored and evaluated for possible infection, agranulocytosis, or NMS.

Seizures. Seizures associated with clozapine are dose related. The vast majority of clozapine-induced seizures are tonic-clonic seizures. Dosages higher than 600 mg/day are associated with greater than 5% risk of seizures. Because of this risk, dosage greater than 600 mg/day is not recommended unless the client has failed to respond to a lower dose. Sound judgment to discontinue or continue clozapine should be used if the client has a seizure. An anticonvulsant may be considered. However, carbamazepine should be avoided because of increased risk of agranulocytosis. Drugs that may increase risk of seizures, such as bupropion (Wellbutrin), should be avoided.

Risperidone

Risperidone is a benzisoxazole derivative. It blocks dopamine (D_2) receptors and 5-HT receptors. Risperidone also blocks D_1, D_4, α-1, α-2 and H_1 histamine receptors. Risperidone is effective in treating both positive and negative symptoms.

Clinical Use

The usual dosage range for risperidone is 4 to 8 mg/day in two divided doses. Higher doses increase the chance of EPS and other side effects. It should be titrated slowly, starting with 1 mg daily in divided doses. In the older adult, the dose should be lower, usually starting at 25% to 50% of usual adult dose. When titration is complete, a once a day dose given at bedtime can be used. For older clients, the bedtime dose may not be appropriate because of the risk for falls. Bedtime doses

may also not be appropriate for clients who experience agitation and insomnia. Compared to other atypical antipsychotics, risperidone has fewer anticholinergic side effects and may be preferred for older clients (Ranier et al., 2001).

Side Effects

Common side effects are insomnia, hypotension, agitation, and headache. Hyperthermia may occur, especially in older clients.

Extrapyramidal Side Effects. Risperidone has a lower incidence of EPS compared with conventional antipsychotics. Administering an anticholinergic drug such as benztropine can be helpful.

Tardive Dyskinesia. The incidence of risperidone-associated tardive dyskinesia is less than with conventional antipsychotics, but this does occur. Clients should be monitored.

Cardiovascular Effects. Hypotension may occur from α-adrenergic blockade. Older clients should be cautioned in order to prevent falls.

Weight Gain. Weight gain has been associated with risperidone, but is not as significant as with clozapine or olanzapine.

Hyperprolactinemia. Risperidone is associated with a rise in prolactin levels.

Olanzapine

Olanzapine is a thienobenzodiazapine. It is an atypical antipsychotic with greater D_2 and weaker D_4 and α-adrenergic blockade. Structurally olanzapine is similar to clozapine, but does not have the risk of agranulocytosis. Olanzapine is effective in treating positive and negative symptoms of schizophrenia. It is also approved for use as monotherapy for bipolar disorder in manic episodes. It is effective in the treatment of schizoaffective disorders.

Clinical Use

The recommended starting dose is 5 to 10 mg daily at bedtime and may be titrated to 20 mg/day. The rapidly disintegrating olanzapine tablet is particularly useful in clients who are noncompliant.

Side Effects

Sedation and Anticholinergic Side Effects. Sedation is common because of the drug's H_1-blocking properties. Doses are commonly taken at bedtime. Anticholinergic side effects are not as significant, with dry mouth being most common.

Weight Gain. Weight gain is a significant side effect of olanzapine. Weight gain, increase in cholesterol and triglycerides levels, and hyperglycemia have been associated with olanzapine use (Meyer, 2001) as have adult-onset diabetes mellitus and diabetic ketoacidosis. Adult-onset diabetes mellitus has been reported to occur between 5 weeks and 17 months after initiation of olanzapine therapy. Discontinuation of olanzapine may be warranted (Zobor et al., 2002).

Seizures. Risk of seizure with olanzapine use is approximately 0.9%. Clomipramine (Anafranil) and other drugs such as bupropion and clozapine, which may induce seizures, should be avoided.

Hyperprolactinemia. High prolactin levels are associated with higher doses of olanzapine.

Quetiapine

Quetiapine is a dibenzothiazapine derivative with weak affinity for serotonin 5-HT_{1A}, 5-HT, dopamine D_1, D_2, histamine H_1, adrenergic α-1, and α-2 receptors. Quetiapine has no appreciable affinity for cholinergic muscarinic and benzodiazepine receptors.

Clinical Use

The recommended initial dose of quetiapine is 25 mg twice a day, with increases in increments of 25 to 50 mg twice or three times a day on the second or third day, as tolerated, to a target range of 300 to 400 mg daily on the third or fourth day. Subsequent titration should generally occur in no less than 2 days with 50-mg increments. The usual dosage range for treatment of schizophrenia is 150 mg to 750 mg/day. Doses greater than 800 mg/day are not recommended.

Side Effects

Sedation. Sedation is due to the H_1-antagonistic effect. Sedation and psychomotor slowing are dose dependent, and clients become more tolerant to this side effect with time.

Cardiovascular Effects. Because of the α-1 adrenergic antagonism, orthostatic hypotension with symptoms of dizziness, tachycardia, and syncope is common. Hypotension may occur especially during the initiation of quetiapine. Quetiapine should be avoided in clients with cardiovascular diseases or other illnesses predisposed to hypotension. Postural hypotension is common during the initial titration period and can be minimized by a slower titration of 25 mg twice a day, smaller dosage increments, or a return to the previous dose titration. Older clients should be carefully monitored to prevent falls.

Cataracts. Development of cataracts has been rarely associated with quetiapine. It is recommended that the client receive an ocular examination to detect possible cataract formation at the initiation of therapy and regularly thereafter.

Weight Gain. Weight gain is not as significant with quetiapine as with olanzapine.

Cholesterol and Triglycerides Elevations. Elevated cholesterol and triglyceride levels have been associated with quetiapine and occur with and without weight gain. Cholesterol and triglyceride levels should be monitored regularly with these clients.

Ziprasidone

Ziprasidone is a benzisothiazoyl piperazine derivative. Ziprasidone is a serotonin (5HT)-2$_A$/dopamine D_2 antagonist. It is also a 5HT-$_{1A}$ agonist and therefore has greater protection against adverse EPS. Ziprasidone also inhibits norepinephrine reuptake.

Clinical Use

The recommended starting dose of ziprasidone oral capsule is 20 mg twice a day to be taken with food. It should be titrated with increments of 20 mg every 2 days up to 80 mg twice a day. An increase in dose over 80 mg twice a day is not recommended.

Ziprasidone for injection is indicated for the treatment of acute agitation for clients with schizophrenia when the use of ziprasidone is appropriate and when a rapid control of agitation is needed. *Psychomotor agitation* is defined in DSM-IV-TR as "excessive motor activity associated with a feeling of inner tension" (APA, 2000). Schizophrenic clients experiencing agitation frequently manifest behaviors that interfere with their diagnosis and care (e.g., threatening behaviors, escalating or urgently distressing behavior, or self-exhausting behavior). Ziprasidone injection may be used to control acute agitation.

New Products

Ziprasidone Injection. Ziprasidone injection has been approved by the Food and Drug Administration (FDA) and became available in the U.S. market in September 2002. It is the first atypical antipsychotics available as an injection (Tandon, 2000).

Preparation of Administration

Ziprasidone is available as a single-dose vial, which requires reconstitution before administration. Any unused portion must be discarded, as the reconstituted drug is not stable for future use. A 1.2-ml amount of sterile water for injection should be added to the vial. The vial should be shaken vigorously until the drug is dissolved. The resulting volume in the vial is 1.5 ml, and each milliliter of reconstituted ziprasidone contains 20 mg. The major disadvantage of ziprasidone injection is its cost.

Risks and Contraindications

Because of ziprasidone's dose-related prolongation of the QT interval and the known association with fatal arrhythmias with QT prolongation by some other drugs, it is contraindicated in clients with a known history of QT prolongation (including congenital QT syndrome), recent acute myocardial infarction, or uncompensated heart failure (Glassman and Thomas Bigger, 2001).

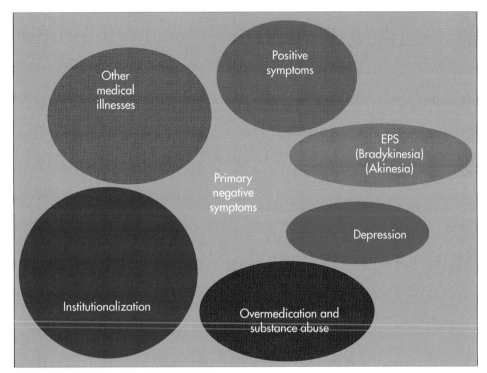

FIGURE 20-2. Primary negative symptoms.

Ziprasidone should be avoided in combination with other drugs that are known to prolong the QT interval. Certain circumstances may increase the risk of occurrence of torsades de pointes and/or sudden death in association with the use of drugs that prolong the QT interval, including (1) bradycardia; (2) hypokalemia or hypomagnesemia; (3) concomitant use of other drugs that prolong QT interval, including quinidine, sotalol, other class Ia and III antiarrhythmics, mesoridazine, thioridazine, chlorpromazine, pimozide, pentamidine, tacrolimus, and others; and (4) presence of congenital prolongation of the QT interval.

Side Effects
The most common side effects are GI discomfort, including nausea, dyspepsia, constipation, diarrhea, and dry mouth. CNS side effects include drowsiness, akathisia, dizziness, EPS, dystonia, and hypertonia. Cardiovascular side effects include tachycardia and postural hypotension. Dermatologic side effects include rash and fungal dermatitis. Other side effects include abnormal vision and upper respiratory infections.

Side effects associated with intramuscular injections include pain at the injection site, headache, postural hypotension, bradycardia, nausea, constipation, dizziness, drowsiness, and sweating.

Inappropriate Use of Atypical Antipsychotics
- Combination with another atypical antipsychotics
- High doses: may increase side effects and may be more expensive

Figure 20-2 describes the negative symptoms overlapping depression, EPS, overmedication and substance abuse, institutionalization, other medical illnesses, and positive symptoms.

SUMMARY
In general, antipsychotic medications should be administered initially in divided doses to minimize side effects and to determine the client's ability to tolerate the medication. Once an effective dose has been established, the dosage regimen should be simplified to once a day dosing. Studies have shown that client medication adherence and compliance improve with daily dosing or less frequent dosing.

In general, antipsychotic medications are well absorbed in the GI tract. To improve adherence and compliance, liquid doses are available, and olanzapine is available in an oral rapidly disintegrating tablet form, which readily dissolves on the tongue. It is generally not necessary to obtain blood samples to determine the drug concentration in the blood. However, serum levels are indicated in specific situations, such as lack of response despite titration to a normal dose range after an adequate trial period (6 weeks), severe or abrupt adverse drug reactions when client is seriously ill, or when lack of client compliance is suspected.

ANTIDEPRESSANTS
The first modern antidepressant medication, marketed in 1958, was imipramine. This tricyclic compound is a modification of the structure of the antipsychotic chlorpromazine.

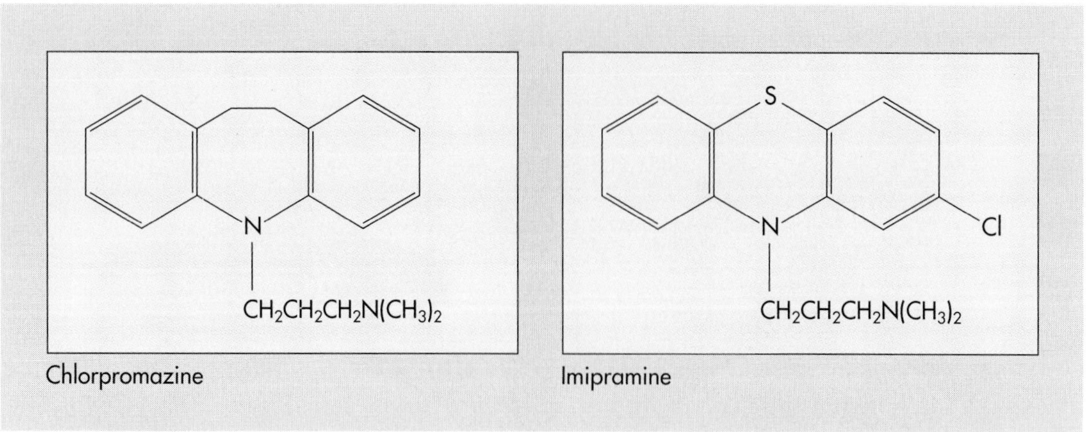

FIGURE 20-3. Chlorpromazine and imipramine are referred to as tricyclics because of their three-ring chemical structure.

The reason imipramine and similar drugs are called *tricyclics* can be readily seen by the compound's three-ring chemical structure (Figure 20-3). Dr. Roland Kuhn, a Swiss psychiatrist, originally administered imipramine to clients with schizophrenia and found no clinical efficacy. Astute observation and the persistence of Dr. Kuhn, who studied imipramine in clients with depression, quickly led to proving imipramine's efficacy in the treatment of depression. This success served as the catalyst for the search for additional antidepressant medications exhibiting improved efficacy and reduced side effects. At the same time, advances in the understanding of the role of serotonin in depression pointed toward a new class of antidepressants, the serotonin selective reuptake inhibitors (SSRIs).

INDICATIONS

The antidepressants have many therapeutic uses, but the primary approved use is to treat major depression as defined by DSM-IV (Katon and Sullivan, 1990). Antidepressants are also effective in the treatment of anxiety, OCDs, panic disorders, bulimia, anorexia nervosa, posttraumatic disorder syndrome, bipolar depression, social phobia, irritable bowel syndrome, enuresis, neuropathic pain, migraine headache, attention deficit/hyperactive disorder, smoke cessation, and autism.

BIOLOGIC THEORY

The biologic theory says that depression is caused by a decreased amount or inadequate function of the catecholamine neurotransmitters norepinephrine and/or serotonin. Antidepressant drugs affect the responses of these neurotransmitters. Presynaptic neurons synthesize these neurotransmitters, which are incorporated into vesicles. The action of the various antidepressants cause the vesicles to release their contents into the synapse. After they are released, neurotransmitters cross the synapse and impact receptors on the postsynaptic neuron. Most of the neurotransmitters are taken back into the presynaptic neuron to conserve this valuable resource. Then they reenter

the synthesis process and are incorporated into the vesicles for future use. The cyclic antidepressants partially block reuptake of norepinephrine and serotonin. Initially, this results in increased amounts of neurotransmitter in the synapse, which reduces the number of receptors on the postsynaptic membrane. This change in receptor density, called downregulation, can take several weeks to occur and is temporarily associated with the antidepressant response (Figure 20-4).

According to the biologic theory, a client who fails to respond therapeutically to an antidepressant may respond more favorably to a different antidepressant. It makes sense to switch to an antidepressant that more specifically affects the neurotransmitter that is associated with the client's depressed state. Even with the strength of the biologic hypothesis, a single theory cannot fully explain the etiology of depression. The efficacy of medications and the ability to measure the complex effects of neurons offer important clues toward better understanding of the causes of depression.

MAJOR CLASSES OF ANTIDEPRESSANTS
Selective Serotonin Reuptake Inhibitors

SSRIs remain first-line drug therapy for the treatment of depression (Celexa, 2000) because of their safety and favorable adverse effect profile. Unlike the tricyclic antidepressants (TCAs), there has been no fatality associated with an overdose of an SSRI. Escitalopram oxalate (Lexapro) is the newest SSRI approved by the FDA to be marketed in the United States (Lexapro, 2002).

SSRIs work by inhibiting the reuptake of 5-HT. This results in an increase of 5-HT concentrations in the synapse. There are six SSRIs approved by the FDA, including the newest escitalopram; more are being studied. Except for fluvoxamine, which is approved for use in anxiety, all the SSRIs are approved for the treatment of major depression disorder. All SSRIs are effective in the treatment of panic

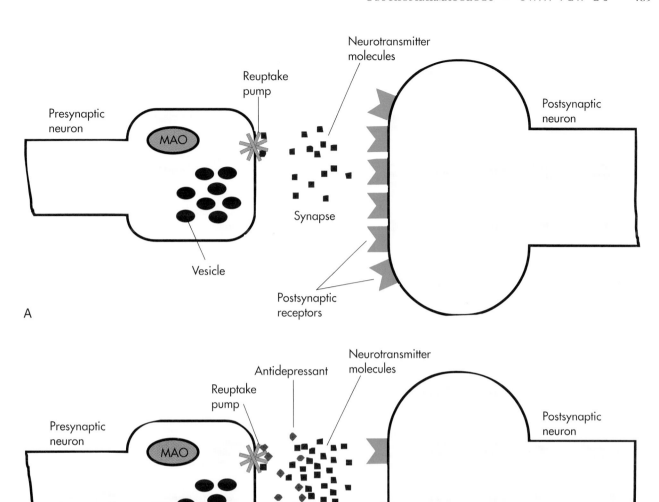

FIGURE 20-4. Neurotransmitter responses to antidepressant therapy. **A,** In the depressed state, sparse amounts of neurotransmitter are available in the synapse of a depressed person. **B,** With treatment, the reuptake of neuro-transmitter is blocked by the antidepressant drug *(in red).* The result is increased amounts of neurotransmitter in the synapse, and, finally, after several weeks the postsynaptic receptors have decreased (i.e., downregulated), which is associated with resolving depression. For the sake of clarity, this drawing omits numerous receptors and postsynaptic intracellular mechanisms that may ultimately prove to be important components of the pathophysi-ologic substrate of depression and antidepressant response.

disorders, OCDs, bulimia nervosa, social phobia, and post-traumatic stress disorders.

1. Citalopram (Celexa)
2. Escitalopram (Lexapro)
3. Fluvoxamine (Luvox)
4. Fluoxetine (Prozac)
5. Paroxetine (Paxil)
6. Sertaline (Zoloft)

Efficacy

The efficacy among SSRIs is similar. Choosing a particular antidepressant depends on the client's acceptance and toler-ance to the adverse effects and, to a lesser extent, cost. Ad-verse effects differ among the SSRIs mainly because of their differing affinities for the 5-HT receptor subtypes, including 5-HT_{2A}, 5HT_{2C}, 5-HT_3, and 5-HT_4. Some clients may toler-ate one antidepressant better than another, so it is important to assess the client thoroughly before choosing a particular drug. To maximize client acceptance and compliance with these medications, monitoring side effects is important and must be continued for the duration of therapy.

Half-Lives

The half-lives of SSRIs differ; this difference should be considered when choosing a particular dosing schedule. For example, fluoxetine has the longest half-life and an active metabolite, norfluoxetine, which prolongs the drug effect. This enabled the development of a **sustained-release** fluoxetine formulation that allows the client to take the drug once a week (Claxton et al., 2000). This is a convenient dosing schedule and should improve client compliance.

Cost

The cost of SSRIs should be taken into consideration. Fluoxetine is now available in generic formulation, although Prozac is the only fluoxetine that is available in a sustained-release formulation suitable to be taken once a week. Paroxetine is available in a sustained release, Paxil CR, but still requires a once a day dose. There is a slight advantage in using Paxil CR, as the slow-release formulation helps to reduce GI upset, but there appears to be no advantage compared to the regular Paxil formulation in the clinical setting, and Paxil CR cannot be cut or split in half to save cost.

Pill splitting or *cutting* can reduce the overall cost of some of the SSRIs. For example, paroxetine 20-, 40-, or 60-mg tablets are priced comparably regardless of the dose. By splitting or cutting in half the higher dose tablet, such as using half tablet of 40 mg for a 20-mg dose, the client can substantially reduce the cost of the medication.

Serotonin Syndrome

SSRIs are subject to a variety of drug interactions because of a complex metabolism process. The potential drug interactions of SSRIs with other drugs that also affect serotonin may lead to the serotonin syndrome, which can be life-threatening. Interacting drugs include monoamine oxidase inhibitors (MAOIs), dextromethorphan, meperidine, and sympathomimetics. The clinical signs of serotonin syndrome include confusion, hypomania, restlessness, myoclonus, hyperreflexia, diaphoresis, shivering, tremor, and diarrhea.

Serotonin syndrome is treated in an acute care hospital setting by the following:

- Discontinuation of medications causing the increase in serotonin
- Supportive measures such as cooling blanket for hyperthermia, benzodiazepines (e.g., clonazepam) for myoclonus (sudden twitching of muscle or muscle parts without any rhythm or pattern), anticonvulsants for seizures, and antihypertensives for increased blood pressure

Adverse Effects of Selective Serotonin Reuptake Inhibitors

The most common side effects are mild. They may be more severe at the initiation of treatment, but lessen or become more tolerable with time. These include GI upset, insomnia, restlessness, irritability, headache, and sexual dysfunction (Fava and Rankin, 2002). If sexual dysfunction is significant, switching to an antidepressant not associated with sexual dysfunction, such as bupropion or nefazodone, should be considered.

SSRIs have been associated with EPS including akathisia, dystonia, and bradykinesia. The SSRIs are not lethal in overdose; this is considered an advantage over other antidepressants such as the TCAs, especially for the client with suicidal risk.

Discontinuation of Therapy

A withdrawal syndrome can occur and the SSRI should be tapered off gradually over 2 to 4 weeks. Symptoms of the withdrawal syndrome include severe headache, GI upset, dizziness, impaired concentration, flulike symptoms, insomnia, and anxiety. Table 20-5 lists side effects of all antidepressants with nursing interventions.

Tricyclic Antidepressants

- Amitriptyline (Elavil)
- Clomipramine (Anafranil)
- Desipramine (Norpramin)
- Imipramine (Tofranil)
- Nortriptyline (Aventyl)
- Protriptyline (Vivactil)
- Trimipramine (Surmontil)

The tricyclics (TCAs) were the first widely used antidepressants to treat depression; however, they have an unfavorable adverse effects profile. With the emergence of the SSRIs, the TCAs have become second-line therapy. This class of antidepressants acts by blocking the reuptake of 5-HT and norepinephrine.

The tertiary amines are frequently metabolized to secondary amines, and the secondary amines are more potent in blocking the reuptake of norepinephrine. This is why the use of tertiary amine TCAs also produces norepinephrine response even though they are primarily active with blocking serotonin reuptake.

TCAs also act on other receptors. These actions contribute to the adverse effects, including antihistaminic, anticholinergic, and effects on cardiac conduction.

Anticholinergic Side Effects

All TCAs have substantial anticholinergic side effects, such as dry mouth, blurred vision, GI upset, constipation, and urinary retention. Among the TCAs, desipramine and nortriptyline have the least intense anticholinerigic side effects. All tricyclics are very sedating and are usually taken at bedtime. Because they can cause cardiotoxicity, an ECG is recommended before the initiation of therapy and should be re-

Table 20-5 Side Effects of Antidepressants With Nursing Interventions

Side Effect	Nursing Interventions
Anticholinergic Effects	
Dry mouth	Offer sugarless gum and candy, artificial saliva. For persistent problems treat with pilocarpine 1% rinse and spit (4 drops of 4% pilocarpine and 12 drops water) or bethanechol (Duvoid, Urecholine) 5 mg sublingual or 10-30 mg qd-bid.
Blurred vision: disturbance of presbyopia (near vision), far vision usually preserved	Ask if vision prescription is current; try pilocarpine 1% eye drops or bethanecol 10-30 mg tid.
Urinary retention	When not caused by benign prostatic hypertrophy (BPH) may be treated with bethanecol 10-30 mg tid.
Constipation	Prevention: encourage fluids (medication givers may offer), fruits and vegetables, mild physical exercise (walks). Treat with bulk-forming laxatives (e.g., Metamucil 1-2 tablespoons qAM or docusate 100 mg qd-bid). Avoid stimulant laxatives when possible; if needed, limit duration to avoid laxative dependence. Or treat with bethanecol 10-30 mg qd-bid.
Anticholinergic delirium (also known as atropine psychosis)	Monitor for agitation restlessness, psychotic signs and symptoms, myoclonic jerking. May occur with or without peripheral anticholinergic signs. Hold anticholinergic drugs. Physostigmine 5 mg IV can rapidly reverse but requires life-support backup and cardiac monitoring.
α-Blockade	
Orthostatic hypotension	Consider other contributing factors such as low-salt diets, restricted fluid intake, dehydration. Antihypertensive medications may exacerbate. Advise client to change positions slowly, dangle feet 1 minute in sitting position when rising from prone; sit immediately when lightheaded. Offer support hose, exercise to strengthen calf muscles to improve venous return.
Sexual Dysfunction	Obtain a clear history that the complaint does not predate the depression or medication use.
Decreased libido	Neostigmine 7.5-15 mg 30 minutes before anticipated intercourse.
Impaired erection	Often an anticholinergic problem; change to less anticholinergic drug or try bethanecol.
Priapism	Rare disorder associated with trazodone. Prolonged painful, nonsexual erection. Medical urgency treated with epinephrine injections to the corpus cavernosa. May require surgical intervention leading to permanent impotence.
Impaired ejaculation	May require switching drug. Try Neostigmine 7.5-15 mg 30 minutes before anticipated intercourse.
Inhibition of orgasm	Less serotonergic drug. Try cyproheptadine 4 mg qd. Note that cyproheptadine, a serotonin antagonist, has caused loss of antidepressant efficacy in some clients. The addition of buproprion has been used successfully.
Hematologic	
Agranulocytosis	Exceedingly rare allergic reaction usually occurring in the first 3 months of treatment. Monitor for fever, sore throat, mucosal ulceration, weakness. Discontinue drug, change to different chemical class.
Petechia, ecchymosis, easy bruising, bleeding	Associated with selective serotonin reuptake inhibitor (SSRI) effect on platelet. May occur with normal or decreased platelet counts. Discontinue drug. Monitor CBC, dizziness, lightheadedness.
Other	
Weight gain	Associated with cyclic antidepressants and monoamine oxidase inhibitors. Recommend diet and exercise. Treat with diuretics (e.g., hydrochlorothiazide for edema).
Weight loss	Associated with SSRI; rarely clinically significant.
Tremor	Advise caffeine may exacerbate. Determine degree of interference with daily activities. Propranolol 10-20 mg tid-qid may be useful.
Antidepressant withdrawal	Anticholinergic rebound can result in GI upset, cramps, diarrhea. Educate client on potential withdrawal symptoms. When discontinuing, taper slowly over several weeks. SSRI withdrawal symptoms include nausea, lightheadedness, dizziness, faintness, fatigue, parasthesias, flulike syndrome. Taper slowly.

From Andrews JM, Nemeroff CB: Contemporary management of depression, *Am J Med* 97(6A):24S, 1994; modified from Pollack MH, Rosenbaum JF: Management of antidepressant-induced side effects: a practical guide for the clinician, *J Clin Psychiatry* 48(1):3, 1987.

peated periodically. TCAs can cause orthostatic hypotension. Clients, especially older inidivduals, should be instructed to rise slowly to prevent falls. Another disadvantage of TCAs is the risk of fatality with an overdose, particularly in clients with suicidal risk.

Monitoring Parameters

Therapeutic blood level monitoring is useful to confirm that the administered dose is maintaining serum drug concentration within the effective range and to prevent toxicity and serious adverse effects.

Box 20-5	Time Course of Response to Antidepressants

First Week
Decreased anxiety
Improved sleep
Client often unaware of these changes

1 to 3 Weeks
Increased activity, sex drive, self-care
Improved concentration, memory
Psychomotor retardation resolves

2 to 4 Weeks
Relief of depressed mood
Less hopelessness
Suicidal ideation subsides

Box 20-6	Dietary Restrictions for Clients Taking Monoamine Oxidase Inhibitors

Prohibited
Aged cheeses
Ripe avocados
Ripe figs
Anchovies
Bean curd/fermented beans
Broad beans (fava/Italian)
Yeast extracts and yeast-derived vitamin supplements
Liver
Delicatessen meats (especially sausage)
Pickled herring
Meat extracts (Marmite, Borvil)
Fermented foods
Chianti and sherry

Allowed with Moderation
Beer and ale (tyramine content varies with brand and can be especially high in imported beers and some nonalcoholic beers)
White wine/distilled spirits
Cottage cheese, cream cheese
Coffee (<2 cups/day)
Chocolate
Soy sauce (tyramine content varies with brand)
Yogurt and sour cream
Spinach, raisins, tomatoes, eggplant, plums

Discontinuation of Therapy

TCAs should be tapered for discontinuation. Abrupt withdrawal can lead to a withdrawal syndrome with GI complaints, dizziness, insomnia, and irritability. The dose should be reduced by 25 to 50 mg/week to minimize withdrawal symptoms. Box 20-5 explains the time course of response to antidepressants.

Monoamine Oxidase Inhibitors

Iproniazid, an antitubercular drug in the 1950s, was a MAOI. Some clients receiving iproniazid were noted to become euphoric. This observation ultimately led to the use of MAOIs as antidepressant agents. The use of MAOIs has been limited as a result of the side affects and dietary modifications. Thus investigation for antidepressant agents continued.

Mode of Action

The neurotransmitters norepinephrine, serotonin, and dopamine are chemically described as monoamines. In the CNS these molecules are synthesized inside the presynaptic neuron. Maintenance of cellular homeostasis requires a mechanism to degrade monoamines. Monoamine oxidase is an enzyme found in the mitochondria of cells that participates in the normal process of degradation of these amines; MAOIs inhibit this enzyme. This inhibition initially results in increased availability of these neurotransmitters. As with other antidepressants, these initial neurotransmitter increases result in postsynaptic receptor downregulation that is temporally related to antidepressant response.

Clinical Use and Efficacy

MAOIs are indicated in the treatment of atypical (novel) depression, major depression without melancholia, or depressive disorders resistant to TCAs. Atypical depression is characterized by hypersomnia, hyperphagia, anxiety, and the absence of vegetative symptoms. In addition, MAOIs have been used with variable success in the treatment of other disorders such as certain anxiety disorders, eating disorders, and some pain syndromes (e.g., migraines).

MAOIs are rapidly absorbed, metabolized in the liver, and have average half-lives of approximately 24 hours. A majority of individuals metabolize MAOIs relatively slowly. This metabolic difference among individuals results in wide variation with respect to required doses for efficacy and sensitivity to side effects at a given dose. There is no clinically available test for this metabolic rate. Thus many clinicians begin MAOI therapy with a 10- or 15-mg test dose. Vital signs and complaints of side effects are monitored closely before beginning titration.

Contraindications to the use of MAOIs include cerebrovascular defects, major cardiovascular disease, and pheochromocytoma (tumor of the adrenal medulla). Older clients do not tolerate MAOIs well, so use is uncommon in individuals over 65 years old. MAOIs have been known to worsen symptoms of Parkinson's disease, induce manic states in bipolar clients, and exacerbate psychotic symptoms in clients with schizophrenia. Clients with diabetes may require adjustment of their hypoglycemic medication. MAOIs are contraindicated in pregnancy.

The use of MAOIs requires additional considerations. As with cyclic antidepressants, initial dosing must be titrated to give clients time to tolerate side effects. Table 20-6 lists initial and maintenance dosing ranges. Clients taking MAOIs must comply with a tyramine-restricted diet (Box 20-6) and must avoid stimulant medications to prevent the risk of a potentially fatal hypertensive crisis. Thus the client's ability to

Table 20-6   Antidepressant Dosing

Generic (Trade Name)*	Starting Dose (mg/day)	Maintenance Dose (mg/day)	FDA Indications
Cyclic Antidepressants			
Tricyclics			
Amitriptyline (Elavil, Endep)	25-50	100-300	
Clomipramine (Anafranil)	25	100-250	
Desipramine (Norpramin)	25-50	100-300	
Doxepin (Sinequan)	25-50	100-300	
Imipramine (Tofranil)	25-50	100-300	
Nortriptyline (Aventyl)	25-50	100-300	
Maprotiline (Ludiomil)	50	100-225	
Protriptyline (Vivactil)	10	15-60	
Trimipramine (Surmontil)	25-50	100-300	
Tricyclic Dibenzoxazepine			
Amoxapine (Asendin)	50	100-400	
Triazolopyridines			
Nefazodone (Serzone)	200	300-600	
Trazodone (Desyrel)	50	150-500	
Piperazinoazepine			
Mirtazapine (Remeron)	15	15-45	
Monoamine Oxidase Inhibitors			
Phenelzine (Nardil)	15	15-90	
Tranylcypromine (Parnate)	10	10-40	
Serotonin-Selective Reuptake Inhibitors†			
Citalopram (Celexa)	20	20-40	Depression only
Fluvoxamine (Luvox)	50	100-300	Obsessive-compulsive disorder only
Fluoxetine (Prozac)	5-20	20-80	Obsessive-compulsive disorder, bulimia nervosa
Paroxetine (Paxil)	10-20	20-50	Obsessive-compulsive disorder, panic
Sertraline (Zoloft)	50-100	50-200	Obsessive-compulsive disorder, panic
Indolamine			
Bupropion (Wellbutrin)	200	300-450	
Phenylethlyamine			
Venlafaxine (Effexor)	75	150-350	

*Use about half the dose for the elderly.

†Note FDA indications in addition to depression.

comply with dietary and medication restrictions is an important consideration before initiating therapy. Response to therapy may take 3 to 6 weeks. Except in emergencies, discontinuations should be tapered.

Side Effects

Orthostatic hypotension is a common initial and sometimes persistent side effect of MAOIs. Dangling feet on rising, changing positions slowly, wearing support stockings, and increasing fluid and salt intake can be effective treatments. A caffeinated drink in the morning may be useful as long as vital signs are monitored initially. Edema, sexual dysfunction, and weight gain are also common and can lead to drug

discontinuation. Complaints of insomnia occur with all MAOIs. Moving the last dose of the day to an earlier time may be helpful. Complaints of confusion or feeling drunk may indicate an excessive dose. Although these drugs do not have direct effects on cholinergic receptors, anticholinergic-type side effects (e.g., dry mouth, urinary hesitancy, constipation) are seen. Paresthesias (numbness, prickling, tingling feelings) may be caused by MAOI-induced pyridoxine (vitamin B_6) deficiency and is treated with oral pyridoxine.

Avoiding certain foods is essential when clients are taking MAOIs. Dietary tyramine is a precursor in the synthesis of norepinephrine. In the presence of an MAOI, foods high in tyramine (an amino acid by-product formed by the bacterial breakdown of tyrosine in fermented foods) can lead to a sharp increase in available norepinephrine and potentially fatal hypertensive crisis. Tyramine is not the only factor in food that can interact with MAOIs. For instance, fava beans contain dopamine, which can affect blood pressure in the presence of MAOIs (see Box 20-6). Previously, dietary restrictions for MAOIs were extensive and made compliance unlikely. Estimates of compliance with an MAOI diet have been as low as 40%. Yet, for several reasons, there are not an overwhelming number of MAOI hypertensive reactions. Foods, different brands of prepared foods, and a client's susceptibility to this interaction all vary widely. For instance, although a cup of coffee may elevate blood pressure and cause headaches in some clients, others taking MAOIs benefit from a cup of coffee as an adjunct to treat hypotension on awakening. Thus client education should consist of simple, clear, written and verbal instructions to absolutely avoid certain foods. Warnings of other foods that may cause problems in some clients or when taken in large quantity should be reviewed. Dietary restrictions should be maintained for 2 weeks after MAOIs are discontinued. All clients need to know the warning signs of hypertensive crisis, which include headache, stiff neck, sweating, nausea, and vomiting. Clients with such symptoms should seek medical attention immediately.

Many drugs can also interact with MAOIs and can lead to a hypertensive crisis or dangerous hypotension. These drugs are listed in Box 20-7. Many over-the-counter medications may be dangerous when taken with MAOIs, including diet pills, nasal decongestants, asthma medications (including inhalers), and cough suppressants (dextromethorphan). Literally hundreds of over-the-counter and prescription combination products under many different brand names contain sympathomimetics that are unsafe to use with MAOIs. Therefore every client taking an MAOI must be educated to consult a physician, dentist, nurse, or pharmacist before taking any additional medication. Although hypertensive events

are generally more dangerous and more common, the response to a sympathomimetic medication or dietary indiscretion can be hypotension rather than hypertension. Whether a hypotensive or hypertensive reaction ensues is a function of the overall adrenergic tone of the client and is not predictable.

Treatment for hypertensive crisis may be started with nifedipine (Procardia, Adalat) 10 mg. Absorption from oral administration is extremely rapid, and reductions of blood pressure may be seen in a matter of minutes. Vital signs should be monitored every 10 to 15 minutes until the client is stable. Other therapies that have been used include the α-adrenergic blockers phentolamine (Regitine) 5 mg intravenous, and chlorpromazine 50 mg PO.

Clients who fail to respond to a non-MAOI antidepressant should usually wait at least 2 weeks before starting an MAOI. An important exception to this is fluoxetine. Because of the long half-life of fluoxetine and its active metabolite norfluoxetine (approximately 7 to 10 days), clients discontinuing fluoxetine should wait at least 5 weeks before starting an MAOI.

Drug-Drug and Drug-Food Interactions

MAOIs have significant drug-drug and drug-food interactions. They are not first-line agents and are reserved for refractory depression.

Drug interactions can be significant. Many of the over-the-counter drugs such as cold and cough preparations contain sympathomimetics and must be avoided. Combinations with other antidepressants such as TCAs are contraindicated because hypertensive crisis may occur. Other antidepressants, if used in combination, must be used with extreme caution and monitored closely. When switching from MAOI to another antidepressant, a 2-week washout period is needed. When switching from another antidepressant, it is necessary to wait 2 weeks after the antidepressant is stopped before starting a MAOI. In the case of fluoxetine, which has a longer half-life, a 6-week interval is recommended.

In general, this class of medication is not suitable for clients with suicidal risk and/or inability to follow the rigid regimen of diet restrictions.

Client Education

Careful and thorough client education and monitoring are required. Clients must be instructed to avoid foods high in tyramine (Hedberg, Gordon, and Glueck, 1966) and be extremely cautious in taking other medications, especially over-the-counter cold and cough medications.

Monoamine Oxidase Inhibitor Withdrawal Syndrome

MAOIs should not be discontinued abruptly. Abrupt withdrawal symptoms may include nausea, sweating, palpitation, nightmares, hallucinations, delirium, and paranoid psychosis.

Box 20-7	Drugs to Avoid When Taking Monoamine Oxidase Inhibitors

Antiasthmatics
  Theophylline and inhalers containing epinephrine or β-agonists (e.g., albuterol [Proventil, Ventolin])
Antihypertensives
  Methyldopa (Aldomet), guanethidine (Ismelin), reserpine
Anesthetics with epinephrine
Allergy, hayfever, cough and cold products, decongestants, diet pills (many combination over-the-counter products; look for inclusion of phenylpropanolamine, ephedrine, phenylephrine, dextromethorphan)
Buspirone (BuSpar)
Meperidine (Demerol)
Serotonin selective reuptake inhibitors
  Fluoxetine (Prozac), sertraline (Zoloft), paroxetine (Paxil), fluvoxamine (Luvox), nefazodone (Serzone)
Yohimbine (Yocon)

OTHER ANTIDEPRESSANTS
Venlafaxine

Venlafaxine is often referred to as a serotonin norepinephrine receptors inhibitor (SNRI). Unlike TCAs, it does not affect other receptors that cause the undesirable adverse effects such as anticholinergic and antihistaminic side effects.

Because venlafaxine affects both serotonin and norepinephrine, it is often used in clients with less than optimal response to an SSRI (Thase, Entsuah, and Rudolph, 2001). It is also used in anxiety disorders (Gelenberg et al., 2000).

Formulations and Dosage

Venlafaxine is available in regular and sustained-release formulations (Prod Info Effexor, 2002). Regular tablets must be given two or three times a day. Venlafaxine XR, the sustained-release formulation, can be administered once a day. If the client cannot tolerate a single sustained-release dose, the dose can be divided to reduce side effects such as GI upset. The initial dose of regular release venlafaxine is 50 to 75 mg/day, administered in two or three divided doses with food. The dose may be increased by 75-mg increments every 4 days. Doses beyond 225 mg do not usually demonstrate increased efficacy; however, severely depressed clients may need up to 350 mg/day. The maximum recommended dose is 375 mg/day (Prod Info Effexor, 2002).

For the sustained-release formulation, the initial recommended dose for venlafaxine XR is 37.5 mg/day administered with food. The maximum recommended dose 225 mg/day (Prod Info Effexor, 2002).

Side Effects

The most common adverse effect is GI upset, which can be more significant in older clients. Venlafaxine can cause increases in blood pressure and should be used with caution in clients with uncontrolled hypertension. The increase in blood pressure is dose related. Other side effects are similar to those associated with the SSRIs, including insomnia, restlessness, headache, and irritability.

Nefazodone

This drug is chemically related to trazodone, but pharmacologically there are some differences. The drug is also referred to as a serotonin antagonist reuptake inhibitor (SARI). It is a 5-HT antagonist and also blocks 5-HT and norepinephrine reuptake.

Half-Life

The half-life is shorter and the drug must be taken two or three times a day. There is no extended formulation.

Dosage

The initial dose of nefazodone is 200 mg/day administered in divided doses of 100 mg twice a day. The dose may be increased by 100 to 200 mg/day (in two divided doses) at intervals of no less than 1 week, depending on client response and

tolerance. In clinical trials the effective dosage range was 300 to 600 mg/day (Prod Info Serzone, 2001). Clients with major depression have responded to a wide range of doses of nefazodone (100 to 600 mg/day in two or three divided doses) in clinical trials (Feighner et al., 1989; D'Amico et al., 1990). The highest dose of nefazodone administered in these trials was 750 mg/day (D'Amico et al., 1990). Meta-analysis of dosing data from pooled clinical trials indicated that most clients responded to nefazodone doses of 300 to 500 mg/day (Archibald, 1989; Balon, 1994). The recommended maximum daily dose for nefazodone is 600 mg (Balon, 1994).

Side Effects

The most common side effects are sedation, GI upset, dry mouth, constipation, and light-headedness. Sexual dysfunction is not a side effect of nefazodone; nefazodone is a viable alternative for clients experiencing sexual dysfunction as a result of SSRI therapy.

In 2002 the FDA issued a "black box warning" as a result of an increased risk of hepatoxicity associated with nefazodone. Fatality has occurred in a small percentage of clients. Hepatic function must be monitored and use of nefazodone should be avoided in clients with impaired hepatic function.

Drug Interactions

Nefazodone is metabolized by the enzyme cytochrome P450 3A4. This enzyme metabolizes the largest number of drugs used therapeutically. Significant drug interactions with many drugs can occur. Psychoactive drugs metabolized by 3A4 include alprazolam, diazepam, carbamazepine, and sertraline. Nonpsychoactive drugs metabolized by 3A4 include nifedipine, verapamil, protease inhibitors, tamoxifen, testosterone, cortisol, progesterone, and cyclosporine.

Potent 3A4 enzyme inhibitors include ketoconazole and the macrolide antibiotics such as erythromycin and clarithromycin. Nefazodone is contraindicated in combination with terfenadine because of enzyme inhibition and cardiotoxicity.

Saint John's Wort, an herbal antidepressant, has significant drug interactions with nefazodone, which diminishes the effectiveness of Saint John's Wort.

Trazodone
Mechanism of Action

Trazodone is an SSRI, and it also blocks serotonin ($5HT_{2A}$) receptors.

Therapeutic Use

Because of its sedative effects, trazodone is used as an agent to counteract insomnia.

Dosage

The therapeutic dosage range is 50 to 600 mg/day. Most clients respond to a dosage of 100 to 300 mg/day in single or divided daily doses (Rawls, 1982). The manufacturer recommends that therapy be initiated at a dose of 150 mg/day in divided doses and increased gradually, as needed, every 3 to 4 days in increments of 50 mg. Outpatient doses should not exceed 400 mg/day in divided doses. Inpatients may receive up to 600 mg/day in divided doses, but this dosage should not be exceeded. Clients should be maintained on the lowest effective dose (Prod Info Trazodone, 1998).

Side Effects

Sedation is a frequent and often intense side effect. Therefore trazodone is currently used as a hypnotic and an antidepressant adjunctive therapy to SSRI to counteract insomnia. The most frequent cardiovascular side effect during therapy is postural hypotension, which may be accompanied by syncope, especially in clients taking concomitant antihypertensive therapy (Rakel, 1987; Spivak et al., 1987). Adjustment of antihypertensive medication may be necessary if administered concurrently (Prod Info Trazodone, 1998).

A rare but serious side effect is priapism. *Priapism* is painful, persistent, abnormal penile erection, unaccompanied by sexual stimulation. This is an emergency and requires prompt medical attention.

Client Education

Sedation and the risk of fall, as well as orthostatic hypotension should be discussed with the client. Male clients should be warned of the potential serious side effect of priapism.

Bupropion
Mechanism of Action

Bupropion has inhibitory effects on dopamine and norepinephrine reuptake, and lesser effect on serotonin reuptake. It is commonly referred to as a norepinephrine-dopamine reuptake inhibitor (NDRI). The exact mechanism is unknown.

Half-Life and Dosing Schedule

Bupropion has a short half-life and must be dosed three times a day. An extended-release product is available and can be dosed once a day. The recommended initial dose of bupropion is 200 mg/day, administered as 100-mg doses once in the morning and once in the evening (Prod Info Wellbutrin, 2001). The recommended initial dose of bupropion sustained release is 150 mg given as a single daily dose in the morning. If the initial dose is tolerated, an increase to 150 mg twice a day is recommended as early as Day 4 (Prod Info Wellbutrin SR, 2001). To prevent the risk of seizure and adverse effects such as dystonia, the maximum single dose of bupropion SR is limited to 150 mg/dose and 450 mg/day, and the non-SR is 100 mg/dose. Minimum interval of dosage is 8 hours for SR formulation and 4 hours for non-SR formulation (Prod Info Wellbutrin, 2001).

Side Effects

Common side effects include nervousness, headache, and insomnia. Seizure is a significant risk; the dose must be titrated and the dosing schedule closely followed. Another common side effect is dystonia.

Other Therapeutic Uses

The drug is helpful with reducing cigarette and alcohol and drug craving (Chengappa et al., 2001). Zyban is the brand name of bupropion as labeled for use as an adjunct therapy for cigarette smoking cessation (Bupropion, 1997). Bupropion is an antidepressant often used in association with alcohol and drug detoxification and rehabilitation.

Mirtazapine
Mechanism of Action

Mirtazapine increases both norepinephrine and serotonin in the synapse. It also blocks serotonin receptors (Davis and Wilde, 1996).

Dosage

The recommended starting dose is 15 mg/day as a single dose. The dose should preferably be given in the evening before sleep. The effective dose range appears to be 15 to 45 mg/day. Dosage changes should not be made in less than 1- to 2-week intervals (Prod Info Remeron, 2000).

Other Uses

Mirtazepine, 15 mg orally, has been given the night before gynecologic surgery to reduce insomnia and to minimize presurgical anxiety.

Side Effects

The major side effects are sedation and weight gain (Gorman, 1999). Interestingly, sedation is more prominent with a lower dose. Weight gain is significant and can be used effectively in older clients. Other side effects include constipation. Serious but rare side effects include neutropenia, agranulocytosis, and hepatotoxicity. Regular monitoring parameters should include complete blood count and liver function tests.

AUGMENTATION THERAPY IN TREATMENT OF MAJOR DEPRESSIVE DISORDER
Psychostimulants
Dextroamphetamine and Methylphenidate

Psychostimulants such as dextroamphetamine and methylphenidate are not FDA approved for treatment of depression. The efficacy for adult treatment has not been determined because of a lack of controlled studies. Dextroamphetamine has been documented as effective in the treatment of depression with low energy in AIDS clients (DSM-III-R). In another study, dextroamphetamine was effective for treatment of poststroke depression. Researchers retrospectively evaluated 17 clients with poststroke depression treated with either dextroamphetamine or methylphenidate during a 5-year period (Masand et al., 1991). A total of 82% of clients improved on psychostimulants; 47% of clients demonstrated a marked or moderate improvement in depressive symptoms. No significant difference in efficacy existed between the two agents. Clients improved quickly within the first 2 days. Only three clients discontinued the psychostimulant treatment because of side effects. In another study, dextroamphetamine was used successfully to improve depression and low energy in 24 clients with AIDS (Wagner, Rabkin, and Rabkin, 1997).

Methylphenidate or dextroamphetamine may be used occasionally as antidepressants; both have been effective for treating depression in some older clients. The dose range is 5 to 40 mg/day for methylphenidate and 10 to 30 mg/day for dextroamphetamine.

Not all clients are suitable for treatment with these drugs, especially clients with potential for drug abuse. These drugs should also be avoided in clients already nervous, anxious, or psychotic.

Lithium

Lithium is indicated in refractory or treatment-resistant depression. Therapeutic blood level monitoring is required. Lithium should be used with caution in older clients and in clients with renal impairment.

Thyroid Therapy

Levothyroxine (T_4) is used. Thyroid function tests must be monitored.

Herbal Supplements

Saint John's Wort is a mild antidepressant commonly used in Europe and is gaining popularity in the United States. Caution is indicated when using Saint John's Wort in conjunction with antidepressants, as many drug-drug interactions are still being studied (Johne et al., 2002).

Nonpharmacologic Intervention
Electroconvulsive Therapy

Electroconvulsive therapy (ECT) involves the use of a series of electrically induced seizures to produce a clinical remission for clients suffering from severe major depression, schizophrenia, or mania. See Chapter 19 for more information on ECT.

BIPOLAR DISORDERS

DRUGS USED IN THE TREATMENT OF BIPOLAR DISORDERS

This section describes the role of lithium, valproate, carbamazepine, and other anticonvulsant mood stabilizers in the treatment of bipolar disorders. Many of the anticonvulsant mood stabilizers have risks of adverse drug reactions and drug interactions (Frances, Docherty, and Kahn, 1996).

Lithium

Lithium is a monovalent cation with antimanic, antipsychotic, and antidepressant activity. Lithium has been used in the treatment of bipolar mania for more than 50 years. It is most effective in the treatment of pure mania but is less ef-

fective in the treatment of mixed state (Bipolar Disorder, 1999).

Therapeutic Dosage Regimen

Lithium is usually started in low divided doses to minimize side effects. The dose is titrated according to response and the appearance of side effects, until serum lithium concentration is within the range of 0.5 to 1.2 mEq/L (Tohen and Grundy, 1999). A typical starting dose is 300 mg three times a day, depending on the client's age and weight. A typical optimal therapeutic dose for acute mania treatment is usually 1800 mg/day. The therapeutic range of serum lithium concentration for acute treatment is 0.8 to 1.2 mEq/L. For maintenance treatment, the dose is usually 900 to 1200 mg, and a therapeutic range of 0.6 to 0.8 mEq/L is generally acceptable. At this range side effects are usually tolerable, and there is therapeutic efficacy to prevent relapse. Lithium is dispensed through a variety of products (Table 20-7).

On a given dose regimen, lithium levels achieve a steady state after 5 days. Because of its narrow therapeutic index, lithium levels should be checked periodically at steady state and after each dose increase. It is appropriate to check lithium levels more frequently when rapid titration is needed, such as in the treatment of acute mania, and when toxicity is suspected. As levels reach the upper limits of the therapeutic range, they should be checked more frequently to minimize the risk of toxicity.

Older clients are more at risk for lithium toxicity, and the dose should be adjusted with the upper end of the therapeutic range of approximately 0.6 mEq/L.

In addition to monitoring serum lithium levels, other baseline and periodic monitoring should include the following: renal function, thyroid function, urinalysis, complete blood count with differentials, serum electrolytes, ECG, and weight. It is advisable to perform a pregnancy test for women of childbearing age before initiating lithium therapy. Renal function test should be ordered every 2 to 3 months

Table 20-7	Lithium Products	
Generic	**Trade Name**
Capsules	
150 mg lithium carbonate	
300 mg lithium carbonate	Eskalith, Lithonate
600 mg lithium carbonate	
Tablets (Scored)	
300 mg lithium carbonate	Eskalith, Lithane
Extended-Release Tablets	
300 mg lithium carbonate	Lithobid
450 mg lithium carbonate	Eskalith CR
Syrup	
Lithium citrate syrup 8 mEq/5 ml*	Cibalith-S syrup

*300 mg of lithium carbonate = 8.12 mEq of lithium.

during the first 6 months of therapy. Thyroid function tests should be ordered every 3 months during the first 6 months of therapy. Subsequently these tests should be performed once every 6 to 12 months, depending on the client's condition or change, such as breakthrough symptoms, increased side effects, or other clinical changes.

Pharmacokinetics

Absorption of oral lithium is rapid, with peak serum concentrations occurring in 30 minutes to 1 hour. The elimination half-life is about 24 hours and is prolonged in older clients and in clients with renal impairment. In all, 90% to 98% of a dose is excreted as unchanged drug in the urine. Box 20-8 describes lithium baseline monitoring.

Side Effects and Toxicity

As many as 75% of clients treated with lithium experience some side effects. Lithium toxicity is closely related to serum lithium levels but can also occur when levels approach the upper end of the therapeutic range. Some side effects are minor or can be reduced by lowering the dose. Side effects that are correlated to peak serum levels, such as tremor, can be reduced by changing to a slow-release formulation or by changing to a single bedtime dose. At levels less than 1.5 mEq/L and within therapeutic range, nausea, vomiting, diarrhea, polyuria, polydipsia, fine tremor, weight gain, hypercalcemia, and hyperkalemia can occur. Other persistent effects include exacerbation of acne, alopecia, weight gain, exacerbation of psoriasis, and increase in white blood cell count. At levels between 1.5 and 2 mEq/L, severe GI effects and neurotoxicity such as unsteady gait, lethargy and sedation, coarsening of tremors, confusion, and slurred speech can occur. At levels greater than 2 mEq/L, severe toxicities appear, including cardiovascular collapse (arrhythmias, atrioventricular block, bradycardia, and myocarditis), seizures, coma, and death. Adverse effects that appear during chronic use include hypothyroidism and, less frequently, renal tubular atrophy, interstitial fibrosis, and glomerular sclerosis.

Strategies for Management of Side Effects. Some of the strategies that have been used to manage persistent side effects include use of β-blockers to treat tremor, diuretics for polydipsia, polyuria or edema, topical antibiotics, or another acne preparation for acne. GI upset may be managed by changing the dose to a slow-release formulation or controlled-released formulation, or by giving lithium with meals.

If a diuretic is used, lithium dose should be reduced (sometimes up to 50%) because of increased intrarenal reabsorption induced by the diuretics. In addition, it is advisable to monitor electrolyte balance, in particular sodium and potassium. Amiloride is a potassium-sparing diuretic that does not alter the lithium level. The starting dose is 5 mg twice a day, and amiloride may have advantages over thiazide diuretics.

Lithium may induce hypothyroidism. Thyroid function tests should be performed and levothyroxine should be prescribed for these clients as appropriate.

Box 20-8	Lithium Baseline Monitoring

Vital signs
Weight
Blood chemistry (electrolytes)
Blood urea nitrogen/creatinine
Complete blood count with differentials
Urinalysis
Thyroid function test
Electrocardiogram
Pregnancy test (for women of childbearing age)

Exacerbation of psoriasis may be treated with dermatologic preparations. However, in some cases discontinuation of lithium is required.

Strategies for Managing Severe Toxicity and Overdose. As the serum level increases to greater than 2.5 mEq/L, the risk of permanent neurologic impairment is significant. It is important therefore to reduce the serum level rapidly. Hemodialysis is the only reliable method to rapidly reduce the serum level and is more effective than peritoneal dialysis. In acute poisoning, hemodialysis is required with lithium levels over 6 to 8 mEq/L, whereas hemodialysis is required at lithium levels above 4 mEq/L for those who have been on long-term therapy. Hemodialysis should be used when a client is more susceptible to underlying medical illness, or when a client deteriorates rapidly and is showing clinical signs of intoxication such as coma, convulsions, cardiovascular collapse, or respiratory failure. Clients should be monitored continuously, especially in the case of an overdose of sustained-release lithium, as manifestation of symptoms may be delayed. Box 20-9 describes serum lithium levels and side effects.

Clinical Use
Acute Treatment

- *Manic or mixed episodes:* Lithium has been proved effective for acute and prophylactic treatment of both manic and depressive episodes in clients with bipolar disorders. The first-line treatment is to combine lithium or valproate with an antipsychotic. For less ill clients, monotherapy with lithium, valproate, or an antipsychotic (atypical antipsychotic such as olanzapine or risperidone) is used. Benzodiazepines may be helpful as a short-term adjunctive treatment.
- *Rapid cycling:* For clients who have rapid cycling bipolar disorder (with four or more mood disorder episodes within 12 months), valproate plus an antipsychotic may be preferred over lithium.
- *Alternative therapy:* Carbamazepine or oxcarbazepine may be used instead of lithium or valproate.
- Antidepressants should be tapered or discontinued.
- Psychosocial therapy should be used in combination with pharmacotherapy.

Box 20-9   Serum Lithium Levels and Side Effects

Transient effects and mild toxicity:
    Fine tremor
    Gastrointestinal upset
    Mild polyuria, polydipsia
    Muscle weakness, lethargy
Persistent effects:
    Fine tremor
    Mild polyuria, polydipsia
    Increased white blood cell count
    Nontoxic goiter, hypothyroidism
    Exacerbation of psoriasis
    Acne
    Alopecia
    Weight gain
Effective acute treatment and prophylaxis—0.5-1.2 mEq/L
Moderate toxicity—lithium level >1.5 mEq/L:
    Coarsening of tremor
    Reappearance of gastrointestinal symptoms
    Confusion
    Sedation, lethargy
As levels increase:
    Ataxia
    Dysarthria
    Mental status deterioration
Severe toxicity—lithium level >2.5 mEq/L:
    Seizures
    Coma
    Death
    Cardiovascular collapse

Other Uses of Lithium

Lithium is also indicated for acute treatment of major depressive disorder, prevention of recurrent major depression, and treatment of cluster headaches.

Client Education

Client education should address potential side effects of lithium, as well as potential drug interactions. Clients should be counseled to avoid a salt-restricting diet, as well as potential drug interactions with thiazide diuretics, angiotensin-converting enzyme inhibitors, nonsteroidal antiinflammatory drugs, and cyclooxygenase-2 inhibitors.

Valproate

Divalproex, valproate, and valproic acid formulations are available in several dosage forms as different salts of valproate. Valproate is the common compound that is measured in the plasma.

Valproate is indicated for the treatment of manic episodes and is the first-line treatment for rapid cycling of bipolar disorder. It is more effective than lithium in treating bipolar disorder with prominent depressive symptoms. It is also effective in adjunctive treatment of schizoaffective disorder (Bogan, Brown, and Suppes, 2000).

Absorption, Distribution, Metabolism, and Excretion

Valproate is rapidly absorbed orally, with peak serum concentrations occurring within 4 hours. Therapeutic serum concentrations range from 50 to 125 μg/ml. Valproate is highly protein bound (i.e., approximately 90%). The cerebrospinal fluid levels are about 10% of corresponding serum levels. The elimination half-life is 6 to 17 hours. Valproate is metabolized extensively in the liver and excreted in the urine.

Dosage and Titration Regimen

It is generally advisable to start with a dose of 20 to 30 mg/kg per day in hospitalized clients. This can be administered on a divided dose regimen. After a serum level is obtained, the dose can be adjusted to a serum level of 50 to 125 μg/ml.

In the outpatient setting or in older clients, a starting dose of 250 mg three times a day may be used and titrated upward in 250-mg increments every few days up to a dose of 60 mg/kg per day and a serum concentration of 50 to 125 μg/ml. Once the client is stable, it is advisable to simplify the dose to once or twice a day to enhance client compliance.

Extended-release divalproex (Depakote ER) is available for once a day dosing. The bioavailability is 15% lower, so the dose may need a small adjustment upward. The extended release is also better tolerated.

Side Effects

Minor side effects include sedation and GI distress. These occur early in treatment and typically resolve with continued treatment or dose adjustment. Divalproex has a wider therapeutic range than lithium. Inadvertent overdose is uncommon, and accidental or intentional poisoning is less likely to be lethal than with lithium, making it a preferred choice over lithium for older clients. In rare incidences, however, valproate can cause serious adverse effects.

Common dose-related side effects include (1) sedation; (2) GI distress, nausea, vomiting, diarrhea, dyspepsia, and anorexia; (3) benign transaminase elevation; (4) osteoporosis; and (5) tremor. These side effects are often transient. Other side effects that are persistent include hair loss, increased appetite, and weight gain. Mild, asymptomatic leukopenia and thrombocytopenia may occur, but usually return to normal when therapy is discontinued.

Hepatotoxicity. Clients with a history of hepatic disease are at higher risk for hepatotoxicity. Hepatic failure has occurred mostly in children 2 years old or younger receiving multiple drug therapy. Life-threatening pancreatitis has been reported in both children and adults shortly after initial use and after several years of use. Baseline liver function tests are indicated before initiation of valproate therapy. Clinical signs of hepatotoxicity and laboratory levels of liver enzymes should be monitored.

Transient and mild elevation of liver enzymes, up to three times the upper limits of normal, do not require discontinuation of valproate. Transient elevated level of ammonia may also be common with valproate therapy. The dose of valproate may be reduced, and the client should be monitored carefully.

Persistent GI Distress. Indigestion, heartburn, and nausea are common side effects of valproate therapy. Taking the dose with food, or a reduction in dose, or change of formulation to divalproex instead of using valproic acid is generally helpful. Administration of a histamine-2 antagonist such as famotidine (Pepcid) may be helpful. If vomiting and severe abdominal pain develop, serum amylase level should be monitored, and the client should be carefully evaluated for pancreatitis.

Tremor. Essential tremor is a common side effect of valproate that can be reduced with dose reduction or by administering a β-blocker such as propranolol (40 to 160 mg in divided doses).

Sedation. This is a common side effect and is more prominent at the initiation of therapy. A more gradual titration may be needed. The once a day bedtime dose using an extended-release valproate may be useful.

Hematologic Effects. Mild leukopenia (total WBC count >3000/mm^3) is usually reversible on dose reduction or discontinuation. Mild cases of thrombocytopenia can be reversed with discontinuation, but more serious cases have occurred. For clients receiving anticoagulation therapy, an appropriate test of clotting function should be monitored closely.

Serious Adverse Effects. Rare, idiosyncratic, but potentially fatal adverse effects with divalproex include fatal hepatic failure, pancreatitis, and thrombocytopenia. Monitoring parameters include hepatic function and complete blood count on a regular basis, usually every 6 months.

Potential Drug-Drug Interactions

Valproate displaces highly protein-bound drugs from their binding sites, resulting in the increased blood levels of the drugs displaced. An example is the drug interaction of valproate with lamotrigine. Valproate interferes with the metabolism of lamotrigine by competing with the glucuronidation enzyme sites in the liver. As a result, valproate increases lamotrigine blood level twofold.

Client Education

Client education should include management of minor side effects as well as the signs and symptoms of hepatic and hematologic side effects. Clients should be advised to report these potentially serious side effects promptly.

Other Uses

Valproate is an anticonvulsant and is effective in the treatment of grand mal, petit mal, myoclonic, and temporal lobe seizures. The drug is much less effective for focal or com-

plex partial seizures. It is also indicated for prophylaxis of migraine headache and as an adjunctive therapy for pain management.

Carbamazepine

Carbamazepine and oxcarbazepine (Trileptal) are indicated as an alternative treatment for acute bipolar mania in lieu of lithium or divalproex.

Mechanism of Action

Carbamazepine is structurally related to imipramine, a TCA. It enhances GABA activity in the brain and inhibits glutamate and aspartate activity.

Carbamazepine possesses psychotropic effects and is less sedating than most anticonvulsants. The drug elevates mood in some depressed clients and is a second-line treatment for bipolar disorder. Although effective in psychiatric disorders, carbamazepine does not have a neurochemical profile resembling that of a classic antipsychotics. However, data suggest that carbamazepine may decrease dopamine turnover without directly blocking dopamine receptors.

Absorption, Distribution, Metabolism, and Excretion

Carbamazepine has a unique pharmacokinetic profile. Metabolism is known to occur via cytochrome P450 3A4 enzyme. Initially it has a half-life of approximately 36 hours. However, carbamazepine induces its own metabolism during treatment; this is complete within 3 to 5 weeks. After this period the half-life is about 24 hours. For this reason, the steady state is not reached until about 4 weeks after initial therapy. Also, with increasing carbamazepine doses in children, a dose-dependent autoinduction process occurs.

The therapeutic drug concentration of carbamazepine is 4 to 12 μg/ml.

Extended-release capsules taken every 12 hours provide steady-state plasma levels comparable to immediate-release tablets taken every 6 hours at the same milligram dose. Box 20-10 gives information on time to peak concentration for the various types of carbamazepine.

Absorption is as follows:
Oral, tablet: 70% to 79%
Oral, solution: 95.9%

Food increases bioavailability; therefore it is recommended that carbamazepine be given with food. Total protein binding is 76%. Unbound drug decreases with increasing total concentrations.

Box 20-10	Time to Peak Concentration for the Various Forms of Carbamazapine (Tegretol)

Immediate-release tablets: 4 to 5 hours
Chewable tablets: 6 hours
Extended-release tablets: 3 to 12 hours
Oral suspension (liquid): 1.5 hours

Dosage Regimen and Monitoring Parameters

Carbamazepine dose ranges from 200 to 800 mg/day. The dose is usually started at the lower end of the range and titrated upward according to response and side effect tolerance. In clients over 12 years old, carbamazepine is usually initiated at 200 to 600 mg/day in divided doses. Usual titration is to increase the dose by 200 mg/day. In hospitalized clients with acute mania, the dose can initially be titrated faster. Rapid titration may cause an increase in side effects such as drowsiness, dizziness, ataxia, and diplopia. Serum levels should be determined 5 days after a dose change, or sooner if toxicity is suspected. The maintenance dose range is 1000 to 1600 mg/day. Doses greater than 1600 mg/day are not recommended.

Baseline laboratory orders should include a complete blood count (CBC) with differential and platelet count; a hepatic panel with lactate dehydrogenase, serum glutamic-oxaloacetic transaminase, serum glutamate-pyruvate transaminase, bilirubin, and alkaline phosphatase; and renal function test. A pregnancy test is recommended for women of childbearing age.

Side Effects and Toxicity

Overdoses or undetected excessive accumulation of carbamazepine can be fatal. Signs of carbamazepine toxicity include dizziness, ataxia, sedation, and diplopia. Acute toxicity can result in stupor or coma. Treatment includes gastric lavage and management of symptoms.

Rare, idiosyncratic, but potentially fatal side effects include agranulocytosis, aplastic anemia, thrombocytopenia, hepatic failure, exfoliative dermatitis (e.g., Stevens-Johnson syndrome), and pancreatitis. Other serious side effects include cardiac conduction disturbances.

A CBC with differential and platelet count, as well as liver function tests are recommended every 2 weeks during the first 2 months of therapy. If the results of the tests are normal, the tests can be done every 3 months thereafter. However, whenever there are signs or symptoms of hepatic, hematologic, or dermatologic reactions, laboratory tests should be done more frequently.

Management of Side Effects. Minor side effects such as nausea can be managed by taking carbamazepine immediately before or after meals, by dividing the doses throughout the day, by changing to a sustained-release form, or by using a histamine-2 antagonist such as famotidine. Cimetidine (Tagamet) is not recommended because of potential drug-drug interactions.

Sedation and dizziness can be managed by decreasing the dose or shifting the dose to bedtime.

Client Education

It is important to counsel clients to monitor for signs and symptoms of hematologic and hepatic abnormalities so that they can be reported promptly. If a rash occurs, the client should be instructed to notify the physician promptly.

Drug-Drug Interactions

Carbamazepine induces the metabolism of many drugs, including its own, through induction of cytochrome P450 oxidation and conjugation. There are many drug interactions. Erythromycin, calcium channel blockers, and SSRIs may increase carbamazepine levels, whereas carbamazepine may decrease the levels of many other drugs including antipsychotics, some steroids, oral contraceptives, thyroid hormones, benzodiazepines, TCAs, and anticonvulsants.

Concomitant use of clozapine may increase the risk of aplastic anemia and should be avoided. Concomitant use of lithium may cause an acute state of confusion.

Oxcarbazepine

Oxcarbazepine has been shown to be as effective as carbamazepine in the treatment of bipolar disorder and is better tolerated. It should be considered an alternative for clients unable to tolerate carbamazepine, including those with hypersensitivity, although caution is advised in these clients (Bulau, Stoll, and Froscher, 1987).

Mechanism of Action

Oxcarbazepine is the 10-keto (10, 11-dihydro-co-oxo-carbamazepine) analog of carbamazepine.

Risks

Hyponatremia is a *major* concern with oxcarbazepine therapy, and may limit its use as an anticonvulsant and antineuralgic. The use of oxcarbazepine in diabetes insipidus has also been suggested, although data to support this use are not available (Pendlebury, Moses, and Eadie, 1989). The mechanism is thought to be due to an antidiuretic hormonelike action on the kidney. Most cases of hyponatremia are asymptomatic, although confusion and an increase in seizure frequency have been observed in some clients. Hyponatremia with oxcarbazepine occurs most commonly in older clients and during administration of high doses of the drug (Kloster et al., 1998; Van Amelsvoort et al., 1994; Steinhoff et al., 1992; Pendlebury, Moses, and Eadie, 1989; Houtkooper et al., 1987; Zakrzewska and Patsalos, 1989; Johannessen and Nielsen, 1987; Nielson et al., 1988).

Side Effects

Headache, drowsiness, dizziness, ataxia, tremor, abnormal gait, fatigue, sedation, encephalopathy, and oculogyric crises are described with administration of oxcarbazepine. Sedation, difficulty in concentration, and memory impairment are also associated with its use.

Hyperlipidemia, antidiuretic hormone effects, and altered reproductive hormones on thyroid function, as well as weight gain and effects on thyroid function are described with the administration of oxcarbazepine. Use of oxcarbazepine has been associated with decreases in T_4 hormone, but not in T_3 or thyroid-stimulating hormone (MICROMEDEX, 2003).

Lamotrigine

Lamotrigine has been studied in bipolar depression and in rapid cycling bipolar disorders. It has been found to be effective for both types of bipolar disorder (Botts and Raskind, 1999).

Dosage Titration and Risk

The initial dose of lamotrigine is 25 mg once a day and is increased in 25-mg increments every other week. When the client is taking valproate in addition to lamotrigine, the dose of lamotrigine should be reduced by half because of drug interaction. Lamotrigine requires a slow titration; the titration schedule must be followed to minimize the risk of skin rash. Approximately 5% of clients develop a maculopapular rash and approximately 0.1% develop Stevens-Johnson syndrome, which is often fatal.

Side Effects

Common side effects include headache, dizziness, GI distress, and blurred or double vision.

Drug Interactions

Significant drug interactions include interactions with valproate.

Gabapentin

Gabapentin (Neurontin) is a GABA analog. Gabapentin has been used for adjunctive therapy as a mood stabilizer (Neurontin, 1999) and for the treatment of partial seizures. It is also being used for social phobia. Gabapentin has many other uses, including adjunctive therapy in alcohol detoxification, anxiety disorder, cluster headache, dystonia, essential tremor, headache, migraine prophylaxis, myalgias, neuropathic cancer pain, nicotine withdrawal, obsessive-compulsive behavior, phantom limb syndrome, and pain management.

Absorption, Distribution, Metabolism, and Excretion

The bioavailability of gabapentin decreases with increasing dose. Its bioavailability is approximately 60% when dosed at 400 mg every 8 hours; bioavailability is reduced to 35% at a dose of 1200 mg every 8 hours.

Less than 35% of gabapentin is protein bound. The drug is not metabolized but is excreted unchanged in the urine.

Dosage

The maintenance dose is 300 to 600 mg three times a day. The maximum time between doses should not exceed 12 hours. The maximum dose is 800 to 1200 mg three times day. Gabapentin should be discontinued gradually to avoid rebound phenomena. Total daily dose is adjusted for renal function. Dose should be adjusted if the creatinine clearance is below 60 ml/min. The recommended dose is 300 mg twice a day for creatinine clearance of 30 to 60 ml/min and 300 mg/day for creatinine clearance of 15 to 30 ml/min.

Risks

Gabapentin is contraindicated in clients with pancreatitis and should be used cautiously in clients with renal impairment (Ramsay, 1994). If the drug is used, the dose should be adjusted accordingly. The dose should be titrated and tapered slowly to avoid rebound phenomena and precipitation of status epilepticus.

Side Effects

Hematologic side effects include leukopenia. Cardiovascular side effects include hypertension, vasodilation, and edema, including peripheral edema and facial edema.

Endocrine effects include fluctuations in blood sugar levels, so caution must be exercised in dosing diabetic clients. Weight gain associated with gabapentin use has been reported.

The most common side effects reported affect the CNS: ataxia, dizziness, involuntary movements, mania, neuropathy, pruritic rash, seizures, and somnolence. Other CNS adverse effects include fatigue, headache, diplopia, impaired concentration or memory, nystagmus, abnormal speech, and tremor.

Topiramate

Topiramate is a sulfamate-substituted monosaccharide and is indicated for treatment of epilepsy. Topiramate is an anticonvulsant and is used as an adjunctive therapy for partial seizures and generalized tonic-clonic seizures. It is not used as monotherapy for bipolar disorder but may be useful as an adjunctive therapy. Topiramate is also used in the treatment of binge eating, bulimia, cluster headache, trigeminal neuralgia, and Tourette's syndrome.

Absorption, Distribution, Metabolism, and Excretion

Topiramate is well absorbed after oral doses; peak serum concentration occurs in 2 to 4 hours. Food alters the rate of absorption, but not significantly. Topiramate is minimally bound to protein. The drug is not metabolized and is excreted unchanged in the urine.

Dosage

Topiramate dosage should be titrated slowly, with an initial dose of 50 mg/day for the first week and increased in 50-mg increments per week until a dose of 400 mg/day (in two divided doses) is reached. Slower titration is necessary to minimize side effects, primarily impaired cognitive function (Martin et al., 1999). Other side effects such as dizziness and drowsiness are also minimized with a slow titration.

The dosage of topiramate is 11 to 35 mg/kg/day for children 5 years or younger and 5.5 to 16.5 mg/kg/day for children 6 to 12 years old. The clearance of topiramate is 50% greater in children, which results in a shorter half-life. In children topiramate has a faster elimination rate, which results in a 30% lower plasma concentration as compared to adults. Topiramate has significant drug interactions with enzyme-inducing anticonvulsants. These result in an increased clearance rate and shorter half-life.

The dose must be adjusted in clients with renal impairment. In clients with creatinine clearance of less than 70 ml/min, 50% of the usual dose is adequate. The clearance of topiramate is decreased by 42% with creatinine clearance of 30 to 69 ml/min and by 54% with creatinine clearance of less than 30 ml/min.

Risks

Topiramate should be used with caution in clients with renal impairment, and the dose adjusted (Bialer, 1993). Topiramate may cause acute myopia and secondary close-angle glaucoma and should not be used in clients with glaucoma. Topiramate should be slowly tapered to avoid the risk of precipitating seizures.

Side Effects

Anemia has been reported with topiramate use. Cardiovascular effects include hypertension, postural hypotension, vasodilation, arrhythmias, palpitations, atrioventricular block, and bundle block.

The most common side effects of topiramate include drowsiness, dizziness, ataxia, speech disorders and related speech problems, psychomotor slowing, nystagmus, fatigue, nervousness, confusion, language problems, anxiety, and cognitive problems. Auditory hallucination has been reported.

NEW DRUG THERAPY IN THE TREATMENT OF BIPOLAR DISORDERS

Several newer anticonvulsants are being used in the treatment of bipolar disorders.

Tiagabine

Tiagabine is a GABA inhibitor for the treatment of partial epilepsy. Tiagabine binds to sites associated with the GABA uptake carrier. The result is that tiagabine blocks GABA uptake into presynaptic neurons, permitting more GABA to be available for receptor binding on the surfaces of postsynaptic cells. Tiagabine also possesses anxiolytic and analgesic properties, and is reported to have minimal effects on cognitive function.

Absorption, Distribution, Metabolism, and Excretion

Tiagabine has a bioavailability of 90%. The drug should be taken with food, which may slow its absorption rate. It is 96% protein bound. Tiagabine is metabolized in the liver, mainly by the enzyme cytochrome P450 3A. Tiagabine is excreted in the urine and feces: 25% is excreted in the urine and 63% in the feces.

Dosage

The usual adult dose for tiagabine is 32 to 56 mg/day in two to four divided doses. Dose adjustments may be needed in the presence of hepatic disease.

The recommended initial dose for adolescents 12 to 18 years old is 4 mg once a day and increased by 4 mg at the end of the first week. The dose may be increased by 4 to 8 mg in weekly increments.

Risks

Tiagabine should be used with caution in clients with liver disease. The dose should be tapered slowly to avoid rebound phenomena. There are many drug interactions with tiagabine. If generalized weakness occurs, tiagabine may need to be discontinued.

Side Effects

Cardiovascular effects include chest pain, hypertension, palpitation, tachycardia, edema, and peripheral edema. The most common side effects of tiagabine therapy include dizziness, difficulty with concentration, drowsiness, anxiety, and tremor. Depression is common, and other psychiatric symptoms may include aggression, emotional lability, and hallucinations. Tinnitus has also been reported. A significant number of clients (20% to 24%) experienced asthenia during clinical trials. About 1% of clients have significant weakness leading to falls or inability to walk. Common GI side effects include nausea, vomiting, and diarrhea. Tiagabine is also frequently associated with rhinitis.

Drug Interactions

There are many drug interactions with tiagabine, including drug interactions with carbamazepine, cimetidine, digoxin, erythromycin, and fosphenytoin. Herb-drug interactions reported to be associated with tiagabine include evening primrose oil and ginkgo.

Zonisamide

Zonisamide is a broad-spectrum anticonvulsant. It has not been studied in the treatment of bipolar disorder.

Mode of Action

The exact mode of action for zonisamide is not thoroughly understood, but may involve blockade of sodium and T-type calcium channels and the inhibition of carbonic anhydrase (Prod Info Zonegran, 2000). It is a structurally unique anticonvulsant. It lacks the ureide moiety common to many compounds in this class and is a sulfonamide derivative. Zonisamide does not potentiate the synaptic activity of GABA, but instead facilitates dopaminergic and serotonergic neurotransmission (Prod Info Zonegran, 2000).

Indications and Clinical Uses

Zonisamide is indicated as an adjunctive therapy for partial seizures in clients unresponsive to other anticonvulsants. The initial dose of 100 mg/day is titrated every 2 weeks to a daily dose of 200 to 400 mg, with a daily maximum dose of 600 mg.

Levetiracetam

Levetiracetam is a broad-spectrum anticonvulsant. It has not been studied in the treatment of bipolar disorders. It is used as monotherapy and as adjunctive therapy for the treatment of partial seizures in adults. Initial dose for the adjunctive treatment of partial onset seizures is 500 mg twice a day. Doses may be increased by 1000 mg/day every 2 weeks. The maximum recommended daily dose is 3000 mg. Dose adjustments are recommended in the presence of renal failure.

TREATMENT OF MANIA

The first step in treating mania includes the use of a mood stabilizer such as lithium or valproate. Atypical antipsychotics have been effective in treating mania, and olanzapine has been approved by the FDA for this use.

Several factors must be considered in selecting a particular mood stabilizer for treatment of mania including the client's past experience and success with a particular drug, family history of response, acceptance of side effects, concomitant medical problems, and other concurrent medications.

For clients with agitation associated with mania, a benzodiazepine is often added to the initial treatment regimen until the client is stabilized. High-potency benzodiazepines such as lorazepam and clonazepam can be used. Alprazolam is not used because its antidepressant effect may precipitate mania.

Atypical Antipsychotics for Mania

The atypical antipsychotics have been used to effectively treat mania. The atypical antipsychotics used include olanzapine, clozapine, quetiapine, risperidone, and ziprasidone. Currently olanzapine is FDA approved for this indication. The atypical antipsychotics are replacing haloperidol and conventional or typical antipsychotics. When haloperidol is used, a mid range dose is often adequate for treatment. A typical dose of haloperidol is 10 to 15 mg/day.

Combination of Mood Stabilizers

Lithium is sometimes combined with valproate for effective treatment of bipolar disorder in the manic phase. Use of valproate in combination with carbamazepine is generally best avoided because of drug interactions. If there are no other alternatives and the combination of valproate and carbamazepine must be used, the dose of valproate must be increased and the dose of carbamazepine must be lowered because of their mutual drug interactions.

Bipolar Depression

Treating bipolar depression is different from treating unipolar depression. The first attempt should be optimization of the mood stabilizer. Lithium is still the therapy of choice. Thyroid function tests should be monitored. Clinical signs of hypothyroidism include depression, which should be treated with thyroid hormone replacement therapy. If an antidepressant is to be used, the client should be carefully monitored, as this may predispose the client to mania. In general, SSRIs and bupropion are thought to be safer and TCAs should be avoided.

MAINTENANCE THERAPY AND LIFELONG INTERVENTION

Because clients with bipolar disorder are faced with the prospect of requiring lifelong medication therapy, the noncompliance rate is high. The goal of maintenance therapy is to prevent recurrence, and there is a fine balance between optimal therapy and client acceptance. The risk of relapse is high on discontinuation of a mood stabilizer, and the client often becomes refractory to treatment, even when the same drug is resumed. Therefore it is important to educate the client on the need for prophylactic treatment despite the lack of symptoms. To avoid noncompliance with medication, an acceptable level of side effects must be attained. A lithium dose between 0.8 and 1.0 mEq/L is an optimal level for maintenance therapy, but usually causes side effects. There are attempts to maintain a level of 0.4 to 0.6 mEq/L to reduce the side effects and correspondingly improve client compliance.

ANXIETY DISORDERS

Anxiety disorders are among the most prevalent psychiatric conditions. OCD is ranked tenth among the leading causes of disability in the United States and worldwide, costing billions of dollars in disability and lost wages. There is strong association between alcohol and drug abuse and anxiety disorders (Kushner, Sher, and Beitman, 1990). Direct and indirect costs of anxiety disorders in 1998 were estimated at $63.1 billion.

GENERALIZED ANXIETY DISORDER

Generalized anxiety disorder (GAD) is characterized by excessive worry, poor concentration and insomnia, and generally by an unidentifiable cause. Symptoms last more than 6 months, and the client may not be able to function in daily life. The lifetime prevalence is 5% (Kendler et al., 1992). Treatment options include antidepressants, benzodiazepines, and buspirone.

Antidepressants

Venlafaxine is an FDA-approved antidepressant drug for generalized anxiety disorder. The sustained-release formulation, Venlafaxine XR, is commonly used because of better compliance with the less frequent dosing schedule. It has a somewhat more rapid onset than other antidepressants. Other first-line drugs include SSRIs such as paroxetine, the TCA imipramine, nefazodone, and mirtazapine. Bupropion, an antidepressant with insignificant serotonin activity, is ineffective. The onset of action of these drugs is typically within 4 weeks.

The advantage of antidepressants over benzodiazepines is that these drugs are also effective for clients suffering major depression and other comorbid anxiety disorders. Other advantages include lower potential for abuse. The disadvantage compared to benzodiazepines includes longer onset of action (4 weeks versus 1 week or less) and less efficacy for physical or somatic symptoms of anxiety.

Antidepressant doses for GAD are similar to those for major depression. Gradual titration minimizes side effects and increases client compliance. Adverse effects of SSRIs and venlafaxine include GI upset, insomnia, irritability, headache, and sexual dysfunction. Imipramine has the side effects of TCAs, that is, anticholinergic effects, drowsiness, and dizziness. Nefazodone can cause drowsiness and liver toxicity.

Benzodiazepines

Clonazepam, lorazepam, and alprazolam are all FDA approved for use in GAD. The longer-acting benzodiazepine, clonazepam, is desirable because of its ease of dosing. It is given once or twice a day. The advantage of

benzodiazepine is its rapid onset (1 week or less). Disadvantages include cognitive impairment, decreased coordination, potential drug abuse, and withdrawal symptoms. In general, shorter-acting benzodiazepines are more difficult to taper and potentially cause more problems with withdrawal.

Buspirone

Buspirone is a 5-HT$_{1A}$ receptor partial agonist. It requires two or three times a day dosing. It is effective in generalized anxiety disorder, but does not appear to be effective in panic disorder.

The major disadvantage of buspirone is its longer onset, usually 2 to 4 weeks. Initial therapy includes the addition of benzodiazepines until the effect of buspirone is seen. Table 20-8 describes the therapeutic modalities of hypnotic and anxiolytic agents.

Table 20-8 Hypnotic and Anxiolytic Agents

Generic Name	Trade Name	Approved Indication	Approx. Benzodiazepine Equivalency (mg)	Active Metabolite	Usual Dosage Range (mg/day)	Half-Life Hours
Barbiturates						
Amobarbital	Amytal	Hypnotic	NA	—	100-200	8-42
Butabarbital	Butisol	Hypnotic	NA	—	50-100	34-42
Pentobarbital	Nembutal	Hypnotic	NA	—	100-200	15-48
Phenobarbital	Luminal	Hypnotic	NA	—	100-200	80-120
Secobarbital	Seconal	Hypnotic	NA	—	100-300	15-40
Benzodiazepines						
Alprazolam	Xanax	A, AD, P	0.5	No	0.75-4 (A) 4-10 (P)	12-15
Chlordiazepoxide	Librium	A, AW, PS	10	Yes	25-200	5-30
Clonazepam	Klonopin	LGS	2.5	No	1-6*	20-50
Clorazepate	Tranxene	A	7.5	Yes	7.5-90	20-80
Diazepam	Valium	A, PS, SE	5	Yes	2-40	20-80
Estazolam	ProSom	Hypnotic	2	No	1-2	10-15
Flurazepam	Dalmane	Hypnotic	15	Yes	15-30	8-40
Halazepam	Paxipam	A	20	Yes	20-160	10-20
Lorazepam	Lorazepam	A, PS	1	No	0.5-10	10-20
Oxazepam	Serax	A, AD, AW	15	No	30-120	5-20
Prazepam	Centrax	A	10	Yes	20-60	20-80
Quazepam	Doral	Hypnotic	2	Yes	30-50	30-50
Temazepam	Restoril	Hypnotic	15	No	15-30	10-20
Triazolam	Halcion	Hypnotic	0.25	No	0.125-0.25	1.5-5
Nonbarbiturate, Nonbenzodiazepine						
Buspirone	Buspar	A	NA		10-60	2-4
Chloral hydrate	Noetec	Hypnotic	NA		500-2000	8-11
Diphenhydramine	Benadryl	Hypnotic	NA		25-100	3-9
Doxylamine	Unisom	Hypnotic	NA		25-100	8-12
Ethchlorvynol	Placydyl	Hypnotic	NA		500-1000	18-20
Zolpidem	Ambien	Hypnotic	NA		5-10	1.5-4

A, Anxiety: AD, anxiety associated with depression; AW, alcohol withdrawal; LGS, Lennox-Gastaut syndrome (seizures); P, panic disorders; PS, psychotic disorders; SE, status epilepticus.
*Dosed up to 20 mg/day for seizure.

PANIC DISORDER

Panic disorder is characterized by periods of intense fear and persistent worry about impending doom. This is commonly associated with multiple physical complaints, fear of public places, specific phobias (examples are bridges, heights, or any environment that the client has associated with the fear of impending doom) and development of agoraphobia and depression. Lifetime prevalence is approximately 3.5%

Antidepressants

The SSRIs as a class are all effective in treating panic disorder. Paroxetine and sertraline are FDA approved, but effective first-line treatment includes all SSRIs. Initial dosing is at 50% of the usual dose and then titrated slowly upward. This approach is crucial for client tolerance, as research has shown that clients with panic disorder are initially very sensitive to the SSRI side effects, and these reactions can be confused with worsening of the anxiety. TCAs, particularly imipramine and clomipramine, are effective. It is important to start with a low dose for tolerability. MAOIs such as phenelzine (Nardil) are effective, but these drugs have many drug-drug and drug-food interactions and should be used with caution.

Benzodiazepines

Alprazolam offers rapid relief at a dose range of 2 to 6 mg/day that may be increased up to 10 mg/day. Clonazepam at a dose range of 1 to 4 mg/day or diazepam, 40 mg/day, have been shown to be effective. Clonazepam is longer acting and can be used on a once or twice a day schedule.

Anticonvulsants

Divalproex or gabapentin is used only for treating refractory panic disorders. The dose for divalproate is 500 to 2250 mg/day. Therapeutic blood level monitoring is recommended to minimize side effects. Gabapentin doses of 600 to 3600 mg/day have been used. Side effects of gabapentin include sedation, dizziness, and headache. Gabapentin has few known drug interactions.

Other anticonvulsants such as carbamazepine are being studied for this indication.

Beta-Blockers

Propranolol is sometimes used to block the peripheral symptoms of panic disorders.

OBSESSIVE-COMPULSIVE DISORDER

OCD has a lifetime prevalence of 2% to 3%, but clients can be severely affected in their daily functions. The disorder is characterized by obsessive or intrusive repetitive thoughts that one cannot control. Compulsions are ritualistic behaviors (e.g., washing hands). Clients suffering from OCD require both pharmacotherapy and nonpharmacologic interventions. Nonpharmacologic interventions include cognitive-behavioral approaches using exposure and response prevention. Drug therapy is effective but requires long-term continuation of therapy to prevent relapse.

Antidepressants

SSRIs and clomipramine are effective in treating OCD. SSRIs are preferred because of their more advantageous adverse effect profile and better client compliance. Fluvoxamine, fluoxetine, paroxetine, and sertraline are all effective. The choice of a particular SSRI depends on side effects and client tolerance. Potential drug interactions should also be considered.

Drug Interactions

Fluvoxamine is the only SSRI that has potent inhibitory effects on the CYP_{1A2} enzyme. Significant drug interactions are with clozapine, TCAs, and theophylline; dose reduction of these drugs are recommended. Fluvoxamine also inhibits CYP 2C19 and CYP 3A4, and dose reduction of several drugs, including alprazolam, is necessary.

Tricyclic Antidepressants

Clomipramine is effective for the treatment for OCD, whereas other TCAs, such as desipramine and imipramine, are not. Clomipramine has the usual side-effect profile of the TCAs including sedation, anticholinergic side effects, orthostatic hypotension, sexual dysfunction, and seizure risk. TCAs are second-line therapy.

Augmentation Therapy

Cognitive behavioral therapy is an important nonpharmacologic intervention. Other augmentation therapy includes the use of (1) dopamine blocking agents, (2) buspirone, (3) lithium, and (4) clonazepam.

Dopamine Blocking Agents

Haloperidol has been found to be effective as an adjunct to fluvoxamine for OCD associated with tics. Olanzapine is currently being studied for use in OCD.

Buspirone

Buspirone, 10 mg three times a day, has been studied as an adjunct. Lithium and clonazepam have been tried and further studies are needed.

POSTTRAUMATIC STRESS DISORDER

The lifetime prevalence of posttraumatic stress disorder (PTSD) is thought to be up to 8%. The disorder is characterized by reexperiencing a traumatic event and avoidance of stimuli that approximate the original traumatic event (Foa, Davidson, and Frances, 1999a).

Antidepressants

SSRIs are effective treatment as a class (Foa, Davidson, and Frances, 1999b). Drug selection is based on client preference, side-effect profile, and client tolerance. Nefazodone and bupropion are also effective. TCAs and MAOIs are effective but generally not used because of their side-effect profile and drug and food interactions.

The use of a combination of different drug classes may be needed.

Benzodiazepines

Benzodiazepines are effective treatment for PTSD. Clonazepam has been used and is effective to reduce flashbacks and nightmares. The major issues with the use of benzodiazepines are tolerance and dependence. There is also risk in the client with alcohol abuse because of additive depressant effects.

Mood Stabilizers

Lithium, divalproex, and carbamazepine have been studied as an adjunct therapy for explosiveness, irritability, and other symptoms associated with PTSD.

GENERALIZED SOCIAL PHOBIA (SOCIAL ANXIETY DISORDER)

Social anxiety disorder (SAD) is characterized by anxiety resulting from fear of scrutiny by others, embarrassment, or humiliation, when the fear is disproportionate and unrealistic. A high incidence of alcohol abuse and depression is associated with social phobia, as clients are often isolated. SAD is the most common anxiety disorder, with a lifetime prevalence of 13% (Boyd et al., 1990).

Antidepressants

The SSRIs, including paroxetine, fluoxetine, fluvoxamine, sertraline, and citalopram, are considered first-line treatment for SAD. Dosing of SAD is similar to that for major depressive disorder. Slow titration increases client compliance and tolerability. The onset of therapeutic effect is about 4 weeks, with optimal effects in 8 to 12 weeks.

Nefazodone may be an option if sexual dysfunction is a significant side effect. Nefazodone is contraindicated in clients with hepatic impairment.

Benzodiazepines

Clonazepam and alprazolam have been found effective.

Gabapentin

The effective dose is 900 to 3600 mg/day. Side effects are sedation, dizziness, and dry mouth.

HERBAL THERAPY
Kava

Kava (*Piper methysticum*) is an herb that has anxiolytic and sedative properties. It is available as a root extract in capsule form. The recommended dose for treating anxiety is 100 to 125 mg dried kava root extract, taken three times a day. It is also available in tablet form as a purified kavalactone, and the dose is 50 to 70 mg three times a day. As a tincture, the usual dose is 30 drops with water three times a day.

Side Effects

Kava was thought to be relatively mild and safe. Recently literature has warned of kava-associated hepatitis, cirrhosis, and liver failure. Other side effects include altered judgment, altered motor reflexes, GI upset, skin rash, and visual disturbances.

Herb-Drug Interactions

Kava is associated with interactions with several drugs including barbiturates, benzodiazepines, dopamine agonists, alcohol, and MAOIs. There is added risk with combinations of other hepatotoxic drugs.

Valerian

Valerian (*Valeriana officinalis*) has anxiolytic and hypnotic properties. It has been used for treatment of mild to moderate insomnia and restlessness and tension.

Valerian is available as a capsule, extract, tincture, and tea. The dose for anxiety relief is 220-mg valerian extract three times a day.

Side Effects

Hepatotoxicity with long-term use has been reported. Side effects include sedation and withdrawal symptoms similar to those associated with benzodiazepines.

CLIENT EDUCATION

- Educate the client that anxiety disorder is a treatable illness, and is not a personal weakness or failure.
- Educate the client regarding the different types of medications that are effective, the side-effect profiles, precautions, and contraindications.
- Encourage clients to participate in the decision-making process when choosing therapy.
- Medications generally take several weeks to achieve maximal effects. The clients should be encouraged to continue the medications even though immediate effect is not seen.
- Nonpharmacologic interventions, when appropriate, should be encouraged.
- Advise the client of potential drug interactions. Clients should be advised to report to the physician or health care professional if they are taking other medications and herbal remedies, whether these are prescription drugs or over-the-counter drugs.
- Counsel the client regarding the risk of mixing alcohol with these medications, especially benzodiazepines.
- Counsel the client to avoid driving or operating machinery, as many of these drugs cause drowsiness and sedation.

SUMMARY

Pharmacotherapy for anxiety disorders is moving away from benzodiazepines toward the serotonergic antidepressants, particularly the SSRIs and venlafaxine. SSRIs and venlafaxine have better safety profiles and do not have the risk of substance abuse, tolerance, and dependence associated with the benzodiazepines. The disadvantage is their slow onset of action. Benzodiazepines are still widely prescribed because of their rapid onset of action and the lack of of sexual dysfunction.

HYPNOTICS

Benzodiazepines

Triazolam

Pharmacokinetics. Triazolam (Halcion) has a short half-life and a fast onset of action. It is indicated for use with the client who has difficulty falling asleep.

Temazepam

Pharmacokinetics. Temazepam (Restoril) has an intermediate half-life with a slow onset of action. It is indicated for the client who awakes early and cannot stay asleep.

Flurazepam

Pharmacokinetics. Flurazepam (Dalmane) has a long half-life with a fast onset of action. It is good for both difficulty in falling asleep and staying asleep. The disadvantage is rebound insomnia.

Nonbenzodiazepine Hypnotics

Zolpidem (Ambien) and zaleplon (Sonata) are the newest nonbenzodiazepine hypnotics. They are structurally unrelated to benzodiazepines and do not appear to have abuse potential. They possess minimal muscle relaxant, anticonvulsant, or anxiolyitc properties. Advantages over benzodiazepines include lack of rebound insomnia, lack of development of dependence, and lack of adverse withdrawal effects. The main disadvantage of zolpidem and zaleplon is their high cost compared to the benzodiazepines hypnotics.

Zolpidem

Zolpidem is an oral imidazopyridime sedative-hypnotic agent.

Pharmacokinetics. Onset is within 30 minutes, and the duration is 3 to 5 hours. It is rapidly absorbed. The half-life of the drug is 2.5 to 5 hours. It is metabolized to inactive compounds (Greenblatt et al., 1998).

Dose. The usual dose is 10 mg immediately before bedtime; the dose for older adults is 5 mg. Repeating the dose is not recommended. The therapy should be limited to 7 to 10 days, and the client should be reevaluated if longer duration is needed.

Side Effects. Dizziness, headache, GI upset, nausea, and mild anterograde amnesia have been reported. For dose over 10 mg/day, there is risk of hallucinations.

Drug Interactions. Zolpidem is highly protein bound. Food decreases absorption. The use of other CNS depressants, including alcohol, should be avoided.

Zaleplon

Zaleplon is a nonbenzodiazepine hypnotic agent.

Pharmacokinetics. Zaleplon is a short-acting pyrazolopyrimidine hypnotic with a rapid onset of action. Onset is within 30 minutes and the duration is 2 hours. The half-life is 1.1 hours. Because of its short onset and short half-life, zaleplon is useful for treating insomnia that occurs in the middle of the night and early morning (Elie et al., 1999).

Dose. The recommended dose for the treatment of insomnia is 10 mg before bedtime. A 5-mg dose is sufficient for a small or low-weight client or for an older adult. The dose may be repeated once.

Side Effects. Dizziness and headache are common.

Other Agents Used for Sleep

Trazodone

Mechanism of Action. Trazodone is a serotonin reuptake inhibitor that blocks serotonin receptors. The dose as a hypnotic is 50 to 200 mg at bedtime.

Pharmacokinetics. There is delayed onset, with a long half-life of 6 hours and longer for older adults and obese clients. Side effects are sedation and orthostatic hypotension. Priapism, which is a rare but serious adverse effect, may occur.

Trazodone is preferred over benzodiazepines for clients on drug or alcohol detoxification programs or when benzodiazepines should be avoided.

Chloral hydrate

Mechanism of Action. The mechanism of action of chloral hydrate (Noctoc) is unknown. The active metabolite is trichloroethanol, which possesses hypnotic effect and is responsible for cross-tolerance.

Pharmacokinetics. Rapid onset is 30 minutes. The half-life is 8 to 11 hours. The duration of effect is 4 to 8 hours.

Dose. The recommended dose is 500 to 1000 mg at bedtime, with a maximum dose of 2 g.

Side Effects. Side effects include GI upset, nausea, vomiting, ataxia, confusion, headache, hallucinations, and rash. Alcohol should be avoided in all clients.

Diphenhydramine

Diphenhydramine is available over the counter. Many over-the-counter sleep remedies contain diphenhydramine, including Nytol, Sominex, and Unisom. It is an antihistamine and an H_1-receptor antagonist.

Pharmacokinetics. Diphenhydramine is metabolized in the liver.

Dose. The recommended dose is 25 to 50 mg at bedtime. Maximum dosage is 300 mg/day.

Side Effects. Tolerance may develop after 2 weeks. This drug should be avoided in older adults because of its anticholinergic side effects.

Melatonin

Melatonin (MICROMEDEX, 2003) is a *N*-acetyl-5-methoxy-tryptamine. It is a naturally occurring hormone secreted by the pineal gland and is a by-product of serotonin metabolism. The dose is 0.3 to 5 mg at bedtime. It is often used to counteract jet lag.

Melatonin is not an herbal product; however, it is commercially available in combination with other herbal remedies. Side effects include drowsiness and daytime fatigue. Other CNS drugs should be avoided when taking melatonin.

Herbal Products

Kava. The dose used as a hypnotic is 60 to 120 mg dried extract (MICROMEDEX, 2003).

Valerian. The dose being used as a hypnotic is 400 to 900 mg at bedtime. Because of its slower onset, valerian needs to be taken 1 hour before bedtime (MICROMEDEX, 2003).

Barbiturates

The use of barbiturates has dramatically decreased because of the many safer and better hypnotics now available. Their dosages and half-lives are listed in Table 20-8.

DRUG TREATMENT IN AGGRESSIVE AND VIOLENT BEHAVIORS

Aggressive and violent behaviors are frequently seen in clients with a wide spectrum of underlying disorders. Brain injury, brain trauma, dementia, mental retardation, and seizure disorders are some of the underlying disorders that lead to aggressive and violent behaviors. CNS infections and drug abuse could also lead to aggressive behaviors. Clients with schizophrenia and personality disorders may often display these behaviors.

TREATMENT

Careful diagnosis should always precede treatment to avoid overuse and misuse of medications. Although no medications have been approved by the FDA specifically for aggression, many medications are being used, primarily for the following two purposes:

1. To use sedating medication in an acute situation to calm the client so that client will not harm self or others.
2. To use medication to treat chronic aggressive behaviors.

FACTORS INFLUENCING THE CHOICE OF MEDICATIONS

Factors most important in the selection of an initial emergency medication include availability of an intramuscular injection, liquid formulation, speed of onset, and previous history of response (Allen et al., 2001a).

ACUTE AGITATION AND AGGRESSION

Sedating medications are commonly used to treat the acute situation. It is important to select a sedating medication that is limited in duration to avoid oversedation and potential adverse effects. Antipsychotics or benzodiazepines are commonly used. Treatment should not exceed 4 weeks. When a client requires more than 4 weeks of treatment, the approach should be changed to that for chronic treatment.

Antipsychotics

Antipsychotics are commonly used to treat acute aggressive and violent behaviors. Often it is the sedating property of the antipsychotics that produces the calming effect for the client. Antipsychotics may cause side effects such as akathisia, which can be mistaken as increased irritability and agitation. The atypical antipsychotics are becoming more commonplace in the treatment of aggressive behavior and have fewer side effects. The disadvantage of using atypical antipsychotics is that only ziprasidone is available in intramuscular injection and it is very expensive. All of the atypical antipsychotics are effective, and the choice depends on the client's condition and the side-effects profile of each drug. For example, olanzapine should be avoided in clients with diabetes and when there is concern with weight gain, quetiapine is preferred for clients with a history of EPS, and risperidone is preferred for older clients and clients who are delirious because this drug produces fewer anticholinergic side effects (Allen et al., 2001c).

Haloperidol

In clients with brain injury and acute aggression, low-dose haloperidol should be used. The recommended dose is 1 mg orally or 0.5 mg intramuscularly, with repeated injections every hour until aggression is controlled. Once a client is not aggressive for 48 hours, the dose of haloperidol should be gradually tapered, with a decreasing daily dose schedule of 25% until discontinuation is achieved.

In clients with dementia and schizophrenia, risperidone can be used (Ranier et al., 2001). Low-dose risperidone of 0.5 to 1 mg should be used, and the doses should be smaller for older adults with dementia.

Trazodone, a sedating antidepressant, has been used to treat older adult clients with sundowning syndrome and aggressive behaviors. A low dose of 50 to 100 mg may be tried.

Benzodiazepines

The sedating properties of benzodiazepines are helpful in the management of acute agitation, aggressiveness, and violent behavior. Another advantage of the benzodiazepines is their quick onset of action. There have been reports of benzodiazepines causing violent and aggressive behaviors, but these are rare.

Lorazepam is the most common benzodiazepine in use. It can be administered orally or by injection. It is commonly used in combination with antipsychotic medication such as haloperidol. Other sedating agents used include valproate, chloral hydrate, and diphenhydramine.

CHRONIC AGGRESSION

When a client continues to exhibit aggressive behavior for more than several weeks, the choice of medication to counteract aggressive behaviors should be guided by the client's underlying condition. For example, when aggression is related to schizophrenia, antipsychotic medication may be used. When aggression is related to mania, lithium or valproate may be used. When aggression is related to seizure disorder, carbamazepine or valproate may be used.

Antipsychotics

Antipsychotics should not be used solely for treatment of aggressive behavior but rather to treat the underlying condition.

Buspirone

Buspirone, an antianxiety agent, has been shown to be effective in treating aggressive behavior. The initial dose is 5 mg twice a day, which is increased by 5-mg increments every 3 to 5 days. The full effect may not be seen for several weeks, and the effective dose may be as high as 45 to 60 mg/day.

Anticonvulsants

Carbamazepine and valproate have been used to treat bipolar disorders and associated aggressive behavior because of their antikindling properties. Carbamazepine has been shown to be effective in reducing aggressive behavior associated with dementia. Lithium may also be useful in treating aggression associated with mania.

Antidepressants

Trazodone has been used in the treatment of aggression associated with organic mental disorders. Other antidepressants such as the SSRIs have also been used. The dose range of the antidepressants used to treat aggression is the same as that used for treatment of depression.

Antihypertensive Medications

The β-blocker propranolol has been used to treat aggression related to organic brain syndrome. Major side effects of propranolol include lowering of blood pressure and heart rate. It should be noted that β-blockers may cause depression.

SPECIAL CONSIDERATIONS FOR CHILDREN

If antipsychotic medication is needed, a low-dose atypical antipsychotic such as olanzapine or risperidone may be used (Allen et al., 2001b).

CHAPTER SUMMARY

■ Atypical antispychotic medications have improved efficacy over conventional antipsychotics in the treatment of negative symptoms. They are both effective in treating schizophrenia.

■ Response to antipsychotic medication is heterogeneous and varies among clients.

■ In general the sequence of response time is as follows: positive, affective, cognitive/perceptual, and negative.

■ Neuroleptic malignant syndrome (NMS) can be a fatal response to any antipsychotic medication, and is most frequently associated with conventional antipsychotics. It is important to recognize NMS and to treat it early. Careful diagnosis is warranted.

■ A great majority of clients respond to pharmacologic treatment. Failure rates may be due to inadequate dosing or length of trial of antidepressants.

■ Antidepressants may cause change in energy levels.

■ Suicidal ideation may persist, so clients are at the highest risk to act on suicidal impulses during the early stage of treatment.

■ Pharmacotherapy for depression has risk. Therefore knowledge of toxicity and efficacy is important for optimal therapeutic response.

■ Adjunctive therapy such as antipsychotics is often used with lithium for bipolar disorder.

■ Antianxiety medications such as benzodiazepines are an adjunct to therapy for short-term use. They may be additive in the long term.

■ Selective serotonin reuptake inhibitors (SSRIs) are first-line treatment for depression and many anxiety disorders.

■ Anticonvulsants are useful in treating bipolar disorders and as adjunctive therapy for pain and other uses.

■ Herbal therapy is commonly used. Caution should be taken with drug-drug interactions. The physician should be consulted.

REVIEW QUESTIONS

1. Neuroleptics are used to treat schizophrenia disorders because they:
   a. Help the serotonin uptake.
   b. Block dopamine receptors.
   c. Prevent the binding of norepinephrine at the receptor sites.
   d. Assist the neurotransmitters to communicate with each other.

2. A 40-year-old client diagnosed with schizophrenia is exhibiting muscle rigidity, fever, and confusion. The nurse assesses that these may be symptoms of:
   a. Delirium tremens
   b. Agranulocytosis
   c. Neuroleptic malignant syndrome
   d. Tardive dyskinesia

3. A 30-year-old client is hospitalized for major depression. He has been taking Zoloft for the past week and has ver-

balized increased energy and improved sleep. The highest priority question the nurse should ask is:
   a. "Are you experiencing any side effects such as dizziness, dry mouth, or irritability?"
   b. "Are you feeling ready for discharge?"
   c. "Do you feel like you should talk to the physician about changing medications?"
   d. "Are you having any thoughts of killing yourself?"

4. A client diagnosed with bipolar disorder complains of nausea, vomiting, diarrhea, thirst, and coarsening hand tremors. The nurse's first response should be:
   a. Suggest that he discuss this with his physician.
   b. Hold his lithium, call the physician for an order to obtain a lithium level, and monitor the client.
   c. Give him some Compazine.
   d. Call his physician to increase the lithium, as it doesn't seem to be working.

5. Which statement demonstrates that the client diagnosed with generalized anxiety disorder is showing improvement:
   a. "I keep feeling like something bad is going to happen. I can't leave my room right now."
   b. "I can't get out of bed. I feel foggy."
   c. "I can't sit still. I feel restless."
   d. "I'm finally able to sleep. I think I'll go to group today."

REFERENCES

Allen MH et al: Guidelines 12: Choice of oral atypical antipsychotic for an agitated, aggressive client with a complicating medical condition: treatment of behavioral emergencies, Expert Consensus Guideline Series. A postgraduate medicine special report, White Plains, NY, 2001a, Expert Knowledge System, website: www.psychguides.com.

Allen MH et al: Treatment of behavioral emergencies, Expert Consensus Guideline Series. A postgraduate medicine special report, White Plains, NY, 2001b, Expert Knowledge System, website: www.psychguides.com.

Allen MH et al: Guidelines 10: Initial medication strategies for a violent and unmanageable child: treatment of behavioral emergencies, Expert Consensus Guideline Series. A postgraduate medicine special report, White Plains, NY, 2001c, Expert Knowledge System, website: www.psychguides.com.

American Psychiatric Association: *Diagnostic and Statistical Manual of Mental Disorders*, Fourth Edition, Text Revision. Washington, DC, American Psychiatric Association, 2000.

Archibald J: Do patients know enough about epilepsy? *Nurs Times* 89(1):48-49, 1993.

Balon R: Fluoxetine for cocaine dependence in methadone maintenance, *J Clin Psychopharmacol* 14(5):360-361, 1994.

Berkow R, editor: *The Merck manual of diagnosis and therapy*, ed 16, 1992, Merck and Co.

Bialer M: Comparative pharmacokinetics of the newer antiepileptic drugs, *Clin Pharmacokinet* 24:441-452, 1993.

Bipolar disorder: management of acute mania in adults. In Manolakis PG: *Guide to drug treatment protocols: a resource for creating and using disease-specific pathways*, Washington, DC, 1999, American Pharmaceutical Association.

Bogan AM, Brown ES, Suppes T: Efficacy of divalproex therapy for schizoaffective disorder, *J Clin Psychopharmacol* 20(5):520-522, 2000.

Botts SR, Raskind J: Gabapentin and lamotrigine in bipolar disorder, *Am J Health Syst Pharm* 56:1939-1944, 1999.

Boyd JH et al: Phobia: prevalence and risk factors, *Soc Psychiatry Psychiatr Epidemiol* 25(6):314-323, 1990.

Bulau P, Stoll KD, Froscher W: Oxcarbazepine versus carbamazepine. In Wolf P et al, editors: *Advances in epilepsy*, vol 16, New York, 1987, Raven Press.

Bupropion (Zyban) for smoking cessation, *Med Lett Drugs Ther* 39(1007):77-78, 1997.

Celexa, citalopram Product Information, Inc, St Louis, 2000, Forest Pharmaceuticals.

Chengappa KNR et al: Bupropion sustained release as a smoking cessation treatment in remitted depressed clients maintained on treatment with selective serotonin reuptake inhibitor antidepressants, *J Clin Psychiatry* 62(7):503-508, 2001.

Claxton A et al: Client compliance to a new enteric-coated weekly formulation of fluoxetine during continuation treatment of major depressive disorder, *J Clin Psychiatry* 61:928-932, 2000.

D'Amico MF et al: Placebo-controlled dose-ranging trial designs in phase II development of neftazodone, *Psychopharmacol Bull* 26(1):147-150, 1990.

Davis R, Wilde MI: Mirtazapine: a review of its pharmacology and therapeutic potential in the management of major depression, *CNS Drugs* 5:389-402, 1996.

Drugs that may cause psychiatric symptoms, *Med Lett* 44(1134):59-62, 2002.

Effexor XR, venlafaxine Product Information, Wyeth-Ayerst Laboratories, Philadelphia (PI revised 09/2000) reviewed 01/2001.

Elie R et al: Sleep latency is shortened during 4 weeks of treatment with zaleplon, a novel nonebnzodiazepine hypnotic, *J Clin Psychiatry* 60(8):536-544, 1999.

Fava M, Rankin MA: Sexual functioning and SSRIs, *J Clin Psychiatry* 63(suppl 5):13-16, 2002.

Feighner JP et al: A placebo-controlled inpatient comparison of fluvoxamine maleate and imipramine in major depression, *Int Clin Psychopharmacol* 4(3):239-244, 1989.

Foa EB, Davidson JRT, Frances A: *Treatment of posttraumatic stress disorder*, Expert Consensus Guideline Series, White Plains, NY, 1999a, Expert Knowledge System, website: www.psychguides.com.

Foa EB, Davidson JRT, Frances A: Treatment of posttraumatic stress disorder. Preferred medications for Guideline 3: Selecting A Specific Medication Strategy, Expert Consensus Guideline Series, White Plains, NY, 1999b, Expert Knowledge System, website: www.psychguides.com.

Frances A, Docherty JP, Kahn DA, editors: The expert consensus guideline series: treatment of bipolar disorder, *J Clin Psychiatry* vol 57 (suppl 12A), 1996.

Gelenberg AJ et al: Efficacy of venlafaxine extended release capsules in nondepressed outclients with generalized anxiety disorder: a 6-month randomized controlled trial, *JAMA* 283:3082-3088, 2000.

Glassman AH, Thomas Bigger JT: Antipsychotic drugs: prolonged QTc interval, torsades de pointes, and sudden death, *Am J Psychiatry* 158(11):1774-1782, 2001.

Gorman JM: Mirtazapine: clinical overview, *J Clin Psychiatry* 60(suppl 17):9-13, 1999.

Greenblatt D et al: Comparative kinetics and dynamics of zaleplon, zolpidem and placebo, *Clin Pharmacol Ther* 64:553-561, 1998.

Hedberg DL, Gordon MW, Glueck BC: Six cases of hypertensive crisis in clients on tranylcypromine after eating chicken livers, *Am J Psychiatry* 122:933-937, 1966.

Hermesh H et al: High serum creatinine kinase level: possible risk factor for neuroleptic malignant syndrome, *J Clin Psychopharm* 22:252-256, 2002.

Houtkooper MA et al: Oxcarbazepine (GP 47.680): a possible alternative to carbamazepine? *Epilepsia* 28(6):693-698, 1987.

Johannessen AC, Nielsen OA: Hyponatremia induced by oxcarbazepine, *Epilepsy Res* 1(2):155-156, 1987.

Johne A et al: Decreased plasma levels of amitriptyline and its metabolites on comedication with an extract from St. John's wort, *J Clin Psychopharmacol* 22:46-54, 2002.

Katon W, Sullivan MD: Depression and chronic medical illness, *J Clin Psychiatry* 51(suppl):3-11, 1990.

Kendler KS et al: Generalized anxiety disorder in women. A population-based twin study. *Arch Gen Psychiatry* 49(4):267-272, 1992.

Kramer TA: Dopamine system stabilizers, *Medscape Psychiatry Mental Health eJournal* vol 7, no 1, 2002.

Kushner MG, Sher KJ, Beitman BD: The relation between alcohol problems and the anxiety disorders, *Am J Psychiatry* 147(6):685-695, 1990.

Lexapro (Escitalopram) Product Information. Forest Pharmaceuticals, Inc, St Louis, 2002.

Martin R et al: Cognitive effects of topiramate, gabapentin, and lamotrigine in healthy young adults, *Neurology* 52:321-327, 1999.

Meyer JM: Novel antipsychotics and severe hyperlipidemia, *J Clin Psychopharmacol* 21:369-374, 2001.

MICROMEDEX Healthcare Series vol 115. 1974-2003 Thomson MICROMEDEX.

Murray CJL, Lopez AD: *The global burden of disease*, Cambridge, Mass, 2000, Harvard University School of Public Health & World Health Organization, 2000.

Neurontin, gabapentin Product Information. Parke-Davis, Morris Plains, NJ, 1999.

Nielson CP et al: Polymorphonuclear leukocyte inhibition by therapeutic concentrations of theophylline is mediated by cyclic-3',5'-adenosine monophosphate, *Am Rev Respir Dis* 137(1):25-30, 1988.

Pendlebury SC, Moses DK, Eadie MJ: Hyponatremia during oxcarbazepine therapy, *Hum Toxicol* 8(5):337-344, 1989.

Ramsay RE: Clinical efficacy and safety of gabapentin, *Neurology* 44(Suppl 5):S23-S30, 1994.

Ranier MK et al: Effect of risperidone on behavioral and psychological symptoms and cognitive function in dementia, *J Clin Psychiatry* 62(11):894-900, 2001.

Rawls WN: TrazodoneB, *Intell Clin Pharmacol* 16:7-13, 1982.

Reid CD: Chemical photosensitivity: another reason to be careful in the sun, *FDA Consumer Magazine,* 1996.

Schatzberg AF, Nemeroff CB: *The American Psychiatric Press textbook of psychopharmacology*, ed 2, 2001, American Psychiatric Publishing.

Spivak B, Radvan M, Shine M: Postural hypotension with syncope possibly precipitated by trazodone, *Am J Psychiatry* 144:11, 1987.

Steinhoff BJ et al: Hyponatremic coma under oxcarbazepine therapy, *Epilepsy Res* 11(1):67-70, 1992.

Tandon R: Introduction-(Ziprasidone), *Br J Clin Pharmacol* 49(suppl 1):1S-3S, 2000.

Taylor DM: Prolongation of QTc interval and antipsychotics, *Am J Psychiatry* 159(6):1062; discussion 1064, 2002.

Thase ME, Entsuah AR, Rudolph RL: Remission rates during treatment with venlafaxine or selective serotonin reuptake inhibitors, *Br J Psychiatry* 178:234-241, 2001.

Tohen M, Grundy S: Management of acute mania, *J Clin Psychiatry* 60(suppl 5):31-34, 1999.

Van Amelsvoort TH et al: Hyponatremia associated with carbamazepine and oxcarbazepine therapy: a review, *Epilepsia* 35(1):181-188, 1994.

Wagner GJ, Rabkin JG, Rabkin R: Dextroamphetamine as a treatment for depression and low energy in AIDS patients: a pilot study, *J Psychosom Res* 42(4):407-411, 1997.

Wang PS et al: Clozapine use and risk of diabetes mellitus, *J Clin Psychopharmacol* 22:236-243, 2002.

Zakrzewska JM, Patsalos PN: Oxcarbazepine: a new drug in the management of intractable trigeminal neuralgia, *J Neurol Neurosurg Psychiatry* 52(4):472-476, 1989.

Zobor P et al: Antipsychotic-induced weight gain and therapeutic response: a differential association, *J Clin Psychopharmacol* 22:244-251, 2002.

21

Complementary and Alternative Therapies

Ruth N. Grendell

OBJECTIVES

- Describe the philosophic differences between alternative and traditional (conventional, allopathic) therapies.

- Discuss the influence of mind-body interrelationships on wellness and health promotion.

- Identify the current alternative therapies used in treatment of physiologic and psychologic health problems, particularly chronic disease management.

- Discuss the nurse's role in providing holistic nursing care.

- Discuss the challenges for nurses in providing care to an ever-increasing diversity of cultural groups entering the Western health care system.

- Discuss the impact of alternative therapies on the nurse's role in applying therapeutic interventions.

- Describe incorporation of alternative therapies in the plan of care.

- Discuss client education concerning concurrent use of alternative therapies and traditional (conventional, allopathic) therapies.

- Discuss the impact of alternative therapies on nursing practice, education, and research.

The biomedical model is based primarily on the following assumptions: (1) the scientific method of identifying causes of **disease** and implementing curative treatments to correct aberrant physiology; (2) infections are defined by the germ theory; and (3) **illness** prevention is based on proper hygiene, public sanitation, and personal lifestyle choices (Schlosser, 1999). In contrast, the focus of the **holistic** or alternative care model is on strengthening one's inner resistance to disease and "healing from within," or enhancing the body's innate healing powers (Kreitzer and Jensen, 2000). Although **nursing** has been strongly influenced by biomedical practices, it also has deep roots in the holistic perspective that considers the impact of all intrapersonal, interpersonal, and environmental interactions as contributing factors to a person's well-being or illness (American Holistic Nursing Association [AHNA], 2002).

Some alternative medical practices have been incorporated into **conventional/traditional medicine**, particularly in pain management and treatment of chronic illness, anxiety, depression, and disease prevention. This chapter describes the contrast in philosophies and treatment modalities between biomedical and holistic models of care and selected alternative therapies and their significance to the practice of nursing.

ALTERNATIVE THERAPY FIELDS

Complementary/alternative medicine (CAM) covers a broad range of healing philosophies, approaches, and therapies and their accompanying theories and beliefs. More than 1800 approaches to healing have been identified (Kreitzer and Jensen, 2000). Some therapies are based on physiologic principles of traditional medicine, whereas others arise from concepts that are in contrast to the accepted medical practices. In 1992 Congress established the Office of Alternative Medicine (OAM) under the direction of the National Institutes of Health (NIH) to evaluate the effectiveness of alternative therapies. In 1998, OAM became the National Center for Complementary and Alternative Medicine (NCCAM). Regional centers for objective, evidenced-based research on alternative therapies are located throughout the nation (NCCAM, 2002; Forbes, 2000). The NCCAM has classified complementary/alternative therapies into seven broad categories: (1) alternative medicine systems; (2) mind-body interventions; (3) pharmacologic- and biologic-based therapies; (4) herbal medications; (5) diet, nutrition and supplements, and lifestyle changes; (6) manipulative and body-based methods; and (7) energy therapies (including biofeedback and bioelectromagnetics). More than 600 CAM therapies are grouped within this continually evolving taxonomy (Pelletier, 2000). The list of CAM practices is constantly being revised as a result of gradual acceptance of some CAM modalities by the medical profession and insurers. Selected CAM therapies are listed in Box 21-1.

HISTORICAL OVERVIEW
Ancient Cultural Beliefs

In ancient times illness was often believed to be punishment for sin or at the whim of the gods—a matter of fate; healing came through purification of the body by incantations and

---

Box 21-1 Alternative Therapy Fields and Selected Examples

Mind-Body Interventions
Meditation
Prayer
Yoga
The arts: music, dance, drama, art, literature, and humor
Psychotherapy
Hypnosis

Alternative Systems of Medical Practice
Traditional Chinese medicine
  Acupuncture
Ayurvedic medicine
Homeopathic medicine
Naturopathy
Environmental medicine
Culture-based community medicine (folk medicine)

Pharmacologic and Biologic Treatments
Vaccines and medicines not yet approved by mainstream medicine
  Animal cartilage
  Chelating chemicals

Diet, Nutrition, Supplements, and Lifestyle Changes
Vitamins, minerals, and supplements
Designer diets—macrobiotic, cancer, weight reduction
Food elimination diets—allergy detection
Vegetarian
Ethnic-based diets

Bioelectromagnetics
Light therapy
Bone growth stimulation
Magnet therapy

Manual Healing Methods
Osteopathy
Chiropractic
Massage
Acupressure
Foot reflexology
Therapeutic touch

Herbal Medications
Chinese herbals
European
American

---

the use of herbs. Evil spirits were believed to cause illnesses and adverse events; good spirits intervened on the behalf of an individual or group. Animal sacrifices were made to appease the gods, and spirits became part of healing rituals. In some countries, however, laws were also passed to regulate the practices of hygiene, sanitation, and preservation of food to protect people from disease.

Hippocrates (400–377 BC), known as the father of modern medicine, introduced beliefs that **health** was not controlled by the gods but was dependent on the harmony, or balance, between the body, the mind, and the environment. He used a patient-centered approach to treat the whole person. The dominant beliefs in most Asian countries considered that this balance between human beings and nature could be attained by finding inner peace and spiritual contentment and by understanding and practicing the interactive powers of the mind and body. In many cultures healers were priest-physicians referred to as holy men, or shamans, and the care they provided was referred to as shamanistic medicine (Ellis and Hartley, 2000; Weil, 2000).

Biomedicine Model Concepts

Conventional Western medicine is based on a worldview strongly influenced by Cartesian dualism (separation of mind and body) and Newtonian physics of the seventeenth and eighteenth centuries. "Disease occurs when the parts break down" (Forbes, 2000). Science and technology revolutionized the practice of medicine and facilitated a greater understanding of human biology and methods of intervention in disease and illness. Standardized treatments and the care regimen are tailored to the client's match with a disease category of defined signs and symptoms. These technically oriented interventions are geared toward rapid results in reversing the deteriorative physiologic disease process and to prolong life (Parkman and Ullrich, 2000). In turning to technology, however, Western medicine lost touch with its own historical roots of treating the whole person (Weil, 2000). Weil states that conventional medicine is also *physician centered,* granting the caregiver the authority for making decisions and placing the client in a passive, somewhat powerless position that limits the client's responsibility in the recovery process.

Holistic Model Concepts

In contrast, the holistic perspective is more concerned with healing of the total person rather than the cure of a specific disease. Each person is viewed as uniquely separate from another human being and is *more* than the sum of the individual parts—what affects one aspect affects all (Parkman and Ullrich, 2000; Dossey and Dossey, 1998). In addition to examining physical symptoms, the clinician considers the influence of cultural and genetic factors, past and current experiences, family structure, and role functions on the person's perception of health and illness and the use of coping mechanisms. Many therapies are used as preventive measures rather than treating disease symptoms. Research indicates that many of the CAM therapies, such as diet, exercise, and **stress**-reduction therapies, are particularly effective in preventing and managing chronic disease processes (Pelletier, 2000). Individuals are encouraged to take active responsibility for their own health and participate in the recovery process when illnesses do occur. A change in attitude and lifestyle, a sense of control and peace, and decreased anxiety can indicate healing even though the particular disease is not cured. Multiple methods may be incorporated into the individualized plan of care. Many alternative therapies are based

---

> ### Box 21-2   Common Themes of Alternative Therapies
>
> Humans have innate recuperative powers.
> Religious and spiritual values are important to the state of health.
> Self-esteem and purpose of life are positive influences in the healing process.
> Thoughts, feelings, emotions, values, and perceived meanings affect physical function.
> Most therapies rely on diet, exercise, relaxation techniques, lifestyle, and attitude changes.
> Focus is on the total person—physical, emotional, mental, and psychosocial health.
> Illness is viewed as an imbalance; interventions are directed toward restoring balance.
> Energy is the force needed to achieve balance and harmony.

on Oriental and Far Eastern beliefs and practices. Some unifying themes among the several alternative therapies include a person's inherent recuperative ability, the importance of self-esteem, and the influence of spiritual and emotional beliefs on health. Treatment methods are based on maintaining or restoring a balance within all aspects of the individual. A detailed listing of themes is provided in Box 21-2.

Rise in Dominance of the Biomedical Model

Before the 1800s, biomedicine and alternative medicine coexisted and competed on a somewhat equal basis. During the latter part of that century, however, the biomedical model was validated as superior because of the scientific discovery of microbes as the cause of many infectious diseases and the development of methods to eradicate those causes. Disease cure rates rose, and favorable surgical outcomes soon followed through the use of proper aseptic techniques and new anesthesia discoveries. Another significant event that legitimized biomedicine was the research report by Abraham Flexner in 1910 that indicated the need for standards in education and licensing of physicians. Philanthropic funding of medical education institutions quickly halted any financial assistance to the schools with the nonmedical, nonscientific curricula.

As a result of the rising dominance of the biomedical model, the credibility of alternative therapies were questioned. These practices were soon relegated to the fringes of health care and often referred to as quackery. Although chiropractic and osteopathic practices continued, others such as homeopathy and naturopathy were almost forgotten (Tedesco and Cicchetti, 2001). Yet today, more than 40% of Americans have reported using alternative therapies; worldwide, more than 90% of the population use them (Parkman and Ullrich, 2000). Although CAM therapies are widely accepted in Europe and other countries, most U.S. health care professionals often ignore the fact that people use many alternative methods in managing their illnesses (Ellis and Hartley, 2000; Pelletier, 2000), although this view is changing.

Merging Philosophies

Renewed interest in mind/body interactions gained momentum in the mid-twentieth century. The discovery that some people exposed to pathogens did not become ill led researchers to challenge the existing biologic theory and to explore other possible influencing causes. Subsequent epidemiologic studies revealed that diet, smoking, and environmental pollution were strongly associated with increased incidences of lung cancer; widowed persons had higher death rates than married persons in the same age-group; socioeconomic factors had impact on disease; and certain religious groups had fewer reports of illness and death from specific diseases. The technologies of modern biomedicine could not provide explanations. The strong possibility of a cause-effect relationship between the environment and mind, spirit, and body in health and illness encouraged further investigation. These findings indicated that many chronic conditions are the result of common lifestyle risks (smoking, diet, being sedentary, stress) that are not amenable to the one-dimensional solutions prescribed by conventional medicine.

Psychoneuroimmunology (PNI), a relatively new field, is the study of a person's psychobiologic factors and their interaction with the stress response and influence on health outcomes. Arousal of the hypothalamic-pituitary-adrenal axis affects the nervous, endocrine, and immune systems. Prolonged exposure to stress and high anxiety levels have been linked to lowered immunity, whereas a greater resistance to illness has been associated with lower stress and anxiety. The PNI model provides a framework for screening risk factors of health problems including stress stimuli, sociodemographic factors, lifestyle behaviors, and health history (Ruiz, 1999).

Scientists, then, explored the age-old mind/body healing modalities of other societies, particularly Oriental medicine. As a result, acupuncture, meditation, relaxation techniques, massage, and other related interventions have been integrated into mainstream health care. Some medical schools have included courses in CAM in the curriculum. Additional research has been undertaken, and several articles have been published (Pelletier, 2000; Dossey and Dossey, 1998). However, progress in integrating CAM into mainstream medicine may be slowed because of regulatory and reimbursement measures, values and misconceptions still held by many traditional practitioners, and the lack of large-scale clinical trials to demonstrate the effectiveness of CAM.

CURRENT ISSUES
The Changing Complexion of Health Care

Modern medicine has become so expensive that it is straining the economy of the United States and many other developed nations, putting itself beyond the reach of much of the world's population, particularly for long-term regimens. Chronic and degenerative illnesses, including cardiovascular disease, cancer, diabetes, arthritis, and depression, are reaching epidemic proportions (Pelletier, 2000). Nearly 70% of the U.S. health care budget is spent on treatment of persons with chronic diseases, and costs will escalate, as the baby-boomer generation grows older. Approximately 160 million people in the United States are covered by managed care, and almost $1 trillion is spent annually on treatment of disease, illness, and injury (including health products purchased at retail stores). An estimated increase to $2 trillion is predicted by 2005 (Zerwekh, 2000).

Unfortunately, biomedical treatments and advanced technology can also have adverse consequences. Microbes have become resistant to medications. Some chronic diseases that still defy scientific interventions have replaced infectious diseases as the major cripplers and killers. Side effects of many of the new "wonder" drugs can have devastating psychologic and physiologic effects.

Consumer confidence in conventional treatment methods has deteriorated, and citizens are turning to legislators to bring about change in the health care system. Reasons given for the growing dissatisfaction include the spiraling costs and restrictions imposed by managed care and health maintenance organizations and consumer desire to have more control in health care decisions. Health care reform requires a focus on disease prevention and health promotion rather than on disease treatment (Pelletier, 2002; Ellis and Hartley, 2000). Exposure to the various alternative therapies through the merger of cultures and abundant information provided by the media has a strong influence on the public's acceptance and use of alternative therapies. Information on health care is covered almost daily by the media and is easily accessible on the Internet. Articles frequently appear in popular magazines, and many bookstores have substantial space allocated to self-help books that have become best sellers. Convenience and fewer side effects from natural substances, less invasive techniques, the possibility of an overall decrease in cost, and the ability to choose are appealing alternatives to traditional medicine (Snyder and Lindquist, 2001; Parkman and Ullrich, 2000).

According to a landmark national study by Eisenberg et al. (1993), of 1539 respondents over 18 years old, approximately 70% to 90% used at least one alternative therapy during the previous year. Participants also reported using both traditional and alternative therapies for chronic conditions with or without informing their medical care providers. Approximately one third of the respondents used over-the-counter (OTC) drugs, and 50% used vitamins and nutritional supplements. The study revealed that $14 billion was spent in out-of-pocket expense by these respondents using alternative remedies for treatment of chronic diseases, with the average number of visits to alternative care clinicians exceeding the average number of visits to traditional care providers. The majority of respondents were in the 25- to 49-year age group, had college educations, and were in a higher-than-average income bracket. Among the chronic conditions reported were back problems, digestive disturbances, headaches, allergies, asthma, hypertension and cardiovascular problems, diabetes mellitus, cancer, arthritis, and substance abuse, particularly alcohol. According to a 1997 update of this study, there was an almost 10% increase in the use of these therapies and an expenditure of more than $22 billion (Eisenberg et al., 1998).

Barriers to Acceptance of Alternative Therapies

Although alternative practices have been in vogue for centuries in Europe, Asia, and the Far East, therapeutic results have primarily been reported via anecdotal reports, so the rigor of the research methods has been questioned. The traditional Western medical world continues to call for clinical studies conducted within strict, controlled parameters. The U.S. Food and Drug Administration (FDA) has also expressed great concern over the lack of guidelines to ensure purity and dosage accuracy of herbal remedies and supplements (Kreitzer and Jensen, 2000). Currently these substances are exempt from FDA approval. There is also a concern over claims that one substance can be a cure-all for many health problems. The FDA continues to argue for the right to regulate these products. Another great concern is the validity of media reports and the credentials of the report writers. There is no effective control of the more than 15,000 health care information sites on the Internet (Zerwekh, 2000).

The tremendous costs for investigation are prohibitive for many advocates of alternative therapies; thus many methods will not be tested. Additional barriers are the heavy reliance on high-technology treatments by society, the dependence on pharmaceuticals, and state laws that limit the practice of medicine or the healing arts to those with professional medical licensure. Political lobbying and advertising influence of drug manufacturers is another major barrier, although most pharmaceutical companies produce OTC compounds that are attractive substitutes to costly prescriptive medications.

Many barriers are typical of those encountered by innovative proposals that challenge any current traditional practices. Additional concerns focus on the dangers of self-diagnosis, potential and critical delay in seeking appropriate medical care, the potential interactions during the concurrent use of herbal and other drugs with prescribed medications, and the detrimental effects of not informing health care providers about the use of CAM products. The scientific research projects at NCCAM have produced a notable shift in thinking by mainstream medical practitioners. Because the use of CAM is continuing to increase, the medical community and consumers deserve to know which therapies have demonstrated effectiveness and which have not (Pelletier, 2000) (Box 21-3).

A past director of NCCAM cautions that some advocates of CAM view it as a religion and tend to believe that all CAM therapies are superior to any form of conventional medicine. CAM has limitations and can be harmful if used improperly. Western medicine also includes some practices that have not been validated by research. "To avoid a double standard, all therapeutic interventions should be held to the same rigorous standards of evidence-based medicine" (Pelletier, 2000).

Impact of the *Healthy People 2000* Report

As early as the 1970s, the rising costs of medical care led several physicians and educators to see the need for integrating technical sophistication with humanistic values. The debate over quality-of-life issues required a focus on changes in education of the public and the profession. Alternative strategies evolved, such as permitting family members to assist in patient care in intensive care units, creating a homelike atmosphere during labor and delivery, presenting health education programs, and establishing self-help support groups. Health appraisal questionnaires were made available in health care facilities, and illnesses were used as "creative opportunities" for instruction on self-care. A limited number of alternative therapies, including acupuncture and stress reduction measures, were introduced into the system (Snyder and Lindquist, 2001; Leonard and Plotnikoff, 2001; Kreitzer and Jensen, 2000).

Health care reform became a major issue in the 1980s, and as a result, several nationwide studies were conducted. The *Healthy People 2000* report published under the auspices of the U.S. Public Health Department in 1990 contained three major goals: (1) to increase healthy life span for all Americans, (2) to reduce the discrepancies in care provided among Americans, and (3) to provide access to preventive services for all. Primary, secondary, and tertiary levels of illness/disease prevention were referred to as healthy lifestyle practices, early screening and treatment, and rehabilitation measures to inhibit complications. These protective and preventive measures required active participation by both individuals and health care providers. The report also targeted specific needs of several high-risk groups, including infants, children, ethnic and low-income groups, and older adults. The amount of progress in meeting these goals was included in the *Healthy People 2010* report. Ongoing research will monitor incidence of health and illness. Statistical indicators of a healthy population include evidence of physical activity, obesity, tobacco and substance abuse, responsible sexual behavior, mental health, injury and violence, environmental quality, and immunizations. (The nurse plays a primary role in health promotion and education. Consider these indicators as you learn about human responses to health and illness.)

EXPLORING EFFECTIVENESS OF ALTERNATIVE THERAPIES
The Informed Client

As mentioned earlier, physician control over disease information may be ebbing as consumers become more active in decisions about their methods of treatment. Many people are turning to therapies that address them as whole beings (Zerwekh, 2000). The Internet is commonly used by self-

Box 21-3 Examples of Ongoing Research Funded by the National Center of Complementary and Alternative Medicine (NCCAM) and Safety Warnings

NOTE: Many of the studies are longitudinal and require several months or years to produce results. Large-scale, long-term, randomized clinical trials are the gold standard of biomedical research (Pelletier, 2000). Preliminary findings have been reported on some of the studies. Warnings have been issued regarding safety of some herbals. The following list is a sample of the many ongoing and proposed research studies at various research centers throughout the nation. The web site was last modified June 13, 2002.

Arthritis Centers in New York and Maryland

(1) Clinical and basic research on the efficacy and long-term results, safety, cost-effectiveness of acupuncture on osteoarthritis of the knee; (2) mind-body therapy on fibromyalgia symptoms; (3) electroacupuncture for pain and inflammatory conditions; and (4) effects of herbal combinations on immune processes.

Age-Related Disease Centers in Indiana and Alabama

Botanical studies of efficacy of polyphenols of soy, grapes, green tea, and several herbs as treatments for cardiac, cancer, osteoporosis, and cognitive decline.

Women's Health Center at Chicago

Study of effectiveness of 10 herbal supplements for women's health. Center will develop an interactive web site and education programs are planned.

Adult Disease Center at Los Angeles

Research on efficacy of (1) yeast-fermented rice on reduction of cholesterol, (2) green tea for reduction of congestive heart failure, (3) soy for decrease in tumor growth, (4) effects of St. John's Wort for mild depression, and (5) study of other dietary supplements.

Ayuverdic Medicine Center in Tucson, Arizona

Specific research on efficacy of ginger, turmeric, and boswellia for inflammatory diseases (including arthritis and asthma).

Center at Johns Hopkins University in Maryland

Research on (1) antioxidant effects of herbs on cancer cells, (2) use of soy and tart cherry extract on pain, (3) effects of PC-SPES (Chinese herb mix) for treatment of prostate cancer (four studies have been placed on hold and the product has been recalled), (4) impact of spiritual practices on disease recurrence and neuroendocrine-immune process of African-American women with breast cancer. A pediatric center will study effects of herbals on recurrent abdominal pain, otitis media, and cerebral palsy.

Cardiovascular Center at Ann Arbor, Michigan

Validation of (1) hawthorn extract for congestive heart failure; (2) reiki biofield energy healing techniques in diabetic peripheral vascular disease and neuropathy; (3) spirituality measures for outcomes of coronary artery bypass graft (CABG) patients; (4) *Qi Gong* on post-CABG pain, healing, and outcomes.

Alerts/Warnings

After evidence-based studies, several safety alerts have been issued by the Agency for Healthcare Research and Quality. Some herbals may be harmful as a result of certain health problems and their interactive effects with other herbals and medications. Web site was updated June 2002. Examples are:

- *Ephedra (Ma huang)* used for weight loss, to increase energy, and enhance athletic ability. The amphetamine-like effects are harmful for persons with hypertension, hyperthyroid, cardiovascular problems, glaucoma, depression, diabetes mellitus, prostate hypertrophy, and retention.
- *Kava (Piper methysticum)* is a member of the pepper family and is used for insomnia, stress, and anxiety reduction. It has been linked with hepatitis and cirrhosis.
- *Garlic* is popular for use in reducing cholesterol levels. It is harmful when combined with drugs for treatment of AIDS. It reduces saquinavir by 50%.
- *St John's Wort* should not be used with protease inhibitors such as indinavir.
- *Bioterrorism protection herbals* have been advocated by some as protection against virulent infections spread by biologic weapons. The Centers for Disease Control and Prevention states there is no scientific basis for this practice. Anthrax and smallpox progress too rapidly for the immune system to counteract them via the use of any complementary and alternative medicine dietary supplement.

Box 21-4 Evaluation Strategies of Medical Resources on the Web

Questions to Ask:
- Who establishes and maintains the site?
- Who finances the site?
- What is the purpose of the site?
- Where does the information come from?
- What is the basis for the information? Is it research based? Are references listed?
- How is the information selected?
- Is the information current? When was the site last updated?
- Are there links to other sites? How were these sites chosen?
- What information does the site collect from you? Why?
- How does the site interact with visitors to the site?

Adapted from NCCAM website: www.nccam.nih.gov.

help and discussion groups for the exchange of information and has provided a pooling of current expertise about a variety of health problems that often goes beyond current information known by the practicing health care provider. However, the validity of information must be evaluated. Box 21-4 describes how to evaluate Internet sources. Broadcasts of documentary films and programs in health education and fitness have also enhanced public awareness of developments in health care and alternative therapies, as well as self-care options.

The Nurse's Role

The health of individuals, families, and communities is a major focus of nursing, with consideration for the effect of the individual's health status, health beliefs, and interactions with self, others, and the environment. Several practice models have been developed to guide the nurse in carrying out these practices. All of the models are designed around a holistic view of the client, giving consideration to the ability for adapting and coping with life events, the impact of social and cultural values on health/illness beliefs, and personal responsibility for healthy outcomes (Leonard and Plotnikoff, 2001; Zerwekh, 2000). It is important for the nurse to create an environment that promotes partnership with clients in all phases of the nursing process (Parkman and Ullrich, 2000). "Holistic nursing is a way of thinking, reflecting, and practicing" (Frisch, 2001).

The AHNA has published standards for holistic practice, and several resources are available through the several nursing specialty groups (Frisch, 2001; Snyder and Lindquist, 2001). Nurses often integrate CAM techniques with the traditional medical practices such as teaching breathing and visualization strategies in managing pain and reducing stress. Serving as teacher and facilitator empowers the client (Parkman and Ullrich, 2000).

APPLICATION OF SELECTED ALTERNATIVE THERAPIES: AN OVERVIEW

During the last 30 years there has been a major effort to identify strategies to assist individuals in coping with both acute diagnoses and chronic psychologic and physiologic health problems, as well as managing sudden and long-term life changes. The greatest benefits of CAM therapies have been in promoting healthy lifestyles and in the management of chronic illnesses and diseases (Pelletier, 2000).

Mind-Body Interventions

Meditation

The relaxation response to meditation consists of a wide range of beneficial physiologic and psychologic effects, including lowered heart and blood pressure rates, decreased serum levels of adrenal corticosteroids, increased immunity to disease, a sense of calmness and peace, and mental alertness. Meditation therapies include biofeedback, visual imagery, and other stress-reduction measures, including yoga and progressive relaxation techniques. Originally, meditation was considered a religious practice (i.e., saying prayers, reciting scripture, saying the rosary, or concentrating on a religious symbol). Meditative techniques can be taught, and a number of audiotapes have been designed to facilitate mastery of concentration. Guidelines for meditating include a routine of selecting a special time and place, assuming a comfortable position, using deep breathing and progressive relaxation exercises, and focusing attention on a chosen mental image (Kreitzer and Jensen, 2000; Parkman and Ullrich, 2000).

Prayer

Prayer differs from meditation in that it involves communication with God, or a superior being, who is believed to answer the prayer. Prayer can be an individual or group action, or an intercessory prayer conducted by other people without the knowledge of the individual for whom the prayers are said. The laying on of hands and anointing the ill person with oil while praying for healing is an ancient form of intercessory prayer. Prayer can be silent or spoken, conversational or formal, or a recitation of a favorite psalm. Illness can interfere with an individual's ability to pray because of feelings of isolation, guilt, grief, or anxiety. Prayer is one of the therapeutic tools nurses use when providing spiritual care to allay a client's distraught feelings. Many hospitals have chaplains to support clients and their families of all faiths (Schlosser, 1999). "Each of these threads—religion, ethnicity, and culture is woven into the fabric of each person's particular response to treatment and healing" (Spector, 2000).

Yoga

Living a balanced life is central to yoga principles. The use of specific body postures, breath control, minimizing stimulation of the senses, leading a simple life, and directed meditation are achieved through daily practices. Concentration on purity of body and mind, self-restraint and contentment with life, studying relevant literature, and daily dedication to a higher being are the means to attain that balance. Originally practiced in India, yoga has become a popular practice as a part of health enhancement and as a therapy for people with chronic diseases (Pelletier, 2000).

Biofeedback

Biofeedback is a technique that initially uses electrical equipment to assist persons in gaining conscious control over body processes that normally are thought to be beyond voluntary command. It is often combined with controlled breathing techniques and/or meditation to provide individuals information about their bodies they are unaware of. Electrodes that are attached to the affected area send information into a monitoring device, which emits a signal to alert the person to changes in a particular body function (e.g., an increase or decrease in muscle tension).

By watching the device, clients can learn to use mental processes to control that particular body action. A therapist instructs the client in the mental exercises during a series of sessions. Eventually the client is able to practice the exercises without the aid of the machine. Biofeedback has been used in the treatment of multiple physical, cognitive, and behavioral symptoms. Among these are hypertension, temperature control, gastrointestinal activity, substance abuse, stress, sleep disorders, migraine headaches, and other vascular disorders (Kreitzer and Jensen, 2000; Pelletier, 2000).

Use of the Arts

The use of music, dance, drama, literature, humor, and art is part of environmental therapy. Quiet background music provides a soothing atmosphere and can be a distracting medium during times of stress and pain. Music is often used in intensive care units, in birthing rooms, during dental procedures, and even as a stimulus for people with lowered levels of consciousness. Mood music allows the listener to express emotions and feelings through dancing, singing, and creative thinking (Young-Mason, 2002; McCaffrey and Locsin, 2002).

Dance is an expression of joy and celebration throughout the world. It has been used as a means to increase self-esteem and body image; lessen depression, fear, and isolation; and express emotions. Art has often been used with children and adults for expression of their feelings about stressful situations and unconscious concerns about their illnesses. Art expression has been a psychotherapy tool in geriatric centers, with children and adolescents, in hospices, in alcohol treatment programs, and in prisons. Books, poetry, and religious writings can be inspirational and can cause a person to become immersed for long periods in the reading situations. Journals and diaries are also forms of expressing one's emotions and have been referred to as *process meditation* and a conversation with the self. Duran (2000) discussed the use of drama, quilting, and story telling as therapeutic tools used by women for centuries.

Humor

Humor and laughter are also used for expressing emotions, relieving tensions and anxiety, and coping with painful or unpleasant situations. Laughter can have positive effects on cognitive ability, respiratory and heart rates, blood pressure, and muscle tension (Kreitzer and Jensen, 2000). Humor rooms supplied with videocassettes and audiotapes, books, cartoons, and artwork have been created for clients, families, and agency staff encouraged the use of humorous artwork on bulletin boards in patient rooms and staff work areas. Minden (2002) conducted a qualitative study of humor as a focal point of therapy for hospitalized male forensic (criminal) psychiatric patients. Under supervision, student nurses held humor groups over a 16-week clinical rotation with a total of 10 rotation time frames. Interview findings indicated enhanced physical, psychologic, and social health. More than half of the men felt an increased sense of spiritual well-being. In his classic book *Anatomy of an Illness* (1979), Norman Cousins, a famous journalist, wrote about the value of humor in relieving the severe pain he experienced from ankylosing spondylitis by stating that a "good belly laugh" allowed him to be pain free for at least 2 hours at a time. Cousins wrote that humor healed him.

Exercise

The benefits of physical exercise are well known. It can bring a general sense of health and vitality, increase respiratory and cardiovascular efficiency, and promote a longer life. People who exercise often sleep better and have improved appetites; exercise is now considered a major factor in self-care (Pelletier, 2000). People with disabilities can perform even simple exercises. Special Olympics for wheelchair athletes is an excellent example of using exercise to enhance the self-image and general health.

Animal-Assisted Therapy

This discussion of mind-body interventions would not be complete without the mention of using companion animals to induce the relaxation response and enhance emotional and physiologic well-being. Studies have shown a reduction in hypertension, heart rate, and social isolation when pets are introduced as a treatment modality. Studies have also shown the benefits to the morale of staff and caregivers. Individuals who are blind, deaf, or paralyzed have used companion animals to assist in accomplishing activities of daily living. Acute and long-term health care agency policies have been altered to allow pets into intensive care units, pediatric wards, hospices, rehabilitation units, and geriatric and other areas. Nurses have been active supporters of animal-assisted therapy (Cole and Gavlinski, 2000).

Psychotherapy and Hypnosis

A variety of social support and self-help groups have implemented many of the psychologic methods such as multiple therapy approaches and cognitive, behavior, and body-oriented therapies to bring about beneficial effects for the participants. Groups are commonly used as adjunct therapy for substance abuse control, weight loss, cancer, grief counseling, and caregiver support.

Hypnosis has been in use since the eighteenth century as a deep relaxation technique and has become a useful tool in the treatment of substance addiction, pain control, fears, and phobias. It has also been used successfully before anesthesia induction, as a means for reducing hypertension, and for dietary management. Hypnosis involves the use of mental images, concentration, use of repetitive words or sounds, and total relaxation. Hypnosis produces an altered state of consciousness that permits the person to focus concentration with minimal distraction. Education in self-hypnosis through the aid of guided audiotapes tailored to meet the individual's specific problem has been used for self-therapy at home (Pelletier, 2000).

Bioelectromagnetics

Concepts of magnetic field therapy relate to the electrical currents that exist within and external to the body, the influence of external currents on the body, and the result of physical and behavioral changes (Zerwekh, 2000). Examples are the electromagnetic energies produced by x-rays, television, microwaves, and light rays. Prolonged exposure to such fields can produce hazardous effects. However, scientists have also discovered that lower-level energy frequencies can be beneficial in designing diagnostic and treatment tools.

Nonthermal electromagnetic fields, which do not cause heating of tissues, have been used for bone repair, nerve stimulation, and wound healing; as electrostimulation via acupuncture needles for stimulation of the immune system; and for neuroendocrine modulations. Unipolor magnets have been used for pain relief, particularly of arthritis. Magnets can be taped to various areas of the body, inserted inside shoes, and placed in mattress covers. Anecdotal accounts have yielded favorable responses (Kreitzer and Jensen, 2000). A new clinical trial by NCCAM (2002) is examining the effectiveness of electrostimulated acupuncture on minimizing delayed nausea after cancer chemotherapy that occurs 24 hours to 5 days posttreatment.

Alternative Systems of Medical Practice

Alternative systems include traditional Oriental medicine; acupuncture; Ayurvedic, homeopathic, naturopathic, and environmental medicines; and anthroposophically extended medicine (which builds on naturopathy, homeopathy, and modern scientific medicine).

Traditional Chinese Medicine

A variety of therapies are practiced within traditional Chinese medicine (TCM), including acupuncture and acupressure, massage, herbal medicine, *qigong*, and *Tai Chi* (a slow-motion dancelike martial art) (see Understanding and Applying Research box). Variations of TCM are practiced in Japan, Korea, and Vietnam. Oriental medicine centers on the diagnosis of disturbances of *qi*, (pronounced "chee") or the vital energy, and the balance between *yin* and *yang* (female and male, cold and hot, dark and light) forces.

UNDERSTANDING and APPLYING RESEARCH

The pain of chronic arthritis that is often ignored and undertreated affects millions of older adults. The purpose of this pilot study was to determine the effect of the age-old Chinese practice of *Tai Chi* in reducing arthritic pain. *Tai Chi* integrates meditation with slow aerobic exercise movements that promote flexibility and muscle strengthening.

A convenience sample of ambulatory community-based men (n = 2) and women (n = 14) 68 to 87 years old diagnosed with arthritis were randomly assigned to the *Tai Chi* experimental group or a control group (with no change in their daily activities). Eight persons in the experimental group attended 10 weekly, 1-hour *Tai Chi* classes. The number of exercises was increased over several sessions. Participants were encouraged to practice the exercises daily whenever possible. All participants recorded their current pain from 0 (no pain) to 10 (worst possible pain) on a weekly basis. Both groups recorded pain and perception of health before and after the study. A significantly greater decrease in pain was reported in the *Tai Chi* group than in the control group. Analgesic use was comparable between the groups. There was no difference in perceptions of health; however, the small sample size limits the ability to generalize the findings of the study to the general population.

Suggestions for future studies included a larger sample size, including persons with weekly average pain intensity scores higher than 3; rating average pain the week before the study; and asking participants to keep daily logs of pain scores and analgesic use throughout the study. Although the study findings show promise, further research is needed before recommending *Tai Chi* for pain relief and perception of health.

Adler P et al: The effects of *Tai Chi* on older adults with chronic arthritis pain, *J Nurs Scholarsh* 32(4):377, 2000.

Diagnostic procedures consist of observing facial expressions and body movements, careful listening and questioning, and palpating body pulses. The relationship of physical and emotional behaviors is used to plan a range of traditional therapies. The most frequent methods used in the United States are acupuncture and massage.

Acupuncture. Acupuncture is a process in which small needles are inserted at selected energy points of the body that correspond to energy pathways, or meridians, that traverse from the body surface to inner organs. Its purpose is to activate the *qi* and achieve a balance when imbalance exists. The needles can be heated and attached to mild electrical current or be twirled by hand to cause vibrations. Numerous studies have revealed the positive effects of acupuncture on a wide range of disorders, including gynecologic, mental, and neural problems and substance addiction. Its effectiveness in pain control and anesthesia is attributed to the release of endogenous opioids (endorphins) that are produced within the central nervous system. Acupuncture is one of the most thoroughly researched and documented alternative medical practices (Parkman and Ullrich, 2000; Pelletier, 2000).

Ayurveda/Ayurvedic Medicine

Ayurvedic (science of life) medicine originated in India and dates back thousands of years. This method may use a combination of therapies including meditation, yoga, massage, herbs, aromatherapy, and biofeedback. The body is viewed as a pharmacy that can make its own natural drugs to heal itself.

The human body is also considered a microcosm of the universe, endowed with principles, or *doshas*, that interact in maintaining balance. The basic nature (*prakriti*), or genetic code, and the relationship among the *doshas* remain unaltered throughout a person's life. Each *dosha* has a principal location in the body. Emphasis is placed on the interdependence of health and the quality of the person's sociocultural life. When any imbalance occurs, a restoration of balance of the internal environment is achieved through proper diet and lifestyle. A recent study funded by the NIH Alternative Medicine Branch demonstrated the positive effects of Ayurvedic practices with healthy adults (Pelletier, 2000).

Homeopathic Medicine

Homeopathic medicine is based on the belief that a drug that produces certain disease symptoms in a healthy person can provide a cure for a sick person experiencing the same symptoms. Diluted substances are used to elicit a cure (e.g., a very dilute solution containing poison ivy compound may be prescribed for a skin rash). The medication must be shaken vigorously or "potentized" for the greatest effectiveness as the solution picks up energy from the dissolved substance. These products are used for acute and chronic health problems, as well as for health promotion.

The homeopathic drug market has become a multimillion-dollar industry. The FDA currently regulates the remedies, and drugs manufactured by reputable pharmaceutical companies are listed in the *Homeopathic Pharmacopoeia of the United States.* Some are sold as OTC drugs; products used for serious conditions require dispensing by a licensed practitioner (Tedesco and Cicchetti, 2001).

Naturopathy

Naturopathy is primarily used by a small group of physicians who have been educated in the sciences and have received specialized training in the disciplines of alternative medicine. They use an eclectic selection of herbs, homeopathy, nutrition, TCM, hydrotherapy, and manipulative therapy in conjunction with modern scientific medical diagnostic methods and standards. Naturopathy focuses on self-healing, and health care is tailored to the individual's needs. The basic principles include use of therapies that do no harm, the physician's primary role as teacher, establishing and maintaining an optimal health and balance, treatment of the whole person, prevention of disease through a healthy lifestyle, and therapeutic use of nutrition (Pelletier, 2000).

Environmental Medicine

Allergy treatment was the original impetus for the development of environmental medicine in the 1940s. Scientists noted that the sensitivity and allergy symptoms of some individuals were improved when certain foods or chemicals, molds, dust, pollens, and other substances were eliminated. Emotional stress was also identified as a source of immune system dysfunction. The person's environmental history became an important component in the diagnostic process by providing a chronologic account of etiologic circumstances leading to the health problem. The elimination of health hazards from the environment has become a major health issue. Examples include the removal of asbestos building insulation materials, instillation of devices for recapture of gasoline fumes and smog emissions on automobiles, removal of certain pesticides from the market, and elimination of preservatives and color additives from foods, medicines, and nutrition supplements.

Culture-Based Community Medicines

The many culture-based practices, or folk medicine, follow naturalistic methods; and a spiritual healer or shaman usually provides religious rituals, which are a major component. Symbols such as prayer wheels, sand paintings, meditation, wearing amulets, group singing, chanting, and dancing ceremonies are part of the healing rituals. On the Navajo reservation, modern hospitals and the shaman's healing room are under the same roof. Some people believe that spells cast by the witch doctor have sometimes proved to be more powerful than Western medicines (Leonard and Plotnikoff, 2000; Parkman and Ullrich, 2000).

Manual Healing Methods

Included in manual healing methods are osteopathic and chiropractic medicines, massage, reflexology, and the techniques of pressure point and other various touch therapies.

Osteopathy and Chiropractic Medicines. These practices involve manipulation of soft tissues and joints. Both require specialized education and licensure to practice. Osteopathic practices are considered to be mainstream medicine by much of the public, and the practitioner often is the primary health care provider. Chiropractic practitioners study the relationship between pressure, strain, or tension on the spinal cord and the ability of the neuromusculoskeletal system to act efficiently. Manual adjustments of the spine to correct alignment are a mainstay of treatment. Some insurance carriers have now approved chiropractic medicine, and the most recent center has been established by NCCAM to study its effects (NIH, 2002).

Massage. More than 80 different forms of massage therapy have been identified. These forms vary from gentle stroking to deep kneading, rubbing, and percussion. Most massage is done with the hands; however, the forearms, elbows, and feet are sometimes used. The primary purposes of massage therapy are to produce muscle and total-body relaxation and increased circulation. Massage techniques, at one time, were included in the fundamental nursing courses. Touch, which is the basic medium of massage therapy, is a form of communication and caring (Kreitzer and Jensen, 2000).

Acupressure. The same meridian points used in acupuncture are manipulated in pressure point therapies. The fingertips are used to apply pressure to more than 600 designated points in soft tissues. Acupressure can be used both as a diagnostic tool and as treatment. The sessions can last up to an hour, with the recipient spending equal time lying in the prone and dorsal positions for a total body treatment. The therapist also places a strong emphasis on mind-spirit-body balance in counseling the client. *Shiatsu*, a Japanese form, is similar to acupressure, with pressure being applied by the palm of the hand, as well as the fingers.

Foot Reflexology. Reflexology, which originated in Egypt, is also referred to as zone therapy. This technique is based on the premise that the feet (and hands) are mirrors of the body, with reflex points that correspond to glands, organs, and other structures in the body. (The feet are considered to be more responsive to massage than the hands.) Massage of a reflex point (without the use of oil, cream, or lotion) stimulates the corresponding organ in that zone. The main goal is to provide relaxation by removing tension in a zone area (*Journal of Reflexology* on-line; Zerwekh, 2000).

Therapeutic Touch. Healing through touch can be traced back to early civilizations. Nurses have practiced various forms of therapeutic touch for many years. Benefits of contact touch such as massage have recently been identified as providing a sense of spiritual balance, relieving mental and emotional tension and anxiety, improving blood flow, easing pain, and stimulating the immune system.

Therapeutic touch also refers to a noncontact technique derived from the laying on of hands associated with Far Eastern, European, and religious philosophies. This method is based on a theory that the release of excess energy from the healer assists the ill person in the healing process. The basic principles can be learned, and workshops have been offered throughout the country. Healing touch is a similar technique and became a certificate program of the American Holistic Nurses' Association in 1993 (Kreitzer and Jensen, 2000; Zerwekh, 2000).

Pharmacologic and Biologic Treatments

Pharmacologic and biologic alternative therapies consist of a variety of drugs and vaccines that have not yet been included in mainstream medicine. Some are designed to stimulate the immune system to ward off diseases and may consist of older herbal remedies. All are considered to be nontoxic. One example is shark and other animal cartilage used as treatment for acquired immunodeficiency syndrome (AIDS), cancer, and arthritis. Cartilage is believed to inhibit tumor growth by cutting off the blood supply to the tumor, suppressing autoimmune reactions, and promoting wound

healing. Ethylene diamine tetraacetic acid (EDTA) is a chemical that binds with metallic ions and is used as a treatment for lead poisoning and other toxic metals. It is now being proposed as treatment for ridding the body of free radicals and thus removing fat deposits from artery walls and improving cardiovascular circulation. A total of 70 studies have yielded positive results; however, the American Heart Association and other organizations do not endorse its use (Turner, 2001).

Herbal Medicine

The use of herbal and plant medicine is an ancient practice worldwide. Tree barks, plant roots, berries, leaves, resins, seeds, and flowers have all been ground into powders, mixed with solutions, brewed in teas, and used singly or in combination as the treatment of ailments (Box 21-5). Herbal remedies are used by one third of adult Americans (an estimated 60 million people). In all 64% of the world's population relies on herbal remedies. More than 1500 herbs are marketed in the United States (Parkman and Ullrich, 2000; Pelletier, 2000).

Records of herbal medicines appeared in Egypt extending back to 2000 BC, in Greece and Rome at the time of Aris-

---

Box 21-5   Examples of Herbs and Food Herbals Used as Alternative Therapies and as the Basis for Allopathic Traditional Medicines

Most of the herbs come from tropical rain forests; others are derived from the sea, and still others come from countries around the world. Flowers, seeds, leaves, woods and barks, vines, tubers, roots, and even grasses have been the basis of alternative and traditional allopathic medicine therapy. (Over one fourth of traditional medicines are based on plant properties.) Different portions of a plant or tree may have different properties and different concentrations and also can be used for different purposes. These products can be used as inhalants, taken internally, added to bathwater, or applied externally. The following is a small list of examples:

- *Analgesics:* Meadowsweet, poplar (balm of Gilead) tree, willow tree (aspirin), wintergreen, oil of clove (used in dentistry), feverfew, nutmeg (for migraine), marijuana (nausea and pain for cancer patients and people with AIDS)
- *Narcotics:* Belladonna, celandine, nightshade, opium poppy
- *Aromatics:* Allspice, angelica, anise, avicena, camomile, ginger, juniper, lavender, mint, nutmeg, pennyroyal, rosemary, wormwood, pine and balsam woods, cinnamon (as incense); used as relaxants, for bronchodilator effects, etc.
- *Stimulants:* Marijuana, nutmeg, peyote, Scotch broom for euphorics and hallucinogens; ginseng (American and Asian) for mental and physical energizer—also considered a panacea for its variety of healing properties; belladonna for atropine effects on the central nervous system
- *Sedatives:* Celery, feverweed, hops, Indian pipe, lavender, monkshood, wild black cherry, mountain laurel, passion flower, peach tree, peony, periwinkle, heliotrope (valerian)
- *Antidepressant/antianxiety agents:* Borage, St. John's Wort, lobelia (in correct dosage), rosemary, pasqueflower, aromatics

- *Antiaging agents:* Ginkgo biloba (increases circulation)
- *Antiseptics:* Garlic (also used to reduce cholesterol), onion, wintergreen, camphor
- *Diaphoretics:* Seneca snakeroot
- *Antioxidants:* Ginger, spices (Indian)
- *Cardiotonics:* Foxglove (digitalis), lily of the valley, *Strophanthus* (ouabain)
- *Ophthalmic agents:* Calabar bean (physiostigmine) used for glaucoma
- *Antihypertensives:* Parsley, skullcap, garlic, hawthorn, wild black cherry, seneca snakeroot (rauwolfia)
- *Contraceptive agents:* Mexican yam—diosegenin that can be converted to progesterone (Syntex)
- *Muscle paralyzing agents:* Strychnos toxifera produces a powerful poison—curare (used to create intercostal muscle paralysis during surgery)
- *Antineoplastic agents:* Yew tree bark (paclitaxel), rosy periwinkle (vincristine, vinblastine); used for childhood leukemias and Hodgkin's disease
- *Gastrointestinal agents:* Papaya for dyspepsia, liquorice flower (carbenoxolone) as treatment for peptic ulcer
- *Antidiarrheal agents:* Opium poppy (paregoric)
- *Cathartics:* Ricinus communis (castor oil)
- *Dermatologic agents:* Aloe vera, wintergreen (ointment)
- *Antibiotic agents:* Fungi (penicillin), iris versicolor (antisyphilitic), lobelia (antisyphilitic)
- *Antimalarials:* Chinchona bark or Peruvian bark (quinine)—also used as antiarrhythmic
- *Antiviral agents:* May apple (used for venereal warts and AIDS)

totle, in the Muslim world, in India, and in the Orient. Each culture compiled a *materia medica*—a listing of drugs and their uses. The American Indians contributed a vast array of herbals to the Colonial American medicine formulary, and herbals continued to be a mainstay of medical practices for many years. Today, herbal products can be marketed only as food supplements, and some are considered to be potentially dangerous by the FDA and other regulatory agencies. No safety guidelines have been established. Nevertheless, the public is purchasing alternative medicines at a greater rate than ever before and adopting many remedies from other cultures.

The formulas of Chinese medicine are based on the correct ratio or balance of a variety of *food herbs* that are harvested and prepared at an appropriate time to enhance their effects. Food herbs are composed of plants (85%), animals (12%), and minerals (3%). The various herbal ingredients are mixed according to the diseases caused by imbalance of *yin* and *yang* rather than the chemistry makeup of the herb. *Yin* and *yang* characteristics and their related properties of cold and heat are used to categorize diseases and medicines. These mixtures are used as supplements to a well-balanced diet and are often prescribed in conjunction with daily exercise and positive thinking, in the belief that a balanced body is a result of a balanced life. Many Chinese herbal stores have captured a large share of the U.S. alternative medicine market.

Examples of commonly used herbs worldwide are *Ginkgo biloba,* echinacea, saw palmetto, *Prunus africanum,* ginseng, and St. John's Wort. Both European and Oriental varieties of *Ginkgo biloba* are used to increase circulation, particularly to bring oxygen to the brain and to retard the effects of aging. European studies have shown its effectiveness for improvement in mental alertness, increased circulation to the extremities, lowered cholesterol, and improved blood flow to the retina. Echinacea, or purple coneflower, is prized for its antiseptic properties and ability to stimulate the immune system, particularly against infections such as flu, colds, and wound healing. Saw palmetto berries and *P. africanum* have become popular treatments for benign prostatic hypertrophy. Ginseng root has been used as a tonic in China for more than 3000 years. It has also been used as an antistress agent and to alter circadian rhythms and amounts of circulating corticosterone. *Hypericum,* the principal ingredient of St. John's Wort, has been termed "nature's Prozac" because of its popular use as an antidepressant (Parkman and Ullrich, 2000; Pelletier, 2000). Examples of natural herbal remedies new to the U.S. market include black cohosh for menopausal symptoms; mental acuity formula, a combination of vitamins and herbs for mild memory problems; probiotic pearls, a dietary supplement with acidophilus and *B. longum* to promote healthy intestinal flora; and pantethine plus, a triple action combination formula to enhance

the breakdown of fat and cholesterol (Rite Care Pharmacy, on-line, September 2002). Additional herbal remedies appear in Box 21-5.

Aromatherapy was initially used in Egypt to relieve pain. Today it is being used for relaxation or as an adjunct to stress reduction measures. More than 300 essential plant oils are currently in use as inhalants, for massage and compresses or as additions to bathwater, and candles. The burning of aromatic woods was used in ancient times to purify the air; incense is still used today as part of healing ceremonies. Other examples include birch oil as an antiinflammatory agent, lavender for headache relief, rosemary added to vaporizers for relief of congestion, and peppermint for nausea relief and as an antipyretic and respiratory stimulant. Aromatherapy is included in Ayurvedic therapy (Parkman and Ullrich, 2000).

Diet and Nutrition

Diet and nutritional needs are integral to both traditional and alternative therapies. Today's affluent diet, which is high in animal fats, refined carbohydrates, and partially hydrogenated vegetable oils, contributes to many of the current health problems in the United States. Alternative healthy diets and a change in lifestyle have been included in educational information to prevent or correct obesity, cardiovascular disease, and diabetes and other chronic health problems. Vitamins and other food supplements are frequently added to the health maintenance plan. Recent studies include research on the value of the antioxidant vitamins C, E, and β-carotene in the prevention of cataracts and cancer, and on the effects of vitamin C and nicotinic acid as replacement therapy for psychiatric clients receiving electroconvulsive and tranquilizer therapy. Megadoses of niacin have been shown to aid in reducing serum cholesterol. Nutritional supplements are given to offset the effects of medicines prescribed for people with AIDS (Parkman and Ullrich, 2000; Pelletier, 2000).

Several diets have been developed as specific treatments for diseases. Macrobiotic cancer diets are based on Oriental beliefs of creating a balance of *yin* and *yang.* Research by environmental medicine scientists has helped to identify potential food antigens such as chemical additives and natural food substances. Food elimination diets have been used to reduce sensitivity to certain substances and hasten recovery from allergic responses. These diets have also been used in the treatment of children with attention deficit/hyperactivity disorder (Pelletier, 2000). Health care providers must be sensitive to ethnic and cultural diets when planning health care activities. Some of these diets may pose health risks because of a lack of essential ingredients or interaction with prescribed medications. Incorporating familiar foods into the diet may also facilitate a person's recovery, and substances in the diet may actually facilitate healing.

CHAPTER SUMMARY

- A stigma continues to be attached to alternative methods; the scientific community often labels alternative methods as a hoax, witchcraft, or magicoreligious practices, and attributes results to placebo effects. Nevertheless, nurses must become knowledgeable about the many methods that clients from diverse cultural and ethnic backgrounds use to manage their lives and be nonjudgmental about these practices.

- Taking a comprehensive history, documenting the findings, and sharing them with others on the health care team are important steps in the plan of care.

- Public education regarding the potential harmful effects of concurrent use of alternative and prescription medicines and the need to inform their health care providers is essential. People must also understand the consequences of self-diagnosis, self-treatment, and delay in seeking help.

- The AHNA suggests that alternative and traditional therapies can complement each other in providing holistic care, and it urges nurses to become familiar with the alternative methods and to incorporate them into the plan of care whenever possible.

- The concepts of caring and healing, as well as commitment to global health are integral components of nursing.

- The nurse attends to a wide range of human experiences and responses to health and disease, and in the provision of a caring relationship, promotes healing and health maintenance.

- The goal of holistic nursing is to enhance the healing of all aspects of the whole person. The nursing profession is qualified to perform independent and interdependent actions that are largely technical such as teaching, administration, and research. It is dynamic and evolutionary, humanistic, and a discipline that is fundamentally based on scientific and theoretical knowledge and founded on moral, ethical, and spiritual values.

- Concepts of health and illness are deeply embedded. Cultural competency requires an awareness of one's own values and those of the healthcare system. Nurses are frequently called on to support decisions that may differ from their own cultural norms and values. Culturally incompetent care challenges the belief system of clients and their families, causes undue stress, and inhibits the healing process. Efficient and effective clinical care in cross-cultural circumstances is defined as a new competency for all nurses.

REVIEW QUESTIONS

1. A 55-year-old client is hospitalized after having a heart attack. Which nursing intervention demonstrates that the nurse is treating the client holistically?
   a. Takes frequent vital signs and discusses the importance of diet
   b. Discusses with the client lifestyle patterns and teaches relaxation techniques for stress, stresses the importance of diet and exercise, and suggests mind-body interventions such as yoga or meditation
   c. Explains that the client needs to have more faith in God to get better
   d. Arranges for a dietitian to review client's new low-cholesterol, low-fat, and low-sodium diet restriction

2. One of the advantages of alternative medicine is that:
   a. It gives the client more control over own treatment.
   b. It allows other companies to benefit besides pharmaceutical companies.
   c. The methods don't require scrupulous research before using them.
   d. It is more cost-effective for low-income families.

3. An appropriate alternative method for a client who has anxiety, difficulty sleeping, and headaches is:
   a. Immitrex.
   b. Limiting the intake of caffeine.
   c. Individual psychotherapy.
   d. Meditation.

4. The core principle of Oriental medicine involves:
   a. The influence of external currents on the body.
   b. The balance of *qi* (energy) and *yin* and *yang* (female and male forces).
   c. Hypnosis and deep relaxation techniques.
   d. The use of electrical equipment to assist the client to gain control over own body.

5. The nurse assesses a client and asks what medications the client is taking including herbal and over-the-counter medication. The client identifies St. John's Wort. The nurse knows that the client is taking this for:
   a. Anxiety.
   b. Pain.
   c. Depression.
   d. Memory recall.

REFERENCES

Adler P et al: The effects of Tai Chi on older adults with chronic arthritis pain, *J Nurs Scholarsh* 32(4):377, 2000.

American Holistic Nursing Association: Mission statement. On-line, website: www.ahna.org, 2002.

Cole K, Gavlinski A: Animal-assisted therapy: the human-animal bond, *AACN Clin Issues: Adv Pract Acute Crit Care* 11(1):139-149, 2000.

Cousins N: *Anatomy of an illness as perceived by the patient,* New York, 1979, WW Norton.

Dossey B, Dossey L: Body-mind-spirit: attending to holistic care, *Am J Nurs* 98(8):35-38, 1998.

Duran D: Integrated women health holistic approaches for comprehensive care (review), *AORN J* 74(5):683-689, 2000.

Eisenberg DM et al: Unconventional medicine in the United States—prevalence, costs, and patterns of use, *N Engl J Med* 328(4):246-252, 1993.

Eisenberg DM et al: Trends in alternative medicine use in the United States, 1990-1997, *JAMA* 280(18):1569-1575, 1998.

Ellis K, Hartley C: *Nursing in today's world: challenges, issues and trends,* Philadelphia, 2000, Lippincott.

Forbes M: Complementary and alternative therapies in nursing and health care. In Zerwekh J, Claborn J, editors: *Nursing today: transitions and trends,* ed 3, Philadelphia, 2000, WB Saunders.

Frisch N: Nursing as a context for alternative/complementary modalities, *Online Journal of Issues in Nursing,* 6(2), 2000, website: www.nursingworld.org/ojin/topic15/50c15_2.htm.

Frisch N: Standards for holistic nursing practice: a way to think about our care that includes complementary and alternative modalities, *Online Journal of Issues in Nursing* 6(2), 2001, website: www.nursingworld.org/ojin/topic15/50c15_2.htm.

Journal of Reflexology, website: www.LookSmartWorld.com.

Kreitzer M, Jensen D: Healing practices: trends, challenges, and opportunities for nurses in acute and critical care, *AACN Clinical Issues* 11(1):7-16, 2000.

Leonard B, Plotnikoff G: Awareness: the heart of cultural competence, *AACN Clinical Issues* 11(1):51-59, 2001.

McCaffrey R, Locsin R: Music listening as a nursing intervention: a symphony of practice, *Holistic Nursing Practice* 16(3):70-77, 2002.

Minden P: Humor as focal point of therapy for forensic psychiatric patients, *Holistic Nursing Practice* 16(4):775-786, 2002.

National Center for Complementary and Alternative Medicine, website: www.altmed.od.nih.gov/nccam

Parkman C, Ullrich S: *Keeping current on age-old practices: a complementary and alternative medicine guide for nurses,* Sunnyvale, Calif, 2000, Nurseweek Pub.

Pelletier K: *The best alternative medicine,* New York, 2000, Simon & Schuster.

Rite-Care Pharmacy: Homeopathic medicine, website: www.LookSmartWorld.com.

Ruiz RJ: Psychoneuroimmunology and preterm birth: a holistic model for obstetrical nursing practice and research, *MCN Am J Matern Child Nurs* 24(5):230-235, 1999.

Schlosser S: Social, cultural and spiritual aspects of health care. In Berger K, Williams M, editors: *Fundamentals of nursing,* Stamford Conn, 1999, Appleton & Lange.

Snyder M, Lindquist R: Issues in complementary therapies: how we got to where we are: *Online Journal of Issues in Nursing* 6(2), 2001, website: www.nursingworld.org/ojin/topic15/50c15_1.htm.

Spector R: *Cultural diversity in health and illness,* Upper Saddle River, NJ, 2000, Prentice Hall.

Tedesco P, Cicchetti J: Like cures like: homeopathy, *Am J Nurs* 101(9):43-50, 2001.

Turner J: Chelation therapy. *Gale encyclopedia of alternative medicine,* 2001, website: www.LookSmartWorld.com.

Young-Mason J: Music therapy: a healing art, *Clin Nurse Spec* 16(3):153-154, 2002.

Weil A: Introduction. In Pelletier K: *The best alternative medicine,* New York, 2000, Simon & Schuster.

Zerwekh J: Contemporary health care delivery: trends and economics. In Zerwekh J, Claborn J, editors: *Nursing today: transitions and trends,* ed 3, Philadelphia, 2000, WB Saunders.

SUGGESTED READINGS

Fadiman A: *The spirit catches you and you fall down,* New York, 1997, Farrar, Straus & Giroux.

Gaydos H: Complementary and alternative therapies in nursing education: trends and issues. *Online Journal of Issues in Nursing,* 2001, website: http://www.nursingworld.org/ojin/topic15/50c15_5.htm.

ONLINE RESOURCES

American Association of Oriental Medicine: www.aaom.org
American Chiropractic Association: www.amerchiro.org
American Holistic Nurses' Association: www.ahna.org
Homeopathic Educational Services: www.homeopathic.com
Spirituality&Health: www.spiritualityhealth.com
Healthy People 2010: www.healthypeople.gov

22

Crisis: Concepts and Interventions

Susan Selverston

OBJECTIVES

- Describe the historical context of crisis intervention and new directions in the field.

- Describe individual crisis triggers (external and internal).

- Discuss the potential psychologic effects of disasters and terrorism.

- Describe approaches to treating disaster threats and disaster victims.

- Discuss crisis assessment, intervention, planning, and prevention strategies, including assessment "in the field" and "in the office."

- Describe barriers to effective crisis intervention.

The word **crisis** can be understood in several ways. A crisis may be viewed as a disturbing event, a threat to well-being, or an opportunity for change and growth. An individual's interpretation of the threat depends on past experience and learning and prior outcomes to similar threats. That interpretation and experience of the event may be considered the crisis. Based on the individual's perception of the event, prior learning, memory, and interpretation of the event, the mental/emotional response to the triggering event may be adaptive (a positive outcome) or maladaptive (a negative outcome). When accompanied by a negative expectation, hopelessness and helplessness occur and the resulting strategies for coping will likely be unsuccessful (Ursin, 2002).

Crisis intervention is a brief therapy, initiated as soon as possible after the crisis event or crisis response occurs. In either situation, the goal of therapy is to assist the client to expect a successful outcome of the challenge and to assist with practical coping strategies. With this type of intervention the client stands a better chance for positive responses to similar future stressors (Ursin, 2002).

Using a biopsychosocial model, the nurse evaluates the objective and subjective threats, both external (tangible) and internal (intangible). The client's mental, emotional, and physical responses to the threats are determined to be adaptive or maladaptive. Adaptive responses are supported, and maladaptive responses are treated with supportive counseling, education, and appropriate linkage to other agencies. When necessary, interventions are tailored to the client's needs, considering basic needs first, the client's resources, and the ability to engage in therapy.

Although the past focus of crisis intervention has been primarily on the individual, groups of people who experience natural and man-made (artificially induced) disasters are also extremely vulnerable. Terrorist acts at home (Oklahoma City bombing, 1995), biologic attacks such as anthrax exposure through the mail, school shootings in the United States (Santana HS, 2002; Columbine HS, 1999) and abroad (Dunblane, Scotland, 1996; Gutenberg HS, Erfurt, Germany, 2002), and of course the events of September 11, 2001 give crisis intervention broader significance. Potential terrorist methods being anticipated and planned for include biologic warfare agents such as anthrax, botulism, plague, smallpox, and others. Chemical agents such as sarin gas, mustard gas, and other toxic or irritating gases, along with disaster planning for explosions, fires, nuclear accidents or attacks, and rescue and relief work, are being addressed at all levels of government. Examples of a new effort to prepare for disasters are everywhere. For example, the Federal Emergency Management Agency (FEMA) has worked to prepare for responses to terrorism after the Oklahoma City bombing (Natural Hazards, November, 2001). Researchers at the Stanford University Center on Stress and Health are studying people's responses to attacks on the United States, using the Internet to collect data (Graham, 2001). The National Institute of Mental Health (NIMH) funded four grants between September 11, 2001 and April 2002 in response to the terrorist attacks through its Rapid Assessment Post Impact of Disaster program, as well as six supplemental grants to existing studies focusing on posttraumatic stress disorders (PTSDs). The overall goal for the research funded by NIMH is to "yield information helpful to the design of large-scale studies on prevention and treatment of mental illnesses resulting from exposure to mass violence" (*NIH News release*, 2002).

Integrated assessments, which take into account physical and emotional responses to threats and trauma, may become the new crisis intervention models. New studies of the psychobiology of stress and PTSDs will contribute knowledge to current treatment planning. Studies of the effects of terrorism on groups of people, based on the frequent amount of recent tragedies and the future potential for these events, will also influence the direction of this evolving field.

HISTORICAL CONTEXT

Claude Bernard (1813-1878), a noted French biologist, provided the theory of physiologic equilibrium (stability of the *milieu interior*). The term for this process, **homeostasis**, was coined by the American experimental physiologist Walter Cannon. **Equilibrium** is a natural state of balance, achieved by the interaction between an internal, biologic feedback system and the external environment that acts to maintain the body within a normal range of functioning. The physiologic concepts of equilibrium and homeostasis are often used as a metaphor to understand psychiatric functioning and crisis theory, although the relationship between the physiologic and psychologic principles is not exact. Equilibrium in both psychiatric and physiologic terms implies a steady state that is as close as possible to the optimal level of health for the organism.

A crisis may better be understood as a threat to the "familiar," and the term *equilibrium*, if used in psychology, should refer to *that familiar state of being* rather than a specific mood or mental status. By viewing a crisis as a radical threat to the norm, it is easier to understand why even a positive situation, such as the birth of a child, or winning the lotto, for example, may provoke a crisis. Hans Selye (1978) explained that an apparent positive event may equally cause a stress response *(eustress)* as a negative event *(distress)*. Alternatively, the crisis response may be viewed as a mismatch between actual reality and what is expected or desired (Ursin, 2002).

Karen Horney, a psychoanalyst of the social psychology school, contributed the concept of the biopsychosocial approach to diagnosis and treatment. Her theory of holistic psychology maintains that a person's emotional/mental makeup not only is a product of early childhood impulses and experiences, but also is formed by interactions with the external world (Kaplan and Sadock, 1998). The common nursing goal, to understand the person as a whole by assessing both internal and external factors, is particularly important in crisis intervention.

Abraham Maslow's hierarchy of needs contributes to crisis theory, in that survival needs must be met in order for higher needs to be addressed. The concept of higher versus lower needs is not meant to rank them in importance or complexity, but simply to suggest that they are built on one another. The idea of a hierarchy of needs has physiologic correlates, such as in the neurologic development of an infant, in which motor control progresses from head to toe. Crisis intervention theory, then, includes the assessment and treatment of needs in logical order, with basic needs being included in the formulation of a plan of action to assist the client to attain a higher level of functioning (see Figure 2-2).

Brief therapy (as opposed to long-term treatment) evolved from the early work of Freud, who only later in his career insisted that long-term analysis was necessary for effective treatment. Soon after Freud's death in 1939, Alexander and French in Chicago challenged the assumptions that only long-term analysis was effective, and promoted brief therapy once again (Budman and Gurman, 1988). Around the same time, Budman and Gurman (1988) report that Eric Lindemann and his colleagues studied the psychologic symptoms of the survivors after the Coconut Grove fire in Boston on November 28, 1942. Lindemann et al. from Massachusetts General Hospital played an active role in helping survivors who had lost loved ones in the disaster. Lindemann's studies of psychologic symptoms surrounding the fire led him to believe that helping bereaved people through the mourning process early on could prevent later psychologic difficulties. From his experience working with grief reactions, Lindemann proposed that grief may be "normal" or "morbid" (abnormal) depending on the preexisting vulnerabilities of the person. He believed that brief therapy could be helpful to both victims and their families.

Beginning in the 1960s through the end of the twentieth century, the cost of health care rose dramatically, and brief therapy was favored for its cost-effective benefit. Therapists who used cognitive-behavioral approaches were able to quantify and thus demonstrate significant therapeutic gains using brief therapy techniques. The general focus of these models is on identifying the client's maladaptive ways of thinking and acting, and then teaching ways to correct the maladaptive thoughts or behaviors (see theoretic perspectives in this text for a review). However, no specific cognitive-behavioral therapeutic technique among the many variations showed better results than another. Therefore the use of a flexible selection of cognitive-behavioral techniques is favored over adherence to one particular formula or model (Budman, 1988).

The twenty-first century brings new ways to deliver crisis intervention other than face-to-face counseling. On-line chat capabilities are immediate ways to communicate by computer, and technology is available to view the person on a TV-like screen while "chatting." It has been stated that e-mail and face-to-face crisis intervention brief therapy share similar goals and interventions, with a few interesting differences. Computer-based therapy usually occurs in private practice rather than in agency-based practice. On a web site, there is greater disclosure of professional interests, treatment philosophy, and resumes than may be allowed by agency practice. Professional qualifications are thus far unregulated on computer-based services. Payment for computer services is almost always self-pay, but only sometimes self-pay at an agency that accepts third-party payments. Finally, it may be more difficult to refer to appropriate local supporting resources, as the provider on the computer may be far from the client and unfamiliar with local supports. In addition, it is possible to gain general information and advice on any subject, including all kinds of mental and emotional problems. Some web sites are designed for professionals, some for lay persons, and others for both groups.

CRISIS
Definitions and Description

A crisis response is the painful, frightening human experience that occurs when one is faced with an overwhelming threat to one's equilibrium, or one's familiar state of being. A rise in anxiety is experienced, physiologic arousal occurs, and concentration and normal daily functioning are often impaired. The individual tries familiar coping mechanisms, but these fail to return the situation to normal, and the person feels unable to meet the challenge. The crisis is a personal admixture of the internal or external triggering event, the meaning of that event to the person, the person's resources, and the person's past experiences coping with similar events (Aguilera, 1998).

A crisis is not a discrete diagnostic category. Many psychiatric disorders may be associated with a crisis, the most common being depressive disorders, anxiety disorders, and more specifically, adjustment disorder and PTSD. An adjustment disorder is typically thought to be an unexpected or abnormal response to a normal event. By contrast, in PTSD, the event is considered abnormal and the response is expected, or at least quite understandable. Some types of crisis are normal responses to normal events, as may occur in a phase-of-life event such as extreme grief with the death of a loved one. In all cases, however, *the response to the stressor is inadequate to remove the threat to one's safety,* be it an actual or a perceived threat, or an expected or unexpected response. Thus a crisis response may be understood as an internal state that may happen to both healthy and unhealthy individuals, in normal or abnormal circumstances, that is acutely painful, frightening, and may be demoralizing.

Although the state of being in crisis is similar regardless of the cause, it is helpful to understand the stimulus when treating the crisis state, as certain types of triggers have predictable consequences. A significant subgroup of victims of traumatic events, for example, may suffer difficulty mastering the environment, problems in relationships with others, and difficulty in feeling that life has purpose. Common symptoms also include hypervigilance, sleep problems, intrusive memories, and emotional withdrawal (Flannery and Everly, 2000).

External (Situational) Crises

An *external stressor* is one that is apparent to another observer and viewed as something that is likely to cause a threat to safety, or well-being, such as a real threat to physical health or the ability to obtain food, clothing, or shelter. Loss of a job, discovery of a spousal affair, death of a loved one, and a threat of death as a result of a serious medical condition affect "real" survival as well as survival of one's self-image and self-esteem. Sometimes, physical, real-world problems can be solved and the crisis response appears settled. Psychiatric symptoms may surface later, however, so anticipatory teaching remains important in any type of crisis intervention.

External stressors may affect individuals or groups of people, with some differences between the experience and treatment of these two subtypes. **Disasters** affecting large numbers of people may trigger a crisis response in some but not all of those affected. Disasters can be natural, as a tornado or flood that destroys a town, or artificially induced, such as a threat of **bioterrorism** or intentional contamination of the air with poisonous gases.

Internal (Subjective) Crises

Internal stressors are severe threats to well-being that are not so obvious to the outside observer. Examples of internal stressors are a new illness that represents aging and loss, a broken promise that represents profound abandonment, and a workplace flirtation or breach of loyalty that results in profound guilt and fear. An internal stressor may also be a threat to a deeply held belief or a loss of faith. Brief psychodynamic therapy often assists the client to understand a current crisis in the context of prior experience.

Phase-of-life events are the normal and predictable changes that happen to all humans over time. Adolescence, work choice, parenthood, midlife, retirement, and old age represent some of these changes. Stress and sometimes a crisis often accompany the phase in normal individuals. Each phase brings with it challenges, expectations from others, internalized images of what and how to be, and losses. Aging, for example, eventually brings loss of strength, mobility, elasticity, balance, reduced memory, slower thinking, and other declining faculties. Self-worth must be redefined as one is challenged by, and successfully or unsuccessfully passes through, life's continuum. By redefining one's criteria for measuring self-worth, one brings a closer match between the actual self and the expected reality, and stress is reduced. The thought "I am successful only as long as I am strong and healthy" is a problem if one is sick and weak. However, the belief that "I am successful because my children love me and I have contributed to others" is compatible with being in ill health and maintaining self-worth.

Disasters

The last decade in the United States brought shocking news of natural and artificially made disasters. However, the hijacking and intentional crash of commercial airplanes into the World Trade Center and the U.S. Pentagon were possibly the most disturbing public events witnessed by U.S. citizens in this country. There followed at all government levels a keen awakening of the need for policies, procedures, and general information about terrorism and responding to disaster. Multiple research questions are being investigated, including these examples from the *Natural Hazards Observer* (November 2001) that will affect future roles of mental health clinicians: How do emergency management organizations respond when many of their members are among the victims? How can diverse religious organizations contribute during such distressing times? What are the policy implications in terms of trade-offs between freedom and security? What ethnic issues arise after an act of terrorism? And significantly, how do public and private organizations communicate and cooperate after an event of this magnitude?

Bioterrorist events differ from natural disasters, according to Robert E. De Martino, MD, a speaker at a 3-day summit meeting organized by Substance Abuse and Mental Health Services Administration (SAMHSA) (Goodman, 2000). Bioterrorist events are less predictable and more drawn out over time. The losses are human and material, and the ultimate amount of damage in bioterrorist attacks is unclear, as opposed to fires or floods, in which the damage is visible and obvious. At present, the art and science of dealing with terrorism in its various forms is still under construction. "Readiness for future attacks demands continuous planning for the unimaginable" (Goodman, 2000).

The following list of symptoms was compiled by the American Academy of Experts in Traumatic Stress in 1999 as a parent information sheet for crisis response in the schools, but it provides a useful list of common *immediate* responses to any traumatic event:

- Shock
- Numbness
- Denial
- Dissociative behavior
- Confusion
- Disorganization
- Difficulty making decisions
- Suggestibility

The most common psychiatric problem after such events is PTSD. Children may suffer from regressed behavior, increased fears, decreased academic performance and poor concentration, increased oppositional behavior, irritability and aggression, emotional lability, and depression.

Being in a traumatic experience and surviving it may have an inoculating effect. In a study of 50 children involved in motor vehicle accidents, 14% suffered PTSD symptoms and 10% developed a specific phobia. Although the severity of physical injury predicted for significantly more PTSD symptoms, previous accident experience predicted for fewer PTSD symptoms (Keppel-Benson, 2002).

On another positive note, it seems that disasters transform people's behavior from isolation to increased interaction with others after the first response of shock and disbelief. Persons tend to feel empathy, or sometimes survivor guilt. Individual identities are set aside and for a time the focus is on the community. Altruism emerges. People set aside their own work to help others (*Natural Hazards Observer*, November 2001).

Although it is true that not everyone who experiences a traumatic event suffers from PTSD symptoms, the risk is high. The NIMH estimates that about 30% of Vietnam veterans developed PTSD at some point after the war. The risk for women is more than twice that for men, and there is frequent concurrent depression, anxiety, and substance abuse (NIMH Publication 01-4597).

Systematic, psychologic **debriefing** for emergency personnel began as an effort to prevent PTSD in emergency personnel. Methods for debriefing are described in the next section. Different versions of this method of crisis therapy have been used in expanded venues, including schools, and in the aftermath of disasters. Training of medical and nonmedical personnel in debriefing skills is increasing for government and private organizations that respond to public emergencies. Although the original aim of *preventing* PTSD by using debriefing methods is not clearly proven, other benefits to the client are valuable and include the opportunity to triage persons needing further psychiatric care, to make referrals to appropriate resource agencies, and to provide timely emotional support in close proximity to the event.

METHODS OF CRISIS INTERVENTION

The *crisis approach to problem solving* involves (1) an assessment of the individual and the problem, (2) planning of therapeutic intervention, (3) intervention, (4) resolution of the crisis, and (5) anticipatory planning (Morley, Messick, and Aguilera, 1967). Crisis counseling after exposure to a traumatic event may include brief psychodynamic psychotherapy, cognitive-behavioral therapy, and sometimes reexposure or hypnotherapy. In addition, antidepressant medications once limited to endogenous depressions (i.e., those depressions without obvious external cause) are frequently offered to assist with adjustment disorders, anxiety, and PTSD. Other medications, such as benzodiazepines or sedative/hypnotics, may be used for short-term relief. The severity and type of symptoms, more than the diagnostic category, determine whether a referral for medication is indicated. In general, when medication is indicated, the combination of medication and interactive therapy is thought to be better than either modality alone.

In disaster work the external stressor may be obvious, but the meaning to the individual may be unspoken and therefore must always be assessed. For example, a person with solid financial resources, fire insurance, and many friends and relatives may react differently to losing a house to a fire than a young, uninsured couple who put all of their assets into their home.

Principles

Psychologic debriefing, or a variant termed *critical incident stress debriefing*, fits well with existing models of crisis intervention. Flannery and Everly (2000) outlined generally agreed on *principles of intervention* in cases of psychologic trauma as follows:

- Immediate (timely) intervention
- Stabilizing the victims with a semblance of order and routine

- Facilitating understanding of the event by gathering facts, listening, and teaching
- Using available resources to help with independent functioning
- Encouraging self-reliance

Components

The *components of intervention* outlined by Irving and Long (2001) are:

- Establishing rapport
- Asking the client to objectively describe the event
- Encouraging emotional expression and making sense of the experience
- Providing education about stress reactions and how to **cope**
- Giving follow-up referrals

A multicomponent approach involves individuals in crisis counseling, group debriefings, staff and victim support groups, staff and victim family counseling, and, when indicated, professional referrals (Irving and Long, 2001; Flannery and Everly, 2000). A substantial amount of information in the literature suggests that the value lies not in the specific tools used but more in the emotional support rendered, the education provided, and in the screening for vulnerable persons needing additional psychiatric care (Arendt and Elklit, 2001; Deahl, 2000).

Assessment in the Field

The phrase *in the field* usually refers to work done outside a controlled, planned care setting such as a hospital or clinic. Field work as it relates to mental health may include case finding at homeless shelters or encampments, collaborative work with law enforcement responders to 911 crisis calls, or responding to physical disasters. Relatively new to the literature, and pertinent to nurses, field work is an approach to crisis intervention that integrates both physical and psychiatric needs (Lerner, 2002). A summary of how to approach someone who may have a simultaneous physical and emotional threat to safety while the traumatic event is taking place appears in Box 22-1.

Other types of field assessments occur when a clinician is part of law enforcement teams. In many cities efforts are made to combine the expertise of mental health professionals with law officers when responding to calls that may involve mentally disordered clients. Both partners are trained to deescalate angry or violent persons, and the mental health partner offers additional expertise in psychiatric assessment. When determining appropriate disposition of the client, the following components are essential:

- Ensuring safety
- Building rapport
- Evaluating for medical and substance-related problems
- Using crisis intervention techniques

Careful evaluations are meant to reduce unnecessary violence between the client and the officer or others, and to provide appropriate treatment to clients who might otherwise go to jail. In the best circumstances these teams coordinate with other community providers to create care plans based on collected observations of "high-profile" individuals, who are often resistant to conventional treatment and are often contacted by the law as a result of citizen complaints. On the other hand, special challenges arise when agencies with competing administrative agendas ask their professionals to work together. The future of many types of crisis work, but especially field work, lies in the effective collaboration of providers from many disciplines and organizations, and in the ability to put the needs of clients above the individual organizational politics (see Nursing Care in the Community box).

Assessment in the Office

It is often a temptation to begin counseling a person who appears in crisis without doing a thorough assessment. However, a careful history and examination will yield a direction for brief therapy that is closer to the real needs of the client. Crisis intervention focuses on the immediate problem, tak-

ing into account the context in which the problem exists. The following components are addressed:

- *Physical safety principles* should govern the environment in which any psychiatric assessment will take place, particularly when persons may be experiencing a crisis. The exit should be of equal distance to client and nurse. No loose objects (potential weapons) should be within reach of a client. An alarm buzzer or some emergency call system should be within easy reach. As with any psychiatric assessment, physical appearance and behavior of the client are briefly assessed, noting hygiene, dress, grooming, level of agitation or control, and stated intentions to harm self or others. At the same time alcohol may be noted on the breath, or there may be other signs of possible intoxication, or of serious medical conditions. Although not typically done in outpatient psychiatric settings, obtaining *vital signs* is a simple, quick, and useful tool that should be used as part of the initial biopsychosocial assessment.

- A *medical history form* should be completed in advance of the interview if possible, and should be reviewed early in the interview. The history should be reviewed and the client observed for physiologic disturbances or problems with mobility (see Chapter 6 for more detailed discussion). A list of medications taken by the client, both prescribed and over the counter, psychiatric and medical, should be carefully noted, along with related dosing information. Consideration is given to potential effects of medications on mood and mental status, as well as interactions between medications and street drugs or alcohol. Crisis clinics may include a drug screen of urine and a breath test for alcohol as routine or as-indicated assessment measures.

- *Introduction and boundaries.* The first visit establishes direction for future sessions when more than one session is necessary and should focus on resolution of symptoms. Clients often have an idea that therapy is nondirective and long-lasting. Crisis therapy is short term, making it essential to explain the number of visits the client can expect and to establish achievable goals for that period of time. It is helpful to explain that questions may be asked of the client about past experiences as a way to understand present issues, but most of the time will be spent looking at the present problems and future expectations.

- *Chief complaint.* The nurse begins intervention by asking, "What brings you here today?" The nurse gently directs the client to identify, first broadly and then more definitively, the reason for the visit, the current symptoms (specific thoughts, mood, functional impairment) that brought the client in, and the precipitating event of the crisis.

- *History of present illness or situation.* What led up to the crisis, and how has the crisis disrupted the indi-

NURSING CARE IN THE COMMUNITY: Crisis Intervention

Crisis intervention acts as a lifeline to the public. A skilled crisis nurse acts as the gatekeeper for the entire mental health system and activates the law enforcement network in emergency situations. The nurse must often make decisions that have a direct impact on the life or death of clients in the community when assessing an individual's danger to self or others. The entire community could be considered along with the client.

Psychiatric mental health nurses working in the community are especially warranted in catastrophic situations such as fires, floods, or earthquakes, both for those who have been traumatized by the event itself and for those who have lost significant others in the tragedy. Victims of the event may have a psychiatric diagnosis that is intensified by the event. They may experience delusions in which they believe they are responsible for the disaster and may not be amenable to rational reassurance. Immediate psychiatric assessment and intervention are necessary to help these individuals manage the effects of the trauma through personal comfort and medication. Hospitalization may also be necessary.

Friends and relatives of trauma victims may also be adversely affected by an overwhelming emotional response that requires psychiatric intervention. They should be given brief reassurances, referred to a community contact, and provided with information about the possible duration of their symptoms.

The nurse must be able to triage the needs of the individual, as well as the community, and may also offer support to individual clients who are expressing fear, loneliness, and other stress-related problems. Some callers may need to check in daily with familiar workers and become well known to crisis service personnel. Strategies focus on identifying an immediate precipitant, evaluating the client's personal safety, and working with him or her to reestablish emotional equilibrium.

Interventions range from giving referrals to programs such as Alcoholics Anonymous and suggesting private therapists, to common-sense advice about daily crises. It is routine to counsel a heartbroken lover, a recently discharged patient with adjustment difficulties, or a parent whose child has become estranged through behaviors such as drug abuse. Some people call crisis centers as proxies for friends or family members who are too upset or disorganized to be coherent.

Although a psychiatrist is always on call for consultation and orders, the crisis nurse must be familiar with the most recent diagnostic manual and be capable of making assessments based on sparse information. He or she must be aware of personal limitations yet be able to take responsibility for rapid independent actions, which may include calling emergency medical technicians (EMTs, paramedics) or the police. As in other community situations, it is safer to err on the side of caution than to hesitate because of fear of intruding on individual clients.

vidual's life and others? What are the individual's strengths, what coping skills have been successful in the past, and what coping skills are being used presently?

- *Family/social history.* Are there others in the family with psychiatric or substance abuse problems? Briefly, what type of family was the client raised in, and what is the current living situation? Who and what resources are currently available to the individual?
- *Mental status.* What is the appearance and grooming? Altered thought processes or altered mood may become apparent during the history-taking. The medical examination may help to rule out physical causes for altered mental status. Always note orientation, admissions of hallucinations (ask, even if you think the client will say "no"), delusions, and thoughts of suicide or homicide. Assess attention, concentration, and fund of knowledge. Is there a normal fund of knowledge? Are there any peculiarities of speech (rapid or slow, loud or soft)? Is the client considered a "reliable historian"? How is the client's insight (i.e., understanding of the symptoms and behavior)? How valid is the client's judgment—what the client actually would do in a given situation demanding emergency action? What did the client do that demonstrates presence or absence of judgment? What has the client's mood been over the past few weeks or months? What is the mood at the moment (affect)? Is the client in control of impulses during the interview? In the past? The more descriptive the report, the more useful it will be.

- *Past medical and psychiatric history.* Was this person ever hospitalized? Why? When? Is there a relationship between then and now? What vulnerabilities are suggested here? Was the person ever arrested? Why? Is he or she currently on parole or probation? Was the person discharged from the military with an honorable or less-than honorable discharge? What happened?
- *Drug and alcohol history.* Phrase questions in a neutral language but in a way that makes it easy to admit to use. Do not ask if someone uses street drugs. Ask, "When did you last experiment with any substances? When was your last alcoholic beverage? How tall was the beer?" A neatly groomed and attractive person may well have a serious drug or alcohol dependence; income level and social status do not protect a client. Avoid assumptions. Review the list of prescription medications provided by the client and consider substance abuse when there are other hints such as getting controlled substances from several physicians. Was the person ever in a drug or alcohol treatment program?
- *Cultural and spiritual issues.* What aspects of a person's ethnicity, religion, beliefs, or experiences with own and other cultures may influence the perception of the crisis or the ability to cope? Are there other relevant cultural issues?
- *Strengths and supports.* What personal resources and supportive resources are available? What successes has the person achieved that can be built on? Look toward family, friends, religious affiliations, community shelters or crisis houses, self-help groups, and drug

and alcohol detoxification centers. Provide a phone number for a crisis hotline.

- *Coping skills.* Has anything like this ever happened before? How does the individual usually manage problems and unhappiness? What has been tried thus far to solve this crisis, and what has worked (adaptive coping) and not worked (maladaptive coping) in the past? Work with the client to remember past successes.
- *Global Assessment of Functioning (GAF).* Use of the **GAF score**, a rating scale from 0 to 100 used to estimate global functioning, provides a simple and useful estimate of overall functional severity, and also serves as a baseline to measure future improvement (APA, 2000). When staff are trained and skilled in the use of the GAF, there is reasonably good reliability of rating scores. See Chapter 6 for more detail concerning GAF.
- *Other criteria.* Other common assessment tools that may be used in conjunction with the preceding interview tools are brief questionnaires that clients fill out. These include the Beck Depression Inventory, Second Edition (BDI-II; Beck, Steer and Brown, 1996), the Beck Anxiety Inventory (Beck, 1993), and the Trauma Symptom Inventory (Breire, 1995). These are but a few of the reliable, valid, and often used assessment instruments. Typically, assessment instruments are given at the beginning and end of therapy to measure progress, both as a concrete therapeutic tool and as a measure of efficacy of the professional's interventions.
- *Collateral information.* Information given by others to the mental health provider is collateral information and can be a significant piece of a thorough assessment. Clients who are ashamed or in denial of their symptoms, or fearful of rehospitalization, may greatly minimize their disabilities. Further, with serious mental illness comes poor insight, difficulty thinking and in verbalizing thoughts, distractibility, dysattention and poor concentration, and poor impulse control, all of which may impede the process of gathering facts. Families and others who interact with and observe the client may reveal critical information that, when incorporated into the assessment of a crisis, may prevent serious errors and shed realistic light on the situation. Although psychiatric professionals cannot reliably predict whether someone will harm self or others, the wise use of collateral information may prevent tragic consequences for the client and others.

PLANNING AND EXECUTING THERAPEUTIC INTERVENTION
General Approach to Crisis Intervention

1. Listen, observe, and ask questions to understand and categorize the nature of the crisis.
2. Decide the order and type of interventions, putting tangible threats before perceived, intangible threats. (The removal of an actual danger may allay the immediate emotional response, but be aware of the potential for PTSD later.)
3. Coordinate with other agencies. This approach is essential, particularly in large-scale disasters with tangible threats such as fires, earthquakes, and war or acts of terror. Be familiar with resources that offer support with basic needs such as food, clothing, shelter, and financial support. Have pamphlets available with referral information.
4. Anticipate future needs related to the crisis and develop a plan with the client for meeting these needs.

As the nurse begins to sort through and categorize the issues with the client, a *structure and form* to the crisis is developed that offers reassurance to the client. The act of *sorting and categorizing* may in itself reduce the initial feeling of being overwhelmed and out of control, both for the client and the nurse. Creating a positive expectation of crisis resolution should be kept in mind as the ultimate therapeutic goal.

Therapeutic note: The nurse may feel guilty when interrupting or redirecting the interview with a very emotionally expressive client or fear that the client will be offended or harmed by the interruption. In fact, the opposite may be true. Once clients have had an opportunity to tell their stories, perseveration on the stressful event may be countertherapeutic and they generally are relieved by being redirected by a confident and caring therapist who offers both support and information, and engages the client in rational thought or healthy diversion.

After gathering information to understand the presenting problem and something about the person's strengths, explore the person's interpretation or perception of events. For example, the external stressor may be "my husband beat me," but the person may feel that "I am worthless and no man will ever love me." External stressors may also involve needing a place to live, hiding from the perpetrator, and arranging care for the children. Planning should target specific functional abilities and disabilities, as well as general disturbances in mood, using supportive and cognitive/behavioral approaches. A set number or range of numbers of sessions available to the client should be discussed with the client to give further focus to the planned interventions.

Explore the client's current and past coping skills and mechanisms. Adaptive strategies that are being used should be reinforced and encouraged. Old strategies that worked in the past may be remembered and tried again. New coping methods are sought, and frequently the person devises some new, highly original methods. This phase of intervention provides the opportunity for learning new skills and for growth.

Maladaptive strategies, such as excessive sleep, avoidance of others, and use of drugs or alcohol, should be reviewed and discussed with the client to explore the relative benefits and liabilities. The nurse should be prepared to support the client with nonpunitive, noncritical approaches, but also continue to teach and encourage adaptive efforts.

CASE STUDY

Laura, a 36-year-old single mother of an 8-year-old girl, entered the clinic for a "refill on her medications to sleep." She is a new client who lost her job as a clerk, as well as her health insurance, 2 months ago. She had been seeing a private therapist for "stress" and sleep problems after she had been asked out on a date by her male supervisor about 6 months ago. She believed she was fired because she turned him down, but he did not pursue her after the first invitation, and she could not prove a claim of harassment. She was told she was fired because of her work performance, which had severely declined over the last 4 months. Laura admitted that this was true, as manifested by difficulty concentrating, depressed mood, 20-pound weight gain, lack of sleep, increased distractibility, and lately, hearing her name called when no one is there. She stated, when asked directly, that she "only smokes a little marijuana at night to relax, and only drinks a few beers on weekends." She had never been hospitalized and never been arrested. She was taking an antidepressant daily but would run out of it in 2 weeks. Her self-esteem plummeted after losing her job, and she now fears she is unable to care properly for her child. She forgot to pick her up at the bus stop twice last week and imagined that she would be responsible for her daughter being kidnapped or murdered as a result of her negligence. She was having passive suicidal thoughts of running off the freeway while driving, but said she wouldn't really do that.

Critical Thinking
1. What is Laura's presenting problem from her viewpoint, and how does that compare with her functional disabilities?
2. What survival/safety issues need to be addressed?
3. What therapeutic approaches will help?
4. What future planning should be included?

Assist the individual to see a cause-and-effect relationship between the stressor and the response. What may be obvious to others may not be to the person suffering. "I wonder if your lack of sleep and nervousness over the past week relates to the fact that you feel so alone and vulnerable since you were physically attacked?" Expect ambivalence or resistance as a normal part of therapy, as therapy is an implied demand for a personal change that may be upsetting or frightening, or too challenging at the time (see Case Study).

Brief therapy planning assumes that the time between and after the clinical sessions is as important as the actual clinical contacts. The time is viewed as an occasion for client work such as the use of adaptive strategies. Examples are keeping a journal, talking with appropriate people about the situation, and asking for help when necessary (Bloom, 2001). Adaptive strategies that are being used should be reinforced and encouraged. Talking more with friends and family, increasing regular exercise, planning recreation time each day, and correcting negative thoughts and replacing them with hopeful ones are other examples of tasks to practice.

Cognitive therapy is one excellent approach for brief interventions. For example, it can be helpful to someone who perseverates on a stressful thought to set aside "worry time" each day. This is a cognitive strategy in the category called *prescribe-the-symptom*. By knowing that you will set aside at least 1 hour a day to worry, you can allow yourself to stop worrying until that time each day. Keeping a log of "successful worrying" for that hour to share with the therapist lends credence to this technique and helps the client gain mastery over obsessive, negative thinking.

The nurse is prepared to offer a wide array of community resources to enhance individual crisis therapy if necessary when brief therapy ends. The nurse helps the client to find situational supports to provide companionship, to monitor for safety if needed, to assist with activities of daily living, and to help with any other needs related to the initial stressor or the maladaptive reaction to it. Significant others may also provide comfort by offering "unconditional positive regard" as proposed by Carl Rogers (see Chapter 19) and help the person preserve or regain self-esteem that was threatened or decreased as a result of the loss of control.

Future planning should target specific **functional disabilities** and anticipate needs that may be more prominent later on. The number of sessions that will be available to the client should be explained early in therapy. This helps the client to focus on the planned interventions. If needed, a referral for psychiatric evaluation follows the nurse's assessment when a possible need for medications exists. A crisis hotline number should be made available to the client.

In disasters or trauma, friends and relatives of victims may also be adversely affected. They also should be given brief reassurances, educated about the possible type and duration of their symptoms, and referred to community contacts.

RESOLUTION OF THE CRISIS
The Summary
As the client's **coping abilities** improve and positive changes occur, the changes may be summarized to allow the person to reexperience and reconfirm the progress that was made. If initial assessment tools were used to measure aspects of the person's functioning, these may be readministered to illustrate progress. The nurse engages the client in this process rather than merely summarizing the therapeutic events herself.

The Open Connection
Assistance is given as needed in making realistic plans for the future. There is discussion of ways in which the present experience may help in coping with future crises. In terminating therapy, it should be underlined for the client that although not all conflicts or problems have been resolved, substantial success has led to overcoming a crisis, and work continues when therapy ends.

Anticipatory Planning
The nurse asks the client what he or she would do if this or a similar event occurred in the future. This is a time for the client to reiterate what was learned in the process and to hypothetically plan for unanticipated events.

BARRIERS TO EFFECTIVE CRISIS INTERVENTION

Failures To Learn From Experience

Some people find themselves in similar crisis situations more than once, appearing to make the same mistakes over and over. When a threatening situation exists, coping activities that were used in the past are tried first. Unfortunately, learning new coping behaviors does not always follow a failure to cope. In part, repeated mistakes result from learning to expect failure, based on one's prior experiences. To learn new behaviors often takes strong motivation, an ability to think logically about the problem, tolerance for change (flexibility), willingness to change, and, most important, confidence or hope. It is this optimism, facilitated by trained professionals, that determines successful crisis resolution.

Existing Mental Disorder

At the extreme end of a crisis continuum, a **psychiatric emergency** poses an immediate threat to safety. Initial support may be medications (antipsychotic and/or antianxiety), a period of time to allow the severe arousal to subside, and/or nonmedical interventions designed to deescalate a situation. Persons with cognitive impairments resulting from major mental illness or injury, or substance intoxication, and persons with cognitive distortions will have greater difficulty resolving a crisis because of their impaired ability to think clearly and use their executive functions (reasoning, judgment) to control their behaviors. The challenge for the professional is to maximize the client's ability to think clearly and calmly before engaging in problem-solving behavior.

It is important to avoid compounding an emergency by creating further trauma whenever possible. When a crisis reaches the level of requiring forced intervention (i.e., restraint and a locked psychiatric unit), an additional crisis for the client may be the perception of being a hostage to the medical system (Mason, 2000). Careful and adequate training of staff in the art of deescalation and in the use of physical restraints when needed can reduce the psychologic and physical harm to both clients and staff and promote the client's sense of safety.

Secondary Gain

Another barrier to effective crisis intervention may be a competing goal of the client that rewards the client for being in crisis. Known as *secondary gain,* these competing motivations are often not obvious to the client or therapist until some time has passed, and progress in therapy is noted to be unusually slow. Typically, brief therapy does not directly address this issue in the time allotted, unless by some combination of skill and luck, the therapist becomes aware of the problem and has time to address it.

History taking provides important clues to issues of secondary gain. For example, a dependent person, or a person with histrionic or borderline traits, who is often ignored by an aloof partner, may have learned to gain sympathy and attention only when behaving in an extreme way, such as a suicide attempt or gesture. Various dramatic situations may be unconsciously created to achieve the goal of having a certain effect on someone else. In these cases, effective crisis intervention may be met in a hostile or defeating way by the client who is in crisis as a tool to gain some other reward. With adequate motivation and skilled therapy, the client may be led to connect the crisis-seeking behavior with the hidden needs and may be guided to more adaptive ways to meet these needs.

Therapist-Client Boundary Problems

Staff members who are exposed to stressors that remind them of their own problems may be less effective in assessing and treating someone in a similar crisis. *Overidentification* or *countertransference* are reactions to the client that in part may come from issues within the therapist. Some examples of this problem may lie with reporting clients to adult or child protection agencies, or to the police in the case of domestic violence, or in Tarasoff (duty to warn) situations (see Chapter 4). These laws, which vary from state to state, mandate that confidentiality be broken by the provider when the safety of others outweighs the individual's right to privacy. Caring nurses wanting to support their client may be reluctant to follow these reporting laws in favor of maintaining rapport. This decision-making process is often painfully colored by one's own need to be liked and accepted by a client; therefore consultation with peers or supervisors is highly recommended when reporting responsibilities arise.

In addition to personal issues interfering with therapy, a therapist exposed to mass trauma may be at risk for PTSD, depression, and other psychiatric sequelae. Those who respond first to disaster are among the most vulnerable to emotional and substance abuse disorders, according to SAMHSA (Goodman, 2002). Close attention is needed to build in safeguards for the welfare of responders to any crisis situation, including disasters. Rest and support for the therapist are essential elements of crisis planning.

DEMANDS ON THE PSYCHIATRIC NURSE WORKING IN CRISIS INTERVENTION

The crisis nurse must be familiar with the most recent diagnostic manual and be capable of making assessments based on information gathered from the client and others known to the client. He or she must be aware of personal limitations and boundaries. There should be an ability to take responsibility for rapid independent actions, which may include cooperative linkage with a variety of other agencies and organizations, including emergency intervention by police. Finally, the nurse should be flexible and up to date on current research on crisis intervention.

CHAPTER SUMMARY

- Crisis intervention theories are in transition since the advent of terrorist threats to the United States. New studies focus on the efficacy of debriefing models, and on understanding the relationships of different types of threats to a crisis response.
- Crisis intervention strategies focus on identifying an immediate precipitant, evaluating the client's personal safety, enhancing positive coping skills to reestablish emotional equilibrium, and planning for the future. The instillation of hope is an essential aspect of effective therapy.
- The new focus may be on an integrated model that includes assessment and treatment of actual physical threats, as well as psychologic threats to equilibrium. Assessments and interventions must include a biopsychosocial view.
- Victims of life-threatening events may have a psychiatric diagnosis that is worsened by the event; conversely, a psychiatric illness may make a person less able to cope with a crisis stressor. Early intervention and referral in disasters will likely lessen the amount and severity of symptoms later on.
- Psychiatric mental health nurses working in the community are especially needed in catastrophic situations such as fires, floods, or earthquakes, for both those who have been traumatized by the event itself and those who have lost significant others in the tragedy. However, first responders are at the most risk for psychiatric problems after trauma, and plans for care of caregivers should be a priority for agencies providing crisis services to the community.

REVIEW QUESTIONS

1. A 40-year-old client is diagnosed with Parkinson's disease. He becomes worried that he will consequently become disabled and not be able to work or support his family. He worries that he will not be able to send his two daughters to college. He begins drinking alcohol excessively to cope with the pressures and the loss of his ability to be independent in the future. The nurse assesses that the client is:
   a. In a situational crisis
   b. In a state of equilibrium
   c. Reflecting on the situational event
   d. Perceiving the event in a distorted way

2. A 20-year-old client is having difficulty adjusting to becoming a father. He has not bonded with his newborn son and frequently stays out late at night drinking with his friends. This is an example of:
   a. Situational crisis
   b. Maturational crisis
   c. Adventitious crisis
   d. Cognition crisis

3. A 35-year-old mother seeks grief counseling after her 8-year-old daughter was raped and murdered. The client tearfully verbalizes that she hates the man who did this to her. She explains that the man is currently being tried for the murder and that she doesn't know what she will do if he is not found guilty. The highest priority nursing response is:
   a. "Have you talked to a psychiatrist about taking some medication to help you cope?"
   b. "Do you have support from your family and friends?"
   c. "What do you need to help you cope?"
   d. "Are you thinking of killing yourself or anyone else like the man who killed your daughter?"

4. Caucasian police officers brutally assault an African-American suspect. The community is plagued with racial hatred and violence. Which is the best nursing diagnosis?
   a. Fear
   b. Powerlessness
   c. Ineffective community coping
   d. Risk for other-directed violence

5. Which statement of a client who suffered a plane crash demonstrates that the client is coping with the crisis?
   a. "I can't ever fly in a plane again."
   b. "I keep having nightmares. I can't eat or sleep."
   c. "I feel guilty that I survived and other people didn't."
   d. "It's been so hard, but I'm starting to sleep better. I've been going to a support group, which helps."

REFERENCES

Aguilera DC: *Crisis intervention: theory and methodology*, St Louis, 1998, Mosby.

American Psychiatric Association: *Diagnostic and Statistical Manual of Mental Disorders*, Fourth Edition, Text Revision. Washington, DC, American Psychiatric Association, 2000.

Arendt M, Elklit A: Effectiveness of psychological debriefing, *Acta Psychiatr Scand* 104:423-437, 2001.

Beck A, Steer R, Brown G: *Beck Depression Inventory*, ed 2, San Antonio, 1996, The Psychological Corporation.

Beck A: *Beck Anxiety Inventory*, San Antonio, 1993, The Psychological Corporation.

Bloom B: Focused single-session psychotherapy: a review of the clinical and research literature, *Brief Treatment and Crisis Intervention* 1:75-86, 2001.

Breire J: *Trauma symptom inventory professional manual*, Odessa, 1995, Psychological Assessment Resources.

Budman S, Gurman S: *Theory and practice of brief therapy*, New York, 1988, Guilford Press.

Deahl M: Psychological debriefing: controversy and challenge, *Aust NZ J Psychiatry* 34:929-939, 2000.

Flannery RB, Everly Jr GS: Crisis intervention: a review, *Int J Emerg Ment Health* 2:119-125, 2000.

Goodman D: Responding to terrorism: recovery, resilience, readiness. In *SAMHSA News,* Rockville, Md, 2000, Office of Communications, Department of Health and Human Services.

Graham S: 9/11: The psychological aftermath, *Sci Am Explore* pp 1-5, 2001, website: www.scientificamerican.com/explorations/2001/111201/anxiety.

Irving P, Long A: Critical incident stress debriefing following traumatic life experiences, *J Psychiatr Ment Health Nurs* 8:307-314, 2001

Kaplan HI, Sadock BJ: *Kaplan and Sadock's synopsis of psychiatry: behavioral sciences, clinical psychiatry*, ed 8, Philadelphia, 1998, Lippincott, Williams & Wilkins.

Keppel-Benson J: Post-traumatic stress in children following motor vehicle accidents, *J Child Psychol Psychiatry* 43:203-212, 2002.

Lerner M: An overview of acute traumatic stress management, *Trauma Response* 8:3-5, 2002.

Mason T: Managing protest behavior: from coercion to compassion, *J Psychiatr Ment Health Nurs* 7(3):269-275, 2000.

Morley W, Messick J, Aguilera D: Crisis: paradigms of intervention, *J Psychiatr Ment Health Serv* 5(6):531-544, 1967

Natural Hazards Observer, Dane S, editor: vol 26, University of Colorado at Boulder, November 2001, website: HAZCTR@spot.colorado.edu.

NIH News Release: NIMH awards new grants in response to terrorist attacks of September 11, 2001, website: www.nih.gov/news/pr/apr2002/nimh-18.htm.

NIMH Publication #01-4597, http://www.nimh.nih.gov October 2001.

Selye H: *The stress of life*, New York, 1978, McGraw Hill.

Ursin H, Eriksen H: *The cognitive activation theory of stress*, Bergen, Norway, 2002, Department of Biological and Medical Psychology; University of Bergen, website: hege.eriksen@psych.uib.no.

SUGGESTED READINGS

Andrews E: 18 die in German school rampage. *San Diego Union Tribune*, pp A-1, A-13, San Diego, 2002.

Bandura A, Adams NE, Beyer J: Cognitive processes mediating behavioral change, *J Pers Soc Psychol* 35:125-139, 1977.

Caplan, G: *An approach to community mental health*, New York, 1961, Grune and Stratton.

Caplan G: *Principles of preventive psychiatry*, New York, 1964, Basic Books.

Clancy G: *Emergency psychiatry service handbook of agitated and violent patients,* 2000, Internet Publisher: The University of Iowa.

Gale C et al: Implications for training of violent acts by patients against psychiatric registrars, *Australas Psychiatry* 8:345-348, 2000.

Kubler-Ross E: *On death and dying*, New York, 1969, MacMillan.

McFarlane A: Traumatic stress in the 21st century, *Aust NZ J Psychiatry* 34:896-902, 2000.

Neese R: Evolutionary origins and functions of the stress response. In Press A, editor: *Encyclopedia of stress*, New York, 2000, Academic Press.

Norris G: Cognitive-behavioral assessment and treatment of maladaptive help-seeking behavior in a patient with schizophrenia, *Aust NZ J Psychiatry* 34:688-691, 2000.

Regehr C: Crisis debriefing groups for emergency responders: reviewing the evidence, *Brief Treatment and Crisis Intervention* 1(2):87-100, 2001.

Sadock B: *Comprehensive textbook of psychiatry*, Philadelphia, 2000, Lippincott Williams & Wilkins.

Selye H: *Stress without distress*, New York, 1956, New American Library.

Shenold C: *Bioterrorism: today's fear, tomorrow's reality,* Sacramento, 2001, CME Resource.

Stevens B, Ellerbrock L: *Crisis intervention: an opportunity to change*, ERIC Clearinghouse on Counseling and Student Services ERIC Identifier: ED405535, 1995, Internet.

ONLINE RESOURCES

American Academy of Experts in Traumatic Stress, www.aaets.org
American Red Cross: www.redcross.org
Centers for Disease Control and Prevention: Public Health Emergency Preparedness and Response: www.bt.cdc.gov
Disaster Relief: www.disasterrelief.org
Environmental Protection Agency: Chemical Emergency Preparedness and Prevention: www.epa.gov/swercepp
National Institute of Mental Health: www.nimh.nih.gov
Substance Abuse and Mental Health Services Administration: www.samhsa.gov
US Department of Energy: www.energy.gov
US Department of Health and Human Services: www.hhs.gov

PART IV AGGRESSIVE BEHAVIORS

23

Violence: Abuse, Neglect, and Rape

Joan C. Urbancic

KEY TERMS

OBJECTIVES

- Consider various theories of family violence for application to nursing practice.

- Discuss conditions that discourage a battered woman from leaving her violent situation.

- Discuss the role of "control" in the etiology of domestic violence.

- Compare the child physical offender with the child sexual offender.

- Describe the common characteristics of victims of family violence.

- Construct examples of how women who are raped are revictimized by society.

- Apply the nursing process in the care of victims of family violence.

Since September 11, 2001, we, as a nation, have become acutely aware of our vulnerability to terrorism and future disasters including biochemical warfare. Nurses, doctors, and other health professionals across the nation are becoming involved in the planning and coordination of initiatives to address worse case scenarios for these future disasters. The Centers for Disease Control and Prevention is concentrating on combating smallpox, anthrax, plague, botulism, and other potential biologic weapons. There are an increasing number of studies that examine the most effective way to train clinicians to respond to terrorists and bioterrorism. Experts have also become more aware of how such terrorism can permanently affect the psychologic, biologic, and social realities of American citizens. Therefore our sense of security and safety and our belief in our invulnerability have been severely challenged by terrorism, and it is sometimes difficult to focus energies elsewhere.

FAMILY VIOLENCE

At the same time, the terrorism in our homes among family members continues at profound levels. Although the incidence of homicides has declined in recent years, the percentage of murdered women who are killed by their intimate partners remains stable at approximately 30% since 1976 (Dawson, 2001). There also has been a dramatic increase in teen involvement in homicides both as victims and perpetrators (Fox and Zawitz, 2001). Fifty percent of offenders are less than 25 years old and most commonly use handguns as the weapons of destruction. The primary cause of death for both African-American and Caucasian male teenagers in the United States is gunshot wounds. Suicide remains the third leading cause of death among children and adolescents.

Despite the decline in homicides, the United States remains the most violent of all industrialized nations, and this violence is one of the most urgent social problems of contemporary American society. Criminal justice experts claim that the family is the birthplace of violence and that interpersonal violence is usually perpetrated by a close friend or family member of the abused. The beliefs that people are safe in their own homes and that family violence is rare are myths that are difficult to dispel. A woman is much more likely to be beaten, raped, and/or murdered by a partner or ex-partner than by a stranger. Approximately 1.5 million women and 800,000 men in the United States are victims of intimate partner physical and/or sexual abuse each year (CDC, 2001). Experts estimate that 10 million children are exposed to marital/woman battering each year (Burnett, 2001; Holden, Geffner, and Jouriles, 1998).

Violence against women affects their family members, as well as society. Research indicates that 28% to 70% of children who are exposed to woman battering are also physically and sexually abused and suffer multiple consequences,

both short and long term, which include posttraumatic stress, social, cognitive, emotional, and behavioral problems. Rarely do the children receive assistance or support to deal with their trauma (Burnett, 2001; Gelles, 2000; Graham-Bermann and Levendosky, 1998; Holden, Geffner, and Jouriles, 1998).

All family members are at much greater risk of being abused by another family member than by a stranger. Family violence that occurs in multiple generations in the same family is called **transgenerational violence**. In 1997 more than 3 million (3,195,000) children were reported to child protective service agencies in the United States for child abuse and neglect (Wang and Daro, 1998). Children are much more likely to be sexually abused by a family member than by someone who is unknown to them. Abuse occurs in all age groups. Each year 2 million older persons are typically abused by their own children or spouses (Wolf, 1995).

Reports are now available on violence in gay and lesbian relationships. Burnett (2001) reported that 11% of lesbians are assaulted by their female partners compared with 30.4% of women who reported being assaulted by their male partners. Approximately 15% of gay men reported being assaulted by their male partner compared with 7.7% of men who reported being assaulted by their female partner.

Studies that examine battered women's experiences when they seek health care services reflect the failure of health care professionals to address family violence. In general, these studies (Glass, Dearwater, and Campbell, 2001; Rodriguez et al., 1999; Stark and Flitcraft, 1996) report a lack of assessment, intervention, and responsiveness by doctors and nurses in the treatment of battered women.

Nursing and medical organizations have all addressed the need to prepare doctors, nurses, and other health care professionals to effectively screen and intervene in the lives of victims of domestic violence. In 1992 the Joint Commission on Accreditation on Healthcare Organizations (JCAHO) mandated policies and procedures for the assessment, treatment, and referral of victims of violence. In 1998 the Health Resources and Services Administration published an action plan to prevent family violence. Most recently the prestigious Institute of Medicine published a document on family violence entitled *Confronting Chronic Neglect: The Education and Training of Health Professionals on Family Violence* (2001). This document indicts educational institutions for not adequately preparing health care professionals to address family violence.

Because nurses interact with families and individuals in a wide variety of settings, they are frequently the first to identify and therapeutically intervene with those experiencing family violence. A question remains as to why nurses often do not intervene therapeutically in family violence. Some explanations include lack of knowledge, stereotypes, prejudices, and poor role models as factors. According to a study by Limandri and Tilden (1996), nurses often feel frustrated because of the ineffectiveness of the system of protective services. Certainly nurses are not exempt from violence in their own lives. Ellis (1999) reported that 58% of the registered nurses in her study had experienced domestic violence in their personal lives. For nurses to confront violence in the lives of others may be too painful a reminder of what is or has occurred in their own lives.

Although it is recognized that "intimate partner abuse" may at times be mutual, the National Violence Against Women survey (NVAW) (Tjaden and Thoennes, 1998) confirmed numerous other studies that indicated that women are much more likely to be assaulted by an intimate partner than men are. The findings from the NVAW survey also confirmed data from the National Crime Victimization Survey (NCVS, 1994). These two national surveys contradict some research by others who claim that men and women are equally at risk for physical assault by their intimate partners (Straus and Gelles, 1986; Morse, 1995). In the NVAW telephone survey of 8000 men and 8000 women, 76% of the women reported being raped or physically abused as an adult by a male partner, whereas only 18% of men reported being abused by their female partners. Repeated studies indicate that women usually do not initiate the violence and, when they are violent toward their partners, it is often in self-defense (Gelles,1997; Kurz, 1993; Stark and Flitcraft, 1996). Because of their lack of power and authority in many families, women are much more vulnerable to battering and abuse. Therefore the abuse experienced by a battered woman is not merely an exchange of blows with her male partner, but a pattern of abuse characterized by coercive control over all aspects of her life that is repetitive, extensive, and escalating over time, with minimal or no provocation. Indeed, the batterer many not use physical violence frequently because he is able to batter psychologically and control his partner's behavior through constant intimidation, isolation, insults, and threats. This coercive control is often reflected in homicide rates of women in the United States and Canada when they try to leave their batterer. Although homicide rates appear to be declining among intimate partners, the statistics continue to be alarming, with women murdered far more often than their male partners. Over 50% of solved murders of women were perpetrated by their intimate partners, whereas only 6% of the men were killed by their intimate partners (Dawson, 2001). According to the U.S. Department of Justice statistics in 1999, 32% of women victims were murdered by their male partners, compared to 3.6% of males who were murdered by their female partners.

DEFINITIONS OF VIOLENCE AND ABUSE

A major problem in the field of domestic or family violence has been the difficulty in developing useful and clear definitions of violence and abuse. It is accepted that psychologic abuse can sometimes be more harmful than physical abuse.

Therefore it is critical to use a broad, holistic approach in the assessment of family violence. For the purpose of this discussion, the definition of **domestic violence** is a "learned pattern of harmful behaviors used by one person in an intimate or family relationship including children, siblings, and the elderly." The purpose of these behaviors is to control the behavior of one's partner or family members. Violent behaviors include, but are not limited to, physical and sexual assault, psychologic abuse, emotional abuse, isolation, threats and intimidation, economic control, and stalking.

THEORIES OF FAMILY VIOLENCE

Several models attempt to explain family violence (Box 23-1); no single model is able to fully explain this phenomenon. Various statistics on family violence are listed in Box 23-2 on p. 522.

The Psychiatric Mental Illness Model

This model focuses on the individual characteristics of the abuser or survivor to explain the phenomenon at hand. In the past, a person who severely injured a child was considered to be psychotic or mentally disturbed; however, when the victim was a woman, she (rather than the abuser) was the fo-

---

Box 23-1	Etiologic Theories Related to Family Violence

Psychiatric/mental illness model

Social learning theory
Aggression as a learned, not instinctual, behavior
Family role modeling
Desensitization to violence through repeated exposure via the media

Sociologic theory
Unemployment
Poverty
Crime
Teenage pregnancy
Isolation

Anthropologic theory
Sexual inequalities
Social organization
Cultural patterning

Feminist theory
Explanatory utility of constructs of gender and power
Analysis of the family as a historically situated institution
Importance of understanding and validating women's experiences
Empowerment of women

Box 23-2   Epidemiology for Violence

Battered Women

1.8 million wives in the United States are abused every year by their husbands.

25% to 50% of all women are abused by their intimate partners at least once.

20% to 25% of women who seek treatment in emergency rooms are there because of battering injuries.

2% to 8% of these women identified abuse as the cause of their injuries.

7% to 17% of pregnant women experience physical abuse by their partners.

Physically Abused Children

2 million children are seriously abused each year by their parents and caregivers.

Of these, 1000 die from results of these injuries.

25% of the 2 million abused children are physically abused; 20% are sexually abused; 55% are neglected.

25% of the 2 million abused children are less than 5 years old; 60% are between ages 5 and 14 years old.

Children less than 3 years old are at a greater risk for fatal abuse than are older children.

Abused and neglected children are at greater risk for later delinquency, adult criminality, and violent crimes than are nonabused or non-neglected children.

Sexually Abused Children

50% of psychiatric clients have histories of physical and sexual abuse.

The average age at which child incest begins is 6 years, with an average duration of 7 years.

Rape

Only one in 10% to 20% of rapes are reported to the police.

More than 90% of rape victims are women.

20% of female college students are raped at some time during their college education.

The most common age group for rape victims is 16 to 25 years.

In 84% of rape cases, the victim is acquainted with the perpetrator.

Only 5% of rapists were psychotic when they raped their victims.

In 90% of rape cases, victims and perpetrators are of the same race.

cus of attention and was judged to be mentally defective (masochistic) for remaining with the abuser. Recently the spotlight turned to a closer examination of the characteristics of the abuser instead of placing blame on the victim. Within the psychiatric model, the causative factors in family violence are defects in the abuser such as mental illness, alcohol and drug abuse, and personality disorders. Interventions focus on treating the mental disorder or personality characteristics of the abuser. External factors are not the focus of this model. The psychiatric model is very popular and is commonly used because it is comforting for society to believe that it is the "abnormal or deranged" person who abuses others or chooses to remain in an abusive relationship (Gelles and Cornell, 1990). Because most people do not

consider themselves mentally ill, they neither question their potential for abuse nor examine their behavior if they are abusive.

Social Learning Theory

Psychologist Albert Bandura's **social learning theory** model (1973) is based on classic research on aggression. This model combines components of behavioral and sociologic theories. Contrary to earlier writings by a variety of people, Bandura's model of social learning theory states that aggression is a learned behavior rather than instinctual. Although Bandura recognizes that neurophysiology can produce aggressive behavior, he maintains that the biologic mechanisms depend on appropriate stimulation for activation and that even when activated, aggressive behavior is still under cognitive control.

Bandura's research showed that children learn how to behave by observing the role models in their own families. Values, attitudes, and behaviors are shaped and developed by significant others in a child's life. The way parents cope with stress, anger, and frustration becomes a powerful lesson for the impressionable child.

Because family role models are usually the ones to which children are exposed, children assume that family behavior is normal and acceptable even though it may be highly violent and abusive. Physical discipline by parents gives children the message that punishment is necessary to enforce rules and gain compliance. In addition, the use of violence or physical force is reinforced because of the power derived from its use. In addition to role modeling in the family, children learn aggressive behavior through direct experience, practice, and observation of other mediums of violence. Support for the social learning theory is seen in repeated generational patterns of family violence. Although exposure to family violence does not guarantee that the pattern of violence will be repeated in subsequent generations, it does increase the child's risk of using violent behavior in adulthood.

Much has been written about the influence of television, films, music, and other media to promote violence. Based on multiple studies, the American Medical Association (1996) issued a document that stated violence in the media (1) encourages aggressive behavior through modeling, (2) disinhibits aggressive acting-out behaviors by repeated exposure, and (3) desensitizes people to violence around them. The desensitization to violence results in people becoming apathetic or unimpressed with the impact of violence on others. Research studies also suggest that repeated exposure to media violence increases feelings of insecurity, distrust, and suspicion of others. In classic studies, Bandura (1973) and other researchers who replicated his work, acknowledged that the vast majority of people do not act out the violence that they observe in the media; however, the majority of people who are heavy television viewers of violence perceive the world as a dangerous, unsafe place. Believing that the world is unsafe may predispose some people to misinterpret social cues and respond as though they are under attack when they are not.

Sociologic Theory

Sociologic models recognize the influence of neurophysiologic and psychologic factors, but their focus is on environmental and socioeconomic forces that underlie violence. Like social learning theory, sociologists reject the notion that aggression is instinctual. According to these theories, conditions such as unemployment, crime, poverty, isolation, teenage pregnancy, and stress are of major concern in addressing violence in families. Many sociologists view violence in families as gender neutral; that is, both sexes play out a role in the problem. This stance is criticized by feminists because it minimizes the impact of male domination and power.

Anthropologic Theory

Cultural attitudes and definitions of abuse and violence vary significantly from one society to another. Some societies may view particular behaviors by its members as violent, whereas other societies may not. This lack of agreement on the perception of violence and abuse makes it difficult to establish a universal definition of family violence that is culturally acceptable to various societies.

Feminist Theory

Multiple studies report that batterers are characterized by patriarchal attitudes that include an excessive need to control and dominate their partners. Feminist researchers claim that these patriarchal values are the underlying basis for violence against women (Campbell and Humphreys, 2003; Draucker, 2002; Stark and Flitcraft, 1996). According to these researchers, violence is a central component of male social standing in Western culture. Men's relationships with women are characterized by disdain, control, dominance, and treatment of women as commodities and sexual objects. Typically the male with strong needs to dominate and control believes it is his right and responsibility to control and beat his wife and children because they are his property to do with as he pleases.

THE BATTERED WOMAN

Battering is the most common cause of injury to women in the United States. Although some women escape from their abusive partners, many remain in a violent relationship that gradually escalates in frequency and severity.

One out of every 10 women in any health care setting is abused by her male intimate partner, but Emergency Department (ED) presentations for domestic violence are higher. In one study that examined ED records retrospectively, physicians found that only 2.8% of the women who were treated in the ED were described as abused on their medical records, even though 25% were actually there be-

cause of battering injuries (Stark and Flitcraft, 1996). In another study of 440 physicians, the majority were screened for intimate partner violence with injured clients, but only 10% of physicians screened new clients and 11% screened prenatal clients. Burnett points out that this finding is highly significant because 77% of women in violent relationships who seek emergency medical care are not seeking care for their physical trauma. Instead, the women have chronic complaints related to ongoing domestic violence symptoms.

Among pregnant women, 7% to 21% experience physical abuse by their partners (Warshaw, 1989). In a study by Parsons and Harper (1999), intimate partners perpetrated 36.4% of homicide-related maternal deaths. Effects of physical abuse on the pregnant woman can be direct or indirect. Direct effects include low birth weight, preterm labor, preterm infants, and infant injury and death. These researchers report that indirect effects of physical abuse have a more profound effect on women's health than do direct effects. Indirect effects include chronic pain, depression, high anxiety, use of drugs and alcohol, and suicide attempts.

A number of studies examining the experiences of battered women in the health care system document (1) the failure of doctors and nurses to make direct inquiries as to how the women received their injuries, even when women wanted to provide this information; (2) subtle blaming and pejorative labeling of the women; and (3) unnecessary or inappropriate dispensing of medication such as tranquilizers (Burnett, 2001; Rodriguez et al., 1999; Stark and Flitcraft, 1996).

DEFINITION OF THE BATTERED WOMAN

The term *battered woman* is used in this chapter to mean a woman who is battered by her intimate partner, including a lesbian partner. A woman is in greatest danger when she attempts to leave the controlling mate. Although it is recognized that violence exists between homosexual couples, this discussion focuses on the most common type of domestic violence, the male abuser and the abused female.

When describing the battered woman, violence, or battering, is not limited to physical abuse. One survivor lived under the constant threat of a loaded gun frequently pressed to her temple by her abuser, but she never received a bruise on her body. Such psychologic abuse is devastating. Other battered women report that over time the physical abuse actually ends but profound psychologic abuse continues. This happens because the threat of violence is so terrorizing to the woman that this threat alone becomes the controlling force. For this reason, advocates for battered women define this form of domestic violence as physical, psychologic, and sexual abuse that is primarily directed at women by men for the purpose of maintaining power and control over the women (Box 23-3).

Battered women represent all ethnic, religious, and socioeconomic groups. However, middle and upper socioeco-

Box 23-3   Behaviors of the Abuser

Economic abuse—strict control of money (even when the woman earns it), food, clothing, transportation, and other resources

Sexual abuse, including marital rape and forcing the woman to participate in sexual activities against her will

Threats and intimidation, including threats of taking the children from the woman or hurting them or other family members

Threatening to injure or kill family pets

Isolating the woman from any support system, including her family, friends, and health care professionals

Constantly demeaning and insulting the woman

Intentionally breaking material objects to terrorize the woman

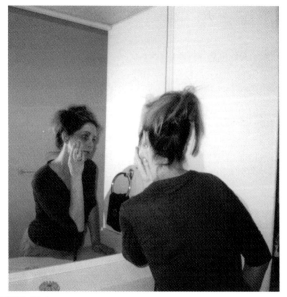

FIGURE 23-1. Physical abuse is the most common cause of injury to women in the United States. Battering occurs in all ethnic, religious, and socioeconomic groups. Although the batterer is unprovoked, the woman is made to feel it is her fault.

nomic women can more easily hide their abuse. Material resources allow middle class and upper class women to be seen by a private physician who is more likely to keep their secret or ask no questions. Most women who are seen in shelters for battered women are those without other options (Figure 23-1).

THE BATTERER

Too often batterers are portrayed as males who have temporarily lost control, usually under provocation. This loss of control is frequently blamed on alcohol or drugs. Actually, batterers abuse their partner whether drunk or sober, but may use drunkenness as an excuse. Despite numerous studies on the characteristics of batterers, no evidence supports the belief that the typical batterer is an alcoholic or is mentally ill. Usually batterers are described by fellow workers as average, normal males who give no hint of the abusive behavior they demonstrate in the privacy of their own homes. Few batterers have criminal records or have physical altercations with others outside of their homes. Such physical abuse against a stranger would result in arrest and incarceration, but the privacy of their homes protects batterers and continues to do so as society turns a blind eye. Batterers learn that there are few if any consequences to their abusive behaviors. The privacy and secrecy in which abuse toward women occurs are the main reasons that abuse is perpetuated.

THE NURSING PROCESS

ASSESSMENT

Assessment of the battered woman begins with the nurse's critical examination of own beliefs and biases about battering. For example, if the nurse believes that a woman has brought the problem on herself for not leaving the abusive relationship, then this attitude, consciously or unconsciously, will most likely be communicated to the battered woman. The nurse's attitude and resulting interactions may revictimize the woman.

Because holistic assessments are the foundation of the nursing process, culture is an important consideration in that assessment. Culture often defines how the battered woman interprets and responds to the violence that has been perpetrated against her. Understanding the battered woman's culture is also critical for developing a treatment plan. Culture is also an important determinant of whether the battered woman seeks assistance from community resources such as the police and shelters. Some ethnic women are isolated and unaware of community resources for abuse, are suspicious of caregivers outside of their own cultural group, and fear being ostracized by their cultural group if they reach out to the broader community. Most battered women's shelters make a concerted effort to reach out to women of all colors and ethnic groups. When caring for a client from a minority culture, it is the nurse's responsibility to learn about the client's culture to provide culturally sensitive care. Questions about the woman's culture are appropriate but must be presented in a sensitive, respectful way so that the woman understands that the nurse is concerned and is intent on learning more about the woman's values and customs to provide effective holistic nursing care.

An understanding of culture is as important when working with the male batterer as it is when working with the battered woman. Before treatment strategies can be planned for the abuser, his cultural attitudes, values, and beliefs must be acknowledged and respected. No cultural beliefs and traditions, however, can be accepted or tolerated at the expense of another person's health and well-being. Because physical abuse, including rape, of women by the partners is common, it is critical to ask about physical, sexual, and emotional abuse in the histories of all women. The nurse must also ask if the abuser hits the chil-

NURSING CARE IN THE COMMUNITY   Survivors of Violence

Survivors of trauma may be of any age, gender, or nationality. They share a bond in that their ability to enjoy fully functional lives has been altered by a disruptive event, be it experiencing molestation as a child, rape as an adult, or armed conflict in war. The event may involve family members or strangers and be life threatening or totally demeaning. The responses of family, friends, or society may be problematic.

The nurse in the community setting, who works with such a disparate group of clients, must be extremely flexible and accepting. As in other emotional disturbances, the presence of a strong supportive network is critical. Debriefing a traumatic incident requires a team effort in which the nurse may play a role as the individual counselor, hearing every detail, or the group facilitator, helping the victims begin to repattern their lives and social interactions. The relationship will be more ongoing than a crisis intervention in the controlled hospital environment.

Assessing the truth in such a situation is often difficult because a molester, rapist, or batterer is usually involved, who may still be threatening to the survivor and perhaps to anyone assisting. Nurses may feel angry at or fearful of the perpetrator and must carefully monitor personal reactions to the situation. Other professions, including child protective services or the police, may become involved, and communication channels must be clear and overt. There is no margin for error when dealing with such a po-

tentially volatile situation as a parent molesting a child or a husband battering his wife.

Survivors of combat are often diagnosed with posttraumatic stress disorder. These persons often lead lives that are estranged from mainstream society and complicated by drug/alcohol abuse. They may respond to questions with anger toward any type of proffered help and require prolonged, specialized counseling before they are willing to participate in group therapy. The community psychiatric mental health nurse may encounter these persons in homeless shelters or living on the street. The nurse must be able to tolerate frequent rebuffs before any sort of therapeutic relationship is established. Patience and a sense of humor in a tension-filled situation may often be the keys to effective interaction.

The nurse working in the community may encounter victims with a strong sense of entitlement who will emphasize their victimization to get special treatment. These individuals will quickly exhaust even the most patient mental health professional. The nurse must know the system of entitlements well and must circumscribe the client's expectations. Such clients must be offered what is available and told that no more will be forthcoming, despite their distress or anger. Such a situation often requires a concerted effort from other mental health disciplines, so that one person does not have to bear the brunt of the client's irritation.

---

dren. Protective services must be notified if the children have been abused.

A complete physical examination must be conducted on every woman who is suspected of being battered, including a neurologic examination and x-ray studies if necessary to determine the existence of previous injuries. Because battering during pregnancy is one of the major causes of complications of pregnancy, nurses need to assess for it. Even older widows may have serious unresolved issues relating to abusive relationships with their deceased husbands. Many battered women report a myriad of physical problems without disclosing the source of violence. Because they have been programmed to believe that somehow they provoked the violence, they feel guilty and ashamed. Nevertheless, if asked directly and under appropriate conditions, most women will disclose the nature of their injuries. These conditions include being respectful and sensitive to the woman's disclosures and informing her that she is not at fault and that no human being has the right to abuse another. In addition, the nurse must provide a safe environment that is conducive to disclosure (see Nursing Care in the Community box). The first step is to separate the woman from her abuser. On many occasions it will be obvious that the woman's partner is determined to remain with her. Separation must occur even if it means calling security for assistance. Often more indirect tactics can be used such as sending him to the admitting desk to give additional information.

During assessment and when taking the woman's history, it is recommended that the nurse begin with the least sensitive questions and gradually progress to the more sensitive ones. Questions should be simple and direct and re-

flect the language and terms that the woman herself uses (see Nursing Assessment Questions box). The Nursing Research Consortium on Violence and Abuse has developed a simple four-item questionnaire, which was adapted by Campbell and Humphreys (1993) for taking general case history (Box 23-4). These questions may be followed by additional questions.

When women do present with current physical trauma, a delay in seeking treatment and/or an illogical explanation for the injury are cues that may indicate abuse. Often, abused women seek treatment for indirect effects of their violent relationships. Complaints may reflect the stress of these violent relationships and/or residual pain from past injuries. Often, the woman appears depressed, anxious, and fatigued. The battered woman typically has more chronic, pain-related, vague complaints than her nonbattered counterpart. Health history may indicate frequent accidents and other traumatic injuries such as lacerations, bruises, and fractures. Spontaneous abortions, suicide attempts, and substance abuse also may be reported.

Other potential indicators of abuse may be identified in the family history. The following potential indicators relate to the woman's partner:

- Very strict disciplinarian
- Belief in physical punishment
- Child abuse
- Alcohol and drug abuse
- Extremely possessive and jealous
- History of violence in his family of origin
- Unemployed
- Seeks to isolate family members

NURSING ASSESSMENT QUESTIONS
For the Battered Woman

1. We often see women who have been hurt by their partners. Is your partner responsible for your injuries?
2. Has your partner ever hurt you?

3. Have you noticed any pattern to this behavior such as an increase in frequency and severity?
4. Does he threaten to use or has he ever used a weapon to hurt you?

Box 23-4	General Case History Questions for the Abused

1. Have you ever been emotionally or physically abused by your partner or someone important to you?
2. Within the last year, have you been hit, slapped, kicked, or otherwise physically hurt by someone? If yes, by whom and how many times?
3. Within the last year, has anyone forced you to have sexual activities? If yes, who and how many times?
4. Are you afraid of your partner or anyone else listed above?

Box 23-5	Physical Indicators of Possible Abuse

General Appearance

Anxious and frightened, depressed and passive, ashamed and embarrassed, poor eye contact, weight problems, looks to partner for answers, partner does all of the talking, partner exhibits smothering and extremely possessive behavior

Skin

Contusions; abrasions and minor lacerations; scars; burns, particularly on breasts, arms, abdomen, chest, neck, face, and genitals

Musculoskeletal

Fractures and sprains, especially of distal versus proximal bones (e.g., skull, facial bones, extremities), dislocated shoulder, and evidence of old fractures

Genital/Rectal

Evidence of vaginal/anal rape such as bruising, edema, and bleeding; also evidence of direct kicks or punches

Abdominal

Internal bleeding or other injuries; chronic pelvic pain

Neurologic

Acute stress disorder, hyperactive reflexes, chronic headaches and backaches, paresthesias from old injuries

---

Box 23-5 presents the most important physical examination indicators of wife/woman abuse.

The nurse must accurately document all statements the woman makes. Open-ended questions that reflect what the woman is disclosing should be used so that she feels in charge of the interview. Documented information must include the name of the abuser and when and how the abuse occurred. When possible, the nurse should record the woman's exact words because such documentation is legally powerful. The nurse must also ask if the abuser hits the children. Protective services must be notified if the children have been abused.

A detailed description of the woman's injuries is documented in the narrative, and a body chart diagram should be used to indicate the location and type of injury. The nurse should ask the woman if she was forced into sexual acts against her will and then examine her for anal and vaginal tears. If there is a possibility of marital rape, the nurse follows the rape protocol and uses an evidence collection kit. If possible, a *sexual abuse nurse examiner (SANE)* is called in to intervene. The nurse also assesses the woman for sexually transmitted diseases (STDs) and documents all laboratory and x-ray results. At least two photographs should be taken of each trauma area, but the woman must sign a consent form first. The nurse should place one set of photographs in the woman's record with identifying data on the back that includes the date, woman's name, hospital number, and name of photographer. Because of the possibility of future legal proceedings, the nurse should request a safe address from the woman where the second set of photographs can be mailed.

It is crucial to reassure the woman that the documentation is confidential and that her partner will not be allowed access to it without her permission (unless it goes to court, at which time the documentation becomes public record). Retaliation by the batterer is always a major concern for the abused woman. However, the woman should understand that she has the right to access her records and that these will be valuable to her in child custody cases or if she chooses to file charges against the abuser.

Walton-Moss and Campbell (2002) cautioned against the use of such terms as *abuse* and *battering* because many abused women do not have this image of themselves. Direct questions are more helpful, such as "Did someone hit you?" It is also important to understand that the woman may love her partner and desperately wants to believe him when he promises that it will never happen again.

It is imperative to assess the woman's potential danger in cases of domestic violence. Information about the pattern of abuse and if it has increased in severity and frequency is vital. Other critical signs that indicate increased danger are that the abuser has a weapon, has been violent outside the house, is a substance abuser, has been stalking the woman, and has threatened suicide/homicide. At times the woman may contemplate suicide. It is well documented that the battered woman is at greatest risk of harm when she tries to leave her abuser (Walton-Moss and Campbell, 2002; Gelles, 1997). Therefore the woman must become aware of this risk, and the nurse must assist her to develop a safety plan. Such a plan typically involves providing the woman with phone numbers of nearby shelters, crisis lines, and community resources. The woman should also be referred to the local crime victims compensation board.

NURSING DIAGNOSIS

The following nursing diagnoses are examples of those that are relevant to the case study on Nina (see Case Study). They are based on information identified in the case study. However, all nursing diagnoses are formulated from information obtained during the assessment phase of the nursing process. The accuracy of the diagnoses depends on a careful, in-depth assessment. Based on the information that was provided, can you identify additional nursing diagnoses?

- Pain related to injuries sustained by battering as evidenced by difficulty breathing deeply and sleeping (multiple fractures)
- Risk for injury related to present and past abuse by husband
- Anxiety and fear related to threat of further battering
- Ineffective family coping related to abuse by husband and denial by wife

DSM Diagnoses

The DSM-IV-TR has not assigned a diagnosis for the battered woman. Stark and Flitcraft (1996) recommended the DSM-IV designation of "physical abuse of adult" because although it is a psychiatric diagnosis, it is nonstigmatizing and allows the woman access to resources. Some researchers and clinicians maintain that posttraumatic stress disorder (PTSD) is an appropriate diagnosis for many battered women who are repeatedly and severely abused (Briere, 1996; van der Kolk, McFarlane, and Weisaeth, 1996). The battered-woman syndrome is a description of what happens over time to the battered woman. This syndrome, as described by Walker (1994), has been allowed in courtrooms in all states as a defense in cases in which battered women have murdered their abusers.

OUTCOME IDENTIFICATION

The following outcome criteria are derived from the nursing diagnoses identified in the case study on Nina. These outcomes are the expected behaviors that Nina will demonstrate as a result of her plan of care. Stabilizing Nina's physical condition and securing her safety are the immediate short-term goals.

Client will:
- Report a decrease in her pain resulting from injuries sustained during her abuse.

CASE STUDY

Nina was brought to the Emergency Department by her husband to whom she has been married for 10 years. Her husband was very attentive to her, spoke reassuringly, and appeared very concerned about Nina's condition. According to her husband, a day ago Nina slipped as she was getting out of the bathtub. When she slipped, she bumped her head on the faucet and then fell on her arm. As her husband spoke, Nina sat quietly with her head down. She cradled her right arm and appeared to be in severe pain. Her right eye was red and swollen shut, and she seemed to have some difficulty breathing. Despite protests from her husband, the nurse interviewed Nina separately from her husband in a private consultation room. Although the nurse inquired directly whether Nina's husband had beaten her, Nina denied the abuse. A complete physical and neurologic examination was performed by the physician and a series of x-ray films were taken. When Nina returned from the radiology department, she was told by the physician that she had fractures of the wrist, facial bones, and several ribs. Nina was also informed that the x-ray films indicated multiple old, healed fractures of the ribs and pelvic girdle. The nurse spent time explaining to Nina how unlikely it was for her injuries to result from a fall in the bathtub. The nurse also reassured Nina that nothing she could have done would deserve such abuse by another person. Nina finally acknowledged that her husband had abused her, but insisted she had no intention of leaving him because he was a good husband. According to Nina, the only time her husband is abusive is when she fails to fulfill her domestic responsibilities and therefore provokes him into losing his temper and beating her. Nina has no children and no family nearby, except for a younger sister who is currently overwhelmed with her own family problems. Nina is psychologically and economically dependent on her husband and has no means of financial or psychologic support.

Critical Thinking

1. What is the first priority for the nurse who suspects abuse when assessing a woman?
2. How should the nurse respond to the shame, guilt, and self-blame of the battered woman?
3. What should a nurse do if he or she becomes angry and rejecting with a battered woman who is in denial about being battered?
4. If you suspected that your neighbor was in an abusive situation, what signs would you look for in the relationship?

- Demonstrate no difficulty breathing and verbalize feeling more relaxed.
- Demonstrate less fear and anxiety by being able to discuss her abuse and explore possible options for resolving it with the nurse.
- Verbalize an awareness of her increasingly dangerous situation because her abuse has intensified over time.
- Discuss with the nurse the implications for herself, her spouse, and other family members if she remains in the present abusive situation and explore with the nurse alternative means of family coping.
- Demonstrate an awareness of the need for safety by taking steps to protect herself in the future.
- Explore the possibility of pursuing litigation against her husband and requesting a restraining order if her husband is not jailed.

- Devise plans to secure her safety in case of future threats of abuse.
- Take advantage of community resources that increase her self-esteem and independence and become involved with an outreach group for battered women.

PLANNING

The plan of care for any survivor of violence should focus on addressing critical physical problems, securing the immediate safety of the victim, examining the implications of the abuse on the woman and other family members, and discussing future plans for safety. In the case of a battered woman such as Nina, who acknowledges the abuse only when confronted by the nurse, all possible options must be explored because she may need to use them in the future. The nurse should develop the care plan with the client and recognize that any effort to impose personal beliefs on the battered woman is fated for failure. Instead, the battered woman needs reassurance that she is capable of making appropriate decisions for herself—even if her decision is to return to her abuser. It is only through empowerment, not threats and intimidation, that the woman is most likely to develop the strength to make independent decisions that foster growth.

IMPLEMENTATION

Once the battered woman's physical condition has been stabilized, it is critical to assess her future safety and collaboratively explore her fears, anxieties, and concerns. Despite the need to leave the abusive situation, the woman may strongly believe that she has no other option except to return. If the woman chooses to return to the batterer, it is important to respect this decision. Making a decision to leave the batterer is usually a gradual process. However, it is critical that the woman realize that she has options. The nurse may serve as the key factor in a beginning awareness that other options do exist.

At present, all states have laws that provide some level of protection for survivors of domestic violence, and there is a definite trend across the country to pass further legislation to ensure this protection. The reality is, however, that there is a large gap between the actual laws and their implementation by the police and criminal justice system. In some localities police are mandated to arrest the abuser if there is evidence of probable violence. In many states the police must provide the battered woman with information on local shelters, domestic violence crisis lines, and her legal rights. However, the police may not always respond appropriately, so it is important that the nurse be able to inform the battered woman of her legal rights.

In recent years, some women's rights advocates and criminal justice experts have been debating mandatory reporting laws on domestic violence (Walton-Moss and Campbell, 2002). Women's rights advocates claim that mandatory domestic violence reporting laws discourage bat-

tered women from seeking treatment for their injuries because the women fear that their situation will be reported to the police and consequently place her in even greater danger with her abuser. Because some women are not ready to deal with the police, being forced to do so could be nontherapeutic and disempowering and even increase their danger of abuse. If no mandatory reporting laws exist, then the police should not be notified unless the woman consents. Although some professionals choose to maintain confidentiality if the battered woman requests it, the deciding factor on reporting is the degree of danger that the woman faces.

Nursing Interventions

Primary prevention for woman abuse begins with identifying families at risk and changing societal views toward wife abuse. Nurses must become politically active to promote social, economic, and psychologic independence for all women. Societal acceptance of violence against women as portrayed in films, television, magazines, and music must not be tolerated. Nurses must become more knowledgeable about factors such as poverty, drugs, gun control, and unemployment, which increase the risk of domestic violence, and must work with other members of the community to establish public policy and programs to address these issues.

Secondary prevention of woman battering involves early case finding and decisive intervention. Specific nursing interventions depend on the stage that the battered woman is in, because a woman in denial about the abuse requires a different strategy than one who is determined not to return to the relationship. In relationships where the abuse is just beginning and is mild, it may be possible to work with the marital dyad when both partners choose to do so. In these cases, the male accepts all responsibility for the abuse and the counseling focuses on preventing any further abuse. In many situations the advanced practice nurse is the appropriate professional to work with the battered woman.

Tertiary prevention is required when the woman has been repeatedly abused, as in the case of Nina. In such instances the focus is on assisting the abused woman to overcome the physical and psychologic effects of the abuse and to prevent future abuse. Because the abuser frequently threatens and harasses the woman when she attempts to leave, it may be difficult for her to follow through. Frequently, these women seek assistance from local shelters that can provide safety and counseling. Nurses are often in the position to provide support and counseling to battered women in shelters. The nursing interventions identified in Table 23-1 relate to the case study describing Nina, who requires tertiary prevention measures in an Emergency Department setting.

EVALUATION

Evaluation is a critical component of the nursing process. It is especially critical with the battered woman because inadequate or inappropriate nursing interventions may result in more serious abuse or even death for the woman. Nurses

Table 23-1 Nursing Interventions for Battered Women

Interventions	Rationales
Report abuse to police.	Provide for safety
Provide medications to relieve pain and anxiety.	Relieve her pain and reduce anxiety
Discuss validity of the woman's anxiety.	
Encourage the woman to discuss events leading to past and present abuse.	Reduce her guilt and shame
Point out the increasingly violent nature of the relationship and concern for her safety.	
Insist that no person has the right to abuse another.	
Explore effectiveness of her current coping skills and suggest additional skills.	Increase her independence and effective coping skills
Focus on strengths, endurance, and abilities.	Increase her self-esteem
Discuss destructive societal expectations of women.	
Discuss frequency of woman abuse.	
Explore family and/or friends as support possibilities.	Increase her awareness of potential support
Discuss potential for using community resources (e.g., shelters and/or hotlines and police).	
Describe current laws on domestic violence.	Increase her awareness of abuse implications
Explore implications of pressing charges against the batterer.	
Explore meaning of potential relationship loss.	
Explore various options for the future.	
Provide fact sheet on domestic violence.	Identify long-term goals
Provide referrals.	
Develop a safety plan with critical papers, money, clothing, and other essentials to be set aside for emergency exits.	
Offer to be available for further questions.	Provide continuity of care

who work in settings where battered women seek treatment must be knowledgeable about the many different responses that may occur in the battered woman. Correct evaluation of outcomes and interventions depends on this recognition. Once a complete nursing care plan is developed, the evaluation is based on achievement of client goals.

CHILD ABUSE

Based on data collected from each state, the National Center on Child Abuse and Neglect conducted three surveys (1980, 1988, 1996) on child maltreatment in the United States (Gelles, 1997). The latest survey indicated that agencies identified 2.9 million maltreated children in the year that the survey was last taken. Based on this total, 620,000 children were physically abused, 302,000 were sexually abused, 536,400 were emotionally abused, and 1,442,000 children were neglected. The National Center on Child Abuse and Neglect report that the rate of child victims has been declining from 15.3 victims per 1000 children in 1993 to 11.8 victims per 1000 in 1999. Unfortunately, protective service agencies have been able to investigate only 28% of the maltreated children under the Harm Standard" and 33% under the Endangerment Standard."

Researchers have only recently begun to document the effects of domestic violence on children. Barnett, Miller-Perrin, and Perrin (1997) identify four general areas of ad-

verse effects: (1) immediate trauma, (2) adverse effects on development, (3) living under high stress, and (4) exposure to violent role models. Overall, children exposed to domestic violence demonstrate more behavioral and emotional problems, cognitive deficits, and health problems than nonexposed children; as adults, the exposed children experience a wide variety of long-term psychologic effects as well. Finally, children who are exposed to marital violence are themselves at high risk for battering by the abuser (Gelles, 1997).

In the 1940s the introduction of x-ray technology dramatically facilitated the identification of abused children. During this time, some physicians began to notice patterns of healed fractures in small children. It was not until 1962, however, when the classic article, "The Battered Child Syndrome" (Kempe et al., 1962), was published that child abuse was thrust into the public consciousness. In 1974 the U.S. government established the National Center on Child Abuse and Neglect. By that time, mandatory reporting requirements for child abuse and neglect were instituted in all 50 states.

Social science research indicates that the majority of parents use physical punishment to discipline their children. Gelles and Cornell (1990) claimed that spanking is the most common form of family violence in the United States. Straus, an eminent sociologist who researches family violence, has been condemning corporal punishment of children for many years (Straus, 2000; Straus, Sugarman, and

Giles-Sims, 1997; Straus, 1994). He found that corporal punishment remains a strong predictor of antisocial behavior for as long as 2 years after the punishment. Straus emphasized that spanking legitimizes and condones the use of violence and contributes to other societal violence by teaching children that "might makes right." Parents tend to discipline their children the way they were disciplined as children, and they often insist that the only language a child understands is physical punishment. It is difficult to change repeated generational patterns of family discipline, even though social science research finds no potential benefit from physical punishment as discipline and much to condemn it. Parents need to be reminded that any physical punishment that leaves bruises on a child is inappropriate and in some states would be considered abusive and subject to prosecution.

DEFINITIONS OF CHILD ABUSE AND NEGLECT

Definitions of **child abuse** and **child neglect** vary from state to state and among clinicians and researchers. The federal definitions of child abuse and neglect are contained in the Child Abuse Prevention and Treatment Act (CAPTA), and they provide the minimum guidelines that each state must use in their own definitions. According to CAPTA, child abuse and neglect are defined as: "at a minimum, any recent act or failure to act on the part of a parent or caretaker, which results in death, serious physical or emotional harm, sexual abuse or exploitation, or an act or failure to act which presents an imminent risk of serious harm" (Legal Information Institute, 1995). Thus the definition includes acts of omission as well as commission and exploitation. Despite the variation in state definitions, it is clear that nurses and other health care professionals must conduct holistic assessments and search for all types of abuse and neglect while recognizing that psychologic abuse is always present to some degree in all abuse and neglect. Indeed, abuse that leaves no physical scars has the potential for disrupting normal growth and development of children even more seriously than the physical. **Child psychologic abuse** includes behaviors that are rejecting, degrading/devaluing, terrorizing, isolating, corrupting, exploiting, denying essential stimulation or availability, and unreliable and inconsistent parenting (Briere, 1992).

THEORETIC FRAMEWORKS OF CHILD ABUSE

No single theory explains the causation of child abuse. It is generally recognized that many complex interacting factors are involved that place children at risk for abuse. Box 23-6 summarizes the various theories of child abuse and neglect.

THE ABUSED CHILD

Younger children, especially those under 3 years old, are at greater risk for fatal abuse than are older children. Because younger children are more fragile than older ones, the fatal-

ity risk is increased. Earlier studies report that premature infants and handicapped and developmentally disabled children are also at higher risk. Sullivan and Knutson (2000) reported that children with disabilities are 3.4 times more likely to be abused than their nonabused peers. National studies (Gelles, 1997; Sedlak and Broadhurst, 1996) indicate that child abuse actually decreases as a child gets older and plateaus by age 14 years. Female children are more likely to experience physical, emotional, and sexual abuse than are males, although males are at greater risk for more serious injuries and emotional neglect.

The greatest concern is the alarming increase in the incidence of child abuse and neglect. Sedlak and Broadhurst (1996) conducted the Third National Incidence Study of Child Abuse and Neglect (NIS-3) and reported a 67% increase in abused and neglected children since the 1986 NIS-2. If one compares the NIS-3 data to the first NIS report in 1980, the increase in child maltreatment has increased by 149%. Although two different measures of abuse and neglect were used for the NIS studies, both indicated a dramatic increase in child maltreatment over the years of these studies. It is important to note that data from the NIS estimates are based on reported cases; therefore it is assumed that the actual number of cases is much higher.

In a discussion of the long-term consequences of childhood abuse, researchers report that abused and neglected children are at greater risk for later delinquency, adult criminality, and violent crimes than are children in the control groups. Abused and neglected children also have more intellectual deficits, learning disabilities, drug and alcohol abuse, and psychiatric problems (Barnett, Miller-Perrin, and Perrin, 1997; Gelles, 1997). In recent years researchers have begun examining how severe abuse affects brain functioning. In particular, they have found that victims are often "primed" to overreact to stress. This state of chronic hyperarousal is the basis for three common outcomes of childhood abuse: PTSD, depression, and irritable bowel syndrome (Kendall-Tackett, 2000).

Box 23-6	Etiologic Theories Related to Child Abuse

Biologic Theory
Parents who were abused as children are at risk for abusing their own children.

Social Learning Theory
Family teaches and accepts violent behavior.
Violence is glorified in the media.
Violence is accepted in families, schools, and churches.

Environmental Theory
Socioeconomic class
Unemployment
Stressful life events

THE CHILD PHYSICAL ABUSER

Research on the characteristics of child physical abusers describes them as immature, lacking in self-esteem, and having unrealistic expectations of children, poor impulse control, and minimal or no external support systems. In cases of physical abuse, 76% of the perpetrators were males and 40% were females. In cases of neglect, females accounted for 87% versus 43% by males (Sedlak and Broadhurst, 1996). When analyzing the likelihood of males versus females as child abusers, it must be considered that mothers are frequently the only adults in the household or at least the most common caregiver.

THE NURSE'S ATTITUDE IN CHILD ABUSE

When nurses work in settings where they may encounter abusive families, it is critical that they take time to assess their own attitudes and feelings before interacting with these families. Humphreys and Ramsey (1993) described three typical reactions by the nurse: (1) horror that parents could perpetrate abuse on their children, (2) denial of the abuse, and (3) fantasies of saving or rescuing the child. None of these responses are helpful to the child, family, or nurse because each interferes with meeting the therapeutic needs of the child and the family, and thus interferes with providing effective nursing care.

If the nurse has a history of abuse in his or her own family, acknowledging the present abuse may initiate some powerful reexperiencing of his or her own abuse. Sometimes the realization of child abuse is so repugnant that nurses may use avoidance to protect themselves. If nurses believe that they are the only ones who are capable of helping the child, they deny parents the opportunity to understand how their behavior has affected the child and how they must change if the family is to survive and become functional. It is important for nurses to accept that most families, given the necessary conditions, have the potential for abusing and neglecting their children.

THE NURSING PROCESS

ASSESSMENT

The following discussion focuses on the nurse's responsibilities in making a holistic assessment of the abused child. Areas of assessment include physical and emotional abuse and neglect of the child. Assessment of the sexually abused child is covered in the next section.

History

It is the nurse's responsibility to identify abuse and neglect and to intervene in a nonjudgmental and nonthreatening manner. An open, honest attitude with parents is much more likely to gain cooperation and trust than a hostile, blaming one. Direct, honest questions are necessary. All states require nurses and other health care professionals to report any suspicion of child abuse to protective service. Failure to report may constitute a misdemeanor.

Typically the history format first focuses on parental concerns, then on general family history, and finally on the present concern (see Nursing Assessment Questions box). This progression moves from the least to the most threatening issue and affords the nurse the opportunity to establish rapport with the parents before requesting information about the most sensitive issue—the possibility of abuse.

When taking the history, the nurse is alert for discrepancies between the parental explanation of the child's injuries and the physical findings. An example of a discrepancy could be the parents' claim that they have no knowledge of how the child broke his or her femur. The nurse should suspect child abuse when fractures of the femur are diagnosed without some history of significant trauma, such as a car accident. Other clues include parental delay in seeking treatment for the child's injuries, failure to use hospitals closer to home, the child's history of multiple injuries, reluctance by parents to give a history, or discrepancies in the histories that each parent gives. To identify inconsistencies in the history, each parent should be interviewed separately. Whenever possible, children should also be interviewed separately from parents, although children may often deny abuse in an effort to protect parents out of feelings of loyalty or fear of retaliation.

It is often extremely helpful to observe the parent-child relationship while taking the history. Taking the history also allows the nurse to role model appropriate child-rearing skills and allows parents to express their fears, concerns, and problems.

All physical findings should be documented on the child diagram on the history form and direct quotations of the parents should be included whenever possible (Box 23-7). At present, photographs are being used more extensively, although they are not a substitute for a detailed

NURSING ASSESSMENT QUESTIONS

For Parents Who Are Suspected of Child Abuse

1. Is there anything in particular that you would like to share about your child or your family as we begin this history?
2. Does your child have any particular health or behavior problems?
3. Have any of your other children ever had similar injuries?
4. How did your child receive these injuries?

history and physical examination. State laws vary regarding authorization for taking photographs without parental consent. Therefore nurses who work in settings that provide care for children should familiarize themselves with state laws.

Box 23-7   Physical Indicators of Possible Child Abuse and Neglect

General Appearance
Excessive fearfulness and watchfulness
Disheveled and malnourished
Failure to thrive

Multiple Injuries
No history of significant trauma

Skin
Unexplained bruises, welts, and scratches in various stages of healing (different colors)
Regular patterns of bruises and welts such as bite marks or marks from electrical cords
Untreated infected wounds
Lacerations from rope burns; especially on the neck, wrists, ankles, and torso
Bruises on buttocks, genitalia, thighs, side of the face, trunk, and upper arms

Burns
Small round cigarette burns (infected insect bites resemble cigarette burns)
Immersion burns (even boundaries that are glovelike, socklike, or symmetric; accidental burns are asymmetric with splash marks)
Patterned burn marks (e.g., from an iron or grill)

Fractures
Fractures in infants younger than age 1 year
Fractures of femur, humerus, posterior ribs, skull, and long bones and any uncommon fractures

Head Injuries
Skull fractures and subdural hematomas (leading cause of death among abused children)
Brain hemorrhages or contusions without external signs of injury (e.g., shaken baby syndrome)
Alopecia caused by hair pulling

Abdominal Injuries
Ruptured liver or spleen
Ruptured blood vessels
Kidney, bladder, or pancreatic injuries
Injuries to jejunum or duodenum

Injuries to Eyes, Ears, Nose, and Mouth
A wide variety of injuries including missing teeth, bruising, perforation of tympanic membrane, epistaxis and nasal fractures, retinal hemorrhage or detachment corneal abrasions, and periorbital hematomas

Other Types of Abuse/Neglect
Munchausen's syndrome by proxy
Deprivational syndromes

NURSING DIAGNOSIS

Nursing diagnoses in a situation such as described in the case study of Marilee must include the parents because the identified client is an infant who depends on her parents for care and nurturance (see Case Study). Therefore the following diagnoses relate to both parents and child. Multiple nursing diagnoses may be identified; the following diagnoses are examples. Nursing diagnoses are formulated from information obtained during the assessment phase of the nursing process. The accuracy of the diagnoses depends on a careful, in-depth assessment.

Family-Related Diagnosis
- Impaired parenting related to inexperience with care giving, unrealistic expectations, marginal family adaptation, social isolation, lack of resources, and poverty

Child-Related Diagnoses
- Disturbed sensory perception related to cerebral trauma (subdural hemorrhage)
- Fear related to physical and emotional abuse
- Anxiety related to physical and emotional abuse

OUTCOME IDENTIFICATION

The nurse derived the outcome criteria for Marilee from the diagnoses that were formulated in collaboration with her parents. These outcomes are the expected behaviors

---

CASE STUDY

Eighteen-month-old Marilee was brought to the Southside Hospital Emergency Department by her parents, Betty and Jim Brown. Although the Browns live on the north side of town, they chose to bring their daughter to the Southside Hospital. Marilee was unconscious when she arrived at 7:00 AM. The physical examination revealed no external signs of trauma on the body except for bruises on the child's upper arms, which resembled grip marks. The Browns reported that Marilee was put to bed the night before in the usual manner but that this morning they were unable to arouse her. The Browns were unaware of any trauma or significant event that could account for their daughter's unconscious state. Both parents were teenagers and clearly agitated about their infant daughter's condition. Mr. Brown refused to have his wife interviewed without him. During the interview and history taking, Betty sat across the room crying softly while Jim answered the nurse's questions. The young couple stated that they are estranged from their own parents and rarely see them. Mr. Brown is currently unemployed.

Critical Thinking
1. What is the first priority for the nurse and health care team in this scenario?
2. What criteria make this young couple at risk for child abuse?
3. How would you establish trust with this young couple?
4. If you suspect child abuse, how would you protect the future safety of this child?
5. Why is an understanding of child developmental stages a critical component of effective parenting?

that Marilee and her parents will demonstrate as a result of the implementation of the plan of care and the nursing interventions.

For Marilee the first priority is the short-term nursing goal of stabilizing her critical physical condition, the subdural hemorrhage that resulted from vigorous shaking by her father. This outcome will be demonstrated by Marilee's renewed ability to respond to stimuli; that is, Marilee will be able to respond to sounds, sights, touch, motion, and smell at the same developmental level she had before her injury. She will recognize her parents, be able to ambulate, and tolerate a light diet.

The nursing diagnoses of fear and anxiety related to Marilee's abuse involve the long-term nursing goal of helping her reestablish the trust of her father and mother.

Outcome Identification for an Abused Child
Client will:
- Demonstrate trust by being receptive to her father and not exhibiting any fear of him. This outcome depends on her father's outcome.

Outcome Identification for an Abusing Parent
Client will:
- Attend parenting classes to improve knowledge and understanding of normal growth and development in children.
- Learn positive parenting skills and use them consistently with his daughter.
- Cooperate with protective services when they investigate him for the alleged abuse.

PLANNING
In all child abuse cases the primary concern is the health and safety of the child. Because Marilee is experiencing a medical crisis, the first priority is to stabilize her physical condition. Next, steps must be taken to secure her short- and long-term safety and to support the family in meeting these goals. Because the child's future health and safety depends on her family, it is critical that the nurse establish a trusting relationship with the family and collaborate on developing goals that are mutually acceptable. At times mutually agreed-on goals in child abuse cases may be difficult to achieve because many parents firmly believe that "sparing the rod spoils the child." However, children are sometimes punished because parents are ignorant of normal child development and interpret the child's inability to achieve parental demands as obstinacy or disobedience. Therefore classes in basic child growth and development are a critical component in addressing the needs of families who abuse or neglect their children. Child discipline and anger-control classes are also important in preventing future child abuse.

IMPLEMENTATION
All too frequently in child abuse cases, the child's physical trauma is addressed without addressing the underlying problem of the abuse. Hospitals and agencies that provide primary care are mandated by the JCAHO to identify clients who are abused and to provide treatment and referrals for them and their families. This mandate usually requires a concerted and collaborative effort by the health care team. The nurse is usually in an optimal position to coordinate this effort. In particular, the nurse must secure the physical and psychologic safety and health of the child, assist the parents to understand the consequences of their abusive behavior, and develop strategies with the parents that will prevent any recurrence of abuse.

When nurses plan interventions for abusive families, they must go beyond the focused family and think in terms of primary prevention for all families, that is, from families that appear normal through high risk. Potential settings for educating and identifying parents are hospital obstetric and pediatric units, substance abuse programs, health clinics, schools, churches, and the community at large. Because of their access to families in their own homes, community health nurses are in an excellent position to assess, teach, and model parenting skills and intervene on the primary prevention level before child maltreatment occurs.

Nursing Interventions
Primary prevention is focused on identifying families at risk and implementing interventions directed at preventing abuse. For Marilee, the nursing interventions are on the secondary prevention level because abuse has already occurred; the present focus is on addressing this current crisis and preventing future occurrences of abuse. In tertiary prevention the child is removed from the home because the safety of the child cannot be secured there. The goal is to maximize the future potential of the child within the constraints of the existing damage. The nursing interventions listed in Table 23-2 focus on secondary prevention for Marilee.

EVALUATION
Because nursing care of this family is necessary after hospital discharge, the nursing evaluation continues throughout the nursing involvement with the family. Evaluation focuses on family achievement of identified goals. The nurse conducts a final evaluation when the public health nurse determines that the family has achieved their goals and there is minimal risk for child abuse.

INTRAFAMILIAL SEXUAL ABUSE OF CHILDREN

The most commonly cited study of the incidence of childhood sexual abuse is derived from Diane Russell's classic work (1986), which includes a random sample of 953

Table 23-2 Nursing Interventions for the Physically Abused Child

Nursing Interventions (Secondary Prevention)	Rationales
Develop a trusting relationship with parents. Be direct and open but supportive. Obtain a holistic history, including the stresses and problems the family is experiencing.	Provide environment for parents that facilitates their sharing the sequence of events leading to abuse.
Explore how events that led to abuse might be altered in the future. Explore alternative strategies for child care problems. Discuss basic child growth and development. Provide parents with basic materials on child growth and development. Have parents apply child development principles. Discuss need for parenting classes. Discuss strategies for anger control. Discuss reporting laws on child abuse.	Problem solve and educate on how to avoid similar scenarios in the future. Gain parental agreement to cooperate with protective services.
Explain child welfare function of protective services. Take steps to inform protective services. Observe parent-child interactions unobtrusively. Involve parents in child care during hospitalization when appropriate. Discuss physical impact of abuse with parents. Discuss short- and long-term psychologic effects of child abuse. Provide referral to postdischarge public health child nursing. Public health nurse will coordinate services and monitor parental progress. Public health nurse will role model and assist parents to apply principles learned in parenting classes in their own lives. Have father discuss how he will maintain anger skills. Teach mother to intervene if father exhibits negative parenting. Assist parents to develop social support systems. Explore community resources with family.	Role model providing care and support for child. Have parents verbalize their understanding of abusive behavior on child. Support parents in the prevention of future abuse. Involve parents in child care classes. Demonstrate anger control skills. Prevent isolation of problem and expand support system.

women. Russell reported that approximately one third of her sample were sexually abused as children; 16% of this sample were incestuously abused by a relative before the age of 18 years. Wyatt's (1985) study corroborated Russell's results with female subjects. Other studies reported that sexual abuse to male children is 15% to 20% (Briere, 1992; Jacobson and Herald, 1990). Finkelhor's (1994) research with college students indicated that 20% of females and 5% to 10% of males were sexually abused as children. Results of a Gallup Poll (1995) indicated that 23% of surveyed adults claim that they were sexually abused during their childhood by an adult or an older child.

The NIS-3 (Sedlak and Broadhurst, 1996) indicated that under the more stringent measure of Harm Standard, sexual abuse increased from 119,200 in 1986 to 217,700 in 1993 (83% increase). Using the less stringent of measure of Endangerment Standard, the incidence of child sexual abuse increased 125% to 300,200 children. Females were sexually abused approximately three times more than male children under both measurement standards, which is consistent in both the NIS-3 and NIS-2 estimates. Throughout this discussion on childhood sexual abuse, the pronoun *she* is used in reference to the child victim; however, it is recognized that male children are also victims of sexual abuse. Also, the term *sexual abuse* is used interchangeably with *incest,* be-

cause most childhood sexual abuse is perpetrated by a relative or someone the child knows and trusts. Many studies (Eilenberg et al., 1996; Henley and Kristiansen, 1997; Jacobson and Herald, 1990) indicated that at least 50% of psychiatric clients and women in the criminal justice system have histories of physical and sexual abuse. Many experts claim that sexual abuse is the worst kind of child abuse because it is hidden and therefore more difficult to detect and address.

DEFINITION OF INTRAFAMILIAL SEXUAL ABUSE

Traditionally intrafamilial sexual abuse, or incest, has been defined as sexual intercourse between blood relatives who are too close to marry. However, incest is no longer defined in such restricted terms, because intercourse with small children is not typical and a multitude of other exploitative sexual activities do occur that can be equally traumatic for the child. In addition, many researchers and clinicians no longer restrict the offender to a blood relative. At present, many clinicians and researchers use the quality of the relationship between the perpetrator and the child to determine whether the abuse was incestual. If the perpetrator is in a caregiver or surrogate parent role to the child, many consider such abuse incestual. Examples of such relationships include stepfathers, mothers' boyfriends, grandmothers' boyfriends, close family friends, close neighbors who might baby-sit, priests, ministers, rabbis, scout leaders, and teachers. Because such people assume a position of trust, nurturance, and protection for the child, the potential for trauma is great because of the betrayal of trust. Because children do not have the cognitive, physical, and psychologic maturity to understand the implications of the sexual activity and because the perpetrator is always in a powerful position, the children are unable to give true consent. Therefore children must be viewed as victims, and the adults must always be viewed as the responsible party in sexually abusive activity.

The recent 2002 disclosures by victims who were sexually abused as children and adolescents by priests is a prime example of how sexual abuse is usually hidden and victims are left alone to deal with the guilt and shame. When the abuse by priests was reported, efforts by the Catholic church hierarchy focused on keeping the abuse a secret rather than on meeting the needs of the victims and protecting future victims from abusive priests. Since these allegations have been made public, priests who are identified as perpetrators are dismissed from active participation with any potential victims.

The Child Abuse Prevention and Treatment Act (CAPTA) defines sexual abuse as "the employment, use, persuasion, inducement, enticement, or coercion of any child to engage in, or assist any other person to engage in, any sexually explicit conduct or simulation of such conduct for the purpose of producing a visual depiction of such conduct" (Legal Information Institute, 1995). The CAPTA definition recognizes the abuse inherent in pornography. A general definition of **childhood incest** is any type of exploitative sexual experience between relatives or surrogate relatives before the victim reaches 18 years old (Urbancic, 2003).

Exploitative actions involve behaviors that the perpetrator uses for his/her sexual gratification with the child. This includes disrobing; nudity; masturbation; voyeurism; fondling; digital or object penetration; and oral, anal, or vaginal penetration. In the typical incestual relationship, the abuse begins very gradually with gentle fondling and gradually escalates over time, often progressing to vaginal or oral penetration. Initially some children may derive pleasure and gratification from the attention and the sexual activity and may actually seek out the abuser. It must be remembered that children are capable of experiencing sexual pleasure when stimulated sexually and that this is a natural physical and biochemical response to the stimulation. Sometimes children feel very special to be the object of such focused attention, particularly if their emotional needs have not been met by others and if the sexual activity provides them with feelings of pleasure, love, and attention. Despite the pleasurable aspects of the abuse, however, children usually feel confused and ashamed and in adulthood may find that the pleasurable memories of the abuse become the basis for serious guilt and shame. Such feelings can be difficult to overcome because the adult survivor believes she or he gave consent and does not view the

activity as abusive. It cannot be overemphasized that the adult is always the responsible person, regardless of how the child responds. It is the adult's task to nurture, set boundaries, and teach age-appropriate behaviors rather than to exploit children for their own sexual gratification (Urbancic, 2003).

HISTORICAL AND THEORETIC PERSPECTIVES ON INCEST

Herman (2000) stated that it was not until the rise of the feminist movement in the late 1970s that it became clear that the most common PTSDs were not those of men in war but of women in everyday life. At this time, adult female survivors of childhood sexual abuse began to speak out, establish self-help groups, and document their abuse experiences. Clinicians began to publish anecdotal works on their experiences with survivors of childhood sexual abuse. As late as 1975, however, Henderson reported in the *Comprehensive Textbook of Psychiatry* that incest rarely occurred and was of little consequence when it did occur.

Since the late 1970s and early 1980s, research on childhood sexual abuse has exploded. Consequently, we have a much better understanding of long-term effects of sexual abuse, as well as effective treatments. The study of psychologic trauma has been helpful in understanding the long-term effects, and today it is commonly recognized that many survivors of sexual abuse share the same symptoms as war hostages who have been exposed to severe, extended, and repeated trauma.

CHARACTERISTICS OF THE INCESTUAL FAMILY

Research on intrafamilial sexual abuse indicates that these families are highly dysfunctional, although overtly they may appear quite normal. Studies do not find a correlation with incest and characteristics such as socioeconomic status, culture, race, and ethnicity. Rather, incest seems to cross all boundaries.

Within incestual families, multiple forms of abuse are likely to be present including physical and other forms of psychologic/emotional abuse. Most incestual families are described as **enmeshed**, which means that they are relatively isolated from those outside the family and tend to focus most of their energies on relationships within the family. Boundaries within the family are poorly defined and are characterized by excessive dependency on each other for physical, social, and psychologic needs. Role reversals often occur. One example is the abused child assuming a caregiver role for the parents and other family members. It must be emphasized, however, that no single pattern can accurately describe the complexity of the incestual family.

Offenders

Characteristics of offenders are primarily based on research of those cases that are examined within the criminal-justice system and therefore are more serious abuse cases. Most cases of sexual abuse are never reported, so these criminal cases are not representative of all offenders. More recently researchers have begun to focus on nonincarcerated offenders.

At present, experts recognize that child sexual offenders are diverse populations that are difficult to classify. They vary in age, occupation, income, marital status, and ethnic group. Some researchers are also beginning to study the female perpetrator, because they believe that this group is more common than studies indicate (Barnett, Miller-Perrin, and Perrin, 1997), although the NIS-3 data showed that males were perpetrators in 89% of cases compared to 12% by females. Existing research on female perpetrators indicate that they are often accomplices to males or to a general pattern of abuse among all family members (Elliot, 1993).

Criminal justice experts have expressed great concern in recent years because of the decreasing age of offenders (Barnett, Miller-Perrin, and Perrin, 1997; Sedlak and Broadhurst, 1996). More juveniles are being identified as offenders, and they demonstrate more violent behavior than do typical adult offenders. In addition, more of these juvenile offenders are prepubescent and include growing numbers of female offenders. These juvenile offenders range in age from 5 to 19 years and represent all ethnic, racial, and socioeconomic classes; 90% are males. The majority of adult offenders report beginning their deviant sexual behavior during adolescence.

There is a critical need for research to identify typologies of sexual offenders and nursing interventions that are effective. Most sexual offenders do not have psychiatric illnesses. They are appropriate for treatment only if they acknowledge that they are guilty of the offense, express remorse, and recognize their need for treatment. However, it is unusual for offenders to express concern for their victims or have any remorse (Herman, 2000).

Characteristics of the Nonoffending Parent

When the abuser is the father, the mother is typically blamed for failing to satisfy her husband's psychologic and sexual needs, of being rejecting and dominating, and of expecting her daughter to assume the role of lover with the father, and be caregiver to both parents. The literature has also blamed the mother for being absent when the incest occurred, even if she was working to support the family. In addition, when the child discloses the abuse to the mother, it has been claimed that the mother commonly denies that the abuse occurred or blames the child for initiating or encouraging it.

Although these have been common themes in the literature, little or no research exists to support the contentions. In fact, recent research suggests that the majority of nonoffending mothers believe their children and take steps to protect them by notifying protective services. Deblinger et al. (1993) reported that mothers of children who are sexually abused by partners are more likely to be battered by the abusive partners than are mothers of children abused by other relatives or nonrelatives. Consequently, these researchers suggested that it is more appropriate to view these battered mothers as secondary victims of abuse rather than colluders and deniers. In addition, they find that the vast majority of mothers believe their children's reports of being abused.

Many nonoffending mothers are initially shocked and unable to believe their child's claim of being sexually abused by the mother's partner. It is especially devastating to the woman if she loves and trusts her partner, because she must now cope with her partner's betrayal in addition to her child being violated and traumatized. It is much simpler and less painful to believe that it did not occur. Nevertheless, many mothers who are initially in shock experience a process involving a crisis of disbelief and/or ambivalence that is followed by gradual acceptance and eventual dedication to healing the child's trauma, as well as their own. It is probably most accurate to recognize that a variety of scenarios exist with regard to the nonoffending mother and that it is inappropriate to try to categorize the complexity of the nonoffending mother according to any one particular pattern or description.

Sexually Abused Children

Most of the research on child victims of sexual abuse has been directed toward female children. Much less is known about the male child victim. Typically, the incest victim is the oldest daughter in the family, and often when she is able to extricate herself from this role, the next daughter replaces her. Some research indicates that the average age when the incestual relationship begins is 8 or 9 years. In Urbancic's study (1993) the average age of the child when the incest began was 6 years, with an average duration of 7 years. The NIS-3 data indicated a very low rate of sexual abuse for children under 2 years, but for children 3 years and older the rate of abuse was relatively constant.

Often the secret is never revealed; however, at other times the child may disclose the incest to a close friend or trusted relative. Sometimes the child discloses the incest during a family argument when her acting-out behavior is being criticized by her parents. Although acting-out behavior by the child is common, there is no unique pattern of behavior that might indicate the presence of abuse. In fact, sometimes the victim is a model child in every way.

Effects of Sexual Abuse on Children

Barnett et al. (1997) and Herman (2000) emphasized that frequently physical, psychologic, and sexual abuse are combined and the resulting combined effects are extremely traumatic. However, Briere and Herman emphasized that even when the effects of other abuse are considered and analyzed in research studies, sexual abuse effects are still significant and usually a key issue. This is a crucial point because some writers discount the trauma of childhood sexual abuse and insist that it is the chaotic family, not the sexual abuse, that is the core problem. In an extensive review of the literature

(Kendall-Tackett, Williams, and Finkelhor, 1993), researchers concluded that no single core of symptoms exist as a common denominator among sexually abused children. Instead, a multitude of symptoms have been identified.

Symptomatology seems to depend on a complex blend of factors including developmental age of the child when the abuse occurs; maternal support; individual coping skills; positive influences that may neutralize the abuse; severity, duration, and frequency of the abuse; relationship to the abuser; and degree of force. However, symptoms can be serious and extend throughout childhood and beyond. The most common childhood symptoms are sexual acting-out behaviors and PTSD. Other commonly experienced symptoms and behaviors in abused children include anxiety, fear, depression, somatic complaints, aggressive antisocial behavior, withdrawn behavior, school learning problems, and hyperactivity. Sexual acting-out behaviors are evidenced by the child's preoccupation with sexual play behavior with dolls and other children, inserting objects into anal and vaginal openings, compulsive masturbation, sexual knowledge beyond her age, and promiscuity. Many of the symptoms are developmentally specific, so one cannot generalize all symptoms across all age groups.

Long-Term Effects of Childhood Sexual Abuse

Just as there is no specific profile for the sexually abused child, there is no one profile for the adult survivor. Researchers have repeatedly found that for many victims, serious long-term effects do result from childhood sexual abuse. Although a range of effects can occur, sexual abuse seems to compound psychiatric problems across a broad range of symptoms including depression, suicide, dissociation, anxiety disorders, hallucinations and delusions, and somatization (Wilson, Friedman, and Lindy, 2001). The most common psychosocial problems of survivors who seek treatment are PTSD, self-damaging behavior, mood disturbances, interpersonal problems, and sexual difficulties. Sexual difficulties include rape, prostitution, compulsive sexuality, and confusion about sexual orientation.

For many survivors of childhood sexual abuse, complex PTSD is a reality that is characterized by a reexperiencing of the trauma via flashbacks and recurrent dreams (Foa, Keane, and Friedman, 2000; van der Kolk, McFarlane, and Weisaeth, 1996; Wilson, Friedman, and Lindy, 2001). Other symptoms of PTSD include numbing or constricted affect, memory problems, difficulty concentrating, irrational guilt and shame, constant vigilance and hyperarousal, sleep problems, and anxiety attacks. The traumatic memories can be experienced through the senses of smell, touch, taste, sight, or sound. Thus the survivor may experience an overwhelming sense of terror when some cue in the environment triggers such a sensory memory. For example, the survivor is exposed to someone who resembles her abuser and she experiences an overwhelming sense of fear, panic, and dread. Because she is unaware of the connection between her powerful reaction and this person as a trigger to her abusive childhood experience, she is unable to give a logical explanation for her reaction and may fear that she is "going crazy."

On many occasions survivors report recurring physical symptoms for which no organic cause can be found. Recently clinicians, researchers, and survivors have begun to relate many of these symptoms to specifics of the abuse. These symptoms are referred to as *body memories*. Women who report being forced into oral sex tended to describe such symptoms as absent gag reflex, teeth clenching, difficulty swallowing, and severe biting of the inside of the mouth. Women who were penetrated vaginally or rectally often report pelvic or rectal pain or severe pain during intercourse. Other body memories are represented by symptoms such as heavy pressure on the chest and difficulty breathing (abuser lying on top of child) and periodic numbness of the hand (hand that masturbated the abuser). It is also likely that many survivors have had multiple unsuccessful surgeries to treat these symptoms, because the survivor and the health care professional are unaware of the relationship between these physical symptoms and the abuse (Urbancic, 2003).

Most survivors in Urbancic's clinical practice report having difficulty trusting others and feeling isolated, different, depressed, vulnerable, and helpless. Most also complain of low self-esteem and feeling deep shame and guilt. Thus a wide variety of symptoms are reported by adult survivors of childhood sexual abuse, leaving no doubt that there can be and often are serious repercussions from such experiences. Fortunately, treatment for adult survivors of childhood sexual abuse has improved dramatically over the last 10 years. With the recognition of common mental health problems such as PTSD, depression, dissociation, and anxiety disorders can often be successfully treated with antidepressants and interactive therapy. Therapy methods have also improved and a variety of modalities now exist that include art and music therapy, anger work, grounding exercises, imagery and relaxation, journaling, group therapy, drama groups, and eye movement desensitization and reprocessing.

THE NURSING PROCESS

ASSESSMENT

As with the assessment of other victims of violence, the nurse should begin with an assessment of her own assumptions, beliefs, and attitudes about childhood sexual abuse. Nurses who believe that the child is responsible in any way for the sexual abuse find it difficult to be supportive toward the child. The nurse must be comfortable when speaking with the child about the abuse so that an attitude of discomfort is not conveyed to the child. Children are adept at picking up nonverbal cues, and the nurse's discomfort may be interpreted by the child as a sign that she should not talk about the abuse or that she is not believed.

Box 23-8   Physical, Behavioral, and Psychosocial Indicators of Possible Childhood Sexual Abuse

General Appearance
Varies from normal to anxious, fearful, and depressed

Probable Physical Examination Indicators
Bruises, lacerations, or bite marks on breasts, neck, buttocks, extremities, and oropharynx
Presence of sexually transmitted disease, including human immunodeficiency virus
Presence of adult pubic hair and semen
Edema, abrasions, petechiae, and erythema of genital area
Lacerations to vagina or anus
Alterations and/or enlargement of hymenal orifice
Dysuria caused by periurethral trauma
Rectal fissures, chafing and erythema, bruising, lacerations, and perianal scarring
Semen in the oropharynx and/or nasopharynx
Scar tissue of labia minora, hymenal membrane, and anus

High-Risk Family History Indicators
Substance abuse in caregivers
History of abuse in parents
Domestic violence
Inadequate impulse control/mental illness in caregivers
Alleged offender with sexual dysfunction and/or poor coping skills, poor social skills
Socially isolated family
Sexual abuse of sibling

Behavioral Indicators
Disclosure and spontaneous discussion of the abuse
Preoccupation with drawing genitals or anxious avoidance of anything to do with genitals/sex
Inappropriate sexual play behavior with dolls or other children, compulsive masturbation, inserting objects into vagina and/or anus, sexualized kissing, fondling genitals of others, and imitating intercourse
Dissociation
Avoidance of particular people
School/learning problems

Possible Psychosocial Indicators
Increased anxiety, fears, depression, low self-esteem
Multiple somatic complaints
Signs of posttraumatic stress disorder
Antisocial behavior, promiscuity, substance abuse
Running away, self-destructive behavior

As with all nursing assessments, a holistic approach is essential (Box 23-8). Because childhood sexual abuse trauma is highly complex and is affected by multiple interacting factors, it is important to gain as much information as possible without subjecting the child to unnecessary and repeated probing and questioning. Most often the nurse encounters the sexually abused child in the Emergency Department or outpatient clinic. Often, the mother or other caregiver brings the child to a medical facility to determine if the child has been sexually abused. Whenever there is a suspicion of childhood abuse, a complete physical examination must be given.

The primary objective is to establish a trusting relationship with the child so that she is as comfortable as possible in relating relevant events and cooperating with the physical examination. It is important to assess the relationship between the caregiver and the child to determine if the child is more comfortable with or without that person. Usually younger children do not want to be separated from their caregiver, whereas older children may be too inhibited to disclose in front of the caregiver for a variety of reasons, such as fear of being blamed by family members, disbelieved, or instrumental in the family break-up. Sometimes the child may retract her disclosure in an effort to protect the abuser with whom she may have a love/hate relationship. Finally, the developmental age of the child is an important factor in her ability to successfully provide data about the abuse; the younger the child, the less able she is to describe events and understand the interviewer's questions.

The majority of children who have been sexually abused do not display any physical signs of abuse because the most common type of abusive activity is fondling, and it seldom leaves physical manifestations. The occurrence of oral copulation or mock intercourse is also difficult to physically document unless the child is examined within a short time after the activity. Giardino et al. (2002) reported that even serious physical injuries from sexual abuse can heal without any significant residual signs. Even with a history of vaginal or anal penetration, abnormal medical findings are reported in only 5.5% of cases (Heger et al., 2002).

In addition to the lack of physical evidence, the sexually abused child may not display any signs of emotional trauma and she may deny, retract, and be inconsistent in her description of the abuse. Caregivers often interpret this behavior to mean that the abuse did not occur and the child is lying. The significance of absent physical or emotional signs must be clearly explained to the child's caregivers. Conversely, multiple emotional/psychologic indicators may be present; however, because many of these signs can also reflect other problems, their presence alone is not a conclusive sign that sexual abuse has occurred. The diagnosis of sexual abuse is difficult and challenging because there is no single profile or set of symptoms that guarantees its presence. Many of the following signs and symptoms must be viewed only as potential indicators of sexual abuse, whereas others are highly probable indicators. Detailed psychosocial protocols and guidelines for health care professionals who interview and evaluate children for sexual abuse have been developed by the American Professional Society on Abused Children (APSAC) Task Force (2002). Guidelines for evaluation of physical signs of sexual abuse have been published by Giardino et al. (2002). The indicators addressed in Boxes 23-7 and 23-8 are derived from these two sets of guidelines and from clinical observation.

NURSING ASSESSMENT QUESTIONS
For the Sexually Abused Child

1. Who do you like to play with best of all?
2. What kind of fun things do you and (name) do together?
3. What kinds of games do you and (name) play when mom isn't around?
4. Are there any games that you and (name) play that you don't like?

Clearly, the meaning of any child's acting-out behavior needs to be explored. Such behavior in abused children usually reflects the anger, confusion, and sense of betrayal that the child is experiencing and is unable to discuss. Although many abused children are able to act out their feelings through rebellious and delinquent behavior, others withdraw, blame themselves, become guilt ridden, and continuously try to be a "better" or "good" child. Such children may function at a high level in school and even be praised and admired for what appears to be mature behavior because they often assume major responsibility for adult caregiver roles in their homes. Finally, some children with abusive histories do not exhibit signs of trauma during childhood but do exhibit them later in life, whereas others seem to escape trauma from abuse throughout their life. As previously discussed, the presence of sexual abuse trauma depends on a wide variety of complex factors, in particular, the degree to which the child receives validation, protection, and support after disclosure is crucial to the resolution of the trauma.

The assessment of child sexual abuse should include a physical examination, interviews with the child and family members, outside information from sources such as teachers and baby-sitters, and psychologic tests if needed.

In general, the interview with the child should take place in an environment in which the child feels safe and comfortable. As with all sensitive topics, questions should begin with the least sensitive and most positive topics and progress to the most sensitive and direct ones. Initial questions are meant to gain the trust of the child and assist her or him to relax and become more spontaneous. The developmental age of the child is a critical factor in the type and level of question that is used; therefore all techniques must be modified according to the child's needs. Small children may have difficulty with nondirective, open-ended questions. Interviewers must be extremely cautious *not* to use leading questions. An example would be, "Daddy likes to tickle your bottom, doesn't he?"

The nurse's role is to provide comfort and safety for the child. Thus the immediate physical and psychologic needs of the child must be determined and addressed. Once these needs have been addressed, it is always critical for the nurse and other health care professionals to make a determination as to whether the child will be safe if returned to her home.

Eventually the child must be asked directly about the possibility of sexual abuse. In a nonemergency situation, questions such as those in the Nursing Assessment Questions box could be used with a small child whose father, stepfather, or other male caregiver is suspected of the abuse.

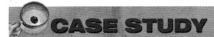

CASE STUDY

Suzy is a 5-year-old female who was brought to the Emergency Department by her mother and stepfather, Mr. and Mrs. Jones, because she was bleeding from the vagina. Mrs. Jones reported that while she was bathing Suzy in the tub, the phone rang, so she left Suzy for a few minutes to answer it. Mr. Jones claims that he went in to check on Suzy when he heard her crying and found her standing in the tub crying and bleeding from the vagina. Mr. and Mrs. Jones maintained that Suzy tried to get out of the tub but slipped and injured herself on the tub faucet. No other persons were in the home at the time of the accident. Suzy was obviously distressed and unable to give a history. She clung to her mother and would not allow anyone, including her stepfather, to touch her. On physical examination Suzy was found to have lacerations of the hymenal membrane and vaginal wall, trauma to surrounding perineal area, and old scarring.

Critical Thinking

1. What are the possible mechanisms for the injury that Suzy received?
2. How would you best prepare Suzy for her physical examination?
3. What kind of questions and comments would be appropriate and helpful to Suzy?
4. How can the nurse structure the environment so that Suzy will feel more safe?

NURSING DIAGNOSIS

The following nursing diagnoses are based on data identified in the case study on Suzy (see Case Study). Nursing diagnoses are formulated from the information obtained during the assessment phase of the nursing process. The accuracy of the diagnoses depends on a careful, in-depth assessment.

- Pain related to injuries sustained from sexual abuse
- Anxiety and fear related to further abuse
- Risk for injury related to sexual abuse by stepfather (increased chances of recurrence and possible prior incidents of sexual abuse by stepfather)
- Disabled family coping related to sexual abuse by stepfather and mother's possible denial as evidenced by the mother's inability to protect her daughter

OUTCOME IDENTIFICATION

Outcome criteria for Suzy are derived from the nursing diagnoses that were identified earlier. These outcomes are the expected behaviors that Suzy and her mother will demonstrate as a result of the plan of care.

For Suzy the first priority is addressing the physical trauma of the sexual abuse, which is the hymenal and vaginal laceration and localized trauma to the perineal area. Presence of scar tissue indicates prior abuse. Depending on the extent of damage and bleeding, Suzy may require surgical repair of her injuries. Based on her plan of care, the first outcome will focus on stabilizing her physical condition. The second priority will be to ensure that the abuse will not recur and the child will be protected in the future.

Outcome Identification for Child Sexual Abuse

Child will:

- Report a decrease in pain and anxiety.
- Verbalize an awareness that she will be protected in the future and that no one will be allowed to injure her again.
- Discuss her present perceptions, distortions, and fears with the nurse.

Child and parent will:

- Follow through on referral sources for herself and her family. Because Suzy's abuse was ongoing and severe, she will require an individual therapist.
- Participate in individual or group therapy. Many organizations exist that conduct groups for survivors, nonoffending parents, offenders, and siblings in families in which sexual abuse has occurred. All family members need to be assessed for the level of their therapy needs.
- Mother will attend parenting classes because she will require assistance in learning how to nurture, support, and protect her daughter in the future.

DSM-IV-TR does recognize sexual abuse of the child. Many adult survivors have been identified as experiencing PTSD, but symptoms for both children and adult survivors of abuse vary greatly, and no single profile has been identified that would clearly describe sexual abuse survivors. However, sexual abuse can be reported under the DSM-IV-TR Axis IV, which focuses on psychosocial and environmental problems.

PLANNING

The plan of care for the abused child begins with stabilizing the child's physical needs, securing the child's safety, and addressing the child's psychologic needs (Table 23-3). Because the child depends on the parents for the continuation of these goals outside of the hospital, the family system must also be assessed. In the case study on Suzy, the stepfather is the suspected abuser; therefore it must be clearly established that the stepfather will not have access to his stepdaughter and that the mother is capable of nurturing and protecting her child in the future. Police and protective services reports must be completed by the attending staff.

IMPLEMENTATION

Nurses need to be educated about the signs and symptoms of childhood sexual abuse so that they are able to recognize them and take swift action in all potential cases. Because the child's safety is critical, nurses should be knowledgeable about the laws in their state and the policies and procedures of their institution for caring for all survivors of abuse, especially children who are the most vulnerable. In severe cases such as Suzy's, the stepfather is removed from the home. Nurses are often the coordinators who ensure that protective services and law enforcement agencies are notified and that treatment referrals are made and are followed through. Usually treatment is mandated by the court after investigations by protective services and the criminal justice system are made.

Types of long-term treatment depend on the child's developmental level and the mother's potential for supporting and protecting the child in the future. With a younger child, play therapy is often used because the child often has difficulty verbalizing feelings about her abuse. Group therapy with other young children is also useful because common fears and misperceptions can be addressed. As the child becomes able to repeatedly address these fears and misperceptions, they will gradually be resolved. Group therapy with other children is also a powerful modality for teaching self-assertive behavior and how to self-protect in the future.

Table 23-3 Nursing Interventions for the Sexually Abused Child	
Nursing Interventions	**Rationales**
Call police and protective services.	Provide for safety needs
Provide medication prn; reassure child that she is safe and that no one will hurt her again.	Relieve the child's pain and anxiety
Encourage her to talk about her fears and concerns.	Allow expression of feelings
Reassure her that she is not to blame and that her abuser did a bad thing to hurt her.	Reduce guilt
Verify that the appropriate agencies have been notified and will follow through.	Coordinate contact of appropriate agencies
Document the mother's responses in terms of supporting her child and being committed to protecting her child in the future.	Assess and strengthen the mother's coping abilities
Provide support and educate about potential resources (e.g., treatment centers, role of social services and criminal justice system).	
Educate the mother about the signs and symptoms of abuse that the child may exhibit and how to support her.	
Assess the mother for her ability to cope with possible feelings of grief and betrayal.	

Adult survivors have a multitude of treatment modalities that have recently become available including antidepressant medications to treat depression, anxiety, and complex PTSD. Practice guidelines from the International Society for Traumatic Stress Studies (Foa, Keane, and Friedman, 2000) provide evidenced-based practice interventions for PTSD in both children and adults. These research guidelines indicate that cognitive behavioral therapy is effective in addressing the distorted guilt, blame, shame, and low self-esteem that survivors of childhood sexual abuse experience. Group therapy that incorporates cognitive behavioral interventions is also a powerful modality. Somatic techniques are helpful in treating the psychobiology of the PTSD through body-mind integration exercises. These modalities include hypnotherapy, eye movement desensitization and reprocessing, imagery and deep breathing, art therapy and body-focused therapy, and thought field therapy (Chu, 1998; Phillips, 2000; Rothschild, 2000; Wilson, Friedman, and Lindy, 2001).

EVALUATION

Ongoing evaluation of the client and family outcomes reveals the efficiency of the nursing interventions and is critical to ensure that the child is protected and supported to recover from the trauma of the abuse. In addition, an ongoing evaluation of the caregiver is needed to determine if this person is following through with the plan of care and to address any problems that may arise. A reliable evaluation of the mother's motivation and ability to support and protect her child requires both short- and long-term assessment. Sometimes the mother may become involved with another partner who is at high risk for child abuse. Thus the mother must be able to confront her own behavior and the decisions she makes with regard to the safety of her children.

ELDER ABUSE

Elder abuse is the last area of family violence to break through public awareness and consciousness. Because it is the most recent family violence phenomenon to gain public attention, it is also the least researched and least understood. In the last 10 years a growing body of knowledge has developed on the issue of elder abuse that has dispelled some of the earlier beliefs about this type of family violence. The first medical publication about elder abuse appeared in the *British Medical Journal* in 1975. The phenomenon of "granny battering" was described. The emerging belief was that elder abuse was the result of stressed caregivers who occasionally became overwhelmed and beat their unruly parents. Victim blaming was implicit in this explanation. Just as abused children and battered women are blamed for provoking or somehow initiating the abuse, so too the older adult "asked for it."

Because of demographic changes in the United States, an ever-increasing number of older adults are living much longer and accounting for a greater proportion of the population. This large block of older citizens has caused heightened pub-

lic interest in the concerns of the aged. Older citizens have also become more political, with organizations such as the Association for Retired Persons and the Grey Panthers. However, because so many older adults are isolated and depend on the people who abuse them, it has been difficult to accurately describe and explain the parameters of this hidden problem. In 1998 the National Center on Elder Abuse (NCEA) conducted the first national incidence study on elder abuse. According to the results of this survey 5% of people over 60 years old in the United States were victims of abuse and/or neglect during that year (approximately 500,000 older adults).

Even when abuse is clearly documented, older adults frequently refuse to acknowledge it. According to the NCEA survey (1998), for each case of reported elder abuse and/or neglect five cases go unreported. As with other victims of abuse, older adults feel too ashamed and guilty to disclose the abuse and frequently believe that somehow they provoked or deserved the abuse. Because their abusers are frequently family members, older adults may hesitate to report abusive incidents for fear of possible institutionalization or loss of the only home they know. Furthermore, as with the battered women and abused children, older adults may have strong feelings of affection and loyalty to their abusers.

DEFINITION OF ELDER ABUSE

The NCEA (2001) recognizes three categories of elder abuse: (1) domestic elder abuse, (2) institutional elder abuse, and (3) self-neglect or self-abuse. The category of self-abuse/self-neglect accounts for 25% of all elder abuse and neglect and typically involves older people who are depressed, confused, and extremely frail. Definitions by states vary according to state laws.

This discussion focuses on six types of domestic elder abuse as described by NCEA:

1. *Physical abuse* is described as the use of physical force that may cause physical pain, injury, or impairment. Besides physical force, this category also includes inappropriate use of drugs and physical restraints and force-feeding.
2. The NCEA describes *sexual abuse* as nonconsensual sexual contact of any kind with an older person.
3. *Emotional or psychologic abuse* involves inflicting pain or distress through verbal or nonverbal acts. Examples include humiliating or harassing the older person, treating the person like a child or forcing isolation.
4. The NCEA defines *neglect* as the refusal or failure to fulfill any part of a person's responsibilities to an elder. Neglect includes the failure by the fiduciary to provide care.
5. *Abandonment* refers to the desertion of the elder by the person who has the responsibility for providing care for the elder.
6. The last type of abuse is *financial or material exploitation*. It is defined as the illegal or improper use of the older person's funds, property, or resources.

Box 23-9	Etiologic Factors Related to Elder Abuse

Biologic Theory
Psychopathology of the abuser

Social Learning Theory
Dependency (financial and relational)
Social isolation
Transgenerational violence

Environmental Theory
External stress

Neglect was the most common type of reported abuse (49%), followed by emotional abuse (35%), financial abuse (30%), and physical abuse (26%).

The Abused Elder

The NCEA defines the older adults as persons over 60 years old. Women are disproportionately represented as victims (67.3% of all reported abuse) compared to male victims (32.4% of all reported abuse) even though women account for only 56% of the population over 60 years old. The median age of abused elders is 77.9 years (excluding self-neglecting elders), with people over 80 years old being the most vulnerable victims.

The Abuser

Recent research indicates that the most likely person to abuse elders is the person who lives with them—a son, daughter, or spouse. According to the NCEA survey, children of the victim comprise the largest category of perpetrators (47%) followed by spouses (19%), other relatives (9%), and grandchildren (8.6%).

THEORIES ON ELDER ABUSE

Although many theories seek to explain elder abuse, no single theory is completely adequate (Box 23-9). Sengstock and Barrett (1993) identify three main foci for theories on elder abuse: abuser characteristics, situational stress, and family relationships. Pillemer (1986) identified five risk factors for elder abuse, which can be articulated within the three foci of Sengstock and Barrett: (1) psychopathology of the abuser, (2) external stress, (3) dependency, (4) social isolation, and (5) transgenerational violence.

Elder abuse is frequently compared with child abuse because in both cases neglect is common. With elder abuse, however, elders continue to have the rights of adults unless they are declared incompetent by a judge. Therefore decisions cannot be legally forced on the elder as they can with children. Elders have the right to choose to remain in a particular environment, even when it is obvious that they are being abused or neglected.

THE NURSING PROCESS

ASSESSMENT

As with other types of family abuse, it is critical to interview the elder apart from the caregiver. In the hospital it is quite easy to simply assert that hospital policy mandates that clients be seen alone. If the nurse is conducting the interview at home, it may be much more difficult to gain access to the elder; nurses may even jeopardize their own safety by insisting on privacy. In these cases, suspected abusers must be assessed for their potential to harm nonfamily members. This assessment must determine whether the abuser is a substance abuser or has a history of mental illness and/or violence because these factors may further compromise the nurse's safety. Sometimes it is possible to identify a family member who is trusted and is able to provide the nurse with an opportunity to visit the elder, as well as to ensure the safety of the nurse. Having another nurse present during a home visit is always an option, but at no time should nurses intentionally place themselves in dangerous home-visit situations.

It is not uncommon for both the abuser and the abused to maintain secrecy about the abuse. As with other types of family violence, abusers frequently threaten their victims with harm if they disclose the abuse. Even without threats of retaliation, however, a great deal of time often lapses before the abused elder is comfortable disclosing the mistreatment. Reluctance is usually due to shame, self-blame, or fear of abandonment, institutionalization, and serious consequences for the abuser. Box 23-10 identifies physical indicators of actual or potential elder abuse. Many of these symptoms are present with normal aging. Therefore as with other types of family violence, the nurse must do a comprehensive assessment and consider the physical symptoms within the broader context of the client's life history (see Nursing Assessment Questions box).

Besides possible physical signs and symptoms of elder abuse and neglect, it is also necessary to assess the older adult for signs of exploitation and/or abandonment. Signs of *exploitation* include complaints by elders or evidence of misuse of their money, loss of control over their finances, material goods taken without consent or approval, and unmet financial needs that are inconsistent with their actual financial status. Signs of *abandonment* include reports by elders or evidence of being left alone and helpless for extended periods without adequate assistance.

NURSING DIAGNOSIS

The following nursing diagnoses are based on the assessment data gathered by the nurse who interviewed and examined Marjorie (see Case Study). These diagnoses represent a few of the possibilities that might be relevant for similar cases. Nursing diagnoses are formulated from the information obtained during the assessment phase of the nursing process see. The accuracy of the diagnoses depends on a careful, in-depth assessment.

NURSING ASSESSMENT QUESTIONS
For the Abused Elder

1. Are you happy living with your _____?
2. Can you tell me about your financial assets and how they are managed?
3. Whom do you turn to when you are feeling down?
4. How are family disagreements handled in your household?
5. Has anyone ever hurt you or touched you when you didn't want to be touched?

Box 23-10	Physical Indicators of Actual or Potential Elder Abuse/Neglect

General Appearance
Anxious, fearful, and passive
Poor eye contact
Looks to caregiver for answers
Poor hygiene and inappropriate dress
Underweight or malnourished
Physically handicapped
No glasses, false teeth, or hearing aid despite need

Skin
Contusions, abrasions, burns, and scars in various stages of healing
Decubitus ulcers, urine burns
Rope marks

Abdominal/Rectal
Distended
Internal bleeding
Fecal impactions

Musculoskeletal Fractures
Evidence of old, healed fractures
Current fractures and sprains
Limited range of motion
Contractures

Genital/Urinary
Vaginal lacerations, bruises, and infections
Urinary tract infections

Neurologic
Slurred speech
Confusion

- Decreased cardiac output and activity intolerance related to change in health status (congestive heart failure)
- Depression related to physical illness, loss of role functioning, and lack of social support
- Moderate to severe anxiety related to change in health status and role functioning
- Ineffective family coping related to alcohol abuse by caregivers and caregiver role strain
- Disturbed personal identity related to changes in health status and role functioning

No diagnosis in the DSM-IV-TR is currently appropriate for the abused older person.

CASE STUDY

Eighty-year-old Marjorie Jones is brought to the Emergency Department by her daughter and son-in-law and is anxiously holding her chest and gasping for breath. Marjorie is currently on medication for congestive heart failure. She is underweight, dehydrated, without dentures, and has poor hygiene. When asked about her missing dentures, she states that they have been lost for several months and that no one has been able to find them. After receiving medical treatment to stabilize her heart condition, Marjorie begins to feel much better and is able to give a brief history to the nurse in the privacy of her hospital room.

Marjorie appears depressed and withdrawn, and had difficulty making eye contact. She states that because of her inability to maintain her own apartment any longer, she moved in with her daughter and son-in-law 18 months ago. Until that time Marjorie had a full life with her widowed friends and had participated in social activities. She had had a part-time housekeeper since her husband died 5 years ago, and she had been able to maintain her independence quite well until she developed congestive heart failure.

Marjorie reports that life is quite different for her now that she is no longer independent. She states that she is having a difficult time adjusting to being "so dependent" and that she "misses her friends." She denies ever being hurt by anyone. After gentle questioning, Marjorie gradually admits having difficulty living with her daughter and son-in-law because of their alcohol abuse. Although neither has harmed her physically, they have discouraged her friends from visiting her and have continually demanded exorbitant room and board payments. Recently, she has noticed that some of her jewelry has disappeared. Marjorie is left alone for long periods, sometimes for an entire weekend, which is frightening to her because she is physically unable to provide for her own needs and has no access to the telephone. In addition, she becomes dyspneic periodically and experiences chest pressure.

Critical Thinking
1. What is the first priority for the nurse in the care of an older person who may be a victim of abuse, neglect, or exploitation?
2. What is the best way to assist an older client like Marjorie to disclose feelings, concerns, and fears?
3. What type of mistreatment has Marjorie been experiencing from her daughter and son-in-law?
4. What characteristics require assessment in Marjorie's daughter and son-in-law?

OUTCOME IDENTIFICATION

Outcome criteria for this section are based on the nursing diagnoses derived from the Case Study on Marjorie. These outcomes are the expected behaviors that someone like Marjorie will demonstrate or achieve as a result of the implementation of the plan of care and the interventions. Because Marjorie came to the Emergency Department with severe cardiac distress, the first priority is stabilizing her congestive heart failure so that she can regain normal cardiac output as evidenced by normal vital signs, freedom from chest pain and dyspnea, and decreased anxiety and fear. The remainder of Marjorie's nursing diagnoses relate to her psychosocial needs, including her depression. Because of her change in health status and her dependency on caregivers who are exploitative and neglectful, Marjorie is feeling helpless, frightened, and depressed.

Outcome Identification for Elder Abuse

Client will:

*   Explore options that may exist in relation to her home situation. Because Marjorie is an adult, she cannot be forced to leave her children's home or press charges against them. If there are mandatory reporting laws in Marjorie's state, her children's abusive behavior will have to be reported.
*   Verbalize feelings about her change in health care status, her dependency on her children, the treatment she has received from her children, and available options for dealing with these concerns.

PLANNING

As with other victims of family violence, securing safety is a major aspect in the plan of care for abused older adults. In the case of Marjorie, stabilizing her congestive heart failure had to be achieved before her abusive home situation could be assessed and before a plan of care for this aspect of her life could be established. Because most states have mandatory elder abuse reporting laws, it is critical that nurses and other health care professionals remain open to the possibility of elder abuse whenever there are potential indicators for it. As noted earlier, many times older adults will deny the existence of the abuse; therefore it is necessary to establish a trusting relationship with older clients to facilitate disclosure. Sengstock and Barrett (1993) suggested that the establishment of trust is the most critical component in planning the care of the abused client. In particular, they warned about being critical of the abuser because older adults are most likely to strongly defend their loved ones, despite the abuse they have experienced. Because nurses have time constraints in such settings as Emergency Departments and clinics, it can be difficult to establish the trust necessary to facilitate disclosure by older abused clients. Nevertheless, the nurse is often in the best position to assess and identify abused clients. Thus the plan of care should include the nurse's taking time to communicate concern, compassion, and a desire to explore options and resources, which can determine whether clients disclose critical information or continue to suffer in silence.

IMPLEMENTATION

As with other cases of family violence, the nurse is often called on to function as the coordinator of care. In Marjorie's case, the nurse may need to work closely with the social worker to develop and implement the plan of care. Because the nurse has frequent opportunities to discuss Marjorie's problems with her, she will be a key person in assisting Marjorie to identify her feelings, recognize her strengths, realistically assess the situation, and explore all possible options before making decisions. Thus the nurse is in a position to address the total biopsychosocial, spiritual, and cultural needs of the client.

Nursing Interventions

As previously mentioned, nursing interventions focus on meeting the biopsychosocial, spiritual, and cultural needs of the client. Thus the nurse can assist Marjorie to accept the limitations of her congestive heart failure and encourage her to optimize her self-care abilities. The highest nursing priority is to balance safety and autonomy. It is also important to assist Marjorie to learn about the community resources that are available to her in terms of maximizing her mental and physical health. Marjorie will require assistance dealing with the guilt and shame she feels about being a burden to her daughter and son-in-law and the abuse they mete out. A plan must be made with the family if Marjorie insists on remaining with them. This plan must clearly explain the family's obligations, Marjorie's rights, and the consequences of abusive or neglectful behavior in the future. As Marjorie's care requirements increase, the potential for greater abuse increases proportionately. Ongoing monitoring and evaluation are necessary, a role that is becoming more important for nurses as they provide ever-increasing amounts of care for older clients in their homes.

The home health care nurse must be prepared to provide counseling, referrals, support, and education to older clients and their families (Table 23-4). Sometimes the caregiver may be in desperate need of stress management techniques, general information on the aging process, basic nursing care principles, and community agencies that provide assistance for older adults. Providing such support may dramatically ease the burden of caring for the older relative and prevent the occurrence of abuse and neglect.

EVALUATION

Evaluating the effectiveness of the outcomes and nursing care plan for elders who have been abused is important because the abuse may continue and even escalate if older clients choose to return to the abusive environment. In a situation like Marjorie's, the potential for escalating abuse is significant because she will probably require increasing assistance from dysfunctional caregivers who are at high risk for continuing the abuse as a result of their substance abuse. However, nurses often are not in a position to follow up with clients once they leave the hospital.

Table 23-4 Nursing Interventions for the Abused Elderly

Nursing Interventions	Rationales
Monitor the client's response to decreased cardiac output.	Support return of normal cardiac output
Monitor the client's response to medications.	
Provide reassurance and support.	
Educate the client about medications and limitations.	
Monitor the client for increased depression and suicide potential.	Reduce the client's sense of helplessness and grief; increase feelings of control
Explore with the client the reasons for feelings of helplessness and grief.	
Discuss the client's capabilities and strengths.	
Explore options that provide the client with increased control.	
Explore ways for the client to increase self-care.	
Explore the client's feelings related to family abuse.	Increase the client's awareness of feelings related to abuse by family
Explore the client's options for remaining with family versus alternate living arrangements.	Increase the client's awareness of options relating to living arrangements
Coordinate referrals.	
Show respect for the client's decisions.	
Evaluate the caregiver's motivation for seeking and using assistance.	Evaluate the caregiver's motivation and ability to provide care in the future
Evaluate family's coping skills.	
Evaluate possible substance abuse by caregiver.	
Evaluate the caregiver's willingness to acknowledge and work on family problems.	

Sengstock and Barrett (1993) claimed that certain clues can be helpful in determining whether the nursing interventions will be successful. These include the willingness of the older client to acknowledge the abuse and the willingness of the older client and the abusive family members to accept outside interventions and/or removal of the elder from the abusive environment. Although many resources for the older client exist in most communities, the family cannot be assisted if they deny the existence of the abuse. Like battered women, older clients may experience multiple occasions of abuse before they gradually make the decision to leave their abusive environment.

RAPE

Although not generally regarded as a type of family violence, rape is an important topic that merits discussion in this chapter. As with all personal violence, rape continues to be a serious social problem in the United States and the world. According to the National Violence Against Women survey (Tjaden and Thoennes, 1998), rape is a crime committed primarily against young women, although males are also raped. In this study the researchers interviewed 8000 women and 18% of the sample reported either experiencing a rape or an attempted rape. In the majority of cases, the women (54%) were less than 17 years old when the rape occurred. In another national survey of women, Kilpatrick, Edmunds, and Seymour (1992) found that 683,000 women are raped yearly and 84% of the victims fail to report the rape to the police. Koss (1993) reported that women who are

incarcerated and those with a history of psychiatric inpatient treatment have a much higher prevalence of reported rape.

In a classic study by Koss, Gidycz, and Wisnewski (1987), 27.7% of college women reported being victims of rape or attempted rape, and 7.7% of college men admitted being perpetrators of sexually assaultive behavior. In 84% of rape cases the victim is acquainted with the offender. Thus rape by a stranger is the exception rather than the rule. Furthermore, the physical violence perpetrated by husbands and boyfriends on their intimate female partners is similar to violence perpetrated by strangers (Stermac, DuMont, and Dunn, 1998).

In their national survey, Tjaden and Thoennes (1998) interviewed both women and men about their experiences with sexual assault. According to their results, 1 out of 6 U. S. women and 1 out of 33 U.S. men were victims of rape or attempted rape. Not only were women the victims much more frequently than men, but they were more likely to be seriously injured during their sexual assault and, if raped before age 18 years, more likely to be physically and sexually revictimized in adulthood.

As a result of the growing public concern about female sexual assault and feminists' demands for action to prevent this violence, many states have passed laws to protect rape victims and more aggressively prosecute rapists. In addition, stronger federal policies for prosecuting perpetrators of sexual harassment and assault have forced corporations and universities to develop policies and procedures for addressing sexual harassment and sexual assault. Despite the positive steps that have been taken in recent years to support rape victims, prosecute offenders, and prevent sexual assault, victim blaming persists. Instead of placing blame on the rapist where it belongs, victims are blamed and revictimized in a myriad of ways. The following scenarios are common examples of victim blaming and revictimization.

- If a woman cannot provide evidence of resisting a rapist, she is often accused of consenting to the sexual activity.
- If the woman was drinking, she is often viewed as causing her own rape.
- If the woman was dressed sensually or was out late at night, she was "looking for it."
- If the woman acted friendly to the rapist, she "led him on or seduced him."
- If the rapist spent money on the woman, she "owed" it to him.

No one has the right to verbally or physically force another into sexual activity against his or her will. If a person says "no," that means "no," even if he or she said "yes" first, then changed his or her mind later. Research indicates that programs on rape education can be effective in changing attitudes and myths about rape in college students (Lonsway, 1998).

DEFINITION OF RAPE

The traditional legal definition of **rape** is forced penile-vaginal penetration against the will of the woman. In the last few years, this traditional definition has been expanded by most states and the federal government to include cunnilingus, fellatio, anal intercourse, or any intrusion of any part of a person's body (Koss, 1993). Nonconsent involves physical force, the threat of physical force, or the inability of the victim to consent for reasons such as age, developmental disability, or intoxication.

Rather than in a dark alley, rapes most commonly occur on dates, at parties, and at other social functions. Although society may believe that rapists are "sick or psychopathic," research has not clearly described general personality patterns for rapists. A growing body of research indicates that many males are sexually aggressive and force their partners into sex. A common male attitude is that women exist to satisfy males; therefore consent is unnecessary. Scully and Marolla (1993) discussed several decades of research on male sexual aggression and concluded that such behavior is viewed as "normal." By not addressing the sexually aggressive behavior of many males and by maintaining the myth that all rapists are "sick," society avoids its responsibility to examine most rapes within the context of learned and socially sanctioned male behavior.

CHARACTERISTICS OF A RAPIST

A common myth about rapists is that most are males of color. Botash, Braen, and Gilchrist (1994) reported that most perpetrators and victims are Caucasian; in 90% of cases victims and perpetrators are of the same race. Rapists have an average age of 31 years, with juveniles accounting for 19% of rape arrests. In approximately 34% of cases, the rapist was intoxicated by alcohol or drugs. Approximately 28% of rapes/sexual assaults are reported to the police. Of this 28%, the likelihood of the rapist being imprisoned is 16%. Therefore 19 out of 20 rapists will do no prison time for their crime (National Crime Victimization Survey, 2000).

Although research has focused on individual characteristics of rapists rather than group behavior, in recent years more attention has focused on fraternities on college campuses as a rape-prone social context. Martin and Hummer (1993), in their study on fraternities and rape on campus, concluded that fraternities provide a physical and sociocultural context that encourages the sexual coercion of women. These researchers acknowledge that not all fraternity men are rapists. Nevertheless, they insist that because of the type of men that are recruited, the social expectations of these organizations, and the lack of university or community supervision, the incidence of rape increases in fraternities. Recently date rape drugs such as Rohypnol and GHB (γ-hydoxybutyrate) are being used more often in the social scene. The perpetrators add the drug to a woman's drink without her knowledge, thereby rendering her helpless to protect herself. Furthermore, these drugs have an amnesia effect so that the victim is uncertain as to what happened once the drugs wear off.

EFFECTS OF RAPE ON THE VICTIM

Many rape victims experience devastating effects from their rape. In the past, rape was frequently viewed as unwanted sex with few if any negative consequences. At present, society is much more aware of the serious short- and long-term effects of rape.

In a literature review of the psychologic consequences of rape, Resick (1993) reported that 1 month after the rape a majority of women continued to experience significant fear, depression, sexual dysfunction, and social adjustment problems. Most women reported a decrease of symptoms after 2 to 3 months. About one third of women continued to experience distress 3 to 6 years after the rape. Resick reported that the symptoms in this third of the women became chronic and generally involved PTSD, depression, anxiety, sexual dysfunctions, and social adjustment problems. In addition, rape victims reported feeling more anger, hostility, and confusion than nonvictims and were more likely to use alcohol and drugs.

Prior psychologic functioning and life stressors are reported to be important in the development of long-term effects of rape. Resick (1993) reported that preassault, assault, and postassault factors may all influence the psychologic functioning of the rape victim. Many rape victims continue to experience PTSD after sexual assault and most likely will require antidepressant medication and cognitive-behavioral therapy. Other possible interventions include imagery rehearsal for nightmares, group therapy, and spiritual counseling (Chang, Skinner, and Boehmer, 2001; Dunmore, Clark, and Ehlers, 2001).

Although victims have a variety of responses to rape, it is always a traumatic experience and requires immediate attention and support from health care professionals to facilitate recovery. Evidence of the rape must be gathered and documented; laboratory tests for pregnancy and sexually transmitted diseases must be completed. Research indicates that the risk of human immunodeficiency virus from rape is approximately 1 in 500, whereas the risk of other STDs is 3.6% to 30% (Resnick, Acierno, and Kilpatrick, 1997). Therefore treatment must include prophylaxis for pregnancy and STDs and referral of the victim to an experienced counselor or rape crisis center.

As with the care of all victims of family violence, nurses are often in a position to assist victims of rape. It is incumbent on the professional nurse to accept responsibility for becoming knowledgeable and skillful in assisting rape victims. This assistance may take a variety of forms including identification of the perpetrator, support for disclosure, and therapeutic interventions to facilitate recovery of this often neglected population. In recent years significant advances have been made in the examination and care of rape victims, and much of this improvement is due to SANE. The SANE program is a component of a new nursing specialty, forensic nursing, which is dedicated to the application of nursing science to the administration of justice (Hutson, 2002; Ledray, 2001). SANE programs have proliferated across the country and have resulted in improved services, increased reporting, improved evidence collection, improved prosecution rates, and a high-quality continuum of care for sexual assault survivors.

CHAPTER SUMMARY

- Violence and abusive behaviors are major public health concerns.
- Because nurses assume many roles in a variety of settings, they are in prime positions to advocate and intervene for those who are victims of family violence.
- Interpersonal violence is more likely to be done by someone the victim knows.
- Battering is the most common cause of injury to women in the United States.
- Domestic violence is generally defined as physical, psychologic, and sexual abuse primarily directed at women by men for the purpose of maintaining control and power.
- Emotional and psychologic abuse can be just as devastating as direct physical abuse.
- Most child physical and sexual abuse is perpetrated by an adult the child knows.
- Actions that ensure protection and safety for the victim are the most important nursing interventions in abusive situations.
- Elder abuse is becoming a greater public concern because the number of older persons in the population is growing.

REVIEW QUESTIONS

1. A client walks into the doctor's office complaining of headaches. She is accompanied by her husband who answers the physician's questions despite the physician asking the client the questions. The client avoids eye contact, has a depressed affect, and her shoulders are slumped. The nurse assesses that the client may be:
   a. Suffering from major depression.
   b. A battered wife.
   c. Afraid to be with people.
   d. Experiencing migraine headaches.

2. A 24-year-old client is admitted to the ED with a broken wrist, swollen and bruised eye, and a fractured jaw. The client agreed to tell the nurse what actually happened if she promised not to tell anyone. The client admitted that her husband abused her and that he has abused her in the past, approximately four to five times, but only when he was drunk. The most appropriate nursing intervention would be:
   a. Treat her physical injuries, suggest she talk to a counselor, but keep the client's secret to maintain trust.
   b. Ask her to bring her husband so that he can get a referral for therapy.
   c. Report the abuse to the police.
   d. Have her talk to another victim of domestic violence.

3. An 8-year-old client is referred by the client's teacher for individual therapy. The client has been aggressive at school and has missed many days of school; the teacher recently found bruises on his back. The best short-term goal would be:
   a. The client will develop a trusting relationship with the therapist.
   b. The client will be free from aggressive behavior.
   c. The parents will attend parenting classes.
   d. The client will consistently attend school.

4. High-risk factors for childhood sexual abuse include:
   a. Undereducated parents.
   b. Low-income families.
   c. Multiple siblings.
   d. Parents who were sexually abused as children.

5. A 75-year-old female client is admitted to the hospital for pneumonia. The nurse observes that her clothes are old and dirty and have holes. She also has decubiti on her sacral area. The best question to asses for the possibility of abuse would be:
   a. "How long have you lived with your son?"
   b. "How much money do you have in your bank account?"
   c. "Describe a typical day at home—what you have to eat, what you do during the day, and what time you bathe."
   d. "Who buys your clothes for you?"

REFERENCES

American Medical Association: *Physician guide to media violence,* Chicago, 1996, AMA.

American Professional Society on Abused Children Task Force: *Guidelines for psychosocial evaluation of suspected sexual abuse in young children,* Chicago, 2002, The Task Force.

Bandura A: *Aggression: a social learning analysis,* Morristown, NJ, 1973, Prentice Hall.

Barnett OL, Miller-Perrin CL, Perrin R: *Family violence across the lifespan: an introduction,* Thousand Oaks, Calif, 1997, Sage.

Botash AS, Braen GR, Gilchrist VJ: Acute care for sexual assault victims, *Patient Care* 28:112, 1994.

Briere J: *Child abuse trauma,* Newbury Park, Calif, 1992, Sage.

Briere J: *Therapy for adults molested as children: beyond survival,* New York, 1996, Springer.

Burnett, LB: Domestic violence, *EMedicine Journal* 2(7), 2001, retrieved 4/12/02 from website: www.emedicine.com/emerg/topic153.htm.

Campbell JC, Humphreys, J: *Family violence in nursing practice,* Philadelphia, 2003, JB Lippincott.

Campbell JC, Humphreys J: *Nursing care of survivors of family violence,* St Louis, 1993, Mosby.

Centers for Disease Control and Prevention: Intimate partner violence fact sheet. National Center for Injury Prevention and Control Home Page, 2001, retrieved /12/02 from website: www.cdc.gov/ncipc/factsheets/ipvfacts.htm

Chang BH, Skinner KM, Boehmer U: Religion and mental health among women veterans with sexual assault experience, *Int J Psychiatr Med* 31 (1):77-95, 2001.

Chu JA: *Rebuilding shattered lives. The responsible treatment of complex post-traumatic and dissociative disorders,* New York, 1998, John Wiley.

Dawson M: *Intimate partner homicide,* Ottawa, Canada, 2001, Research and Statistics Division, Department of Canadian Justice.

Deblinger E et al: Psychosocial characteristics and correlate of symptom distress in nonoffending mothers of sexually abused children, *J Interpersonal Violence* 8:155, 1993.

Draucker C: Domestic violence: the challenge for nursing. *Online Journal of Issues in Nursing* 7, (1), 2002, retrieved /12/02 from website: www.nursingworld.org/ojn/topic17/tpc17_1.htm.

Dunmore E, Clark DM, Ehlers A: A prospective investigation of the role of cognitive factors in persistent posttraumatic stress disorder after physical or sexual assault, *Behav Res Ther* 39(9):1063-1084, 2001.

Eilenberg J et al: Quality and use of trauma histories obtained from psychiatric outpatients through mandated inquiries, *Psychiatr Serv* 47:165, 1996.

Elliot M: *Female abuse of children,* New York, 1993, Guilford.

Ellis JM: Barriers to effective screening for domestic violence by registered nurses in emergency departments, *Crit Care Nurs Q* 22(1):27-41, 1999.

Finkelhor D: Current information on the scope and nature of child sexual abuse, *Future Child* 4(2):21-53, 1994.

Foa EB, Keane TM, Friedman MJ: *Effective treatments for PTSD,* New York, 2000, Guilford Press.

Fox JA, Zawitz MW: Intimate partner homicides, US Department of Justice Statistics. Bureau of Justice. Statistics. 2001, retrieved 8/1/02 from website: www.ojp.usdoj.gov/bjs

Gelles RJ: Public policy for violence against women, *Am J Prev Med* 19 (4):298-301, 2000.

Gelles RJ: *Intimate violence in families,* Thousand Oaks, Calif, 1997, Sage.

Gelles RJ, Cornell CP: *Intimate violence in families,* Newbury Park, Calif, 1990, Sage.

Giardino A et al: *Sexual assault: victimization across the life-span,* Maryland Heights, Mo, 2002, GW Medical Publishing.

Glass N, Dearwater S, Campbell J: Intimate partner violence screening and intervention, *J Emerg Nurs* 27(2):141-149, 2001.

Graham-Bermann SA, Levendosky AA: Traumatic stress symptoms in children of battered women, *J Interpersonal Violence* 13:111, 1998.

Heger A et al: Children referred for possible sexual abuse: medical findings in 2384 children, *Child Abuse Negl* 26:645-659, 2002.

Henderson J: Incest. In Freedman AM, Kaplan HI, Sadock BS, editors: *Comprehensive textbook of psychiatry,* Baltimore, 1975, Williams & Wilkins.

Henley J, Kristiansen C: An analysis of the impact of prison on women survivors of child sexual abuse, *Women and Therapy: A Feminist Quarterly* 20:29-44, 1997.

Herman J: *Father-daughter incest,* New York, 2000, Basic Books.

Holden GW, Geffner R, Jouriles EN: *Children exposed to marital violence: theory, research and applied issues,* Washington, DC, 1998, American Psychological Association.

Humphreys J, Ramsey AM: Child abuse. In Campbell J, Humphreys J, editors: *Nursing care of survivors of family violence,* St Louis, 1993, Mosby.

Hutson LA: Development of sexual assault nurse examiner programs, *Nurs Clin North Am* 37:79-88, 2002.

Institute of Medicine (IOM): *Confronting chronic neglect: the education and training of health professionals on family violence,* Washington, DC, 2001, National Academy Press.

Jacobson A, Herald C: The relevance of childhood sexual abuse to adult psychiatric inpatient care, *Hosp Community Psychiatry* 41:154, 1990.

Kempe CH et al: The battered child syndrome, *JAMA* 181:17, 1962.

Kendall-Tackett K: Physiological correlates of childhood abuse: chronic hyperarousal in PTSD, depression, and irritable bowel syndrome, *Child Abuse Negl* 24:799-810, 2000.

Kendall-Tackett K, Williams LM, Finkelhor D: Impact of sexual abuse on children: a review and synthesis of recent empirical studies, *Psychol Bull* 113:164, 1993.

Kilpatrick DG, Edmunds CN, Seymour AK: *Rape in America: a report to the nation.* Charleston, SC, 1992, National Victims' Center.

Koss MP: Detecting the scope of rape, *J Interpersonal Violence* 8:198, 1993.

Koss MP, Gidycz KA, Wisnewski N: The scope of rape: incidence and prevalence of sexual aggression and victimization in a national sample of higher education students, *J Consult Clin Psychol* 55(2):162-170, 1987.

Kurz D: 18 Social science perspectives on wife abuse: current debates and future directions. In Bart PB, Moran EG, editors: *Violence against women,* Newbury Park, Calif, 1993, Sage.

Ledray L. Forensic evidence collection and care of the sexual assault survivor: The SANE-SART response. *Violence Against Women Online Resources.* August, 2001, retrieved July 4, 2002 from website: www.vaw.umn.edu/FinalDocuments/Commissioned Docs/ForensicEvidence.pdf.

Legal Information Institute. *The Child Abuse Prevention and Treatment Act (CAPTA).* US Code Collection, Title 42, Chapter 67-Subchapter I, Sec.510g. 1995, retrieved 7/5/02 from website: www.4law.cornell.edu/uscode/42/5106g/html.

Limandri BJ, Tilden VP: Nurses' reasoning in the assessment of family violence, *Image J Nurs Sch* 28:247, 1996.

Lonsway KA: Beyond "No means no": outcomes of an intensive program to train peer facilitators for campus acquaintance rape education, *J Interpersonal Violence* 13:73, 1998.

Martin PY, Hummer RA: Fraternities and rape on campus. In Bart PB, Moran EG, editors: *Violence against women,* Newbury Park, Calif, 1993, Sage.

National Center on Elder Abuse: (1998). The national elder abuse incidence study: Final report September 1998, retrieved 11/08/01 from website: www.a0a.gov/abuse/report/default.htm.

National Center on Elder Abuse. (2001). *The basics: What is elder abuse?* retrieved on 11/8/01 from website: www.elderabusecenter.org/basic/index.html.

National Crime Victimization Survey. Bureau of Justice Statistics, U.S. Department of Justice, 2000, retrieved 7/04/02 from website: www.ncpa.org/studies/s229/s229.html.

Parsons LH, Harper MA: Violent maternal deaths in North Carolina, *Obstet Gynecol* 94(6):990-993, 1999.

Phillips M: *Finding the energy to heal,* New York, 2000, Norton.

Pillemer KA: Risk factors in elder abuse: results from a case-control study. In Pillemer KA, Wolf R, editors: *Elder abuse: conflict in the family,* Dover, England, 1986, Auburn House.

Pillemer KA, Finkelhor D: The prevalence of elder abuse: a random sample survey, *Gerontologist* 28:51, 1988.

Resick P: The psychological impact of rape, *J Interpersonal Violence* 8:223, 1993.

Resnick HS, Acierno R, Kilpatrick DG: Health impact of interpersonal violence 2: medical and mental health outcomes, *Behav Med* 23:65-78, 1997.

Rodriguez MA et al: Screening and intervention for intimate partner abuse, *JAMA* 282:468-474, 1999.

Rothschild B: *The body remembers: the psychophysiology of trauma & trauma treatment,* New York, 2000, Norton and Company.

Russell D: *The secret trauma,* New York, 1986, Basic Books.

Scully D, Marolla J: Riding the bull at Gilley's: convicted rapists describe the rewards of rape. In Bart EP, Moran G, editors: *Violence against women,* Newbury Park, Calif, 1993, Sage.

Sedlak AJ, Broadhurst DD: The third national incidence study of child abuse and neglect. National Clearinghouse on Child Abuse and Neglect Information. September, 1996, retrieved 4/13/02 from website: www. calib.com/nccanch/pubs/statinfo/niss3.cfm.

Sengstock MC, Barrett S: Abuse and neglect of the elderly in family settings. In Campbell JC, Humphreys J, editors: *Nursing care of survivors of family violence,* St Louis, 1993, Mosby.

Stark E, Flitcraft A: *Women at risk: domestic violence and women's health,* Thousand Oaks, Calif, 1996, Sage.

Stermac L, DuMont J, Dunn S: Violence in known-assailant sexual assaults, *J Interpersonal Violence* 13:398, 1998.

Straus MA, Gelles R: Societal change and change in family violence from 1975 to 1985 as revealed by two national studies, *J Marriage Family* 48:465-479, 1986.

Straus MA, Sugarman DB, Giles-Sims: Spanking by parents and subsequent antisocial behavior of children, *Arch Pediatr Adolesc Med* 151:761, 1997.

Straus MA: *Beating the devil out of them: corporal punishment in American families,* Lexington, Mass, 1994, Lexington Books.

Straus MA: Corporal punishment and primary prevention of physical abuse, *Child Abuse Negl* 24:1109-1114, 2000.

Sullivan PM, Knutson JF: Maltreatment and disabilities: a population-based epidemiological study, *Child Abuse Negl* 24:1257-1273, 2000.

Tjaden P, Thoennes N: *Prevalence, incidence, and consequences of violence against women: findings from the National Violence Against Women survey,* Washington, DC, 1998, National Institute of Justice.

Urbancic J: Intrafamilial sexual abuse. In Campbell J, Humphries J, editors: *Nursing care of survivors of family violence,* St Louis, 1993, Mosby.

Urbancic J: Intrafamilial sexual abuse. In Campbell J, Humphries J, editors: *Family violence in nursing practice,* Philadelphia, 2003, Lippincott.

van der Kolk BA, McFarlane AC, Weisaeth L: *Traumatic stress: the effects of overwhelming experience on mind, body, and society,* New York, 1996, Guilford Press.

Walker LE: *Abused women and survivor therapy,* Washington, DC, 1994, American Psychological Association.

Walton-Moss B, Campbell J: Intimate partner violence: implications for nursing, *Online Journal of Issues in Nursing* 7(1):1-17, 2002.

Wang CT, Daro D: *Current trends in child abuse reporting and fatalities: the results of the 1997 annual fifty state survey,* Chicago, 1998, Prevent Child Abuse America.

Warshaw C: Limitations of the medical model in the care of battered women, *Gender Sociology* 3:506, 1989.

Wilson JP, Friedman MJ, Lindy JD: *Treating psychological trauma & PTSD,* New York, 2001, Guilford Press.

Wolf R: Abuse of the elderly. In Gelles R, editor: *Visions 2010: families & violence, abuse and neglect,* Minneapolis, 1995, National Council on Family Relations.

Wyatt GE: The sexual abuse of Afro-American and White-American women in childhood, *Child Abuse Negl* 9:507, 1985.

ONLINE RESOURCES
Intimate Partner Abuse

National Coalition Against Domestic Violence: www.ncadv.org

US Department of Justice Office on Violence Against Women: www.ojp. usdoj.gov/vawo/

Minnesota Center Against Violence and Abuse: www.mincava.umn.edu/link

National Domestic Violence Hotline: www.ndvh.org

Family Violence Prevention Fund: www.fvpf.org

Child Abuse and Neglect

National Clearinghouse on Child Abuse and Neglect Information: www.calib.com/nccanch

Child Welfare League of America: www.cwla.org

American Professional Society on the Abuse of Children: www.apsac.org

Elder Abuse

National Center on Elder Abuse (NCEA): www.elderabusecenter.org

Clearinghouse on Abuse and Neglect of the Elderly (CANE): http://db.rdms.udel.edu:8080/CANE/index.jsp

American Society on Aging: www.asaging.org

National Committee for the Prevention of Elder Abuse (NCPEA): www. preventelderabuse.org

National Fraud Information Center: www.fraud.org

Rape

The National Women's Health Information Center: Sexual Assault and Abuse: www.4woman.gov/violence/violence.cfm?page=95

Violence Against Women Online Resources: www.vaw.umn.edu

Sexual Abuse Nurse Exams Information: www.forensic-science.com/course_description/fs207.html

24 Suicide

Pamela E. Marcus

KEY TERMS

cognitive rigidity (p. 552)
comorbidity (p. 556)
conscious suicidal
  intention (p. 559)
imminence (p. 558)
lethality (p. 558)
parasuicidal behavior
  (p. 558)
perturbation (p. 552)
suicide (p. 551)
suicidal ideation (p. 559)
suicidology (p. 552)
unconscious suicidal
  intention (p. 559)

OBJECTIVES

- Analyze the scope of suicide by age, gender, ethnicity, socioeconomic status, and familial factors.

- Compare and contrast biologic, psychologic, and sociologic theories regarding the etiology of suicide.

- Distinguish between suicidal ideation, gesture, threat, attempt, and successful suicide.

- Discuss key elements in the assessment of suicide risk.

- Apply the nursing process for suicidal clients and their families.

- Construct a nursing care plan for a client admitted to the psychiatric care unit with depression and suicidal ideation.

- Describe the responsibility of mental health professionals in protecting clients from self-harm.

- Discuss the role of parents and significant adults in observing self-destructive clues in youth and in offering guidance and assistance.

Suicide, the act of taking one's own life, is a major public health and mental health problem in the United States. A total of 28,332 Americans died from suicide in 2000; this represents a rate of 10 deaths for every 100,000 people. It is the eleventh leading cause of death in this country. In 1999 the number of deaths by suicide was nearly double the rate of homicides in that same year. **Suicide** is the third leading cause of death for adolescents and young adults between the ages of 10 and 24 years. The suicide rate for the older population is growing faster than the rate for any other age group. It is anticipated that this rate will increase as more individuals enter their older years (Center for the Advancement of Health, 2002).

Suicidal thoughts, threats, and attempts often precede clients' search for mental health treatment in a variety of settings. Imminent risk for suicide is one of the leading criteria for medical care of clients admitted to psychiatric hospitals. Health professionals in all disciplines increasingly are being called on to assist with assessing suicide risk and ensuring that clients receive prompt intervention to provide physical and psychologic safety. Nurses are strategically positioned to contribute to these efforts by the nature of the broad scope of their practice in multiple health care settings.

HISTORICAL AND THEORETIC PERSPECTIVES

World history includes many references to suicide as a religious, psychologic, or social phenomenon. Suicide was considered both a spiritual offense and a legal offense against the king in Europe, dating back to 673 AD. Individuals who committed suicide were not allowed a Christian burial, and all of their possessions were forfeited to the king unless it was determined that the suicide was a result of madness or physical illness (Celo-Cruz, 1992). Shakespeare wrote of suicide in *Romeo and Juliet* and in *Macbeth*. Suicides increased after the stock market crash in 1929 and during the Great Depression as people took their own lives rather than face financial ruin and humiliation. Japan's kamikaze pilots of World War II elevated suicide to a high cultural level as they sacrificed their lives for their country and their religious principles. Recently, suicide bombers have caused causalities in the Middle East, as did the pilots who flew suicidal terrorist missions into the World Trade Center, Pentagon, and Pennsylvania on September 11, 2001, to make a political statement against the United States.

Throughout history, suicide has served as a solution to the disappointments and obstacles that people have faced. It was not until the late 1800s that pioneers such as Durkheim, a sociologist, and Freud, a psychoanalyst, began to study the phenomenon from theoretic viewpoints.

Sociologic Theory

Durkheim, in his classic work of 1897, classified the social and cultural aspects of suicide into four subtypes: anomic, egoistic, altruistic, and fatalistic (Durkheim, 1951). He defined anomic suicides as acts of self-destruction by individuals who have become estranged from important relationships in their groups, especially as this estrangement relates to their standard of living (e.g., the suicides after the 1929 stock market crash). Durkheim characterized egoistic suicides as self-inflicted deaths of individuals who are influenced to turn against their own conscience (e.g., the suicide of a devout Catholic adolescent after she has had an abortion forbidden by her religion). Altruistic suicides are defined as self-inflicted deaths based on obedience to a group's goals that override the person's own best interests (e.g., the terrorist pilot incidents on September 11, 2001). Durkheim defined fatalistic suicides as self-inflicted deaths resulting from excessive regulation (e.g., the suicides of felons who hang themselves in prison to escape oppression).

Psychoanalytic Theory

Freud viewed suicide from a psychoanalytic viewpoint. At the 1910 psychoanalytic meeting on suicide in Vienna, he described self-destruction as hostility directed inward toward the internalized love object (Freud, 1920; Stekel, 1967). These early formulations ignored other critical feeling states, such as shame, hopelessness, helplessness, worthlessness, and fear. Later Freud incorporated many accompanying psychologic and sociologic clinical features, such as guilt, into his views about suicide (Litman, 1967). Freud identified the following features of human life that he believed made each individual somewhat vulnerable to suicide:

- The death instinct, the splitting of the ego when the individual is unable to assume mastery over his or her instincts and has to conform to others' wishes or die
- The influence of group institutions, such as family and society, that require compliance from each member of the group through guilt

Psychoanalytic theorists who followed Freud have added their own perspectives to the notion of suicide. Menninger described several sources of suicidal impulses: the wish to kill, the wish to be killed, and the wish to die. According to Jung, the suicidal person holds an unconscious wish for spiritual rebirth after feeling that life has lost its meaning. Adler identified the importance of inferiority, narcissism, and low self-esteem in suicidal acts. Horney believed suicide to be a solution for someone experiencing extreme alienation of self as a result of great disparity between the idealized self and the perceived psychosocial self (Weiss, 1966).

Interpersonal Theory

Sullivan broadened the theoretic knowledge base of suicide by emphasizing the importance of interpersonal relationship factors. According to him, persons can never be isolated from the interactions of significant people in their lives (Sullivan, 1931). Therefore Sullivan believed, the suicidal act should be understood within the context of the perceptions of the suicidal person by his or her significant others. He viewed suicide as evidence of failure to resolve interpersonal conflicts (Sullivan, 1956).

These classic sociologic, psychodynamic, and interpersonal theories formed the foundation for the major contemporary etiologies that followed.

ETIOLOGY

The contemporary, scientific, and humane study of suicide, called **suicidology**, began in the early 1960s when several important events occurred.

The Center for Studies of Suicide Prevention was established at the National Institute of Mental Health in 1966. The American Association of Suicidology was founded in 1967. The *Bulletin of Suicidology*, the first professional journal devoted to the study of self-destruction phenomena, began publication in 1967. There was an increase in the number of suicide prevention centers, from 3 in 1958 to more than 100 in 1968. The 1910 Viennese psychoanalytic meetings on suicide were reconvened at the first annual conference of the American Association of Suicidology in Chicago in 1968. Shneidman and his colleagues led the discussion of innovations in the prevention of suicide. Currently, there is a telephone number, 1-800-SUICIDE, that can be used throughout the country to provide counseling and crisis intervention for individuals who are suicidal. The American Association of Suicidology sponsors research and clinical competence by certifying Crisis Hotlines to join the 1-800-SUICIDE network.

Biologic Factors

The structure and chemistry of the brain have been studied most thoroughly in relation to affective or mood disorders (see Chapter 10). Neurotransmitters, or certain chemicals in the brain that regulate mood, have been identified (e.g., serotonin, dopamine, norepinephrine, and γ-aminobutyric acid [GABA]). Recently, research with adults has suggested that irregularities in the serotonin system are found in suicidal clients. In a 1994 study by Nielson and colleagues, the major metabolite of serotonin, 5-hydroxyindoleacetic acid (5-HIAA), which is found in cerebrospinal fluid, was studied in conjunction with the genotype, tryptophan hydroxylase (TPH). This was the first report to implicate a specific gene in the predisposition to certain antisocial and suicidal behavior that was postulated to be regulated by serotonin (Nielson et al., 1994). Currently there are no medications that specifically affect suicidal behavior. However, medications that regulate serotonin levels are effective in the treatment of mood disorders that often accompany suicidal ideation (see Chapters 10 and 20).

Another psychologic factor is the neurobiologic correlation of depression and suicide. Suicide is most often correlated with depression, and as depression resolves, suicide risk diminishes. The biologic changes in depression can be correlated with alterations in specific areas of the brain (see Chapters 3 and 10).

- *Mood*: Sadness and dysphoria are associated with limbic lesions that can be moderated with dopamine.
- *Affect*: Separate motor systems of the limbic and brainstem regions of the brain influence control of the face and facial expressions and the muscular responses associated with emotional affect (e.g., crying).
- *Motivation*: Changes in the pleasure response, which is moderated by dopamine and dopamine antagonists, are correlated with motivational levels.
- *Cognitive content*: Frontal lobe dysfunction is thought to be related to feelings of hopelessness and worthlessness, both of which are precursors to suicidal thoughts.

The explosion of knowledge in psychobiology requires that nurses integrate the psychophysiologic aspects of illness with the behavioral sciences in their own nursing practice.

Psychologic Factors

Intrapsychologic and interpersonal theories continue to dominate the psychologic view of suicidal behavior. Contemporary etiologies include:

- Self-directed aggression or self-destruction as an act of murder directed at the love object toward whom the person feels ambivalent, leading to states of isolation and loneliness
- Death as an atonement for wrongdoings
- Death as a way to recapture the lost love object
- Suicidal death as a secondary result of the major depressive processes
- Suicidal ideation and parasuicidal behavior resulting from abandonment anxiety

Most psychodynamic theorists after Freud have theorized that depression follows the loss of a significant love object and leads to feelings of helplessness, hopelessness, guilt, and diminished self-esteem. Suicide can serve as a way to end those painful feeling states. This model emphasizes the functioning of the psyche and the reporting of subjective experiences.

Cognitive theory adds to the understanding of suicidal episodes by emphasizing the role of particular thought patterns: negativism, self-worthlessness, and a bleak view of the future. **Cognitive rigidity**, the inability to identify problems and solutions, has been hypothesized as a factor in suicide when accompanied by stress (Rudd et al., 1994).

Shneidman (1985) developed the term **perturbation**, defined as a determination of an individual's level of distress and rated on a scale of 1 to 9. Perturbation refers to how upset, disturbed, or perturbed the individual is. Shneidman (1985), building on his 35 years of work as a suicidologist, lectured about the common psychologic features of suicide. He defined suicide as a "response to an inner decision that the pain is unendurable, intolerable, and unacceptable. It is an unwillingness to endure that pain rather than the pain itself." He outlined the 10 psychologic commonalities of suicide from his studies (Box 24-1).

Feelings of abandonment and abandonment anxiety are important to understand to prevent a suicidal gesture in

Box 24-1   Psychologic Commonalities of Suicide

1. The common *purpose* of suicide is to solve a problem. The health care professional must assist the suicidal person in identifying the life problem that needs to be solved or changed.
2. The common *goal* of suicide is the cessation of consciousness (i.e., death).
3. The common *stimulus* of suicide is intolerable psychologic pain, along with the decision not to experience that pain.
4. The common *stressor* in suicide is frustrated psychologic needs, such as achievement, affiliation, aggression, autonomy, dominance, harm avoidance, shame avoidance, nurturance, order, or play.
5. The common *emotions* of suicide are helplessness and hopelessness.
6. The common *cognitive state* is ambivalence.
7. The common *perceptual state* is constriction with pain, frustration of needs, and helplessness.
8. The common *action* of suicide is aggression or exiting the scene.
9. The common *interpersonal act* is the communication of intention.
10. The common *consistency* in suicide is lifelong patterns of failure, stress, duress, and threats to self-esteem.

From Schneidman E: *Definition of suicide,* New York, 1985, John Wiley & Sons.

Box 24-2   Etiologic Factors Related to Suicide

Biologic Factors
- The neurotransmitters—principally serotonin, dopamine, norepinephrine, and γ-aminobutyric acid (GABA)—have been linked through extensive research to emotional responses.
- Serotonin plays a major role in regulating mood and influences the occurrence of depression and suicidality.
- Genetic influences are being found; a specific gene has been implicated in the predisposition to suicide.
- Others have found that dimensions of depression, such as mood, affect, motivation, and cognitive content, are correlated to alterations in specific brain structure.

Psychologic Factors
- Self-directed aggression
- Unresolved interpersonal conflicts
- Negativistic thinking patterns
- A reduction in positive reinforcement

Sociologic Factors
- Isolation and alienation from social groups
- Biopsychosocial influences

clients with interpersonal disturbances, especially in individuals with borderline personality disorder (Linehan, 1993; Masterson, 1976) (see Chapter 12).

In addition, the development of behavioral approaches based on learning theory contributed to the understanding and treatment of mental health problems. Interventions for suicidal ideation based on learning theory are directed toward decreasing unpleasant events and increasing pleasant events. Tension-reducing relaxation techniques, stress management skills, and rehearsal of problem-solving techniques are valuable adjuncts to reducing depression and suicidal behavior.

Sociologic Factors

Contemporary sociologists have reinforced Durkheim's earlier work on suicide. Contemporary social scientists have supported the idea that alienation from social groups after disruption of family, community, or social relationships leads some individuals to attempt or commit suicide (Maris, 1985; Richman, 1986). In a prospective study of almost 100,000 women from 1970 to 1975 in Norway, sociologists Hoyer and Lund (1993) found empiric support for Durkheim's notion that marriage and parenthood lead to a lower suicide rate for women.

Thus the findings of sociologic studies have provided added dimensions to the biologic and psychologic explanations of suicidal behavior. A more holistic approach is to consider a biopsychosocial model that integrates all of these schools of thought in explaining such complex human concepts as suicide (Box 24-2).

EPIDEMIOLOGY
Prevalence

Suicide and suicidal behavior are found among persons of all ages (including young children), among both sexes, and among all ethnic groups and socioeconomic levels (Box 24-3). Wilson (1994) reported that suicide accounts for nearly 1% of all deaths in the world. The Hungarians and Finns have suicide rates two to three times those of the United States and most of Europe. Interestingly, that figure holds true even when persons of those nationalities emigrate to other countries, suggesting some biologic influence. In 2000, 28,332 people died by suicide in the United States. This statistic places suicide as the eleventh cause of death in America; 1500 individuals in the United States attempt suicide daily, with 80 successful suicides (Center for the Advancement of Health, 2002).

Age

The two most vulnerable age groups for suicide are older adults and youths between 15 and 24 years old.

Older Adults. Rates of suicide are highest among the older population, age 65 years and greater. Older adults have suicide rates 50% higher than those of the nation as a whole. In a recent study in England, older individuals with severe vision disorders, neurologic disease, and cancer had a greater probability of committing suicide. In this study men were more likely to commit suicide if they had a serious illness (Waem et al., 2002).

Shneidman (1985) suggested that the high suicide rates among older adults represent failure to adapt to significant

Box 24-3 Epidemiology of Suicide

Age, Gender, and Ethnicity

- Of the 28,332 completed suicides in the United States annually, the majority are Caucasian males of all ages.
- The two groups most at risk are youth ages 15 to 24 years (with suicides increasing at the fastest rate in African-American men ages 19 to 24 years) and Caucasian men over age 65 years (with suicides increasing at the fastest rate in men in the 85+ age group).
- Native-American adolescent males and Hispanic females are high-risk groups among ethnic minority populations.
- Females in general attempt more suicides than males.

Socioeconomic and Familial Factors

- Suicide crosses all socioeconomic levels.
- Affluent, educated overachievers are as vulnerable to suicide as people at the poverty level who are unemployed, undereducated, living in substandard housing, and often the victims of crime.
- Prolonged family disruption and familial predisposition to depression and suicide, biologically or as a learned behavior from other family members, contribute to the incidence rates.
- Family turmoil, disturbed parent-child relationships, physical and sexual abuse by family members, and hostile and rejecting parental attitudes have been found to promote suicidal behavior.

Co-occurrence With Related Health Issues

- Suicidal behavior is strongly associated with psychiatric disorders.
- Mood disorders, substance abuse, schizophrenia, borderline personality disorder, and panic disorders have a co-occurrence with high-risk suicidal behavior.
- Depression remains as the single best predictor of suicide risk in all ages.
- Suicide is the leading cause of death during the first 10 years of the course of schizophrenic illness.
- The research is mixed on the correlation of suicide with panic disorders, but it is thought by most to be associated with suicide risk, especially when panic disorder coexists with obsessive-compulsive disorder or phobias.
- Independent of another specific psychiatric diagnosis, alcohol use and abuse are highly correlated with most suicidal acts, especially among youth. It is underdiagnosed and underreported among older adults.
- Similarly, chronic physical illness contributes to suicidal behavior. Physical health problems, such as heart disease, hypertension, obesity, and diabetes, were found in more than half of the outpatient clients who committed suicide in several studies. Older adults are particularly prone.

losses, inability to endure emotional pain, and pessimistic attitudes toward the aging process that are related to loneliness, illness, rejection by family and society, sudden termination of meaningful work, disruption of long-standing relationships, and feelings of emptiness. As the population ages and seniors become the dominant subgroup, suicide may increasingly become a major public health problem. A study relating to suicidal thought and self-transcendence found that older clients who experienced a loss of meaning in their lives were at greater risk for suicide completion, especially

if they had lost the will to live (Buchanan, Farran, and Clark, 1995).

Youth. Young people ages 15 to 24 years have a suicide rate of 1.2 deaths out of every 100,000 individuals. The 1999 statistics showed 242 individuals from the age of 10 to 14 years old completed suicide in the United States. This places suicide as the third leading cause of death for youth, after accidents and homicides. As many as 11% of all high school students have made at least one suicide attempt; 12% of deaths in adolescents were due to suicide (Center for the Advancement of Health, 2002).

Although there are few studies related to suicide rates for children under the age of 15 years, some statistical and anecdotal studies have chronicled successful suicide attempts in this age group. Children as young as 2½ years old have attempted suicide. Wolk and Weissman (1996) studied data from 226 individuals who had been depressed as children to determine the rate of suicidal behavior. They concluded that 4% of these individuals had completed suicide and that 37% of the individuals who had depression as children had reported suicide attempts. The authors found that 16% of the group who had anxiety disorders as children had attempted suicide and that 6% of individuals in the normal control group had attempted suicide. This study emphasizes the importance of childhood depression as a risk factor to assess in order to decrease the potential for suicide attempts in individuals, especially during adolescence.

Gender and Ethnicity

National suicide rates tend to obscure the importance of gender and ethnicity in defining the scope of suicidal behavior. Caucasian suicide rates are approximately twice those of non-Caucasian rates as a whole. Although the high suicide rates of older Caucasian men have been highlighted, it is important to note that suicide rates for African-American men have tripled during the last 25 years among the 85+ age group.

After older Caucasian men, African-American young adult men have the next highest rate of suicide. Males commit suicide at rates three to four times those of females. Although Caucasian and African-American women have comparatively low completed suicide rates, females have the highest rate of suicide attempts (Valente, 1989). Females have generally been found to make three to four times as many attempts, and the female Hispanic suicide attempt rate is higher than that of any other ethnic minority group in the United States (Heacock, 1990).

African-Americans and Hispanics rank below the midrange when compared with the suicide rates of other reporting nations of the world. In the United States, Hispanic and Asian rates of suicide are similar to those of Caucasians. However, there are very few publications detailing the incidence of suicide among Hispanic youth. One article points out that the Hispanic population is not homogeneous and that what may be characteristic of one subgroup may not be of another. For example, rates vary among Puerto Ricans, Dominicans, Cubans, and Mexican-Americans (Smith et al., 1985). Zayas (1978), in an early study, noted that several cultural factors have a bearing on suicide attempts among Hispanic adolescent females, including socioeconomic disadvantages, traditional gender roles, socialization, acculturation, cultural identity, and intergenerational conflict.

Another infrequently studied ethnic group is Native-Americans. This oversight is particularly alarming in that Native-Americans are often noted to be the ethnic group with the highest suicide rates in the United States, according to the American Association of Suicidology. When studying Native-Americans, it is important to note tribal group differences. Epidemiologic research focusing on Native-American suicide factors warrants a higher profile.

Socioeconomic Status

Suicide crosses all socioeconomic levels. In fact, studies show that poverty and unemployment contribute to high suicide rates and, conversely, that a high gross national product per capita and a high quality of life with associated stresses also contribute to suicidal behavior. Yang et al. (1992) studied the sociologic and economic theories of suicide and found high unemployment rates to be positively related to suicide rates. They argued that people's expectations of decreased future income because of unemployment lead to an increased probability of suicide. Zayas (1978) found that socioeconomic disadvantages such as poverty, substandard housing, unemployment, crime, victimization, poor health care, and poor education contributed to the high rate of suicidal behavior among Hispanics. By contrast, Lester (1984) demonstrated that nations with a higher quality of life and income also had higher suicide rates but for different reasons. A high quality of life leaves fewer external events on which to blame one's misfortune and failures, and thus inner-directed aggression may occur. Yang et al. (1992) have postulated that economic prosperity produces a social environment that is conducive to suicidal behavior: urbanization, often a by-product of prosperity, leads to a decline in social cohesion or an increase in social isolation, and a quickened pace of life increases stress for individuals. Thus both economic well-being and poverty can create circumstances leading to the choice of suicide as a solution to stressful events.

Familial Influences

Suicidal behavior is frequently a symptom of prolonged and progressive family disruption and dysfunction. In addition, significant changes in the family, such as divorce; death of a spouse, parent, or child; and social isolation contribute to high suicide rates.

The family is most influential in the lives of children and adolescents and contributes to the incidence of suicidal behavior in those age groups. A suicidal adolescent may feel estranged from family members and may experience rejection and a loss of love. Actual physical or psychologic loss,

CLINICAL ALERT

Adolescents who completed suicides experienced the loss of their mothers by suicide before their own deaths more often than those who attempted suicide. A careful family history and a record of previous attempts are critical to the thoroughness of the nursing assessment and the determination of suicide risk.

Of special note is that young children and older adults are less likely to have an explicit plan, thus making the assessment of risk more difficult.

as in death, separation, or emotional distancing from the family, is thought to be one of the most significant factors in the high incidence of adolescent suicides (Husain, 1990).

There is a familial predisposition to suicide in that many suicidal adolescents often have histories of suicidal behavior among their immediate and extended families. Those adolescents who completed suicide more often lost their mothers by suicide before their own deaths than did those who attempted suicide. Suicidal behavior becomes a learned familial adaptation to problems and stressors.

Familial cultural values also are strong factors in suicidal behavior. For example, in Hispanic families, family honor and family centeredness and cohesiveness are variables that buffer against suicidal behavior or contribute to it. Hispanic youth may experience conflict between traditional Hispanic values and the values of the dominant culture. Intergenerational tension, language barriers, and role conflicts may contribute to mental health problems. Adolescents who can relate positively to the main culture and still have positive relationships with their family members who have more traditional values are often sheltered from such problems.

Co-occurrence With Related Health Issues

Suicidal behavior is strongly associated with the occurrence of psychiatric disorders and other health-related problems (see Box 24-3). Psychiatric illness, alcohol and other drug use and abuse, and medical illnesses are important adjuncts to suicidal events. Tanskanen et al. (1998) studied smoking and suicidal behavior. They found that individuals who smoked cigarettes had a 43% higher risk of having mild to severe suicidal ideation, as compared with a nonsmoking sample of individuals.

Suicidal ideation and completion often occur when individuals feel hopeless about their problems. In the study by Waem et al. (2002) of older adults with health problems, the population was rated depending on the severity of the illness. They discovered that serious illness or disability increased the risk for suicide completion, particularly in men. In this study sample, individuals with mood disorders as well as physical illness had a higher probability of suicide.

Psychiatric Disorders

The presence of a diagnosable mental disorder increases the risk for suicide, regardless of age. The **comorbidity** of mood disorder and substance abuse increases the probability of suicide. The risk for completed suicide secondary to a mental disorder is higher in men than in women. Beautrais et al. (1996) found that 90.1% of their research population had an emotional illness at the time of their suicide attempt. The most commonly identified emotional illnesses in this study were mood disorder, substance abuse, conduct disorder or antisocial disorder, and nonaffective psychosis.

Depression. The single best predictor of suicidal thinking is the presence of a mood disorder. Research indicates that 30% to 70% of all completed suicides are related to depression. Other studies indicate that persons specifically diagnosed with major depressive disorder commit 10% to 15% of completed suicides. Depression is a major factor for persons attempting suicide as well.

Schizophrenia. Another diagnostic category linked with suicide is schizophrenia. Suicide is the leading cause of premature death in that population, with an estimated 10% incidence of suicide in the first 10 years of the illness and a 15% lifetime incidence (Nyman and Jonsson, 1986; Thornton et al., 2001). One study reported that clients with schizophrenia expressed high levels of subjective stress and feelings of hopelessness, loneliness, and dissatisfaction with social relationships (Cohen et al., 1990). Since schizophrenia most often has its onset in late adolescence or early young adulthood, the high-risk period for suicide is in the 20- to 30-year age group. Other risk factors that are associated with suicide completion in this population are active psychotic symptoms, depression, and a history of prior suicide attempts. Women have a higher completion rate after an acute exacerbation of the illness, as well as depressive symptoms and the use of alcohol (Heilä et al., 1997). This population must be carefully evaluated and reevaluated for suicide risk, particularly during the first 10 years of the illness.

Panic Disorder. When assessing the individual for suicidal potential, it is important to assess the person with a panic disorder for the possibility of suicidal ideation. There is a high comorbidity of suicidal behavior with panic disorder, major depression, and substance abuse (Lepine et al., 1993). Evidence supports that panic disorder, in conjunction with phobias and obsessive-compulsive disorders, is a risk factor for suicide and suicide attempts (Sakinofsky et al., 1991).

Some researchers have concluded that clients with panic disorder have an increased risk for suicide attempts comparable to that of clients with major depression and are at greater risk than persons without a psychiatric disorder (Johnson, 1990).

Borderline Personality Disorder. DSM-IV-TR criteria for borderline personality disorder include "recurrent suicidal behavior, gestures, or threats, or self-mutilating behavior" (APA, 2000). Often the individual with this disorder experiences suicidal behavior when there is a loss or a perceived loss (Gunderson, 1984; Masterson, 1976). Brodsky et al. (1997) studied the relationship between the characteristics of individuals with borderline personality disorder and their suicidal behavior. These authors found the trait of impulsivity to be an important risk factor for suicide attempts. It is therefore imperative that the nurse assess the client for impulsive behavioral patterns. This study also found that individuals with a history of childhood abuse have a higher possibility for self-destructive behaviors (Brodsky et al., 1997).

Alcohol and Other Drugs

Of special clinical relevance is the high concurrence of alcohol and other drug use with suicidal behavior. In a clinical review of eight clients who committed suicide less than 60 days after discharge from one of two psychiatric hospitals from 1988 to 1993, all had been drinking or using other drugs at the time of the completed suicides (Barbee, 1993).

One study of 93 outpatient clients who completed suicide found that the majority of them were young, male, had a history of drug and alcohol abuse, and had a primary diagnosis of depression. Of the outpatient clients who completed suicide, 62% used drugs, as compared with 18% of all outpatient clients (Earle et al., 1994). In another study exploring differences in patterns of cocaine and alcohol use before completion of suicide, there were differences in age, sex, and race among the study population. Of the individuals who used cocaine before completed suicide, 94.6% were male, with 51.4% African-American and 43.2% Caucasian. The Caucasian adolescents used either alcohol and cocaine or both before completing suicide (50% of the study population) and 41.7% used alcohol before the suicide attempt. African-American adolescents in this study did not use any substance before the suicide attempt (86.7%) (Garlow, 2002). Drugs contribute to poor, impulsive decisions that can lead to high-risk, self-injurious behaviors. A high percentage of alcohol- and drug-related automobile accidents among teens may be suicide attempts (Barbee, 1993).

Medical Illnesses

Physical health problems have been identified as a component of the profile for persons at risk for suicidal behaviors because of their co-occurrence with depression. The Medical Outcomes Study, one of the first major national studies

---

CLINICAL ALERT

Conflicting findings among researchers may lead nurses and other clinicians to overlook the possible lethality of clients with panic disorder, obsessive-compulsive disorder, and phobias. A careful suicide assessment is required to ensure that this possibility is considered because clients with anxiety disorders may develop depression that could result in suicidality (see Chapters 9 and 10).

Box 24-5   Risk Factors for Suicide

- *Age.* Persons most at risk for suicide are youth ages 15 to 24 years and older adults age 65 years and older, with those 85 years and older being the most vulnerable.
- *Sex.* Men by far have a greater incidence of completed suicides. Women have a higher rate of suicide attempts and gestures.
- *Race/ethnicity.* Suicide rates for Caucasians are twice those of non-Caucasians. However, rates for African-American men over age 85 years are increasing faster than those for any other group. Second most at risk are young African-American and Native-American males.
- *Physical and emotional symptoms.* High-risk indicators are serious depression, significant changes in weight, serious sleep disturbances, extreme fatigue and loss of energy, self-deprecation, anger, feelings of hopelessness, and preoccupation with themes of death and dying. Serious depression is often the precursor to suicidal behavior.
- *Suicide plan.* The presence and nature of the suicide plan are the most critical factors in assigning suicide risk. A plan clearly signals forethought and intent and often helps determine the level of lethality. Plans that are more precise, detailed, and explicit about the method to be used in the suicide act indicate high risk. If the method described is highly lethal (e.g., a gunshot to the head versus an overdose of pills), and if the method is readily available, the risk is elevated even more. Add alcohol and other drugs, poor impulse control, and limited time for rescue attempts, and the risk reaches a critical level. Plans often include instructions regarding the distribution of possessions and may mention the intent to join a deceased loved one in afterlife, especially if the loved one had committed suicide.
- *History of previous attempts.* The majority of persons who complete suicides have made previous suicide attempts (see Understanding and Applying Research box on p. 558).
- *Social supports and resources.* The availability of a support system for a suicidal person often determines the outcome of an emotional crisis. This "life line" of caring, support, confrontation, and limit setting, as appropriate from family, friends, and community resources, assists suicidal persons in choosing other alternatives in solving their problems. Real or perceived lack of support systems or failure to use the support system that is available significantly increases the risk for suicide.
- *Recent losses.* One of the major emotional determinants of suicidal behavior is real or perceived losses, separations, or abandonment. Unresolved grief reactions can lead to depression and suicidal behavior.
- *Medical problems.* Persons who suffer painful, debilitating, acute or chronic conditions, or terminal illness are of special concern for suicide risk.
- *Alcohol and other drugs.* These substances are often lethal companions to suicidal acts. Drugs may lower inhibition, heighten depression, and quicken impulsivity. It is generally thought that at least 50% of adolescents are legally drunk at the time of their death by suicide and that an even higher percentage have a history of recent alcohol or other drug abuse.
- *Cognition and problem-solving ability.* The inability to adequately identify problems and corresponding solutions greatly contributes to the choice of suicide as a solution to problems.

status. Each jurisdiction has rules and regulations that govern involuntary psychiatric admission; however, care is provided on an inpatient setting, usually for 72 hours, depending on specific state statutes. This allows clinicians to hospitalize these individuals for an evaluation of risk and to determine appropriate treatment recommendations. These clients' rights are protected to prevent exploitation and punishment (Monahan et al. 1996). Those judged not to be imminently in danger of hurting or killing themselves may choose less restrictive treatment options such as partial hospitalization programs or outpatient programs. In some states involuntary outpatient treatment is used to assist an individual who has demonstrated a risk over time to harm self or others. This involuntary outpatient treatment usually involves an outpatient structured program and medication administration. An advance directive is generally drawn up that gives the individual choices in care, such as where the individual wants to be hospitalized, any specified practitioner that can provide care during the crisis period, and any adverse reactions to medications that have been experienced in the past. The combination of requests outlined in the advance directive and the legal statutes mandating care provide a level of safety for the individual at risk (APA, 1999). *Any suicidal thoughts or behaviors, whether ideation, threat, gesture, or attempt, indicate an emergency situation and require prompt assessment and intervention.* Suicide risk and imminence usually decrease after support systems are established for those at risk and the cry for help has been answered.

Ideation versus Intent

Suicidal ideation, or thinking about suicide without clear intent, places a person at lower risk than a person who intends or proposes to die through a suicidal act. There are two categories of intention: conscious and unconscious. **Conscious suicidal intention** is usually characterized by various aspects of awareness:

- Awareness of the outcomes or anticipated results of the suicidal behavior
- Awareness of others' responses to suicide threats or attempts
- Awareness of the lethality index of the chosen method
- Awareness of rescue possibilities (i.e., part of the plan includes various avenues of rescue, or the plan is designed so that rescue is difficult or remote; the latter is a more lethal attribute than the former)

Unconscious suicidal intention is often more difficult to assess because it requires a higher level of skill and knowledge of psychodynamic theory. Often, there is a cluster of symptoms characteristic of the dynamics of self-destruction: depression, anxiety, guilt, hopelessness, hostility, and dependency, along with fantasies symbolic of death, hurting others, killing oneself, failure, and hopelessness. The motivation to hurt or kill oneself is outside of awareness yet is often expressed by extreme risk-taking behaviors. For example, some platform parachutists who jump from low heights off stationary objects such as buildings, towers, or cliffs may have unconscious wishes to hurt themselves or end their lives under the guise of an "extreme sport." Others may seek dangerous occupations such as skyscraper workers, bridge builders, and high-wire artists without nets as metaphors for suicidal wishes. Some persons may place themselves in dangerous, vulnerable situations that result in their deaths at the hands of others (e.g., victim-precipitated homicides). Some psychiatric clients unconsciously manipulate others through suicide threats or attempts and unconsciously arrange to be found or rescued. Unfortunately, the rescue plans may fail, resulting in completed suicides.

It is important to listen to the communication of intent among suicidal persons. Often individuals who were higher risk and have completed suicides communicated their intent

<table><tr><td>Box 24-6   Severity Index for Suicide Risk</td></tr></table>

1. *Suicidal ideation.* No risk of suicide.
2. *Mild thoughts of suicide.* Fleeting thoughts of suicide, for example, "This is stupid, don't think like that; you have much to do yet, like raising your child." The client tells you that he/she is not going to make any suicide attempt. The client has support systems in his/her life and is able to identify a purpose for living.
3. *Moderate thoughts of suicide.* The client thinks about suicide as an option for solving his/her problems. The client describes the feeling of wanting to go to sleep and never wake up. The client has no explicit plans for suicide. He/she states that he/she does not want to die, so much as escape from a sense of being overwhelmed by problems. The client has support people in his/her life, but the client does not utilize them because he/she feels that "he/she is a burden to others." Religious beliefs are a deterrent to a suicidal gesture or threat.
4. *Advanced thoughts of suicide.* The client makes a suicidal gesture, not necessarily lethal (a small overdose, cutting wrists), or has more intrusive thoughts of suicide, and tells the psychotherapist or nurse that he/she is suicidal. The client is able to write own contract for safety; however, the client is initially hesitant to do so. The client does not use a support system, starts to give things away, does not buy needed items, and checks insurance policies. The client rationalizes religious beliefs. This client needs hospitalization to prevent a lethal suicide gesture.
5. *Severe thoughts of suicide.* The client wants to die and cannot identify any other solution but suicide. The client cuts off communication with others and isolates self from others. The client may demonstrate an increase in energy after deciding on the details of suicide, including the means of death and the place and time death will occur. The client may not disclose the plan to the psychotherapist or nurse because he/she may intervene and prevent the suicide attempt. If the client is experiencing auditory hallucinations, he/she will not tell the psychotherapist or nurse about the commanding voices because the voices are demanding that the client not disclose the suicidal ideas. The client has begun to question and rationalize his/her relationship with God, if any, and may state that he/she is not worthy in God's eyes. The client experiences intrusive thoughts of death and suicide throughout most of his/her thought process.

Data from Green E, Katz J, Marcus PL: Practice guidelines for suicide/self-harm prevention. In Green E, Katz J, editors: *Clinical practice guidelines for the adult patient,* St Louis, 1995, Mosby.

in advance only to their significant other. Individuals who are at moderate risk of suicide communicated by threatening suicide to family members or health care providers. The degree of severity can be anticipated by listening to the extent of the suicidal thoughts of the individual, as well as the feelings of hopelessness and the availability of a method to carry out the suicidal plan (Box 24-6).

Nurses should carefully observe and listen for direct and indirect communication regarding clients' suicidal intent. They should listen not only for the words, but also for the underlying themes that the words refer to or symbolize. Although a suicidal intent may seem manipulative in terms of the individual's reason for this action, it should never be ignored. *Suicidal intent accompanied by imminence represents a high level of lethality.*

Chosen Method and Accessibility

The third determinant of lethality is perhaps the most critical. The method and its availability determine the outcome of the suicidal behavior. One is more likely to seriously injure or kill oneself if there is an easily accessible means or method.

Persons who complete suicide tend to engage in only one high-lethality act through violent methods: using firearms (the most prevalent high-lethality method used in the United States), piercing of vital organs, hanging, jumping from high places, or using carbon monoxide poisoning. Men who complete suicides are more likely to select more violent means and use guns or knives or hang themselves; women are more likely to jump from high places or overdose. Nonfatal attempters tend to engage in multiple, low-lethality acts and use self-poisoning by pill ingestion (the most common method for suicide attempts), followed by wrist cutting. These methods allow time for rescue because of the slowness of their physiologic actions. Most who attempt suicide use the same method for repeated suicide attempts.

Accessibility to dangerous weapons raises the suicide risk. The increase in youth suicide rates is in proportion to the increased use of firearms. The most rapid increase in firearm suicides has been in the 15- to 24-year age range. Because of the increasing availability of firearms and other weapons, it is important for parents to be aware of the activities and peers of their children. Any clues or signs of self-

CLINICAL ALERT

Asking suicidal clients and their family members about their access to dangerous weapons must be a part of the nursing assessment. Many will verify that there are guns and other dangerous weapons in the home that are easily accessible. If the clients are experienced in firearms use (e.g., policemen, military personnel, or hunters), the risk for suicide rises sharply. Provisions must be made at the end of the assessment to secure the weapons and have family and friends remove them from the home or from automobiles and trucks. Usually, a physician's order is required before dangerous weapons are returned to the at-risk client.

destructive behavior or any verbalizations regarding violence toward self and or others should be investigated by parents and significant adults so that help and guidance can be offered, which may prevent a possible tragedy.

Suicidal clients in psychiatric hospitals or on psychiatric units in general hospitals are high suicide risks. Hospitals report a wide range of 20 to 90 completed suicides per 100,000 client years. The most vulnerable periods for attempts are within the first 24 hours after admission and as discharge approaches. Close observation is required as clients move from one suicide precaution level to another. Remember that *a sudden brightening of affect or lifting of depression may signal that the client has resolved his or her ambivalence about living or dying, has made the decision to commit suicide, and is awaiting the opportunity.* Some clients have attempted or completed suicide while they were not on suicide precautions at all. Observation of all clients at least every 15 to 30 minutes, whether or not they are suicidal, is vital in detecting early clues to self-destructive behavior.

Hanging is the most prevalent suicide method used in hospital settings and is lethal. Sharp objects are usually not available to clients, as part of the safety program of the unit. However, sheets, towels, belts, cords, plastic garbage bags, shoestrings, and articles of clothing have been used to create nooses. Other clients may "cheek" their psychotropic medications and use them later in overdose attempts. Some chronically suicidal clients who sneak sharp objects into the hospital are prone to cutting attempts, usually of the wrists or antecubital areas of the arms. Clients diagnosed with borderline personality disorders or dissociative disorders are prone to these attempts. Searching the client on admission and when returning from off-ground passes is an important safety intervention to detect contraband such as razors, knives, pieces of glass, and aluminum cans.

It is not possible to prevent all suicides, even in the most secure facilities such as psychiatric hospitals and jails, but *close observation and continued reassessment of suicide risk minimize the chances of completed suicides.* Mental health professionals have an obligation to protect clients from harming themselves, just as parents and significant adults must be responsible for youth who demonstrate signs of self-destructive behavior requiring prompt intervention.

PROGNOSIS

Suicidal behavior is a treatable mental health problem. The prognosis for many suicidal clients is related to the severity of their accompanying mental disorder. Because most suicidal behavior is correlated closely with major depressive disorders, effective treatment of depression results in a rapid reduction in suicide risk. The majority of clients with depression who are treated with antidepressant medications demonstrate increased improvement or complete remission of their depressive symptoms according to the Clinical Practice Guidelines (Cummings, 1993). Clients with schizophrenia and panic disorder who maintain therapeutic blood levels of the prescribed psychotropic medications also have a

favorable response and a positive outcome related to reduction in suicide risk (see Chapter 20 for further information about medication).

DISCHARGE CRITERIA

Discharge criteria are necessary guidelines for both the client and the nursing staff and lead to a completion of treatment goals. The admission assessment establishes the groundwork for discharge criteria. Without an accurate, thorough, and knowledgeable assessment and appropriate treatment plan, effective interventions and timely discharge activities can be delayed. Discharge criteria help to establish time frames in which goals are achieved, designate areas of responsibility and accountability by way of documentation, and meet specific institutional, professional, certifying, legal, or funding requirements.

Discharge criteria for the suicidal client must include:
- Indications that the client is no longer imminently suicidal
- Determination that the client's living environment is safe for his or her return
- A consistent, available support system for the client to determine whether he or she is feeling self-destructive
- A commitment from the client to use psychotherapy to understand the crises that precipitated the suicidal ideation and/or attempt
- An agreement by the client to use a suicide hotline (1-800-SUICIDE) or call a supportive friend or family member if suicidal ideation is experienced again

THE NURSING PROCESS

ASSESSMENT

The nursing assessment is a critical step toward ensuring the client's safety. Accurate assessment, continuing throughout the course of hospitalization, helps the nurse provide appropriate intervention and discharge planning. Determining an individual's risk for self-harm requires a thorough evaluation of factors that contribute to suicidality (e.g., a mental status examination and an evaluation of the client's support resources).

The initial assessment helps determine the presence of specific risk factors. Noting the presence of symptoms does not necessarily mean that a client is suicidal. However, recognizing a cluster of certain symptoms within a given time frame is necessary to accurately assess suicidal intent (see Nursing Care in the Community box on p. 562).

When assessing the client's potential for suicide, the nurse will observe for the following:
1. The observable behavior of the client. A calm client may be highly suicidal, whereas an agitated client may not be dangerous. Although appearances can be deceiving, increased perturbation (Shneidman, 1985, 1996) often signals an imminent suicide attempt and

NURSING CARE IN THE COMMUNITY   Suicide

Everyone working in mental health recognizes that it is standard proce-dure to assess all individuals experiencing depression for suicidality and the ability to agree to a no-harm contract with his or her mental health professional. Evaluation is based on the lethality of the suicide plan and the availability of the means to carry it out. The community mental health nurse's personal knowledge of the client's family and lifestyle and the abil-ity to offer access to the mental health system are distinct advantages. The nurse's availability on an extended basis may help to establish credibility with clients so that agreements are based on relationships and trust.

It is important to consider the individual in the context of daily life, which is also an advantage of being in the community. The older individ-ual, living alone, may be at high risk for suicidal acts, as are young per-sons newly diagnosed with a major psychiatric illness. Assessment can be made, not only on the basis of the client's demographics, but also on the basis of interviews with the persons in the client's support system. The in-terview should be focused on the appearance of the vegetative signs of depression, as well as religious orientation, personal habits, and medica-tion compliance. The capability of the person, especially his or her ability to organize, is significant. Those who seem to be improving are often at increased risk, as they are better able to plan and implement a lethal at-tempt. Other elements that must be considered as risk factors are the dis-inhibiting effects of certain medications and the mind-altering effects of substance abuse.

Assessment of suicidality remains a difficult issue in the community, because many clients desire the security of the hospital psychiatric unit and have found that expressing suicidal intent leads to admission. They have become adept at manipulating the system to get what they feel they need without making an effort to change themselves.

Although the community mental health nurse may recognize system abuse by certain clients, preserving life remains a central duty no mat-ter how frequently the client has used suicidality as a ploy to enter the hospital. Each situation must be individually evaluated, and all options must be explored regardless of a client's past behavior. The nurse's paramount role is as an advocate for the client. Sometimes the human contact and focused attention, along with a personalized no-harm con-tract, will make a difference in the client's feeling of despair, isolation, and subsequent suicidal behavior. A partial hospitalization or intensive outpatient treatment program may offer enough individual support. At other times, only the constraints imposed by hospitalization will prevent suicide.

---

is characterized by impulsivity, restlessness, exces-sive motor agitation, and a brightening of affect. With some clients, however, withdrawal, apathy, irri-tability, and immobility may intensify with suicidal-ity. Suicides do occur in hospitals. It is important that nurses consistently monitor a suicidal client's behav-ior, affect, and interactions with others. Lethality lev-els can increase during hospitalization, particularly as depression lifts and discharge becomes imminent.

2. *The history from the client.* Careful scrutiny some-times reveals precipitating events that contribute to current self-destructive thoughts. It is important to determine why the client is feeling suicidal at this time. In gathering the client's history, the nurse may identify self-defeating coping patterns and past ex-periences that have negatively affected the client's self-esteem. Making note of significant anniversary dates may help to predict a future suicide attempt.

3. *Information from friends or relatives.* Useful infor-mation regarding the client's history can be obtained from friends or relatives. Often it is helpful to inter-view the client and family together and separately (in case the friend or relative is hesitant to speak openly in front of the client). The nurse should assess how family members and friends feel about the client's suicidal behavior. Family members who are angry, disgusted, or frustrated with the self-destructive client may actually provoke the client to complete a plan of suicide.

4. *History of suicidal gestures or attempts.* The suicide attempt is often used as a way of coping with painful feelings. People who have used this coping style in the past are at greater risk for using it again.

5. *The mental status examination.* Disturbance in con-centration, orientation, and memory suggests possi-ble organic brain syndrome, which may reduce the client's impulse control and increase the potential for self-harm. Disturbance in thought processing, evi-denced in command hallucinations, places the client at greater risk to act destructively.

6. *The physical examination.* A physical examination should always be conducted when there are obvious signs and symptoms of substance abuse (e.g., im-paired attention, irritability, euphoria, slurred speech, unsteady gait, flushed face, psychomotor agitation, needle tracks), previous suicide attempts (e.g., scars on wrists), or debilitating medical conditions, in-cluding chronic pain.

7. *The nurse's intuition.* The nurse's own feelings of uneasiness, anxiety, or unexplained sadness may be the only clues that a seemingly calm client is barely able to refrain from acting on suicidal impulses. Al-though these feelings may be described as intuition, research suggests that "intuitive feelings" tend to be based on previous experiences in similar client care situations (Aguilera, 1998). Nevertheless, if the nurse does not "feel right" about a client, this impor-tant source of information should not be ignored.

Nurses can use the questions in the Nursing Assessment Questions box to determine the client's risk for suicide.

The following discussion refers to the Case Study. The nurse knew the first task of assessment was to make psy-

NURSING ASSESSMENT QUESTIONS
Suicide

1. Is the client hopeless? Does the client see no prospects for the future? No solutions to his/her problems?
2. Has the client made a recent suicide attempt? Are the client's suicide attempts severe or multiple? Does the client show impulsivity?
3. Are suicide attempts increasing in frequency or lethality? Is the client obsessing or fantasizing about suicide or death?
4. Does the client have insomnia with suicide ruminations at night that continue into the early morning hours?
5. Is the client anxious? Are there any symptoms of panic or posttraumatic stress disorder (PTSD)?
6. Does the client have bipolar disorder, postpartum psychosis, or psychotic depression? Is the client experiencing pathologic grief, especially with command hallucinations, guilt or other co-morbid conditions (e.g., chemical dependency, alcoholism, or personality disorder)?
7. Is there a history of suicide by a relative or close friend? Is the client isolated? Does the client lack resources and available family?

8. Does the client have detailed suicidal plans? Are lethal means available to the client for suicide, such as a gun or other weapon?
9. Did the client leave a suicide note or give away valued possessions?
10. Is the client becoming increasingly frustrated with therapy, illness, or problems? Is the client feeling powerless and unable to learn how to cope?
11. Has the client been offered electroconvulsive therapy (ECT) and demonstrated ambivalence over it? Has the client interpreted the recommendation as an admission of failure and hopelessness versus a positive solution?

A "yes" answer to any one of these questions suggests that the client must be assessed carefully by the treatment team for possible admission to a locked facility, with suicide precautions instituted as per policy.

Developed by the Committee for Suicide Assessment, Sharp Mesa Vista Hospital, San Diego, California.

chologic contact with the client. She planned to listen to how Jeff viewed his situation and then communicate her understanding of his thoughts and feelings. The nurse realized that it was important to establish rapport and trust with Jeff. She believed that the client-centered approach, developed by Rogers (1961), would facilitate open communication and in turn assist her in more accurately assessing Jeff's risk for suicide (see Chapter 19 for further information about Carl Rogers).

The nurse used empathic listening techniques by listening for both facts and feelings (i.e., what happened and how the client felt about it). The nurse demonstrated caring and interest by using reflective statements so that Jeff knew the nurse had heard what he had been saying.

When feelings were obviously present but not yet expressed, the nurse would gently comment, "I sense how upset you are by the way you are speaking. It seems like you are also angry and frustrated about what has happened."

Psychologic contact is not always made solely through verbal communication. Sometimes, nonverbal, physical contact is quite effective. A gentle touch on the forearm or placing an arm around a shoulder can have an important calming effect and signify human concern as well.

The nurse demonstrated concern for Jeff by offering him a tissue when his eyes filled with tears. The nurse not only recognized and acknowledged his feelings, but also responded in a calm, controlled manner, resisting the tendency to become anxious, angry, or depressed because of the intensity of the client's feelings. During the assessment of Jeff, the nurse included the questions in the Nursing Assessment Questions box on p. 564.

After a suicide attempt, an individual may continue to be at high risk for attempting suicide again. When clients are

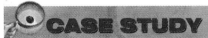

CASE STUDY

Jeff, age 24 years, had been hospitalized at age 18 years after overdosing on tricyclic antidepressants. At the time, Jeff's suicide attempt seemed to be linked to the end of a 2-year relationship with his girlfriend. Since the initial episode of major depression, Jeff successfully graduated from college and, after the sudden death of his father, returned home to live with his mother. Soon, however, he began to feel frustrated and inadequate when unable to find employment commensurate with his educational background and intellectual capabilities. Jeff was forced to accept a part-time position that paid minimum wage and lacked benefits. When his steady girlfriend suddenly relocated to another state, he felt rejected and abandoned.

Jeff's mother, who noticed that he had become more withdrawn and isolative, was concerned that Jeff might be self-destructive. After finding a loaded pistol lying on a table alongside Jeff's bed, Jeff's mother phoned the local mental health crisis intervention center to discuss her concerns about her son's behavior. While talking with the intake nurse, she added that Jeff had recently instructed her to donate his body organs to medical science if "anything should happen" to him.

The nurse requested that Jeff come to the center for an immediate assessment to determine his risk for suicide.

Critical Thinking

1. What information did the nurse gather during the phone conversation with Jeff's mother that alerted her to his need for an immediate suicide assessment? Why is this information pertinent to suicidal ideation?
2. What other factors will the nurse consider when assessing Jeff's risk for suicide during the face-to-face evaluation?
3. Identify one factor noted in the assessment that may help reduce Jeff's risk for self-harm.

NURSING ASSESSMENT QUESTIONS
Suicide

1. What does the client understand about why his mother suggested he come to the center for a mental health assessment? *To determine if the client will validate his mother's concerns or deny that a problem exists*
2. What was Jeff's intention in having a loaded gun lying next to his bed? Did he intend to kill himself or someone else? *Asking directly about a client's intentions can decrease anxiety and feelings of humiliation and shame*
3. Has Jeff taken antidepressants or mood-stabilizing medications in the past? Currently? Have medications used in the past been effective in improving Jeff's mood and lowering his lethality level? Does he have access to other lethal means of suicide?
4. When was the last time Jeff used alcohol or other drugs? When was he last intoxicated? *Clients who use alcohol and other drugs are at*

higher risk to complete a suicide attempt; increased impulsivity, disorientation, and confusion, which often accompany drug and alcohol use, place people at higher risk for suicide*
5. With whom does Jeff share his feelings? *To determine if Jeff has a trusted and reliable support system; if so, the lethality level could be lower*
6. What were the circumstances surrounding his father's death? Is there a history of depression or suicide on either side of Jeff's family? *To determine the nature of Jeff's father's death, family history of depression, or family style of coping, all of which increase the risk of suicide*
7. The nurse asked Jeff's mother: "How do you feel about Jeff's thoughts of suicide?" *To determine if Jeff's mother is a support resource for him*

admitted to the hospital after a suicide attempt, ongoing assessments are necessary to determine whether the person continues to be at high risk.

NURSING DIAGNOSIS

Suicidal clients are frequently admitted to psychiatric units, Emergency Departments, and intensive care units of general medical hospitals. Suicide attempts can occur before or during hospitalization. Hangings, medication overdoses, and jumps from high places are frequent methods of suicide in hospitals. An accurate nursing diagnosis based on a thorough, ongoing assessment is necessary when identifying and prioritizing the client's needs for nursing interventions.

A complete nursing diagnosis is individualized and related to the client's behaviors and nursing needs. Validation of the nursing diagnosis with the client is required. However, the client may deny suicidal intent or the need for extra precautions. In the case of the diagnosis of risk for suicide or risk for self-directed violence, caution is recommended in determining the level of risk. *It is best to err on the side of caution when diagnosing suicidality than to allow serious injury or death to occur.*

Nursing Diagnoses Related to Suicide

Primary diagnosis:
- Risk for suicide
- Risk for self-directed violence

Secondary diagnoses may include:
- Ineffective coping
- Hopelessness
- Powerlessness
- Chronic low self-esteem
- Social isolation
- Disturbed thought processes

Collaborative Diagnoses

Clients with chronic mental illness are at higher risk for suicide. Several medical diagnoses include a group of symptoms that relate to the nursing diagnosis of risk for suicide and risk for self-directed violence.

Major depression and bipolar disorder are affective disorders that may include the symptoms of suicidal ideation, plans, gestures, and recurring suicide attempts.

Schizophrenia, with associated psychotic features such as delusions and command hallucinations, can also manifest as life-threatening behaviors. Hostile voices may direct the client to kill himself or herself.

Mental disorders resulting from a medical condition (such as substance abuse) may involve increased suicide risk if the client is repeating negative or self-defeating patterns. The client may be subject to an increased potential for self-directed violence when attempting to deal with stress by using alcohol or other drugs, demonstrating impulsive behavior, or having limited adaptive responses, mood swings, or confusion.

Indirect, self-destructive behaviors, sometimes identified as passive forms of suicide, are exhibited in the medical diagnoses of anorexia nervosa, bulimia nervosa, and noncompliance with medical treatment.

Clients with personality disorders such as borderline personality disorder, antisocial personality disorder, or schizotypal personality disorder may have a potential for suicide completion, especially if there is another Axis I diagnosis or if substance abuse is involved (see Collaborative Diagnoses table).

OUTCOME IDENTIFICATION

Outcomes are derived from the nursing diagnoses and are defined as anticipated, expected client behaviors or responses that are achieved as a result of nursing interventions. Outcomes must be stated in clear behavioral or measurable terms.

COLLABORATIVE DIAGNOSES

DSM-IV-TR Diagnoses*	NANDA Diagnoses†
Major depression, single episode	Risk for self-directed violence‡
Major depression, recurrent	Risk for suicide Ineffective coping
Major depression with psychotic features	Chronic low self-esteem Hopelessness Powerlessness
Bipolar disorder	Disturbed thought processes Defensive coping Impaired social interaction Impaired verbal communication
Schizophrenia	Disturbed sensory perception Disturbed thought processes Social isolation
Mental disorders caused by a general medical condition	Ineffective coping Self-care deficit

*From American Psychiatric Association: *Diagnostic and Statistical Manual of Mental Disorders*, Fourth Edition, Text Revision. Washington, DC, American Psychiatric Association, 2000.

†From NANDA International (2003). NANDA Nursing Diagnoses: Definitions and Classification 2003-2004, Philadelphia: NANDA.

‡Risk for violence and risk for suicide may be present in all DSM-IV-TR diagnoses listed above.

Client will:
- Remain safe and free from self-harm.
- Verbalize an absence of suicidal ideation/plan/intent.
- Verbalize a desire to live and list several reasons for wanting to live.
- Agree to write and sign a no-self-harm contract with the nursing staff, attending psychiatrist, or individual therapist as an agreement between the client and the team.
- Agree to inform staff immediately if suicidal feelings/thoughts recur.
- Display brightened affect with broad range of expression and spontaneity and cheerful content of speech that reflects a hopeful, optimistic attitude.
- Initiate social interactions with peers and staff (individually and in groups).
- Use effective coping methods to counteract feelings of hopelessness.
- Express a sense of self-worth. Meet own needs through clear, direct methods of communication.
- Verbalize realistic role expectations and goals for meeting them.

- Demonstrate absence of psychotic thinking (e.g., delusions, command hallucinations directing self-harm).
- Make plans for the future that include follow-up psychotherapy and prescribed medication compliance.
- List several friends or supportive individuals (such as a clergy member) or use a suicide hotline (1-800-SUICIDE) to prevent a possible suicide attempt when experiencing increased suicidal thoughts.

PLANNING

The nurse's awareness of a client's risk for suicide and the recurrent nature of suicide attempts warrant a plan of care aimed at saving lives and restoring biopsychosocial stability. The plan of care for the suicidal client emphasizes a reduction in the risk of self-destructive behaviors by monitoring client behaviors and providing a safe environment, promoting the client's feelings of self-worth and hope, improving coping skills, limiting social isolation, and building self-esteem.

IMPLEMENTATION

Primary nursing responsibilities involve the prevention of suicide. The nurse must recognize and effectively intervene in the potentially lethal behaviors of clients at risk. This process involves a continuing assessment of lethality factors to determine the client's risk level while working with the client to restore hope, connect with support resources, and develop positive alternatives to assist in improved coping.

Nursing Interventions

The following interventions must be consistently implemented with all hospitalized suicidal clients.

To provide safety and prevent violence:
1. All unit precautions for preventing suicide should be strictly enforced. This includes vigilantly maintaining a safe environment by:
    a. Routinely counting silverware and all other sharp objects before and after the client's use
    b. Having awareness of the client's whereabouts at all times
    c. Providing one-to-one supervision for the client as warranted, based on assessment of the client's current lethality level
    d. Planning so that the unit is always covered by experienced staff, especially at staff mealtimes, breaks, vacations, change of shift, or unit staff meetings (times during which most suicides occur in hospitals)
    e. Providing a roommate for the suicidal client
    f. Requesting that visitors clear all gifts with staff
    g. Searching the suicidal individual for drugs, sharp objects, cords, shoelaces, and other potential weapons after a return from a pass
    h. Thoroughly assessing the client before any passes to determine the client's current risk level

UNDERSTANDING and APPLYING RESEARCH

No-suicide contracts have been used since the early 1970s as a means of assisting the client to take responsibility for his/her safety. This author reviewed the charts of 577 individuals with diagnoses such as major mood disorder, schizoaffective disorder, or schizophrenia to determine the effectiveness of no-suicide contracts. In the study group, 31 subjects injured himself or herself during the hospitalization. Each of the individuals was on high levels of observation; three clients were under constant observation; one individual was in the seclusion room. A total of 14 out of 31 individuals expressed suicidal intent. No-suicide contracts were used with 20 out of 31 clients. Most of the contracts were verbal.

There were two hypotheses in this study:

1. How does no-suicide contracting affect the likelihood of any self-harm behavior controlling for consistency of nursing assignment, client anxiety at the time of admission, the degree of environmental restriction, and the level of observation?
2. What is the likelihood of suicidal behavior (self-harm behavior with expression of suicidal intent) for clients with no-suicide contracts versus clients without contracts controlling for consistency of nursing assignment, client anxiety at the time of admission, the degree of environmental restriction, and the level of observation?

The study demonstrated that clients with no-suicide contracts were five times more likely to harm self or have suicidal gestures than individual without contracts. Clients with Axis II diagnosis of borderline personality disorder ($n=10$) or mental retardation ($n=2$) were 10 times more likely to harm self than individuals without Axis II diagnosis. Clients that had the same registered nurse assigned during the hospitalization had a lower likelihood of self-harm.

This study demonstrated that no-suicide contracts did not prevent self-harm behaviors. If no-suicide contracts are used, it is important to attend to other risks for suicide. The consistency of assigning a nurse during the course of hospital stay may reduce the risk of self-harm.

From Drew BL: Self-harm behavior and no-suicide contracting in psychiatric inpatient settings, *Arch Psychiatr Nurs* 15:99-106, 2001.

i. Encouraging the client to write a no suicide contract that is used as a means of communication between the staff and the client to promote self exploration and to encourage new methods of asking for assistance when feeling hopeless and isolated. *This indicates to the client the nurse's caring, concern, and consistent follow-through as well as offers the client an opportunity to take charge of self when feeling hopeless and powerless.* NOTE: No-suicide contracts do not preclude the need for constant observation/ supervision (see Understanding and Applying Research box).

2. Being mindful that most suicides occur within 90 days after hospitalization, the nurse must reinforce with families, guardians, social services, or legal authorities the necessity of removing any possible weapons (e.g., guns or drugs) in the person's home environment to a safe location before the client's return home.

3. Because working with suicidal clients is emotionally draining and anxiety producing, the nurse must help create a supportive environment for self and other staff, which includes clinical supervision and informal discussions regarding feelings about suicide, death, hostility, anger, depression, and other painful feelings. Developing an ongoing relationship with a suicidal client is an intense experience in which the client and nurse both examine their feelings about the meaning of life and death. It is an opportunity for the nurse to share a commitment to life, hope, and caring for another person. *Receiving support and supervision enables the nurse to develop this kind of intense, caring relationship so that both the nurse and client experience less anxiety and have increased energy to work toward hope and health.*

To assist in development of improved coping skills:

1. Nurses use specific techniques that include nonjudgmental, empathic listening, encouragement, tolerance of expressions of pain, and flexible responses to client needs.
2. The nurse encourages the client to focus on strengths rather than weaknesses so that the client becomes aware of positive qualities and capabilities that have helped with coping in the past. Nurses provide learning opportunities for improved coping by introducing the client to therapeutic modalities that assist in more positive thinking. *By replacing or substituting irrational, self-deprecating thoughts, beliefs, and images, the client can become more capable of viewing life realistically and rationally.*
3. Nurses help reduce the overwhelming effects of problems by helping clients prioritize their concerns. Breaking the issues down into more manageable parts achieves this goal. The nurse can assist in this process by:
   a. Encouraging the client to prioritize problems from most to least urgent
   b. Supporting the client in finding immediate solutions for the most urgent problems
   c. Postponing finding solutions to those problems that do not require immediate remedy
   d. Encouraging the client to delegate problem solving to others when appropriate
   e. Helping the individual to acknowledge problems that are beyond his or her control
   f. Identifying, defining, and promoting healthy adaptive behaviors in clients
   g. Encouraging continuance of healthy behaviors when improved coping strategies are demonstrated (positive reinforcement)
   h. Encouraging the individual to discuss the feelings generated by ineffective coping (e.g., frustration, anger, inadequacy)
   i. Affirming the client's rational decisions that have been based on accurate judgment

NURSING CARE PLAN

Tiffany, a 15-year-old, was admitted to the adolescent psychiatric unit of a local community hospital after her nurse therapist assessed that she was imminently suicidal. Over the past year Tiffany had become preoccupied with wanting to die. She reported that she had overdosed on analgesics and antibiotics three times in the last 6 months but never told anyone and did not seek medical attention. She reported that she made her first suicide attempt when she was 10 by self-inflicting lacerations to her wrists with a razor blade. Within the past year she had cut her wrists five or six times. Tiffany complained that she felt helpless to change her relationship with her mother, who she felt misunderstood her and from whom she felt alienated. She reported poor school performance, increased irritability, morbid thoughts, decreased appetite, periods of insomnia, low self-esteem, and a history of sexual abuse by a babysitter's boyfriend when she was 8 years old.

During her weekly therapy session, Tiffany announced to her therapist: "I am no longer willing to honor our contract not to harm myself. Nothing is changing at home. My mother hates me and doesn't want me in her life. My stepdad is the only person Mom really cares about outside of herself. I hate how I look, and I hate how I am. I saved most of the pain pills my doctor gave me when I injured my leg." Laughing, she added, "I think there's enough to really put me out of my pain this time."

When questioned further, Tiffany admitted she was planning to kill herself. She indicated that she didn't know exactly when she would attempt to do so but promised, "I am not going to wait much longer."

To provide for her immediate safety, the nurse therapist ordered Tiffany's admission to the hospital.

DSM-IV-TR Diagnoses

Axis I	Major depression, recurrent
Axis II	Developmental reading disorder
	Borderline personality traits
Axis III	Fractured left tibia; healing
Axis IV	Problem with primary support system
Axis V	GAF = 10 (current)
	GAF = 35 (past year)

NURSING DIAGNOSIS: Risk for suicide and risk for self-directed violence. Risk factors: dysfunctional family relationships, ineffective coping style, low self-esteem, effects of sexual abuse, verbalized intent to die, history of several previous suicide attempts, lethal suicide plan, severely depressed mood.

CLIENT OUTCOMES	NURSING INTERVENTIONS	EVALUATION
Tiffany will verbalize an absence of suicidal ideation, intent, plan.	Check the client and room for potentially dangerous items and observe for any secretive behavior. *Protecting the client from self-destructive behavior promotes safety and gives a message of caring and concern.*	On the third day of hospitalization, Tiffany told her primary nurse that she wanted to live. She reported that suicidal ideation had ceased by the fifth day of hospitalization.
Tiffany will express a desire to live and will list several reasons for wanting to live.	Support Tiffany in developing a hopeful attitude. Reinforce her efforts at positive self-evaluation, self-control, and goal-setting *to promote self-esteem and provide hope for change.*	The client reported looking forward to summer vacation. She accepted a job as a veterinarian's assistant. She identified her appearance and intelligence as positive attributes.
Tiffany will make plans for the future that include identification of a viable support system and a daily plan for structured activities with friends and family, routine exercise, weekly therapy sessions, and medication compliance.	Encourage Tiffany to list people she will contact for support and help her develop a daily plan of structured activities that include a health care regimen. *Additional support and success-oriented activities will increase the client's sense of self-worth, decrease feelings of alienation, and lessen the suicide risk.*	Tiffany developed a weekly plan of activities that included a health care regimen and a part-time job. She listed her mother, stepfather, and two friends as people she would talk with.

NURSING DIAGNOSIS: Ineffective coping related to negative thinking patterns, self-defeating behaviors, disturbance in self-concept, multiple stressors, and ineffective support system, as evidenced by self-destructive behaviors, lack of assertive communication, impaired judgment and insight, misdirected anger, and social isolation.

CLIENT OUTCOMES	NURSING INTERVENTIONS	EVALUATION
Tiffany will demonstrate improved coping skills by: Discussing feelings and needs assertively Taking responsibility for feelings and not blaming others Making a written list of healthy coping skills to use in times of increased stress Keeping a daily journal of thoughts and feelings related to her relationships Engaging in efforts to socialize with peers and reestablish communication with family	Teach cognitive and behavioral techniques to assist Tiffany in limiting negative thought patterns and self-defeating behaviors and using more realistic self-evaluations. Encourage attendance at all psychoeducation groups. Review journal daily. Point out any self-defeating thoughts. Role-model assertive communication. *Therapeutic modalities can help the client to identify and replace self-defeating thoughts and behaviors with an improved, healthy coping style.*	Tiffany directly confronted her feelings with others in group, individual, and family therapy. Tiffany labeled and challenged her "thinking errors" in journal work, owned responsibility for her feelings/actions, and progressively stopped accusing or blaming others.

Continued

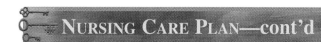

NURSING CARE PLAN—cont'd

NURSING DIAGNOSIS: Compromised family coping related to highly conflicted family relationships, enmeshed relationship with mother, hostile relationship with stepfather, and ineffective communication and parenting skills, as evidenced by distancing behaviors toward client, inability to set consistent limits, and inappropriate parent-child boundaries.

FAMILY OUTCOMES	NURSING INTERVENTIONS	EVALUATION
Family will attend all scheduled family therapies and parent support group, where they will discuss their feelings of fear, guilt, and frustration related to Tiffany's suicide attempts.	Encourage parents to actively participate in Tiffany's treatment. Routinely update parents on any changes in Tiffany's behaviors. Encourage Tiffany and parents to directly confront their feelings. Role-model effective listening skills and assertive communication. *Demonstrating involvement in Tiffany's treatment will convey a message of caring and concern and parents' willingness to make needed changes.*	Parents attended all family groups. Mother planned one afternoon each week for special time with Tiffany. Parents openly discussed feelings with the client and each other. They asked for referral to a parenting skills workshop.
Parents will demonstrate willingness to listen to daughter's concerns and self-doubts. Parents will praise Tiffany when she engages in healthy coping behaviors.	Apprise parents of any changes in Tiffany's behavior. Provide support and reassurance when Tiffany's mood and/or behavior fluctuate. Discuss warning signs of impending decompensation such as increased irritability, isolation, failure to maintain medication regimen, and depressed mood. Inform parents of risk factors after hospitalization (e.g., significant losses or disappointments that forewarn decompensation). Reinforce attempts at improved communication and parenting skills. *Maintaining supportive communication with families enhances the client's support resources, decreases family members' anxiety, and promotes healthy coping.*	Parents reassured Tiffany when she voiced self-doubts. Parents requested involvement in parents' aftercare group after Tiffany's discharge.

j. Reinforcing the client's attempts to make independent decisions

k. Acknowledging the client's demonstrated willingness to implement improved coping behaviors such as assertive communication

l. Responding to delusional statements by stating the reality of the situation without arguing with the client's reality

To enhance family and social support systems:

1. Enlist the family as allies in the client's treatment. *Family attendance at psychoeducation groups and family therapy is crucial in helping the client work through and understand complex and toxic family structures, systems, and dynamics that may contribute to the individual's suicidal feelings.*

2. Determine the degree of available family support that contributes to overall risk management. Inform family members about critical signs that the client may exhibit as depression lifts and discharge occur. Encourage the removal of any lethal weapons from the client's home environment.

3. Provide understanding and encouragement when family members express feelings (e.g., frustration, helplessness, or guilt) and intense affect.

4. Contact social services to assist with any needed vocational and financial support.

5. Refer the client to aftercare groups, support groups, and 12-step groups as needed.

6. Refer the client to a suicide hotline (1-800-SUICIDE) that can be used when the client is feeling overwhelmed and suicidal in the future.

Additional Treatment Modalities

Depending on the client's diagnosis, pharmacologic intervention is often a primary consideration in the treatment of the suicidal client. Antidepressants, anxiolytics, and antipsychotic medications are frequently used, depending on the individual's need, history, and previous response to medication intervention.

Psychotherapeutic interventions may vary and can include insight-oriented techniques, cognitive reframing, and brief, solution-focused crisis interventions.

Electroconvulsive therapy (ECT) may be used with adults whose response patterns reflect a lack of positive response to medication (i.e., *intractable* or *refractory* depression). These adults concurrently present with long-standing histories of severe depression while expressing imminent intent to die. ECT is discussed in detail in Chapter 19.

EVALUATION

An evaluation of the client's response to the plan of care is crucial in working with suicidal individuals. An ongoing, all-encompassing evaluation considers the accuracy of the nursing diagnosis, the appropriateness of the intervention based on the client's response, and the timeliness with which the intervention occurred. Evaluation helps the nurse target areas of outcome that are critical to the client's continued survival. A client's lack of positive response to nursing interventions may indicate a need to alter the interventions, implement other treatment modalities, or reexamine target dates for completion of outcomes.

Deliberate, conscientious evaluation of a suicidal client's response to nursing interventions that are directed toward promoting safety and biopsychosocial stabilization helps ensure the client's continued safety and readiness for discharge.

CHAPTER SUMMARY

■ Suicide is a major public health and mental health problem in the United States.

■ Durkheim classified four subtypes of suicide relating to social and cultural aspects: anomic, egoistic, altruistic, and fatalistic.

■ Etiologies of suicide include biologic factors, which deal with chemical imbalances; psychologic factors, which dominate the understanding of suicide and define the dynamics of intrapsychic, interpersonal, cognitive, and behavioral approaches in explaining suicidal behavior; and sociologic factors, which relate to influences of social groups that contribute to suicide.

■ Around the world, suicide accounts for nearly 1% of all deaths. The United States reported 28,332 in 2000, a rate of 10 deaths for every 100,000 individuals.

■ The most vulnerable groups for suicide are older adults and youths ages 15 to 24 years. Caucasians and men are more likely to be at risk for suicide. Suicide crosses all socioeconomic levels.

■ Suicidal behavior is strongly associated with the occurrence of psychiatric disorders and other health-related problems such as depression, schizophrenia, panic disorders, substance abuse, some personality disorders (such as borderline personality disorder), and medical disorders.

■ Imminence, intent, and the method chosen and its accessibility are the three determinants that indicate the level of lethality and the levels of interventions necessary for safety.

■ Suicidal behavior is treatable.

■ Discharge criteria for the suicidal client must include indications that the client is no longer imminently suicidal, that the client's environment is safe to return to, and that a support system is in place for the client to access.

■ The plan of care emphasizes a reduction in the risk of self-destructive behaviors by monitoring the client's behaviors and providing a safe environment, promoting feelings of self-worth and hope, improving coping skills, limiting social isolation, and building self-esteem.

REVIEW QUESTIONS

1. Regarding suicide, the nurse understands that:
   a. Suicide is more prevalent in poverty-stricken families.
   b. The death of a parent is one of the most significant factors of adolescent suicide.
   c. Older adults are the least likely to commit suicide.
   d. It is very difficult to assess for suicide because the client seldom exhibits any signs.

2. A 14-year-old client reveals that a peer in the partial hospitalization program stated that he was going to shoot himself that night. The nurse requests to speak to the client who verbalized the suicidal threat. The most critical question for the nurse to ask would be:
   a. "Do you have access to a gun?"
   b. "Why do you want to kill yourself?"
   c. "Have you been taking your Zoloft?"
   d. "Did something happen with your parents?"

3. A 20-year-old client was recently hospitalized after taking an overdose of aspirin. The client was started on Paxil 20 mg. What is the most appropriate short-term goal?
   a. The client will be free from suicidal thoughts.
   b. The client will verbalize goals for the future.
   c. The client will verbalize and demonstrate three adaptive coping skills.
   d. The client will verbalize suicidal thoughts to nursing staff.

4. Which statement demonstrates that the client's risk of suicide is low?
   a. "My life isn't worth living."
   b. "I just want to go to sleep and never wake up."
   c. "I know that I have options. I have a lot of people who love me and want to help."
   d. "I don't need to take my medications anymore. I won't be needing them."

5. A 30-year-old client has been taking Zoloft for 2 weeks. He has been brighter and more sociable on the unit. He attempted suicide 1 month ago after his wife left him. The most appropriate nursing intervention would be:
   a. Supervise the client 24 hours/day.
   b. Discuss with the physician when to discontinue suicidal precautions.
   c. Begin discharge planning.
   d. Have the client run group therapy.

REFERENCES

Aguilera DC: Suicide: theoretical concepts. In Aguilera DC: *Crisis intervention: theory and methodology,* ed 8, St Louis, 1998, Mosby.

American Psychiatric Association: *Diagnostic and Statistical Manual of Mental Disorders,* Fourth Edition, Text Revision. Washington, DC, 2000, American Psychiatric Association.

American Psychiatric Association: *Resource document on mandatory outpatient treatment* Washington, 1999, American Psychiatric Association.

Barbee M: Professionally speaking: what are the warning signs for suicidal adolescents? *J Psychosoc Nurs Ment Health Serv* 31:37, 1993.

Barber ME et al: Aborted suicide attempts: a new classification of suicidal behavior, *Am J Psychiatry* 155(3):385, 1998.

Beautrais AL et al: Prevalence and comorbidity of mental disorders in persons making serious suicide attempts: a case-control study, *Am J Psychiatry* 153:1009, 1996.

Brodsky BS et al: Characteristics of borderline personality disorder associated with suicidal behavior, *Am J Psychiatry* 154(12):1715, 1997.

Buchanan D, Farran C, Clark D: Suicidal thought and self-transcendence in older adults, *J Psychosoc Nurs Ment Health Serv* 33(10):31, 1995.

Celo-Cruz M: Aid-in-dying: should we decriminalize physician-assisted suicide and physician-committed euthanasia? *Am J Law Med* 4:369, 1992.

Center for the Advancement of Health, Facts of Life (2002) 7(8), website: www.cfah.org

Cohen L et al: Suicide and schizophrenia: data from a prospective community treatment study, *Am J Psychiatry* 147:602, 1990.

Cummings J: The neuroanatomy of depression, *J Clin Psychiatry* 54:14, 1993.

Drew BL: Self-harm behavior and no-suicide contracting in psychiatric inpatient settings, *Arch Psychiatr Nurs* 15:99-106, 2001.

Durkheim E: *Suicide,* Glencol, 1951, The Free Press (originally published as *Le Suicide* in 1897).

Earle K et al: Characteristics of outpatient suicides, *Hosp Comm Psychiatry* 45:123, 1994.

Freud S: *Mourning and melancholia,* Collected papers, London, 1920, Hogarth Press (originally published in Germany in 1917).

Garlow SJ: Age, gender, and ethnicity differences in patterns of cocaine and ethanol use preceding suicide, *Am J Psychiatry* 159:615-700, 2002.

Green E, Katz J, Marcus P: Practice guideline for suicide/self-harm prevention. In Green E, Katz J, editors: *Clinical practice guidelines for the adult patient,* St Louis, 1995, Mosby.

Gunderson JG: *Borderline personality disorder,* Washington, DC, 1984, American Psychiatric Press.

Heacock D: Suicidal behavior in black and Hispanic youth, *Psychiatr Ann* 20:134, 1990.

Heilä H et al: Suicide and schizophrenia: a nationwide psychological autopsy study on age- and sex-specific clinical characteristics of 92 suicide victims with schizophrenia, *Am J Psychiatry* 154:1235, 1997.

Hoyer G, Lund E: Suicide among women related to number of children in marriage, *Arch Gen Psychiatry* 50(2):134, 1993.

Husain S: Current perspectives on the role of psychosocial factors in adolescent suicide, *Psychiatr Ann* 20:122, 1990.

Johnson J: Panic disorder, comorbidity, and suicide attempts, *Arch Gen Psychiatry* 47:805, 1990.

Lepine J et al: Suicide attempts in patients with panic disorder, *Arch Gen Psychiatry* 50:144, 1993.

Lester D: The association between quality of life and suicide and homicide rates, *J Soc Psychol* 124:247, 1984.

Linehan MM: *Cognitive-behavioral treatment of borderline personality disorder,* New York, 1993, Guildford Press.

Litman R: Sigmund Freud on suicide, *Bull Suicidology* p 11, 1967.

Maris R: The adolescent suicide problem, *Suicide Life Threat Behav* 15:91, 1985.

Masterson JF: *Psychotherapy of the borderline adult: a developmental approach,* New York, 1976, Brunner/Mazel.

Monahan J et al: Coercion to inpatient treatment: initial results and implications for assertive treatment in the community. In Dennis D, Monahan J, editors: *Coercion and aggressive community treatment: a new frontier in mental health law,* New York, 1996, Plenum.

NANDA International (2003). NANDA Nursing Diagnoses: Definitions and Classification 2003-2004, Philadelphia: NANDA.

Nielson D et al: Suicidality and 5-hydroxyindoleacic acid concentration associated with tryptophan-hydroxylase polymorphism, *Arch Gen Psychiatry* 51:34, 1994.

Nyman A, Jonsson H: Patterns of self-destructive behavior in schizophrenia, *Acta Psychiatr Scand* 73:252, 1986.

Richman J: *Family therapy for suicidal people,* New York, 1986, Springer.

Rogers C, editor: *On becoming a person,* Boston, 1961, Houghton Mifflin.

Rudd D et al: Problem-solving appraisal in suicide ideators and attempters, *Am J Orthopsychiatry* 64(1):136, 1994.

Sakinofsky I et al: Problem resolution and repetition of parasuicide: a prospective study, *Br J Psychiatry* 156:395, 1991.

Shneidman E: *Definition of suicide,* New York, 1985, John Wiley & Sons.

Shneidman ES: *The suicidal mind,* New York, 1996, Oxford University Press.

Smith J et al: Comparison of suicide among Anglos and Hispanics in five Southwestern states, *Suicide Life Threat Behav* 15:14, 1985.

Stekel W: Suicide and will. In Freidman P, editor: *On suicide,* New York, 1967, International Universities Press.

Sullivan H: Socio-psychiatric research: its implications for the schizophrenia problem and mental hygiene, *Am J Psychiatry* 10:977, 1931.

Sullivan H: The manic-depressive psychosis. In Perry H et al, editors: *Clinical studies in psychiatry,* New York, 1956, WW Norton.

Tanskanen A et al: Smoking and suicidality among psychiatric patients, *Am J Psychiatry* 155:129, 1998.

Valente S: Adolescent suicide: assessment and intervention, *J Child Adolesc Psychiatr Nurs* 2(1):34, 1989.

Waem M et al: Burden of illness and suicide in elderly people: case-control study, *Br Med J* 324(7350):1355-1358, 2002.

Weiss J: The suicidal patient. In Arieti S, editor: *American handbook of psychiatry,* New York, 1966, Basic Books.

Wells K et al: The functioning and well-being of depressed patients, *JAMA* 262:914, 1989.

Wilson D: *New York Times,* April 9, 1994.

Wolk SI, Weissman MM: Suicidal behavior in depressed children grown up: preliminary results of a longitudinal study, *Psychiatr Ann* 26:331, 1996.

Yang B et al: Sociological and economic theories of suicide: a comparison of the USA and Taiwan, *Soc Sci Med* 34:333, 1992.

Zayas L: Towards an understanding of suicide risks in young Hispanic females, *J Adolesc Res* 2:1, 1978.

SUGGESTED READINGS

Andreasen N: *The broken brain,* New York, 1984, Harper & Row.

Arato M et al: Retrospective psychiatric assessment of 200 suicides, *Acta Psychiatr Scand* 77:454, 1988.

Bongar B: *The suicidal patient, clinical and legal standards of care,* Washington, DC, 1991, American Psychological Association.

Boyd J, Moscicki E: Firearms and youth suicide, *Am J Public Health* 76:1240, 1986.

Egan MP et al: The "no suicide contract": helpful or harmful? *J Psychosoc Nurs Ment Health Serv* 35(3):31, 1997.

Farberow N, editor: *The many faces of suicide: indirect self-destructive behavior,* New York, 1980, McGraw-Hill.

Fawcett J et al: Suicide: clues from interpersonal communication, *Arch Gen Psychiatry* 21:129, 1969.

May P, Dizmang L: Suicide and the American Indian, *Psychiatr Ann* 4(9):22, 1974.

McIntosh J: Older adults: the next suicide epidemic? *Suicide Life Threat Behav* 22:322, 1992.

Mellick E et al: Suicide among elderly white men: development of a profile, *J Psychosoc Nurs Ment Health Serv* 30:29, 1992.

Miller M: *Suicide after sixty: the final alternative,* New York, 1979, Springer.

Shneidman E: Fifty-eight years. In Shneidman E, editor: *On the nature of suicide,* San Francisco, 1969, Jossey-Bass.

Toolan J: Depression and suicide. In Caplan G, editor: *Child and adolescent psychiatry, sociocultural and community psychiatry,* New York, 1974, Basic Books.

Trygstad L: The need to know: biological learning needs identified by practicing psychiatric nurses, *J Psychosoc Nurs Ment Health Serv* 32(2):13, 1994.

Weissman M et al: Suicidal ideation and suicide attempts in panic disorder and attacks, *N Engl J Med* 321:1209, 1989.

ONLINE RESOURCE

American Association of Suicidology: www.suicidology.org

PART V CARE IN THE COMMUNITY

25 Grief and Loss

Charles Kemp

OBJECTIVES

- Discuss four major categories for symptoms of grief.
- Describe three components of the normal grief process.
- Distinguish between symptoms/behaviors of grief and those of depression.
- Analyze the risk for dysfunctional grief reactions in selected high-risk clients.
- Discuss the major goals for intervention in acute grief.
- Evaluate the points of intervention with respect to intervention efficacy.
- Compare and contrast chronic sorrow with other types of grief, and list persons at risk for chronic sorrow.
- Explain how posttraumatic stress disorder can be a feature of dysfunctional grief.
- Apply the nursing process in managing clients experiencing grief.

Grief is the painful psychologic and physiologic response to loss. Although it is most commonly associated with the death of a loved one, grief occurs when there is any significant loss, including loss of self-esteem, identity, dignity, or sense of worth. Grief descends on the client newly admitted to a psychiatric hospital, the client who undergoes mutilating surgery, the parents of an infant with birth defects, the child who changes schools, the victim of violence, the nurse who works with victims of violence, the betrayed lover, and the person who loses a job or retires. Grief comes to everyone. Most nurses are in daily contact with grief—other people's and their own.

This chapter describes grief in the following terms: definitions, responses or manifestations, stages or process, and types of grief, including anticipatory, acute, dysfunctional, and chronic sorrow. Assessment information, diagnoses, interventions, and case studies are included.

The terms **grief, bereavement,** and **mourning** are often used interchangeably and there is sometimes disagreement about their exact meanings (Tomita and Kitamura, 2002).

In some cases a grieving person may benefit from psychosocial or pharmacologic intervention, and in other cases, grief may become pathologic (see later discussion on dysfunctional grief). Although grief is painful, however, it is important to understand that grief and its pain are normal (and, indeed, inevitable) aspects of life (American Psychiatric Association [APA], 2000; Freud, 1917; Lev and McCorkle, 1998).

RESPONSES

Responses to bereavement (loss) may be examined as a range of physical, cognitive, relating, and affective manifestations of pain—the intensity of which are often a surprise to the mourner. Lindemann's seminal study of grief (1944) and other more current studies (Parkes, 2001; Stroebe et al., 2000; Tomita and Kitamura, 2002) identified many of the manifestations of grief, including physical distress, preoccupation with the image of the deceased, guilt, hostile reactions, and disruptions in patterns of conduct. These and other physical and psychologic manifestations can be summarized as follows.

Physical Manifestations

Physical manifestations of grief include weakness, anorexia, feelings of choking, shortness of breath, tightness in the chest, dry mouth, and gastrointestinal disturbances. Fatigue, exhaustion, and insomnia are common. Bereaved persons frequently seek medical assistance for vague symptoms such as chest discomfort or gastrointestinal problems, some of which seem to have no physiologic basis (Steen, 1998). In addition, although grief is seldom a direct cause of illness or death (except for suicide), there is a clear link between grief and increased vulnerability to physical and mental illness, especially myocardial infarction, hypertension, rheumatoid arthritis, depression, alcohol and other drug abuse, and malnutrition (Charlton et al., 2001; Ringdal et al., 2001; Tomita and Kitamura, 2002).

Cognitive Manifestations

Cognitive manifestations center on preoccupation with the persona of the deceased. The involuntary nature and intensity of the preoccupation are surprising and distressing to some. It is common for the preoccupation to take the form of conversations with the deceased (in normal grief, with the recognition that the deceased person is not actually present). Especially with older adults, these conversations may continue for the rest of the survivor's life. Over time, preoccupation usually diminishes, although links with the deceased may be maintained for many years and, in some people, continue until death (Weiss and Richards, 1997). These links may be in the form of remembrances such as treasured things or renegotiated relationships with the deceased. Formerly thought by some to be a symptom that needed resolution, the drive to maintain links between the living and the dead is increasingly recognized as normative behavior (Reisman, 2001; Silverman and Worden, 1992). Indeed, in some cultures (e.g., Chinese and Vietnamese) the failure to maintain formal links with deceased ancestors is thought to be pathologic (Kemp and Chang, 2002). Another common symptom is difficulty concentrating, such as complete lapses of focus or even orientation to time and place. Seeking and longing for the lost person or object are universally experienced. Hallucinations are experienced by some grieving persons. These are most often described as momentary glimpses of the person who died, or brief (two or three words) auditory messages perceived to be spoken by the deceased. In most cases hallucinations diminish within a month or two after the loss and thus may be considered as part of the normal grieving process. In a few cases hallucinations persist, increase in number or intensity, or become derogatory or threatening, such as beckoning the survivor to join the deceased. They are then considered negative hallucinations (pathologic grief), and therapeutic interventions, including hospitalization and/or antipsychotic medications, may be indicated (APA, 2000; Kemp, 1999; Stroebe et al., 2000).

Behavioral and Relating Manifestations

Grief and bereavement figure prominently in the DSM Axis IV dimension of psychosocial and environmental problems. Among the Axis IV problems directly and/or indirectly related to grief and bereavement (APA, 2000) are:
- Death of a family member
- Health problems in a family
- Inadequate social support
- Adjustment to life-cycle transition
- Inadequate finances

Behavioral and relating manifestations of grief include disruptions in patterns of conduct ranging from an inability to perform even basic activities of daily living; to dragging through daily activities; to a restless, disorganized behavior that includes "searching" for that which is lost and obsessive rumination and reminiscence; and overall, an intense sense of isolation (Charlton et al., 2001; Hentz, 2002; Lindemann, 1944; Weiss and Richards, 1997). The old life and patterns lose meaning and satisfaction without the lost object or person, and there does not seem to be a new life or patterns to which the bereaved individual can turn. This loss of relating and meaning is a major etiology of despair or hopelessness.

Affective Manifestations

Affective manifestations of grief are often overwhelming, with sadness, guilt, loneliness, and anger being the most common. Sadness, loneliness, and hopelessness tend to predominate and may, along with other symptoms, meet the criteria for diagnosis of an affective disorder (e.g., major depression or dysthymic disorder). The most common differences between symptoms of bereavement and major depression or dysthymic disorder are that psychomotor retardation, morbid guilt, and suicidal ideation are less common in bereavement and that affective disorders are of longer duration than bereavement (APA, 2000; Hentz, 2002; Nuss and Zubenko, 1992). However, dysfunctional or unresolved grief may result in major depression.

Guilt is a pervasive theme in grief, even in children as young as 2 years (Gibbons, 1992; Jacob, 1996). Many survivors search for their failures or omissions in the relationship, and when significant mistakes are not found, may proceed to magnify whatever small transgressions might exist (Lindemann, 1944). Guilt may be especially troublesome for those whose relationships with the deceased were ambivalent and characterized by unresolved or unexpressed feelings. Survivor guilt is common among people who go through an intense experience (e.g., war) and survive when others do not. A similar guilt is experienced when survivors believe that they should have died instead of the loved one. Grief accompanied by "guilt about things other than actions taken or not taken by the survivor at the time of death," (APA, 2000) sustained loss of self-esteem, and ambivalence about living is an indication that suicide risk is increased and help is needed. Anger is common and may be directed toward the person who died, to family members, to the health care staff, or to God, or it may be turned inward to self.

Anger is generally a response to the anxiety derived from the powerlessness and vulnerability resulting from the death of a loved one and other losses. Anger toward the deceased is common: "How could she do this to me? It's not fair!" Many survivors feel it is "wrong" to feel anger toward a deceased loved one and thus turn the anger inward. Anger turned inward may also reflect a survivor's inability to release the lost person or object. To those who have spent a lifetime suppressing anger, these overwhelming and "wrong" or ego-dystonic feelings are distressing and indicate to some individuals that they are "going crazy." Some need permission to express anger. If the death itself is not enough to engender anger, tending to the business, such as funeral preparations, surrounding the death may result in anger. Death, usually the greatest and most painful loss in life, is seen by some morticians, lawyers, and others only as a point of vulnerability through which survivors can be exploited for profit.

The impulse to use drugs, including prescription drugs and alcohol, may occur or, if the survivor already uses, increase. Bereaved persons with a history of any sort of drug misuse or mental illness are at risk for recurrence or exacerbation of these problems (Carman, 1997).

STAGES AND PROCESS OF GRIEF
Stages

Grief is often described in terms of stages. Although there is variation among the different conceptions, many stage-oriented theories can be summarized as having three basic stages: avoidance (numbing and blunting), confrontation (disorganization and despair), and reestablishment (reorganization and recovery) (Kemp, 1999; Parkes, 2001). Avoidance includes both the initial denial and subsequent brief periods of time when the survivor "forgets," then "remembers" with shock and pain, the losses and grief. Confrontation is the often lengthy period of active mourning and includes the previously discussed most acute physical, cognitive, behavioral and relating, and affective manifestations of grief. Reestablishment occurs, not as a distinct stage but as the *gradual* decrease of symptoms and adjustment to life without that which was lost. The problem with stages is that they tend to be neater in theory than they are in reality and thus may mislead some individuals into thinking that grief is a matter of progressing in an orderly manner through stages and then being finished with grief.

Process
Characteristics

Rather than well-defined stages, it is more helpful to think in terms of a process of common and dynamic responses to grief. Thus a person might initially respond to the death of a loved one with shock and disbelief, followed by protest and despair; go through a period of emotionless cognitive activity (planning the funeral, etc.) interspersed with waves of despair; then experience yearning, despair, and disorganization (sobbing, confusion, wandering); and gradually begin the long, painful, and varied process of rebuilding a life without the person who died. An essential feature of this process is its dynamic, changing nature (Cowles and Rodgers, 1991; Kemp, 1999; Parkes, 2001; Reisman, 2001). Periods of apparently normal functioning, for example, may be interspersed with periods of psychologic distress or symptoms (almost indistinguishable from those of major depression). Countless people say, "It seems like I'm doing fine, and then, for no reason at all, I start crying." (As if some external or practical reason were needed!)

The grief process might include all of the aforementioned responses, phases, or symptoms, or only several of them. There might be no "stage of avoidance" or no period of organized cognitive activity, or very little in the way of resolution, reorganization, or adjustment to the environment in the absence of the deceased. Moreover, when death is ex-

Box 25-1   Summary of Grief Theories

Lindemann
Grief is manifested by predictable psychologic and somatic symptomatology. Acute mourning is characterized by somatic distress, preoccupation with the deceased person's image, guilt, hostile reactions, and loss of patterns of conduct. Dysfunctional or "morbid" grief reactions are defined as distortions of some aspect of "normal grief." The duration of grief and development of dysfunctional grief are largely dependent on the success with which the mourner *works* through the grief.

Kübler-Ross
Elisabeth Kübler-Ross' stages of dying (denial, anger, bargaining, depression, acceptance) are often applied to grief. The initial response to loss may include denial, anger, and bargaining. Denial is characterized by refusal to accept the loss. Anger may initially be directed at the health care staff and then, later in the process, at the person who died. Bargaining and denial are often mixed in a futile attempt to "reverse reality." Depression tends to be the lengthiest phase, and in dysfunctional grief it may become chronic and meet DSM-IV-TR criteria for major depression. Acceptance of the loss is a gradual process that includes aspects of previous stages. As the grief work progresses, acceptance increases.

Bowlby
Grief and loss are characterized first by numbness in which the loss is recognized but not necessarily felt as real. Numbness is followed by yearning and searching, in which the loss is still not fully realized. In the third phase, disorganization and despair, the loss is real, and intense emotional pain and cognitive disorganization occur. Reorganization is the final phase and is characterized by a gradual adjustment to life without the deceased.

Engel
The initial response to loss is shock and disbelief. Awareness of the loss and the meaning of the loss develop during the first year of mourning. Eventually, the relationship is resolved and put into perspective.

Shneidman
Conceptualizing less structure or stages than other theorists in regard to grief, Shneidman views the expression of grief as being dependent primarily on an individual's personality or style of living. An individual who goes through life feeling depressed and guilty is likely to grieve similarly. One who avoids emotional investments with others will also tend to try to avoid grief as well.

Theory Synthesis
Grief tends to occur in several phases. The initial response to loss may be shock, numbness, denial, or other attempts to defend against the reality and pain of loss. This initial phase is followed by painful psychologic and physical disequilibrium—which, in the case of chronic grief, may last indefinitely. The third phase of resolution or recovery is a gradual process in which "the good days begin to outnumber the bad." Ultimately, although not forgotten, the relationship with the deceased is resolved and placed into perspective.

---

pected, the grief process begins before the person dies. Grief occurring before the death or other loss is called anticipatory grief and is discussed later.

A summary of grief theories is provided in Box 25-1.

Grief Work
Stages and process are associated with another common characteristic of grief—work. Named first by Lindemann (1944), **grief work** is the means by which people move through the stages or process of grief (Carpenito, 2002). Grief work is both a struggle to not give in to despair and a willingness to confront the reality of despair. Thus within the grief process, the bereaved person must continue to some extent to move forward with the business of life, which includes paying the bills, making decisions, and at the same time, being able to express the deep, painful emotions of grieving.

Tasks in Grief
There are certain **tasks in grief,** the accomplishment of which helps in the resolution of grief (Carpenito, 2002; Cooley, 1992; Kemp, 1999). These tasks are:
- Telling the "death story" or describing (in detail) events surrounding the death (or loss)
- Expressing and accepting the sadness of grief

- Expressing and accepting guilt, anger, and other feelings perceived as negative
- Reviewing the relationship with the deceased
- Exploring possibilities in life after the loss (e.g., new relationships, activities, sources of support, and so on)
- Understanding common processes and problems in grief
- Being understood or accepted by others

Complicating Factors
Grief work is complicated by several factors. First, it is extremely painful. Many people are surprised at the intensity and depth of the pain experienced in grieving and often make an attempt, consciously or unconsciously, to avoid the distress, often by throwing themselves back into a busy schedule or taking a vacation. Second, the work is inherently contradictory. The pain demands expression, but there is often the fear that if the pain is expressed, the control over feelings will be lost. "I know that if I start crying, I will never stop." Third, both emotion-based coping (such as expressing deep, powerful feelings) and problem-solving coping (such as developing strategies for going on with life) are needed to most successfully complete the work. Finally, in most of the Western world, cultural values support avoiding the expression of grief. For example, self-control is highly

valued, especially by men. There is a tendency to try to rush through grief and get back to work or get on with one's life (or as TV newscasters say, *ad nauseum,* "let the healing begin"). Rituals that formerly helped in individual and community expression of grief are now often brief "celebrations" of the deceased's life or other upbeat and usually brief events. The expression of grief, therefore, is limited to what is "appropriate" in public and then what occurs when the bereaved individual is alone—with the pain.

TYPES OF GRIEF

Types of grief include anticipatory, acute, and dysfunctional, as well as chronic sorrow. There is disagreement about definitions, especially in terms of the time required for resolution of a particular form of grief.

Anticipatory Grief

Anticipatory grief, or premourning, is defined as grief associated with anticipation of a predicted death or developing loss (Ackley, 2002; Heffner and Byock, 2002; Shneidman, 1980). Anticipatory grief may begin with a catastrophic diagnosis when the client and family enter a new dimension of being characterized by a sharp sense of vulnerability. The old and comfortable illusory dimension of being, in which death, suffering, or loss does not exist, then dies, and grief for that life ensues. Here, as in other situations, the grief may be complex. For example, in a family in which a loved one develops dementia, grief may be acute (related to the current condition), ongoing (as the family continuously loses aspects of the loved one), and anticipatory (as the long-term reality of the disorder is clarified).

Early in the development of the anticipatory grief model, anticipatory grief was viewed as an adaptive process that could help resolve relationships and prepare survivors, to some extent, for the anticipated loss. Ideally the realization that loss was approaching would afford the people involved an opportunity to work on interpersonal and spiritual reconciliation and provide support for one another (Parkes, 1998; Rando, 1988). More recently, anticipatory grief has been seen by some clinicians and researchers as being associated with a high incidence of depression (Levy, 1991) or with family withdrawal from the client. There is general agreement that (1) grief begins when a serious physical or mental illness occurs; (2) this grief may be termed anticipatory and involves pain, as do other forms of grief; and (3) a lack of emotional response to serious illness or other loss is an indication that dysfunction or dysfunctional grief is likely (Ackley, 2002; Carpenito, 2002). Thus anticipatory grief may be viewed as normative, and persons experiencing it may benefit from intervention.

Acute Grief

Acute grief, usually referred to simply as grief, is the prototypic painful experience after a loss. Its symptoms and process are described earlier in the chapter. Although there is agreement that acute grief is time limited, an issue that has never been satisfactorily resolved is the question of how long acute (or normal) grief lasts. An early theory is that acute grief lasts approximately 1 year (Shneidman, 1980). More recently the time span for acute grief has been interfaced with the severity of symptoms, severity of trauma or loss, nature of the relationship, and cultural values (APA, 2000; Stroebe et al., 2000; Kemp, 1999). Acute grief does not have a clear ending; gradually the sadness lessens, the pain diminishes, and eventually the mourner moves forward with his or her life—even though complete recovery may never occur (Hentz, 2002; Reisman, 2001; Weiss and Richards, 1997). In some traditional cultures (e.g., East Indian) and among some individuals in certain religions (e.g., Jewish and Hindu), grief may be ongoing and not limited by time (Goodman et al., 1991).

Within the process of healing and moving on, there are times of acute exacerbation—times when some situation or event brings back the pain, and the mourner again feels overwhelmed with grief. Holidays, birthdays, and other significant milestones are obvious events with the potential to rekindle the grief. Other precipitants are less obvious, and thus the mourner is unable to prepare for them. For example, a song, an image, or a smell may occur in an unguarded moment and the sadness returns as powerful as it was in the beginning. These moments of exacerbation also decrease over time.

Dysfunctional Grief

Dysfunctional grief has been described in multiple ways. Lindemann (1944) and a host of contemporary writers and researchers (APA, 2000; Bowlby, 1980; Cowles and Rodgers, 1991; Parkes, 1998; Stroebe et al., 2000) have emphasized normative and dysfunctional aspects of grief. In other words, up to some point, grief is *normal*, and beyond that point, grief is variously considered *dysfunctional, pathologic, complicated,* and more recently, *traumatic* (Horowitz et al., 1997; Jacobs, Mazure, and Prigerson, 2000; Stroebe et al., 2000). Posttraumatic stress disorder (PTSD) is sometimes a feature of dysfunctional grief (Kemp, 1998; Melhem et al., 2001). If depression is the predominant feature of bereavement and is incapacitating 2 months after the loss, the client may be diagnosed as having a major depressive disorder (APA, 2000).

Although there is considerable debate about the details of exactly what constitutes dysfunctional grief, all sources refer to essentially the same phenomenon when describing dysfunctional grief: grief that lasts longer and is characterized by greater disability or other dysfunctional patterns than usual as defined by cultural values. In addition, recent studies (e.g., Piper et al., 2001) have identified levels of severity of dysfunctional grief.

Types of dysfunctional grief (APA, 2000; Hospice and Palliative Nurses Association [HPNA], 1997; Jacobs, Mazure, and Prigerson, 2000; Kemp, 1999; Silverman, Johnson, and Prigerson, 2001; Stroebe, et al., 2000; Parkes, 1998) include:

- *Traumatic grief,* which occurs when there is traumatic loss such as a spouse murdered, a child dying suddenly and unexpectedly, rape, or multiple deaths.

CLINICAL ALERT

The following increase a client's potential for developing dysfunctional grief:

- Premorbid psychiatric history or history of psychosocial trauma
- Social isolation
- Relationship with the deceased that was characterized by unresolved conflict, ambivalence (e.g., "love-hate")
- Relationship with the deceased that was characterized by enmeshment and a high level of introjection, hence difficulty "letting go"
- Person who suppresses grief
- Young age

PTSD is often a concurrent or complicating factor, and the grief/PTSD may be characterized by psychic numbing, intrusive thoughts, avoidance of stimuli, increased arousal, and other aspects of PTSD (Melhem et al., 2001). There may also be distortion, usually exaggeration, of one or more normative components of grief, with anger and guilt being most common. As noted previously the term *traumatic grief* is used by some (e.g., Jacobs et al., 2000) to refer to pathologic or dysfunctional grief.

- *Absent or inhibited grief,* which is characterized by minimal emotional expression of grief and is sometimes related to trauma as noted previously. Absent grief may convert to **delayed grief** and thus be experienced years after the loss. Precipitating factors for conversion to delayed grief often are powerful experiences such as psychotherapy or religious conversion.
- *Conflicted grief,* which may occur when the relationship with the deceased or lost object is characterized by ambivalence or conflict. Initial responses to the loss may be minimal and then intensify rather than diminish over time, and the survivor may feel "haunted" by the deceased. An adult survivor of childhood sexual abuse whose abusing parent dies is an example of a person at risk for conflicted grief.
- *Chronic grief,* which is unending grief after a loss. Chronic grief may be related to the survivor and the deceased having a highly dependent relationship. In other cases chronic grief is a result of (1) severe loss and (2) lack of resources or support to deal with the loss. Chronic grief may be especially common in some cultural groups such as Cambodian refugees or Native-Americans.

In general, dysfunctional grief is associated with unresolved issues in the relationship with the person who died; inhibited expression of grief; lack of social support; the "deritualization" of Western culture (e.g., mourning periods of 1 or 2 days); uncertain loss (e.g., prisoners of war); traumatic loss (e.g., by murder); multiple losses; loss that is seldom discussed (e.g., rape); undervalued loss such as that

felt by some who have had an abortion, miscarriage, or other losses that may not be recognized by others as significant; and by the accumulated effects of current grief on past unresolved grief (Ackley, 2002; Parkes, 2001).

Chronic Sorrow

Chronic sorrow is a form of grief that may include characteristics of other forms of grief but differs in several essential aspects. First, chronic sorrow is a response to *ongoing* loss such as the chronic illness of a loved one. Second, persons experiencing chronic sorrow seldom experience disability such as major depression but typically function at a higher level in activities of daily living than those experiencing other forms of grief (Burke et al., 1992). Persons at risk for chronic sorrow include parents with children who have mental retardation, schizophrenia, or other chronic illness; spouses of persons with long-term chronic illnesses such as multiple sclerosis, alcoholism, or Alzheimer's disease; and persons with similar disorders (Lichtenstein, Laska, and Clair, 2002; Pejlert, 2001; Lindgren, 1996). Still undocumented are the effects on the grief process that result when the etiology of chronic sorrow is removed (i.e., when the disabled person dies).

Grief and Depression

Grief and depression are often compared with one another. Grief, especially dysfunctional grief, also shares characteristics with PTSD, particularly in that both invariably involve loss (Table 25-1).

BEREAVEMENT CARE ACROSS THE LIFE SPAN
Prevention
Before Loss

Grief is a universal experience that may come with or without warning and occurs many times and with varying intensity throughout life. The major psychosocial determinants of pathology in grief are a psychiatric history before the loss and inadequate social support (Silverman, Johnson, and Prigerson, 2001). It follows, then, that grief is best addressed by the primary promotion of mental health, such as family involvement in community and faith activities, improved parenting, and other such efforts to promote mental and spiritual health.

When Loss Is Impending

A second point at which health promotion or disability prevention should be considered in relation to grief work is in the case of terminal illness or other anticipated loss. Interventions in these situations include assisting individuals and families in working toward personal, interpersonal, and spiritual reconciliation—and not necessarily anticipatory grief. Even in the best of relationships, there may be unresolved issues or areas in which growth is possible, and whether or

Table 25-1	Comparison of Grief, Depression, and Posttraumatic Stress Disorder	
Grief	**Depression**	**Posttraumatic Stress Disorder**
Process related to loss.	Relatively static or cyclic affective disorder not necessarily related to loss.	Relatively static anxiety disorder related to trauma. Precipitating event is outside the range of usual human experience.
Symptoms usually appear shortly after the loss.	Symptoms may or may not be associated with an identified loss.	Symptoms often appear years after the trauma.
Depressive symptoms include dysphoric mood of sadness, hopelessness, and despair; anger is common, as are periods of agitation.	Depressive symptoms are similar to but more intense than grief, except that anger is seldom expressed and psychomotor retardation, morbid guilt, and suicidal ideation are more common.	Depressive symptoms are common. Other symptoms include persistent reexperiencing of the trauma (vs preoccupation with the image of the deceased, as in grief). Increased arousal is common.
Physical symptoms cover a wide spectrum. Physical sequelae may include heart disease and other chronic illness.	Physical symptoms are primarily neurovegetative.	Sleep disturbances may resemble those of grief or depression; hypervigilance is common.
Spiritual beliefs may provide meaning or context.	Spiritual beliefs seldom provide context or meaning.	Seldom any relation to spiritual beliefs.

not interpersonal issues are addressed, promoting health in this stage of life includes promoting participation of the *client and family* in care. Clearly, effective participation in care has a positive effect on the grief process after death (although long-term effects are not known for caregivers in Alzheimer's disease, schizophrenia, and other similar chronic illnesses). A variety of means exist for intervention at this point, including individual informal or formal counseling in acute care settings, family support groups, hospice care, and spiritual support. Nurses and other health care professionals should address the health needs of family members, as well as those of clients (see Understanding and Applying Research box).

Preventive grief therapy is offered as a matter of course to survivors in several circumstances. For example, hospice and palliative care programs typically offer bereavement calls or visits at specified intervals to survivors. Many hospice programs also periodically hold seminars and other events or activities for bereaved adults or children. Churches and synagogues hold grief workshops for members and others in the community. These are generally weekend or time-limited groups similar to self-help groups such as I Can Cope and others. Religiously oriented grief activities are also held in some cases in association with significant religious holidays related to death or remembrance.

After the Loss

The third intervention point is after the loss occurs (**postvention**). Intervention at this point may be preventive and directed toward addressing existing problems that are interpersonal in nature or related to normative or dysfunctional grief. The tasks in grief (see earlier discussion) provide a framework for intervention after loss.

UNDERSTANDING and APPLYING RESEARCH

The purpose of this grounded theory study was to explore the experiences of family caregivers after admission of a spouse to a long-term care facility. Although the study was done in Sweden, the experiences of the family carers were clearly universal and thus the study is universally applicable. There is sweetness and sadness in this study. It is about love—where there is nearly always sweetness and sadness; but here the story is about love and loss. Can we research such things? Yes, we can and should.

Placing a loved one in a long-term care facility is often a rather sudden move for which there is little preparation. The move/separation is permanent; and is a highly emotional experience, entailing sadness, loneliness, and isolation. In many cases, the loss and loneliness are largely unacknowledged by formal and informal support networks. It is common for both spouses to attempt to continue their relationship with one another and to create new roles and relationships with facility staff. Also common is for both spouses to hide their anxiety and grief from one another.

"It's more important than anything to me that Olaf is comfortable... as comfortable as he can be...because he has given me so much in life..."

Carers work toward "keeping"—"keeping in touch" and "keeping it special" with the spouse in the facility; and "keeping an eye" on the facility. Relations with the facility are critically important and, unfortunately, not always characterized by equality and openness to communication from the carers.

The authors discuss opportunities for intervention including preparation for and assistance with the decision and move, recognition of and assistance with the emotional distress, and creation of a warm and welcoming environment that encourages and supports an active role for the carers. Strangely, the authors do not directly discuss grief. Yet grief is what the study is about and the authors find the very heart of it in a lovely manner. Can we say that research is lovely? Not often. But this time we can.

Sandberg J, Lundh U, Nolan MR: Placing a spouse in a care home: the importance of keeping, *J Clin Nurs* 10: 406, 2001.

Problem-Oriented Grief Therapy

Grief therapy is offered when a problem—not necessarily dysfunctional grief—exists or is anticipated. Like other of life's unavoidable processes, the difficult and painful transitions in normative grief usually respond to understanding and support. Grief therapy often focuses on emotional responses to the loss and problem solving related to moving forward in life (i.e., undoing bonds of attachment) (Parkes, 2001; Worden, 1982) or finding or reconstructing meaning in the loss or relationship (Neimeyer, 2001).

Emotional issues center around the telling and retelling of the details of the story (of the death and surrounding issues) and the history of the relationship, with emphasis on the experience and expression of the feelings, particularly sadness, anger, guilt, or other troubling feelings (Carpenito, 2002). In earlier phases of the process, the bereaved person may recall only the positive qualities of the deceased. As the mourner progresses through the grief work, both positive and negative qualities of the deceased and the relationship emerge. Problem-focused strategies may address questions of developing support, relationships, and other issues inherent in "the new life" or life after a loved one dies. Family-oriented therapy focuses on improving communications, increasing cohesiveness, and enhancing problem solving (Kissane et al., 1998).

In response to frequent overuse of medications to mask grief, some practitioners discourage the use of anxiolytic or antidepressant medications for bereaved persons. However, even in cases of normal grief, mourners may require short-term use of these medications at certain stages of the grief process. Selective serotonin reuptake inhibitors are the mainstay of therapy in most settings and for most problems of grief, including dysfunctional grief (Casarett, Kutner, and Abrahm, 2001).

Reassurance is an essential component in grief therapy. The absence of cultural norms for expressing or otherwise dealing with grief results in some people feeling as if their grief is the beginning of insanity. Although some will not initially believe it, they need to hear from the nurse that their experience is grief and is normal and not mental illness. The tasks in grief, described earlier, provide a framework for therapy.

Interventions in Dysfunctional Grief

In dysfunctional grief there is often unresolved grief from the past and/or a preexisting psychologic condition that must be addressed as part of the grief therapy. Thus therapy includes the issues noted previously and other interpersonal issues. Often, a central issue in dysfunctional grief is the promotion of the client's ability to express the pain of the grief rather than only the anger or guilt (Ackley, 2002; Carpenito, 2002). It is common for bereaved persons to have ill-defined fantasies of catastrophe if their pain is expressed: "If I ever start crying, I will never stop." Clients with dysfunctional grief are at increased risk for suicide or, to a lesser extent, for hurting others. They may also experience

UNDERSTANDING and APPLYING RESEARCH

The purpose of the clinical investigation was to examine the prevalence of significant loss through the death of another person as well as complicated (or dysfunctional) grief among psychiatric outpatients. Of 729 patients questioned about losses, 55% had suffered the loss of one or more (average three) loved one(s) in their lifetimes. Of these, 235 or about 33% met the criteria for moderate (17%) or severe (16%) complicated grief. Criteria included intrusion or avoidance of loss stimuli, pathologic grief, grief anxiety, and general symptomatic distress. Compared with other psychiatric outpatients, including those who had suffered the loss of loved ones, those with severe complicated grief had significantly higher levels of depression, anxiety, and general symptomatic distress; 33% positive findings in any physical or mental pathology or symptomatology is highly significant. Questions about loss are uncommon in psychiatric interviews, as are patient complaints about loss. Implications of this study include need for loss and grief assessment among psychiatric patients, cost-effective means of treating complicated grief, and preventive measures among bereaved persons.

Piper WE, Ogrodniczuk JS, Azim HF, Weideman R: Prevalence of loss and dysfunctional grief among psychiatric outpatients, *Psychiatr Serv* 52:1069, 2001.

CLINICAL ALERT

The likelihood of suicide attempts and completion is increased in grief, especially dysfunctional grief. The loss of psychosocial support systems is especially significant for men. Sustained loss of self-esteem, blaming self for the death, and ambivalence about living indicate that suicide risk is markedly increased.

physical and mental disorders as previously discussed (see Understanding and Applying Research box).

The client's primary physician, nurse practitioner, or other source of primary health care should be involved or at least kept aware of treatment for several specific reasons. First, it is common for such clients to frequently seek medical care, often for vague or difficult-to-evaluate complaints that are actually somatic expressions of grief. Awareness of dysfunctional grief and ongoing therapy may help health care providers avoid unnecessary tests and treatment. Second, there is significant risk of suicide in dysfunctional grief, and an informed health care provider can be alert to suicidal hints, gestures, and attempts to obtain lethal amounts of medications. All health care professionals involved in the care of a person with dysfunctional grief should be alert to the possibility of the client's seeking help from multiple sources and the potential for lethal medication admixture.

SPIRITUALITY AND GRIEF

All basic spiritual needs or issues may be threatened by the grief experience: meaning, hope, relatedness, forgiveness, and transcendence may fall away and leave the mourner in a

NURSING ASSESSMENT QUESTIONS
Persons Experiencing Grief

1. Describe how it has been for you since [your husband] died.
2. How have you reacted to other major losses in your life?
3. Whom do you depend on when you are having a hard time, like now? Talk about how it is when you ask for help.
4. Let's go over all the prescription and other medicine and vitamins you are taking.

5. How often do you have alcoholic drinks (or other drugs)? When you drink (take drugs), how much do you take, and how does it make you feel?

A question not to ask is, "How are you doing?" Cultural norms are to respond to such questions with "pretty good," "OK," or "fine." These answers are essentially meaningless.

---

spiritual vacuum. The nature of God and previously held beliefs, including any easy answers to life's problems (e.g., that faith protects one from pain), are called into question and may not support the reality of the current feelings. Grief may then be experienced as a test of faith, and the awareness or acknowledgment of anger or other negative feelings may be interpreted as a personal spiritual failure (a source of more guilt).

Although dreams and visions are seen as significant spiritual events in some cultures, in the context of Western cultures they may be discounted as either immaterial or pathologic. There may be reluctance by the grieving individual to discuss these experiences and feelings with family, friends, or clergy. As mourners struggle to find a context for the doubt and confusion that may accompany these experiences, it is important for the nurse to listen with openness, determining how these experiences either confirm or challenge the mourner's spiritual and religious beliefs. Some individuals are confirmed in their traditional beliefs; others see the dissolution of their faith; some find or rediscover a deeper faith (see Chapter 5).

Grief has the potential to transform those who experience it, for better or worse. Grief can be an "invitation to a new life" in which the discontinuity of death/loss and grief can be taken to a "higher continuity" (Carse, 1980), or grief can be a context for retreat into an impoverished life. Interventions in grief are most efficacious when used to promote health and prevent dysfunction. Interventions are less efficacious in the postvention period and least efficacious in treating dysfunctional grief.

THE NURSING PROCESS

ASSESSMENT

Nursing assessment of a person who is bereaved is based on knowledge of normative and pathologic aspects of the grief process, influences on the grief process, and the person's resources. Assessment encompasses (1) the grief experience of the mourner; (2) factors that inhibit or promote working through the grief process, including cultural and religious norms; and (3) the mourner's ability to mobilize cognitive, behavioral, and emotion-based coping strategies. The client's current level of functioning should be assessed, with the understanding that up to a point (about which there is disagreement), impaired functioning is to be expected (see Nursing Assessment Question box).

Physical Disturbances

Physical disturbances in acute grief include weakness, anorexia, shortness of breath, tightness of the chest, dry mouth, and gastrointestinal disturbances such as constipation or diarrhea, abdominal pain, gas, and nausea and vomiting. Cardiovascular and gastrointestinal problems predominate in chronic grief. Vague physical complaints such as unfocused abdominal pain or shortness of breath are especially common in all stages and types of grief.

Cognitive Disturbances

Cognitive disturbances are often focused on preoccupation with images and thoughts of the deceased. This preoccupation may be so pervasive that the bereaved person is unable to carry on with some activities of daily living. The inability to control thoughts is distressing to many mourners. In acute grief these obsessive thoughts are normal; they are simply part of the process. Preoccupation that results in significant disturbance of daily life (e.g., work) is widely considered pathologic after about 1 year past the date of death when the person who died was an adult and 2 or more years past the date of death when the deceased was a child.

Behavioral and Relating Disturbances

Behavioral and relating disturbances may result from the depressive aspects of grief. People who are bereaved may describe themselves as "stopped" and thus unable to participate in relationships (see Case Study on p. 582). There is a tendency in survivors to ruminate about the death and the relationship with the deceased. In at least the earlier phases of the process, talk of the deceased tends to focus only on his or her "good" qualities and ignore the multifaceted nature of the individual. Many people who are bereaved cry with little apparent provocation, which often results in discomfort for the mourner and others. In chronic grief the talk of the death and the relationship tends to be repetitive and superficial rather than progressive and insightful.

CASE STUDY

Mrs. Jones is 70 years old and lives alone in the apartment she shared with her husband for the past 17 years since retirement. Her husband died last month, after a 2-year struggle with prostate cancer. Since her husband's death, Mrs. Jones has felt sad and depressed. She wants to spend time with others but says, "They are happy, and I'm sad, and it's no good for anyone." For the past week, except for "forcing" herself to take her daily walk around the block, Mrs. Jones has spent most of her time alone in her apartment. She has a poor appetite, difficulty sleeping, and feels guilty about "all the things I could have done to help my husband." Most of the other residents in the complex are similar in age to Mrs. Jones, and she is very close to several of them. Her only son lives in another state and has offered to let her move into a bedroom in his home.

Critical Thinking

1. According to your assessment, what type of grief is Mrs. Jones experiencing?
2. From your knowledge of the grieving process, what are three important needs of Mrs. Jones?
3. What personal resources are likely to be most helpful to Mrs. Jones at the present time?

COLLABORATIVE DIAGNOSES

DSM-IV-TR Diagnoses*	Nursing Diagnoses†
Adjustment disorder	Impaired adjustment
Dysthymic disorder	Disabled family coping
Major depressive disorder	Ineffective individual coping
	Ineffective denial
	Interrupted family processes
	Fatigue
	Anticipatory grieving
	Dysfunctional grieving
	Hopelessness
	Disturbed personal identity
	Post-trauma syndrome
	Powerlessness
	Ineffective role performance
	Situational low self-esteem
	Ineffective sexuality patterns
	Disturbed sleep pattern
	Impaired social interaction
	Social isolation
	Chronic sorrow
	Spiritual distress
	Disturbed thought processes
	Risk for other-directed violence
	Risk for self-directed violence

*From American Psychiatric Association: *Diagnostic and Statistical Manual of Mental Disorders,* Fourth Edition, Text Revision. Washington, DC, American Psychiatric Association, 2000.
†From NANDA International (2003). NANDA Nursing Diagnoses: Definitions and Classification 2003-2004. Philadelphia: NANDA.

Affective Disturbances

Affective disturbances are primarily those of sadness or depression, anger, and guilt. Cultural norms of "carrying on" inhibit expression of these feelings. People who are bereaved soon learn that "nobody wants to hear your sad story." Sadness and even feelings of depression are not considered pathologic unless they persist a year or two past the death or include suicidal ideation.

NURSING DIAGNOSIS

Nursing diagnosis of grief or problems occurring in grief may be dysfunctional by the more common approach of identifying problems of a physical or psychologic nature and seeking to alleviate the discomfort. The grief process by itself includes discomfort, and attempts to avoid or eliminate the discomfort, no matter how well intentioned, may impede the grieving process. On the other hand, extreme discomfort may require pharmacologic intervention. The point at which discomfort is classified as extreme or abnormal versus normal has not been defined. Thus an insightful diagnosis may focus on the *expression* of normal feelings (e.g., anger, guilt, sadness) as much as on what feelings exist (see Collaborative Diagnoses table).

Nursing Diagnoses for Acute Grief

- Disturbed personal identity related to change in role and relationships, as evidenced by the inability to establish new patterns of relating to others and the environment after the death of a spouse or loved one
- Situational low self-esteem related to pervasive feelings of guilt and cognitive distortions secondary to guilt, as evidenced by ruminating about inadequacies in the relationship with the deceased and blaming self for all problems in the relationship

- Impaired social interaction related to altered role performance and disruptions in usual patterns of conduct/ interactions, as evidenced by difficulty in adapting to life changes and developing relationships according to the current situation

Nursing Diagnoses for Dysfunctional Grief

- Dysfunctional grieving related to unresolved guilt, as evidenced by frequent references to personal failings in the relationship with the deceased
- Dysfunctional grieving (unexpressed) related to fear of catastrophe if grief is expressed, as evidenced by absence of expression of feelings related to the grief process
- Risk for self-directed violence. Risk factors: feelings of hopelessness and anger and reports and observed incidents of rage over perceived inability to live without the deceased

Nursing Diagnoses for Chronic Sorrow

- Chronic sorrow related to effects of the death of a loved one or experiences of chronic physical or mental illness or disability (e.g., Alzheimer's disease, schizophrenia, mental retardation, cancer), as evidenced by recurring feelings of sadness and grief that vary in intensity over time and may interfere with the person's ability to reach the highest level of personal and social well-being
- Caregiver role strain related to chronic sorrow, as evidenced by caregiver withdrawal from community life to care for a loved one with chronic schizophrenia

OUTCOME IDENTIFICATION

Outcome criteria focus on enhancement of emotional coping skills or methods (e.g., greater expression of feelings of grief) and cognitive and behavioral coping abilities (e.g., strategies to develop more functional patterns of living, appropriate to changed life circumstances).

Client will:

- Verbalize absence of suicidal ideations.
- Express guilty and/or angry feelings related to the death and grief versus suppression of grief.
- Express both positive and negative feelings about the deceased versus idealizing the qualities of the deceased.
- Explore the relationship with the deceased in a multifaceted way that includes both positive and negative aspects.
- Formulate and implement reasonable plans for adapting life and the identified role to present circumstances.
- Participate in at least one social or community activity each week.

PLANNING

The plan of care for a person with acute grief consists primarily of (1) supporting mobilization of the person's personal and community resources, (2) providing normative data about the grief process, and (3) supporting the person in her or his grief work (see Case Study). Each of these is discussed next.

Assistance may be needed in mobilizing resources (e.g., family, friends, and spiritual supports), because individuals often are reluctant to ask for help and resources often do not know how to provide help. In addition, some of the symptoms of grief (e.g., fatigue, sadness, and anger) promote isolation rather than relating. Frequently, if either the bereaved person or his or her support systems can initiate contact, the other will respond appropriately. Too often, however, the mourner and resources exist in isolation, each wishing they knew how to make contact with the other.

Normative data on grief (i.e., explanation of physical, emotional, social, and spiritual difficulties inherent in the grief process) can be provided to both the bereaved and his or her support systems. In a culture in many ways lacking in ritual and tradition, grief may sometimes seem mysterious

CASE STUDY

Mr. and Mrs. Mason have a 26-year-old son, Jim, who has chronic undifferentiated schizophrenia. Jim lives at home most of the year, except when he is admitted to the state hospital (two or three times a year). Jim has never worked, has no friends, is withdrawn most of the time, has violent episodes about once a month, and is noncompliant with medications. The Masons have tried different hospitals (but now they no longer have insurance coverage for Jim), a variety of antipsychotic medications, different therapists, prayer, and alternative therapies, but nothing has changed the course of the illness. Mr. Mason works long hours at an auto parts store, and Mrs. Mason stays home with Jim. Mr. and Mrs. Mason have begun seeing the clinical nurse specialist from the state hospital community outreach program. Their chief complaints as a couple and individually are overwhelming feelings of hopelessness and physical and mental exhaustion. The clinical nurse specialist has diagnosed their problem as caregiver role strain related to chronic sorrow, as evidenced by the caregivers' withdrawal from community life to care for their son with chronic schizophrenia. The nurse has implemented a plan of care that includes (1) weekly couples' counseling, (2) regular family support group in a community facility, and (3) biweekly home visits by an outreach staff member to assist Jim with medication compliance.

Critical Thinking

1. What is your opinion about whether Jim will experience significant improvement in his disorder?
2. Part of the care is directed to the parents. Why are they also receiving care instead of Jim alone, as he is the one who is mentally ill? What might happen with Jim if his parents are no longer able to cope?
3. Discuss potential success in relation to this plan. Are the Masons likely to achieve happiness as a result of receiving care?
4. Discuss each of the following feelings that family members sometimes experience about relatives with chronic mental illness: anger, sorrow, love, disgust, and despair.

and/or pathologic even to those one might expect to be helpful (e.g., clergy). The nurse teaches survivors and others (such as family members) what they might experience in the grief process. Bereavement (survivor) groups are an excellent forum for such teaching.

Supporting the mourner in his or her grief work includes facilitating the telling of how the deceased died and related events and exploring both positive and negative aspects of the relationship with the deceased, positive and negative aspects of the deceased, and cognitive and behavioral coping strategies. Assistance with mobilizing resources and providing normative data is also part of support.

The plan of care for a person with dysfunctional grieving focuses on the specific pathologic condition of the client. Normative aspects of grief are also addressed.

Plans can also be directed toward the community. In community-focused planning the nurse helps churches, synagogues, community centers, hospitals, and other organizations develop self-help groups for bereaved persons. Nurses also serve as facilitators for such groups (see Nursing Care in the Community box on p. 584).

NURSING CARE IN THE COMMUNITY Grief and Loss

Grief and loss may be encountered anywhere in the community. The aging wife may be losing her husband after years of declining health, the young person with schizophrenia may feel the loss of hope for the future, or the mature adult may experience unexpected unemployment. Each person perceives the world as changing dramatically without the prospect of immediate stabilization. The mental health nurse in the community responds to each of these crises with both compassion and practicality. The nurse must assess the client's need to voice emotional pain or to maintain silence. Expressing emotional empathy with the client and acknowledging the pain are not unprofessional as long as the nurse maintains emotional objectivity.

During the initial grief reaction the nurse should encourage expression of memory and emotion. The nurse may also assess the individual's ability to tolerate difficult emotions and use prescribed medication, if appropriate, while assisting the individual in adapting to change and loss. The nurse needs to be sensitive to both the client and the support network to gauge how much intervention is necessary and can be tolerated.

The community is an ideal environment to support the grieving process. The community mental health nurse can ensure that referrals to appropriate support groups are accessed, as well as offer individual comfort and assistance. Rituals that are performed and expressed by cultural preferences should be respected and encouraged. Spiritual counselors such as clergy may be used to offer the client comfort, sustenance, and ceremony for grief.

The time of grieving varies widely among individuals, so the concept of well-delineated, consecutive stages may need to be individualized. Some individuals have difficulty focusing on grieving, and for them the process seems to take longer. A person may appear to have returned to a normal, pregrief state, but still feel numb and anguished inside. The nurse assists by acknowledging the length of the process and educating the family and community to also respect the time necessary for the client's recovery.

The nurse should allow at least a year of follow-up care with both the client and support system to evaluate the client's level of function, food consumption, and sleep patterns. Depending on cultural and other factors (e.g., manner of death), if the client is dysfunctional and depressed for more than 3 to 6 months, the grief may have become pathologic, and thoughts of suicide should be explored. If there are substantial concerns and the client appears to be clinically depressed, the client should be referred to a psychiatrist and may require hospitalization and medication. After a significant loss, client safety is always of major concern.

IMPLEMENTATION

The first priority in planning care for a person with dysfunctional grief is to assess the risk for violence toward self or others. The client's physical health may also be a major concern. The plan includes efforts to work toward resolving the grief through emotional, cognitive, and behavioral means. Chemical dependency presents a major barrier to the individual's goal attainment and must be addressed. Dependence on anxiolytic medications is common. In many cases the approach can be growth oriented rather than directed only to treatment of symptoms.

Nursing Interventions

Bereavement care should ideally take place in the community before the client deteriorates to the extent that hospitalization is required.

1. Assess the client for intent to kill self or others *to ensure safety and prevent violence.*
2. Promote a therapeutic alliance between the client and the nurse. *Developing a working relationship may be difficult because of the client's suppressed feelings. Death and other major losses are often experienced as complete destruction of the certainty and order around which people structure their lives. It is therefore necessary for the nurse to be certain and orderly with respect to following through on all obligations such as schedules and appointments.*
3. Facilitate the client's expression of feelings related to the loss, and validate the feelings already expressed by the client. Also, begin to introduce the possibility of other feelings related to the loss, such as ambivalence. Help the client take an increasingly active role in exploring and understanding the full response to the grief. *Ambivalent feelings are especially difficult for many clients to acknowledge. Many clients are prone to merely repeat feelings and thoughts rather than explore, expand, and understand them. Although some repetition of feelings, concerns, and experiences is unavoidable and somewhat helpful, it is important for the client to understand the full grief response to begin the healing process.*
4. Help the client understand the relationship between self and the lost person or object and to express and understand the grief and attendant feelings. Facilitate a review of the client's relationship with the deceased, and help the client to discuss and understand meanings within the relationship, hopes fulfilled, disappointments, and strengths and weaknesses of the relationship. *It is essential that the client move beyond the grief that is related to the death or loss and begin to understand the full meaning of the relationship, both good and bad.*
5. Facilitate the full expression of grief by assisting the client in linking together the full spectrum of feelings, both positive and negative, regarding the loss and the relationship with the deceased. *It is necessary for the client to remember the deceased as a real human being with both positive and negative qualities, to "let go" of the idealistic image of the person, and begin to move forward without guilt and remorse. Some survivors are more successful at this than others.*
6. Promote interactions with others and offer limited and specific options for the client to increase **social**

NURSING CARE PLAN

Mr. Smith and his wife had been married for 41 years when she died 18 months ago from bacterial endocarditis. Since his wife's death, Mr. Smith has become increasingly seclusive. He expresses extreme anger toward the physicians and nurses involved in his wife's care. Mr. Smith keeps his home exactly as it was when Mrs. Smith was alive. He has not disposed of any of her belongings and has renewed subscriptions to magazines that only Mrs. Smith read. Both Mr. and Mrs. Smith drank heavily but denied alcoholism. They had no children, and their relationship was characterized by frequent verbal and occasional physical abuse. Mr. Smith continues to drink daily. He complains of heart problems and is angry with his physician, who insists that Mr. Smith has only mild hypertension that should respond to dietary changes. Mr. Smith has begun keeping his curtains drawn and denies the need for interpersonal relationships.

DSM-IV-TR Diagnoses

Axis I	Major depression; alcoholism
Axis II	None known
Axis III	Hypertension
Axis IV	Problem with primary support group (death of spouse)
	Problem related to the social environment (living alone)
Axis V	GAF = 45 (current)
	GAF = 45 (past year)

NURSING DIAGNOSIS: Dysfunctional grieving (chronic distorted) related to inability to appropriately express the full spectrum of feelings associated with wife's death, as evidenced by social isolation, projected danger, daily alcohol use, and somatic complaints.

CLIENT OUTCOMES	NURSING INTERVENTIONS	EVALUATION
Mr. Smith will engage in a therapeutic alliance with the nurse.	Visit Mr. Smith's home at a regular time on the same day once each week. *Constancy and dependability are essential in developing productive relationships.*	Mr. Smith agrees to visits.
Mr. Smith will cease intake of alcohol at least 4 hours before and during visits with nurse.	Develop a contract with Mr. Smith in which he agrees to sobriety during visits. *Sobriety is essential to therapeutic relationships and personal growth.*	Mr. Smith maintains sobriety during visits.
	Institute chemical dependency care plan (see Chapter 13).	Mr. Smith enters and continues in a 12-step or other program intended to promote sobriety.
Mr. Smith will express angry, sad, and other feelings concerning his wife's death.	Gradually present Mr. Smith with aspects of his grief experience that will help him uncover his sadness and ambivalence. *Feelings of sadness and ambivalence are threatening to Mr. Smith and should not be introduced too rapidly.*	Mr. Smith is able to express sadness, confusion, ambivalence, and other feelings in addition to anger.
	Recognize the legitimacy of Mr. Smith's anger. Demonstrate acceptance and understanding of the ambivalence and other feelings such as sadness and confusion. *Anger is the means by which Mr. Smith may be expressing other feelings not yet in his awareness. Facilitating other feelings helps to better manage anger and promote resolution of grief.*	Mr. Smith begins to accept the validity of anger and feelings other than anger that may be hidden behind the expression of anger and rage.
Mr. Smith will discuss his hopes (fulfilled and unfulfilled) and his disappointments about his relationship with his wife.	Assist Mr. Smith in reviewing his relationship with his wife, and the hopes each one held, including those fulfilled and those that led to disappointments. *Although Mr. Smith's problems are attributed to his wife's death, they are also, to a great extent, attributable to his relationship with his wife and his difficulty coping with the loss of his wife.*	Mr. Smith discusses his relationship with his wife in realistic terms (neither idealized nor all negative) and expresses both positive and negative feelings about their relationship.
Mr. Smith will grieve in a functional manner for his wife, for their relationship, and for himself.	Facilitate Mr. Smith's linking together all of his feelings and responses related to his relationship with his wife, to his life, and to his current dysfunctional behavior. *This is the full expression of grief.*	Mr. Smith fully expresses his grief.

Continued

support, both individually and in the community. Encourage the client to continue engaging in social relationships—even when, as some mourners say, it feels as if "it's just going through the motions." *It is important for the client to begin to move forward and "join the living," even if it means "going through the motions" at first. With encouragement from family and friends, the client should eventually develop a healthy social life while experiencing (in a healthy sense) both good and bad memories of the deceased.*

NURSING CARE PLAN—cont'd

NURSING DIAGNOSIS: Social isolation related to seclusive behavior patterns secondary to unresolved grief, as evidenced by refusal to engage in interpersonal relationships.

CLIENT OUTCOMES	NURSING INTERVENTIONS	EVALUATION
Mr. Smith will agree to regular visits in his home with the nurse.	Adhere to 30-minute limit for visits; be prompt according to schedule. *Structure in care increases order, understanding, and predictability and will help promote Mr. Smith's developing cognitive coping strategies, such as making realistic plans for the future.*	Mr. Smith tolerates visits and eventually remarks that he looks forward to them.
Mr. Smith participates in one social activity weekly. (Alcohol should not be served or available.)	Give Mr. Smith choices of time-limited social activities that are likely to be enjoyable and convenient for him. *Activities that are enjoyable and sociable are more likely to be repeated; too many choices are likely to be overwhelming; time limits will reduce anxiety.*	Mr. Smith follows through and attends activities, and expresses a favorable response.
Mr. Smith participates in the termination phase of the relationship by increasing his social activities and continuing in his recovery from alcoholism.	Include Mr. Smith in plans for termination by working with him to make plans for increased social activity as the relationship is terminated. Together, the nurse and Mr. Smith should write a schedule for termination that decreases the frequency of visits and ultimately ends the visits. *The therapeutic alliance progresses from collaboration between the nurse and client to the client's achieving independence.*	Mr. Smith (1) participates in planning for termination, (2) initiates additional social activities, and (3) continues in his recovery.

CLIENT AND FAMILY TEACHING GUIDELINES

There is little tradition related to grief in this contemporary technologic society. It is therefore extremely helpful to provide persons who are bereaved with normative data about grief. This should include common:

- Physical responses to grief
- Cognitive responses to grief
- Behavioral responses to grief
- Affective responses to grief

It is helpful to write a list of grief reactions (in layperson's terms) and review the list with the person who is bereaved. The power or intensity of feelings in response to loss is especially important to discuss with the bereaved person.

Collaborative Interventions

A multidisciplinary approach by a team consisting of nurse, psychiatrist, psychologist, social worker, occupational therapist, and other health care providers is not usually necessary, although community resources are an important part of care. Because of the frequency and vagueness of physical complaints, the most important discipline other than nursing is the client's nurse practitioner or physician or other source of primary care.

EVALUATION

The nurse evaluates the client's increasing ability to express feelings and to develop effective coping strategies such as increasing social interactions. It is important for the client to express the full spectrum of feelings that are (1) associated with the loss and (2) related to the relationship with the deceased. Expressing feelings only about the loss itself is not sufficient for successful progress in grief work (see Client and Family Teaching Guidelines box). The nurse should remember that grief is a normal response to loss and that the feelings associated with grief are necessarily painful. The key to successful grief work depends on the individual's understanding of the relationship with the deceased. When that occurs, the client is able to continue the work of investing in new relationships.

CHAPTER SUMMARY

- Grief encompasses all spheres of being. Symptoms include physical, cognitive, behavioral, and affective reactions.
- Although grief is commonly presented in stages, it is more effective to conceptualize grief in terms of a dynamic process in which certain tasks are usually accomplished.
- Grief may be classified as acute, anticipatory, dysfunctional or pathologic, and as chronic sorrow. Types of dysfunctional grief include traumatic grief, absent or inhibited grief, conflicted grief, and chronic grief.
- The potential for dysfunctional grief is decreased in situations where clients have a healthy family life, provide care for the person who is dying, participate in community-oriented bereavement programs, and re-

ceive therapy if they are at risk. Therapy for persons experiencing dysfunctional grief includes facilitating expression of suppressed feelings, mobilizing cognitive and behavioral coping skills, dealing with unresolved aspects of the relationship, and encouraging reentry into socialization and meaning.

REVIEW QUESTIONS

1. A woman who continues to become tearful and has difficulty verbalizing her feelings of sadness with visual reminders of her father who died 11 years ago from a heart attack is experiencing:
   a. Anticipatory grieving
   b. Traumatic grief
   c. Absent grief
   d. Chronic grief

2. A client was just told that he had liver cancer. He states, "I can't believe this is happening to me. I lost my mother to cancer. I can't go through what she went through." The highest priority nursing diagnosis is:
   a. Anticipatory grieving
   b. Ineffective coping
   c. Ineffective denial
   d. Risk for self-directed violence

3. A mother brings her 4-year-old son to the Emergency Department after a car hit him. The doctor tells the mother that her son could not be saved. The highest priority nursing intervention would be:
   a. Bring her to a room to be by herself.
   b. Explain all the medical interventions attempted.
   c. Stay with the client until a support person arrives.
   d. Give her referrals for a grief-counseling group.

4. A client is in the end stage of AIDS. Which statement by the client demonstrates that the client has come to terms with his death?
   a. "When am I going to feel better? I thought that this new research drug would work."
   b. "I'm not ready to go. I haven't done so many things."
   c. "I've made the necessary arrangements. I'm tired, but I'm ready to go."
   d. "I don't understand why this has to happen to me."

5. Grief therapy focuses on:
   a. Preventing the occurrence of anxiety and depression.
   b. Emotional responses to loss and problem solving related to moving forward in life.
   c. Preventing physical symptoms from occurring such as difficulty sleeping or eating or gastrointestinal disturbance.
   d. Discourages the client to express unresolved anger.

REFERENCES

Ackley BJ: Anticipatory grieving. In Ackley BJ, Ladwig GB, editors: *Nursing diagnosis handbook*, ed 5, St Louis, 2002, Mosby.

American Psychiatric Association: *Diagnostic and Statistical Manual of Mental Disorders*, Fourth Edition, Text Revision. Washington, DC, American Psychiatric Association, 2000.

Bowlby J: *Loss: sadness and depression,* vol 3, *Attachment and loss,* New York, 1980, Basic Books.

Burke ML et al: Current knowledge and research on chronic sorrow: a foundation for inquiry, *Death Studies* 16:231, 1992.

Carman MB: The psychology of normal aging, *Psychiatr Clin North Am* 20:15, 1997.

Carpenito LJ: *Nursing diagnosis: application to clinical practice*, Philadelphia, 2002, Lippincott.

Carse JB: *Death and existence,* New York, 1980, John Wiley & Sons.

Casarett D, Kutner JS, Abrahm J: Life after death: a practical approach to grief and bereavement, *Ann Intern Med* 134:208, 2001.

Charlton R et al: Spousal bereavement: implications for health, *Fam Pract* 18:614, 2001.

Cooley ME: Bereavement care: a role for nurses, *Cancer Nurs* 15:125, 1992.

Cowles KV, Rodgers BL: The concept of grief: a foundation for nursing research and practice, *Res Nurs Health* 14:119, 1991.

Engel G: Grief and grieving, *Am J Nurs* 64:93, 1964.

Freud S: Mourning and melancholia. In Strachey J, editor, *The standard edition of the complete psychological works of Sigmund Freud,* vol 14, London, 1917, Hogarth Press.

Gibbons MB: A child dies, a child survives: the impact of sibling loss, *J Pediatr Health Care* 6:65, 1992.

Goodman M et al: Cultural differences among elderly women in coping with the death of an adult child, *J Gerontol* 46:321, 1991.

Heffner JE, Byock IR: Palliative and end-of-life pearls, Philadelphia, 2002, Hanley & Belfus.

Hentz P: The body remembers: grieving and a circle of time, *Qual Health Res* 12:161, 2002.

Horowitz MJ et al: Diagnostic criteria for dysfunctional grief disorder, *Am J Psychiatry* 154:904, 1997.

Hospice and Palliative Nurses Association: *The hospice nurses study guide: a preparation for the CRNH candidate,* ed 2, Pittsburgh, 1997, The Association.

Jacob SR: The grief experience of older women whose husbands had hospice care, *J Adv Nurs* 24:280, 1996.

Jacobs S, Mazure C, Prigerson H: Diagnostic criteria for traumatic grief, *Death Studies* 24:185, 2000.

Kemp C, Chang B-J: Culture and the end of life: Chinese, *J Hospice Palliative Nursing* 4:1, 2002.

Kemp C: Refugee mental health issues, *Refugee health*, web site: www.baylor.edu/~Charles_Kemp/refugee_health.htm, 1998.

Kemp C: *Terminal illness: a guide to nursing care,* ed 2, Philadelphia, 1999, Lippincott–Williams & Wilkins.

Kissane DW et al: Family grief therapy: a preliminary account of a new model to promote healthy family functioning during palliative care and bereavement, *Psycho-oncology* 7:14, 1994.

Kubler-Ross E: *On death and dying,* New York, 1969, Macmillan.

Lev EL, McCorkle R: Loss, grief, and bereavement in family members of cancer patients, *Semin Oncol Nurs* 14:145, 1998.

Levy LH: Anticipatory grief: its measurement and proposed reconceptualization, *Hosp J* 7:1, 1991.

Lichtenstein B, Laska MK, Clair JM: Chronic sorrow in the HIV-positive patient: issues of race, gender, and social support, *AIDS Patient Care STDS* 16:27, 2002.

Lindemann E: Symptomatology and management of acute grief, *Am J Psychiatry* 101:141, 1944.

Lindgren CL: Chronic sorrow in persons with Parkinson's disease and their spouses, *Sch Inq Nurs Pract* 10:351, 1996.

Melhem NM et al: Comorbidity of Axis I disorders in patients with traumatic grief, *J Clin Psychiatry* 62:884, 2001.

Neimeyer RA: Reauthoring life narratives: grief therapy as meaning reconstruction, *Isr J Psychiatry Relat Sci* 38:171, 2001.

Nuss WS, Zubenko GS: Correlates of persistent depressive symptoms in widows, *Am J Psychiatry* 149:346, 1992.

Parkes CM: Bereavement dissected: a re-examination of the basic components influencing the reaction to loss, *Isr J Psychiatry Relat Sci* 38:150, 2001.

Parkes CM: Bereavement. In Doyle D, Hanks GWC, MacDonald N, editors: *Oxford textbook of palliative medicine,* ed 2, Oxford, 1998, Oxford University Press.

Pejlert A: Being a parent of an adult son or daughter with severe mental illness receiving professional care: parents' narratives, *Health Soc Care Community* 9:194, 2001.

Piper WE et al: Prevalence of loss and dysfunctional grief among psychiatric outpatients, *Psychiatr Serv* 52:1069, 2001.

Rando TA: *Grieving,* Lexington, Mass, 1988, Lexington Books.

Reisman AS: Death of a spouse: illusory basic assumptions and continuation of bonds, *Death Studies* 23:445, 2001.

Ringdal GI et al: Factors affecting grief reactions in close family members to individuals who have died from cancer, *J Pain Symptom Manage* 22:1016, 2001.

Shneidman ES, *Voices of death,* New York, 1980, Harper & Row.

Silverman PR, Worden JW: Children's reactions in the early months after the death of a parent, *Am J Orthopsychiatry* 62:93, 1992.

Silverman GK, Johnson JG, Prigerson HG: Preliminary of the effects of prior trauma and loss on risk for psychiatric disorders in recently widowed people, *Isr J Psychiatry Relat Sci* 38:202, 2001.

Steen KF: A comprehensive approach to bereavement, *Nurse Pract* 23:54, 1998.

Stroebe M et al: On the classification and diagnosis of pathological grief, *Clin Psychol Rev* 20:57, 2000.

Tomita T, Kitamura T: Clinical and research measures of grief: a reconsideration, *Compr Psychiatry* 43:95, 2002.

Weiss RS, Richards TA: A scale for predicting quality of recovery following the death of a partner, *J Pers Soc Psychol* 72:885, 1997.

Worden J: *Grief counseling and grief therapy: a handbook for the mental health practitioner,* New York, 1982, Springer.

26

Persons With HIV/AIDS

Gwen van Servellen

OBJECTIVES

- Discuss the prevalence of HIV/AIDS, particularly in vulnerable populations.

- Discuss the prevalence of psychiatric disorders that sometimes predate HIV infection.

- Examine the risk of psychiatric and psychologic morbidity for those coping with HIV/AIDS.

- Distinguish between adjustment disorders and Axis I mood disorders in persons with HIV/AIDS using the criteria of severity of symptoms, treatment, and prognosis.

- Examine potential interactions between behavioral characteristics of persons coping with HIV/AIDS and treatment adherence management.

- Discuss why persons practicing high-risk behaviors may have difficulty changing these behaviors.

- Apply the nursing process for persons with HIV/AIDS.

This chapter identifies and discusses the skills and knowledge needed to provide care to clients experiencing neuropsychiatric syndromes and psychosocial distress related to infection with the **human immunodeficiency virus (HIV)** and **acquired immunodeficiency syndrome (AIDS).** All mental health providers must be HIV/AIDS knowledgeable. To understand the impact of HIV disease on the mental and emotional functioning of clients and their families, it is important to first define HIV disease.

HIV disease has been identified by the U.S. Department of Health and Human Services as a major public health problem in the nation. AIDS, the advanced stage of illness in HIV disease, is fatal. HIV disease is characterized by a defect in the natural immunity against disease, especially against certain **opportunistic diseases/infections** and AIDS-related cancers. Although individuals in the symptomatic state are identifiable by a specific set of signs and symptoms, those who are infected but asymptomatic may go undiagnosed for long periods of time. Neither health care providers nor clients themselves may suspect HIV infection. Because infected asymptomatic individuals are capable of transmitting the disease to others, even if they remain asymptomatic for a long time, HIV disease is unquestionably a serious public health threat.

Both clinical and research evidence indicates that HIV infects the brain and results in central nervous system impairment in some individuals. In addition to the troublesome neuropsychologic and neuropsychiatric consequences of HIV, many more, if not all individuals, experience significant psychologic distress related to awareness of their diagnosis and subsequent adaptation to the consequences of this chronic life-threatening illness. The psychosocial needs of those infected and affected by HIV (families and significant others of those infected) are numerous and present significant challenges to quality of life and the management of treatment adherence in these individuals. Those infected or affected by HIV/AIDS need help in varying degrees to cope with psychologic distress related to the disease. Although this includes care and counsel to those infected, it also includes information and counseling services to those who are coping with an HIV diagnosis in a friend or family member or who are themselves not infected but who are attempting to change high-risk behaviors. Sexual transmission and infection through needle exchange in drug abuse are the primary modes of transmission. Efforts to change these high-risk behaviors are not always immediately successful, because making these changes is exceedingly complex and involves altering behaviors that are not easily discussed or readily changed. As impoverished African-American and Latino subgroups are disproportionately represented in the AIDS community, a focus on culturally held beliefs and needs is critical to successful interventions for prevent and treat HIV.

Psychologic distress, particularly feelings of anxiety and depression, in persons living with HIV or AIDS is of concern to clinicians caring for these individuals for a variety of

UNDERSTANDING and APPLYING RESEARCH

HIV/AIDS is reported to impose significant psychosocial stressors, among which are stigmatization, lifestyle changes, illness-related uncertainty, and existential issues related to diagnosis with a life-threatening chronic illness. The purpose of this study was to measure the impact of a stress management training program on measures of psychologic distress and quality of life in men with HIV disease. The investigators used a 6-month pretest-posttest design to compare the effectiveness of a 6-week stress management program (progressive muscle relaxation training, yoga form stretching with integrative breathing, and mental techniques such as thematic imagery and beginning meditation) on several outcome measures: stress levels, coping patterns, quality of life, psychologic distress, illness-related uncertainty, and CD4 T-lymphocyte levels. At 6 weeks those clients receiving the intervention (stress management training program) appeared to experience in the emotional well-being dimension of the quality-of-life measure. Although changes in other measures were in the predicted direction, indicating improvement, only the emotional well-being subscale was found to be significantly higher immediately after the program. After 6 months, the intervention group had a relative decline in HIV-related intrusive thinking, a measure of illness-related psychologic distress. The investigators concluded that the stress management training program may have buffered illness-related stress over time, the exact mechanism by which is still incompletely understood. It may be that stress management may enhance quality of life and mitigate psychologic distress by virtue of its impact on the sense of personal control and/or optimism clients experience using stress management strategies. Future studies should include measures of personal control and/or optimism.

McCain NL et al: The influence of stress management training in HIV disease, *Nurs Res* 45:246, 1996.

reasons. First, these conditions are negative-affective states reflective of subjective distress and possible maladaptive coping. Further, this subjective distress can significantly alter clients' quality of life in the short and long term. Also, these conditions, when present as enduring clinical syndromes, present with behavioral, somatic, and cognitive features that affect clients' health status and ability to follow medical treatment regimens. Negative affect, irritability, decreased energy and lethargy, altered performance, restlessness and/or interrupted sleep, feelings of helplessness, punitive and self-accusatory evaluations, and persistent fear and worry influence individuals' ability to endure the course of this chronic condition and demanding treatment regimens. These conditions further tax clients' resources and affect their feelings of hopefulness and quality of life. Although suicidal responses in clients with HIV/AIDS may be understandable, this level of hopelessness and any potential risk for suicide can be effectively prevented and should always be included in nursing assessments. Life-threatening illnesses increase the incidence of psychologic distress, particularly depression when the condition is viewed with hopelessness, and anxiety when uncertainty surrounds one's ability to cope and be helped by treatment (see Understanding and Applying Research box).

In HIV/AIDS, as in other life-threatening illness (e.g., advanced cancer), health status carries both primary and secondary implications for quality of life and functional performance. Individuals who are symptomatic are aware of their disease and its potential to impact their lives. Both physical and psychologic symptoms have a direct impact on quality of life but also an indirect impact through the process of secondary appraisal. HIV-related symptoms or the occurrence of opportunistic diseases/infections can be perceived as threatening because of their meaning. For some, these symptoms are a reminder of their vulnerability. In addition, the real or anticipated consequences of these symptoms (e.g., declining role performance, functional deficits, and altered social activities) may also be perceived as threatening. Adaptation during symptomatic HIV disease requires realignment of goal-related activities in order to achieve a positive emotional state. When perceived as being outside the individual's control, physical and psychologic symptoms can be viewed as overwhelming, and this feeling may lead to depression, anxiety, or both. Symptoms can also be perceived as stable (recurrent) and global (affecting many outcomes important to the individual). To the extent that one or more symptoms are perceived as uncontrollable, stable, and global, their occurrence might produce additional psychologic distress.

EPIDEMIOLOGY

The Centers for Disease Control and Prevention (CDC) publishes HIV/AIDS surveillance reports. This publication typically identifies the numbers of full-blown cases of AIDS in the United States reported to the CDC. AIDS surveillance is conducted in all states, the District of Columbia, and U.S. territories. Cases are reported to CDC by using a standard definition and form. As cases of HIV infection are not reportable in many states, the total number of persons in the United States infected with the virus at any one time is unknown and can only be estimated.

As of June 2002, the cumulative number of cases of AIDS in the United States was nearly 800,000 (CDC, 2001). Further, an analysis of AIDS cases in the United States through the year 2000 indicated that AIDS prevalence has increased steadily over time from 1981 through the first half of 2000, although the incidence of AIDS has declined (CDC, 2002). CDC reports on the average 40,000 new cases of AIDS annually. As of December 31, 2000, an estimated 337,731 persons in the United States were living with AIDS (CDC, 2002). In 1996, sharp declines in the incidence of AIDS were observed for the first time; from 1998 to 1999 these declines began to level and from 1999 to 2000, essentially no change in the incidence of AIDS was observed. HIV surveillance data indicate that deaths from AIDS have declined. The number of newly infected cases of HIV infection progressing to AIDS and the number of deaths resulting from AIDS have declined as a result of newly available therapies. Consequently, the number of people living with AIDS has increased. Since 1996, highly active antiretroviral therapy (HAART) has prolonged the interval between the diagnosis of HIV infection and the development of full-blown AIDS. This fact has diminished the capacity of AIDS surveillance data alone to monitor the underlying impact of HIV in the United States. From 1994 to 2000, HIV infection was diagnosed in 128,813 persons in the 25 states that monitor HIV infection (CDC, 2002). Although there has been a decline in cases of HIV infection, patterns and characteristics of these trends raise concern. For example, it was estimated that 25% of those persons diagnosed with HIV infection are not aware of their diagnosis.

In addition, it is important to understand that to derive meaningful predictions of the threat of HIV/AIDS, many different factors that seem to influence the rate of new infections and reportable cases of AIDS must be considered. These factors include a host of demographic characteristics including regional differences, gender, age, ethnicity, and exposure category. Although HIV/AIDS does not discriminate—rural and urban, heterosexual men and women, children, adolescents, and elders are living with HIV/AIDS—some groups are disproportionately affected. Formerly a disease of gay white men in largely urban areas of the United States, HIV/AIDS has permeated most populations, creating a challenge similar to major serious epidemics in history. The number of cases of HIV/AIDS as a result of reported heterosexual transmission is rising at rates surpassing that of homosexual transmission. Although exposure continues to occur through homosexual encounters and injection drug use (blood exposure), the dramatic shift to those reporting heterosexual exposure (particularly among African-American and Latino women) has increased the need to think differently about those at risk for HIV/AIDS.

Cultural Considerations

Once primarily an affliction of gay Caucasian men in major urban epicenters, HIV/AIDS has spread with faster-than-average increases in populations difficult to reach from the perspective of both prevention and treatment. One such shift has been the rising number of newly diagnosed cases of AIDS in rural areas of the United States (CDC, 2002). This shift has occurred even though the number of reported AIDS cases is still lower in rural regions as compared with urban areas, and there has been a steady decrease in the number of AIDS cases nationwide. Attention has focused on this growing problem because the rate of increase in cases has risen faster than that in urban areas, showing an infiltration of the disease into smaller communities. One reason for the rise in reported AIDS cases in rural areas may be that individuals who migrated from rural to urban areas are moving back to rural communities once they have been diagnosed as having HIV infection. This backward migration has raised concern about the adequacy of health care and supportive services in regions where HIV/AIDS may be poorly understood and where specialists are typically not available. Rural communities have been challenged to design shared-care models to improve the care to this underserved population (Mainous et al., 1997).

A second population of concern that has also been difficult to reach is women and adolescent girls. A decade ago, women seemed to be on the periphery of the HIV/AIDS epidemic. They are now at the center of it. As of December 2000, according to the World Health Organization, 16.4 million women were living with HIV/AIDS worldwide, accounting for 47% of the 34.7 million adults living with HIV/AIDS (NIAID, May 2001). Women and adolescent girls accounted for almost one out of five new cases of AIDS diagnosed in 1996 in the United States (USDHHS, 1997). Of the estimated 69,775 adult and adolescent women living with AIDS in December 2001, 40,051 (57%) were exposed through heterosexual contact, and 27,475 (39%) were infected through intravenous drug use (CDC, 2002). One of the groups with the greatest proportionate increase in incidence (12%) is non-Hispanic African-American women with heterosexual risk/exposures (USDHHS, 1997). The number of women with HIV and AIDS has also increased steadily worldwide.

Women with HIV/AIDS are faced with the day-to-day issues of dealing with this profoundly life-threatening illness in themselves and, for many, in their young children and spouses or partners. They are both the infected and affected, coping with their own disease course and the challenges of caring for children who are infected. Clearly, one of the most critical psychosocial concerns in this and other populations is the shock of learning about their HIV status. Women (or for that matter men) who do not perceive themselves to be at risk are less likely to suspect infection and are more likely to delay testing. Once tested, they may have significantly greater difficulty in coming to terms with their infection, having never suspected that they could be infected. In some instances, their partners were also unaware of or hid their HIV serostatus. The sense of stigma and shame attached to their diagnosis can be overwhelming. Addressing the shock and disbelief surrounding their awareness of their diagnosis and their perceived fantasies related to their prognosis has been identified as critical to the care of these populations.

Clients with HIV/AIDS may not trust the traditional medical care establishment or may have trouble accessing it because of a lack of insurance coverage. Many have a world view and perspective about health and illness that is not easily understood or accepted by medical providers. Their socioeconomic and immigration status may have contributed to their lack of access and utilization of available health care resources. To effectively care for these individuals, it is important for the nurse to develop trust and understanding of the individual's perspective on health and attitudes toward conventional treatment. Specifically, it is critical that the nurse understand the client's beliefs, fears, and life goals. Initial acceptance of treatment rests on the degree to which clients feel they can trust the provider. For socioeconomically vulnerable individuals, lack of compliance with treatment may be due to limited resources or competing needs that interfere with ability to access and use services.

In summary, specific characteristic of individuals and populations, including cultural and regional differences in predisposing factors and adaptive behaviors, influence all aspects of health care, from prevention of infection to treatment of late-stage AIDS. Culturally sensitive interventions must take into account subtle, as well as more obvious regional and ethnic characteristics of these populations.

ETIOLOGY OF PSYCHOLOGIC DISTRESS IN HIV/AIDS

In establishing the basis for psychologic distress in clients with HIV disease, it is important to understand various etiologic underpinnings. Psychoneurologic and psychosocial theories are discussed as they explain the etiology of impairment and distress in persons (primarily adults) with HIV disease. The first important consideration, however, is whether the mental disorder and psychologic symptoms predate HIV infection (i.e., Does the individual have a history of moderate-to-severe and persistent mental illness that occurred before the HIV infection?). Some individuals, such as those with major depression, bipolar disorder, injection and noninjection drug use, and alcohol abuse, have engaged in high-risk behaviors that resulted in their becoming infected with HIV. Because early testing and therapy can be extremely effective, these individuals should be closely monitored for their ability to access and use existing HIV treatment services.

The focus of the following discussion is on mood and/or cognitive disorders related to an HIV/AIDS diagnosis, with or without a prior psychiatric illness. The primary DSM-IV-TR diagnoses for review are adjustment disorders with anxiety, depression, and/or disturbance of conduct.

Biologic/Neuropsychiatric Factors

Nervous system disease associated with HIV can take a variety of forms. HIV affects the brain in the form of **AIDS dementia**, the spinal cord as vacuolar myelopathy, and nerve endings as peripheral neuropathy. Soon after the discovery of AIDS, health care providers were puzzled not only by the frequency of cognitive impairment among hospitalized clients, but also by the severity of impairment.

The profound dementia noted in some clients with AIDS seemed disproportionate to the clinical condition, laboratory values, and gross neuropathologic findings present in these clients (Perry and Markowitz, 1986). To confound this discovery even more, the histories of many of these clients revealed that psychologic and cognitive problems predated signs of immune deficiency. It is now known that HIV has a direct effect on the central nervous system and causes a subacute encephalopathy. Cortical atrophy and ventricular dilation have been shown on computed tomography (CT) scans, indicating possible permanent and significant damage to the central nervous system (Perry and Jacobsen, 1986). It is now well understood that HIV (1) easily crosses the blood-brain barrier, (2) is present in the brains of almost all infected persons, and (3) directly or indirectly destroys cells in the nervous system. And, in some individuals it causes a specific HIV-related dementia syndrome.

With this knowledge of histopathology, accurate diagnosis of cognitive and affective changes in clients can be made. Changes in mood can be evidence of clinical depression or represent signs of AIDS-related dementia. Even with organically based changes, the signs and symptoms can be subtle, and laboratory findings may not immediately point to irregularities. The insidious emotional problems tend to mimic functional disorders. Also, initially the neurologic examination, laboratory values, electroencephalogram, cerebrospinal fluid, and CT scan of the brain may appear normal. Additionally confusing is the fact that many of these high-risk and sometimes socially impaired individuals have psychosocial stresses that can explain the emotional distress they exhibit. Differential diagnosis is aided by seropositivity, the absence of a premorbid or family history of psychiatric illness (including substance abuse), positive signs on neuropsychologic testing, and signs of organicity (e.g., imbalance, tremor, avoidance of complex tasks, and sensitivity to drugs and alcohol). Although AIDS dementias vary, they can generally be categorized into two primary types: a dementia chiefly characterized by moderate signs of depression and a more acute psychotic presentation. The first of these is evidenced in apathy, withdrawal, fatigue, hypersomnia, weight loss, anorexia, psychomotor retardation, and subtle cognitive deficits. The acute psychotic presentation can include delusions, hallucinations, psychomotor agitation, mania with grandiosity, and profound cognitive impairment.

AIDS-related moderate to severe cases of dementia have been reported to occur in approximately 7% of clients newly diagnosed with HIV/AIDS and in up to 30% of those with more advanced HIV disease. Recent reports of the effects of HAART have indicated that the prevalence of AIDS dementia may be far less of a concern. Specifically, since the onset of HAART, there has been a significant reduction in the risk for developing HIV dementia. Not only have there been fewer cases of dementia, there appears to be longer life expectancy after onset of HIV dementia.

When clients' impairment is determined to be primarily organically based, the influence of psychosocial phenomena may be present but is not the initial target for intervention. Rather, clients with AIDS-related dementia are treated like clients with other organically based dementias. In summary, nervous system disease is associated with HIV infection. Primary HIV disease carries the potential for neuropsychiatric complications. Behavioral and cognitive symptoms of AIDS dementia are:

- Poor concentration
- Difficulties with problem solving
- Apathy
- Social withdrawal
- Forgetfulness
- Slowness of thought
- Motor deficits tremor, impaired rapid repetitive movements, imbalance, and ataxia

Sometimes these symptoms are accompanied by delirium, delusions, or hallucinations. Symptoms of depression, which include apathy, motor slowing, and attention deficits, are often misinterpreted as early signs of dementia. Clients might also abuse alcohol and/or cocaine and other drugs, which adds to the complexity of understanding the neurologic manifestations of advanced HIV disease. Cocaine psychosis, for example, has been said to closely resemble and mask psychosis caused by HIV (Shaffer and Costikyan, 1988).

Psychosocial Factors

With HIV disease there is a spectrum of disorders in which psychosocial, particularly stress-related, disorders are important. Essentially four categories of individuals may need intervention.

First, there are *those who believe they are at risk for HIV infection but have not gone for testing.* These individuals are "the worried well," some of whom experience ongoing stress, assuming they are indeed seropositive. They tend to exaggerate their risk rather than deny it. They may display low self-esteem, anxiety, uncertainty, and at times irrationality. They may appear somewhat histrionic and indecisive. They may offer clues to their concern, indicating a desire for help. Still, their fear of being seropositive may prevent them from taking care of themselves and confronting their irrationally based concerns.

The second category of individuals needing attention are *those who are asymptomatic but HIV positive.* Although one tends to think of HIV as an acute fatal illness, most clients are either asymptomatic or symptomatic but do not meet the criteria for full-blown AIDS. Even those who have been symptomatic may remain highly functional between symptomatic episodes. After a prolonged incubation period of months or years, most clients will go on to develop AIDS-related symptoms and AIDS. Of primary concern to individuals is the uncertainty they must face on a day-to-day basis.

The third category of individuals are *those who are symptomatic but have not yet developed an AIDS-defining condition.* Early in the epidemic these clients were diagnosed with AIDS-related complex. Symptomatic individuals are not acutely ill but tend to suffer from various AIDS-related conditions and side effects from the antiretroviral medications they are taking.

In studies of symptomatic versus asymptomatic HIV disease, persons with symptoms were reported to exhibit more distress. It was suggested that the prevalence of depressive disorders may increase at later stages of HIV infection before and after AIDS develops (Seth, 1991). A drop in **CD4 count** or a diagnosable opportunistic infection might trigger further fears of impending decline in health or even demise. However, only AIDS-related signs and symptoms, not CD4 count, has been associated with increasing risk of clinical depression (Lyketsos et al., 1996).

The fourth and final category of individuals suffering directly from HIV disease is *clients with full-blown AIDS.* The clinical course of many AIDS-related conditions may be quite varied. Kaposi's sarcoma (KS), a malignant neoplastic vascular proliferation in immunocompromised clients with AIDS, for example, may present as a slowly progressive disease over many years, or a rapidly fulminant progression over weeks to months. Both KS and *Pneumocystis carinii* pneumonia are less frequently observed today than they were before the advent of HAART. With the refinement of medications to combat opportunistic diseases/infections and lower HIV **viral load**, the median survival rate has markedly increased even for those with advanced HIV disease. Available data on the client's disease course, immune status (current CD4 count and viral load), and general health status can offer a clearer prognosis. The depression these clients experience may not be simply a normal grief response about having a fatal illness. For some individuals, a pathologic process characterized by alienation, irrational guilt, diminished self-esteem, and pronounced suicidal ideation may be present. Still, the impact of an entry into AIDS on depression and depressive symptoms needs further study to determine the likelihood that an HIV-specific mood disorder exists (Lyketsos et al., 1996).

Data about suicidal ideation and numbers of suicide attempts in clients with HIV/AIDS are limited. Previous studies have suggested that suicidal ideation is prevalent (Brown and Rundell 1989; Frierson and Lippmann, 1988; Glass, 1988; Kieger et al., 1988; Marzuk et al., 1988; Plott et al., 1989). With the advent of HAART, however, hopefulness has been restored to many who felt powerless over HIV/AIDS. Thus, although declining physical health status may worsen individuals' depression and increase their suicide risk, the advent of new therapies may work to counteract this process. With limited decline in physical health status attributable to new therapies, feelings of hopefulness are possible that may counteract feelings of despair related to one's disease. Hopelessness is seen as an important risk factor for suicide. When it occurs, either in the presence or absence of physical decline, it should be addressed aggressively.

CLINICAL DESCRIPTION

The primary DSM-IV-TR diagnostic condition addressed here is adjustment disorder. Adjustment disorders in HIV/AIDS are also referred to as *severe demoralization syndromes*. These syndromes are to be contrasted with a diagnosis of major depression. Major depression presents with a syndrome of low mood, in which clients complain of persistent sadness or flatness of emotional tone, and anhedonia, in which clients are unable to experience pleasure or satisfaction in things that would ordinarily produce such responses (Angelino and Treisman, 2001). Clients experiencing adjustment disorders with depressed mood may experience some of the same sadness of someone with major depression but usually reports feeling fairly normal when distracted from thinking about the circumstances that cause them distress. When reminded, they experience a welling up of sadness and overwhelming grief (Angelino and Treisman, 2001). Thus adjustment disorders are intimately linked to the overwhelming feelings provoked by the circumstances of living with HIV. Adjustment disorders are coded according to the subtype that best characterizes the predominant

Box 26-1   Adjustment Disorder Subtypes

- With depressed mood
- With anxiety
- With mixed anxiety and depressed mood
- With disturbance of conduct
- With mixed disturbance of emotions and conduct
- Unspecified (maladaptive reactions to psychosocial stressors not classifiable above)

From American Psychiatric Association: *Diagnostic and Statistical Manual of Mental Disorders*, Fourth Edition, Text Revision. Washington, DC, American Psychiatric Association, 2000.

symptoms. See Box 26-1 for specific types of adjustment disorders.

Note that although clients may also display other psychiatric disorders (e.g., a major depressive episode and/or psychoactive substance abuse), adjustment disorders with anxious and/or depressed mood are more commonly diagnosed in clients seeking HIV treatment in community-based primary care clinics. As previously stated, this diagnosis pertains to their reaction to having a serious life-threatening illness. A differentiating and defining feature for adjustment disorder is that the disorder begins within 3 months of onset of a stressor and lasts no longer than 6 months after the stressor or its consequences have subsided. Other recurring disorders (e.g., bipolar illness or recurrent major depression) may also be observed but may predate clients' seroconversion or onset of an HIV-related stressor. The prevalence of previous psychiatric illness and/or substance abuse disorders in HIV-infected individuals is not fully known, but it is believed to be higher than for some community samples based partly on the fact that HIV is transmitted through exposure to infected needles in substance abusing populations. Bing et al. (2001) indicated that the rates of psychiatric and drug use disorders vary depending on the population studied and the comparison groups used. However, depression in HIV clinic populations generally range from 22% to 32%, which is two to three times higher than in general community populations.

In addition to ruling out the presence of another Axis I disorder (e.g., major depressive episode), consideration is given to other diagnostic categories when conducting a differential diagnosis assessment of these clients. These conditions include bereavement reaction, psychologic factors related to a medical condition, posttraumatic stress disorder, stress disorder, and personality disorders. Although diagnostic assessments may vary, substance abuse and bereavement reactions are frequently seen as comorbid conditions in clients whose Axis I diagnosis is either major depressive episode or adjustment disorder with emotional features. Specific HIV-related problems observed on psychiatric hospital admissions are:

- Anxiety and depression related to deteriorating physical health status
- Social rejection related to HIV seropositive status
- Increased drug use as a response to HIV seropositivity

- Shame or guilt concerning stigmatized sexual practices
- Guilt or fear over having put others at risk (including fear of retribution)
- Homicidal ideation toward the presumed party who infected the client

PROGNOSIS

Although the prognosis for resolution of anxiety and depression in clients suffering adjustment disorders is generally good, the case for resolution in persons living with HIV/AIDS is not well documented, primarily because the stresses associated with HIV/AIDS may persist and thus suspend resolution of this condition. Researchers who study the psychologic and neuropsychiatric effects of HIV attempt to isolate crisis points where psychosocial stressors or other precipitants can lead to more serious levels of depression, anxiety, and other psychiatric problems. Because HIV infection is a chronic stressful life event depicted by a series of physical, functional, and psychosocial losses, anxiety and depression are likely to occur intermittently and relate to the psychologic pain accompanying different phases of the disease process. Some experiences may be severe enough to precipitate a dysphoric mood and/or a crisis (Duffy, 1994). Although the concept of "crisis points" seems to be applicable to this population, several considerations are important.

The experience of HIV/AIDS as a crisis is highly variable. Some clients struggle with the disease, and this struggle is evident. Other clients seem to cope well and even seem to find new courage to take on healthier life styles. Thus, assuming that all clients experience the same level of distress denies individual differences in the ways in which people cope with life stress. Caution should be used in generalizing about the inevitability of psychologic distress and what may constitute a crisis for clients.

THE NURSING PROCESS

ASSESSMENT

The psychosocial assessment of a client with HIV/AIDS with a diagnosis of adjustment disorder, anxiety, and/or depression requires a thorough appraisal of primary and secondary nursing diagnoses. The clinical assessment that enables nurses to derive pertinent nursing diagnoses must be all inclusive. Identifying data, current symptoms, and history of the present problem (anxiety, depression, and/or conduct) must be addressed. Specific data about sleep patterns, appetite, and change in weight are important in assessing the severity of the mood disturbance. Details about previous psychiatric contacts (both outpatient and hospitalizations), including precipitating events, will establish any preexisting psychiatric disorders that may place the client at risk for current or future episodes of clinical depression or anxiety.

Data regarding the client's family unit and current social network are particularly relevant. A description of the fam-

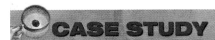
CASE STUDY

Rocio is a 29-year-old Hispanic woman married to José, who is reported to be behaviorally bisexual and HIV positive. Two months ago, Rocio was diagnosed as HIV positive with symptomatic HIV disease. She is positive for AIDS-related fatigue, fevers, nausea, diarrhea, dyspnea, and wasting syndrome. A thorough gynecologic examination reveals that Rocio is in the early stages of cervical dysplasia. The nurse practitioner in the women's clinic asked to have Rocio evaluated by the psychiatric team. She is 5 months' pregnant and has three additional children under age 5 years. Rocio and José are undocumented residents who have lived in the United States for 1½ years. Their primary language is Spanish. When questioned about her pregnancy and her personal health, Rocio sobbed uncontrollably. She explained that she is really worried about her children and what will happen to them. She cannot eat or sleep, and she has not told any friends or family that she is HIV positive, because she is ashamed and worried that they would not be kind to her children if they knew her diagnosis. When distracted from thinking or talking about her diagnosis, Rocio appears optimistic and grateful for the care she is receiving at the clinic.

Critical Thinking

1. What are the client's most immediate problems or needs related to her HIV diagnosis?
2. What assessment data reflect the client's sensitivity to her diagnosis?
3. Why might the client be reluctant to seek the social support she needs?
4. What stressors could contribute to fear, anxiety, a sense of helplessness, and depression?

ily unit of origin, including the family's history of traumatic events, migration, and cultural factors, help to sensitize providers to the contextual nature of the client's responses to his or her illness and the potential for the co-occurrence of posttraumatic stress disorder. These same data about current relationships are also critical because they influence ways in which clients cope with HIV/AIDS and the availability of existing resources (see Case Study).

Social history information is of general importance, but certain data hold special significance. The nature of the client's social network and history of (past and current) sexual practices are important. In many cases, clients are not only living with the personal threat of HIV, but they are also dealing with the possibility of placing others at risk. A diagnosis of HIV brings with it an array of responsibilities to those with whom clients have been intimate. A final area of assessment is the client's previous and current tendencies to inflict personal harm or to harm others. As previously noted, risk for suicide should be seriously evaluated and monitored over time as the course of illness advances. Anger and rage also may be manifested through violent behaviors, homicidal threats or gestures directed at those believed to be the source of infection, and occasionally toward society at large.

Finally, in assessing the basis for psychologic distress, a thorough mental status examination is conducted on all clients. Periodic assessments are done as the disease progresses, with careful attention given to monitoring any adverse findings.

NURSING DIAGNOSIS

Nursing diagnoses are formulated from the data gathered by the nurse during the assessment phase of the nursing process. The accuracy of nursing diagnoses relies on the careful, comprehensive assessment of the client's history, presenting symptoms, behavior, and responses to actual and potential life stressors. The reliability of all informants, whether the sources are clients themselves, their significant others, and/or previous data from charts, is extremely important. Multiple sources of data can confirm information and ensure appropriate assessment and diagnoses.

Nursing Diagnoses for Persons With AIDS Experiencing Adjustment Disorders With Depressed or Anxious Mood

- Anxiety
- Compromised family coping
- Ineffective coping
- Hopelessness
- Ineffective denial
- Noncompliance
- Powerlessness or risk for powerlessness
- Chronic or situational low self-esteem
- Social isolation
- Risk for suicide

  See Collaborative Diagnoses table.

OUTCOME IDENTIFICATION

Outcome criteria are derived from the nursing diagnoses and are the expected client responses to be achieved.

Client will:

- Verbalize absence of suicidal ideation and plans.
- State reduced frequency/intensity of feelings of hopelessness and powerlessness.
- Reduce ineffective denial and engage in a therapeutic alliance with staff to evaluate coping options.
- Initiate social interactions with others with HIV/AIDS (both individually and in groups) to gain information and support about coping effectively with HIV/AIDS.
- Identify barriers or problems that may precipitate exacerbation of the experience of anxiety and/or depression (e.g., perception of inadequate social support or perception of powerlessness over physical symptoms).
- Verbalize clear, goal-directed, short-term plans that are achievable and that focus on problem solving.
- Express improved self-esteem and self-confidence in managing his/her illness and treatment and demonstrate intentions and behaviors to improve antiretroviral treatment adherence.

COLLABORATIVE DIAGNOSES

DSM-IV-TR Diagnoses*	NANDA Diagnoses†
Adjustment disorder	
With depressed mood	Ineffective coping
	Hopelessness
	Powerlessness
	Situational low self-esteem
	Social isolation
	Noncompliance
	Risk for suicide
	Risk for other-directed violence
	Risk for self-directed violence
With anxiety	Anxiety
	Death anxiety
	Ineffective coping
	Noncompliance
With mixed anxiety and depressed mood	(All those in above anxiety and depressed mood categories)
With disturbance of conduct	Defensive coping
	Ineffective coping
	Ineffective denial
	Noncompliance
	Risk for other-directed violence
	Risk for self-directed violence

NOTE: DSM-IV-TR diagnoses of adjustment disorder with mixed disturbance of emotions and conduct, and adjustment disorder, unspecified, are not addressed here, given the overlap with the previous diagnostic subtypes.

*From American Psychiatric Association: *Diagnostic and Statistical Manual of Mental Disorders,* Fourth Edition, Text Revision. Washington, DC, American Psychiatric Association, 2000.

†From NANDA International (2003). NANDA Nursing Diagnoses: Definitions and Classification 2003-2004. Philadelphia: NANDA.

PLANNING

The nurse's awareness of the complexities of living with HIV disease is extremely critical in deriving an appropriate plan of care for the client, the client's family, and his or her friends, partners, or significant others.

For clients who are diagnosed with adjustment disorders, the nurse considers a plan of action that will:

1. Prevent violence toward self
2. Address concerns in a coherent, goal-directed, problem-solving manner
3. Increase social networking that will provide needed information and comfort
4. Monitor adverse effects of stressors on clients' current level of adaptation
5. Use staff in an effective therapeutic alliance when social supports diminish or when social networks cannot provide the technical expertise the client requires

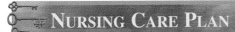
NURSING CARE PLAN

Steve, a 32-year-old Caucasian homosexual man, formerly a travel agent, has been retired for 2 years because of complications from AIDS. He has had a history of depression since his early twenties for which he received outpatient counseling. He sees his physician regularly; currently he has esophageal candidiasis and wasting syndrome. He came to this clinic appointment expressing a great deal of hopelessness about his future. He stated that he didn't want to live anymore and that he was tired of fighting AIDS. When asked if he had thought about suicide or had a suicide plan, he hesitated when stating that he could make it quick and fatal by jumping out of a window.

DSM-IV-TR Diagnoses
Axis I	Major depression, recurrent
Axis II	Deferred
Axis III	Acquired immunodeficiency syndrome (AIDS) with candidiasis and wasting syndrome
Axis IV	Moderate—financial difficulties Inconsistent support system
Axis V	GAF = 50 GAF = 60 (last year)

NURSING DIAGNOSIS: Powerlessness related to responses to treatment of HIV disease and symptoms, as evidenced by verbalization of suicidal thoughts and plans, inability to forecast a positive future, verbalization of powerlessness as a result of physical decline, decreased functioning, and lack of progress in treatment regimen.

CLIENT OUTCOMES	NURSING INTERVENTIONS	EVALUATION
Steve will verbalize absence of suicidal ideation and plans.	Assist Steve to (1)identify his needs and short-term achievable goals, (2) relate these goals to his life tasks, and (3) contract to avoid acting out with suicidal gestures or attempts *to facilitate the client's adaptive coping responses and decrease feelings of loss of control; to help support Steve's goal.*	Steve progressively states optimism about achieving goals within his anticipated life span.
Steve will verbalize increased feelings of personal competence and self-efficacy in relation to managing his symptoms.	Identify with Steve options that he has in controlling his emotional and physical distress (e.g., stress management strategies and ways to cope with fatigue and diarrhea) *to counteract feelings of powerlessness and helplessness that, if not abated, result in hopelessness.*	Steve identifies and begins to implement new strategies for coping with his symptoms. He verbalizes feelings of competence, as identified in the main outcome.
Steve will develop a therapeutic alliance with staff.	Engage Steve in an active problem-solving approach addressing each stressor and discussing appropriate coping options/strategies *to evaluate Steve's coping options/methods.*	Steve regards the nurse as a facilitator and supportive resource. He initiates discussion of stressors and options.
Steve will initiate social interactions with others with HIV to gain information and support.	Offer referrals to Steve regarding support groups and particularly voluntary home care services *to help Steve gain information and support.*	Steve attends support group of his choice or identifies at least one other person with AIDS whom he can talk to on a weekly basis.
Steve will identify barriers or problems associated with exacerbation of his anxiety/depression.	Assist Steve in reviewing what precipitating events and/or thoughts increase his anxiety/depression *to avoid such events, when possible, through increased awareness.*	Steve expressed awareness of recurring stressors that worsen his anxiety and depression.
Steve will verbalize goal-directed plans that are both achievable and solution focused.	Assist Steve in formulating goals that are realistic and achievable. These should be directed toward improving the quality of life and reducing stressors in day-to-day living *to decrease frustration and increase success through goal attainment.*	Steve articulates two or three short-term goals he can realistically commit to with respect to his present condition.

IMPLEMENTATION

The challenges of working and intervening with clients are considerable and multiple. Families and caregivers also are greatly affected and often devastated by both the client's diagnosis and responses to his/her disease. Therefore it is important that families and significant others are considered and included in the interventions when appropriate and with the consent of the client.

For example, significant others who are encouraged to engage in problem-solving coping methods (versus emotion-focused coping) may be more helpful to clients who are trying to minimize the psychologic burden of adapting to their disease. Significant others need to be taught about the disease, its course, and what can be expected over time. Knowledge deficits must be addressed by trained professionals. Support groups for caregivers of persons with HIV/AIDS are available and can be particularly helpful to family and significant others. They provide support and comfort in dealing with anticipated bereavement, fear of contagion, and the stress of caregiving. Support networks of a less formal design also exist to provide assistance for clients and their loved ones through newsletters and drop-in centers.

Nursing Interventions

Clients with HIV/AIDS may have numerous symptoms; consequently, these clients require multiple interventions addressing various aspects of their spiritual, psychosocial, and physical well-being. An integrated multidisciplinary approach to treatment is important. The interventions discussed here are largely in the psychosocial domain, and they are directed toward altering maladaptive individual coping and treating impaired social interactions. Many nursing interventions for HIV parallel interventions used with other illness, particularly life-threatening cancers. People with HIV, however, have unique experiences not always found with other life-threatening illness (e.g., dealing with disease contagion, the stigma and shame associated with their diagnosis, and even feelings of betrayal by those who might have given them HIV). These features of the disease experience cause strong feelings that negatively impact individuals and might even affect their health status and approach to treatment. Successful coping with HIV/AIDS is a priority in maintaining their quality of life over the course of their illness.

The primary category of intervention in the psychosocial domain is to ensure safety of the client and others. The nurse then focuses on facilitating adaptive coping to the multiple stressors that the client will confront. Interventions to enhance effective or adaptive coping include:

- Assist clients to maintain or improve their quality of life.
- Assist clients to manage or contain their feelings of fear, anxiety, grief, guilt, depression, and helplessness.
- Enhance clients' sense of self-worth and positive self-esteem.
- Avert a state of hopelessness and powerlessness.
- Assist clients to satisfactorily adapt their relationships as they are confronted with various stages of dependency on family, significant others, and their health care providers.
- Assist clients to maintain the highest level of functioning possible.
- Assist clients to develop a long-range treatment adherence management plan.

Along these lines nurses can also intervene to help clients cope adaptively to each phase of their HIV disease.

With respect to maintaining or improving clients' quality of life, nurses can intervene to alter the physical discomfort and psychosocial isolation clients experience. They can teach clients to handle pain and fatigue caused by their illness and/or side effects of their HIV antiretroviral therapy regimen. In doing this, they are also helping the client to exert control and minimize feelings of helplessness.

Social support networks are important to clients with HIV/AIDS. Without them, social isolation and loneliness can occur and significantly impact their quality of life. Also, disengagement is a normal process in adjusting to physical decline. The nurse needs to help the client preserve those relationships with friends and family who are capable of meeting the client's dependency needs. Loss of role functioning is usually painful to a client but even more so when supportive relationships, for what ever reasons, are not available to the client.

Containing feelings of anxiety, helplessness, grief, guilt, depression, and fear is also important to maintaining the client's quality of life. Helping the client become informed about HIV disease and treatment options lessens the anxiety many clients experience because it reduces uncertainty surrounding the disease and likely prognosis. The nurse also needs to appreciate that some clients are not comforted by information, and the instruction they provide may not be heard or understood. Teaching needs to be paced and delivered in doses reflective of the individual's receptivity and ability to comprehend both written and verbal instruction.

Supporting clients when they are confronting the multiple losses associated with their disease is comforting and helpful in reducing negative feelings of grief and depression. These anticipated or actual losses include physical decline and loss of social role, income, and supportive relationships. Loss of dignity related to declines in health and/or functional status may also occur. The client's psychologic distress may be reduced if nurses anticipate these losses and prepare clients to cope with these circumstances. Nurses can also supplement clients' resources by providing them with knowledge of social and financial services and counseling assistance.

Helping the client maintain or enhance a sense of self-worth and avert a state of powerlessness and hopelessness in the face of this serious disease requires thoughtful consideration about the ways that clients are affected by their disease. Sometimes the nurse teaches the client how to respond to the curiosity of others. Hiding one's illness and minimizing its effects can be adaptive because it helps clients live as normally as possible despite their symptoms and effects of treatment.

Assisting the client in preserving relationships requires both direct and indirect intervention. Nurses can help clients understand reasons for reactions of family and friends. Less directly, they can assist informal caregivers by teaching them how to respond to the client's reaction to his/her illness and treatment. AIDS caregivers usually are concerned about contagion of the disease. Providing factual information to these caregivers may decrease any tendency they may have to withdraw because of fear of becoming infected with HIV. In cases where clients are sexually active with partners, nurses need to monitor, teach, and support them in adhering to safe sexual practices. The role of the nurse in dealing with persons with HIV/AIDS in the community is summarized in the Nursing Care in the Community box.

A final important category of intervention is related to treatment of acute and subacute syndromes associated with cognitive impairment. Dementia associated with AIDS includes cognitive, motor, and behavioral manifestations. Ini-

NURSING CARE IN THE COMMUNITY — Persons With HIV/AIDS

The continued epidemic of HIV/AIDS in homosexual, heterosexual, and some minority communities presents challenges and opportunities for community mental health nurses. With health care becoming more of a managed system further constrained by capitation, the role of community mental health nurses is changing. Community mental health nurses are no longer bound to the traditions of the past. Instead, these nurses can become partners in community-based care for the majority of clients with HIV/AIDS.

Future long-term management of this chronic infection will involve more outreach efforts by medical and social services. Already, many community-based organizations are involved in the care of these clients. Support groups, social services, housing, nutritional counseling, peer advocacy support and education, occupational therapy, and drug and alcohol counseling are some of the ancillary services available in the community.

The community mental health nurse's role in working successfully with these clients includes identifying one's personal attitudes, beliefs, and values about AIDS, gay lifestyles, drug abuse, and sexuality. Also, a thorough knowledge of AIDS and the biopsychosocial issues associated with HIV disease and treatment is essential.

Nurses can offer much to these clients and their families and significant others. Counseling, brief supportive therapy, and just being a caring presence can make a difference. Anxiety and depression must be addressed with these clients. The potential for suicide should be a concern. Social support, financial resources, housing needs, and possible job loss are other issues that need to be considered.

The nurse must be prepared to work collaboratively with other health care professionals. Teamwork for seamless coordination of all medical and social services and appropriate referrals to other community-based agencies will enhance the care and quality of life for these clients.

Newer drug therapies that suppress viral multiplication have contributed to the prospects of improving the health and quality of life of these clients. The recent announcement of the testing of an AIDS vaccine holds promise. Despite these advances, there is much to be done in the way of caring for and counseling men and women living with HIV/AIDS. Community mental health nurses play an important role in the prevention of the spread of HIV and in enhancing individuals' abilities to manage their illness and maintain the highest level of treatment adherence possible to reduce HIV morbidity and mortality. The initial diagnosis of HIV infection and the delivery of bad news with the worsening of the client's condition can trigger significant sadness and despair. Because of the stigma associated with HIV/AIDS, considerable fear, shame, and even loss of important supportive relationships can occur. Because of the significant stigma attached to the diagnosis, clients infected with HIV may experience so much impairment in their social interactions that they become invisible in their community.

---

tial symptoms are usually memory impairment and concentration difficulties. These symptoms can be overlooked and are frequently confused with symptoms associated with depression. However, clients may complain of forgetfulness, "slowed thinking," and difficulty concentrating when engaged in conversations, watching TV programs, or reading. In some cases poor balance and coordination occur early on. As this syndrome progresses, with no chance of reversal, clients may become dependent on others for completion of activities of daily living. Many clients and their caregivers fear the development of dementia. They may have observed friends whose lives were significantly compromised by AIDS dementia in all areas—cognitive, motor, and behavior. In addition, AIDS dementia is not easily identified, and symptoms can wax and wane, causing a great deal of uncertainty and anxiety. For this reason, early thorough assessment and instruction of the client and caregivers about signs and symptoms are extremely important interventions.

With the advent of new therapies, researchers are hopeful that not only will AIDS dementia decline but that some clients with dementia will regain their lost faculties. Whether these symptoms are reversible and what level of cognitive improvement will result are the subjects of ongoing study.

Nurses working with clients with AIDS who also have dementia participate in the neuropsychiatric assessment of their clients by recording problems related to memory, attention span, concentration, and motor deficits. They provide support to the client, family, and friends who are assuming client care. Caregivers or partners may welcome respite care or home care, depending on the client's functional status and needs. It is important to help clients and their families remember treatment and medication schedules. This may include the use of checklists, bulletin boards, pill boxes, alarms, and other strategies to promote self-care management and ease the burden of care for significant others.

Additional Treatment Modalities

Nursing interventions contribute significantly to the client's ability to cope effectively with HIV disease; however, it is important to keep in mind that other disciplines and therapies play a critical role in the client's ability to deal with psychologic distress related to HIV. Currently accepted treatments of adjustment problems in clients with HIV/AIDS parallel those for other populations with adjustment disorders, but important key differences are addressed in this section regarding pharmacologic intervention, the preferred format for individual counseling, psychosocial support networks specific to persons living with HIV/AIDS and their significant others, and the use of other modes to decrease stress and promote clients' highest level of functioning.

Pharmacologic Intervention

Medical. Formerly the first line of treatment for HIV was prescription of a reverse transcriptase inhibitor (e.g., AZT). This was referred to as monotherapy, as only one agent was involved. With advances in antiretroviral therapies, more complex combination regimens have replaced monotherapy approaches. **Combination antiretroviral therapies** include HAART and mega-HAART. These regimens include combinations of nucleoside reverse transcriptase inhibitors (e.g., didanosine [Videx], stavudine [Zerit], lamivudine [Epivir], and zidovudine [Retrovir]), non-nucleoside reverse transcriptase inhibitors (e.g., efavirenz [Sustiva] and nevirapine [Viramune]), protease inhibitors (e.g., indinavir [Crixivan], lopinavir [Kaletra], and nelfinavir [Viracept]), and a fourth classification, nucleotide analog reverse transcriptase inhibitor (e.g., tenofovir disoproxil fumarate [Viread]). These classifications of drugs work together to interrupt production of new virus. Combination therapies are the most effective treatment available but may cause disabling side effects.

Psychopharmacology. Psychotropic medications can be useful in the treatment of clients with HIV disease. There are no medical reasons to avoid their use. The most commonly used psychotropic medications with clients with HIV/AIDS experiencing moderate to severe distress are antidepressants and anxiolytics. It is generally understood that the best outcome results from the use of medications with combined cognitive behavioral counseling approaches. Counseling and psychotherapy are generally considered to be the standard of care for clients with significant, persistent depression and/or anxiety. Still, in the case of demoralization syndromes (adjustment disorders), some feel that clients may respond well to a relatively unstructured supportive interaction with a caring provider who is not technically trained (Angelino and Treisman, 2001).

Antidepressant medication can be prescribed if the client manifests a significant depressed or anxious condition. Sometimes an antidepressant is initiated prophylactically when new uncontrollable stressors are anticipated. Anxiolytics are prescribed in daily dosages or as needed to reduce the client's anxiety. The choice of antidepressant or anxiolytic and dose of medication often depends on the client's neurovegetative symptoms and underlying physical illness. For example, for an agitated client with gastroenteritis who is also having difficulties with diarrhea because of the disease or complications from treatment, an antidepressant medication with more anticholinergic action may be the best choice. This medication diminishes diarrhea and provides mild sedation and thus works to the client's advantage. In addition to the individual's overall health status and specific emotional distress, the age of the client is important. For example, older adults and adolescents are generally treated with lower doses of psychotropic medications. The first step in antidepressant treatment is to assist the client to consistently take the medication and to use an adequate therapeutic dose (Angelino and Treisman, 2001). Generally physicians begin with low doses of the chosen medication and slowly increase the level to minimize medication side effects. It must be remembered that in addition to the potential side effects clients may experience while on antidepressants, they are also experiencing to varying degrees side effects from their antiretroviral medications. Once the client is on a dose of medication for at least 2 weeks, the client should be reassessed for improvements in mood and the presence of any continuing distressing side effects. With this assessment, decisions can be made about altering or keeping the medications as prescribed.

Complementary Therapies

In the absence of a definitive cure, many clients with HIV have chosen to supplement their treatment programs with complementary therapies or treatments not commonly provided by medical physicians but that may be taken in conjunction with their medical treatment (Ostrow et al., 1997). Complementary therapies in HIV/AIDS include mind-body remedies or herbal supplements aimed at reducing individuals' symptoms or treatment side effects, enhancing immune status, or improving their sense of well-being. Examples of these therapies include, acupuncture, massage, herbs, vitamins, meditation, and stress reduction. With few exceptions, these approaches are believed to be helpful and not harmful. Exceptions are the use of Saint-John's Wort, which has been shown to reduce the blood plasma concentration of indinavir, a protease inhibitor, and garlic supplements, which have been shown to interact with saquinavir, another protease inhibitor. Clients should be cautioned to discuss with their health care provider the use of an herbal or dietary supplement to prevent any adverse effects resulting from interactions with their antiviral treatment regimen.

The stress of HIV infection is chronic and may persist over long periods with acute exacerbations. Attention is drawn to recommended alternative methods of managing stress. Along these lines, there are well-documented techniques (e.g., stress reduction, meditation, and relaxation techniques) that are extremely useful to many persons at various stages of HIV/AIDS. For example, stress management strategies and progressive relaxation exercises can be taught to clients. Stress management manuals and self-help books, as well as brief workshops in the community, are available to help clients learn these techniques. Some of these instructional aids are also on videotape.

The individual's desire to control psychologic distress through alternative methods that may include spiritual practices must be recognized, discussed, and supported. Spirituality as treatment is receiving increased attention, as a growing body of literature suggests that there is an important connection between how one interprets the meaning of his or her illness and the ability to cope with illness and loss. Taking spirituality and prayer into account when assessing individuals' needs and resources and in developing intervention strategies requires a shift in perspective (see Understanding and Applying Research box).

Clients' self-management strategies must be monitored for other reasons as well. Clients must be cautioned that HIV-infected bodies are different from disease-free systems. Weight loss generated by diet changes and physical exercise is usually more of a problem than a desired goal. Unnecessary calorie depletion and calorie burning should be kept at

UNDERSTANDING and APPLYING RESEARCH

The purpose of this study was to describe the manner in which women cope with HIV infection by providing additional data about the prevalence of specific adaptive and maladaptive cognitive and behavioral coping responses and examining whether the prevalence of these responses varied across three ethnic groups (African-American, Caucasian, and Latina women). Women who were 18 years and older, HIV positive, and not currently pregnant were recruited; 53 women were interviewed, all of whom spoke English. In this sample of women, nearly 40% reported clinically significant levels of depressive symptomatology and anxiety on the Brief Symptom Inventory. Compared with normative samples, all infected women, regardless of ethnic group, reported distress levels. Prayer and rediscovery of what is important in life were their most frequent coping responses. Denial (refusal to believe one is HIV positive) and trying to feel better by eating, drinking, smoking, using drugs or medications, etc. were the least often reported means of coping with HIV infection. The study suggests that clinicians should not overlook the importance of spiritual faith and practices in women adapting to HIV infection.

Kaplan MS, Marks G, Mertens SB: Distress and coping among women with HIV infection: preliminary findings from a multiethnic sample, *Am J Orthopsychiatry* 67:80, 1997.

a minimum. The recommendation for exercise should focus on moderation, with the major goal of exercise geared to strength building and resistance training. Adding muscle mass is a good thing; burning calories is not.

EVALUATION

If nursing interventions are successful, the client will show significant signs of improvement in coping ability. If coping ability improves, changes in client mood, behavior, and functional abilities should also improve. Increases in clients' understanding of their illness and treatment will also be evident. A large part of the treatment of persons with HIV/AIDS is individualized teaching to help them regain and maintain a sense of control over their lives, symptoms, and disease.

Effective coping should be evidenced in the outcome criteria addressed in the treatment plan. That is, clients will demonstrate an ability to manage and contain uncomfortable feelings of fear, anxiety, guilt, grief, and depression. Because their ability to manage their symptoms will improve, their sense of self-worth and self-esteem should be enhanced. Relationships with others, especially those in caregiver roles, should have been strengthened by the added instruction and support from the nurse. The client should demonstrate a realistic level of hope as a result of the nurse's efforts to help him/her find meaning in life and set small, realistic goals. Although clients may not consistently experience a strong sense of well-being, they should experience improved quality of life based on increased feelings of cognitive, behavioral, and decisional control. Helping clients achieve a sense of control helps them minimize fear, anxiety, and depression associated with HIV/AIDS and is im-

portant in their ability to cope with illness and loss and manage their adherence to antiretroviral therapy.

CHAPTER SUMMARY

- HIV disease is considered a major public health problem worldwide.
- Persons may be infected with HIV but may be asymptomatic for long periods of time.
- AIDS is the advanced stage of HIV disease.
- AIDS does not discriminate; it occurs in both genders, in all socioeconomic groups, in all ages, and in all ethnic/racial communities.
- AIDS is disproportionately found in certain disadvantaged minorities that traditionally have experienced problems in accessing existing services.
- Shifts in rates of HIV infection in the United States suggest that adolescent girls and women are increasingly vulnerable for HIV/AIDS.
- Dramatic shifts in the numbers of persons living with AIDS have occurred as a result of the advent of effective antiretroviral medication regimens. Consequently, more people are living longer with HIV and must learn to cope effectively with the ongoing impact of their disease and treatment.
- One principal DSM-IV-TR diagnosis among persons with HIV/AIDS is adjustment disorder. This diagnosis must be differentiated from other mood disorders (e.g., major depression).
- Nursing assessment and interventions should be conducted in collaboration with the client and, in some cases, family and/or significant others.
- Psychotropic medications may be helpful for clients experiencing more severe depression or anxiety, especially when coupled with structured or unstructured supportive counseling.
- Complementary therapies, such as stress reduction, relaxation, and spirituality or prayer, have been useful to many clients in various stages of HIV disease.

REVIEW QUESTIONS

1. A 30-year-old client was hospitalized with pneumonia and dehydration secondary to end-stage AIDS. He was confused and delusional. An appropriate nursing diagnosis would be:
   a. Disturbed thought processes
   b. Hopelessness
   c. Powerlessness
   d. Disturbed personality identity

2. A 17-year-old male was informed of his HIV positive status. He tells the nurse, "Well, I know what I need to do now." The highest priority nursing intervention is to:
   a. Offer support groups.
   b. Assess for suicidality and have the client contract for safety.
   c. Discuss the newest medication statistics.
   d. Arrange for him to talk to a social worker.

3. Which statement demonstrates that a client diagnosed with HIV has accepted his illness?
   a. "I think they made a mistake. That happens you know."
   b. "No one will want to come near me now."
   c. "Why didn't I stop taking heroin."
   d. "I'll do what I can to stay healthy. They are discovering new medications all the time."

4. Clients with HIV can use which of the following to help cope with the illness:
   a. Alcohol to numb the pain
   b. Marijuana for nausea
   c. Stress reduction techniques such as guided imagery or meditation
   d. Low-sugar diet

5. A client diagnosed with HIV complains of difficulty concentrating, forgetfulness, and fatigue. The nurse assesses that the client is:
   a. Depressed
   b. Suffering from AIDS dementia
   c. Psychotic
   d. Anxious

REFERENCES

Angelino AF, Treisman GJ: Management of psychiatric disorders in patients with human immunodeficiency virus, *HIV/AIDS CID* 33:847-856, 2001.

American Psychiatric Association: *Diagnostic and Statistical Manual of Mental Disorders*, Fourth Edition, Text Revision. Washington, DC, American Psychiatric Association, 2000.

Bing EG et al: Psychiatric disorders and drug use among human immunodeficiency virus-infected adults in the United States, *Arch Gen Psychiatry* 58:721-728, 2001.

Brown G, Rundell J: Suicidal tendencies in women with human immunodeficiency virus infection, *Am J Psychiatry* 146:556, 1989.

Centers for Disease Control and Prevention: *HIV surveillance report, June 2001*, Atlanta, 2001, U.S. Department of Health and Human Services.

Centers for Disease Control and Prevention, U.S. Department of Health and Human Services: *MMWR*, vol 51, no 27, July 12, 2002.

Duffy VJ: Crisis points in HIV disease, *AIDS Patient Care* 8(1):28, 1994.

Frierson RL, Lippmann SB: Suicide and AIDS, *Psychosomatics* 29:226, 1988.

Glass RM: AIDS and suicide, *JAMA* 259:1369, 1988.

Kaplan MS, Marks G, Mertens SB: Distress and coping among women with HIV infection: preliminary findings from a multiethnic sample, *Am J Orthopsychiatry* 67:80, 1997.

Kieger K et al: AIDS and suicide in California, *JAMA* 266:1881, 1988.

Lyketsos CG et al: Depressive symptoms over the course of HIV infection before AIDS, *Soc Psychiatry Psychiatr Epidemiol* 31:212-219, 1996.

Mainous AG et al: Illustrations and implications of current models of HIV health service provision in rural areas, *AIDS Patient Care STDs* 11:25, 1997.

Marzuk PM et al: Increased risk of suicide in persons with AIDS, *JAMA* 259:1333, 1988.

McCain NL et al: The influence of stress management training in HIV disease, *Nurs Res* 45:246, 1996.

National Institute of Allergy and Infectious Diseases (NIAID), National Institutes of Health: HIV infection in women, *NIAID Fact Sheet*, May 2001.

NANDA International (2003). NANDA Nursing Diagnoses: Definitions and Classification 2003-2004. Philadelphia: NANDA.

Ostrow MJ et al: Determinants of complementary therapy use in HIV-infected individuals receiving antiretroviral or anti-opportunistic agents, *J Acq Immune Defic Syndr and Human Retrovir* 15:115-120, 1997.

Perry S, Jacobsen P: Neuropsychiatric manifestations of AIDS-spectrum disorders, *Hosp Community Psychiatry* 37:135, 1986.

Perry S, Markowitz J: Psychiatric intervention for AIDS-spectrum disorders, *Hosp Community Psychiatry* 37:1001, 1986.

Plott RT et al: Suicide of AIDS patients in Texas: a preliminary report, *Tex Med* 85:40, 1989.

Seth R: Psychiatric illness in patients with HIV infection and AIDS referred to liaison psychiatrists, *Br J Psychiatry* 159:347-350, 1991.

Shaffer HJ, Costikyan DS: Cocaine psychosis and AIDS: a contemporary diagnostic dilemma, *J Subst Abuse Treat* 5:9, 1988.

U.S. Department of Health and Human Services, CDC: Update: trends in AIDS incidence—United States, 1996, *MMWR* 46:861, 1997.

27

Community Psychiatric Mental Health Nursing

Alwilda Scholler-Jaquish

OBJECTIVES

- Discuss the factors that influenced the deinstitutionalization movement.
- Describe the components of community mental health nursing.
- List outpatient treatment options commonly available in community settings.
- Compare and contrast therapy and rehabilitation.
- Discuss the components of case management.
- Explain the impact of managed care on community psychiatric rehabilitation.
- Analyze the key elements of psychiatric home health care.
- Identify factors that contribute to homelessness of people with severe and persistent mental illness.
- Describe the cultural needs of community residents.
- Explore the factors contributing to the incarceration of mentally ill persons.
- Identify the predictors of violence in the mentally ill.
- Apply the nursing process to clients in the community and in the home.

The current emphasis in psychiatric treatment is on outpatient or community-based programs. Community treatment of psychiatric clients occurs on a continuum of care that includes the community hospital, partial hospitalization programs, evaluation and treatment facilities, psychiatric rehabilitation programs, respite care, and a myriad of independent and semi-independent living arrangements. Community psychiatric mental health nursing encompasses a variety of treatment modalities and activities that address the treatment needs of psychiatric clients striving to maintain a stable position in the community.

ROLE OF THE NURSE

The role of the psychiatric nurse specializing in community mental health is to help the client maintain his or her highest level of functioning and independence within the community. The nurse's role is a challenging one. It requires a sound understanding of human behavior and development, psychiatric disorders, and prevailing treatments. Keen assessment skills and insight based on experience and good judgment are necessary. Skills in group and family process are also essential elements for the successful practice of the community psychiatric mental health nurse. In addition, it is critical for the nurse to have an extensive knowledge of the available community resources, the development and maintenance of community networks, the multidisciplinary treatment team process, and working with clients and families to facilitate their adjustment in the community.

Nurses with advanced degrees may work as managers of community mental health centers or programs, consult with staff in residential centers, serve as case managers, practice as clinical nurse specialists, or work in home health agencies providing mental health care (Helwig, 1997; Laskowski, 2001; Worley, 1997b).

HISTORICAL PERSPECTIVE

Before the early 1960s all psychiatric care was administered and received in inpatient settings, primarily state hospitals. State hospitals have been in existence since the late eighteenth century, when the care of the mentally ill was shifted from jails and poorhouses to a more humane setting. In the mid-1800s Dorothea Dix shaped hospital care for mentally ill persons by convincing legislators that caring for the mentally ill was a public responsibility.

In 1955 state hospitals reached a peak hospital census of 559,000 people. In the early 1960s a number of social, political, and economic issues brought attention to the apparent warehousing of chronically mentally ill people in state institutions. For example, in one instance the Joint Commission on Mental Illness and Health report cited the serious overcrowding of state hospitals, the ineffectiveness and debilitating nature of long-term hospitalization, and the high cost of institutional care. The result of this report was the advent of the Mental Retardation Facilities and Community Mental Health Centers Construction Act of 1963. Social and political activists called attention to the appalling conditions

in which human beings were forced to live (*History of mental illness,* no date).

Little was available in the way of treatment except for tranquilizing medications such as chlorpromazine (Thorazine) and electroshock therapy (ECT). New medications were developed that controlled psychiatric symptoms, making community living possible (see Chapter 20). Legal advocates addressed the long-term commitment in mental institutions and initiated concerns about the need for client's rights (*History of mental illness,* no date). During the many years of institutionalization, clients worked for the state hospital in many areas ranging from garden work, farming, food preparation, and janitorial services. Legally, the clients could no longer be allowed to work without being paid for their services.

In 1964 health insurance provided mental health coverage for individuals. The following year Medicare was initiated to provide health care for older adults. Medicaid, designed to provide health care for the poor, was passed in 1966. Collectively these events combined to create deinstitutionalization as costs increased and benefits diminished. Over the next 10 years there was rapid emptying of mental institutions across the country.

Deinstitutionalization

During **deinstitutionalization,** federal dollars were recommended in legislation; however, the enacted legislation was never funded. The goal was to provide community mental health centers to meet the perceived needs of the community with the intention of creating a follow-up care system that would decrease the need for psychiatric hospitalization. Many cities established mental health centers, but they were often underfunded and could not meet the needs of the severely mentally ill persons discharged from state hospitals or the needs of community members. Care for severely mentally ill persons was shifted from large state hospitals to communities. Clients with identifiable family members were discharged to a home they had not known for 20 years or longer. Family members were not enthusiastic about the sudden arrival of a mentally ill person in their home. Those without known family were transferred to half-way houses that were supposed to provide supervision for the residents. However, these facilities were poorly funded and many failed to meet their goal in the first few years. Persons discharged to their family homes or to half-way houses soon wandered off and became homeless. Clients who had been ill cared for in a state institution now wandered the streets without food, shelter, medication, or protection of any kind. More than 100,000 mentally ill homeless were left to roam the streets. In addition to the homeless, tens of thousands of older mentally ill persons and mentally retarded persons of all ages were transferred to nursing homes where the care of the residents was compromised with the drastic change in the milieu. Between 1963 and 1986 the state hospital population decreased by 75%, from 504,000 to 138,000 (Drake and Wallach, 1999; *History of mental illness,* no date; Scholler-Jaquish, 2000).

Deinstitutionalization was both a historical fact and a set of legal mandates governing the treatment of mentally ill persons. The people directly affected by the deinstitutionalization process almost 40 years ago no longer exist. However, the components of the process continue as legal mandates for psychiatric care. Short-term stays in psychiatric facilities have been magnified with managed care plans that require clients to be discharged as soon as their psychotic episodes are under control. Another component is the use of the least restrictive measures to control persons in psychotic episodes. Physical or behavioral restraints can be used only for short-time periods with documented circulation checks every 15 minutes. Admission to a seclusion room requires close supervision and release as soon as the person is able to manage his or her behavior.

Mentally ill persons who are actively psychotic cannot be required to obtain psychiatric treatment unless they pose a threat to themselves or others. A homeless person who is actively hallucinating may be a nuisance, but cannot receive treatment because the person poses no direct threat to others. Another component of this process involves the person's right to determine his or her own treatment. No matter how disturbed a person may be, he or she has the right to refuse medication. In a psychiatric setting, certain medications may be ordered by a physician on a limited basis. In some settings, medication may be administered on an emergency basis by a registered nurse who can obtain the physician's order either before or immediately after the medication has been given. The drug can be given only as a **least restrictive** intervention, and each emergency thereafter requires a physician order as well (JCAHO, 2003) (see Chapter 4).

Psychotropic Medications

In addition to an increased commitment to community care, deinstitutionalization was highly influenced by two other factors. The introduction of phenothiazine and lithium carbonate in the late 1950s for the treatment of mental illnesses made possible the discharge of clients who previously experienced refractory psychosis. Today further development of antipsychotic medications continues to greatly influence the prognosis of psychiatric treatment, leading to rapid and often premature discharge of clients from hospitals.

The community mental health nurse faces a number of issues related to the use and misuse of psychotropic medications. Noncompliance is a complex problem that can be described as "not adhering to the prescribed plan of care." In some instances, the client makes a decision to stop taking their medications. Noncompliance also includes a lack of money to obtain the medications, lack of access, or the belief by clients that the medications are making them worse (Harris and Kellner, 1997; Janicak et al., 1998).

Educating clients and family members about psychotropic medications is a major responsibility of the nurse working in community settings. Information about medications should be clear and brief. It is of the utmost importance for the person to understand the importance of a regular regimen and to be aware of the most serious side effects. Teaching medication compliance and safety is an ongoing process, and the individual's knowledge and needs should be assessed whether the nurse encounters the client on a regular basis or episodically (Harris and Kellner, 1997).

Legal Influences

The deinstitutionalization movement was also highly influenced by a civil rights movement that emphasized the rights of persons to self-determination. Legal decisions during this era made it difficult to commit people to mental institutions against their will. Litigation ensued for more treatment and less restrictive alternatives in the care of mentally ill persons. Treatment, rather than custodial care, became the focus of institutional settings. The U.S. Court of Appeals mandated the "least restrictive alternative to hospitalization" as the guide for the placement of clients, thus discouraging unnecessary hospitalization (see Chapter 4).

Community mental health nurses are continually challenged with legal and ethical issues in their practice. There must always be a signed consent for treatment. Careful documentation of the care provided and the client's response is an essential part of every client contact. Nurses may be liable for failure to warn potential victims when they become aware of a client's self-destructive behavior or actions that could be harmful to others. Nurses must be aware of the state laws in the area in which they practice to meet the challenge of maintaining confidentiality while sharing necessary information about a client. Gray areas occur when the nurse learns of illegal behavior on the part of a client, such as stealing clothes to satisfy a delusion of grandeur or sexual promiscuity in which the client has human immunodeficiency virus (HIV) or hepatitis C. The nurse should develop a trusting relationship with the client and not agree to *never* disclose unsafe behavior. State law may require the reporting of persons who can transmit HIV disease. In these more complex situations, the community mental health nurse must communicate with both the client and the agency to determine an appropriate course of action to protect the client and the community (Kjervik, 1997).

CURRENT COMMUNITY PSYCHIATRIC TREATMENT SYSTEMS

To provide cogent care to clients and families, community psychiatric mental health nurses need to understand the context, diversity, and parameters of psychiatric treatment systems. Systems of care vary from state to state, county to county, and community to community. Community-based psychiatric treatment is often provided by public/private partnerships using grants and government funds, but it also may be provided by private enterprises or government agencies. Home health care for psychiatric clients may be provided by public health or community health nursing departments or by private home health agencies.

Community Mental Health Centers

Legislation to fund **community mental health centers (CMHCs)** was signed into law by President Carter near the end of his term. President Reagan's administration chose not to fund the act and reduced the legislation to providing care for chronically mentally ill persons. The National Institute of Mental Health (NIMH) took the lead in assisting states to define chronic mental illness (now known as severe and persistent mental illness). As a result of these changes, CMHCs provide psychosocial education, psychoeducation, social skills, family and peer support, psychiatric case management, and medication supervision (Worley, 1997b).

Special populations with mental illness also need services. These populations include the homeless mentally ill, the mentally ill in jail, those with mental illness and substance abuse, those with mental illness and AIDS, children with chronic mental illness, and older adults with mental illness. These populations requires the development of programs to effectively manage the specific needs of each group (Worley, 1997a).

Funding

In most states the state hospital system and the community treatment system are funded separately. In some states, mental health funding is distributed from the state directly to treatment providers. Other states distribute mental health dollars to each county government, which in turn distributes the money to treatment providers. Some states have developed a system of regional support networks. A regional support network is an alliance or bonding together of a few counties to share the funding and the burden of mental health care. This approach is particularly advantageous in rural counties, where it is more difficult to secure treatment providers. The more layers of government involved in the distribution of funds, the more money is spent on administrative costs rather than on clients' needs. Local government or administrative offices, however, often have a clearer vision of the actual needs of the community being served, thereby avoiding unnecessary programs.

Many states are now contracting with private health maintenance organizations (HMOs) to finance mental health services for Medicaid and Medicare clients. Documentation is the key to obtaining financial reimbursement for care. A program that is not reimbursed cannot continue to provide care to the most needy of our citizens.

Philosophy

Two separate philosophies currently dominate the organization of mental health care provider systems. These philosophies are sharply debated in urban areas and regional and state hospital catchment areas that have larger populations of persons with severe and persistent mental illness. The central debate of the two philosophies is the issue of *freedom of choice* versus *continuity of care* for psychiatric clients.

Freedom of Choice

Freedom-of-choice advocates argue that all people, regardless of their disabilities, deserve a vast array of treatments from which to choose. In this mode, clients select from different modalities and treatment providers and may receive care at several different agencies. The client is empowered to design his or her own treatment. In the current trend of managed care, these systems operate on the idea of managed competition. An underlying assumption of this system approach is that agencies compete to develop services that will best serve persons with mental disorders. In practice, freedom-of-choice systems have experienced some common problems with client care. Persons with severe and persistent mental illness often have symptoms that affect their behavior, sometimes making them unpleasant or uncooperative and predisposing them to reject treatment. Many agencies do not choose to develop treatment options for severe mental disorders because of the nature of their mission. Consequently, systems may actually have a dearth of services for the people within the system who need the most intervention. Both the provider and the client have the freedom to make decisions. Treatment providers in these systems can refuse to treat a person whose symptoms make the person hesitant to accept treatment, thereby leaving a client who is difficult to treat without services. Combined with these problems is the fact that some severe mental disorders have a primary symptom of withdrawal. Often a client will withdraw from treatment as a result of impaired judgment caused by worsening illness when in fact the treatment actually needs to increase. The severe and persistent mentally ill who are incarcerated also have the right to refuse treatment. In a system built on a myriad of treatment options without a central contact, a client's withdrawal from treatment is less noticeable because of the resulting fragmentation of care.

Continuity of Care

Continuity-of-care advocates argue that persons with severe and persistent mental illness need to have one stable treatment provider throughout all phases and episodes of their illness. The underlying assumption is that some symptoms of mental illness are the very processes that disrupt a person's care and therefore they also need to be treated. Within these systems a central care provider or case manager is responsible for assessment, the securing of treatment, and referral to appropriate services. The majority of the services may or may not be provided by a central care coordinator, but the coordinator has the primary relationship with the client. A disadvantage of this system is that the client may be limited by the coordinator's view of the client's condition, the situation, or the system. A second disadvantage of this system is that when a case manager leaves, the client experiences a major disruption in a primary relationship and may have difficulty continuing treatment or establishing a new relationship. The advantages of this type of system are less treatment fragmentation and the fact that the client has someone to contact with whom he or she can interact and who will act on the client's behalf to coordinate care.

Many systems, whether offering freedom of choice or continuity of care, operate on the concept of *episodes of care,* following the medical model. Under this philosophy the client encounters the system only when his or her symptoms require care, much like the care an individual receives at the medical practitioner's office. The advantage of this model lies in its potential to serve increased numbers of clients because not all clients will require services at the same time. The disadvantage of this model is that primary prevention is not used. Often, clients do not encounter a provider until they need acute intervention. Acute and inpatient intervention is more costly, both to the system and to the client. Generally the more severe the episode of illness, the longer and more difficult the recovery period, resulting in more disruption to the client's life.

Managed Care

Managed care emerged during the 1990s in an effort to stem the spiraling costs of health care. HMOs were originally intended to reduce the cost of health expenses with a small portion dedicated to mental health crisis care. More recently, managed mental health care organizations (MMHCO) have evolved to deliver mental health and substance abuse services. Typically the MMHCOs develop a network of providers that work under cost containment practices used by health care HMOs.

Third-party payer systems hire case managers to review the effectiveness and cost-effectiveness of a client's treatment. This type of utilization review mandates that community mental health nurses clearly describe the needs and benefits of treatment for their clients to validate their need for care. Goal-focused treatment, development of realistic and measurable treatment plans, and organization of care around accepted guidelines and preferred practices are the objectives of client advocacy under managed care (Schreter, 1997).

In some states the managed care program reimburses care providers through a capitated system instead of the fee-for-service system used in previous years. In a fee-for-service system, treatment providers are reimbursed for each service rendered. In a capitated system (**capitation**), a flat fee is assigned for each client. The service provider is reimbursed the flat fee whether the client uses services minimally or maximally. Treatment providers changing to capitated systems must strategize to find cost-effective interventions to decrease the number of interventions needed, or increase the numbers of persons served, in order to survive at the same rate of pay. This approach encourages practitioners to provide less care. Practitioners that determine a need for treatment find that a client's care may be denied (Zubritsky, 1997).

The implications for treatment in community mental health centers are enormous. Some treatment agencies deal with this new payment system by offering more group and less individual therapy. Other treatment agencies use the episodes-of-care model discussed previously.

CULTURAL CONSIDERATIONS IN COMMUNITY MENTAL HEALTH NURSING

There are populations of people who have settled, immigrated, or been displaced to large and small cities throughout the United States. Large cities are multicultural settings with many languages, styles of dress, and responses to mental illness. Community health nurses are challenged to identify the specific populations within their service areas and adapt or develop programs to meet the needs of the identified racial or ethnic group. Large settlements of ethnic minorities require the development of a culturally competent approach to care. This necessitates community involvement, the development of trust, and cultural sensitivity (Huggins, 2003; Kennedy, 1997).

An example of a culturally congruent approach to community mental health care is the Arab-American and Chaldean behavioral health programs in the Detroit area. The staff is bicultural and many are trilingual. Psychiatrists and mental health workers who understand their language and are culturally sensitive provide a high quality of care for their clients. This mental health center also serves the community by providing sensitivity training for the community (Arab-American Chaldean Council, no date).

COMPONENTS OF COMMUNITY PSYCHIATRIC CARE
Community Psychiatric Programs

Research has clearly demonstrated that the combination of treatment programming and medication therapy is more effective for preventing relapse in psychiatric disorders than the use of medications alone (Janicak et al., 1998). Community psychiatric programs are outpatient programs staffed by interdisciplinary teams and are available during the work week. Day treatment programs provide services in 3- to 6-hour time blocks. These programs provide at least one of the basic treatment components of group therapy such as psychoeducational classes, skills training, milieu therapy, and activities. The day treatment programs provide therapy for the client while allowing family members to go to work and conduct necessary personal business. Most clients attend these programs voluntarily, although some individuals may be mandated to the program as a least restrictive alternative to inpatient treatment (see Understanding and Applying Research box on p. 608).

In the field of psychiatric programming, a philosophical distinction is made between therapy and rehabilitation. Both therapy and rehabilitation are vital to the overall treatment of clients who are mentally impaired. Both have philosophical goals of preventing relapse or further deterioration. The distinction is in the focus of treatment. Therapy focuses on reducing the client's discomfort, liabilities, symptoms, and illness to help promote their adjustment in the community. Rehabilitation focuses on developing a person's strengths and assets and improving health by restoring or increasing their functioning in the community. There are four main models of community psychiatric programming: *partial*

UNDERSTANDING and APPLYING RESEARCH

In a study of 12 clinical nurse specialists who worked in outpatient mental health centers, the participants were interviewed and asked to describe difficult client situations. The study emphasized the importance of the nurse-client relationship. Difficulties encountered by the clinical nurse specialists were managed within the context of the established nurse-client relationship. Participants stressed the importance of clinical supervision for validation, insight, and support within the mental health system. The researcher was surprised to learn about the problems the nurses had with intrusive behaviors by the clients including stalking of the nurses and/or their family members.

Laskowski C: The mental health clinical nurse specialist and the "difficult" patient: evolving meaning, *Issues Ment Health Nurs* 22:5, 2001.

hospitalization programs, traditional day treatment, psychosocial rehabilitation/skills training programs, and psychosocial clubhouse models.

Partial Hospitalization Programs

Partial hospitalization programs are the most intensive treatment of the therapeutic models. These programs are one step away from the hospital on the treatment continuum of care and are specifically designed to prevent hospital admissions. The program may reside in a hospital setting or at a mental health ambulatory treatment center. The nature of the program affects reimbursement from government and third-party payers. For example, Medicare reimburses hospital-based partial hospitalization programs at a higher rate than non-hospital-based activities.

Clients enter partial hospitalization programs either when they are discharged from the hospital and are still in a fragile state or when they have become so symptomatic that they require intensive structure and intervention. This is a short-term intervention, and the average stay is 3 weeks to 3 months. Partial hospitalization programs are generally staffed with psychiatric mental health nurses, a psychiatrist, and psychology or social work staff. The treatment regimen includes individual therapy, group therapy, psychoeducation classes, structured activities, and medication monitoring. The goal of the program is to increase the client's functioning to a level that the client can maintain outside the hospital. The focus is on reduction of symptoms that greatly inhibit or prohibit community living. A nurse working in a partial hospitalization program monitors symptoms and mental status, facilitates groups, teaches psychoeducation classes, plans and implements activities, and works with a psychiatrist in monitoring the effects and side effects of medications (Garrison, 1997).

Psychosocial Rehabilitation/ Skills Training Programs

Psychosocial rehabilitation/skills training programs distinguish themselves from other treatment programs by emphasizing different goals. The focus of these programs is for the client to acquire skills that will compensate for the neu-rocognitive and neuropsychiatric deficits caused by mental disorders. The primary assumption of the rehabilitation model is that the client has a deficit in a skilled performance or lacks the skills necessary for living, learning, or work.

There is a basic assumption that the client has the potential for growth and that he or she can develop the skills to make personal choices and to manage their illness. The mental health workers assist clients to normalize relationships with themselves and others to help them successfully integrate into the community. Clients are provided with training and education in how to deal with the "here and now" problems of daily living. They learn by doing and participating in problem solving in the real world. Daily living brings any number of big and small problems that must be successfully managed by the client (Bacon, 1997).

Mental health professionals in these programs do not distance themselves from the clients. Instead, they know their clients by their first names and caregivers are also known by their first names. This informal relationship allows the client to learn skills in relating to others. The staff addresses the client's rights and assists the individual in developing a sense of empowerment. They also work with the client's family and strive to achieve positive outcomes for the client and family (Bacon, 1997).

A nurse working in this environment is responsible for helping the client to identify a specific area of need and then assisting the client in developing a realistic plan of intervention designated to induce a behavioral change. The nurse is also responsible for creating and teaching psychoeducation/skill-building classes that address the neurocognitive needs of the clients (see Case Study).

Case Management

Psychiatric mental health nurses have been involved in the coordination of care for clients with mental illnesses for years. Many services and resources are necessary to meet the multiple needs of persons with severe and persistent mental illness.

Case management is a strategy to coordinate care and reduce fragmented care. Psychiatric case management can be conducted by one case manager or an interdisciplinary team that includes nurses, physicians, and social workers who develop a plan of care for a specific client population. Care coordination is the primary component of all case management models. The focus of case management is to advocate for individuals or families by integrating and coordinating care or multiple services. Goals for case management are multidimensional and include:
- Identification and outreach
- Assessment
- Enhancing client **activities of daily living**
- Service plan
- Monitoring

Case managers locate potential clients and make referrals for appropriate resources. Clients may be referred or may be identified during hospitalization. Case managers monitor the client's symptoms, compliance with medication, and ability

CASE STUDY

Matt is a 43-year-old man with a long history of chronic paranoid schizophrenia. He lives in a government-subsidized apartment and attends the local clubhouse model of treatment 5 days a week. At the clubhouse his primary job is washing dishes and serving food in the cafe. Within the clubhouse setting, Matt is socially appropriate and congenial. He exhibits no positive symptoms of his illness but has residual negative symptoms of blunted affect and compromised hygiene. He had expressed a desire to ride the bus, and the nurse offered to come to his apartment to teach him the bus route from his apartment to the club.

When the nurse arrives at Matt's apartment, she sees that it is a health hazard. Matt's kitchen counters are covered with moldy, dirty dishes adorned with cockroaches. Dirty laundry is piled throughout the house, and there is a strong odor of filth. Matt has hidden salami under the couch because he is afraid that the neighbors will steal it out of his refrigerator. There are cigarette burns on both the couch and the bed. There are no towels in the bathroom, about which Matt is unconcerned because, he says, he does not wash his hands after using the toilet, nor does he bathe.

Critical Thinking

1. What is the nurse's primary concern?
2. How will this affect Matt's treatment plan? Rank the concerns from highest to lowest priority.
3. What resources discussed in this chapter will be useful in Matt's treatment?
4. How will the nurse discuss this with Matt?
5. Knowing the extent of Matt's compromised hygiene, what is the nurse's role in Matt's selection of clubhouse jobs?
6. Does the nurse have an obligation to protect the health of other clubhouse members?
7. What are some interventions that the nurse can develop to help Matt work on this issue without embarrassing him in front of his clubhouse members while still protecting others?
8. What symptoms of schizophrenia in particular will interfere with Matt's ability to understand the connection between his poor hygiene and his work at the clubhouse?

Box 27-1   Why Case Management?

Case management addresses a wide variety of health care issues and needs. As a result, it is often implemented for multiple reasons, including these:

1. Case management focuses on the full spectrum of needs presented by clients and their families; it is client focused. Client and family satisfaction within case management systems is generally high.
2. A strong component of case management is an outcome orientation to care. The goal is to move the client/family toward optimal care outcomes.
3. Case management facilitates and promotes coordination of client care, minimizing fragmentation.
4. Case management promotes cost-effective care by minimizing fragmentation, maximizing coordination, and facilitating client/family movement through the health care system.
5. Case management maximizes and coordinates the contributions of all disciplines within the health care team.
6. Case management responds to the needs of insurers and other third-party payers, specifically those related to outcome-based, cost-effective care.
7. The needs of clients, providers, and payers all receive attention within a case management system. Case management represents a merger of clinical and financial interests, systems, and outcomes.
8. Case management can be included in the marketing strategies of hospitals and other institutions to target clients/families, insurers, and employers.

Modified from American Nurses Association: *Case management by nurses,* Washington, DC, 1992, The Association.

(American Nurses Association, 1994). Some case management programs exceed this recommendation, hiring only master's prepared nurses, whereas others hire bachelor-level psychology and social work majors.

LEVELS OF ASSISTED LIVING

Paramount to the client's adjustment is having a place to live within the community. Maslow's hierarchy of needs identifies food, shelter, and clothing as basic necessities that must be met before a person progresses to higher needs and levels of development (Maslow, 1954) (see Figure 2-2). People with psychiatric disorders are more likely than the average population to live in physically inadequate dwellings in neighborhoods of high crime and to pay a higher percentage of their income on housing (Owen et al., 1996). During the last two decades, communities have developed options along the continuum of community living arrangements to suit the needs of persons with psychiatric disabilities. Persons with severe mental illness who live in an adult family home experience lower rehospitalization rates. Table 27-1 represents living arrangements along a continuum of care.

There are two basic types of residential treatment programs that are supervised by staff 24 hours a day: (1) programs that are supported through foster care or (2) independent living programs. Supervised **adult residential treatment programs** provide on-site staff 24 hours a day for 4 to 16 residents. These

to function on a day-to-day basis. All aspects of a person's life must be assessed to determine the extent of the client's needs and the individual's ability to meet those needs (Worley, 1997a). In one instance, a homeless mentally ill man was provided housing but was living on general assistance (GA-Welfare) of $100 to $200 a month. He was not able to pay his basic utilities or to buy food. This person had an address and a place to live but he had no furniture, utilities, or medication. He went "home" to sleep at night but for all intents and purposes he continued to live as a homeless person—a homeless person with an address. He had no one to advocate for him or his needs.

The case manager advocates for the client and/or the family by coordinating or providing services along the continuum of care. Effective case management has the potential to minimize health care costs to the client, family, and society (Box 27-1). Case managers may be nurses or other mental health professionals. The recommended minimum preparation for a nurse case manager is a baccalaureate degree in nursing with 3 years of appropriate clinical experience

Table 27-1   Community Living Arrangements

			Structured Living Facilities		Intensive Residential Treatment Facility
Independent	Semi-Independent	Adult Family Home	Board-and-Care Homes, Congregate Care Facilities	Skilled Nursing Facilities	
Description of Function					
Lives on own or with others with no need for supervision Has freedom to do as he or she wishes Exhibits responsible behavior Handles responsibilites, duties appropriately	Shares responsibilities with two to four others Has need for minimal structure and supervision Works toward independent living, concentrating on needed skills Needs to live with others for ongoing support	Family-type living situation Does not require as much structure as structured living facilities and intensive residential care Requires 24-hour supervision Has some freedom and independence as appropriate to individual	Structured living facility Does not require as much structure as intensive residential care 24-hour care	Structured living facility Highly supervised 24-hour care	Need for highly structured, treatment-oriented residential living facility 24-hour supervision Different levels of need and care
Client Criteria					
Stable Able to demonstrate most skills needed to live independently satisfactorily Has good activities of daily living (ADL) Able to take medications on own responsibly Structures own time adequately	Able to demonstrate most skills to live independently satisfactorily Able to cooperate with others Has good ADL Able to take medications on own responsibly Structures own time adequately	Demonstrates ability to get along with others Follows house rules and treatment plan (if appropriate) Able to structure own time adequately Has good ADL Able to take own medications appropriately	Able to cooperate with others Follows house rules and structure	Functioning level warrants needed care Unable to provide for self independently Follows facility rules and treatment plan	Poor history of compliance with treatment and community living Need for 24-hour supervision Able to follow rules of facility and treatment plan

programs can be found in group homes, half-way houses, respite programs, or intermediate care facilities. The clients benefit from both staff and peer support. The staff monitors clients' symptoms and manages their medical regimen. There is an emphasis on interpersonal relationships between client and staff and client and peers. The residents participate in communication, prevocational preparation, and life within the facility (O'Neil and Allard, 1997). The staff assists them to obtain entitlements so they can qualify for health care. The clients are taught the basic self-care skills they need to progress to the next level of community living. These skills include how to take medication as prescribed, how to describe medication side effects to their doctor, basic grooming and hygiene, and appropriate interpersonal behavior. Studies indicate the persons with severe mental illness strive for normalcy. They want to be like others and to be independent (Pickens, 1999). Rehabilitation programming in these facilities follows the models of community psychiatric treatment programs described earlier in the chapter.

Congregate care facilities, or board-and-care homes, are group homes for persons with psychiatric illnesses that usu-

ally house 6 to 15 residents. Congregate care facilities provide food, housing, and supervision of medication regimens and daily living skills. Residents of these facilities often receive outpatient care at the local community mental health center. In some communities, the community mental health centers provide free consultation to the congregate care facility. Most congregate care facilities require the resident to be involved in some kind of adjunct treatment.

Adult family homes (supportive housing programs) provide a quieter, more personal living arrangement for clients needing supervision. Also called adult foster homes, these residential facilities are provided by families who agree to "adopt" one or two persons into their home. The client becomes a part of the family structure and is expected to fit into the normal routines of the household. The adult family home provider supervises medication regimens if necessary, expects the client to perform routine tasks of daily living, and assists the client in acquiring services and skills needed to live independently in the community. An adult family home is beneficial to the client who cannot tolerate the larger numbers of persons in congregate care facilities, but may be more difficult for clients who cannot tolerate the increased intimacy involved in being part of a family. A recent study of clients who lived in a homelike setting after discharge from a psychiatric facility described the difficulties clients experienced in trying to conform to a family setting. The clients struggled to make it work and described their feelings of increased competence and self-confidence once they succeeded in their struggle (Pejlert, Asplund, and Norberg, 1999).

Semi-independent living is designated for persons living with two to four other persons in the community with minimal supervision. Clients in these situations generally are assisted by an **independent living skills** staff who systematically teach residents the skills needed for adult independent life such as cooking and budgeting.

HOME VISITS

It is estimated that 70% of mentally ill individuals live in the community. The Health Care Financing Administration determined in 1979 that psychiatric home health care could be reimbursed by Medicare and Medicaid. To be eligible for home care, clients must be homebound, have a demonstrated medical necessity, and require intermittent care. For example, a woman with schizophrenia lives alone in a small apartment. Her auditory, visual, and tactile hallucinations are controlled with bimonthly injections of haloperidol (Haldol). Without the episodic home visits for supervision and monitoring of her medical regimen, this client's symptoms would become so disabling that she would require hospitalization.

Many home health agencies now have a subspecialty to provide psychiatric home health care. Nurses assess clients and their response to treatment. During the visit, the home health nurse assesses the individual's safety in the living environment. In addition, the nurse assesses for any potential risks from other members of the household (Hellwig, 1997). A broad range of psychiatric home visits are reimbursed by third-party payers, with each payer having specific criteria for reimbursement. For example, the requirement for reimbursement by Medicare is that the primary treating professional in the client's overall care is a psychiatrist.

Safety

Psychiatric home visits vary in focus, time spent, intensity, and outcome. It is crucial that the nurse planning a home visit evaluate the potential risks of that visit before the actual interventions are initiated. Risk evaluation always includes the client's history, usual relationship with the nurse, current mental status, and living situation. The nurse may decide to make a visit alone or with another treatment provider. Security personnel may be provided for nurses making home visits in high-risk neighborhoods, especially those in large cities.

Categories of Home Visits

The goals of community psychiatric mental health nursing home visits fall into three basic categories: client engagement, client assessment, and client teaching. Because many clients with mental disorders exhibit primary symptoms of withdrawal or social isolation, it is sometimes necessary to first locate the person out in the community. These home visits are frequently not prearranged with the client because anticipation of a visit may increase the client's anxiety and lead to further exacerbation of symptoms. Also, some clients may avoid a visit, fearing that they might be involuntarily hospitalized. The goal of the visit is to reengage the client with the system of care by bringing the client in contact with the primary case manager or nurse. Some clients are seen in their homes for several months before they agree to engage in treatment at the local mental health center. Assertive outreach as a component of community psychiatric mental health care engages clients who generally resist traditional, office-based treatment (Herinckx et al., 1997) (see Case Study).

CASE STUDY

Ron is a 20-year-old college student who was discharged from inpatient psychiatric services to independent living 2 weeks ago. He was originally brought to the hospital by four of his friends when he became drunk, belligerent, and threatening at a party. His friends reported that Ron's behavior had changed the previous month. Before he was hospitalized, Ron began staying up all night, consuming large quantities of alcohol, and fighting with other dorm residents, and he had gotten two speeding tickets in the previous week. In the hospital he was diagnosed with bipolar I disorder, single manic episode. He was treated with lithium carbonate 300 mg tid and clonazepam (Klonopin) 2 mg hs and discharged with a week's supply of medication. Today the nurse case manager received a call from Ron's apartment manager, who was concerned because Ron had sarcastically said he would just go kill himself when he was asked to turn his music down. The manager reports that other tenants are complaining that Ron makes noise at all hours of the night. The nurse has not seen Ron since his discharge 2 weeks ago and is unable to reach him by telephone.

Nursing Diagnoses
1. Risk for injury related to destructive behaviors and hyperactivity, as evidenced by increased agitation and potentially injurious behavior (drinking alcohol, speeding, fighting)
2. Risk for violence. Risk factors: manic excitement, increased motor activity, and provocative behaviors (e.g., consumes large amounts of alcohol, speeding tickets, and fighting)
3. Disturbed sleep pattern related to manic excitement, as evidenced by staying up all night, hyperactivity, and agitation
4. Impaired social interaction related to manic excitement, as evidenced by dysfunctional interaction with peers and others (e.g., belligerent behavior with peers, threatening others, plays loud music, makes noise all night)

Critical Thinking
1. What factors should the nurse consider when making a decision about a home visit?
2. What assessments need to be done when Ron is seen?
3. How will the nurse assess Ron's personal safety?
4. What other information is needed to complete the nursing assessment?
5. What other DSM-IV-TR diagnoses need to be explored at this point?
6. If Ron refuses to be seen or responds defensively or with denial, how should the nurse respond?
7. How should the nurse proceed in getting help for Ron and also protecting herself?

Schizophrenia

TEACH THE CLIENT:

1. Schizophrenia is a brain disorder that requires both medication and psychosocial therapy.
2. Withdrawal is a common symptom, and it is important to communicate with health care providers when beginning to feel more reluctant or afraid to interact with people.
3. It may take months for symptoms to get under control. Increased involvement in therapy leads to a better outcome.

TEACH THE FAMILY:

1. Schizophrenia is a brain disease that affects 1% of the world's population. The brain disease has nothing to do with how the client was parented.
2. Chronic brain diseases puts special stresses on the family. National organizations for education and support of family members, such as The National Alliance for the Mentally Ill (NAMI), assist families with the emotional burden, decrease isolation, and provide resource information on a local and national level.
3. High levels of expressed negative emotion within the family system may exacerbate symptoms of schizophrenia. It is important for all family members to find appropriate ways to express their grief and deal with conflict.
4. Prescribed medications for the client are important and may require supervision and monitoring by the family to ensure effectiveness and assess symptoms.
5. Local mental health centers and some school districts sometimes provide support groups to parents and to siblings of people with mental disorders.

A home visit is an illuminating part of treatment. Seeing the client within the context of his or her living situation expands the nurse's understanding of the client's overall functioning level. An outpatient clinic provides a location to assess how the client functions in a semipublic environment for a short period of time, whereas a person's home gives the nurse a deeper sense of how the client functions on more fundamental and enduring levels (e.g., with activities of daily living and independent living skills) (see Client and Family Teaching Guidelines box).

Neurocognitive deficits associated with mental illnesses frequently interfere with client learning and, more important, with the process of learning. Some clients are unable to perform a learned skill when the skill setting changes. A home visit is an effective approach for teaching basic independent living skills to clients who experience transfer-of-learning deficits. During home learning, clients have the opportunity to use their own equipment in their own setting, which increases the potential for task retention. The teaching process may need to be repeated if the client changes residences.

HOMELESS MENTALLY ILL

Homelessness is a major problem throughout the country compounded by poverty, unemployment, underemployment, substance abuse, and mental illness. Homeless persons are more likely to be male and to represent the racial or ethnic minority in a specific area of the country. There have been numerous studies to determine the number of homeless persons in each state and major city. These studies detracted from the reasons for homelessness. Although deinstitutionalization played a role in homelessness several decades ago, the current major contributors to homelessness in mentally ill persons is short-term treatment, lack of family support, inability to carry out the activities of daily living, lack of access to care and or medication prescriptions, and exacerbation of psychotic symptoms (Meisler, 1997).

The National Coalition for the Homeless reported that 20% to 25% of any homeless population has severe and persistent mental illness (see Chapter 12). Of the estimated 4 million people with severe mental illness, only 5% are homeless at any given time. Of the homeless mentally ill, many need hospitalization and at least 5% need long-term institutionalization (NCH, 1999).

In his seminal study on homeless in the Chicago area, Rossi (1991) found that the leading cause of homelessness is the failure of the person's social network. The family support was most likely to fail when a dependent male drained the emotional and financial support of the household. This was more apparent when the family was poor and struggling for survival. For the most part, a dependent male is an unwelcome member of any household.

Racial and ethnic differences play a significant role in the family's response to mentally ill members. Some cultural groups are protective of the ill individual, whereas others may soon become exhausted with the care and dependency needs of the ill person. Dependent men are less well tolerated than dependent women. Mentally ill persons with positive psychiatric symptoms may drain the emotional reserve of even the strongest family.

Severely and persistently mentally ill persons may move in and out of homelessness because of exacerbation of symptoms or discontinuation of medications. Attempting to live a homeless existence is difficult even for persons with intact mental health and abilities. There is a need to acquire food, shelter, and protection every day. Persons who are severely and persistently mentally ill find it extremely difficult and often impossible to obtain the most basic necessities of life. Some seek refuge in places that they believe to be safe, such as in tunnels, in caves, under bridges, or in secluded parks. The more disengaged persons become from society as a whole, the more difficult it becomes to offer them needed services (Meisler, 1997).

Contrary to public opinion, homeless persons are not all alike. Unfortunately, public policies and treatment programs are designed to service what they consider to be the "typical" homeless person. The Scholler-Jaquish Intervention Model for Homeless Persons (2000) provides a way to plan care and services to the severely mentally ill homeless according to identifiable needs (Table 27-2). The model is organized in three stages of homelessness and the three levels of public health prevention. The levels of prevention include

Table 27-2	Nursing Intervention Model for Homeless Persons		
	Stage One	Stage Two	Stage Three
Primary prevention	Advocacy Promotion of low-income housing Increase in minimum wage Drug and alcohol education Drug and alcohol treatment programs Access to health care Coping skills Job training AIDS prevention Aggression management Community mental health centers Mental health programs for ethnic and racial minorities Promoting legislation for homeless mentally ill	Advocacy Self-advocacy Preventing violence Interpersonal skills training Anger management Immunizations (flu, pneumonia) Legal assistance programs for homeless Access to health care Access to mental health care Drug and alcohol treatment programs at service centers	Advocacy Multiservice outreach centers Wet detoxification programs
Secondary prevention	Diagnostic services Mental health screenings treatment programs for drugs, alcohol, and mental illness Illness prevention	Monitor psychiatric status Monitor compliance with medical regimen for TB, AIDS Wet detoxification	Mobile treatment programs: provide care for client where they are or in walk-in clinics Monitor changes in physical and/or mental status Monthly antipsychotic medications if accepted Treatment for TB Access to basic nutrition Wet detoxification Nutrition Outreach mental health service
Tertiary prevention	Treatment of chronic mental illness Drug and alcohol treatment programs Case management Symptom management	Treatment for mental illness Treatment for major health problems Wet and dry detoxification programs	

primary, secondary, and tertiary prevention. Primary prevention addresses prevention, health promotion, and education. Secondary prevention includes screening, treatment of illness, and reduction of disability. Tertiary prevention includes rehabilitation and palliative care.

In Stage One the mentally ill homeless are newly diagnosed persons who maintain contact with service providers and family members. These individuals are the most likely to be able to secure a place to sleep and eat. Persons in Stage One are the most amenable to outreach services and treatment.

Homeless persons in Stage Two have few connections with normative society and are more likely to be episodically admitted for acute exacerbations of psychiatric symptoms. The homeless mentally ill in Stage Two are likely to rely on alcohol or drugs to control their psychiatric symptoms. Individuals with bipolar mania are more likely to use alcohol to help control their symptoms. Persons with schizophrenia also use alcohol to reduce the intensity of their hallucinations. Individuals who are depressed are more apt to rely on opiates for relief. The persons in Stage Two may be helped if assistance is readily available, but they may not be able to approach care providers on their own. Or they may be in such a state of distress that they appear frightening to emergency health care workers and are therefore rejected.

The severely mentally ill persons in Stage Three are the most disaffiliated. These individuals have no access to medications, but they may respond to outreach workers who provide food or first-aid measures. These Stage Three homeless mentally ill persons have no relief from their psychiatric symptoms. Providing health care to these individuals requires a creative approach and health care workers who can accept the multiple problems of these very needy human beings (Scholler-Jaquish, 2000).

VIOLENCE AND THE MENTALLY ILL

Violence is a problem for mentally ill persons. Individuals who experience the positive symptoms of visual, auditory, or tactile hallucinations may injure themselves or others during their hallucinatory experiences. Some persons with severe and persistent mental illness experience command hallucinations that instruct them to hurt or kill themselves or others. These individuals need careful monitoring by mental health professionals and family members. Unfortunately, a child or parent with mental illness may kill family members who erroneously believe that they can manage the mentally ill person. Threats or behaviors indicating that risk for violence should be taken seriously may be missed or denied by family members. Unfortunately, in the last decade we have

CLINICAL ALERT

The nurse must be constantly alert to suicidal ideation and intent. The period of highest risk is often the first month out of the hospital after the client has been discharged. Clients with schizophrenia who hear voices (auditory command hallucinations) instructing them to harm themselves are at equal or greater risk than those with depression. One predictor of suicidal risk is a history of previous attempts and the lethality of those attempts.

witnessed an increase of mass murders by mentally ill persons. Community mental health nurses are responsible for protecting themselves, the client, and the family from clients experiencing command hallucinations instructing them to kill their classmates, employees, co-workers, or family members (Arboleda-Florez, Holley, and Crisanti, 1998; Eronen, Angermeyer, and Schulze, 1998; Flannery et al., 1998; Hersh and Borum, 1998).

The predictors of violence include:

- History of past violence
- Drug and alcohol abuse
- Serious mental illness combined with a failure to take medication
- Neurologic impairment
- Paranoid delusions
- Command hallucinations (Treatment Advocacy Center, no date)

Severely mentally ill persons with negative symptoms may be victims of abuse by others. In some instances, mentally disabled persons are victimized by their own family members or care providers. Physically, sexually, or emotionally abused mentally disabled persons are reluctant to tell others for fear of losing the security that they have. Others may try to tell mental health workers and not be understood or believed.

Police officers are called on to deal with mentally or emotionally disturbed persons. In some instances, police officers have been specially trained to respond to psychiatric emergencies. There have been incidents in which police officers have used excessive and even deadly force in dealing with mentally ill persons. Persons attempting suicide have been killed by police officers responding to the reported incidents. Emotionally distraught people carrying knives or other objects have been shot multiple times by police officers. In some very tragic events, persons known to be severely mentally ill have been shot to death by police officers responding to a disturbance. In one instance a woman with psychosis who refused to leave her home for several days was killed by the local police officers when she stepped outside of the house (Amnesty International, 2000).

Community mental health nurses must engage in community education for law enforcement agencies and other emergency responders. The most effective intervention plan is known as the Memphis Plan in which teams of police officers receive special training in crisis intervention. After the situa-

tion is deescalated, the disturbed person is taken to a psychiatric facility instead of to a police department (Amnesty International, 2002).

MENTALLY ILL PERSONS IN JAIL

The incarceration of mentally ill persons is an urgent national problem. As many as 300,000 people with schizophrenia or bipolar disorder are currently incarcerated. These mentally ill persons make up 16% of the total prison population. Many were charged with misdemeanors; a much smaller number were charged with felonies resulting from their disordered thought processes (NCH, 1997; Open Society Institute, 1996; Treatment Advocacy Center, no date). Factors involved in the incarceration of mentally ill persons include homelessness, attitudes of community and police force members, more rigid commitment criteria, and lack of adequate community supports.

Nursing responsibilities in correctional institutions vary and may include:

- Assessing of suicide risk
- Evaluating mental status
- Monitoring effectiveness of medications
- Providing a liaison between the inmates and the community treatment providers
- Providing care when warranted
- Providing general mental health treatment
- Providing education for inmates and prison staff

Nurses working with incarcerated mentally ill individuals may encounter a twofold stigma that is frustrating and tragic. The legal mandate to protect an individual's right to refuse medication applies in prison the same as it does in general society. Unfortunately, when persons who are already unable to think clearly refuse psychotropic medications, the result is one of the tragedies of society. Dorthea Dix, a pioneer in mental health nursing, would be shocked to find prisoners who are uncontrollable in their cells and living in conditions worse than wild animals. The prolonged months or years without the necessary psychotropic medications to help manage psychotic symptoms reduce these people to tragic semblances of human beings.

OTHER COMPONENTS OF COMMUNITY PSYCHIATRIC MENTAL HEALTH NURSING

Community psychiatric mental health nursing frequently involves crisis intervention with individuals as well as with groups of people. Many communities have special multidisciplinary teams of mental health professionals who provide mental health care as a component of disaster relief. Crisis intervention with groups and individuals is covered in Chapter 22.

Clients undergoing a severe exacerbation of psychiatric symptoms may need to be detained in a psychiatric hospital against their will for their own safety or for the safety of the community. Community psychiatric mental health nurses need a thorough understanding of the Involuntary Treatment Act covered in Chapter 4. Also, a thorough knowledge of appropriate nursing interventions and other treatment modalities is essential.

Medication management is a fundamental role of the community psychiatric mental health nurse. Nurses may work in medication clinics or follow-up clinics where the primary identified role is to monitor the effects and side effects of the client's prescribed medication, or they may work in psychiatric rehabilitation programs where medication monitoring is one of many functions. Regardless of the nurse's vocational setting, a strong knowledge of psychopharmacology is required (see Chapter 20).

CHAPTER SUMMARY

- Community psychiatric mental health services have greatly increased since the 1960s.
- Community psychiatric mental health programming is an essential element in the treatment of persons with persistent mental illness.
- Case management is a pivotal role for the community psychiatric mental health nurse.
- Community psychiatric mental health nurses frequently collaborate with or participate in multidisciplinary teams.
- Partial hospitalization programs are designed to assist the client to integrate into society.
- A purpose of a psychiatric home visit is to engage the client in treatment, to assess the client, and/or to teach the client a community-based skill.
- Managed care has a strong influence on the delivery of community psychiatric mental health care.
- A total of 20% to 25% of the homeless population has severe and persistent mental illness.
- The intervention model for homelessness provides a guide for working with mentally ill homeless persons.
- As many as 16% of prison inmates are severely and persistently mentally ill.
- Severely and persistently mentally ill persons may commit acts of violence associated with failure to take medications, a history of violence, paranoid delusions, or command hallucinations.
- Mentally ill persons may be abused by family, care providers, or law enforcement officers.

REVIEW QUESTIONS

1. The focus of the traditional day treatment is to:
   a. Stabilize the client from a crisis.
   b. Provide skills training and psychoeducation.
   c. Conduct research studies.
   d. Cure the client of mental illness.

2. A client who would benefit from case management is a client who:
   a. Is 16 and was recently diagnosed with major depression.
   b. Uses alcohol daily.
   c. Was recently started on clozapine (Clozaril).
   d. Is HIV positive, diagnosed with paranoid schizophrenia and drug dependency, and has had seven hospitalizations in the past 5 years.

3. An appropriate goal for a client in a board and care would be that the client will:
   a. Be responsible for own medication.
   b. Apply for a job.
   c. Comply with medication regimen and complete resident job.
   d. Coordinate a support group for the mentally ill.

4. A 28-year-old male was incarcerated for armed robbery. Before being convicted he used alcohol and drugs and was diagnosed with bipolar disorder. The nurse observes the client to be very loud and boisterous with hyperverbal speech stating that he was wrongly convicted and has spent the past 2 weeks staying up all night to prove it. Based on this assessment, the nurse concludes that the client:
   a. Has stopped taking his lithium.
   b. Needs a new attorney.
   c. Is having difficulty coping with prison.
   d. Needs a support group.

5. The psychiatric nurse visits a client in the community. He was diagnosed with chronic paranoid schizophrenia and has been taking risperidone (Risperdal) 2 mg bid. The nurse evaluates that the client requires some medication education after she observes the client:
   a. Drinking caffeine.
   b. Eating a cheeseburger.
   c. To have gained some weight.
   d. Sunbathing without sunscreen.

REFERENCES

American Nurses Association: *Case management by nurses*, Washington, DC, 1992: The Association.
American Nurses Association: *Statement on psychiatric mental health clinical nursing practice and standards of psychiatric mental health clinical nursing practice*, Washington, DC, 1994, The Association.
Amnesty International: Mentally ill or homeless: vulnerable to police abuse, no date, available online, accessed September 30, 2002, website: www.connix.com/~marpa/amnesty%20international.htm.
Arab-American Chaldean Council: Arab-American and Chaldean behavioral health programs, Author, no date, available online, accessed September 28, 2002, website: www.arabacc.org/BEHAVIORAL.htm.
Arboleda-Florez J, Holley H, Crisanti A: Understanding causal paths between mental illness and violence, *Soc Psychiatry Psychiatr Epidemiol* 33(Suppl 1):S38, 1998.
Bacon RC: Psychosocial rehabilitation. In Worley NK, editor, *Mental health nursing in the community*, St Louis, 1997, Mosby.
Drake RE, Wallach MA: Homelessness and mental illness: a story of failure, *Psychiatr Serv* 50:589, 1999.

Eronen M, Angermeyer MC, Schulze B: The psychiatric epidemiology of violent behavior, *Soc Psychiatry Psychiatr Epidemiol* 33(Suppl 1):S13, 1998.

Flannerry RB et al: Characteristics of violent versus nonviolent patients with schizophrenia, *Psychiatr Q* 69:83, 1998.

Garrison BL: Partial hospital program. In Worley NK, editor: *Mental health nursing in the community,* St Louis, 1997, Mosby.

Harris DE, Kellner NL: Medication management. In Worley NK, editor: *Mental health nursing in the community,* St Louis, 1997, Mosby.

Hellwig K: Home care. In Worley NK, editor, *Mental health nursing in the community,* St Louis, 1997, Mosby.

Herinckx HA et al: Assertive community treatment versus usual care in engaging and retaining clients with severe mental illness, *Psychiatr Serv* 48:1297, 1997.

Hersh K, Borum R: Command hallucinations, compliance and risk assessment, *J Am Acad Psychiatry Law* 26:353, 1998.

History of mental illness (no date), available online, accessed September 30, 2002, website: www.ohiou.edu/~ridges/history.html.

Huggins M: Culture. In Mohr WK, editor, *Johnson's psychiatric-mental health nursing,* ed 5, Philadelphia, 2003, Lippincott Williams & Wilkins.

Janicak et al: *Treatment with antipsychotics: principles and practice of psychopharmacotherapy,* ed 2, Baltimore, 1998, Williams & Wilkins.

Kennedy MK: Cultural competency. In Worley NK, editor, *Mental health nursing in the community,* St Louis, 1997, Mosby.

Kjervik DK: Legal and ethical issues. In Worley NK, editor, *Mental health nursing in the community,* St Louis, 1997, Mosby.

Laskowski C: The mental health clinical nurse specialist and the "difficult" patient: evolving meaning, *Issues Ment Health Nurs* 22:5, 2001.

Liberman RP et al: Skills training versus psychosocial occupational therapy for persons with persistent schizophrenia, *Am J Psychiatry* vol 155, no 8, 1998.

Maslow AH: *Motivation and personality,* New York, 1954, Harper & Row.

Meisler N: Homeless persons with mental illness. In Worley NK, editor: *Mental health nursing in the community,* St Louis, 1997, Mosby.

National Coalition of Homelessness [NCH]: *Criminalization of homelessness: waste and injustice,* 1997, available online, accessed September 30, 2002, website: www.nch.air.net/sn/1997/sept/waste.html.

National Coalition of Homelessness [NCH]: *Mental illness and homelessness,* NCH Fact sheet No 5, April 1999, available online, accessed September 28, 2002, website: www.nationalhomeless.org/mental.html.

O'Neil CA, Allard PS: Residential treatment. In Worley NK, editor, *Mental health nursing in the community,* St Louis, 1997: Mosby.

Open Society Institute, Mental illness in jail. 1996. website: www.soros.org/crime/ Available on line, accessed October 1, 2002.

Owen C et al: Housing accommodation preferences of people with psychiatric disabilities, *Psychiatr Serv* 47(6):628, 1996.

Pejlert A, Asplund K, Norberg A: Toward recovery: living in a home-like setting after the move from a hospital ward, *J Clin Nurs* 8:663, 1999.

Pickens JM: Living with serious mental illness: the desire for normalcy, *Nurs Sci Q* 12:233, 1999.

Rossi PH: *Down and out in America: the origins of homelessness in America,* Chicago, 1991, University of Chicago Press.

Scholler-Jaquish A: Homelessness in America. In Smith CM, Maurer FA, editors: *Community health nursing: theory and practice,* ed 2, Philadelphia, 2000, WB Saunders.

Schreter RK: Essential skills for managed behavioral health care, *Psychiatr Serv* 48:653, 1997.

Treatment Advocacy Center: *Homelessness, incarceration, episodes of violence: way of life for almost half of Americans with untreated mental illness,* (no date), available online, accessed October 3, 2002, website: www.psychlaws.org/GeneralResources/fact2.htm.

Worley NK: Case management. In Worley NK, editor, *Mental health nursing in the community,* St Louis, 1997a, Mosby.

Worley NK: Community mental health centers. In Worley NK, editor: *Mental health nursing in the community,* St Louis, 1997b, Mosby.

Zubritsky CD: Managed behavioral health services. In Worley NK, editor: *Mental health nursing in the community,* St Louis, 1997, Mosby.

SUGGESTED READINGS

Hiday VA et al: Criminal victimization of persons with severe mental illness, *Pscyhiatr Serv* 50:62, 1999.

Laban JK, Blum J: Persons with mental illness in jail. In Worley NK, editor: *Mental health nursing in the community,* St Louis, 1997, Mosby.

28

Persons With Severe and Persistent Mental Illness

Alwilda Scholler-Jaquish

OBJECTIVES

- Describe manifestations of severe and persistent mental illness across the life span.

- Discuss psychologic problems of persons with severe and persistent mental illness and their impact on the client and family.

- Explain how behavioral manifestations of severe and persistent mental illness affect a person's ability to function independently.

- State risk factors for persons with severe and persistent mental illness.

- Examine the relationship between poverty, severe and persistent mental illness, and homelessness.

- Explore the relationship between culture and severe and persistent mental illness.

- Distinguish between the behaviors of institutionalized persons with severe and persistent mental illness and the behaviors of young people with severe and persistent mental illness who have had few experiences with mental health treatment.

- Describe nursing interventions appropriate for individuals with severe and persistent mental illness.

- Apply the nursing process to clients with severe and persistent mental illness.

The impact of severe and persistent mental illness on the individual, family members, care providers, and the community is significant. Although any psychiatric diagnosis can result in a disabling condition, most references to **severe and persistent mental illness** (a psychiatric disorder that persists over time with remissions and recurrence of severe and disabling symptoms) address the concerns of the most severely disabled individuals (Bachrach, 1996; Yap, 2000). Persons with severe and persistent mental illness pose some of the most difficult social, medical, and political problems of our time. The National Institute of Mental Health (NIMH) reports that almost 19% of the population—more than 18 million people—have a major depressive disorder, and that another 2 million are diagnosed with schizophrenia (NIMH, 2002). Each individual with a severe and persistent mental illness will have a different life experience. However, each person lives in a world in which he or she is expected to have relationships with others and to provide for shelter and the necessities of life. The impact of the degree and frequency of psychiatric symptoms affects the ability to function effectively in the world in which the person lives. The public is supportive of the person who recovers from a psychiatric illness and is able to resume normal functions. However, people with severe and persistent mental illness are often shunned by society and isolated from the community (Kaplan and Sadock, 1998).

Nurses are the care professionals who have the most frequent and most consistent involvement with persons with severe and persistent mental illness. Few people are so dependent on the compassionate and professional care provided by nurses as are these individuals and their families. Nurses help persons with severe and persistent mental illness to develop strategies for coping with emotional and behavioral manifestations of their mental disorder. The individual is supported during times of crisis and encouraged during times of remission. Nurses also help family members cope with the challenges of living with this troubled population.

DEVELOPMENT OF SEVERE AND PERSISTENT MENTAL ILLNESS

Persons with these disorders often experience transient and recurrent psychiatric symptoms. Severe and persistent mental illness is diagnosed when it is believed that the person will have some manifestation of the disease process throughout his or her lifetime. The person's symptoms often are passed off as "odd" behaviors ("That's just her way") without recognition that these behaviors are clues to mental illness. Family members may tolerate a wide range of behaviors without clear understanding that an individual may have a psychiatric illness. Even treatment by mental professionals in outpatient or inpatient facilities may not clearly identify the chronicity of the person's illness.

Severe and persistent mental illness is often diagnosed in retrospect. The individual may have had several episodes of symptomatic behavior by the time symptoms have endured persistently enough for a major mental disorder to be confirmed. Looking back at the person's history of behavioral problems and symptoms, a pattern emerges that reveals the chronicity and impact of the mental disorder. Often the episodes were symptoms of a more comprehensive pattern of mental illness (Kaplan and Sadock, 1998; Kouzis and Eaton, 1997).

Diagnostic Features

Persons with severe and persistent mental illness have emotional disorders that interfere with their ability to live and function independently. This definition includes disorders that interfere with the individual's ability to perform activities of daily living, such as those related to personal hygiene and self-care, self-direction, interpersonal relationships, social interactions, learning, recreation, and economic self-sufficiency. The most common psychiatric diagnoses include schizophrenia, mood disorders, delusional disorders, dementia, amnesia, and other cognitive or psychotic disorders. In children, the most common diagnoses include pervasive developmental disorders, autism, childhood schizophrenia, conduct disorders, and mental retardation (American Psychiatric Association [APA], 2000; Kaplan and Sadock, 1998; Scott, 2000).

Young Adults With Severe and Persistent Mental Illness

Some of the components of deinstitutionalization included restriction of admissions to psychiatric facilities, as well as short-term hospital stays (Torrey, 1988). These policies have probably contributed to the development of the new phenomenon known as *young persons with severe and persistent mental illness.* These adults, between ages 18 and 35 years, have the most severe, overt disorders and lack internal controls, rarely take psychotropic medications, and exhibit excessive drug and alcohol abuse (Scholler-Jaquish, 2000b; Torrey, 1996).

It has been suggested that substance abuse is a form of self-medication for severe and persistent mental illness. There is an indication that those with mood disorders are more likely to abuse cocaine, those with schizophrenia are more likely to use alcohol for symptom relief, and those with conduct disorders are more likely to abuse heroin and other drugs. Many of those with severe and persistent mental illness are polysubstance abusers. A recent study suggested that reinforcement techniques may be effective in reducing cocaine use in persons with severe and persistent mental illness (Shaner et al., 1997).

PSYCHOLOGIC MANIFESTATIONS OF SEVERE AND PERSISTENT MENTAL ILLNESS

The person with severe and persistent mental illness has numerous psychologic manifestations. The specific cognitive or behavioral manifestations may be associated with specific mental disorders, as well as with the individual's unique life history.

Disturbed Thought Processes

For the purposes of this chapter, disturbed thought processes is defined as any disruption in the individual's ability to solve problems and think clearly. Disturbances may include hallucinations, delusions, or confusion (NOTE: NANDA [2003-2004] describes hallucinations as disturbed sensory perception). The disturbed thought processes may be transient, recurrent, or permanent. The recurrent and transient disturbances in thought processes are a major difficulty that persons with severe and persistent mental illness face in establishing independent living arrangements. One example is an **idea of influence,** in which the person believes that his or her thoughts are influenced by an external source.

Persons with severe and persistent mental illness have limited coping skills in managing problems of daily living. They also lack skills in communicating their thoughts and emotions to others. Additional stressors can precipitate major disruptions in their ability to cope (Kaplan and Sadock, 1998).

Chronic Low Self-Esteem

Chronic low self-esteem is a common problem for persons with severe and persistent mental illness. Mental illness affects the self-perception and ability to make sense out of life events. The delusions, hallucinations, and other negative symptoms of mental illness affect their memory, perception, and ability to think clearly. These individuals are often excluded from social activities because they look and act differently from others. They thus see themselves as ineffective and helpless; many are very much aware of their own peculiarities. Persons who experience small successes may resist making further attempts for fear of failure or expectations that they could do more (Webster, 2000).

Loneliness

Whether social isolation is self-imposed or results from avoidance of others, people with severe and persistent mental illness are often lonely people. Loneliness occurs when the need for intimacy is not met. Some elements of loneliness include problems with social relationships, inability to make decisions, and a focus on weaknesses in self or others. Persons with severe and persistent mental illness are often unable to express their feelings of loneliness and may withdraw further in fear of rejection. They experience a signifi-

CLINICAL ALERT

Persons with severe and persistent mental illness frequently experience hallucinations, delusions, and depression, which put them at great risk for suicide. Command-type hallucinations (voices instructing the client to kill himself/herself) are especially life-threatening (Torrey, 1995; Kaplan and Sadock, 1998).

cant amount of distress in attempting to describe their feelings of loneliness. Loneliness is difficult for anyone, yet persons with a severe and persistent mental illness are often unable to make the necessary changes in their lives or behaviors to break out of the experience of loneliness. Individuals who live alone or those who live in group settings may experience the same degree of loneliness. Persons with severe and persistent mental illness have demonstrated significantly more loneliness than those who are not mentally ill (Brown, Hamera, and Long, 1996).

Worthlessness and Hopelessness

People who struggle with major mental illness can experience an overwhelming sense of worthlessness and hopelessness. Worthlessness is awareness that one's efforts are ineffectual or insignificant. Feelings of worthlessness diminish the person's self-esteem and increase his or her risk of depression.

Hopelessness is a critical indicator of long-term suicidal risk (Kaplan and Sadock, 1998). It is a feeling that there are few alternatives or personal choices available. The individual is unable to mobilize energy to relieve feelings of futility and despair (Fortinash and Holoday Worret, 2003).

Depression

Depressive episodes can accompany other mental disorders, making the life of the person with severe and persistent mental illness much more difficult. Depression has been defined as "an emotional state, ranging in severity from mild to severe, characterized by discouragement, sadness, worthlessness, psychomotor retardation or agitation, and varying degrees of inability to care for self" (Kaplan and Sadock, 1998).

Depression may be related to the individual's awareness that he or she is unable to cope with the world. Persons who develop severe and persistent mental illness as adults and who have experienced relationships and successes in life should be considered at high risk for suicide during depressive episodes. When depression accompanies schizophrenia or Alzheimer's disease, the risk of suicide increases significantly (see Chapter 10).

Suicide

Suicide has been defined as self-induced annihilation in a person who believes death is the best solution for his or her perceived problem. Suicide attempts in persons with severe and persistent mental illness occur most often in persons with affective (mood) disorders or schizophrenia. Although persons with severe and persistent mental illness may express suicidal ideations while in the hospital, they are more likely to commit suicide after they leave the nursing unit. However, any person with suicidal ideations or a history of suicidal gestures should be considered at high risk for a suicide attempt. Chapter 24 discusses this topic in more depth.

Suicidal behavior is frequently seen in persons with bipolar disorder. Individuals with a dual diagnosis such as bipolar disorder and alcoholism are at a much higher risk for suicidal behavior. Affective disorder, alcoholism, and illicit substance abuse contribute to an increased rate of attempted suicide. It has been suggested that disinhibition resulting from ingestion of alcohol or drugs may result in self-destructive behavior. Disinhibition associated with substance abuse occurring at the same time as the individual experiences dysphoria, agitation, or impulsivitiy, may lead to higher rates of suicidal behavior (Marcus, 2000; Potash et al., 2000).

It is important to explore suicidal clients' fantasies about the consequences of their potential suicide. Their fantasies may include wishes for revenge, power, control, punishment, sacrifice, reunion with the dead, protection of loved ones, or a new life. Persons most likely to act out suicidal fantasies may have lost a loved object, may have received an injury to their self-image, may experience overwhelming feelings of rage or guilt, may have cultural beliefs that suicide is necessary to protect others, or may identify with a suicide victim (Kaplan and Sadock, 1998).

CULTURAL IMPLICATIONS ASSOCIATED WITH SEVERE AND PERSISTENT MENTAL ILLNESS

People in every culture throughout the world develop mental illness (Ahmed, 2000; Israel Mental Association, 1999; Palestinian Counseling Center, 2002; Australian Embassy, 2000). How mental illness is understood varies not only within major cultural groups but within subgroups as well. This discussion is designed to encourage nurses to become culturally sensitive and to provide culturally competent care. A culturally sensitive nurse must be able to recognize that each person is a member of a cultural group who has grown up with certain values and beliefs that were present long before the person became mentally ill. Culturally competent care is a lifelong process as the nurse begins to recognize that food, clothing, relationships, rituals (such as healing ceremonies), language, and behavior hold special meanings for individual cultures. Knowledge of ethnic diversity is essential in the development of diagnoses and treatment plans. The DSM-IV-TR criteria for mental illness may be misleading, as it represents the behaviors of persons who are of the majority culture in the United States (Aponte and Johnson, 2000; Borrows, 2001; Flaskerud, 2000; Gray, 1999; Herrick and Brown, 1999).

People living in the United States represent every racial and ethnic group in the world. Their culture, language, religious beliefs, and customs may vary significantly from those of the dominant culture. Nurses tend to be members of the dominant culture or have adopted the majority attitudes about care and mental illness. It is therefore essential for psychiatric nurses to develop an awareness and sensitivity to the cultural groups represented in their geographic region. In addition to cultural differences, there are genetic differences in the physiologic response to psychotropic medication. There are major differences in the interpretation of psychiatric signs and symptoms by the individual and family mem-

bers. Believing themselves to be possessed by demons, some might seek relief with healing rituals, and if that fails, they may attempt suicide to prevent their family from being affected by the demonic force.

In the United States the largest minority groups include African-Americans, Hispanics, and Asians. Each minority group copes with mental illness differently. The risk of overdiagnosing psychotic disorders in minorities may arise from cultural distance or misunderstanding of symptoms (King, 2001; Williams, 1995). A study of Mexican migrant workers suggests that persons who remained in their cultural groups demonstrated less major mental illness than the Mexican-Americans who had increased rates of acculturation (Alderete et al., 2000). Like Hispanics, Asians represent many different nations, ethnic differences, and languages. Asians may underutilize mental health services based on cultural values and understanding of mental illness (Uba, 1994). All minority groups report racism directed toward their racial or ethnic group.

Individuals differ in the nature and scope of the care they expect from health care professionals. Members of cultural groups that have experienced real or perceived ethnic intolerance or abuse may fear extensive treatment. There may be an intrinsic belief that psychiatric care could be dangerous and the client and family may insist on short-term treatment and seek relief within the practices of their own culture. Psychotherapy is not universally recognized and may be rejected in favor of medications or alternative treatments. The expression of symptoms varies from uninhibited behaviors to almost total withdrawal to avoid detection of the severity of distress experienced by the individual or family. The willingness of family members to be actively involved in the care of a person with severe and persistent mental illness is affected by culture and financial status, as well as by the integrity of the family support system (Aponte and Johnson, 2000; Borrows, 2001; Flaskerud, 2000; Gray, 1999; Herrick and Brown, 1999; Williams, 1995).

Traditional societies may devote little attention to the mental health needs of women and children (Australian-Afghan Consulate, 2000). In developing countries there may be a tendency to treat severe and persistent mental illness with drugs and electroconvulsive therapy (Abbasi, 2000). After the September 11, 2001 terrorist attack in New York City, the political, social, and human conditions in Afghanistan were revealed to the world. Widespread violence, political control, and limitation of individuality are rampant throughout the country. This fundamentalist control was directed to women who for several years were required to live in isolation in their homes. Any deviation from the imposed rules and controls could result in death. Most, if not every member of Afghan society, have experienced poverty and isolation, have been subjected to severe restriction in every aspect of their lives, and have witnessed or experienced torture. Savage killings of citizens or perceived enemies left survivors with the horrors of the dead scattered across the landscape. A large percentage of the Afghan population became refugees to escape the Taliban regime. Mental health problems and psychiatric illness are very high in the Afghan traditional society (Australian Consulate, 2000; Grinfeld, 2002). In many societies the so-called talk therapies would seem irrelevant. In assessing a client's cultural orientation, it is helpful to determine the nature of treatment that is the norm in the individual's culture.

It has been suggested that persons immigrating to the United States have a higher rate of mental illness related to the rate of acculturation (Keyes, 2000). **Acculturation** is the modification or adaptation of traits from another culture. The predominant culture of the United States may be very different than one's country of origin. Persons with severe and persistent mental illness may respond more favorably to behaviors, symbols, or language that are similar to their own cultures.

The psychiatric nurse caring for a person from an unfamiliar cultural group must be careful to avoid behaviors considered inappropriate by that culture. Examples of behaviors that may be considered inappropriate are a female nurse looking directly at a male client, a nurse touching a person (may be interpreted as an assault), and a nurse of the opposite sex caring for a client (may be viewed as offensive by the client and family). One's attire may have special meaning for individuals of different cultures, and attempts to modify clothing on a psychiatric unit by well-meaning nurses may incite anxiety, aggression, or symptom recurrence.

Psychiatric nurses must recognize the importance of being culturally sensitive and providing culturally competent care to members of diverse cultural groups represented in the United States. Despite the cultural differences, members of all societies are subject to the same major mental illnesses such as schizophrenia. In addition to cultural differences in how symptoms are expressed, there may be specific culture-bound psychiatric illnesses that are not recognized in any other culture such as *amok, evil eye,* and *witchcraft* (APA, 2000). Interpreters may be necessary to assess the individual's cognitive function and to enhance communication among the individual, family, and care providers.

Inappropriate psychiatric care may exacerbate symptoms, whereas culturally competent care may assist in helping the individual gain control of his or her life. In multiethnic urban areas psychiatric nurses need to be aware of the differences within the groups with which they work (Castillo, 1996; Lechner, 2000a). Resources for nurses working in multiethnic populations include textbooks on cultural psychiatry (Al-Issa and Tousignant, 1997; Tseng, 2001; Uba, 1994).

BEHAVIORAL MANIFESTATIONS OF SEVERE AND PERSISTENT MENTAL ILLNESS

Persons with severe and persistent mental illness often have difficulty in self-care, personal hygiene, independent living, interpersonal relations, and employment. Assaultive behaviors and criminal activity can alienate them from their fam-

ily and professional mental services. These behavioral manifestations may be present in young children, as well as adults including older adults. The degree of disability determines the extent and nature of the individual's behaviors. Persons with severe and persistent mental illness who are receiving psychotropic medication in an inpatient setting may not exhibit the same level of disability when they leave the hospital and resume living in the community. Persons who are noncompliant with their psychotropic medications may return to problematic behaviors once they return to their previous living situation. It is important to assess the extent and nature of the individual's behavior in the community, as described by the client and his or her family or caregivers.

Activities of Daily Living

Activities of daily living are essential skills needed to live independently. Persons with severe and persistent mental illness often lack basic self-maintenance skills such as personal grooming, table manners, and social interaction skills. Their careless behavior may result from impaired judgment, forgetfulness, or lack of motivation (Bachrach, 1996). The lack of these essential skills interferes with the individual's ability to be accepted in community settings. The inability to function adequately in social settings is a major factor in the poor quality of life that many persons with severe and persistent mental illness experience (Castle, 1997). Persons with schizophrenia often have poor social skills and frequently avoid social encounters (Bachrach, 1996; Kouzis and Eaton, 1997).

Independent Living

During the deinstitutionalization process (when persons with mental illness were released to the community), it was believed that mental deterioration was caused by long-term hospitalization. It was not recognized that many persons with severe and persistent mental illness were not fully capable of living a "normal" life in the community. More important, no one predicted that these individuals would experience significant exacerbations during the course of their disease process, placing a large emotional and financial burden on themselves and the community at large.

Personal survival depends on the person's ability to secure an income, locate a place to live, and maintain interpersonal relationships. Persons who live independently are responsible for obtaining food and clothing and for maintaining their living space. Chronically mentally ill persons

CLINICAL ALERT

Careless behaviors in handling cigarettes, sharp instruments, or hot liquids pose safety hazards to persons with chronic mental illness. These behaviors can be attributed to impaired judgment, forgetfulness, self-neglect, lack of motivation, and reduced sensations as a result of exposure to the cold (Bernheim and Lehman, 1985).

search for a sense of normalcy by seeking their own place and space and by engaging in meaningful activities (Pickens, 1999).

A recent study suggests that persons with severe and persistent mental illness can successfully complete a daily activities check list, which indicates that the individual can live independently given the resources (Brown, Hamera, and Long, 1996; So, Toglia, and Donohue, 1997). Persons with bipolar disorder may be compliant until they experience a manic episode or stop taking their medication (Baker, 2001). A large proportion of the people with severe and persistent mental illness are living impoverished existences and rely heavily on others for financial and personal support (Ware and Goldfinger, 1997). Poverty affects the individual's ability to secure housing, shelter, food, and medication, and to find supportive relationships.

Adherence to Medications

Persons with severe and persistent mental illness may find it difficult to comply with a regular course of psychotropic medications. For some individuals this may be associated with attitudes about taking medications, whereas others may feel so much improvement that they believe they no longer need the medications (Ruscher, de Wit, and Mazmanian, 1997). Medications may be lost or stolen and prescriptions may be difficult to obtain. Persons discharged with a prescription may find the cost prohibitive.

The side effects of medications are one of the primary reasons for discontinuing a prescribed medical regimen (Piazza et al., 1997). The person's ability to remember his or her medications, the dosage, and the need for adherence must be carefully assessed by the health care provider (So, Toglia, and Donohue, 1997). The longer a person is ill and the more educated the person is before the onset of mental illness, the more likely the person will be well informed about his or her medications (Tempier, 1996). Educational programs designed for persons with severe and persistent mental illness may enhance their ability to self-manage their own medications (Hornung et al., 1996; Ruscher, deWit, and Mazmanian, 1997).

Medical Illness in Those With Severe and Persistent Mental Illness

Persons with severe and persistent mental illness are subject to the same medical, surgical, obstetric, and physiologic conditions as the general population. It has been recognized that, as a group, those with severe and persistent mental illness have a much higher rate of morbidity and mortality (Dembling, 1997; Felker, Yazel, and Short, 1996). In some instances the increased number of illnesses may be associated with a lack of knowledge and awareness of the signs and symptoms of common health problems (Getty, Perese, and Knab, 1998).

Some persons with severe and persistent mental illness may not know how to access the health care system when they are ill, and their medical illness may not be recognized

when they do present themselves for medical care. There is an indication that hospitalized psychiatric clients may not receive the same amount of pain medication as other clients (Wise and Mann, 1996). The assessment of the physical and psychiatric conditions of hospitalized clients is important. Many medical conditions may exacerbate or mimic psychiatric disorders. Severe and persistent mental illness results in a higher mortality rate than in the general population as a result of undiagnosed and untreated medical problems and self-destructive behaviors (Dembling, 1997; Felker, Yazel, and Short, 1996).

Employment

Work is a key factor in rehabilitation of persons with severe and persistent mental illness because it provides meaning and organization in their lives. However, many skills are required to obtain a job, such as completing an application, negotiating an interview, or obtaining transportation to the place of employment. Persons with severe and persistent mental illness may never have acquired job skills, or they may not be able to resume their former occupation. Preparations for employment may increase job satisfaction and retention (Lloyd and Bassett, 1997). Once they secure a job, many are unable to retain it for a long period. Retention can be a problem related to forgetfulness, difficulty in self-organization, and poor impulse control. The inability to obtain employment is a major difficulty for the psychiatric client and contributes significantly to the person's poor quality of living (Figure 28-1).

It has been suggested that persons who participate in supported employment that incorporates working and vocational services may be more successful in maintaining employment (Bond et al., 1997).

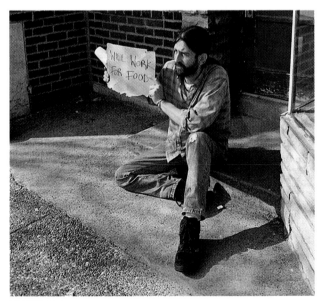

FIGURE 28-1. Persons with chronic mental illness are often unable to maintain regular employment and must rely on others for support. (Copyright Cathy Lander-Goldberg, Lander Photographics.)

Dependent Living With Family

The majority of persons with severe and persistent mental illness live with their families. Changes in the care of clients with severe and persistent mental illness have shifted from a hospital-based program to a community-centered system, and families often serve as extensions of the mental health system (Saunders, 1997). Mental health professionals look to the family as primary support persons for these individuals. Family members are expected to provide care management activities such as assessment, monitoring for compliance with the treatment regimen, and advocacy (Saunders, 1997). However, not all families are strong enough to cope with the demands of the family member with severe and persistent mental illness. Family members may find it difficult to talk about the problems they encounter in dealing with a family member with mental illness. Family secrets are common in these households, as information is withheld from care providers and other family members (Beard and Gillespie, 2001). The person's presence in the home drains financial, emotional, and personal resources. In some cases, the family is also dysfunctional and may be unable to provide the necessary support for the person.

Mentally Ill Parents

There are persons with severe and persistent mental illness who are married and had children before or during the onset of severe psychiatric symptoms. A spouse may be repeatedly hospitalized or maintained primarily on an outpatient basis or may be living with an adult whose behavior is unpredictable and even bizarre. During periods of exacerbation, persons with severe and persistent mental illness may require frequent care and close supervision. The presence of children in the home can result in great stress for everyone concerned (Buist, 1998; Cook and Sliegman, 2000).

Some persons with mood disorders are able to sustain minimal employment; however, they are unable to disguise their disorder from family members, a dilemma that may be confusing for everyone concerned. Children of persons with severe and persistent mental illness are often at risk for mental illness themselves. The mental illness of a parent has a significant effect on the child's development (Hindle, 1998; Powell, 1998). Unstable family life has been correlated with the subsequent development of severe and persistent mental illness in the children. The children may also be at risk for physical abuse. Mental health professionals should closely evaluate the home environment and the ability of family members to successfully cope, as well as determine whether the children are physically and emotionally safe. When parents are unable to care for their children, grandparents may find themselves in the position of raising a second family. Grandparents are increasingly assuming the role of primary care providers for small children as a result of mental illness in their own adult children (Ganache, 2000). Books such as *Daughter of the Queen of Sheba: A Memoir* (Lyden, 1998) describes one woman's experience as a child, care taker, and adult daughter of her mentally ill mother. Books of this na-

ture can serve to inform psychiatric nurses of the issues faced by children who appear to be safe in the home of a mentally ill parent. A number of books provide guidance for family and friends to care for mentally ill family members (Hatfield, Lefley, and Strauss, 1993; Johnson, 1994). Psychiatric nurses may benefit from this text, which is designed to help mental health personnel work with mentally ill parents (Gopfert, Webster, and Seeman, 1996).

Mentally ill parents have many of the same problems as normal parents, with the added burden of dealing with the stressors of their illness. These women are more likely to have been married than women without children. Partners may be one of the stressors that the mother has to cope with in addition to the needs of her children. Mentally ill parents are concerned about their children and the impact their illness may have on their offspring. These mothers may need education about normal childhood development. Almost 50% of the parents with psychiatric disorders also have children with disabilities. Thus the mentally ill parent may be responsible for managing the care and treatment of a mentally ill child (CMHS, 1999). Psychiatric nurses caring for parents need to include the family in the care plan and facilitate support using a multidisciplinary team approach.

Parents of Adult Mentally Ill Children

The behaviors of persons with severe and persistent mental illness may be passive or hostile. Some individuals are **parasitic** (totally dependent on someone else for their every need), apathetic (indifferent to others and surroundings), and live in self-imposed isolation within the family unit. Others may refuse to take medication and reflect profound hopelessness and despair. Delusional thought processes, stereotyped bizarre behaviors, and eating disorders contribute to the disruption of the family living situation (Doornbas, 1997). Hostile, abusive, and assaultive behaviors may also be directed at family members. **Sleep reversal** (a state in which normal sleeping patterns are reversed and the individual sleeps during the day and is active during the night), running away, poor personal hygiene, and property damage are some of the most frustrating behaviors that disrupt the household. Families have reported that the highest burden is coping with the positive and negative symptoms of persons with bipolar disorders (Mueser et al., 1996; Torrey, 2002).

The burden of care for mentally ill adult children may become an increasing burden as the family ages. Parents describe feelings of chronic sorrow, sadness, shame, guilt, dis-

> **CLINICAL ALERT**
>
> Women with severe and persistent mental illness are at great risk for victimization (CMHS, 2000), and children of mentally ill parents are at risk for mental and physical problems (Gopfert, Webster, and Seeman, 1996).

appointment, and losses (Howard, 1998; Pejlert, 2001). When adult children are difficult to manage, the parents may have little control over their behavior. There is no relief from the stress of parenthood as the individual ages and continues to need close supervision.

Resources such as community support and support groups such as local chapters of the National Association of Mental Illness (NAMI) can be helpful to clients and families. In addition, books may be helpful in assisting family members with the ongoing responsibility of a dependent adult (Johnson, 1994; Torrey, 2002; Woolis and Hatfied, 1992). Caring for mentally ill adult children occurs across cultures and is mediated by cultural values and beliefs about mental illness (Donnelly, 2001).

Siblings

The brothers and sisters of severely and persistently mentally ill children are affected in many ways. They are affected by the disruption in the household, as well as from the amount of parental effort required to manage the care of the family member. In some instances children are expected to collaborate with parents in denying the severity of the sibling's illness. Siblings are expected to give up some of their own developmental needs to provide for the needs of their brother or sister. When the mentally ill sibling is prone to assaultive behaviors, their family members and particularly the brothers and sisters may be the target of their behavior. Many times the siblings assume a significant part of the care during childhood and into adulthood. To compensate for the disruptive child, a sibling may strive for perfection or act out in anger and resentment against parents for failing to protect him or her from this unnatural burden. Siblings are expected to assume responsibilities for their troubled family member as they both mature. Both parents and siblings are responsible for the adult mentally ill family member, which can be an exhausting lifelong task. The stress can be difficult to manage as the need for assistance and care continues over the years. Two women have written about their experiences of growing up with mentally ill siblings and the disruptions they experienced in their own lives (Lawrence, 2002; Moorman, 2002).

Psychiatric nurses working with persons who rely on their siblings for assistance need to be aware of the importance of assessing the total family situation. Brothers and sisters may find assistance in support groups for siblings of mentally ill persons. On a positive note, the unique perspective of growing up with a mentally ill person may encourage siblings to advocate for others.

Sexuality

There are numerous sexual and relationship problems associated with severe and persistent mental illness (Bhui, Puffet, and Strathdee, 1997). These persons may have a normal sexual drive but may be unable to discern appropriate sexual responses. Individuals with severe and persistent mental illness may be sexually promiscuous or may be exploited because of their desire for affection and acceptance. These vulnerable individuals are at an increased risk for HIV/AIDS and other sexually transmitted diseases (Carey et al., 1997).

Rape is not uncommon in women with severe and persistent mental illness who may be unable to discern inappropriate sexual advances. Pregnancies may occur during hospitalization, resulting in additional stressors for all concerned (News, 1997). These women are less likely to receive information about menstruation, birth control, or screening for breast or cervical cancer (Ritsher, Coursey, and Ferrell, 1997). They may be subject to unwanted pregnancies and poor prenatal care and are more likely to be exposed to violent behaviors and less likely to have a stable partner (Gold award, 1996; Miller and Finnerty, 1996; Ritsher, Coursey, and Ferrell, 1997).

There may also be inappropriate sexual acting-out behaviors by persons with severe and persistent mental illness. These behaviors increase the risks of exposure to HIV infection (Carey et al., 1997). Individuals may masturbate or expose themselves in ways that are offensive or threatening to others. Efforts to control offensive sexual behavior have included punishment, stigmatization, and chemical castration. The use of medroxyprogesterone (Depo-Provera) can significantly reduce a man's sex drive and render him medically castrated. Although the aggressive behavior is controlled, this treatment raises ethical questions and concerns and is generally not the treatment of choice.

It is important to remember that persons with severe and persistent mental illness may also have sexual preferences. Psychiatric nurses must be aware that the chronically mentally ill persons may also be gay or lesbian and as such require appropriate nursing interventions (Hellman, 1996).

Pregnancy

There are legal and ethical concerns related to pregnancy and the potential effects of psychotropic medications. Antipsychotic medications may affect the fetus; however, withholding medications from a pregnant woman may result in exacerbations of psychotic behavior. Concerns about the expectant mother and unborn infant must be made in collaboration with the mother, psychiatrist, and obstetrician (Jaffe, 2002). If possible, the expectant mother should avoid medications that are known to affect the fetus. An alternative to psychotropic medications is electroconvulsive therapy, which can be safely used throughout pregnancy (Lentz, 1996). Depending on the expectant mother's support system it is advisable to include social workers and a legal advocate to protect the best interests of the fetus and the mother.

Psychiatric nurses working with mentally ill pregnant women need to be aware that pregnancy is a time of turbulent behavior under the best of circumstances (Munroe, 2002). Providing for the safe care of the mother and fetus is challenging for all concerned. Pregnant mentally ill women present a complex set of obstetric, psychiatric, social, family, and legal concerns (Gold award, 1996; Miller and Finnerty, 1996).

One study suggested that postpartum exacerbations may be clustered in families. Nurses caring for pregnant mentally ill women must conduct a careful family history as part of a comprehensive plan of care (Jones and Craddock, 2001).

Violent and Criminal Behavior

Persons with severe and persistent mental illness commit a disproportionate number of violent or criminal acts, which reveals lack of judgment and self-control. These persons may respond with violence to perceived threats (Green, 1997). Violence by a person with severe and persistent mental illness may pose a danger to family members or care providers. Children may be the targets of verbal and physical aggression. Violent behavior often makes community living difficult if not impossible. There is an even greater risk for violence in persons with a dual diagnosis (e.g., when drug and alcohol abuse coexist).

Many persons with severe and persistent mental illness have had extensive contact with the criminal justice system. People with mental illness commit crimes for a variety of reasons, as poor impulse control and acting-out behaviors may result in disorderly conduct, disturbing the peace, and trespassing. Some of these individuals tend to commit more serious crimes, such as shoplifting, petty theft, and prostitution, as a means of survival (Lamb and Weinberger, 1998; Teplin, Abram, and McClelland, 1996).

Some persons with severe and persistent mental illness commit violent crimes that pose a threat to public safety, such as residential burglary, assault, rape, and robbery. Young persons with severe and persistent mental illness who have had little mental health treatment are more likely to be involved in criminal acts of violence. The three primary predictors of violence are a history of past violence, drug and alcohol abuse, and failure to take medication. It is estimated that as many as 1000 people in the United States are murdered each year by persons with severe and persistent mental illness (Torrey, 1996). Unfortunately, murder has become the leading occupational hazard as persons with severe and persistent mental illness act out their anger and delusions against their supervisors and co-workers (Schmitt, 1999).

Many mass murders have been committed by people who experienced hallucinations or delusions coupled with poor impulse control and substance abuse. With the restricted policies for hospitalization, many violent persons are treated for a brief period and then released. Persons with severe and persistent mental illness who commit violent crimes are often delusional. These persons may commit crimes because of command hallucinations, whereby they believe "voices" tell them to perform certain acts. Others commit violent crimes because they are unable to control their impulsive urges (Kaplan and Sadock, 1998; Silva, Leong, and Weinstock, 1997; Torrey, 1997).

Persons with severe and persistent mental illness who commit criminal acts of violence are more likely to be placed in prison than in a psychiatric institution. Even in prison, persons with psychosis are legally allowed to choose whether they will take their medication. The rights of the individual and the goal of freedom of choice often collide with the rights of family members to live without fear of harm to themselves or others.

PERSONS WITH SEVERE AND PERSISTENT MENTAL ILLNESS WHO HAVE SPECIAL PROBLEMS

Within the population of people with severe and persistent mental illness there are subgroups with unique and special problems that affect their ability to respond to psychiatric interventions.

Mentally Retarded Persons With Severe and Persistent Mental Illness

Essential features of mental retardation are an IQ below 70 and impairments in adaptive functioning that began before the person was 18 years old. Behavioral patterns include cognitive deficits revealed in concreteness of thinking and neurologic dysfunction. Persons with mild to moderate retardation are believed to be more susceptible to mental illness. The conflict between the person's expectations and actual abilities may be a source of lifelong stress. In addition to a variety of personality disorders, the person with mental retardation and mental illness can experience affective, as well as psychotic disorders. There are indications that at least 40% of individuals with mental retardation meet the criteria for at least one psychiatric disorder (Kaplan and Sadock, 1998). Depression and psychotic disorders are underreported in persons with mental retardation (Gorman, 1997). A breakdown of central nervous system processing is a common feature in persons with a dual diagnosis of mental retardation and mental illness. Self-stimulating and self-injurious behaviors are often associated with underlying neurologic dysfunction (Gorman, 1997). Treatment for this special population requires an interdisciplinary approach. Psychopharmacology is an important modality used in conjunction with other therapies such as counseling, cognitive therapy, behavior management, social skills training, and activity therapy (Reiss, 1993).

Persons With Sensory and Communication Impairments

Individuals with sensory deprivations may experience many difficulties communicating with others, which is exacerbated by their mental illness. Persons with severe and

---

CLINICAL ALERT

A client who commits a violent act toward an individual just before admission to a hospital is likely to attack that same person within 2 weeks after discharge. Hospital personnel should make an attempt to warn the potential victim, per hospital and regulatory protocols, if the client voices threats before discharge (Tardiff et al., 1997) (see Chapter 4).

persistent mental illness and sensory impairment may be hospitalized much longer and receive less treatment (Fitzgerald and Parkes, 1998). Cases have been reported in which hearing-impaired clients were institutionalized for many years before it became known that the individual's social deficits were not a result of mental illness. Any person with symptoms of severe and persistent mental illness should receive a careful medical evaluation before a final diagnosis is made.

Older Adults With Severe and Persistent Mental Illness

Older adults with severe and persistent mental illness include those who have had mental illness for decades, as well as those whose mental disorder was diagnosed after age 50 years. Older adults who develop severe and persistent mental illness may have an insidious onset that is not immediately noted by their family members or care providers. Depression is a serious problem in older adults and requires appropriate intervention to reduce the risk of suicide. Schizophrenia is usually manifested during the early years of a person's life, and there are many people who have grown old with this condition (Harvey et al., 1997). Nevertheless, schizophrenia may also manifest after age 45 years. Family members of older adults with severe and persistent mental illness may find themselves becoming a primary caregiver in a most difficult situation at a difficult time in their lives (Eliopoulos, 2000b).

Alzheimer's disease and other dementias are the most common causes of mental illness in older adults. As many as 20% of older adults over the age of 80 years suffer some form of dementia. The onset of dementia is insidious and requires careful evaluation and diagnosis (Kaplan and Sadock, 1998; Pace-Murphy, Dyer, and Gleason, 2000). The behavioral changes in older adults with severe and persistent mental illness are disturbing to spouses and adult children. Family members have concerns about the person's safety, as well as his or her memory loss and disorientation. Some older persons may become so agitated that they require intensive treatment (Mintzer et al., 1997). As persons with senile dementia continue to lose cognitive ability, they may strike out in fear at family members, who they no longer recognize. The mental deterioration of the older person may precipitate emotional disturbances in the spouse or adult children. Partial hospitalization may provide an effective method of treatment for individuals with agitated dementia (Shoemaker, 2000).

The exploding population of people over age 65 years was estimated to reach 35 million by the year 2000 and is expected to reach more than 64 million by the year 2030. It is anticipated that there will be 16 million mentally ill older adults by the year 2030. The combined effect of increased costs for extended care facilities and the limitations placed on services by insurance programs result in limited care being provided for the aged with severe and persistent mental illness. This places an increasingly large burden on the adult children. Adult children, especially daughters, are fulfilling most dependence needs of older parents. Not only is the burden of care difficult, but it is often psychologically difficult for the caregiver who is now responsible for the dependent parent. The awareness of the stress and psychologic strain for caregivers has resulted in a variety of educational programs designed to assist them in coping with unexpected life situations (Pruchno, Burant, and Peters, 1997; Seltzer and Li, 1996).

The stress and strain of providing care for a dependent parent affects the entire family system. Male in-laws are more likely to report marital strain than female in-laws. The presence of strong family support and the avoidance of conflict serve to reduce the stress for caregiving family members. Emotional distance and family demands on the caregiver increase the risks for stress and strain for the caregiver, the older person, and the extended family (Lieberman and Fisher, 1999).

Abuse of persons with dementia by their caregivers is believed to be associated with the premorbid existence of family violence. Spouse abuse may continue in the form of maltreatment by care providers (Buttell, 1999). Nurses working with clients with Alzheimer's disease and their families are encouraged to explore the nature of spouse and family relationships before the onset of dementia.

Substance Abuse

Persons with severe and persistent mental illness who are also dependent on one or more substances are among the most difficult to treat in either psychiatric or substance abuse treatment programs. Persons with a **dual diagnosis** (i.e., they have two identified primary psychiatric diagnoses) have a high rate of hospitalization. Many more persons with mental disorders abuse alcohol and drugs than in the general population. The coexistence of drug abuse and mental illness is associated with a more severe course of illness. Substance abuse can distort symptoms and diminish impulse control. Persons with a dual diagnosis often have unstable living arrangements and may act out in violent and criminal behavior. Diminished impulse control can result in increased suicidal behaviors (Potash et al., 2000). They have more difficulty organizing their lives and are prone to homelessness. Persons with severe and persistent mental illness who have a dual diagnosis are more difficult to treat than individuals with one primary psychiatric diagnosis (Riggin and Redding, 2000).

CLINICAL ALERT

Clients with a dual diagnosis of alcoholism and bipolar disorder are at significant risk for suicide (Potash et al, 2000).

CHILDREN AND ADOLESCENTS WITH SEVERE AND PERSISTENT MENTAL ILLNESS

Severe and persistent mental illness is generally considered a diagnosis that occurs in a person's adult years. However, many severe and persistent mental illnesses have their onset in childhood or adolescence. Schizophrenia can develop in children more than 5 years old. Bipolar disorders may be associated with other diagnoses such as conduct disorders. The age of onset of the first episode of bipolar disorder was lower when the child was also diagnosed with attention deficit/hyperactivity disorder (ADHD) than for children without a childhood history of ADHD (Sachs et al., 2000). Although children experiencing manic episodes engage in high-risk behaviors, they do so without intent to cause harm to anyone. Children of bipolar parents may not be identified until their symptoms become more severe (Cogan, 1998).

For the most part, children who develop severe and persistent mental illness at an early age will be severely affected throughout their lives. Many adolescents have manifestations of mental illness that may be recognized retrospectively. Severe and persistent mental illnesses in children and youth have severe, long-lasting, and devastating effects on the children, their families, and society (Angold et al., 1998).

Children With Severe and Persistent Mental Illness

It is difficult to consider the realities of children with severe and persistent mental illness. The word *chronic* may refer to the anticipated length of treatment, a diagnostic category, or a set of behavioral patterns. Some of the symptoms of children with severe and persistent mental illness include interpersonal problems, inability to learn or achieve at school, and behaviors that differ from the norm or are inconsistent with the child's age. These problems are generally longstanding and severe. It is often difficult to distinguish between behaviors of severely disturbed children and behaviors of those who are hearing impaired, sight impaired, or brain damaged (Lechner, 2000b).

Most children with severe and persistent mental illness have no former level of optimal functioning to which they can return, because the basic components of personality functioning have never developed to a level approaching age-appropriate maturity. Unable to develop the prerequisites for growth, children with severe and persistent mental illness tend to have deficits in every area of personality and social functioning (Kaplan and Sadock, 1998). Their lives may be filled with frightening thoughts, constant fear of failure, and overwhelming sadness. They may fear their own aggressiveness or that of others. Children with severe and persistent mental illness may frighten other children or even adults, because they may be viewed as real physical threats. These children may be difficult to be around because of their

demanding, ungrateful, abusive, aggressive, or morose behaviors (Angold et al, 1998).

Psychiatric disorders that occur in childhood include mood disorders, schizophrenia, conduct disorders, and autism (Kaplan and Sadock, 1998). Bipolar disorder is increasingly being diagnosed in young children. The diagnosis is difficult to make, as bipolar disorder may coexist with ADHD and learning disorders (Mohr, 2001) (see Chapter 15).

The self-concept of children with severe and persistent mental illness is poor, as they often view themselves as bad or deficient, and many think of themselves as not entirely human. Their behavioral problems cover a wide range—from almost total withdrawal to acts of aggression toward self or others (Kaplan and Sadock, 1998).

Adolescents With Severe and Persistent Mental Illness

Adolescence is a difficult and tumultuous time for many people. Young people in the midst of life transitions, hormonal changes, and relationship difficulties who also have a psychiatric illness can be challenging to their families and to mental health professionals. The onset of bipolar disorder in adolescence may be associated with conduct disorder. These adolescents may experience disruptions in their lives, including criminal activity, substance abuse, and aggressive and self-destructive behaviors (Hodgman, 1996).

Mental illnesses may not be recognized initially as family members attempt to make sense of the young person's behavior. In some instances the adolescent's peers may be more sensitive and aware of the seriousness of their friend's illness than families or teachers. There is an interesting novel written about a young girl who is cared for by friends as she struggles with schizophrenia (Neufeld, 1999). Family members also struggle with the burden of the adolescent's symptoms, the negative impact of the mental illness on the family members, and their own grief (Doornbas, 1997). Psychiatric disorders that may appear during adolescence include schizophrenia, mood disorders, bipolar disorder, conduct disorder, and substance abuse (Lechner 2000c).

Adolescence is also a time of heightened sexual awareness and sexual drives. Experimenting with sexual activity may be desired yet acted out in inappropriate ways. Adolescent girls may have heightened sexual awareness or may not understand sexual overtures made toward them. Sexual attention may be associated with friendliness on the part of the

CLINICAL ALERT

The mental disorders that are most common in adolescents who attempt or complete suicide are bipolar disorder and schizophrenia. The characteristics of adolescents who attempt or complete suicide are similar; therefore it is critical for nurses to assess for suicidality and intervene early to protect the client (Kaplan and Sadock, 1998).

other person. Pregnancy does occur in severely and persistently mentally ill adolescent girls as a result of contact with other mentally ill persons, perpetrators who take advantage of the girl's lack of awareness, or care providers. There is significant difficulty for all involved when mentally ill young girls have children (Howe and Howe, 2000).

Vocational training can help these young people fulfill their need for meaningful activity in their lives (Lloyd and Bassett, 1997).

HOMELESS PERSONS WITH SEVERE AND PERSISTENT MENTAL ILLNESS

Many homeless persons with severe and persistent mental illness have been institutionalized. However, an increasing number of the homeless are young persons with severe and persistent mental illness who also abuse drugs and alcohol. Reports suggest that as many as 200,000 individuals with severe and persistent mental illness are homeless (Treatment Advocacy Center, 2002). Social conditions such as poverty and unemployment, combined with chronic mental disorders, often result in homeless persons who are unable to maintain stable living arrangements (Scholler-Jaquish, 2000a). Homeless persons with severe and persistent mental illness may also have a primary diagnosis of substance abuse. A significant number have a dual diagnosis, with one or more additional primary diagnoses.

Homelessness among people with severe and persistent mental illness has multiple and often unrelated causes. Economic constraints, unemployment, cutbacks in federal programs, **restrictive admission policies** (limiting the length of stay for inpatient psychiatric treatment), and a lack of adequate low-cost housing facilities are some of the factors contributing to homelessness. A disproportionate number of homeless persons with severe and persistent mental illness are members of racial minorities. Racial minorities vary according to the geographic region. The poor minority members with severe and persistent mental illness have only their families or public institutions to provide care. Dependent adults can place such an enormous burden on their families that often the family is forced to ask the person to leave. When forced out of their family home, these people often have no place to go except the street (Rossi and Wright, 1987; Scholler-Jaquish, 2000a; Torrey, 1996).

Homeless persons with severe and persistent mental illness are among the hardest hit persons in society. Unable to think clearly, unable to make effective decisions, and unable to obtain medications, therapy, or shelter, they wander the streets of modern cities and rural communities. Seager

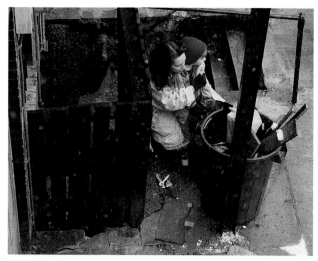

FIGURE 28-2. Many of the homeless are young mothers with young children. (Copyright Cathy Lander-Goldberg, Lander Photographics.)

(1998) wrote about the vulnerability of the homeless mentally ill who have been abandoned to the streets. The quality of life is grim for these individuals who rummage through garbage cans and dumpsters for food. Medical illness, accidental injury, hypothermia, victimization, and murder present continuous risks for the homeless mentally ill (Treatment Advocacy Center, 2002). In one instance, a homeless mentally ill man was sleeping on a secluded bench when a gang of youths doused him with gasoline and set him on fire. The homeless mentally ill are vulnerable to the risk of violence on the streets. In a southern California city, it was recently reported in the news that homeless men were persuaded to fight each other and to engage in destructive, dare-devil acts that were filmed by rogue "film-makers" for the viewing public. The homeless men were compensated for their efforts, but sustained injuries in many cases. The legal system is now involved.

With the increase in poverty and inadequate housing, the number of homeless women has increased. Homeless women tend to be young mothers with young children (Figure 28-2), single adults, or older women with overt psychopathology. Although there has been an increase in homelessness among women, only 15% of all homeless people are female.

It is estimated that 25% of homeless women have a serious mental health problem. One study reported that 41% of these women had a major mental disorder such as schizophrenia or mood disorders, and that another 44% of the same group demonstrated severe anxiety disorders. Unmarried adult homeless women with severe and persistent mental illness tend to have a history similar to the life experiences of men with severe and persistent mental illness. These women have a high rate of alcoholism or substance abuse coexisting with personality disorders or other mental disorders. They may associate with one or more men for companionship and safety, or they may maintain a solitary existence, living in fear of assault and rape. Older homeless women with severe and persistent mental illness are **disaffiliated** (they do not associate with family, friends, or service providers) (Strasser, 1978). They are more likely to have psychotic disorders also associated with alcoholism. The greater the person is disaffiliated from normal society, the greater the distancing from care providers.

PROVIDERS OF CARE FOR PERSONS WITH SEVERE AND PERSISTENT MENTAL ILLNESS

Persons with severe and persistent mental illness may live at home; in a community living arrangement with other persons with mental illness; or in an acute care hospital, psychiatric institution, jail, or nursing home. In each case the nature of the care required differs from the care that is provided. It is important for nurses working with persons with severe and persistent mental illness to be aware of the differences in care available in each of these settings (Shoemaker, 2000).

Psychiatric Institutions

Despite the impact of deinstitutionalization, state mental hospitals still provide more than 50% of all psychiatric inpatient care. The restrictive policies regarding admission criteria and length of stay result in short-term institutionalization. Managed care systems vigilantly restrict inpatient care for psychiatric clients. The urge to contain costs has resulted in minimizing the care for some of society's neediest persons. However, short-term care may be stressful and disruptive to clients with schizophrenia, who account for the largest number (more than 70%) of hospital admissions in any given year.

The psychiatric hospital maintains an important role in the treatment of severe mental illness. It provides a therapeutic, structured environment that is designed to meet the individual's need for care, protection, and control. It may also be an opportunity for the person with severe and persistent mental illness to get away from a stressful situation. When these individuals are in crisis, the psychiatric hospital may be the most appropriate place in which to seek care. It also provides an opportunity for family members to work with the psychiatric treatment team in preparation for discharge.

There is a "revolving door" effect with a significant number of clients who are admitted for short-term hospitalization and discharged when symptoms are being managed on the nursing unit. Thus persons with severe and persistent mental illness may receive only episodic care aimed at controlling symptoms and are then discharged to family members, community programs, or their own care (Saunders, 1997).

General Hospitals

As the state mental hospitals reduced their bed capacity, general hospitals began to increase their number of psychiatric beds (Bellack and Mueser, 1986). Hospital units that had been unlocked began to receive young persons with severe and persistent mental illness, as well as acutely ill psychiatric clients. Persons with severe and persistent mental illness who were untreated or noncompliant in follow-up care were more likely to be psychotic and violent. They often required **restrictive environments** to protect them from harming themselves or others. A restrictive environment helps a client gain control of his or her behavior. The client may be placed in open- or closed-door seclusion during periods of extreme agitation, suicidal ideation, or threats of violence to self or others.

Restrictive commitment policies limit commitment for admission to a psychiatric facility to persons who threaten to harm self or others. These policies have increased the number of persons with severe and persistent mental illness who must rely on general community hospitals for care (Fenton et al., 1998; Gater et al., 1997). There are indications that changes in involuntary commitment laws have prevented people with severe mental illness from gaining access to appropriate psychiatric care. General hospital units have become locked wards to house people with severe and persistent mental illness who were a threat to the safety of others. The restriction of mental health benefits by third-party payers has significantly reduced the amount of time a client may receive care (Sharfstein, Webb, and Stoline, 1998) (see Chapter 4).

Aftercare

Aftercare programs include a variety of community programs and services from partial hospitalization to sheltered living. The types of programs available in a specific community depend on the size and nature of the community, as well as the community's financial constraints. Outpatient clinics are often associated with acute care hospitals. The size of the outpatient programs and the extent of their services depend on the availability of reimbursement for services (Fenton et al., 1998; Gater et al., 1997). Insurance companies limit the number of days of therapy that they will pay for specific disorders.

A variety of community programs have been developed in more recent years. Some include partial care services with day care provided in an acute care hospital and a return to the individual's place of residence at night. Partial care programs place their emphasis on improving the capabilities of persons with severe and persistent mental illness. Other living arrangements include lodgings for four or more people. In some situations a manager visits the residence once a day or at other periodic intervals. Some programs provide for a live-in manager who helps the residents resolve interpersonal or household issues. Assertive community programs have been associated with lower rates of rehospitalization (Gold award, 1997; Klinkenberg and Calsyn, 1996; Gater et al., 1997; Getty, Perese, and Knab, 1998). Community service programs such as mobile outreach and crisis interventions provide access to care for difficult-to-reach persons (Gold award, 1997).

Homeless Shelters

Other types of community programs that provide services to persons with severe and persistent mental illness include homeless shelters, soup kitchens, and substance abuse treatment programs. These individuals may consistently use the same program or go from place to place. Most service providers for the homeless have restrictions on serving individuals who are actively hallucinating, intoxicated, or displaying threatening acting-out behaviors. Persons who are noncompliant with the provider's rules are often refused admission or forced to leave the facility. Thus some of the most out-of-touch persons are turned away from the only places that remain available to them. Persons with severe and persistent mental illness who become disaffiliated from family, health care services, and providers for the homeless often suffer the full ravages of untreated mental disorders. Shelters may provide an evening meal, a change of clothes, and a place to take a shower. However, they have no staff or facilities to deal with psychotic or violent homeless people with severe and persistent mental illness (Scholler-Jaquish, 2000a).

Foster Care

Foster care can be used as a temporary or permanent way of removing the child, adolescent, or adult with severe and persistent mental illness from an unsafe environment. Children with severe and persistent mental illness may be at risk of abusive behavior from parents or siblings. Therapeutic foster care must be carefully selected to ensure that the child is in a safe environment. Adults at risk in their own homes may be removed to foster care to receive appropriate physical care and engage in healthy interpersonal relationships.

Prisons and Jails

Current reports suggest that from 6% to 15% of persons in city and county jails are those with severe and persistent mental illness and that up to 15% of the prison population have severe mental disorders. Many of these offenders have a history of mental illness and are unable to function well in society. A large number of prisoners with severe and persistent mental illness are also homeless (Jordan et al., 1996; Lamb and Weinberger, 1998; Teplin, Abram, and McClelland, 1996). Incarceration of persons with severe and persistent mental illness persons poses serious problems for these individuals, as well as for the prison system.

Some individuals are arrested for minor offenses and may be held in the local jail. Mentally ill persons may be arrested because there are no other facilities available. They are often arrested for minor offenses such as vagrancy, trespassing, disorderly conduct, or failure to pay for a meal. Jails are inadequately prepared to care for the severely mentally ill offender who is able to refuse to take psychotropic medications. The suicide rate among mentally ill offenders is higher than for any other group of offenders (Open Society Institute, 2002).

Family members may find it necessary to have a relative with severe and persistent mental illness arrested for violent or threatening behavior. In some situations, emergency involuntary admissions require that the persons making the arrest or signing the commitment orders must also witness the violent behavior. If that does not happen, the individual may be jailed for his or her mental illness rather than admitted to a psychiatric facility. Many persons with severe mental illness serve long-term prison sentences with a minimal amount of psychiatric treatment. There is reason to be concerned that prison facilities are becoming like the asylums of the past.

Family

The majority of people with severe and persistent mental illness live with their families. Family members are key players in providing community mental health services. They are elected to assume responsibility for the client with little if any support, few resources, and no appreciation. The behaviors associated with severe and persistent mental illness intrude on the lives of the family members and make extraordinary demands of them. The stressors experienced by family members depend on their physical endurance and emotional health, as well as on the nature and intensity of the illness of the individual.

It is important to know that the family structure can provide the greatest support for adults with severe and persistent mental illness; however, it is a position of great responsibility for all concerned. Family providers should be referred to self-help groups or for counseling to maintain their emotional stability. The Client and Family Teaching Guidelines box details information a nurse should provide to the client and family.

Under any circumstance, it is difficult to live with a family member who has a severe and persistent mental illness, whether he or she is hospitalized, acting out, or in an interval between psychiatric symptoms (remission). Nurses working with persons with severe and persistent mental illness must be aware of the needs and concerns of family members.

Health Promotion Activities

Health promotion activities include many forms of education programs and are often described in terms of illness prevention and a means of maintaining wellness. Promotion activities for persons with severe and persistent mental illness are planned to reduce the frequency of exacerbations, increase the individual's ability to live independently, improve medication compliance, improve care practices, increase recognition of signs and symptoms indicating the need for interventions, and help families function more effectively. The next sections describe examples of health promotion activities.

Activities of Daily Living

These activities may be individually designed charts, plans developed with the family and client, or goals established with the individual and caregiver. A schedule of telephone

CLIENT AND FAMILY TEACHING GUIDELINES

Tips for Managing a Crisis

It is important to attempt to reverse any escalation in psychotic symptoms and provide immediate protection and support for the person with severe and persistent mental illness, and for family members.

Warning signs of a crisis include sleeplessness, ritualistic behaviors, increased suspiciousness, and unpredictable outbursts.

Remember that things always go better if you speak softly and in simple sentences. It is uncommon for a person to lose total control of thoughts, feelings, and behaviors.

Accept the fact that this individual is in an "altered state of reality" and may act out in response to hallucinations.

It is imperative to stay calm. Trust your feelings; if you are frightened, take immediate action to protect yourself, according to learned techniques (if you have been instructed in self-protection). Do nothing, however, to aggravate the situation. If you are alone, call for someone to stay with you while professional help is on the way. If it is necessary to call the police, explain that your relative is mentally ill and that you need help during this crisis. (If police know that this is a psychiatric crisis, they are more likely to respond with strategies than if they think that criminal activity is in progress.)

Some simple tips include:

Don't threaten. This may increase fear or increase the risk of assaultive behavior.

Don't shout. If the person isn't listening to you, he or she is probably listening to other "voices" (hallucinations).

Don't criticize. It will only make things worse.

Don't argue with other family members. This is not the time to fix blame or prove a point.

Don't bait the person. This could lead to the person acting on his/her wild threats, and the consequences could be tragic.

Don't stand over the mentally ill person. If the person is seated, seat yourself, as standing may pose a threat.

Avoid continuous eye contact or touching. This may intimidate the person, especially if paranoia exists.

Comply with requests that are not dangerous. This gives the individual a sense of control and may increase cooperation.

Don't block the doorway. However, place yourself between the client and an exit, in the event that you may need to leave the area.

Evacuate. All family members should be evacuated in the event that the person appears to be out of control and there is risk for injury.

---

contacts can provide support and encouragement for persons with severe and persistent mental illness. Such activities help to remind the individual about medications and assess level of functioning.

Medication Education

Nurses must provide and reinforce education about medications, frequency, side effects, and the need for compliance. Individuals with these disorders need to know about the potential side effects of medications and the appropriate action to take when they begin to be troubled by side effects or begin to think about discontinuing their medication.

Family Education

Family education includes the nature of severe and persistent mental illness and the changes associated with long-term health problems. These educational programs should include signs and symptoms of exacerbation (return of symptoms), as well as strategies about how to respond to positive and negative symptoms. Families should be instructed in developing methods for coping with individuals who may become psychotic and/or violent.

Sex Education

Sex education is an essential nursing intervention that includes appropriate sexual behaviors and personal hygiene, as well as the importance of regular gynecologic examinations and recognition of abnormal signs and symptoms. Sexually active men must be taught about the use of condoms and avoiding unsafe sexual behaviors. Women need to know about the risks involved in pregnancy and how to protect themselves from unwanted pregnancy, sexually transmitted diseases, and the potential for violence.

Family Support

Support, encouragement, and assistance in coping with daily life events are essential for families with persons who have severe and persistent mental illness. Spouses play a significant role in the quality of life for their partners. Exacerbations place additional strains on what may already be a difficult life situation. Children of parents with severe and persistent mental illness need assurance that they are not responsible for their parents' illness. They may also need assistance in finding healthy adult role models.

Promotion Programs for the Community

These programs should consider the importance of reintegrating persons with severe and persistent mental illness into the community. School programs should stress recognition of signs and symptoms of mental illness in children and adolescents. Strategies for dealing with children and adolescents who talk about committing destructive acts against themselves or others should be developed (see Chapter 24).

Physicians and nurses providing medical care for clients with severe and persistent mental illness should learn about the person's normal response to pain and discomfort. It is important that persons with severe and persistent mental illness receive appropriate care when they become ill.

PUBLIC POLICY ISSUES

Nurses have opportunities to make an impact on public policies at the local, state, and national levels. National policies relating to persons with severe and persistent mental illness must address the need for programs that are more flexible, comprehensive, and easier to access. There is a critical need for coordinated services with consistent financing at the city and state levels. Treatment programs in general and psychiatric hospitals in particular must be more creative in their approaches to treating clients with severe and persistent mental illness. Individuals who are clearly unable to care for themselves must not be left to roam the streets without treatment and without access to psychiatric care. Persons who pose a threat to society because of their violent behavior require treatment in appropriate mental health facilities rather than criminal intervention that could worsen their condition.

One of the most acute problems facing persons with severe and persistent mental illness is housing, because they vary in their need for supervised living arrangements. Provisions for housing in a variety of settings could be made available, including adult foster care and residential treatment programs. Adequate low-income housing could be made available for persons with severe and persistent mental illness who have low-paying jobs or for those who subsist on entitlements alone. The lack of adequate housing is as severe a problem as the unavailability of adequate care.

Access to care is an increasingly important concern. The individual's ability to access the mental health system may be limited by his or her ability to seek assistance, as well as by a lack of knowledge. Nurses can play an important role in advocating for increased resources for mental health care. In addition, nurses can educate self-help groups and other community groups about the nature and impact of severe and persistent mental illness. The quality of the available mental health care is also a concern for nurses. Short-term, episodic care is not sufficient to provide adequate care for persons with severe and persistent mental illness. Walk-in mental health clinics could be made available for these clients and their families. The clinics could monitor medication compliance, as well as provide individual and/or group psychotherapy. Psychopharmacology alone is not sufficient treatment for persons with severe and persistent mental illness. These individuals must also have access to psychotherapy to assist them with the complexity of their lives and their feelings.

Models for providing mental health services to persons with severe and persistent mental illness vary according to regions of the country and resources available. Mental health professionals have advocated a comprehensive health team approach to address the variety of problems these individuals experience. A treatment team of professionals can provide more and better-coordinated services than mental health specialists working independently of one another.

Special programs can be developed for the care and treatment of homeless persons with severe and persistent mental illness. There are strong indications that available programs such as homeless shelters or soup kitchens can be effective means to reach homeless persons with severe and persistent mental illness. Nurse-managed clinics in shelters and soup kitchens allow for easy access to health care professionals (Scholler-Jaquish, 2000a). These clinics could also distribute psychotropic medications to help homeless persons with severe and persistent mental illness increase their compli-

ance with treatment and improve their ability to function in the world.

THE NURSING PROCESS

ASSESSMENT

When conducting an initial assessment interview with a person with severe and persistent mental illness, it is important to be sensitive to the client's concerns. Establishment of a therapeutic relationship begins with the development of a sense of trust between the nurse and client. The nurse should explain the nature and purpose of the interview and tell the client where the interview will take place and approximately how long it will last. The nurse must allow for as much privacy as possible while using appropriate precautions during the interview, as these clients may have a history of poor impulse control or violent outbursts. It is critical to review client history if available.

Effective assessment provides the nurse with information about the nature of the client's problems. Clients with severe and persistent mental illness often have unidentified medical problems that have been neglected as a result of the individual's dysfunctional life style. It is therefore important to conduct a thorough assessment of these clients, as each person presents a unique set of nursing challenges (Box 28-1) (see Nursing Assessment Questions box on p. 635).

NURSING DIAGNOSIS

Nursing diagnosis is a process used to interpret the data collected during the assessment phase. Nursing diagnoses are statements that describe an individual's health state or alteration in a person's life processes (see Collaborative Diagnoses table on p. 636).

Nursing Diagnoses for Persons With Severe and Persistent Mental Illness

Safety and/or health risks:
- Ineffective health maintenance
- Risk for injury
- Imbalanced nutrition: less than body requirements
- Bathing/hygiene self-care deficit
- Dressing/grooming self-care deficit
- Risk for self-mutilation
- Risk for other-directed violence
- Risk for self-directed violence

Perceptual/cognitive disturbances:
- Anxiety
- Fear
- Hopelessness
- Disturbed personal identity
- Powerlessness
- Chronic low self-esteem
- Disturbed sensory perception (hallucinations)
- Disturbed thought processes (delusions, impaired problem solving)

Box 28-1   Assessment of Clients With Severe and Persistent Mental Illness

Physiologic Disturbances

PHYSICAL INTEGRITY

The nurse will examine the client to determine if there is evidence of impaired skin integrity, such as abrasions, bruises, lacerations, scars, and needle puncture sites. Abrasions and bruises may indicate that the client was subjected to self-inflicted injury or trauma before admission. It is important to determine if the injuries are recent or almost healed, as well as the nature and source of the injuries. When examining abrasions and bruises, it is always important to determine if infection or inflammation is present. If there is a history suggestive of trauma or violence, it is important to carefully inspect the client's body surface for additional injuries.

HORMONAL/METABOLIC PATTERNS

Children with severe mental illness may have inborn errors of metabolism. This information may be obtained through the client's history or from observing the child's physical characteristics. Does the client have a history of diabetes mellitus or kidney disease? Female clients should be assessed for their menstrual patterns. In each of these areas of concern, the nurse needs to know if the client is taking any medications for metabolic or hormonal disturbances.

CIRCULATION

The nurse will assess the client's medical record for indications of neurologic changes and cardiac status.

NUTRITION

Assessment of the client's nutritional history and present status is important, as many of these individuals live a disorganized and confused lifestyle in which their nutritional intake may be significantly altered.

PHYSICAL REGULATION

Assessment of physical regulation includes the client's temperature and the potential for infection. The medication history for persons with severe mental illness is important. It is necessary to know the nature and type of medications that the client has been prescribed, as well as his or her compliance in taking the medications. Disturbances of the immune system should also be evaluated at this time.

OXYGENATION

Assessment of the client's respiratory system includes evidence of dyspnea, cough, or labored breathing. It must be determined if the client smokes, how long he or she has been smoking, and the number of cigarettes smoked each day.

ELIMINATION

It is essential to know if the client has normal elimination habits. The nurse will want to know if the client has difficulties in handling urine or stool, or ritualistic behaviors associated with elimination. The client's urine can also be screened for nonprescription drugs and psychotropic medications.

Mobility Disturbances

ACTIVITY

The nature and extent of the client's activity patterns provide important information for the nurse. The presence of any physical disability such as paralysis or fractures affects the development of the nursing care plan. The nurse needs to know if there are gait disturbances, tremors, or ritualistic behavior associated with moving from place to place. The client with

severe mental illness may demonstrate lethargic movements or may be hyperactive and move rapidly from place to place. Lethargy may be related to major depression or catatonic features of schizophrenia. Hyperactivity may be related to agitation associated with anxiety, hallucinations, paranoid delusions, mania, or other mental or neurologic disorders.

REST

The person with severe and persistent mental illness may have developed sleeping patterns that differ from the norm. Clients may exhibit sleep reversal (sleeping during the daytime and being awake during the night). The nurse should assess the person's ability to fall asleep and remain asleep. Individuals who have difficulty falling asleep may have symptoms of depression or psychomotor agitation. They may be ruminating or obsessing about suicide while awake and may require a more thorough assessment and medications to help them sleep.

RECREATION

Individuals with severe and persistent mental illness may have a significant deficit in diversional activities. The person is often so preoccupied with the symptoms of the mental disorder, or the effort it takes to get through the day, that he or she may lead a dull and uninteresting existence. Too much free time on a client's hands may lead to thought disorders and suicidal ruminations if there is underlying depression. The client needs support in planning activities throughout the day.

ENVIRONMENTAL MAINTENANCE

The nurse's assessment of the client's ability to manage his or her living arrangement provides important cues about the treatment plan, as well as for discharge planning. If the person lives in a group situation, the nurse needs to know the extent to which the client participates in maintaining individual and shared living space.

One of the most important components of this section includes assessing the individual's risk for injury, violence, and the possession of weapons. Persons with severe and persistent mental illness may be at risk for harming themselves or others. Suicide rates are high in these individuals, so the nurse must thoroughly assess for suicidal ideations, gestures, or attempts. In assessing suicidal ideations or attempts, the nurse needs to know what method the individual has used in the past (if there is a history). It is also important to determine the availability of weapons and firearms and the person's access to them.

SELF-CARE

The ability of persons with severe and persistent mental illness to perform activities of daily living, such as personal hygiene and grooming, may be significantly impaired. When these individuals have significant self-care deficits, they may not be able to bathe or clean themselves appropriately.

Communication Disturbances

VERBAL COMMUNICATION

In times of illness and stress, bilingual individuals often resort to their native language or may speak in a combined dialect that seems disordered and confused. The presence of speech impairments related to physical defects provides the nurse with important cues. Verbal symptoms of psychiatric disorders include perseveration, circumstantiality, punning, rhyming, echolalia, mutism, word salad, cryptic language, symbolic references, neologisms, poverty of content, confabulation, and logorrhea.

Continued

Box 28-1　Assessment of Clients With Severe and Persistent Mental Illness—cont'd

NONVERBAL COMMUNICATION

Nonverbal disturbances include posture, manner of dress, and gestures. Persons with chronic mental illness may crouch on the floor, pace back and forth, or retreat from others. Their ability to make and hold eye contact provides the nurse with important cues. Gestures may include ritualistic movements, striking themselves, or striking out at others. Inappropriate sexual behaviors are also important to note, as these individuals may have trouble expressing sexuality appropriately as a result of the pathology of their illness.

Cognitive Disturbances
ORIENTATION

Assessment of the individual's orientation to time, place, person, and situation provides essential data for the plan of care. The person with severe mental illness may be oriented to all parameters or only one. For example, the person may know his or her identity and where he or she is, but not the month or the year. The person may be confused about the diagnosis or not know why he or she is hospitalized or being questioned. Mental confusion can be related to the individual's psychiatric disorder, side effects of medications, dual diagnosis (alcoholism or substance abuse), or physical disorders.

MEMORY

The nurse needs to assess the individual's memory to determine if he or she has intact recent and remote memory. The individual's ability to demonstrate abstract or concrete thinking affects his or her ability to understand and communicate effectively. Problems with recent or short-term memory may signify early dementia or other amnestic or cognitive disorders. Further investigation may be necessary, as many things can affect memory.

PERCEPTION

The person's understanding of the purpose and nature of treatment should also be assessed. Some persons with severe mental illness may not be clear about why they have been admitted to an inpatient unit, and a more thorough explanation by the nurse, in a clear and concise way, may be warranted. Repetition is sometimes necessary.

THOUGHT PROCESSES

The person with severe and persistent mental illness may exhibit one or more thinking disturbances. These may include dereistic and autistic thinking, delusions, thought withdrawal, thought insertion, thought blocking, thought broadcasting, magical thinking, looseness of association, ideas of reference, flight of ideas, ideas of influence, and tangentiality.

Persons with severe mental illness may have well-defined delusions such as paranoid delusions in which they believe that a force is attempting to control their minds or cause them harm. Obsessional thought patterns may take the form of ritualistic behaviors or may be manifested by an obsessive desire to control or possess another person. The nurse needs to demonstrate patience with these clients and provide a safe environment.

Perceptual Disturbances
SENSORY PERCEPTION

The senses include vision, hearing, taste, touch, and smell. Any of these senses can be impaired by physical and mental disorders. Persons with severe and persistent mental illness may have hallucinations involving one or more of the senses. The more common hallucinations in schizophrenia are auditory, and involve the client hearing sounds or voices. The nurse needs to acknowledge the client's hallucinations while presenting a nonthreatening reality.

ATTENTION

The nurse assesses the client's ability to follow directions, as well as follow verbal and visual cues. Evidence of psychiatric disturbance may include distractibility, hyperalertness, inattention, or selective inattention. The individual who demonstrates extreme anxiety or manic behaviors is easily distractible and needs immediate help in focusing.

SELF-CONCEPT

The person with severe and persistent mental illness, almost by definition, has significant disturbances in self-image, self-esteem, and personal identity. Assessment for these disturbances includes statements of negative self-concept and negative self-worth. Cognitive, milieu, and activity therapy can help these clients gain a sense of self-worth.

MEANINGFULNESS

Persons with severe and persistent mental illness may have difficulty finding meaning in a life that seems purposeless and hopeless. These individuals may express hopelessness (feelings and thoughts that their lives will never get better). In addition, they may express powerlessness (they are unable to effect any change in their life situations). When a person expresses feelings of hopelessness and powerless, it is important to immediately assess for suicidal ideations.

Relating Disturbances
ROLE

Each person has certain role expectations congruent with societal norms. The assessment of the person's marital status and relationship with parents, siblings, spouse, children, and others provides significant information about the individual's ability to function in society.

Sexual relationships may be difficult for the individual to maintain. There are wide variations in sexual expression among persons with severe and persistent mental illness. Some individuals may exhibit little interest, whereas others may have difficulty controlling their sexual behaviors. Still others may express sexuality in an inappropriate way, given the nature of their mental illness. These clients may develop a sexual relationship with other clients, which may not always be a positive experience, as both parties are often ill-equipped to handle the responsibility of a mature sexual relationship. Education about human sexuality may be useful for some clients.

SOCIALIZATION

Persons with severe mental illness often have difficulties in maintaining social relationships with others. Their ability to develop a meaningful relationship with people outside their immediate family is often significantly impaired. The age of onset of the mental disorder affects the individual's ability to socialize with others.

Feeling Disturbances
COMFORT/PAIN

The individual's awareness of pain or discomfort is affected by his or her physical condition and the presence of any injuries before hospitalization. Some individuals with severe mental illness may not be able to describe their sense of pain or discomfort and must rely on the nurse or others to be aware of changes that could affect their comfort level. Accrediting bodies, including the Joint Commission of Accreditation of Healthcare Organizations (JCAHO) and the Board of Registered Nurses (BRN), currently consider pain to be the fifth vital sign for all clients.

Box 28-1 Assessment of Clients With Severe and Persistent Mental Illness—cont'd

EMOTIONAL STATES

Persons with severe and persistent mental illness may exhibit signs of mood disturbance such as major depression, anxiety, mania, agitation, and fear. The emotional disturbances are related to the individual's mental disorder(s). Assessing the way the individual is coping with his or her emotional disturbance is important in the plan of care. Anger and aggression may be expressed through sarcasm, fault finding, domineering behavior, and the threat or use of violence, in which case immediate interventions are necessary.

Problem-Solving Disturbances
COPING

Coping mechanisms of persons with severe and persistent mental illness are often inadequate or inappropriate for the situation. Defense mechanisms that may be exhibited include rationalization, conversion, displacement, regression, introjection, projection, denial, disassociation, symbolization, fantasy, or splitting. It is important to note that some defense mechanisms may be necessary for the client's emotional survival at key points in his or her illness.

PARTICIPATION

The individual's ability or willingness to participate in treatment is assessed on admission and on an ongoing basis throughout the hospitalization. Persons with a history of noncompliance may exhibit compliance in a controlled environment. The degree of compliance with the therapeutic regimen can be assessed through nursing observations and frequent communication with the treatment team. At some point, gentle but firm confrontation may be necessary.

JUDGMENT/INSIGHT

Disturbances in judgment and insight are common among persons with severe mental illness. Thought disorders and disorganized living experiences may seriously affect the individual's decision-making ability. These individuals may exhibit indecisiveness or may make poor judgments about themselves and others. The severity of the illness affects the degree of difficulty the person experiences. They may have to be helped with decisions for a period of time.

NURSING ASSESSMENT QUESTIONS
Persons With Severe and Persistent Mental Illness

1. When did you first have trouble managing your own life? *To determine duration of the illness*
2. Did your family have religious preferences? *To determine basic values in the home*
3. What is the place like where you live? *To determine the person's current living situation*
4. Is there a family member who helps you out? *To determine relationship with family members*
5. Are there times when you hear voices talking to you? *To determine presence of auditory hallucinations*
6. (If yes) What do the voices that you hear tell you? *To determine if voices are troubling or threatening, such as command hallucinations*
7. Have there been times when you were so excited you could hardly contain yourself? *To determine the presence of mania or hypomania*
8. Have there been times when you have thought of hurting someone else? *To determine any patterns of violence toward others*
9. Have there been times when you felt life isn't worth living? *To determine the presence of hopelessness or depression*
10. (If yes) Have you ever thought about ending your life? *To determine suicidal intent*
11. (If yes) Are you thinking about that now? *To determine if client is in imminent danger*
12. (If yes) Assure client that nurse/staff will protect client; proceed with usual suicide precautions *to provide safety and comfort* (see Chapter 24).

Problems in communicating and relating to others:
- Impaired verbal communication
- Delayed growth and development
- Ineffective sexuality pattern
- Impaired social interaction
- Social isolation

Disturbances in coping (client and/or family):
- Defensive coping
- Compromised family coping
- Disabling family coping
- Ineffective coping
- Ineffective denial

Client and family teaching needs:
- Deficient knowledge (medication, treatment, symptoms)
- Noncompliance (medication, therapy, aftercare)
- Ineffective role performance

OUTCOME IDENTIFICATION

Outcome criteria for persons with severe and persistent mental illness include short- and long-term client behaviors and responses to treatment. Outcomes will be stated in clear, measurable, and behavioral terms; will be identified as expected or anticipated; and whenever possible will include a time frame in which the client is expected to achieve them. Clients with severe and persistent mental illness vary significantly in the extent and nature of their disorders. The following outcomes are not intended to be all inclusive for clients with chronic mental illness.

Client will:
- Verbalize absence of suicidal ideation or plan.
- Display consistent, optimistic attitude.
- List several reasons for wanting to live.
- Demonstrate self-care appropriate for age.

COLLABORATIVE DIAGNOSES

DSM-IV-TR Diagnoses*	NANDA Diagnoses†
Mood disorders	Impaired verbal
Major depression,	communication
recurrent	Defensive coping
Bipolar disorder,	Disabled family coping
depressed	Ineffective coping
Bipolar disorder,	Ineffective denial
mania	Dysfunctional family
Bipolar disorder,	processes
mixed	Hopelessness
Schizophrenia, catatonic	Risk for injury
type	Imbalanced nutrition: less
Schizophrenia, chronic,	than body requirements
undifferentiated type	Powerlessness
Schizophrenia, paranoid	Bathing/hygiene self-care
type	deficit
Schizophrenia, residual	Dressing/grooming self-care
type	deficit
Substance use disorders	Chronic low self-esteem
(all types)	Disturbed sensory-
Substance abuse	perception
Substance dependence	Impaired social interaction
Alcohol use disorders	Social isolation
(all types)	Disturbed thought processes
Alcohol abuse	Risk for other-directed
Alcohol dependence	violence
	Risk for self-directed
	violence

*From American Psychiatric Association: *Diagnostic and Statistical Manual of Mental Disorders*, Fourth Edition, Text Revision. Washington, DC, American Psychiatric Association, 2000.
†From NANDA International (2003). NANDA Nursing Diagnoses: Definitions and Classification 2003-2004. Philadelphia: NANDA.

- Initiate conversation with staff.
- Demonstrate effective problem-solving skills.
- Express sense of self-worth.
- Demonstrate absence of delusions.
- Engage in positive relationships with significant others or identified support persons.
- Verbalize feeling in control of self and situations.
- Make choices regarding management of care.
- Demonstrate absence of verbal intentions to harm self or others.
- Demonstrate absence of violent or aggressive behaviors.
- Communicate with others using appropriate language, tone, and speech pattern.
- Participate in individual milieu and group activities without disruptions.
- Demonstrate socially appropriate behavior.
- Adhere to prescribed facility regimen.
- Eat adequate amounts of different food groups.

CASE STUDY

A psychiatric nurse who provides consultation for a local homeless shelter brought Jake to the hospital for evaluation and possible admission. The shelter staff asked the nurse to see Jake, who was rocking back and forth on his cot, mumbling incoherently to himself. When the nurse spoke to Jake, he stated his name and date of birth. He said he had been homeless since he was 12 or 13 years old, adding, "My family thought I was strange, and they sent me away. I found a place to stay in a junkyard. The old man who owned the junkyard let me stay there. He brought me food and let me sleep in a room behind his office. I stayed there until last month, when the old man died. I don't have anywhere to go. I can't stand the noise of the radio. The radio plays in my head all of the time. I just wish it would stop."

Critical Thinking
1. What are Jake's most immediate problems?
2. What might the hallucinations be saying to Jake?
3. What nursing diagnoses would be relevant for Jake?
4. What outcome criteria, based on the nursing diagnoses, might be established with Jake?
5. What are three appropriate nursing interventions critical to Jake's situation?

- Stop talking to self.
- Seek staff when hallucinations begin.
- Refrain from harming self or others.
- Demonstrate reality-based thinking in verbal and nonverbal behavior.
- Distinguish boundaries between self and others and the environment.
- Use coping strategies in a functional, adaptive manner.
- Demonstrate absence of overt confusion.
- Demonstrate orientation to time, place, and person.
- Sit through meals or other activities without agitation or restlessness.
- Display control of angry, impulsive emotions.

PLANNING

The nurse's knowledge and understanding of the complexities of providing care to persons with severe and persistent mental illness are essential in the development of a comprehensive plan of care for the individual client. Each person has his or her own history of mental disorders, previous treatment, coexisting medical illness, and current symptoms. Nursing care addresses the short- and long-term needs of the individual and family members when appropriate.

It is important to remember that the individual's altered, disorganized thought process and/or mental deterioration may limit the extent to which he or she participates in the development of a plan of care. Many persons with severe and persistent mental illness have been alienated from their families and live alone or live a homeless existence (see Case Study). For those persons, it may be necessary to include community mental health care providers in the development of the nursing care plan as described in the Nursing Care in the Community box.

NURSING CARE IN THE COMMUNITY   Persons With Severe and Persistent Mental Illness

The community mental health nurse assisting persons with severe and persistent mental illness offers individualized care and family support, and monitors medication adherence and responses. Clients whose illnesses are in remission may have relatively smooth periods of functioning during which they need only minimal contact with the nurse. At these times their strengths should be assessed and encouraged. However, this period may be deceptive, not only for the nurse but also for the client. The client may begin to believe that the need for medication has passed and may discontinue prescriptions without consultation. Unfortunately, when medications are stopped, the person's thought processes often become progressively disorganized. Without a reality check from a supportive person, the mentally ill client may regress to the point of needing involuntary treatment. The nurse in the community must effectively monitor clients' behaviors so that, if possible, acute episodes are avoided. The community mental health nurse must be able to distinguish between chronic low-level functioning and an acute psychotic state. An essential part of the nurse's role involves developing a relaxed and trusting relationship with the client and educating him or her to recognize and report symptoms that generally precede psychosis in order to facilitate early intervention.

Although it is critical to encourage continuity of the nurse-client relationship and promote attachment, it is equally important to connect the client to the outside world with meaningful employment, volunteer work, and constructive recreation. Many persons with mental illness live lives of fearful isolation and require immense amounts of encouragement to venture out of their restrictive environments. Clients need to have confidence in building a long-term relationship with a counselor or case manager who can connect them with a group of peers for work, recreation, or education. These peer groups serve multiple functions of social support, corrective feedback, and integration of individuals into the community. The community mental health nurse will continue to monitor each client, as well as support group cohesiveness and community participation.

UNDERSTANDING and APPLYING RESEARCH

The purpose of this study was to examine the care meanings, expressions, and experiences of one group of chronically mentally ill persons living in the community. Understanding their ideas about care would enable nurses to provide care in a way that could enhance the health and well-being of these people, reduce the frequency and length of hospital stays, and lead to more positive interactions in the community. The study included questions about the shared norms, lifeways, environment, experiences, and care meanings and how this group of people interpreted these concepts. A total of 15 clients, 9 family members, and 15 staff members participated in the study. Data were collected through open-ended interviews and observations over an 11-month period. Data from 54 interviews were analyzed.

The meaning of care was described as listening, doing for others, spending time with others, doing things together, and sensitivity to the feelings of others. An analysis of the data related to values, norms, and lifeways revealed that the group valued respect, genuineness, honesty, and friendliness. A job was seen as a way to become independent. Many of these individuals spent time alone and often borrowed money and cigarettes. Watching television was the most frequent source of entertainment. Participants accepted waiting in line as being normal. The small amount of money they earned was spent on soft drinks, coffee, and cigarettes.

Data related to cultural and social structure factors revealed that money was a constant concern. Experiences with emergency commitments and hospitalization left the participants fearful of the police and fearful of hospitalization. Several of the participants had graduated from high school and others had taken college courses. One person was working on a baccalaureate degree. Some of the participants participated in religious services and others thought it was a way to make one feel comfortable. Religion was also part of the symptomatology of a few of the clients. Eleven of the 15 key informants reported that they had little if any contact with their families. Staff members stated that caring for a mentally ill relative for 20 to 30 years may have resulted in families becoming "burned out." Most of the participants had never been married. Differences between themselves and the dominant culture were apparent to the participants.

Conclusion: The chronically mentally ill who live in the community have identifiable values, norms, and lifeways that set them apart from the dominant culture. Nurses can use this information to design and provide culturally sensitive care to those with severe and persistent mental illness.

George TB: Care meanings, expressions, and experiences of those with chronic mental illness, *Arch Psychiatr Nurs* 16:25, 2002.

IMPLEMENTATION

The plan of care for clients with severe and persistent mental illness varies depending on the nature of the person's mental disorder, age, and physical health status. Although the individual's mental disorder is long term, he or she will be admitted episodically for treatment of the disease process. General hospitals provide short-term care, whereas state psychiatric institutions provide longer term care. Nursing interventions may be applied in either setting; however, achievement of the goals may take much longer for persons with severe and persistent mental illness.

These individuals experience impairment in their physical health, mental status, emotional responses, social status, and spirituality. The nurse providing care for the person with severe and persistent mental illness will be challenged to prioritize a plan that addresses the client's most important needs (see Understanding and Applying Research box). In addition to the manifestations of the disease process, these individuals need assistance with social interactions, self-esteem, knowledge of the disease process, compliance with the treatment regimen, and discharge planning. It is important to consider the individual's priorities when planning care away

NURSING CARE PLAN

Kevin was brought to the Emergency Department and admitted to the general hospital for psychiatric care. He had been treated in this hospital in the past and also had been committed to a state psychiatric hospital three times in the last 10 years.

Kevin was the fourth of six children and appeared to be normal in every respect until he had an onset of psychosis when he was 16 years old. He had lived at home until he was 28 years old and for the last 5 years had been living periodically in partial care facilities and supervised residential housing.

When Kevin ran out of his antipsychotic medication 4 weeks ago, he began to be belligerent and threatened another resident, accusing him of stealing his food. When the resident manager tried to intervene, Kevin became upset and ran away. His family was unable to locate him until they were notified that he was in the Emergency Department.

Kevin had been living on the street and in missions for the homeless since he ran away. The police had been called to a soup kitchen because Kevin was assaultive, noncooperative, and belligerent to the staff and oth-ers. Kevin fought with the police until they were able to restrain him and take him to the hospital. He had been without antipsychotic drugs for almost 1 month.

On admission to the unit, Kevin was actively hallucinating and talking to an unseen presence. His affect was flat and his movements were slow. When approached by the staff or other clients, Kevin ignored them or spoke in a belligerent tone of voice. He has no history of drug or alcohol abuse. He was unkempt, and his clothing was soiled.

DSM-IV-TR Diagnoses

Axis I	Schizophrenia, undifferentiated; chronic with acute exacerbation
Axis II	Deferred
Axis III	Deferred
Axis IV	Severity of psychosocial stressors = 5; serious chronic illness
Axis V	GAF = 30 (current)
	GAF = 50 (past year)

NURSING DIAGNOSIS: Disturbed sensory perception (auditory) related to changes in internal and external stimuli accompanied by impaired ability to respond to stimuli, as evidenced by inattention to surroundings, misinterpretation of environment, hallucinations, and difficulty maintaining conversations.

CLIENT OUTCOMES	NURSING INTERVENTIONS	EVALUATION
Kevin will seek staff when feeling anxious or when hallucinations begin.	Continuously orient Kevin to the nursing unit and to the events and activities that are going on to *present reality.* Use clear, concrete statements and avoid abstract concepts *to help Kevin understand the message.* Reassure Kevin that he is safe and will not be harmed *to help him begin to trust the environment.*	Kevin sought staff when he was feeling anxious and told them how he was feeling.
Kevin will be able to hold conversations without hallucinating.	Focus on real events or activities *to reinforce reality and divert Kevin's attention from his hallucinations.* Describe Kevin's hallucinatory behavior to him *to facilitate disclosure by reflecting on his behavior.* Determine stressors that may trigger the hallucinations *to assist Kevin in beginning to avoid or reduce his hallucinations.*	Kevin held conversations with staff, clients, and family without evidence of hallucinations.
Kevin will refrain from harming himself or others.	Follow hospital's guidelines for administration of emergency medications or behavioral restraint or seclusion, as least restrictive measures (when all else fails), when Kevin is in danger of injuring himself or others *to prevent harm to Kevin or others.* Accept and support Kevin's feelings underlying the hallucinations *to convey understanding and reduce anxiety.* Set limits on Kevin's behavior, when necessary, *to keep the environment safe for all clients.* Encourage Kevin to take medications *to control psychotic symptoms.*	Kevin did not harm himself and was not a threat to others.
Kevin will use techniques and activities to manage stress and anxiety.	Praise Kevin's efforts to use techniques to distract from or manage his hallucinations *to promote repetition of positive behaviors.* Provide a consistent, structured milieu *to promote trust, safety, and a sense of well-being.* Provide group situations in which Kevin can learn and practice activities of daily living *to increase feelings of adequacy.*	Kevin demonstrated effective use of techniques to manage his stress and feelings of anxiety before discharge.

NURSING CARE PLAN—cont'd

NURSING DIAGNOSIS: Social isolation related to negative experiences of aloneness and disturbed sensory-perception, as evidenced by running away from the partial care facility, withdrawal from the environment and others in the environment, noncommunicative manner, flat affect, and minimal or absent eye contact.

CLIENT OUTCOMES	NURSING INTERVENTIONS	EVALUATION
Kevin will say that he is willing to engage in social interaction with others in the environment.	Engage Kevin in meaningful, nonthreatening individual and group interactions every day *to let him know that participation is expected and that he is a worthwhile member of the community.* Act as a role model for social behaviors in one-to-one and in groups *to help Kevin identify appropriate skills.*	Kevin said he was willing to participate in social interactions on the unit.
Kevin will participate in social activities with family and with others on the unit (e.g., meals, games, and crafts).	Help Kevin seek out other clients who have similar interests *to promote more enjoyable socialization.* Praise Kevin for attempts to seek out others with similar interests *to promote continued positive socialization.* Encourage Kevin's family to call him on the telephone and to visit him on the unit. *A strong family network will increase Kevin's social contacts and promote self-esteem.*	Kevin participated in social activities on the unit and had social contact with his family.
Kevin will express pleasure derived from social conversations with other clients, staff, and family.	Provide Kevin with graded activities according to his level of tolerance *to gradually expose him to more complex social interactions.* Provide opportunities for Kevin to go on outings *to encourage a variety of more complex social experiences.* Encourage Kevin to engage in social activities that are within his physical capabilities *to provide him with successful social experiences.*	Kevin expressed pleasure in participating in social activities before discharge.

NURSING DIAGNOSIS: Impaired verbal communication related to inability to use language effectively when interacting with others, disturbed thought processes, and disturbed sensory perception, as evidenced by speaking minimally or not speaking for long periods.

CLIENT OUTCOMES	NURSING INTERVENTIONS	EVALUATION
Kevin will communicate his thoughts in a coherent, goal-directed manner.	Demonstrate a calm, quiet demeanor rather than attempting to force Kevin to speak *to demonstrate acceptance.* Actively listen and observe Kevin's verbal and nonverbal cues during the communication process *to demonstrate an interest in meeting his need.* Anticipate Kevin's needs until he is able to communicate them effectively *to provide for Kevin's safety and comfort.*	Kevin communicated his thoughts and feelings in a goal-directed manner.
Kevin will demonstrate reality-based thought processes in verbal communication.	Encourage Kevin to approach other clients to engage in conversations *to allow him to practice communication skills in a safe setting.* Help Kevin to listen and engage in actual conversations with staff and other clients in individual and group activities *to encourage him to respond to reality rather than listen to his own autistic thoughts.*	Kevin was able to maintain reality-based verbal communication with staff, peers, and family members before discharge.
Kevin will initiate strategies to decrease anxiety and promote meaningful and coherent verbal communication.	Teach Kevin strategies (e.g., deep breathing, replacing irrational or negative thoughts with realistic ones, seeking out a supportive person) to use when he initially experiences impaired verbal communication *to decrease anxiety and to promote more functional speech patterns.* Praise Kevin for his attempts to engage in coherent and meaningful conversations with others *to increase self-esteem and promote functional speech patterns.*	Kevin was able to identify and use effective strategies to control his anxiety and to promote effective verbal communication skills before discharge.

Continued

NURSING CARE PLAN—cont'd

NURSING DIAGNOSIS: Self-care deficit (bathing/hygiene, dressing/grooming) related to disturbed sensory perception and disturbed thought processes, as evidenced by withdrawal from reality (hallucinating) and impaired ability to perform hygiene tasks, dress, or groom appropriately (unbathed and disheveled).

CLIENT OUTCOMES

Kevin will consistently perform personal hygiene and groom and dress appropriately.

NURSING INTERVENTIONS

Assist Kevin with personal hygiene, grooming, dressing, and laundry until he can function independently *to preserve his dignity and self-esteem.*

Establish routines for self-care, adding more complex tasks as Kevin's condition improves *to organize his chaotic world and promote success.*

Praise Kevin for attempts at self-care and each successfully completed task *to increase feelings of self-worth.*

EVALUATION

Kevin performed all self-care activities of hygiene, dressing, and grooming in an appropriate manner before discharge.

from the hospital. If the person's concerns are not addressed, his or her ability or willingness to remain compliant with the treatment plan may be affected. Family members or community mental health care providers must be involved in the discharge planning process to help the client maintain an optimal level of functioning over a period of time.

Nursing Interventions

1. Assess the risk of danger to self and others *to ensure safety and prevent violence.*
2. Encourage the client to alert the staff when self-destructive thoughts occur *to help manage destructive thoughts before acting on them.*
3. Orient the client to the milieu and modify the environment *to reduce situations that provoke anxiety.*
4. Provide positive feedback when the client demonstrates self-control *to ensure repetition of functional behaviors.*
5. Seclude the client during periods of high risk for harming self and others *to provide a safe environment.*
6. Educate family members about symptoms of noncompliance with psychotropic medications or exacerbation of the mental disorder *to promote knowledge, which may enhance compliance.*
7. Educate the family in self-protective actions in relation to the client *to ensure family safety.*
8. Provide nonthreatening reality orientation *to decrease the risk of upsetting the client and initiating harmful reactions.*
9. Instruct the client in recognizing harmful or inappropriate behaviors *to increase the client's self-awareness.*
10. Assess the client for delusions and hallucinations *to determine the level of psychosis.*
11. Interpret the meaning of the hallucination or delusion for the client *to determine the intent.*
12. Instruct the client to alert the staff when hallucinations begin *so that the staff can intervene and minimize their impact.*
13. Teach techniques to stop or reduce hallucinations, such as whistling, hand clapping, and loudly telling them to stop, *to offer the client strategies to manage hallucinations.*
14. Praise efforts at controlling hallucinations *to reinforce the client's functional behavior.*
15. Work with clients to manage hygiene, grooming, and activities of daily living *to increase self-esteem by improving appearance and giving the client the satisfaction of self-help.*
16. Assist in selecting appropriate clothing *to reduce the incidence of ridicule by other clients.*
17. Monitor elimination and bathing patterns and establish a routine *to encourage proper hygiene and prevent injury to the bowel and bladder. Clients with psychosis often have trouble attending to activities of daily living.*
18. Set a regular eating schedule *to remind the client when it is time to eat. Clients with psychosis often forget or refuse to eat and could become physically ill.*
19. Supervise food preparation to ensure safety. *Persons with psychosis may be careless in food preparation.*
20. Assist with regulation of sleep-wake patterns *to promote healthy sleep patterns because clients with chronic mental illness experience irregular sleep-wake patterns.*
    Provide activities to keep the client awake during the day.
    Encourage dressing before breakfast and staying awake all day.
    Promote relaxation at night.
21. Listen actively to the client's verbal and nonverbal communication *to elicit the client's style of communication and to better understand and anticipate the client's needs.*
22. Encourage the client to engage in conversations with others *to promote socialization and decrease isolation.*
23. Teach clients anxiety-reducing techniques when they are experiencing impaired communication *to reduce anxiety when clients are having difficulty expressing themselves.*

24. Praise attempts to speak clearly and effectively *to encourage repetition of the client's clear, expressive behaviors.*

25. Enhance social skills, such as proper communication, eating/table manners, and social activities, *to promote the client's acceptability by others and increase self-esteem.*

26. Act as a role model for effective social interaction *to teach the client effective social skills.*

27. Praise successful social interactions or attempts *to reinforce positive social behavior.*

28. Teach the client and family about the disorder and symptom management *to promote knowledge, which may enhance compliance and reduce guilt.*

29. Arrange private meetings so that the family can express special concerns regarding the client *to clarify confusion about the illness and provide opportunities for expression of feelings.*

30. Teach the family to recognize early behavioral signs and symptoms of the client's failure to take medication *to be able to seek early intervention, promote medication compliance, and reduce recidivism.*

Additional Treatment Modalities

Nurses working with persons with severe and persistent mental illness are involved in collaborative interventions with a variety of mental health specialists and disciplines. These clients require an interdisciplinary approach during hospitalization, for discharge planning, and for follow-up care after discharge.

Psychotropic Medications

Psychotropic medications are administered to reduce the client's psychotic behavior and help control anxiety. The most common medications used for clients with chronic mental illness are the antipsychotic drugs.

Medications such as haloperidol (Haldol) and loxapine (Loxitane) can be used for both acute episodes of psychosis and long-term management of the client with severe and persistent mental illness. There a high rate of extrapyramidal reactions (movement disorders) with haloperidol. Nurses should note any evidence of these side effects and report them immediately to the physician. Newer or atypical antipsychotic medications such as ziprasidone (Geodon), which is currently available in both oral and intramuscular forms, and risperidone (Risperdal), may be effective alternatives to the older or typical antipsychotics. These drugs demonstrate less serious side effects and reduced incidence of troubling symptoms in general. Antianxiety and antidepressant medications are also used for clients with severe and persistent mental illness (see Chapter 20 for further information about medications).

Group, Occupational, and Other Therapies

The client with severe and persistent mental illness will benefit from group therapy in that it offers the client opportunities to enhance communication skills and to express feelings in a nonthreatening setting. The group also provides an acceptable forum for the client to interact with others in a safe environment. Nurses and other therapists serve as role models for social interactions and guide the group dynamics in a fair and meaningful way.

Occupational therapy can help the client with severe and persistent mental illness to coordinate movements and express inner feelings through a variety of art forms. The client can also learn new dressing, grooming, and homemaking skills. The occupational therapist is an important adjunct to the psychiatric mental health nurse, as both the therapist and nurse work together to assess the client's level of functioning from different perspectives. Therapeutic recreation, which includes movement, dance, and other recreational activities, is also a valuable adjunct to nursing in working with these clients, as the activities help clients to get in touch with their feelings and attitudes toward self, others, and the world around them in a nonthreatening way (see Chapter 19).

EVALUATION

The nurse is expected to evaluate changes in client behaviors and responses to treatment and interventions. Outcomes should be stated so that there is a specified time in which the desired behavior will be evaluated. At the time of evaluation, it is important to determine if the client has satisfactorily met the desired outcome or made progress toward achieving the outcome. The date that the outcome is achieved (and that outcome identification is no longer active) is noted. During evaluation, it may be decided that the original outcome identification is no longer applicable because of changes in the client's condition.

CHAPTER SUMMARY

- Severe and persistent mental illness is manifested by acute exacerbations and remissions.
- Persons experiencing severe and persistent mental illness may have one or more mental disorders, which affects every aspect of life.
- These individuals may have difficulty managing their medication, as well as problems organizing their lives on a daily basis.
- Persons do not die from their mental disorder and can have the same life span as any other adult, yet may be at risk for injury or harm as a result of environmental and personal stressors.
- Many of these disorders are first evident during adolescence. Young adults with mental illness are more likely to live chaotic lifestyles associated with undertreated mental disorders and substance abuse.
- Family members of persons with these disorders experience a significant amount of acute and chronic stress.
- Many of these individuals live in impoverished conditions with little or no support from family or friends who have given up on them.

- Persons with severe and persistent mental illness have normal sexual drives and interests, although they may act them out in inappropriate ways.
- There is a high rate of suicide among these individuals.
- Many people with severe and persistent mental illness can be helped to control hallucinations and delusions through an effective medication regimen and steady support system.
- Family members who receive their own support from health care personnel and community groups can learn how to intervene in the client's sensory/perceptual disturbances and prevent violence.
- Cultural values and beliefs affect the individual's perception of a mental illness, presenting symptoms, and response to treatment.
- Mentally ill pregnant women need careful management by a comprehensive health care team.

REVIEW QUESTIONS

1. The biggest relapse behavior for a 20-year-old client who is chronically mentally ill is:
   a. Failure to attend outpatient programs.
   b. Unavailability of state institutions.
   c. Medication noncompliance and alcohol and/or drug use.
   d. Failure to maintain a vocation.

2. A 22-year-old client has been diagnosed with paranoid schizophrenia for the past year. He has been taking olanzapine (Zyprexa) for his symptoms. He has been increasingly depressed with feelings of loneliness because his friends avoid him. He realizes that he will never live a normal life like his friends. The nurse at the outpatient clinic observes that he has been withdrawn and has lost weight. The highest priority nursing intervention at this time would be:
   a. Encourage him to attend groups.
   b. Assess for suicidality.
   c. Review with the client the importance of taking his medications.
   d. Help him to find a job.

3. Predictors of violence in the chronically mentally ill include:
   a. Sexual abuse
   b. Medication compliance
   c. Comorbidity
   d. Previous violent behavior

4. A 30-year-old client with chronic schizophrenia was found wandering the streets, barely clothed, and yelling obscenities. The psychiatric nurse assessed the client in the Emergency Department. Which behavior meets involuntary hospitalization criteria?
   a. The client stopped taking his medication 1 month ago.
   b. The client is homeless.
   c. The client states he hears voices telling him to kill little people.
   d. The client admits to drinking alcohol excessively.

5. A 43-year-old client diagnosed with chronic psychosis becomes agitated and threatens to harm a staff person. The best nursing intervention would be to:
   a. Talk in one-step simple directions and in a calming voice.
   b. Threaten that if he doesn't calm down he will be put into restraints.
   c. Confront the client on how inappropriate his behavior is.
   d. Catch his attention by putting your hands on his shoulders.

REFERENCES

Ahmed SH: Development of mental care in Pakistan past, present and future, 2000. Available, accessed, September 18, 2002, website: www.euro.who.int/MNH/WHD/TechPres_Pakistan1.pdf.

Alderete E et al: Lifetime prevalence of and risk factors for psychiatric disorders among Mexican migrant farmworkers in California, *Am J Public Health* 90:608, 2000.

Al-Issa I, Tousignant M, editors: *Ethnicity, immigration, and psychopathology,* New York, 1997, Plenum Press.

American Psychiatric Association: *Diagnostic and Statistical Manual of Mental Disorders,* Fourth Edition, Text Revision. Washington, DC, American Psychiatric Association, 2000.

Angold A et al: Perceived burden and service use for child and adolescent psychiatric disorders, *Am J Public Health* 88:75-80, 1998.

Aponte JF, Johnson LR: The impact of culture on the intervention and treatment of ethnic populations. In Aponte JF, Johnson LR, editors: *Intervention and cultural diversity,* ed 2, Needham Hts, Mass, 2000: Allyn & Bacon.

Australian-Afghan Consulate: Afghan-Australian relations. Available online, accessed September 20, 2002,website: www.afghanconsulate.net/message_from_baird.htm, June 20, 2000.

Bachrach LL: The chronic patient: patient's quality of life: a continuing concern in the literature, *Psychiatr Serv* 47:1305, 1996.

Baker JA: Bipolar disorders: an overview of current literature. *J Psychiatry Ment Health Nurs* 8:473, 2001.

Beard JJ, Gillespie P: *Nothing to hide: mental illness in the family.* Boston, 2001, The New Press.

Bellack AS, Mueser KT: A comprehensive treatment program for schizophrenia and chronic mental illness, *Commun Mental Health J* 22(3)174, 1986.

Bernheim KF, Lehman AF: *Working with families of the mentally ill,* New York, 1985, WW Norton.

Bhui K, Puffet A, Strathdee G: Sexual relationship problems amongst patients with severe chronic psychoses, *Soc Psychiatry Psychiatr Epidemiol* 32:459, 1997.

Bond GR et al: An update on supported employment for people with severe mental illness, *Psychiatr Serv* 48:335, 1997.

Borrows JA: *The Chippewa experience with the therapy process: stepping stones to healing,* UMI, vol 61, 2001.

Brown C, Hamera E, Long C: The daily activities check list: a functional assessment for consumers with mental illness living in the community, *Occup Ther Care* 10(3):33, 1996.

Buist A: Mentally ill families: when are the children safe? *Issues Mental Health Nurs* 27:261, 1998.

Buttell FP: The relationship between spouse abuse and the maltreatment of dementia sufferers of their caregivers, *J Alzheimer's Dis* 14:230, 1999.

Carey MP et al: Behavioral risk for HIV infection among adults with a severe and persistent mental illness: patterns and psychological antecedents, *Community Ment Health J* 33(2):133, 1997.

Castillo RLL: *Culture and mental illness,* Pacific Grove, Calif, 1996, Brooks/Cole.

Castle LN: Beyond medication: what else does the patient with schizophrenia need to reintegrate into the community? *J Psychosoc Nurs Mental Health Serv* 35(9):18, 1997.

Center for Mental Health Services [CMHS]: Critical issues for parents with mental illness and their families, 1999. Accessed September 23, 2002, website: www.mental.org/publications/allpubs/KEN-01-0109/ch2.asp.

Cogan MB: *Diagnosis and treatment* (on-line), 1998.

Cook JA, Sliegman P: Experiences of parents with mental illness and their service needs, *J NAMI Calif* 11(2):21, 2000.

Dembling B: Datapoints: mental disorders as contributing cause of death in the United States in 1992, *Psychiatr Serv* 48:45, 1997.

Donnelly PL: Korean American family experiences of caregiving for their mentally ill adult children: an interpretive inquiry, *J Transcultural Nurs* 12:292, 2001.

Doornbas MM: The problems and coping methods of caregivers of young adults with mental illness, *J Psychol Nurs Ment Health Serv* 35(9):41, 1997.

Eliopoulos C: Cognitive disorders. In Carson VB, editor: *Mental health nursing: the nurse-patient journey,* ed 2, Philadelphia, 2000b, WB Saunders.

Felker B, Yazel JJ, Short D: Mortality and medical comorbidity amongst psychiatric patients: a review, *Psychiatr Serv* 47:1356, 1996.

Fenton WS et al: Randomized trial of general hospital and residential alternative care for patients with severe and persistent mental illness, *Am J Psychiatry* 155:516, 1998.

Fitzgerald RG, Parkes CM: Blindness and loss of other sensory and cognitive functions, *BMJ* 316(7138):1160, 1998.

Flaskerud JH: Ethnicity, culture, and neuropsychiatry. *Issues in Mental Health Nursing* 21:5, 2000.

Fortinash KM, Holoday Worret PA: *Psychiatric nursing care plans,* ed 4, St Louis, 2003, Mosby.

Ganache G: Grandparents caring for grandchildren when parents have mental illness, *J NAMI Calif* 11(2):32, 2000.

Gater R et al: The care of patients with chronic schizophrenia: a comparison between two services, *Psychol Med* 27:1325, 1997.

George TB: Care meanings, expressions, and experiences of those with chronic mental illness, *Arch Psychiatr Nurs* 16:25, 2002.

Getty C, Perese E, Knab S: Capacity for self-care of persons with mental illnesses living in community residences and the ability of their surrogate families to perform care functions, *Issues Mental Health Nurs* 19:53, 1998.

Gold award: comprehensive prenatal and postpartum psychiatric care for women with severe mental illness, *Psychiatr Serv* 47:1108, 1996.

Gold award: linking mentally ill persons with services through crisis intervention, mobile outreach, and community education, *Psychiatr Serv* 48:1450, 1997.

Gopfert M, Webster J, Seeman, MV, editors: *Parental psychiatric disorder: distressed parents and their families,* Cambridge, 1996, Cambridge University Press.

Gorman PA: Sensory dysfunction in dual diagnosis: mental retardation/mental illness and autism, *Occup Ther Ment Health* 13(1):3, 1997.

Gray GE: Providing mental health services to the African American community, *J Calif Alliance for Mentally Ill* 10(1):24, 1999.

Green SA: Silence and violence, *Psychiatr Serv* 48:175, 1997.

Grinfeld MJ: Mental consequences of conflict neglected, *Psychiatric Times* 19 (4). Accessed September 25, 2002, website: www.psychistrictimes.com/p020401a.html.

Harvey PD et al: Cognitive impairment in geriatric chronic schizophrenic patients: a cross-national study in New York and London, *Int Geriatr Psychiatry* 12:1001, 1997.

Hatfield AB, Lefley HP, Strauss JS: *Surviving mental illness,* New York, 1993, Guilford Press.

Hellman RE: Issues in the treatment of lesbian women and gay men with severe and persistent mental illness, *Psychiatr Serv* 47:1093, 1996.

Herrick C, Brown HN: Mental disorders and syndromes found among Asians residing in the United States, *Issues in Mental Health Nurs* 20:275, 1999.

Hindle D: Growing up with a parent who has a chronic mental illness: one's child's perspective. *Child Family Social Work* 3:259, 1998.

Hodgman CH: Adolescent psychiatric conditions, *Compr Ther* 22:796, 1996.

Hornung WP et al: Psychoeducational training for schizophrenic patients: background, procedure and empirical findings, *Patient Educ Counsel* 29:257, 1996.

Howard PB: The experience of fathers of adult children with schizophrenia. *Issues in Mental Health Nursing* 19:399, 1998.

Howe J, Howe C: When mentally ill children have children, *J NAMI Calif* 11(1):21, 2000.

Israel Mental Association: 1999, Accessed September 25, 2002, website: http://members.tripod.com/Goldin_Yarik/about_amuta_e.htm.

Jaffe DF: Pregnancy pointers for women with NBD. Accessed September 18, 2002. Web site: www.schizophrenia.com/schizoph/NBDpreg.html

Johnson JT: *Hidden victims-hidden healers: an eight stage healing process for family and friends of the mentally ill,* New York, 1994, PEMA.

Jones I, Craddock N: Familiality of the puerperal trigger in bipolar disorder: results of a family study, *Am J Psychiatry* 158:913, 2001.

Jordan BK et al: Prevalence of psychiatric disorders among incarcerated women: convicted felons entering prison, *Arch Gen Psychiatry* 53:513, 1996.

Kaplan HI, Sadock BJ: *Kaplan and Sadock's synopsis of psychiatry: behavioral sciences/clinical psychiatry,* ed 8, Baltimore, 1998, Williams & Wilkins.

Keyes EF: Mental health status in refugees: an integration of current research, *Issues Mental Health Nurs* 21:397, 2000.

King SV: "God won't put more on you than you can bear": faith as a coping strategy among older African American caregiving parents of adult children with disabilities, *J Religion Disabilities* 4(4):7, 2001.

Klinkenberg WD, Calsyn RJ: Predictors of receipt of aftercare and recidivism among persons with severe and persistent mental illness: a review, *Psychiatr Serv* 47:487, 1996.

Kouzis AC, Eaton WW: Psychopathology and the development of disability, *Soc Psychiatry Psychiatr Epidemiol* 32:379, 1997.

Lamb HR, Weinberger LE: Persons with severe mental illness in jails and prisons: a review, *Psychiatr Serv* 49:483, 1998.

Lawrence C: *Looking for Mary Gabriel,* New York, 2002, Dunne Books.

Lechner S: Travelers from many lands. In Carson VB, editor: *Mental health nursing: the nurse-patient journey,* ed 2, Philadelphia, 2000a, WB Saunders.

Lechner S: The child. In Carson VB, editor: *Mental health nursing: the nurse-patient journey,* ed 2, Philadelphia, 2000b, WB Saunders.

Lechner S: The adolescent. In Carson VB, editor: *Mental health nursing: the nurse-patient journey,* ed 2, Philadelphia, 2000c, WB Saunders.

Lentz SK: Electroconvulsive therapy during pregnancy, 1996. Accessed September 18, 2002, website: www.ect.org/resources/pregnancy.html.

Lieberman MA, Fisher L: The impact of dementia on adult offspring and their spouses: the contribution of family characteristics, *J Mental Health Aging* 5:207, 1999.

Lloyd C, Bassett J: Life is for living: a pre-vocational program for young people with psychosis, *Aust Occup Ther J* 44(2):82, 1997.

Lyden J: *Daughter of the queen of Sheba: a memoir,* New York, 1998, Penguin.

Marcus PE: Suicide. In Carson VB, editor: *Mental health nursing: the nurse-patient journey,* ed 2, Philadelphia, 2000, WB Saunders.

Miller LJ, Finnerty M: Sexuality, pregnancy, and childrearing among women with schizophrenia—spectrum disorders, *Psychiatr Serv* 47:502, 1996.

Mintzer JE et al: The effectiveness of a continuum of care using brief and partial hospitalization for agitated dementia patients, *Psychiatr Serv* 48:1435, 1997.

Mohr WK: Bipolar disorder in children, *J Psychosocial Nurs Mental Health Serv* 39(3):12, 48, 2001.

Moorman M: *My sister's keeper: learning to cope with a sibling's mental illness,* New York, 2002, WW Norton.

Munroe H: The impact of schizophrenia on women: a voyage of turbulence. *Women's health matters,* January, 2002. Accessed September 18, 2002, website: www.womensmatters.ca/facts/quick_show_d.cfm?number=333.

Mueser KT et al: Family burden of schizophrenia and bipolar disorder: perceptions of relatives and professionals, *Psychiatr Serv* 47:507, 1996.

NANDA International (2003). NANDA Nursing Diagnoses: Definitions and Classification 2003-2004. Philadelphia: NANDA.

National Institute of Mental Health [NIMH]: Mental disorders in America. Accessed September 18, 2002. Website: www.nimh.nih.gov/publicat/numbers.cfm

Neufeld J: *Lisa, bright and dark: a novel,* New York, 1999, Puffin.

News in mental nursing: sex in the state hospital a continuing headache, *J Psychosoc Nurs* 35(6):6, 1997.

Open Society Institute: Mental illness in US jails. (no date). Accessed September 17, 2002, website: www.soros.org/crime/research_brief_1.html.

Pace-Murphy K, Dyer CB, Gleason MS: Delirium, dementia, and other amnestic disorders. In Palestinian Counseling Center: Accessed September 25, 2002, website: www.pcc-jer.or/affiliations.htm.

Pejlert A: Being a parent of an adult son or daughter with severe mental illness receiving professional care: parents narratives, *Social Care Community* 9:194, 2001.

Piazza LA et al: Sexual functioning in chronically depressed patients treated with SSRI antidepressants: a pilot study, *Am J Psychiatry* 154:1757, 1997.

Pickens JM: Living with serious illness: the desire for normalcy, *Nurs Sci Q* 12:233, 1999.

Potash JB et al: Attempted suicide and alcoholism in bipolar disorder: clinical and family relationships, *Am J Psychiatry* 157:2048, 2000.

Powell J: First person account: paranoid schizophrenia—a daughter's story, *Schizophr Bull* 24:175, 1998.

Pruchno RA, Burant CJ, Peters ND: Understanding the well-being of caregivers, *Gerontologist* 37:102, 1997.

Reiss S: Mental illness in persons with mental retardation, 1993, accessed September 19, 2002, website: www.thearc.org/faqs/mimrqa.html.

Riggin OZ, Redding BA: Substance related disorders. In Fortinash KM, Holoday Worret PA, editors: *Psychiatric mental health nursing,* ed 2, St Louis, 2000: Mosby.

Ritsher JEB, Coursey RD, Ferrell EW: A survey on issues in the lives of women with severe mental illness, *Psychiatr Serv* 48:1273, 1997.

Rossi PH, Wright JD: The determinants of homelessness, *Health Affairs* 6(1):19-32, 1987.

Ruscher SM, de Wit R, Mazmanian D: Psychiatric patients' attitudes about medication and factors affecting noncompliance, *Psychiatr Serv* 48:82, 1997.

Sachs GS et al: Comorbidity of attention deficit hyperactivity disorder with early and late-onset bipolar disorder, *Am J Psychiatry* 157:466, 2000.

Saunders J: Walking a mile in their shoes . . . symbolic interaction for families living with severe mental illness, *J Psychosoc Nurs Ment Serv* 35(6):45, 1997.

Schmitt SM: Criminalizing the mentally ill, *CTOnline,*1999, accessed September 18, 2002, website: www.counseling.org/ctonline/criminalization.htm.

Scholler-Jaquish A: Homelessness in America. In Smith C, Maurer F, editors: *Community nursing: theory and practice,* ed 2, Philadelphia, 2000a, WB Saunders.

Scholler-Jaquish A: Persons with chronic mental illness. In Fortinash KM, Holoday Worret PA, editors: *Psychiatric mental health nursing,* ed 2, St Louis, 2000b, Mosby.

Scott CM: Mood disorders. In Carson VB, editor: *Mental nursing: the nurse-patient journey,* ed 2, Philadelphia, 2000, WB Saunders.

Seager SB: *Street crazy: the tragedy of the homeless mentally ill,* New York, 1998, Westcom Press.

Seltzer MM, Li LW: The transitions of caregiving: subjective and objective definitions, *Gerontologist* 36:614, 1996.

Shaner et al: Monetary reinforcement of abstinence from cocaine among mentally ill patients with cocaine dependence, *Psychiatr Serv* 48:807, 1997.

Sharfstein SS, Webb WL, Stoline AM: *Schizophrenia: questions and answers,* National Institute of Mental Health (on-line), 1998.

Shoemaker N: The continuum of care. In Carson VB, editor: *Mental health nursing: the nurse-patient journey,* ed 2, Philadelphia, 2000, WB Saunders.

Silva JA, Leong GB, Weinstock R: Violent behaviors associated with the antichrist delusion, *J Forensic Sci* 42:1058, 1997.

So YP, Toglia J, Donohue MV: A study of memory functioning in chronic schizophrenic patients, *Occup Ther Ment* 13(1):1, 1997.

Strasser JA: Urban transient women, *Am J Nurs* 78(12):2076, 1978.

Tempier R: Long-term psychiatric patients' knowledge about their medication, *Psychiatr Serv* 47:1385, 1996.

Teplin LA, Abram KM, McClelland GM: Prevalence of psychiatric disorders among incarcerated women. I. Pretrial jail detainees, *Arch Gen Psychiatry* 53:505, 1996.

Torrey EF: *Nowhere to go: the tragic odyssey of the homeless mentally ill,* New York, 1988, Harper.

Torrey EF: *Surviving schizophrenia,* ed 3, New York, 1995, Harper Perennial.

Torrey EF: *Out of the shadows: confronting America's mental illness,* New York, 1996, John Wiley & Sons.

Torrey EF: Stop the madness, *New York Times,* July 18, 1997, accessed September 18, 2002, website: www.psych-.com/madness1.htm.

Treatment Advocacy Center: Many Americans with untreated psychiatric illnesses have nowhere to go, homelessness: tragic side effect of nontreatment (no date), accessed September 18, 2002, website: www.psychlaws.org/GeneralResources/fact11.htm.

Tseng WF: *Handbook of cultural psychiatry,* San Diego, 2001, Academic Press.

Uba L: *Asian Americans: personality patterns, identity, and mental health,* New York, 1994, Guilford Press.

Ware NC, Goldfinger SM: Poverty and rehabilitation in severe psychiatric disorders, *Psychiatr Rehabilitation J* 21(1):3-9, 1997.

Webster MM: Interactive therapies and methods of implementation. In Fortinash KM, Holoday Worret PA, editors: *Psychiatric mental health nursing,* ed 2, St Louis, 2000, Mosby.

Williams DR: African American mental health: persisting question and paradoxical findings, 1995, accessed September 18, 2002, website: www.rcgd.isr.umich.edu/prba/perspectives/spring1995/dwilliams.pdf .

Wise TN, Mann LS: Utilization of pain medication in hospitalized psychiatric patients, *Gen Hosp Psychiatry* 18:422, 1996.

Yap EL: Neurobiological influences. In Carson VB, editor: *Mental health nursing: the nurse-patient journey,* ed 2, Philadelphia, 2000, WB Saunders.

SUGGESTED READINGS

Eliopoulos C: The older adult. In Carson VB, editor: *Mental health nursing: the nurse-patient journey,* ed 2, Philadelphia, 2000a, WB Saunders.

Fordyce E, Taylor D: Thought disorders. In Carson VB, editor: *Mental health nursing: the nurse-patient journey,* ed 2, Philadelphia, 2000, WB Saunders.

Hunter EF: Telephone support for persons with chronic mental illness, *Home Health Nurse* 18:172, 2000.

McCann E: Recent developments in psychological interventions for people with psychosis, *Issues in Mental Health Nursing* 22:99-107, 2001.

Simon C: *Mad house: growing up in the shadow of mentally ill siblings,* New York, 1997, Doubleday.

Tardiff K et al: A prospective study of violence by psychiatric patients after hospital discharge, *Psychiatr Serv* 48:678, 1997.

Teschinsky U: Living with schizophrenia: the family illness experience, *Issues in Mental Health Nursing* 21:387, 2000.

Torrey EF: *Surviving schizophrenia: a manual for families, consumers, and providers,* ed 4, New York, 2001, Quill.

U.S. Public Service: Mental health: culture, race, and ethnicity. A report to the surgeon general. Accessed September 23, 2002. website: www.surgeongeneral.gov/library/mental/cre/execsummary-1.html.

Appendix A
DSM-IV-TR Classification

NOS = Not Otherwise Specified.

An *x* appearing in a diagnostic code indicates that a specific code number is required.

An ellipsis (. . .) is used in the names of certain disorders to indicate that the name of a specific mental disorder or general medical condition should be inserted when recording the name (e.g., 293.0 Delirium Due to Hypothyroidism).

If criteria are currently met, one of the following severity specifiers may be noted after the diagnosis:
Mild
Moderate
Severe

If criteria are no longer met, one of the following specifiers may be noted:
In Partial Remission
In Full Remission
Prior History

DISORDERS USUALLY FIRST DIAGNOSED IN INFANCY, CHILDHOOD, OR ADOLESCENCE
Mental Retardation

Note: These are coded on Axis II.

317	Mild Mental Retardation
318.0	Moderate Mental Retardation
318.1	Severe Mental Retardation
318.2	Profound Mental Retardation
319	Mental Retardation, Severity Unspecified

Learning Disorders

315.00	Reading Disorder
315.1	Mathematics Disorder
315.2	Disorder of Written Expression
315.9	Learning Disorder NOS

Motor Skills Disorder

315.4	Developmental Coordination Disorder

Communication Disorders

315.31	Expressive Language Disorder
315.32	Mixed Receptive-Expressive Language Disorder
315.39	Phonologic Disorder
307.0	Stuttering
307.9	Communication Disorder NOS

Pervasive Developmental Disorders

299.00	Autistic Disorder
299.80	Rett's Disorder
299.10	Childhood Disintegrative Disorder
299.80	Asperger's Disorder
299.80	Pervasive Developmental Disorder NOS

Attention-Deficit and Disruptive Behavior Disorders

314.xx	Attention-Deficit/Hyperactivity Disorder
.01	Combined Type
.00	Predominantly Inattentive Type
.01	Predominantly Hyperactive-Impulsive Type
314.9	Attention-Deficit/Hyperactivity Disorder NOS
312.xx	Conduct Disorder
.81	Childhood-Onset Type
.82	Adolescent-Onset Type
.89	Unspecified Onset
313.81	Oppositional Defiant Disorder
312.9	Disruptive Behavior Disorder NOS

Feeding and Eating Disorders of Infancy or Early Childhood

307.52	Pica
307.53	Rumination Disorder
307.59	Feeding Disorder of Infancy or Early Childhood

Tic Disorders

307.23	Tourette's Disorder
307.22	Chronic Motor or Vocal Tic Disorder
307.21	Transient Tic Disorder
	Specify if: Single Episode/Recurrent
307.20	Tic Disorder NOS

Elimination Disorders

___.__	Encopresis
787.6	With Constipation and Overflow Incontinence
307.7	Without Constipation and Overflow Incontinence
307.6	Enuresis (Not Due to a General Medical Condition)
	Specify type: Nocturnal Only/Diurnal Only/Nocturnal and Diurnal

Other Disorders of Infancy, Childhood, or Adolescence

309.21	Separation Anxiety Disorder
	Specify if: Early Onset
313.23	Selective Mutism
313.89	Reactive Attachment Disorder of Infancy or Early Childhood
	Specify type: Inhibited Type/Disinhibited Type
307.3	Stereotypic Movement Disorder
	Specify if: With Self-Injurious Behavior
313.9	Disorder of Infancy, Childhood, or Adolescence NOS

DELIRIUM, DEMENTIA, AND AMNESTIC AND OTHER COGNITIVE DISORDERS
Delirium

293.0	Delirium Due to . . . *[Indicate the General Medical Condition]*
__.__	Substance Intoxication Delirium *(refer to Substance-Related Disorders for substance-specific codes)*
__.__	Substance Withdrawal Delirium *(refer to Substance-Related Disorders for substance-specific codes)*
__.__	Delirium Due to Multiple Etiologies *(code each of the specific etiologies)*
780.09	Delirium NOS

Dementia

294.xx	Dementia of the Alzheimer's Type, With Early Onset *(also code 331.0 Alzheimer's disease on Axis III)*
.10	Without Behavioral Disturbance
.11	With Behavioral Disturbance
294.xx	Dementia of the Alzheimer's Type, With Late Onset *(also code 331.0 Alzheimer's disease on Axis III)*
.10	Without Behavioral Disturbance
.11	With Behavioral Disturbance
290.xx	Vascular Dementia
.40	Uncomplicated
.41	With Delirium
.42	With Delusions
.43	With Depressed Mood
	Specify if: With Behavioral Disturbance

Code presence or absence of a behavioral disturbance in the fifth digit for Dementia Due to a General Medical Condition:
  0=Without Behavioral Disturbance
  1=With Behavioral Disturbance

294.1x	Dementia Due to HIV Disease *(also code 042 HIV on Axis III)*
294.1x	Dementia Due to Head Trauma *(also code 854.00 head injury on Axis III)*

294.1x	Dementia Due to Parkinson's Disease *(also code 332.0 Parkinson's disease on Axis III)*
294.1x	Dementia Due to Huntington's Disease *(also code 333.4 Huntington's disease on Axis III)*
294.1x	Dementia Due to Pick's Disease *(also code 331.1 Pick's disease on Axis III)*
294.1x	Dementia Due to Creutzfeldt-Jakob Disease *(also code 046.1 Creutzfeldt-Jakob disease on Axis III)*
294.1x	Dementia Due to . . . *[Indicate the General Medical Condition not listed above] (also code the general medical condition on Axis III)*
__.__	Substance-Induced Persisting Dementia *(refer to Substance-Related Disorders for substance-specific codes)*
__.__	Dementia Due to Multiple Etiologies *(code each of the specific etiologies)*
294.8	Dementia NOS

Amnestic Disorders

294.0	Amnestic Disorder Due to . . . *[Indicate the General Medical Condition]*
	Specify if: Transient/Chronic
__.__	Substance-Induced Persisting Amnestic Disorder *(refer to Substance-Related Disorders for substance-specific codes)*
294.8	Amnestic Disorder NOS

Other Cognitive Disorders

294.9	Cognitive Disorder NOS

MENTAL DISORDERS DUE TO A GENERAL MEDICAL CONDITION NOT ELSEWHERE CLASSIFIED

293.89	Catatonic Disorder Due to . . . *[Indicate the General Medical Condition]*
310.1	Personality Change Due to . . . *[Indicate the General Medical Condition]*
	Specify type: Labile Type/Disinhibited Type/Aggressive Type/Apathetic Type/Paranoid Type/ Other Type/Combined Type/Unspecified Type
293.9	Mental Disorder NOS Due to . . . *[Indicate the General Medical Condition]*

SUBSTANCE-RELATED DISORDERS
The following specifiers may be applied to Substance Dependence as noted:
[a]With Physiologic Dependence/Without Physiologic Dependence
[b]Early Full Remission/Early Partial Remission/Sustained Full Remission/Sustained Partial Remission
[c]In a Controlled Environment

^dOn Agonist Therapy

The following specifiers apply to Substance-Induced Disorders as noted:

^IWith Onset During Intoxication/^WWith Onset During Withdrawal

Alcohol-Related Disorders
Alcohol Use Disorders
303.90 Alcohol Dependence^{a,b,c}
305.00 Alcohol Abuse

Alcohol-Induced Disorders
303.00 Alcohol Intoxication
291.81 Alcohol Withdrawal
    Specify if: With Perceptual Disturbances
291.0 Alcohol Intoxication Delirium
291.0 Alcohol Withdrawal Delirium
291.2 Alcohol-Induced Persisting Dementia
291.1 Alcohol-Induced Persisting Amnestic Disorder
291.x Alcohol-Induced Psychotic Disorder
  .5 With Delusions^{I,W}
  .3 With Hallucinations^{I,W}
291.89 Alcohol-Induced Mood Disorder^{I,W}
291.89 Alcohol-Induced Anxiety Disorder^{I,W}
291.89 Alcohol-Induced Sexual Dysfunction^I
291.89 Alcohol-Induced Sleep Disorder^{I,W}
291.9 Alcohol-Related Disorder NOS

Amphetamine (or Amphetamine-Like)–Related Disorders
Amphetamine Use Disorders
304.40 Amphetamine Dependence^{a,b,c}
305.70 Amphetamine Abuse

Amphetamine-Induced Disorders
292.89 Amphetamine Intoxication
    Specify if: With Perceptual Disturbances
292.0 Amphetamine Withdrawal
292.81 Amphetamine Intoxication Delirium
292.xx Amphetamine-Induced Psychotic Disorder
  .11 With Delusions^I
  .12 With Hallucinations^I
292.84 Amphetamine-Induced Mood Disorder^{I,W}
292.89 Amphetamine-Induced Anxiety Disorder^I
292.89 Amphetamine-Induced Sexual Dysfunction^I
292.89 Amphetamine-Induced Sleep Disorder^{I,W}
292.9 Amphetamine-Related Disorder NOS

Caffeine-Related Disorders
Caffeine-Induced Disorders
305.90 Caffeine Intoxication
292.89 Caffeine-Induced Anxiety Disorder^I
292.89 Caffeine-Induced Sleep Disorder^I
292.9 Caffeine-Related Disorder NOS

Cannabis-Related Disorders
Cannabis Use Disorders
304.30 Cannabis Dependence^{a,b,c}
305.20 Cannabis Abuse

Cannabis-Induced Disorders
292.89 Cannabis Intoxication
    Specify if: With Perceptual Disturbances
292.81 Cannabis Intoxication Delirium
292.xx Cannabis-Induced Psychotic Disorder
  .11 With Delusions^I
  .12 With Hallucinations^I
292.89 Cannabis-Induced Anxiety Disorder^I
292.9 Cannabis-Related Disorder NOS

Cocaine-Related Disorders
Cocaine Use Disorders
304.20 Cocaine Dependence^{a,b,c}
305.60 Cocaine Abuse

Cocaine-Induced Disorders
292.89 Cocaine Intoxication
    Specify if: With Perceptual Disturbances
292.0 Cocaine Withdrawal
292.81 Cocaine Intoxication Delirium
292.xx Cocaine-Induced Psychotic Disorder
  .11 With Delusions^I
  .12 With Hallucinations^I
292.84 Cocaine-Induced Mood Disorder^{I,W}
292.89 Cocaine-Induced Anxiety Disorder^{I,W}
292.89 Cocaine-Induced Sexual Dysfunction^I
292.89 Cocaine-Induced Sleep Disorder^{I,W}
292.9 Cocaine-Related Disorder NOS

Hallucinogen-Related Disorders
Hallucinogen Use Disorders
304.50 Hallucinogen Dependence^{b,c}
305.30 Hallucinogen Abuse

Hallucinogen-Induced Disorders
292.89 Hallucinogen Intoxication
292.89 Hallucinogen Persisting Perception Disorder (Flashbacks)
292.81 Hallucinogen Intoxication Delirium
292.xx Hallucinogen-Induced Psychotic Disorder
  .11 With Delusions^I
  .12 With Hallucinations^I
292.84 Hallucinogen-Induced Mood Disorder^I
292.89 Hallucinogen-Induced Anxiety Disorder^I
292.9 Hallucinogen-Related Disorder NOS

Inhalant-Related Disorders
Inhalant Use Disorders
304.60 Inhalant Dependence^{b,c}
305.90 Inhalant Abuse

Inhalant-Induced Disorders
292.89   Inhalant Intoxication
292.81   Inhalant Intoxication Delirium
292.82   Inhalant-Induced Persisting Dementia
292.xx   Inhalant-Induced Psychotic Disorder
.11   With Delusions[I]
.12   With Hallucinations[I]
292.84   Inhalant-Induced Mood Disorder[I]
292.89   Inhalant-Induced Anxiety Disorder[I]
292.9   Inhalant-Related Disorder NOS

Nicotine-Related Disorders
Nicotine Use Disorder
305.1   Nicotine Dependence[a,b]

Nicotine-Induced Disorder
292.0   Nicotine Withdrawal
292.9   Nicotine-Related Disorder NOS

Opioid-Related Disorders
Opioid Use Disorders
304.00   Opioid Dependence[a,b,c,d]
305.50   Opioid Abuse

Opioid-Induced Disorders
292.89   Opioid Intoxication
    Specify if: With Perceptual Disturbances
292.0   Opioid Withdrawal
292.81   Opioid Intoxication Delirium
292.xx   Opioid-Induced Psychotic Disorder
.11   With Delusions[I]
.12   With Hallucinations[I]
292.84   Opioid-Induced Mood Disorder[I]
292.89   Opioid-Induced Sexual Dysfunction[I]
292.89   Opioid-Induced Sleep Disorder[I,W]
292.9   Opioid-Related Disorder NOS

Phencyclidine (or Phencyclidine-Like)–Related Disorders
Phencyclidine Use Disorders
304.60   Phencyclidine Dependence[b,c]
305.90   Phencyclidine Abuse

Phencyclidine-Induced Disorders
292.89   Phencyclidine Intoxication
    Specify if: With Perceptual Disturbances
292.81   Phencyclidine Intoxication Delirium
292.xx   Phencyclidine-Induced Psychotic Disorder
.11   With Delusions[I]
.12   With Hallucinations[I]
292.84   Phencyclidine-Induced Mood Disorder[I]
292.89   Phencyclidine-Induced Anxiety Disorder[I]
292.9   Phencyclidine-Related Disorder NOS

Sedative-, Hypnotic-, or Anxiolytic-Related Disorders
Sedative, Hypnotic, or Anxiolytic Use Disorders
304.10   Sedative, Hypnotic, or Anxiolytic Dependence[a,b,c]
305.40   Sedative, Hypnotic, or Anxiolytic Abuse

Sedative-, Hypnotic-, or Anxiolytic-Induced Disorders
292.89   Sedative, Hypnotic, or Anxiolytic Intoxication
292.0   Sedative, Hypnotic, or Anxiolytic Withdrawal
    Specify if: With Perceptual Disturbances
292.81   Sedative, Hypnotic, or Anxiolytic Intoxication Delirium
292.81   Sedative, Hypnotic, or Anxiolytic Withdrawal Delirium
292.82   Sedative-, Hypnotic-, or Anxiolytic-Induced Persisting Dementia
292.83   Sedative-, Hypnotic-, or Anxiolytic-Induced Persisting Amnestic Disorder
292.xx   Sedative-, Hypnotic-, or Anxiolytic-Induced Psychotic Disorder
.11   With Delusions[I,W]
.12   With Hallucinations[I,W]
292.84   Sedative-, Hypnotic-, or Anxiolytic-Induced Mood Disorder[I,W]
292.89   Sedative-, Hypnotic-, or Anxiolytic-Induced Anxiety Disorder[W]
292.89   Sedative-, Hypnotic-, or Anxiolytic-Induced Sexual Dysfunction[I]
292.89   Sedative-, Hypnotic-, or Anxiolytic-Induced Sleep Disorder[I,W]
292.9   Sedative-, Hypnotic-, or Anxiolytic-Related Disorder NOS

Polysubstance-Related Disorder
304.80   Polysubstance Dependence[a,b,c,d]

Other (or Unknown) Substance–Related Disorders
Other (or Unknown) Substance Use Disorders
304.90   Other (or Unknown) Substance Dependence[a,b,c,d]
305.90   Other (or Unknown) Substance Abuse

Other (or Unknown) Substance–Induced Disorders
292.89   Other (or Unknown) Substance Intoxication
    Specify if: With Perceptual Disturbances
292.0   Other (or Unknown) Substance Withdrawal
    Specify if: With Perceptual Disturbances
292.81   Other (or Unknown) Substance–Induced Delirium
292.82   Other (or Unknown) Substance–Induced Persisting Dementia

292.83	Other (or Unknown) Substance–Induced Persisting Amnestic Disorder
292.xx	Other (or Unknown) Substance–Induced Psychotic Disorder
.11	With Delusions[I,W]
.12	With Hallucinations[I,W]
292.84	Other (or Unknown) Substance–Induced Mood Disorder[I,W]
292.89	Other (or Unknown) Substance–Induced Anxiety Disorder[I,W]
292.89	Other (or Unknown) Substance–Induced Sexual Dysfunction[I]
292.89	Other (or Unknown) Substance–Induced Sleep Disorder[I,W]
292.9	Other (or Unknown) Substance–Related Disorder NOS

SCHIZOPHRENIA AND OTHER PSYCHOTIC DISORDERS

295.xx	Schizophrenia

The following Classification of Longitudinal Course applies to all subtypes of Schizophrenia:

Episodic With Interepisode Residual Symptoms (*specify if:* With Prominent Negative Symptoms)/Episodic With No Interepisode Residual Symptoms
Continuous (*specify if:* With Prominent Negative Symptoms)
Single Episode in Partial Remission (*specify if:* With Prominent Negative Symptoms)/Single Episode In Full Remission
Other or Unspecified Pattern

.30	Paranoid Type
.10	Disorganized Type
.20	Catatonic Type
.90	Undifferentiated Type
.60	Residual Type

295.40	Schizophreniform Disorder
	Specify if: Without Good Prognostic Features/With Good Prognostic Features
295.70	Schizoaffective Disorder
	Specify type: Bipolar Type/Depressive Type
297.1	Delusional Disorder
	Specify type: Erotomanic Type/Grandiose Type/Jealous Type/Persecutory Type/Somatic Type/Mixed Type/Unspecified Type
298.8	Brief Psychotic Disorder
	Specify if: With Marked Stressor(s)/Without Marked Stressor(s)/With Postpartum Onset
297.3	Shared Psychotic Disorder
293.xx	Psychotic Disorder Due to . . . *[Indicate the General Medical Condition]*
.81	With Delusions
.82	With Hallucinations

___.___	Substance-Induced Psychotic Disorder *(refer to Substance-Related Disorders for substance-specific codes)*
	Specify if: With Onset During Intoxication/With Onset During Withdrawal
298.9	Psychotic Disorder NOS

MOOD DISORDERS

Code current state of Major Depressive Disorder or Bipolar I Disorder in fifth digit:

1 = Mild
2 = Moderate
3 = Severe Without Psychotic Features
4 = Severe With Psychotic Features
    Specify: Mood-Congruent Psychotic Features/Mood-Incongruent Psychotic Features
5 = In Partial Remission
6 = In Full Remission
0 = Unspecified

The following specifiers apply (for current or most recent episode) to Mood Disorders as noted:
[a]Severity/Psychotic/Remission Specifiers/[b]Chronic/[c]With Catatonic Features/[d]With Melancholic Features/[e]With Atypical Features/[f]With Postpartum Onset

The following specifiers apply to Mood Disorders as noted:
[g]With or Without Full Interepisode Recovery/[h]With Seasonal Pattern/[i]With Rapid Cycling

Depressive Disorders

296.xx	Major Depressive Disorder
.2x	Single Episode[a,b,c,d,e,f]
.3x	Recurrent[a,b,c,d,e,f,g,h]
300.4	Dysthymic Disorder
	Specify if: Early Onset/Late Onset
	Specify: With Atypical Features
311	Depressive Disorder NOS

Bipolar Disorders

296.xx	Bipolar I Disorder
.0x	Single Manic Episode[a,c,f]
	Specify if: Mixed
.40	Most Recent Episode Hypomanic[g,h,i]
.4x	Most Recent Episode Manic[a,c,f,g,h,i]
.6x	Most Recent Episode Mixed[a,c,f,g,h,i]
.5x	Most Recent Episode Depressed[a,b,c,d,e,f,g,h,i]
.7	Most Recent Episode Unspecified[g,h,i]
296.89	Bipolar II Disorder[a,b,c,d,e,f,g,h,i]
	Specify (current or most recent episode): Hypomanic/Depressed
301.13	Cyclothymic Disorder
296.80	Bipolar Disorder NOS
293.83	Mood Disorder Due to . . . *[Indicate the General Medical Condition]*

Specify type: With Depressive Features/With
Major Depressive-Like Episode/With
Manic Features/With Mixed Features

___.___ Substance-Induced Mood Disorder *(refer to Substance-Related Disorders for substance-specific codes)*
Specify type: With Depressive Features/With
Manic Features/With Mixed Features
Specify if: With Onset During
Intoxication/With Onset During
Withdrawal

296.90   Mood Disorder NOS

ANXIETY DISORDERS

300.01   Panic Disorder Without Agoraphobia
300.21   Panic Disorder With Agoraphobia
300.22   Agoraphobia Without History of Panic Disorder
300.29   Specific Phobia
Specify type: Animal Type/Natural
Environment Type/Blood-Injection-Injury
Type/Situational Type/Other Type
300.23   Social Phobia
Specify if: Generalized
300.3   Obsessive-Compulsive Disorder
Specify if: With Poor Insight
309.81   Posttraumatic Stress Disorder
Specify if: Acute/Chronic
Specify if: With Delayed Onset
308.3   Acute Stress Disorder
300.02   Generalized Anxiety Disorder
293.84   Anxiety Disorder Due to . . . *[Indicate the General Medical Condition]*
Specify if: With Generalized Anxiety/With
Panic Attacks/With Obsessive-Compulsive
Symptoms

___.___ Substance-Induced Anxiety Disorder *(refer to Substance-Related Disorders for substance-specific codes)*
Specify if: With Generalized Anxiety/With
Panic Attacks/With Obsessive-Compulsive
Symptoms/With Phobic Symptoms
Specify if: With Onset During
Intoxication/With Onset During
Withdrawal
300.00   Anxiety Disorder NOS

SOMATOFORM DISORDERS

300.81   Somatization Disorder
300.82   Undifferentiated Somatoform Disorder
300.11   Conversion Disorder
Specify type: With Motor Symptom or
Deficit/With Sensory Symptom or
Deficit/With Seizures or Convulsions/With
Mixed Presentation

307.xx   Pain Disorder
.80   Associated With Psychologic Factors
.89   Associated With Both Psychologic Factors and a General Medical Condition
Specify if: Acute/Chronic
300.7   Hypochondriasis
Specify if: With Poor Insight
300.7   Body Dysmorphic Disorder
300.82   Somatoform Disorder NOS

FACTITIOUS DISORDERS

300.xx   Factitious Disorder
.16   With Predominantly Psychologic Signs and Symptoms
.19   With Predominantly Physical Signs and Symptoms
.19   With Combined Psychologic and Physical Signs and Symptoms
300.19   Factitious Disorder NOS

DISSOCIATIVE DISORDERS

300.12   Dissociative Amnesia
300.13   Dissociative Fugue
300.14   Dissociative Identity Disorder
300.6   Depersonalization Disorder
300.15   Dissociative Disorder NOS

SEXUAL AND GENDER IDENTITY DISORDERS
Sexual Dysfunctions
The following specifiers apply to all primary Sexual Dysfunctions:
Lifelong Type/Acquired Type
Generalized Type/Situational Type
Due to Psychologic Factors/Due to Combined Factors

Sexual Desire Disorders
302.71   Hypoactive Sexual Desire Disorder
302.79   Sexual Aversion Disorder

Sexual Arousal Disorders
302.72   Female Sexual Arousal Disorder
302.72   Male Erectile Disorder

Orgasmic Disorders
302.73   Female Orgasmic Disorder
302.74   Male Orgasmic Disorder
302.75   Premature Ejaculation

Sexual Pain Disorders
302.76   Dyspareunia (Not Due to a General Medical Condition)
306.51   Vaginismus (Not Due to a General Medical Condition)

Sexual Dysfunction Due to a General Medical Condition

625.8	Female Hypoactive Sexual Desire Disorder Due to . . . *[Indicate the General Medical Condition]*
608.89	Male Hypoactive Sexual Desire Disorder Due to . . . *[Indicate the General Medical Condition]*
607.84	Male Erectile Disorder Due to . . . *[Indicate the General Medical Condition]*
625.0	Female Dyspareunia Due to . . . *[Indicate the General Medical Condition]*
608.89	Male Dyspareunia Due to . . . *[Indicate the General Medical Condition]*
625.8	Other Female Sexual Dysfunction Due to . . . *[Indicate the General Medical Condition]*
608.89	Other Male Sexual Dysfunction Due to . . . *[Indicate the General Medical Condition]*
___.__	Substance-Induced Sexual Dysfunction *(refer to Substance-Related Disorders for substance-specific codes)*
	Specify if: With Impaired Desire/With Impaired Arousal/With Impaired Orgasm/With Sexual Pain
	Specify if: With Onset During Intoxication
302.70	Sexual Dysfunction NOS

Paraphilias

302.4	Exhibitionism
302.81	Fetishism
302.89	Frotteurism
302.2	Pedophilia
	Specify if: Sexually Attracted to Males/Sexually Attracted to Females/Sexually Attracted to Both
	Specify if: Limited to Incest
	Specify type: Exclusive Type/Nonexclusive Type
302.83	Sexual Masochism
302.84	Sexual Sadism
302.3	Transvestic Fetishism
	Specify if: With Gender Dysphoria
302.82	Voyeurism
302.9	Paraphilia NOS

Gender Identity Disorders

302.xx	Gender Identity Disorder
.6	In Children
.85	In Adolescents or Adults
	Specify if: Sexually Attracted to Males/Sexually Attracted to Females/Sexually Attracted to Both/Sexually Attracted to Neither
302.6	Gender Identity Disorder NOS
302.9	Sexual Disorder NOS

EATING DISORDERS

307.1	Anorexia Nervosa
	Specify type: Restricting Type; Binge-Eating/Purging Type
307.51	Bulimia Nervosa
	Specify type: Purging Type/Nonpurging Type
307.50	Eating Disorder NOS

SLEEP DISORDERS
Primary Sleep Disorders
Dyssomnias

307.42	Primary Insomnia
307.44	Primary Hypersomnia
	Specify if: Recurrent
347	Narcolepsy
780.59	Breathing-Related Sleep Disorder
307.45	Circadian Rhythm Sleep Disorder
	Specify type: Delayed Sleep Phase Type/Jet Lag Type/Shift Work Type/Unspecified Type
307.47	Dyssomnia NOS

Parasomnias

307.47	Nightmare Disorder
307.46	Sleep Terror Disorder
307.46	Sleepwalking Disorder
307.47	Parasomnia NOS

Sleep Disorders Related to Another Mental Disorder

307.42	Insomnia Related to . . . *[Indicate the Axis I or Axis II Disorder]*
307.44	Hypersomnia Related to . . . *[Indicate the Axis I or Axis II Disorder]*

Other Sleep Disorders

780.xx	Sleep Disorder Due to . . . *[Indicate the General Medical Condition]*
.52	Insomnia Type
.54	Hypersomnia Type
.59	Parasomnia Type
.59	Mixed Type
___.__	Substance-Induced Sleep Disorder *(refer to Substance-Related Disorders for substance-specific codes)*
	Specify type: Insomnia Type/Hypersomnia Type/Parasomnia Type/Mixed Type
	Specify if: With Onset During Intoxication/With Onset During Withdrawal

IMPULSE-CONTROL DISORDERS NOT ELSEWHERE CLASSIFIED

312.34	Intermittent Explosive Disorder
312.32	Kleptomania

312.33	Pyromania
312.31	Pathologic Gambling
312.39	Trichotillomania
312.30	Impulse-Control Disorder NOS

ADJUSTMENT DISORDERS

309.xx	Adjustment Disorder
.0	With Depressed Mood
.24	With Anxiety
.28	With Mixed Anxiety and Depressed Mood
.3	With Disturbance of Conduct
.4	With Mixed Disturbance of Emotions and Conduct
.9	Unspecified

Specify if: Acute/Chronic

PERSONALITY DISORDERS

Note: These are coded on Axis II.

301.0	Paranoid Personality Disorder
301.20	Schizoid Personality Disorder
301.22	Schizotypal Personality Disorder
301.7	Antisocial Personality Disorder
301.83	Borderline Personality Disorder
301.50	Histrionic Personality Disorder
301.81	Narcissistic Personality Disorder
301.82	Avoidant Personality Disorder
301.6	Dependent Personality Disorder
301.4	Obsessive-Compulsive Personality Disorder
301.9	Personality Disorder NOS

OTHER CONDITIONS THAT MAY BE A FOCUS OF CLINICAL ATTENTION
Psychologic Factors Affecting Medical Condition

316	. . . [Specified Psychologic Factor] Affecting . . . [Indicate the General Medical Condition]

Choose name based on nature of factors:

Mental Disorder Affecting Medical Condition
Psychological Symptoms Affecting Medical Condition
Personality Traits or Coping Style Affecting Medical Condition
Maladaptive Health Behaviors Affecting Medical Condition
Stress-Related Physiologic Response Affecting Medical Condition
Other or Unspecified Psychologic Factors Affecting Medical Condition

Medication-Induced Movement Disorders

332.1	Neuroleptic-Induced Parkinsonism
333.92	Neuroleptic Malignant Syndrome
333.7	Neuroleptic-Induced Acute Dystonia
333.99	Neuroleptic-Induced Acute Akathisia
333.82	Neuroleptic-Induced Tardive Dyskinesia
333.1	Medication-Induced Postural Tremor
333.90	Medication-Induced Movement Disorder NOS

Other Medication-Induced Disorder

995.2	Adverse Effects of Medication NOS

Relational Problems

V61.9	Relational Problem Related to a Mental Disorder or General Medical Condition
V61.20	Parent-Child Relational Problem
V61.10	Partner Relational Problem
V61.8	Sibling Relational Problem
V62.81	Relational Problem NOS

Problems Related to Abuse or Neglect

V61.21	Physical Abuse of Child *(code 995.5 if focus of attention is on victim)*
V61.21	Sexual Abuse of Child *(code 995.5 if focus of attention is on victim)*
V61.21	Neglect of Child *(code 995.5 if focus of attention is on victim)*
___.__	Physical Abuse of Adult
V61.12	(if by partner)
V62.83	(if by person other than partner) *(code 995.81 if focus of attention is on victim)*
___.__	Sexual Abuse of Adult
V61.12	(if by partner)
V62.83	(if by person other than partner) *(code 995.83 if focus of attention is on victim)*

Additional Conditions That May Be a Focus of Clinical Attention

V15.81	Noncompliance With Treatment
V65.2	Malingering
V71.01	Adult Antisocial Behavior
V71.02	Child or Adolescent Antisocial Behavior
V62.89	Borderline Intellectual Functioning

Note: This is coded on Axis II.

780.9	Age-Related Cognitive Decline
V62.82	Bereavement
V62.3	Academic Problem
V62.2	Occupational Problem
313.82	Identity Problem
V62.89	Religious or Spiritual Problem
V62.4	Acculturation Problem
V62.89	Phase of Life Problem

ADDITIONAL CODES

300.9	Unspecified Mental Disorder (nonpsychotic)
V71.09	No Diagnosis or Condition on Axis I
799.9	Diagnosis or Condition Deferred on Axis I
V71.09	No Diagnosis on Axis II
799.9	Diagnosis Deferred on Axis II

MULTIAXIAL SYSTEM

Axis I	Clinical Disorders
	Other Conditions That May Be a Focus of Clinical Attention
Axis II	Personality Disorders
	Mental Retardation
Axis III	General Medical Conditions
Axis IV	Psychosocial and Environmental Problems
Axis V	Global Assessment of Functioning

From American Psychiatric Association: *Diagnostic and Statistical Manual of Mental Disorders,* Fourth Edition, Text Revision. Washington, DC, American Psychiatric Association, 2000.

Appendix B

American Nurses Association Standards of Psychiatric-Mental Health Nursing Practice

STANDARDS OF CARE
Standard I. Assessment
The psychiatric-mental health nurse collects patient health data.

Standard II. Diagnosis
The psychiatric-mental health nurse analyzes the assessment data in determining diagnoses.

Standard III. Outcome Identification
The psychiatric-mental health nurse identifies expected outcomes individualized to the patient.

Standard IV. Planning
The psychiatric-mental health nurse develops a plan of care that is negotiated among the patient, nurse, family, and health care team and prescribes evidence-based interventions to attain expected outcomes.

Standard V. Implementation
The psychiatric-mental health nurse implements the interventions identified in the plan of care.

Standard Va. Counseling
The psychiatric-mental health nurse uses counseling interventions to assist patients in improving or regaining their previous coping abilities, fostering mental health, and preventing mental illness and disability.

Standard Vb. Milieu Therapy
The psychiatric-mental health nurse provides, structures, and maintains a therapeutic environment in collaboration with the patient and other health care clinicians.

Standard Vc. Promotion of Self-Care Activities
The psychiatric-mental health nurse structures interventions around the patient's activities of daily living to foster self-care and mental and physical well-being.

Standard Vd. Psychobiological Interventions
The psychiatric-mental health nurse uses knowledge of psychobiological interventions and applies clinical skills to restore the patient's health and prevent further disability.

Standard Ve. Health Teaching
The psychiatric-mental health nurse, through health teaching, assists patients in achieving satisfying, productive, and healthy patterns of living.

Standard Vf. Case Management
The psychiatric-mental health nurse provides case management to coordinate comprehensive health services and to ensure continuity of care.

Standard Vg. Health Promotion and Health Maintenance
The psychiatric-mental health nurse uses strategies and interventions to promote and maintain health and prevent mental illness.

The following interventions (Vh-Vj) may be performed only by the APRN-PMH.

Advanced Practice Interventions Vh-Vj
Standard Vh. Psychotherapy
The APRN-PMH uses individual, group, and family psychotherapy, and other therapeutic treatments to assist patients in preventing mental illness and disability, treating mental health disorders, and improving mental health status and functional abilities.

Standard Vi. Prescriptive Authority and Treatment
The APRN-PMH uses prescriptive authority, procedures, and treatments in accordance with state and federal laws and regulations, to treat symptoms of psychiatric illness and improve functional health status.

Standard Vj. Consultation
The APRN-PMH provides consultation to enhance the abilities of other clinicians to provide services for patients and effect change in the system.

Standard VI. Evaluation
The psychiatric-mental health nurse evaluates the patient's progress in attaining expected outcomes.

STANDARDS OF PROFESSIONAL PERFORMANCE

Standard I. Quality of Care

The psychiatric-mental health nurse systematically evaluates the quality of care and effectiveness of psychiatric-mental health nursing practice.

Standard II. Performance Appraisal

The psychiatric-mental health nurse evaluates one's own psychiatric-mental health nursing practice in relation to professional practice standards and relevant statuses and regulations.

Standard III. Education

The psychiatric-mental health nurse acquires and maintains current knowledge in nursing practice.

Standard IV. Collegiality

The psychiatric-mental health nurse interacts with and contributes to the professional development of peers, health care clinicians, and others, as colleagues.

Standard V. Ethics

The psychiatric-mental health nurse's assessments, actions, and recommendations on behalf of patients are determined and implemented in an ethical manner.

Standard VI. Collaboration

The psychiatric-mental health nurse collaborates with the patient, significant others, and health care clinicians in providing care.

Standard VII. Research

The psychiatric-mental health nurse contributes to nursing and mental health through the use of research methods and findings.

Standard VIII. Resource Utilization

The psychiatric-mental health nurse considers factors related to safety, effectiveness, and cost in planning and delivering patient care.

From American Nurses Association: *Statement on the scope and standards of psychiatric-mental health nursing practice,* Washington, DC, 2000, American Nurses Publishing.

Appendix C
Classification Systems: NIC and NOC

NURSING INTERVENTIONS CLASSIFICATION
Definition, Purpose, and Progress

Nursing Interventions Classification (NIC), now in its third edition, is the first comprehensive standardized language that describes the treatments performed by nurses. The classification was researched and developed from 1987 through 1995 by the members of the Iowa Intervention Project Research Team, and its work was published in 1992, 1996, and most recently in 2000. The NIC taxonomy was first introduced in the second edition and has now been updated to include 486 interventions that nurses do for clients, both collaborative and independent, and including direct and indirect care. This is a significant number when compared with the 433 interventions in the second edition and the 336 interventions in the first edition. In the 2000 edition, the taxonomy includes 7 domains and 30 classes. A new community domain containing two new classes has been added, as well as a new child-rearing class in the family domain. Each intervention has a label name, a definition, a list of activities that a nurse might need to carry out the intervention, and a brief list of background readings. The activities can be selected and modified as required to meet the specific needs of the individual or the population. The background readings do not include a complete reference list for each intervention, but rather they are places for nurses to begin. The readings represent a few sources that were used in the development of the intervention's definition and activity list and provide support that this intervention is used by nurses. NIC can be used to communicate a common meaning across settings, and yet provide a way for nurses to individualize care. It can be used in all specialties by both new and practicing nurses. A new feature in the 2000 edition is specialty area core interventions as identified by 39 specialty organizations. NIC interventions can be physiologic, such as airway suctioning and decubitus ulcer care, or psychosocial, such as anxiety reduction and assisting the client with coping skills. NIC interventions are effective in the treatment of physical or psychiatric illnesses, such as hypertension or cognitive disturbances, respectively. They are equally effective in preventing various types of illnesses, such as fall prevention or prevention of self-harm. NIC interventions are also used in health promotion, such as education about the health hazards of smoking, the value of good nutrition, and the importance of stress reduction. NIC continues to identify and refine nursing

actions from groups of data found throughout current nursing texts and literature and includes them in the NIC taxonomy where they are systematically organized, with clear rules and principles for each intervention. As in previous editions, a form is provided in the 2000 edition for nurses to submit suggestions for new or revised interventions and to participate in consistent improvement of the NIC classification (McClosky and Bulechek, 2000).

Strengths of NIC

- Comprehensive
- Research based
- Developed inductively based on existing practice
- Reflects current clinical practice and research
- Has easy-to-use organizing structure (domains, classes, interventions activities)
- Uses language that is clear and clinically meaningful
- Has established process and structure for continued refinement
- Has been field tested
- Accessible through numerous publications
- Linked to NANDA nursing diagnoses, Omaha system problems, and NOC outcomes
- Recipient of national recognition
- Developed at same site as outcomes classification
- Translated into several languages (McCloskey and Bulecek, 2000)

NIC and NANDA Linkage

Linkages between NIC interventions and NANDA diagnoses have been updated in the 2000 edition and include the new NIC interventions and the new diagnoses in the 1999-2000 NANDA publication. Although NIC can be used without NANDA, the linkage will facilitate intervention selections for the many NANDA users. This is important, as NANDA is widely endorsed by nurses and is a major part of clinical decision making in nursing practice, as indicated in this text and other nursing texts and journals (McCloskey and Bulecek, 2000).

History of NIC Research Methodology

In the initial development of NIC, time-proven research methods were used by the Iowa team to distinguish and refine the most relevant intervention labels from the myriad associated activities that accompanied the nursing problems or nursing diagnoses. A two-round Delphi questionnaire was used in expert surveys, and responses from the first round of questions were used to modify the questionnaire during the second round. Fehring's research methodology was adapted for use with interventions and yielded intervention content validity scores with critical and supporting activities. Typically, most textbooks that were researched included several hundred of these "interventions," and quite often these actions were a combination of assessment and treatment activities, as well as a mixture of nurse-initiated and physician-initiated actions. During content analysis, the team discovered that each intervention label had anywhere from one to several hundred associated activities. Also, the lists of interventions for the same diagnosis varied enormously from one text to another. The process was such that groups of related intervention labels were ultimately selected as a result of an in-depth investigation process by nursing professionals. Lists of accompanying activities were computer generated, and participants were asked to create each activity according to the extent to which it was characteristic of the label (McCloskey and Bulechek, 1996).

NURSING OUTCOMES CLASSIFICATION
Definition, Purpose, and Progress

Nursing Outcomes Classification (NOC), now in its second edition, presented its first comprehensive, standardized language to describe client outcomes responsive to nursing interventions in 1997 and most recently in 2000. The classification was developed by members of the Nursing-Sensitive Outcomes Classification team, which began its research in August 1991. The second edition of NOC currently contains 260 outcomes, significantly more than the 190 outcomes published in the first edition. Fifty-seven new outcomes for individual patient and family caregivers and seven family-level and six community-level outcomes have been added to the new edition. The new edition also includes a taxonomic structure for the classification and a description of how the structure was developed. Outcomes include indicators (e.g., observable client states, behaviors, or self-reported perceptions) that nurses can use to assess the effects of the interventions. Each outcome has a label (name); a definition; a set of indicators that describe specific patient, caregiver, family, or community states related to the outcome; a 5 point Likert-type measurement scale; and selected references used in the development of the outcome. Although indicators and measurement scales are encouraged, the goal of the research team is to standardize the label name and definition for each outcome, both of which help nurses to evaluate and quantify patient status in relation to a particular outcome. The evaluation of the reliability and validity of the scales is incomplete, yet feedback from clinicians using the outcome measures in clinical settings has been positive. The need for nursing to define the patient outcomes responsive to nursing care has continued to increase since the first published text. The growth of managed care and the emphasis on cost containment continue to raise concerns about outcome effectiveness and the quality of health care (Johnson, Mass, and Moorhead, 2000).

In the first edition the nursing-sensitive outcomes were presented as neutral concepts reflecting a client's physical state, such as mobility or hydration, or psychologic state, such as coping or grieving. The team contended that neutral outcomes can be measured on a continuum, which differs from discrete goals, which are either met or unmet. The team believed then and now that this neutral state helps nurses identify and analyze outcomes recently achieved for specific client populations, as well as to identify realistic standards of care for specific populations. For example, clients can be aggregated in myriad ways, such as by nursing or medical diagnoses, or by service unit or illness acuity; and the difference in outcomes achievement can be analyzed by client characteristics such as age, gender, or functional states. The NOC method of outcome selection is considered more effective than the usual practice, which is to set one standard or select a single goal for all clients regardless of individual characteristics, which tends to produce ineffective outcomes attainment (Johnson and Maas, 1997).

Strengths of NOC

- Comprehensive
- Research based
- Developed inductively and deductively
- Grounded in clinical practice and research
- Uses clear, clinically useful language
- Outcomes can be shared by all disciplines
- Optimizes information for the evaluation of effectiveness
- Tested in clinical field sites
- Dissemination emphasized
- Linked to NANDA nursing diagnoses and NIC interventions (Johnson, Maas, and Moorhead, 2000)

NOC and NANDA Linkage

The 2000 edition of the NOC publication offers clear examples of linkage between NOC and the new nursing diagnoses in the 1999-2000 NANDA publication. NOC lists suggested outcomes and additional associated outcomes for several NANDA diagnoses, both physiologic and psychologic in nature. Linkages indicate that NOC is clearly influenced by NANDA, and continues to work with NANDA and other time-honored taxonomy classification systems, to help nurses achieve quality client outcomes in today's challenging and dynamic health care environment.

History of NOC Research Methodology

The research team conducted two pilot studies, published in the 1997 edition, to test content validity in measuring nursing-sensitive outcomes and indicators. Client satisfaction was included in the methodology. A literature review revealed client satisfaction with the following items:

- Safety
- Physical environment
- Availability of and access to care
- Providing client rights
- Caring
- Technical aspects of care
- Meeting physical needs
- Continuity of care
- Functional state
- Teaching/counseling
- Communication
- Symptom management
- Finances (Johnson and Maas, 1997)

SUMMARY

The development of the NIC and NOC classification systems was clearly influenced by NANDA, whose standardization of a taxonomic structure for the classification of nursing diagnoses began in 1973, was formalized in 1982, and continues to develop and evolve into the twenty-first century. All three classifications strive to develop and refine a standard language that assists nurses in making quality decisions for health care practices and policies while challenged by managed care and cost containment. NIC, NOC, and NANDA are comprehensive companions that significantly influence the teaching of diagnostic reasoning, critical thinking, and the continued development and refinement of nursing theory and knowledge. The 2000 editions of NIC and NOC were published before the newest edition of NANDA diagnoses, NANDA Nursing Diagnoses: Definitions & Classification 2003-2004 (2003), which are included in this text.

REFERENCES

Johnson M, Maas M, editors: *Nursing outcomes classification (NOC)*, St Louis, 1997, Mosby.

Johnson M, Maas M, Moorhead S, editors: *Nursing outcomes classification (NOC)*, ed 2, St Louis, 2000, Mosby.

McCloskey JC, Bulechek GM, editors: *Nursing interventions classification (NIC)*, ed 2, St Louis, 1996, Mosby.

McCloskey JC, Bulechek, GM, editors: *Nursing interventions classification (NIC)*, ed 3, St Louis, 2000, Mosby.

NANDA International (2003). NANDA Nursing Diagnoses: Definitions and Classification 2003-2004. Philadelphia: NANDA.

Appendix D
Answers to Review Questions

Chapter 1
1. a
2. c
3. b
4. b
5. d

Chapter 2
1. b
2. c
3. c
4. b
5. c

Chapter 3
1. c
2. d
3. b
4. b
5. a

Chapter 4
1. b
2. a
3. c
4. a
5. d

Chapter 5
1. b
2. a
3. c
4. a
5. c

Chapter 6
1. d
2. a
3. c
4. b
5. d

Chapter 7
1. b
2. c
3. b
4. d
5. a

Chapter 8
1. d
2. c
3. b
4. a
5. b

Chapter 9
1. c
2. d
3. c
4. a
5. b

Chapter 10
1. b
2. c
3. d
4. a
5. b

Chapter 11
1. c
2. a
3. d
4. c
5. b

Chapter 12
1. b
2. c
3. d
4. d
5. b

Chapter 13
1. c
2. d
3. c
4. a
5. d

Chapter 14
1. a
2. c
3. b
4. d
5. b

Chapter 15
1. b
2. c
3. b
4. d
5. a

Chapter 16
1. d
2. b
3. c
4. b
5. a

Chapter 17
1. c
2. b
3. a
4. c
5. d

Chapter 18
1. c
2. b
3. a
4. c
5. d

Chapter 19
1. a
2. c
3. b
4. c
5. d

Chapter 20
1. b
2. c
3. d
4. b
5. d

Chapter 21
1. b
2. a
3. d
4. b
5. c

Chapter 22
1. a
2. b
3. d
4. c
5. d

Chapter 23
1. b
2. c
3. a
4. d
5. c

Chapter 24
1. b
2. a
3. d
4. c
5. a

Chapter 25
1. d
2. d
3. c
4. c
5. b

Chapter 26
1. a
2. b
3. d
4. c
5. b

Chapter 27
1. b
2. d
3. c
4. a
5. d

Chapter 28
1. c
2. b
3. d
4. c
5. a

Glossary

Abstinence   Voluntary refraining from a behavior or the use of a substance that has caused problems in psychosocial, biologic, cognitive/perceptual, or spiritual/belief dimensions of life, especially with regard to food, alcohol, or drugs.

Abuse   A maladaptive pattern of substance use leading to problems in psychosocial, biologic, cognitive/perceptual, or spiritual/belief dimensions of life (Chapter 13).

Acculturation   Adapting or modifying cultural values and beliefs to accommodate living in a new culture (Chapters 5, 28).

Action potential   A wave of electrical depolarization that travels down a neuron to transfer information; when the impulse reaches the end of the neuron, it stimulates the production and release of chemical compounds called neurotransmitters (Chapter 3).

Acting-out   The expression of internal affective states through external activities and behaviors, which are often destructive and/or maladaptive.

Activities of daily living (ADLs)   The set of activities used in routine daily lives, such as personal hygiene, grooming, eating, and recreation (Chapter 27).

Activity theory   Theory states that maintaining an active lifestyle and social roles offsets the negative effects of aging (Chapter 8).

Activity therapy   Action-oriented process with the goal of increasing awareness of feelings, behaviors, perceptions, and cognition to maximize function and reduce pathology (Chapter 19).

Acquired immunodeficiency syndrome (AIDS)   The advanced stage of HIV disease. HIV causes AIDS. HIV becomes AIDS when an individual's T-cell count reads low (below 200/mm^3) or opportunistic infections appear that indicate the immune system is weakened (Chapter 26).

Acute grief   The initial response to loss. Although it diminishes over time, acute grief may last for as long as several years, primarily depending on the meaning of the lost person or object for the survivor (Chapter 25).

Adaptation   The adjustment of an individual to changing life conditions (Chapter 8).

Adaptive   The ability to adapt to change in internal or external circumstances or conditions (Chapter 1).

Adjunct therapy   An action-oriented process with the primary intention of fostering adaptation and productivity for the purpose of minimizing pathology and promoting the maintenance of health.

Adjustment disorder   Short-term disturbances in mood or behavior with nonpsychotic manifestations resulting from identifiable stressors. The severity of the reaction is not predictable by the severity of the stressor (Chapter 18).

Adult developmental theory   A theory that although persons may complete developmental tasks of childhood, they continue to evolve as maturity progresses. Adulthood is divided into four age categories, and central themes of adult experience and development are articulated (Chapter 18).

Adult family home   A living arrangement in which a family takes one or two boarders into their home to be a part of the family (Chapter 27).

Adult residential treatment program (ARTP)   A 24-hour care facility with staff on duty to provide care for 4 to 16 residents who require more structure than is required in halfway houses or group homes (Chapter 27).

Adverse drug reaction   An unintended effect of a medication resulting in severe, unwanted symptoms or consequences.

Affect   Outward, bodily expression of emotions, ranging through joy, sorrow, anger, etc. *Blunted affect:* Restricted expression of emotions. *Flat affect:* Lack of outward expression of emotions. *Inappropriate affect:* Affect that is not congruent with the emotion being felt (e.g., laughing when sad). *Labile affect:* Rapid changes in emotional expression (Chapters 10, 11).

Affective instability   Rapidly fluctuating moods in which the individual is emotionally reactive to external events and lacks coping skills to manage feeling states (Chapter 16).

Ageism   Systematic stereotyping and discrimination against the elderly (Chapter 8).

Agnosia   The loss of comprehension of auditory, visual, or other sensations, although the senses are intact (Chapters 11, 14).

Agonist   A chemical that results in stimulation of activity of the target receptor.

Agoraphobia   Fear of open spaces or public spaces, related to feelings of loss of control, which may be associated with panic (Chapter 9).

Agranulocytosis   A drop in the production of leukocytes, specifically the neutrophil cell line, leaving the body defenseless against bacterial infection (Chapter 20).

Agraphia   The loss of the ability to write (Chapter 14).

AIDS dementia   A progressive neurologic syndrome caused by a subacute chronic HIV encephalitis. Cognitive impairment indicative of damage to the central nervous system is evidenced in these clients (Chapter 26).

AIDS wasting syndrome (AWS)   During the later stages of AIDS, clients may experience significant weight loss. A condition of an unexplained weight loss of 10%, along with chronic diarrhea, fatigue, or unexplained fever, and a loss of muscle mass, may occur during the later stages of AIDS.

Akathisia   Literally, *not sitting*. A syndrome caused by dopamine-blocking drugs characterized by both motor restlessness and a subjective feeling of inner restlessness (Chapter 20).

Alcoholism   A chronic, progressive, and potentially fatal biogenic and psychosocial disease characterized by impaired control over drinking, tolerance, and physical dependence that leads to loss of control, distorted thinking, and other social consequences (Chapter 13).

Alexithymia   A condition in which individuals have difficulty recognizing and describing their emotions. The term literally means *no words for feelings*. Individuals with eating disorders often have a restricted emotional life (Chapter 16).

Allele   Small defects or variations in genes (Chapter 3).

Allopathic   The health beliefs and practices that are derived from the scientific models of the present time and involve the use of technology and other modalities of present-day health care, such as immunization, proper nutrition, and resuscitation.

Alpha₁ blockade   The process of inhibiting $alpha_1$-receptors that may result in orthostatic hypotension and reflex tachycardia.

Alter ego   A function of the therapist to reflect back the client's attitudes and feelings without including the client's negative connotations.

Alzheimer's disease   A neurodegenerative disease characterized by progressive, irreversible, and lethal structural damage to the brain due to the presence of beta-amyloid proteins and leading to loss of cognitive functions and symptoms of progressive dementia (Chapter 14).

Ambivalence   Simultaneously holding two different attitudes, emotions, thoughts, or feelings about a person, object, or situation (Chapter 11).

Amygdala   The part of the limbic system that modulates common emotional states such as feelings of anger and aggression, love, and comfort in social settings (Chapter 3).

Analysis   Taking apart collected data to examine and interpret each piece and identify variations from typical behaviors or responses; discovering patterns or relationships in the data that may be cues or clues that require further investigation; one cognitive process involved in diagnostic reasoning (Chapter 6).

Anhedonia   The loss of pleasure and interest in activities previously enjoyed or in life itself (Chapter 10).

Anorexia nervosa   An eating disorder classified in DSM-IV-TR, characterized by self-starvation, weight loss below minimum normal weight, intense fear of being fat even when emaciated, distorted body image, and amenorrhea in females (Chapter 16).

Antagonist   A chemical that causes inhibition of activity of the target receptor.

Anticholinergic delirium   Toxic effects of anticholinergic drugs characterized by confusion, perceptive disturbances, sleep disturbance, increased or decreased psychomotor activity, and change in level of consciousness. Also called atropine psychosis, this syndrome may present as a psychotic state (Chapter 20).

Anticipatory grief   Grief experienced before death or loss occurs (e.g., when a loved one has a terminal illness) (Chapter 25).

Antiretroviral therapy   The use of drugs, such as AZT, ddI, and ddC. These drugs, often administered to clients via drug trials, treat the major opportunistic diseases associated with AIDS. Treatment with antiretroviral therapy can significantly affect the progression of AIDS by preventing opportunistic infections.

Anxiety   A vague, nonspecific feeling of uneasiness, tension, apprehension, and sometimes dread or pending doom. Anxiety occurs as a result of a threat to one's biologic, physiologic, or social integrity arising from external influences. It is a universal experience and an integral part of human existence (Chapter 9).

Anxiolytic   Anxiety-reducing effects such as those resulting from antianxiety medications (Chapter 9).

Aphasia   *Expressive aphasia*: The inability to speak or write. *Receptive aphasia*: The inability to comprehend what is being said or written (Chapter 14).

Appraisal   As related to crisis, the ongoing perceptual process by which a potentially harmful event is distinguished from a potentially beneficial or irrelevant event.

Apraxia   The loss of the ability to carry out purposeful, complex movements and to use objects properly (Chapter 14).

Art medium   Materials or technical methods used for artistic expression (Chapter 19).

Art therapy   The use of the creative process for psychotherapeutic value and rehabilitation (Chapter 19).

Assent   To agree, concur, or yield (Chapter 15).

Assimilation   To become absorbed into another culture and to adopt its characteristics (Chapter 5).

Association cortex   The part of the cerebral frontal lobe that performs many of the activities that make us human, such as reasoning, planning, working memory, insight, inhibition, and judgment; the area of the brain most responsible for personality (Chapter 3).

Attending   Being attentive to a client's verbal and nonverbal behaviors by using words and behaviors that illustrate that the nurse is listening (Chapter 19).

Atypical antipsychotics   Antipsychotic medications that have an improved negative symptom response with minimal extrapyramidal symptoms, as they block serotonin more than dopamine. They are also known as *novel* antipsychotics, although terms used to describe these drugs are still evolving (Chapter 20).

Atypical depression   Depression with features that include hypersomnia, weight gain, mood reactivity, and sensitivity in interpersonal relationships (Chapter 10).

Autism   A pervasive developmental disorder characterized by marked impairment of social and cognitive abilities (Chapter 15).

Autistic thinking   Disturbances in thought due to the intrusion of a private fantasy world that is internally stimulated, resulting in abnormal responses to people and events in the real world (Chapter 11).

Autodiagnosis   Self-examination of one's own thoughts, feelings, perceptions, and attitudes about a particular client (Chapter 1).

Autonomy versus shame and doubt   Erikson's term for the second developmental crisis. Parental encouragement toward self-sufficiency in basic tasks of toileting, dressing, and feeding foster autonomy. Thwarted efforts by overcontrolling or undercontrolling parents result in the polar opposite, or shame and doubt. Shame is rage turned against the self. Doubt is an internal feeling of badness.

Axon   The part of the neuron that transmits signals from the neuron's cell body to connect with other neurons and cells (Chapter 3).

Basal ganglia   An area of the central nervous system made up of cell bodies and that is responsible for motor functions and association (Chapter 3).

Battering   Physical, sexual and/or mental abuse of women by intimate partners or those with whom they have been intimate (Chapter 23).

Battered women   Women who are abused physically, mentally, or emotionally by their male intimates or those with whom they have been intimate.

Behavior modification   Type of therapy that focuses on modifying observable behavior by manipulating the environment, the behavior, or the consequences of a behavior (Chapter 15).

Behavioral reorganization   A new way of viewing development, emphasizing that new developmental capabilities are fit together and organized into previous capabilities in an orderly, patterned, and predictable fashion and build in a cumulative manner from earlier capabilities in a direction of greater complexity.

Bereavement   The objective state following loss, especially of a loved one; the state of grieving (Chapter 25).

Binge eating disorder (BED)   A pattern of binge eating without the purging characteristic of bulimia nervosa. BED is commonly known as compulsive overeating. It is included in DSM-IV-TR as a proposed diagnosis for further study (Chapter 16).

Bioavailability   The amount, usually described as a percentage, of a drug administered that reaches the blood.

Bioterrorism   A threat of a disaster caused by biologic or chemical weaponry (Chapter 22).

Bipolar disorder   A mood disorder characterized by episodes of mania and depression (Chapter 10).

Blackout   Loss of memory of events that occur after the onset of the causative agent or condition such as the ingestion of alcohol or drugs (Chapter 13).

Body image disturbance   A perceptual disturbance in the way individual's body shape, size, weight, and proportions are subjectively perceived and experienced. Typically, persons with anorexia complain of feeling "fat" or see their stomach/hips/thighs as fat when they are clearly underweight (Chapter 16).

Body knowledge   An *embodied* knowledge that allows a person to recognize familiar and unfamiliar mental, emotional, and body mechanisms—a sense of balance/imbalance changes.

Boundary   Distinguishing and separating the self from others by clarifying the limits and extent of the nurse's responsibilities and duties in relationship to the client and others (Chapter 19).

Boundary violations   Going beyond the established therapeutic relationship standards (Chapter 7).

Breach of duty   Failure to perform by act of commission or omission within scope of practice and adhere to defined standard of care (Chapter 4).

Bulimarexia   An obsession with thinness, dieting, and a compulsive cycle of bingeing and purging. This syndrome is now labeled bulimia nervosa.

Bulimia nervosa   An eating disorder classified in DSM-IV-TR, characterized by recurrent episodes of binge eating subjectively experienced as out of control, followed by inappropriate compensatory behavior to prevent weight gain, such as self-induced vomiting; overuse of laxatives, diuretics, or diet pills; fasting; or excessive exercise. Also present is excessive preoccupation with body shape and weight (Chapter 16).

Capitation   A system of reimbursement whereby a set amount of money is designated for each client regardless of the amount of services provided for the client (Chapter 27).

Case finding   The methodic and deliberate identification of people of any age who are ill and in need of care or who are at risk for incurring illness and injury.

Case management   Clinical coordination of inpatient and outpatient treatments designed to support the client's highest level of functioning. Services include crisis intervention, supportive counseling, consultation/collaboration with multidisciplinary treatment providers, medication, and mental status monitoring (Chapter 27).

Catastrophic reaction   A sudden or gradual negative change in the behavior of clients with dementia caused by their inability to understand and cope with stimuli in the environment (Chapter 14).

CD4 count   The CD4 lymphocyte count (T4 cell count) is the most commonly used marker to determine HIV progression. HIV attacks CD4 cells that help fight infections (Chapter 26).

Central nervous system   A division of the human nervous system containing the brain and spinal cord (Chapter 3).

Cerebral cortex   The thin layer of gray matter that makes up the surface of the two cerebral hemispheres; the area where information related to sensation, speech, thinking, voluntary motor function, and perception is merged (Chapter 3).

Cerebrum   The largest structure in the central nervous system; can be subdivided into right and left hemispheres and contains four main lobes (Chapter 3).

Challenge   An actual or potential task or undertaking that by its very nature may be difficult yet stimulating (Chapter 2).

Chemical restraint   The use of psychotropic drugs and sedatives to reduce or eliminate psychiatric symptoms. Symptom management through medication as part of the client's standard treatment plan is another way to describe chemical restraint and is the currently accepted description (Chapter 28).

Childhood incest   Any type of exploitative sexual experience between relatives or surrogate relatives before the victim reaches the age of 18 years (Chapter 23).

Child neglect   Harm or threatened harm to a child's health or welfare by a parent, legal guardian, or any other person responsible for the child's health or welfare through failure to provide adequate food, clothing, shelter, or medical care, or by placing the child's health or welfare at unreasonable risk (Chapter 23).

Child physical abuse   Injury inflicted on a child that can range from minor bruises and lacerations to severe neurologic trauma and death. Psychologic abuse is also included (Chapter 23).

Child psychologic abuse   Rejection, degradation/devaluation, terrorization, isolation, corruption, exploitation, denying essential stimulation to a child, and unreliable and inconsistent parenting (Chapter 23).

Chronic mental illness   A psychiatric disorder that persists over time with remissions and recurrence of severe, disabling symptoms.

Chronic sorrow   Grief in response to an ongoing loss, such as a long chronic illness in a loved one (Chapter 25).

Chronically mentally ill   Persons who have manifested the symptoms of chronic mental illness.

Clear and convincing evidence   A burden of proof that requires more than that used in a civil proceeding and less than that used in a criminal proceeding. Civil proceedings call for merely a preponderance of evidence, whereas criminal proceedings require proof beyond a reasonable doubt (Chapter 4).

Clinical pathway   A standardized format used to provide and monitor client care and progress by way of the case management, interdisciplinary health care delivery system. (Also known as critical pathway, care path, or Care Map) (Chapter 6).

Closure   The last stage in psychodrama or movement/dance therapy in which the experience is analyzed to promote insight and a sense of finality. (Also known as *sharing*) (Chapter 19).

Codependence   A relationship in which the actions of a member of the family or close friend or colleague of an alcohol- or drug-dependent person tend to perpetuate the person's dependence and thereby retard the process of recovery. The term is also now used figuratively to describe the way in which the community or society acts as an enabler of alcohol or drug dependence, or other areas of dysfunction (e.g., family, gambling, spending) (Chapter 13).

Codependency   An emotional, psychologic, and behavioral pattern of coping that an individual develops as a result of prolonged exposure to a dysfunctional pattern of behavior within the family of origin. The individual experiences difficulty with identity development and setting functional boundaries, which lead to taking care of others rather than self.

Cognition   Awareness and subjective meaning of an event.

Cognitive rigidity   The inability to adequately identify problems and corresponding solutions (Chapter 24).

Cognitive symptoms   Difficulties in concentration, memory, and learning (Chapter 11).

Cognitive theory   Theory that explains how thought processes are structured, how they develop, and their influence on behaviors (Chapter 8).

Cognitive triad   A pattern of thinking noted in depressed people and characterized by (1) a negative self-assessment, (2) a negative view of the present, and (3) a negative view of the future.

Cohort   A group united by one or more common factors.

Collegiality   Working within a body of associates or colleagues (e.g., a team of home care providers).

Combination antiretroviral therapies   Complex regimens for treating HIV/AIDS. Replaced previous monotherapy approaches (Chapter 26).

Commitment   Court ordered evaluation certifying that an individual is to be confined to a mental health facility for treatment (Chapter 4).

Communication   A reciprocal process of sending and receiving messages between two or more people and their environment; the vehicle for establishing a therapeutic relationship (Chapter 7).

Community-linked health care   Care provided by public and/or private partnerships using grant and government funds.

Community mental health center   An outpatient facility that provides multiple mental health treatments and programs for people in a specified area (Chapter 27).

Comorbid   More than one psychiatric diagnosis occurring at the same time in the same individual (Chapter 12).

Comorbidity   The co-occurrence of two or more psychiatric or other disorders, which may be due to a causal relationship between the two, an underlying predisposition to both, or the disorders may be unrelated. Depression is a common comorbid disorder in clients with eating disorders. Different theories exist about the association between eating disorders and mood disorders (Chapters 16, 24).

Complementary/alternative medicine (CAM)   CAM covers a broad range of healing philosophies, approaches, and therapies. It generally is defined as those treatments and health care practices not taught widely in medical schools, not generally used in hospitals, and not usually reimbursed by medical insurance companies (National Center for Complementary and Alternative Medicine, NCCAM). Additional terms include holistic *therapies* and *integrative medicine* (Chapter 21).

Compensatory developmental task Developmental tasks that deal with replacing losses with some other mechanism (e.g., developing new skills or hobbies after retirement).

Competency to stand trial The ability of an individual to understand the charges and their consequences, to understand the nature and object of the legal proceedings, and to advise an attorney to assist in the defense (Chapter 4).

Compulsion An unremitting, repetitive impulse to perform a behavior, such as hand washing, checking, cleaning, or putting things in order; or mental acts, such as praying, counting, or repeating words silently. The goal of the behavior is to prevent or reduce anxiety or distress, not to provide pleasure or gratification. Compulsive acts often occur to reduce the distress that accompanies an obsession or to prevent some dreaded event or situation (Chapter 9).

Concentrated care Also called *intensive* care. Home care services delivered during a crisis, usually on a short-term basis, and designed to meet a specific, acute need.

Concrete operational period Piaget's term for the third stage of cognitive development whereby the child begins to think and reason in logical ways about the present and the past.

Confidentiality The right of the psychiatric client to keep information from people outside the health care team (Chapter 7).

Congregate care facility (*also* board-and-care homes) A group home specializing in housing mental health clients. Group homes have 24-hour staffing and management, but not necessarily nursing staff. Some homes offer more monitoring of clients than others (Chapter 27).

Congruence Consistency of agreement between verbal and nonverbal behavior (Chapter 7).

Conscious suicidal intention A state of awareness characterized by a desire to bring about one's own death (Chapter 24).

Continuity theory Theory that promotes the premise that people become "more like themselves" as they age, maintaining continuity of habits, beliefs, and values (Chapter 8).

Contraband Any objects that are prohibited by law, or the rules of a facility. On an acute care psychiatric unit this includes illegal drugs, dangerous objects such as knives, guns, or anything that may prove harmful to clients on that unit (Chapter 15).

Conventional antipsychotics Antipsychotic medications associated with dopamine blockade, resulting in extrapyramidal symptoms. They are also known as *traditional* antipsychotics, although terminology for antipsychotics is evolving (Chapter 20).

Conventional/traditional medicine (Also known as *Western medicine, mainstream medicine, orthodox medicine, allopathic medicine, biomedicine*) The primary medicine practiced in the United States. The major focus is on the biologic mechanisms of disease, ruling out potential causes, then forming a diagnosis and treatment of a specific disease (Chapter 21).

Conventional morality Kohlberg's second stage of morality whereby moral decisions consider the perspective of the victim and are first based on a desire for approval from others to avoid guilt, and later based on defined rights, assigned duty, rules of the community, and respect for authority.

Conversion reaction A repression of an emotional problem by replacing it with a physical symptom. Most often involves the sensory organs or voluntary nervous system.

Cope To adapt to a threat to integrity using a variety of tools, including adaptive (useful) and/or maladaptive (ineffective) maneuvers. One can cope internally via changes in thinking or psychologic defense mechanisms, or externally, via actions (Chapter 22).

Coping Various strategies used consciously or unconsciously to deal with stress and tensions arising from perceived threats to psychologic integrity. It is the process of attempting to solve life problems.

Coping abilities An individual's ability to respond to a challenge or threat; an expectation of a favorable outcome. May lead to adaptive or maladaptive outcome (Chapter 22).

Corpus callosum A large bundle of white matter that connects the right and left sides of the cerebral cortex (Chapter 3).

Countertransference The nurse's feelings and responses to a client that are associated with a significant person in the nurse's life. Although countertransference may be a natural part of therapy, the nurse needs to be aware of it and manage it to avoid behaving inappropriately toward the client (Chapters 7, 19).

Creativity The ability to apply original ideas to the solution of problems; the development of theories, techniques, or devices; or the production of novel forms of art, literature, philosophy, or science.

Crisis (1) An event that threatens well-being such as sudden death in the family or an earthquake; (2) a response to an event, where the person interprets the event as a threat to well-being, or to one's normal state of being. The interpretation of a threat leads to attempts to cope with the threat; (3) failed attempts to meet a threat, resulting in an assumption that the threat cannot be remedied; that is, the crisis begins when coping efforts fail (Chapter 22).

Crisis intervention Therapeutic techniques for helping individuals experiencing a crisis.

Crisis theory A theory that examines conscious coping abilities and unconscious defense mechanisms and how they help or inhibit interaction with the individual. Crises are separated into three categories: maturational, situational, and adventitious.

Critical thinking   An intellectual, disciplined process of actively and skillfully conceptualizing, applying, analyzing, synthesizing, and evaluating information through observation, experience, reasoning, and communication, as a guide to belief or action (Chapter 6).

Cross-tolerance   A tolerance to other drugs that develops after exposure to only one agent (e.g., tolerance to alcohol is accompanied by cross-tolerance to volatile anesthetics or barbiturates) (Chapter 13).

Cultural competence   Standard of practice that ensures the caregiver accepts and recognizes multiple aspects of cultural diversity among individuals and helps them receive information that they understand (Chapters 5, 28).

Culture   The collective process of acquiring shared beliefs, dominant patterns of behavior, values, and attitudes learned through socialization (Chapter 5).

Debriefing   Traumatic events may cause a variety of impressions and responses among individuals who all experience the same event. To debrief is to share, as a group, one's recollection of events in a nonjudgmental atmosphere. Debriefing may have several purposes: to learn from and avoid repeating the event, to share and thus support individual reactions to the event, and to avoid posttraumatic stress effects by facilitating open communication at an early stage after a trauma (Chapter 22).

Decanoate   Decanoic (10 carbon) acid ester, which is linked to the antipsychotics fluphenazine and haloperidol to create the long-acting antipsychotics. Dissolved in sesame oil and injected intramuscularly or subcutaneously, the decanoate is cleaved as the rate-limiting pharmacokinetic step to release the active drug.

Defense   A means or method of protecting oneself; an unconscious mental activity or mental structure (e.g., a defense mechanism) that protects the ego from anxiety.

Defense mechanisms   Also known as ego defenses. Automatic and semiautomatic mental processes to protect the ego (person) against anxiety resulting from feelings and impulses that threaten psychologic harm, conflict, or exposure, for example, denial and repression (Chapter 9).

Defensive functioning   Actions that may operate on an unconscious level (automatic mental mechanisms such as denial, repression, projection) or on a conscious level (learned techniques such as humor, altruism, sublimation). Defensive activity serves to protect the individual from anxiety (Chapter 1).

Deinstitutionalization   Discharge from the psychiatric institution or hospital into the community. Specifically refers to the discharge of severely mentally ill clients with long-term hospitalizations into less-structured care during the 1960s (Chapter 27).

Delayed grief   Grief that is not expressed or experienced until well after a loss, often as a result of circumstances such as being focused on survival (as among refugees) (Chapter 25).

Delirium   A disturbance of consciousness and a change in cognition that develop over a short period of time and tends to fluctuate during the course of the day, characterized by disorientation to time and place; reduced ability to focus, sustain, or shift attention; incoherent speech; and continual aimless physical activity (Chapter 14).

Delusions   False beliefs that are fixed and resistant to reasoning (Chapter 11).

Dementia   A global impairment of intellectual (cognitive) functions (e.g., thinking, remembering, reasoning) that usually is progressive and of sufficient severity to interfere with a person's normal social and occupational functioning (Chapter 14).

Dendrites   The part of the neuron designed to collect incoming signals from other neurons and send the signal to the neuron's cell body (Chapter 3).

Denial   Avoidance of reality that threatens an individual's self-concept. Denial is demonstrated by ignoring or deemphasizing the importance of an event, observation, or feeling. At times, denial helps one survive life stressors (Chapter 9).

Dependency ratio   The number of individuals below the age of 18 years and over the age of 64 years who are dependent on those persons ages 18 to 64 years.

Depersonalization   Feelings of unreality or alienation. Individuals experiencing depersonalization have difficulty distinguishing themselves from others. Depersonalization may occur in extreme anxiety (Chapter 9).

Depo-Lupron leuprolide   A synthetic analog of naturally occurring gonadotropin-releasing hormone. It inhibits gonadotropin secretion, thus suppressing testicular testosterone.

Depo-Lupron medroxyprogesterone acetate   A medication used in the adjunctive treatment of sexual disorders; a sexual appetite suppressant; lowers testosterone level to a prepubescent level.

Depo-Provera (medroxyprogesterone acetate)   A medication used in the adjunctive treatment of sexual disorders; a sexual appetite suppressant; lowers testosterone level to a prepubescent level (Chapter 17).

Depression   A dysphoric or depressed mood state. The relatively normal symptom of feeling somewhat depressed, or "sad" or "blue," must be distinguished from the diagnosis of major depression that is more severe, and in addition to depressed mood includes several other symptoms (changes in appetite, weight, sleep, activity, libido, energy; thoughts of death or suicide, and more) (Chapter 10).

Derealization   The feeling that the surrounding world is not real or is distorted.

Dereism   A loss of connection with reality and logic that occurs just before autistic thinking noted in schizophrenia. Thoughts become private and idiosyncratic (Chapter 11).

Designer drugs   Illegal drugs used at all-night parties, called raves or trances. Designer drugs include GHB, ketamine, ecstasy, and others (Chapter 13)

Detoxification   The removal of toxins or poisons from a person. Treatment that assists the individual in withdrawing from the physical effects of substances (Chapter 13).

Devaluation   A method of coping whereby a person deals with emotional conflict or stressors by attributing exaggerated negative qualities to self or others (Chapter 12).

Developmental contexts   The necessary circumstances that must exist for development to occur; some circumstances are related to nature (genes, inheritance), and others are related to nurture (environment).

Dichotomous thinking   A cognitive distortion common to people with eating disorders in which an individual views a situation as all or nothing, black or white, all good or all bad. If a situation is less than perfect, it is perceived as a failure (Chapter 16).

Disaffiliated   A person who does not associate with family, friends, or service providers (Chapter 28).

Disaster   An extreme external stressor, threatening the basic needs of a group people. A disaster may be natural or created by humans (Chapter 22).

Disease   A term used to describe altered body functions and a condition that places limitations on daily activities with the presence of recognizable disease symptoms. It is a result of the inability to adapt to certain stressors. Formerly it was believed that a specific disease had one particular cause. Today, it is known that the individual's physical and psychologic responses are affected by multiple stimuli and interactions with their environments (Chapter 21).

Disengagement theory   The process of mutual withdrawal between the aging individual and society (Chapter 8).

Disorientation   A loss of familiarity with place, time, and person (Chapter 14).

Dissociation   The separation of an overwhelming event from one's conscious awareness; a prominent defense mechanism in dissociative identity disorder (formerly known as multiple personality disorder) (Chapter 9).

Distress   A subjective response to internal or external stimuli that are threatening or perceived as threatening to the self.

Diurnal variation   Feeling worse or more depressed in the morning and better in the evening.

Domestic violence   Learned behaviors used by one or more persons in an intimate or family relationship for the purpose of controlling the behavior of others. Violence may take the form of physical, psychologic, sexual, or emotional abuse; intimidation; threats; isolation; economic control; or stalking.

Double   The individual in psychodrama who operates as the *inner voice* of the protagonist to express repressed thoughts, feelings, and conflicts.

Double-bind   A situation in which contradictory messages are given to one person by another, demanding a response or choice between two opposing alternatives (Chapter 11).

Dual diagnosis   A term used when the individual has two identified primary psychiatric diagnoses, most commonly used when one diagnosis is drug or alcohol related. For example, the person may have both a substance-related disorder and a mood disorder (Chapters 13, 28).

Duty to Warn   The legal obligation of a mental health professional to warn an intended victim of potential harm from a client with mental illness (Chapter 4).

Dynamic   Refers to an active and energetic state; the capacity or ability to change; as opposed to static, fixed, stationary (Chapter 2).

Dysarthria   Difficulty in articulating words; this is especially frustrating because the client knows what words to use but has trouble forming them (more commonly found in vascular dementias and strokes) (Chapter 14).

Dysfunctional grief (also termed pathologic, complicated, or traumatic grief)   Grief expressed to a significantly greater or lesser intensity over a significantly longer or shorter time than is culturally expected. It may manifest itself in serious physical and/or emotional disabilities (Chapter 25).

Dysphoria   Depressed, sad mood (Chapter 10).

Dysthymia   Chronic, low-level depression lasting more than 2 years that may lead to more severe depression if untreated (Chapter 10).

Dystonic   Pertaining to unstable states or to some disorder.

Eclectic approach   Selecting or choosing from various sources and not following any one system. In therapy, refers to use of several different modalities together, when treating clients (Chapter 1).

Ego   Freud's word for the self, whose major role is to find safe and appropriate ways for needs (instincts) to be met (gratified) in the external world. Lies mostly in the conscious.

Ego defenses   Automatic psychologic processes that keep out the threat of internal and external stressors and dangers or deny awareness to protect the self. (Also known as defense mechanisms or mental mechanisms.)

Ego dissonance   Inconsistency between attitudes and behaviors.

Ego dystonic pedophile   A person who is cognitively aware that his or her behavior is inappropriate and is truly affected by this, which may lead to seeking treatment (Chapter 17).

Ego state   A coherent set of feelings developed by the child's organization of similar life experiences and accompanied by a related set of coherent and observable behavior patterns. There are three ego states defined in transactional analysis: parent, adult, and child.

Ego syntonic pedophile   A person who is cognitively aware that his or her behavior is inappropriate, but is not troubled by this so will not seek treatment (Chapter 17).

Elder abuse   Includes psychologic or emotional neglect, psychologic or emotional abuse, violation of personal rights, financial abuse, physical neglect, and direct physical abuse to persons over 65 years old (Chapter 23).

Electroconvulsive therapy (ECT)   A type of biologic therapy performed with the client under general anesthesia, most often used to treat major depression, in which a brief electrical stimulus is applied to the brain, producing a seizure (Chapter 19).

Empathy   Projecting sensitivity and understanding of another's feelings and communicating the understanding in a way that the client comprehends (Chapter 7).

Enabler   One who supports someone to continue on a path of substance abuse by providing excuses for or helping the affected individual avoid the consequences of his or her behavior (Chapter 13).

Enactment   The action portion in psychodrama in which a scene or sequence of events is portrayed (Chapter 19).

Encopresis   The repeated passage of feces into inappropriate places (e.g., clothing or floor), whether involuntary or intentional (Chapter 15).

Endogenous agonist/antagonist   A substance that occurs naturally in a cell or tissue that stimulates or inhibits a receptor (e.g., dopamine, GABA).

Enmeshed   A pattern seen frequently in dysfunctional families, where members have diffuse rather than clear boundaries, lack clear role definitions, and are excessively involved in each others lives. This makes it difficult to individuate and separate, which is a necessity for healthy functioning (Chapters 13, 23).

Enmeshed families   A pattern of family relationships in which children are pressured to conform to parental expectations rather than express their individuality. Overinvolvement among family members, discouragement of outside relationships, and blurring of boundaries occur (e.g., a mother will "feel" her daughter's emotions) (Chapter 16).

Enuresis   The repeated voiding of urine into bed or clothing, whether involuntary or intentional (Chapter 15).

Equilibrium   A state of balance (Chapter 22).

EROS-CTD system   The only FDA-approved treatment for female sexual dysfunction. It is a small, battery-operated device that increases blood flow to the clitoris and external genitalia (Chapter 17).

Estradiol   Endocrine testing for the female determines the level of estradiol in the bloodstream. Estradiol levels may reflect the level of sexual desire.

Ethnicity   A specific cultural group's sense of identification associated with its common social and cultural heritage (Chapter 5).

Ethnocentrism   The tendency of members of one cultural group to view the members of other cultural groups in terms of the standards of behavior, attitudes, and values of their own group; belief in the superiority of one's own group (Chapter 5).

Ethnomethodology   The study of people in context, through inductive, qualitative methods.

Eustress   A nonspecific stress response associated with desirable events such as marriage, birth of a child, job promotion, etc., from the Greek word *eu* or *good*.

Euthymia   A mood that is normal and level (Chapter 10).

Evaluative responses   Responses that place a determined or conclusive value on a person, object, situation, or event, for example, "good" or "bad," "nice" or "mean," "pretty" or "ugly" (Chapter 2).

Evidence-based practice   Nursing practice that is proven effective by virtue of having undergone research versus being accepted merely on opinions, or because of a history of having been done a certain way for a long time (Chapter 1).

Expert witness   A person with education and experience on a specialized subject who is qualified as an expert and allowed to testify, thereby assisting the jury in understanding technical information (Chapter 4).

External vacuum pump   A cylindric vacuum pump applied to the penis. When operated, it brings blood into the penis and traps it there, thus improving erection.

Extrapyramidal motor system   A collection of nerve fibers responsible for much of the involuntary motor functioning of the central nervous system; can be adversely impacted by drugs used to treat psychiatric illness (Chapter 3).

Extrapyramidal side effects (EPS)   Movement-related side effects caused by the dopamine blockade of antipsychotic medications, most notably the older, traditional types. They are collectively known as extrapyramidal symptom(s) or EPS (Chapter 20).

Extrapyramidal symptoms (EPS)   The collective term used to describe the motor side effects of dopamine-blocking medications. EPS includes acute dystonia, akathisia, parkinsonism, and tardive dyskinesia.

Faith   Belief, confidence, or trust in anything, which is not necessarily based on proof, or substantiated by actual fact. May refer to a religion, or spiritual belief (Chapter 5).

Faulty information processing   Fixed and rigid patterns of thinking that block the contextual aspects of a situation and are characteristic of depressed people.

Feedback   The measure by which the effectiveness of the message is gauged (Chapter 7).

Feminist theory   Includes four major dimensions of wife abuse: (1) the explanatory utility of the constructs of gender and power, (2) the analysis of the family as a historically situated institution, (3) the crucial importance of understanding and validating women's experiences, and (4) the use of scholarship for women.

Fetal alcohol syndrome (FAS)   A set of congenital psychologic, behavioral, and physical abnormalities that occur in infants whose mothers consumed high amounts of alcohol during pregnancy (Chapter 13).

Figure-background formation   The concept that an organism's foremost need or specific interest will define the reality of the moment.

First-pass effect   Refers to the process of orally administered drugs, when absorbed, first passing through the liver, where substantial percentages of the administered dose may be metabolized before the drug is distributed to the tissues.

Fissures   Grooves on the surface of the brain that extend deep into the brain (Chapter 3).

Flight of ideas   The shifting from one idea to another without completing the previous idea, or an abrupt change of topics, expressed in a rapid flow of speech. Although most commonly seen in the manic phase of bipolar disorder, it may be noted in schizophrenia and is often confused with the looseness of associations (LOA) most often manifested in schizophrenia, in which thoughts are more fragmented (Chapters 10, 11).

Forensic psychiatry   A branch of psychiatry that studies individuals who commit crimes and enter the court system, some of whom are incarcerated.

Formal operations period   Piaget's term for the fourth stage of cognitive development whereby the child learns to think in abstract and hypothetical ways about future events and learns to develop strategies for solving complex problems.

Frontal lobe   The largest of the four lobes of the cerebrum; responsible for motor function, higher thought, memory, and judgment (Chapter 3).

Frustration   A state of being upset that results from ones ideas, plans, or actions being thwarted, negated, blocked, or discarded (Chapter 2).

Functional disabilities   Difficulties with normal, day-to-day activities, resulting from a mental or physical deficit (Chapter 22).

GAF score   Global Assessment of Functioning. The fifth axis (assessment category) in the DSM IV-TR that describes a person's overall functioning in society. A measure of pre-crisis and current level of functioning (Chapter 22).

Generativity   In Erikson's personality theory, the positive outcome of one of the stages of adult personality development; the ability to do creative work or to contribute to the raising of one's children. The opposite of stagnation.

Generic approach   A method that focuses on the characteristic course of the particular kind of crisis rather than on the psychodynamics of each individual in crisis.

Genuineness   A quality of an effective nurse that encompasses openness, honesty, and sincerity (Chapter 7).

Gerontology   The scientific study of the aging process involving multiple disciplines and settings.

Gray matter   Brain tissue composed of nerve cell bodies and dendrites (Chapter 3).

Grief   The dynamic natural response to loss. Grief affects physical, cognitive, behavioral, emotional, social, and spiritual aspects of the individual (Chapter 25).

Grief work   The intense psychologic effort to (1) fully express the feelings associated with grief, (2) understand the relationship with the deceased, and paradoxically, (3) carry on with essential activities of daily living (Chapter 25).

Gyri   Raised convolutions visible on the cerebral cortex surface (Chapter 3).

Half-life   The time required for the serum concentration of a drug to decrease by 50% (Chapter 13).

Hallucination   A subjective disorder of perception in which one of the five senses is involved in the absence of external stimuli (Chapter 11).

Hardiness   A sense of mastery or self-confidence needed to appropriately appraise and interpret health stressors.

Health   The absence of disease; a state of total well-being. The various definitions imply that health is dynamic, with the focus on a healthy lifestyle. Health has been referred to as a condition of adjustment, or adaptation, to physical, psychologic, social, and environmental changes. A person's *health status* refers to that status at a given point in time. For some individuals, health is defined in terms related to the ability to work (Chapter 21).

Heritage consistency   The observance of the beliefs and practices of one's traditional cultural belief system (Chapter 5).

Hippocampus   The area located in the inside fold of the temporal lobe below the thalamus; the site of the intersection between the storage of memories and their reproduction of emotional coloring (Chapter 3).

Holism   A term with various interpretations and meanings. In the broadest sense, holism refers to a belief system in which persons are unified, complex, interdependent systems with interrelated physical, mental, emotional, spiritual, and social dimensions (Chapter 18).

Holistic   Of or pertaining to holism, a philosophy that states that in nature individuals function as complete units that cannot be reduced to the sum of their parts. Holistic medicine refers to the comprehensive and total care of each client, in which all needs (physical, emotional, social, spiritual, economic) are considered and treated (Chapter 21).

Homeopathic   Health beliefs and practices derived from traditional cultural knowledge to maintain health, prevent changes in health status, and restore health.

Homeostasis   The way the body, using feedback mechanisms, maintains a stable internal environment, despite changes in the external environment (Chapter 22).

Human genome   All of the genes carried on human chromosomes (Chapter 3).

Human immunodeficiency virus (HIV)   HIV was first recognized as a virus infecting humans in 1981. HIV attacks the human immune system so that, over time, the body has less ability to ward off infectious diseases. HIV causes AIDS (Chapter 26).

Humanistic nursing   A view of nursing as an interactive process, developed by nursing theorists, Patterson and Zderad, that occurs between two persons—one needing help and the other willing to give help (Chapter 9).

Hypochondriasis   A long-standing dependency. A preoccupation with the "sick role." A fear or belief that one has a serious illness in spite of medical reassurances to the contrary.

Hypomania   The mood of elation with higher-than-usual activity and social interaction; not as expansive as full mania (Chapter 10).

Hypothalamus   The part of the limbic system that rests deep within the brain and helps regulate basic human functions such as sleep-rest patterns, body temperature, and physical drives of hunger and sex (Chapter 3).

Id   The basic level of the personality that lies in the unconscious and consists of primitive drives and instincts aimed at self-preservation.

Idealization   The tendency of a person with borderline personality disorder to idealize persons or groups beyond their capabilities when they are meeting that person's needs (Chapter 12).

Idea of influence   A delusional belief that one's thought processes are being influenced by an external source such as radar, space aliens, or another person (Chapter 28).

Ideas of reference   Incorrect interpretations of incidents and external events as having a particular or special meaning specific to the person.

Identified client   In family therapy, the member of the family (or group) whose behavior is seen as causing the problem for the family (or group).

Identity versus role confusion   Erikson's term for the fifth developmental crisis. Self-assurance of the previous stage leads to the adolescent's gaining a self-identity and the development of an ability to determine where the adolescent fits in society. Failure to develop a self-identity leads to role confusion, poor self-confidence, and alienation.

Illness   Sickness, disease, or ailment. Illness has been labeled as an unexpected stressful event in individuals' lives that can interrupt them from fulfilling their usual tasks or roles. Illness is often perceived to be a crisis event. The terms *illness* and *disease* are often used synonymously; however, the disease process may be present without the person feeling ill, such as a lump in the breast that has not yet been detected. *Chronic illness* is a health problem with symptoms or disabilities requiring long-term management that affect persons across the life span.

Imminence   The likelihood that an event will occur within a specific time period (Chapter 24).

Incidence   The frequency of occurrences of a specific disorder within a designated time period; number of new cases.

Independent activities of daily living (IADLs)   Activities an individual requires to function in the community (e.g., shopping, preparing meals, transportation).

Independent living skills   Activities required to maintain independent adult life (e.g., meal preparation, shopping, transportation, paying bills). Independent living skills are closely related to activities of daily living but require a higher level of skill and problem-solving ability (Chapter 27).

Indifference   Refers to the nurse's disconnected or aloof lack of concern. A separation from the client's needs or situation.

Individual approach   The individual approach differs from the generic approach in its emphasis on assessment, by a professional, of the interpersonal and intrapsychic processes of the person in crisis.

Industry versus inferiority   Erikson's term for the fourth developmental crisis. From the initiative achieved in the previous stage, the child develops an ability to master learning and develop peer relationships that lead to self-assurance or industry. Failure to master academic and social pursuits leads to inferiority and hinders attempts to try new things.

Inference   The interpretation of behavior, assumption of motive, and formation of a conclusion before having all the information (Chapter 2).

Initiative versus guilt   Erikson's term for the third developmental crisis. Self-sufficiency allows the child to undertake and plan tasks and join with others in cooperative efforts resulting in increased initiative. If the child's desire to show initiative causes excessive conflict in the family, guilt results.

Insight   The ability to perceive oneself realistically and understand oneself.

Institutionalization   Placing or confining persons with mental disorders in state-run facilities, such as residential treatment programs designed to treat such disorders (Chapter 28).

Interactive context of behaviors   Behavior is shaped and reinforced by interaction with one's social system while the social system is being shaped and reinforced by the same interaction.

Intermediate care   Short-term home care services designed to assist the client and family in achieving a planned, higher level of functioning.

Interoceptive deficits   The inability to correctly identify and respond to bodily sensations. Individuals with eating disorders are often out of touch with their bodies and either fail to recognize or mistrust physical sensations such as hunger, satiety, fatigue, or pain, as well as emotional states (Chapter 16).

Interpersonal communication   Communication between two or more persons containing both verbal and nonverbal messages (Chapter 7).

Interpersonal theory   A theory of human development framing interpersonal behaviors and relationships as the central factors influencing child and adolescent development across six "eras" (Chapter 8).

Intoxication   The physiologic state of being poisoned by a drug or other toxic substance (Chapter 13).

Intracorporal injections   Injections of various medications into the right and left corpus cavernosum to improve erection.

Intrapersonal communication Communication occurring within oneself that can be functional or dysfunctional (Chapter 7).

Intrapsychic Pertaining to the mind or mental process.

Intuition Insight into a situation without the benefit of critical analysis. (Also known as *intuitive reasoning*) (Chapter 6).

Isolation A feeling of aloneness with perceived social rejection or lack of support from others during a crisis.

Judgment An opinion or a conclusion that may affect or influence another person's life circumstances or situations (Chapter 1).

Key statement A key statement is one that is continually brought up by the client in conversation; one that the client stresses or emphasizes; or one that is *not said* or is deliberately omitted even though the topic is a known problem or conflict, given the client's history (Chapter 19).

Kindling The creation of electrophysiologic sensitivity in the brain from stress that results in alteration of neural functioning (Chapter 10).

Label A word or phrase that describes a person or group. Usually has a negative connotation for clients with psychiatric disorders and signifies a stereotype that is detrimental for the individual (Chapter 1).

Learned helplessness The perception that events are uncontrollable, leading to apathy, helplessness, powerlessness, and depression (Chapter 10).

Least restrictive A therapeutic intervention or treatment that is applied when all other less intrusive methods have been tried and were unsuccessful. Example: Initiating seclusion and restraint because talking to the client or reducing environmental stimulus did not prevent the client's behavior from escalating to a point of self-harm or harm to others (Chapter 27).

Least restrictive alternative Providing the least restrictive treatment in the least restrictive setting for a mental health client (Chapter 4).

Legal duty Something that an individual is required to do by law (Chapter 4).

Lethality The potential for causing death related to the level of danger associated with the suicidal plan along a continuum from low to high probability (e.g., a cut on both wrists versus a gunshot wound to the head) (Chapter 24).

Libido The energy of the instincts held in the id.

Life span The maximum length of survival genetically fixed for each species.

Life stages The framework for several theories of adult development that divide life span into a series of sequential transitions (Chapter 8).

Limbic system A group of structures found deep in the brain; responsible for modulation of instincts, drives, needs, and emotions (Chapter 3).

Locus of control An aspect of personality that deals with the degree of control one perceives over one's own destiny. *Internal locus of control* refers to the ability to actively control one's own destiny. *External locus of control* refers to the inability to control one's own destiny.

Loosening of associations (LOA) Thought disturbance in which the speaker rapidly shifts expression of ideas from one subject to another in an unrelated manner. Most commonly noted in schizophrenia (Chapter 11).

Loss A process characterized by a series of overlapping stages that include common psychologic and behavioral manifestations of recognition, adjustment, and resolution (Chapter 18).

Lovemap A term coined by John Money that refers to an idiosyncratic image in the mind-brain that depicts the idealized lover and lovemaking activities.

Lupron-Depot (leuprolide) A synthetic analog of naturally occurring gonadotropin-releasing hormone. It inhibits gonadotropin secretion, thus suppressing testicular testosterone (Chapter 17).

Machismo Compulsive masculinity characterized by a man's excessive need to control and dominate his wife at all costs.

Maintenance care Home care services provided when the client has reached a stable, higher level of functioning such as surveillance, client and family education, and emotional support. Concentrated and intermediate care is performed by skilled providers, and maintenance is performed by less skilled providers.

Maladaptive The opposite of adaptive. Signifies a response that may result in unfavorable circumstances, situations, or conditions for an individual who is unable or unwilling to adapt to meet standards that are accepted by the medical or social communities (Chapter 1).

Mandatory outpatient treatment An individual is legally required to undergo mental health treatment in an outpatient setting, generally due to noncompliance and/or alleged propensity for dangerous acts (Chapter 4).

Mania An elevated, expansive, or irritable mood accompanied by hyperactivity, grandiosity, and loss of reality (Chapter 10).

Medium Method by which a message is sent, which can be written, verbal, or tactile (Chapter 7).

Melancholic depression Severe depression characterized by anhedonia, feeling worse in the morning, weight loss, and psychomotor retardation (Chapter 10).

Message The information (feelings or ideas) being sent and received (Chapter 7).

Metabolism The biotransformation of a drug molecule into a new molecule.

Metabolite The result of biotransformation of a drug. Although most metabolites tend to be pharmacologically inactive and less toxic, there are important exceptions (e.g., fluoxetine is metabolized into the active metabolite norfluoxetine; ethanol is metabolized into the more toxic acetaldehyde) (Chapter 20).

Metamemory One's self-perceptions of memory changes.

Metaneeds   As the physiologic and safety needs are met, the need for belonging and love emerges.

Milieu therapy   Re-creates a community atmosphere on an inpatient hospital unit, a partial hospitalization unit, or a day treatment setting to facilitate interaction between client peers to identify and problem solve issues that occur while relating to others (Chapter 12).

Mirroring   A technique in psychodrama and movement/dance therapy in which one individual imitates the behavior patterns of another to show the person how other people perceive and react to him or her.

Mood   A feeling state reported by the client that can vary with external and internal changes (Chapter 10).

Moral development   Encompasses moral judgment or reasoning processes and involves making decisions about right or wrong actions in a particular situation (Chapter 8).

Motor cortex   The part of the frontal lobe responsible for controlling voluntary motor activity of specific muscles (Chapter 3).

Mourning   The social expression of grief (Chapter 25).

Movement   Kinesthetic behavior in which individuals communicate by the use of body motions rather than formal language.

Movement/dance therapy   The therapeutic use of movement (kinesics) as a process that expands the emotional, cognitive, and physical integration of the individual (Chapter 19).

Music   The science or art of assembling or performing intelligible combinations of tones in an organized, structured form.

Music therapy   The use of music as a therapeutic goal, such as restoring, maintaining, or improving mental and physical health (Chapter 19).

Negative symptoms   A syndrome that includes flat affect, poverty of speech, poor grooming, withdrawal, and disturbance in volition (Chapter 11).

Neologism   Invention of words to which meanings are attached (Chapter 14).

Neuritic plaques   Insoluble deposits of protein and cellular material outside the neuron (Chapter 14).

Neurofibrillary tangle   Insoluble twisted filaments that accumulate inside the neuron (Chapter 14).

Neuroleptic   Literally, *to clasp the neuron*; the term used to describe antipsychotic medications (Chapter 20).

Neuroleptic malignant syndrome (NMS)   A rare but potentially lethal toxic reaction to dopamine-blocking drugs that presents with a constellation of symptoms, including fever, automatic instability, increased muscular rigidity, and altered mental status (Chapter 20).

Neuron   A nerve cell, the elemental functioning unit in the brain; composed of a cell body, an axon, and connecting dendrite branches (Chapter 3).

Neuropsychiatric   The combination of two words (*neurology* and *psychiatry*) represents two separate areas of study and practice that have merged into one. Neuro-

psychiatry has burgeoned since the "decade of the brain" —the 1990s and represents new biologically based methods for diagnosing, treating, and researching psychiatric disorders that have proven successful in bringing science closer to answers about etiology and treatment (Chapter 1).

Neurotransmission   The process by which electrochemical signals are sent throughout the brain (Chapter 10).

Neurotransmitter   A chemical substance released by presynaptic cells when stimulated that functions to activate postsynaptic cells and thus cause them to act as messengers in the central nervous system. Common neurotransmitters are acetylcholine, dopamine, norepinephrine, serotonin, and gamma-aminobutyric acid (GABA) (Chapter 3).

Neuroplasticity   The dynamic nature of neuronal tissue that allows for alteration in both the structure and function of the brain (Chapter 3).

Neutrality   The manner in which the nurse interacts with the client that shows respect and acceptance regardless of the client's appearance or behavior (Chapter 2).

Nihilism   Belief that existence is senseless and useless (Chapter 10).

Nocturnal penile tumescence   A test that uses a strain gauge around the penis to depict the pattern of arousal while the client sleeps (Chapter 17).

Nonadrenergic   A neuronal system or neuron that manufactures and/or responds to norepinephrine.

Nonverbal communication   Nonverbal behaviors displayed by individuals during the process of an interaction (Chapter 7).

Norms   The standards of behavior, attitudes, and perceptions that a group has for its members. Norms represent the shared expectations of appropriate behavior (Chapter 19).

Nuclear family   A family made up of the parental dyad and the individual's siblings.

Nursing   Nursing has many definitions. The American Nurses Association (ANA) Social Policy Statement (1995) defines nursing as the diagnosis and treatment of human responses to actual and potential health problems. The statement emphasizes the nurse's role in addressing a wide range of human experiences and responses to health and disease and the provision of a caring relationship that promotes healing and health maintenance. It is the application of nursing science and theory and the integration of the art of nursing that create environments that facilitate healing. The goal of holistic nursing is nursing practice that enhances healing the whole person from birth to death (Chapter 21).

Nursing Interventions Classification (NIC)   The first comprehensive standardized classification of treatments performed by nurses; developed in 1987 by members of the Iowa Intervention Project research team (Chapter 6).

Nursing Outcomes Classification (NOC)   The first comprehensive standardized classification used to describe patient outcomes that are influenced by nursing; developed in 1991 by the Iowa Outcomes Project. Outcomes include indicators such as patient states, behaviors, and self-reported perceptions (Chapter 6).

Object constancy The ability to maintain a relationship regardless of frustration and changes in the relationship (Chapter 12).

Object relations The stability and depth of an individual's relations with significant others as manifested by warmth, dedication, concern, and tactfulness (Chapter 12).

Objectivity The state of remaining free from bias, prejudice, and personal identification in an interaction with another person (Chapter 1).

Obsessions Persistent ideas, thoughts, impulses, or images about death, sexual matters, religion, or any themes that lead to the person's efforts to resist them. They result in marked anxiety or distress (Chapter 9).

Occipital lobe A division of the cerebrum that is responsible for visual functioning (Chapter 3).

Occupation The goal-directed use of time, energy, interest, and attention to foster adaptation and productivity, to minimize pathology, and to promote the maintenance of health.

Occupational therapy The application of goal-directed, purposeful activity in assessing and treating individuals with mental, physical, or developmental disabilities (Chapter 19).

Old, old (the) Persons over 85 years old (Chapter 18).

Opportunistic diseases Diseases that typically appear in clients with AIDS, especially when their T-cell count declines are called opportunistic diseases. They include such diseases as toxoplasmic encephalitis, cryptococcosis, cytomegalovirus (CMV), *Pneumocystis carinii* pneumonia (PCP), and less frequently observed cancers (e.g., Kaposi's sarcoma). Highly active antiretroviral therapies have been shown to reduce the incidence of HIV-related opportunistic diseases as well as extend life (Chapter 26).

Organismic self-regulation The concept that once the need is satisfied, it will recede and allow the emergence of the next need.

Overselect A behavior commonly noted in children with psychiatric disorders. The child tends to be so specific about the stimuli that he or she selects to respond so that it appears as if there is no response at all.

Oxytocin Possible prosexual peptide with known influence on milk expulsion, contractions during labor, and orgasm. May have positive sexual effects (Chapter 17).

Pain A subjective feeling of discomfort as indicated by the client, generally on a scale of 1 to 10 (1-3 = mild) (4-6 = moderate) (7-10 = severe). Pain is considered a fifth vital sign by the accrediting bodies of The Joint Committee on Accreditation of Healthcare Organizations (JCAHO) and The Board of Registered Nursing (BRN).

Panic A circumscribed period of extreme anxiety. During panic one's perceptions are distorted and the ability to inte-grate and separate environmental stimuli is impaired (Chapter 9).

Panic attacks Discrete periods of panic that are characterized by several cognitive and physiologic symptoms (Chapter 9).

Paradigm A side-by-side example to show a clear pattern.

Paranoia A mental disorder characterized by persecutory thoughts or delusions (Chapter 14).

Paraphilias Sexual deviations/disorders presenting with inappropriate sexual fantasies involving deviant sexual acts, inappropriate sexual urges, and acting-out of these fantasies and urges (Chapter 17).

Parasitic One's total dependence on someone else for one's every need (Chapter 28).

Parasuicidal behavior Suicidal gestures and attempts that are unsuccessful and of low lethality (e.g., superficial cutting of the wrists) (Chapter 24).

Parietal lobe A division of the cerebrum that functions as a processing center (Chapter 3).

Penile-brachial index (PBI) A test that determines the difference between the penile and brachial blood pressure that assesses vascularization to the penis (Chapter 17).

Penile plethysmograph A diagnostic test that determines a person's arousal pattern and level of arousal. This test may reveal the source of the client's arousal and the degree of its significance.

Performance inadequacy The fear of beginning nurses that they will not know what to say to help clients resolve their problems.

Peripheral nervous system A division of the nervous system that includes all nerves not in the brain or spinal cord and includes the cranial nerves (Chapter 3).

Perseveration A disturbance in thought association that is manifested by repetitive verbalizations or motions, or persistent repetition of the same idea in response to different questions. Perseveration is commonly seen in clients with schizophrenia or dementia (Chapters 11, 14).

Personality traits Behaviors and enduring patterns of perceiving, relating to, and thinking about the environment and oneself that are exhibited in a wide range of social and personal contexts (Chapter 12).

Persons with severe and persistent mental illness Persons who manifest the symptoms of severe and persistent mental illness (Chapter 28).

Perturbation A determination of an individual's level of distress, developed by Shneidman and rated on a scale of 1 to 9. Refers to how upset, disturbed, or perturbed the individual is (Chapter 24).

Pervasive developmental disorders A collection of disorders in which the child experiences deficits in a broad range of developmental areas (Chapter 15).

Pheromones Airborne odorous chemicals (that are often unconscious) that may influence bonding and sexual attraction (Chapter 17).

Phobias   A group of disorders primarily characterized by avoidance of a specific situation or escape, if that situation is unexpectedly encountered (Chapter 9).

Physical dependence   A physiologic state of adaptation to a drug or alcohol, usually characterized by the development of tolerance to drug effects (Chapter 13).

Pleasure principle   The goal of experiencing pleasure while avoiding pain. This principle represents the id's goal in the personality to satisfy a person's innate needs and instincts.

Plethysmography   A diagnostic test for males and females that may help determine arousal patterns and level of arousal and assesses blood flow to the genitals (Chapter 17).

Positive affirmation   A self-supporting message that reinforces confidence and enhances performance.

Positive cognitive set   The belief that success is possible and that one can achieve what one believes.

Positive regard   Acceptance of and respect for a client (Chapter 7).

Positive symptoms   A syndrome that includes hallucinations, increased speech production with loose associations, and bizarre behavior (Chapter 11).

Postconventional morality   Kohlberg's third stage of morality in which moral decisions reflect underlying ethical principles that consider societal needs and are first based on a sense of community respect and disrespect and later based on principles of justice, the reciprocity and quality of human rights, and respect for the dignity of human beings as individuals.

Postvention   Grief therapy after a death occurs but before a pathologic condition develops (Chapter 25).

Poverty of thought   A psychopathologic thought disturbance in schizophrenia. The client's inability to think logically and sequentially is reflected in *poverty of content speech,* which is vague, repetitive, and disconnected (Chapter 11).

Preconventional morality   Kohlberg's first stage of morality whereby moral decisions are self-centered and the child's behavior is first based on avoidance of punishment and later based on a desire to gain rewards or benefits.

Premorbid   The period just preceding the onset of a mental illness. Characteristics of the personality may indicate the type of disorder that may occur (Chapter 11).

Premotor area   The part of the frontal lobe responsible for coordinated voluntary movement of multiple muscles (Chapter 3).

Preoperational period   Piaget's term for the second stage of cognitive development whereby the child remains egocentric, is oriented in the present, and only guesses about cause and effect.

Pressured speech   Rapid speech with an urgent quality.

Prevalence   The number of cases of a specific disorder in a normal population at a given point in time; the number of existing cases.

Primary prevention   Prevention efforts that focus on reduction of the incidence of mental disorders within the community. It is directed toward occurrence of mental health problems with emphasis on health promotion and prevention of disorders.

Primary process thinking   Prelogical thought that aims for wish fulfillment. It is associated with the pleasure principle characteristic of the id portion of the personality (Chapter 11).

Privileged communication   Communication between a professional and a client that is confidential and protected from forced disclosure in court unless authorized by the client. The privilege is delegated by statutes in the various states (Chapter 4).

Problem solving   The process involved in discovering the correct sequence of alternatives leading to a goal or to an ideational solution.

Prodromal symptoms   Early symptoms, such as a deterioration in functioning, that may mark the onset of a mental illness (Chapter 11).

Projection   The process whereby a person deals with his or her emotional conflicts or stressors, both internal and external, by unconsciously and falsely attributing to another person his or her own unacceptable feelings, impulses, or thoughts.

Projective identification   Projecting one's emotional conflicts and stressors to another who does not fully disavow what is projected. The individual remains aware of his or her own affects or impulses but misattributes them as justifiable reactions to the other person (Chapter 12).

Protagonist   The individual, in psychodrama, who presents and acts out his or her emotional problems and interpersonal relationships.

Protective factors   Factors that help an individual guard against risks. May be internal (capacity to tolerate stress) or external (a caring responsive teacher) (see Risk Factors, Chapter 1).

Protein binding   The holding of a drug in the blood by circulating protein molecules. The percentage of a drug that is protein bound varies widely. The percentage of a drug that is protein bound is not pharmacologically active until released.

Psyche   The mind as the center of thought processes, emotions, and behavior.

Psychiatric emergency   A psychiatric crisis that threatens the personal health or safety of the client or others and requires intervention (Chapter 22).

Psychiatric rehabilitation/skills training program   Outpatient program designed to address cognitive, social, and functional deficits caused by mental illnesses (Chapter 27).

Psychodrama   Guided, dramatic action used to examine problems or issues identified by an individual, for the purpose of enhancing physical or emotional well-being, increasing learning, and developing new skills (Chapter 19).

Psychoeducation   A type of therapy that educates the client with a paraphilic disorder to identify situations/objects that may trigger inappropriate sexual activity and develop awareness of relapse prevention strategies and the importance of treatment compliance (Chapter 17).

Psychologic morbidity   The prevalence of psychologic impairment in a specific population. With respect to AIDS, psychologic morbidity refers to the prevalence of emotional distress and syndromic conditions in persons with AIDS (PWAs).

Psychologic dependence   The compulsive use of substances, leading to a state of craving a drug or alcohol for its positive effect or to avoid negative effects associated with its absence (Chapter 13).

Psychomotor agitation   Agitated motor activity (Chapter 10).

Psychomotor retardation   The slowing of physiologic processes, resulting in slow movement, speech, and reaction time (Chapter 10).

Psychosexual theory   Theory that views the child's development as a biologically driven series of conflicts and meeting gratification needs that proceeds through a series of stages (Chapter 8).

Psychosis   Inability to recognize reality, bizarre behaviors, or inability to deal with life's demands (Chapter 11).

Psychosocial theory   Erikson's eight stages in a person's social development. Each stage is marked by a particular type of crisis resulting from the ego's attempt to meet the demands of social reality (Chapter 8).

Psychosomatic illness   Pertaining to a physical disorder that is notably influenced or caused by emotional or mental factors involving the mind and the body.

Psychotropic   Literally, *mind nutrition*. The term used to describe drugs that affect the central nervous system (Chapter 20).

Purging   The use of self-induced vomiting and/or the abuse of laxatives, diuretics, syrup of ipecac, diet pills, or enemas to avoid weight gain following a binge. One or more of these behaviors, as well as periods of fasting and excessive exercise during an episode of bulimia nervosa, may be used (Chapter 16).

Rape   The act of physically forcing sexual intercourse (Chapter 23).

Rave   Raves and trance events are generally nightlong dances, often held in warehouses. Club drugs, sometimes referred to as designer drugs, are often used by teens and young adults who participate in nightclub, bar, rave, or trance scenes (Chapter 13).

Reality principle   The goal of postponing immediate gratification until a suitable object for this satisfaction is found. The ego is ruled by this principle.

Receiver   The individual who both receives and interprets the message (Chapter 7).

Receptors   Protein molecules located in the cell walls of tissues that receive chemical stimulation resulting in stimulation or inhibition of activity of the target cell.

Sexual recidivism   Chronic, repetitive acting out of sexual behaviors considered to be unacceptable that have or have not resulted in criminal conviction (Chapter 17).

Recreation   To create again by some form of play, amusement, or relaxation.

Recreational therapy   (also known as *therapeutic recreation*) A type of therapy that uses play to restore, remediate, or rehabilitate to improve functioning and independence, and reduce or eliminate effects of illness or disability (Chapter 19).

Refractory   A term used when an individual is not responsive to medication or other types of treatment, generally requiring new or different therapeutic measures (Chapter 20).

Reframing   A technique of changing the viewpoint of a situation and replacing it with another viewpoint that fits the facts equally well but changes the entire meaning.

Regressive developmental task   Developmental tasks that focus on adjustments to physical, psychologic, and functional changes resulting from aging.

Relapse   The resumption of a pattern of substance use or dependency after a period of sobriety or abstinence (Chapter 13).

Relapse prevention   A means of helping the chemically dependent individual maintain behavioral changes over a prolonged period of time (Chapter 13).

Religion   An organized system of beliefs about the cause, nature, and purpose of life, often expressed through the belief in or worship of divine beings (Chapter 5).

Repression   The involuntary exclusion of a painful, threatening experience. Begins in infancy and continues throughout life. Underlies all other defense mechanisms but also operates as its own defense mechanism (Chapter 9).

Residual symptoms   Minor disturbances that may remain after an episode of schizophrenia but do not include delusions, hallucinations, incoherence, or gross disorganization (Chapter 11).

Resistance   The inability, whether conscious or unconscious, to accept change; the denial of new problems (Chapter 7).

Restrictive admission policies   A component of the deinstitutionalization process that limits the length of stay until symptoms are under control (Chapter 28).

Restrictive commitment policies   A component of the deinstitutionalization process that limits commitment to a psychiatric facility to cases where there is a threat to harm self and/or others (Chapter 28).

Restrictive environment   An environment that restricts activity of a client to help the client regain control of his or her behavior. The individual may be placed in open-door or closed-door seclusion during periods of extreme agitation, suicidal ideations, or threats of violence to self or others (Chapter 28).

Rewards   Something received (or given) in return for service, merit, or intervention (Chapter 2).

Risk factors   Certain identified internal characteristics or external influences that are present before a disorder occurs. An individual is more vulnerable to develop a disorder when these factors are present (Chapter 1). (See *protective factors*.)

Rites of passage   Rituals such as puberty, marriage, birth, and death that facilitate maturational development; associated with life transition. These rites commonly consist of three stages: separation, transition, and incorporation (Chapter 8).

Roles   Expected social behavior patterns generally determined by an individual's status in a particular group. Peplau identified four roles for the psychiatric mental health nurse: (1) resource person, (2) counselor, (3) surrogate, and (4) technical expert (Chapter 19).

Safeguards   Relapse prevention strategies used to assist the individual in developing control over inappropriate sexual acting-out (reoffending) behaviors.

Safety   The sense of security developed within the therapeutic relationship when the responsibilities and expectations of each party are clearly defined. Safety develops from knowing the boundaries of a relationship and acting within them (Chapter 19).

Schemata   The cognitive set of the self and world through which situations are perceived, coded, and interpreted (Chapter 10).

Schizoaffective disorder   A disorder closely associated with schizophrenia, with a typical age of onset in early adulthood, although it can occur any time from adolescence to late adulthood. Essential to the diagnosis is an uninterrupted period of illness during which there is an episode of either major depression, mania, or a mixed episode; delusions or hallucinations for at least 2 weeks in the absence of prominent mood symptoms; and mood symptoms throughout most of the illness (Chapter 11).

Seasonal affective disorder (SAD)   A type of mood disorder that occurs at a regular time each year (Chapter 10).

Secondary gain   Any benefit, such as personal attention, sympathy from others, or escape from unwanted responsibilities, as a result of illness. Individuals with eating disorders may experience secondary gain when family or friends pay a great deal of attention to their eating behavior (e.g., preparing special meals or making special arrangements in an attempt to encourage them to eat) (Chapter 16).

Secondary prevention   Prevention efforts directed toward reducing the prevalence of mental disorders through early identification and treatment of problems. This stage occurs after the problem arises and aims at shortening the course or duration of the episode.

Selective attention   The ability to discriminate and focus on relevant information.

Selective gene expression   Activation of a specific gene through alterations in brain chemistry and messenger RNA (Chapter 10).

Self-actualization   A concept developed by Maslow as an ongoing actualization of potentials, capacities, and talents as fulfillment of a mission, and as a greater knowledge and acceptance of one's own intrinsic nature (Chapter 8).

Self-system   Sullivan's term for the system that infants develop to cope with anxiety associated with the interpersonal process of need satisfaction and security. The individual develops self-appraisal as a result of significant others' responses to actions of the individual. Actions that cause anxiety result in "bad-me" self-appraisals. Actions that cause no anxiety result in "good-me" self-appraisals. Actions of disapproval cause severe anxiety, emotional withdrawal, and "not-me" self-appraisals.

Sender   The individual who initiates the transmission of information (Chapter 7).

Sensate focus   A learned exercise developed by Masters and Johnson that involves concentrating on the sensations produced by touching (Chapter 17).

Sensorimotor period   Piaget's term for the first stage of cognitive development in which children use their senses and motor skills to manipulate the environment and develop the ability to differentiate self from objects.

Serostatus   The presence or absence of HIV antibodies in the bloodstream. HIV status is determined through laboratory tests and is either seropositive or seronegative.

Seroconversion   The term used to signify that HIV antibodies are discernible in the individual's laboratory blood tests. A person who was previously exposed to the HIV virus and showed no presence of the virus but subsequently tests positive for the virus has experienced seroconversion.

Serum level monitoring   The process of obtaining blood samples to determine drug concentration (Chapter 20).

Severe and persistent mental illness   A psychiatric disorder that persists over time with remissions and recurrence of severe and disabling symptoms (Chapter 28).

Severe and persistent   This term is currently widely accepted and replaces the term *chronic* when referring to unremitting or frequently recurring symptoms of certain psychiatric disorders (schizophrenia) that continue to distress an individual and interfere with function throughout life (Chapter 1).

Sick role   A set of social expectations that an ill person meets, such as (1) being exempt from usual social role responsibilities, (2) not being morally responsible for being ill, (3) being obligated to "want to get well," and (4) being obligated to seek competent help.

Side effect   An undesired nontherapeutic and often predictable consequence of medication. Frequently diminished with time. Contrast with adverse drug reaction (Chapter 20).

Sleep reversal   A state in which normal sleeping patterns are reversed; the individual sleeps during the day and is active during the night (Chapter 28).

Sobriety   The state of complete abstinence from alcohol and/or other drugs of abuse (Chapter 13).

Social learning   The process by which children acquire the behaviors they need to survive and function in society. The behaviors result from repeated interactions in their environments (Chapter 8).

Social learning theory   Bandura's theory that aggression is not instinctual but a learned behavior (Chapter 23).

Social support   The presence of other individuals who are able to give understanding, encouragement, and other assistance in life, especially during difficult times (Chapter 25).

Socialization   The process of being raised within a culture and acquiring the characteristics of the given group (Chapter 5).

Solutions   The answer(s) to a problem (Chapter 2).

Somatic complaints   Expressions of grief, depression, resentment, or other internal feelings that are manifested instead as bodily pain and discomfort. Often children, adolescents, and adults describe biologic symptoms for what are actually psychiatric disorders or dysfunctional responses to life crises (Chapter 15).

Somatization   The conversion of mental states or experiences into bodily symptoms associated with anxiety.

Spirituality   The effort to find purpose and meaning in life through a search for the sacred (Chapter 5).

Splitting   Keeping the positive and negative aspects of self or others separate from each other. An individual who uses the unconscious defense mechanism of splitting cannot tolerate ambiguity; therefore people, events, or ideas are either good or bad, right or wrong, black or white, but not gray (Chapter 12).

Spontane   A dopaminergic agonist, Apomorphine, that is in the final stages of FDA approval as a remedy for erectile dysfunction. This is a sublingual tablet that exerts its action through central pathways (Chapter 17).

State disorders   The diagnoses made on Axis I. These diagnoses constitute behavior patterns that are not as pervasive or long-lasting as trait disorders (Chapter 12).

Static   Fixed, stationary, unchanging. Opposite of dynamic (Chapter 2).

Stereotypes   To form an oversimplified, standardized opinion of a person or group of people that is often determined without adequate information (Chapter 1).

Stigma   Social reproach. Attitudinal devaluation and demeaning by society of an individual or group of people with disabilities or disorders who are judged, labeled, alienated, and thought incapable of fulfilling valued social roles or contributing to society (Chapter 1).

Stress   (1) A term that refers to both a stimulus and a response. It can denote a nonspecific response of the body to any demand placed on it, whether the causal event is negative (a painful experience) or positive (a happy occasion). (2) A state produced by a change in the environment that is perceived as challenging, threatening, or damaging to the person's dynamic equilibrium. (3) The wear and tear on the body over time. (4) Psychologic stress has been defined as all processes, whether originating in the external environment or within the person, that demand a mental appraisal of the event before the involvement or activation of any other system (Chapters 9, 21).

Subjectivity   Emphasizing one's own moods, attitudes, and opinions in an interaction with another person (Chapter 1).

Suicide   The act of taking one's own life (Chapter 24).

Suicide ideation   Thoughts of suicide including *one or more* plans and thoughts about how it would be to end one's life (Chapter 24).

Suicide ideators   Those persons who experience suicidal thinking on a consistent basis.

Suicidology   The scientific and humane study of human self-destruction (Chapter 24).

Sulci   Shallow grooves in the surface of the cerebrum running between gyri (Chapter 3).

Sundowner's syndrome   The confusion and irritation common in dementia clients at the end of the day, probably resulting from general tiredness and an inability to process any more information after a long day of struggling to interpret their environment correctly.

Sundowning   A behavioral disorder associated with an increase in confusion and agitation that occurs in the evening hours (Chapter 14).

Superego   The portion of the mind, differentiated from the ego, that contains the traditional values and taboos of society as interpreted by the child's parents and that becomes part of the self. Lies in the preconscious.

Sustained release   Medications designed to provide slow, controlled dissolution, which allows longer dosing intervals (Chapter 20).

Synthesis   Combining several parts of relevant data into a single piece of information; comparing behavioral patterns with learned theories or typical patterns of behavior to identify strengths and seek explanations for symptoms; one cognitive process involved in diagnostic reasoning (Chapter 6).

Syntonic   Pertaining to a state of stability.

Tardive dyskinesia (TD)   A syndrome of abnormal, involuntary movements occurring after months or years of treatment with neuroleptic drugs that block dopamine type 2 receptors. These movements are often described as oral, buccal, lingual, or masticatory, but can occur throughout the body (Chapter 20).

Tasks in grief   Tasks or activities common in the psychosocial experience of grieving. Accomplishing these tasks helps resolve grief (Chapter 25).

Taxonomy   A classification of known phenomena under a hierarchical structure (Chapter 6).

Temperament   Objective differences in the intensity and duration of arousal and emotionality generally thought to be a product of biologic constitution (Chapter 10).

Temporal lobe   One of the four lobes of the cerebrum responsible for hearing and receiving auditory information (Chapter 3).

Teratogen   Substances that causes developmental malformations in the fetus (Chapter 13).

Tertiary prevention   Prevention efforts that have the dual focus of reduction of residual effects of the disorder and rehabilitation of the individual who experienced the mental disorder.

Testosterone   A sex steroid responsible for sexual drive useful in the treatment of some male and female sexual dysfunctions (Chapter 17).

Thalamus   Part of the limbic system and primarily a regulatory structure that relays all sensory information, except smell, from the peripheral nervous system to the cortex of the central nervous system (Chapter 3).

Theme development　The part of movement/dance therapy in which a specific issue or feeling is actively being explored.

Themes　Repeated patterns of interactions the client experiences in relationships with self and/or others (Chapter 19).

Therapeutic alliance　A goal-oriented, purposeful relationship between a professional member of a treatment team and a client, in which each agrees to work together to help the client resolve problematic areas in the client's life. In nursing this is the *nurse-client relationship* (Chapter 1).

Therapeutic communication　Verbal and nonverbal communication that takes place between the nurse and client. The content signifies "what" is being discussed. The content has meaning and focuses primarily on the client's concerns. The process refers to all aspects of meta-communication, or "how" the client and nurse communicate and the intent of each message (Chapter 7).

Therapeutic milieu　An environment designed to promote emotional health that is based on the assumption that the clients are active participants in their own lives and therefore need to be involved in the management of their behavior and environment (Chapter 19).

Therapeutic play　Age-appropriate play activities used purposefully by the nurse for assessment, intervention, and promotion of normal growth and development in children (Chapter 15).

Therapeutic relationship　A personal relationship that is established to help one of the participants deal more effectively and maturely with some difficulty in life. It is a goal-directed, client-centered, and objective relationship (Chapter 19).

Thought blocking　The abrupt interruption in the flow of thoughts or ideas resulting from a disturbance in the speed of associations (Chapter 11).

Tic　A sudden, rapid, recurrent, nonrhythmic, stereotyped movement or vocalization that is considered irresistible but is often suppressible for short periods (Chapter 15).

Titration　An incremental adjustment of medication dose to allow for tolerance to side effects. For example, many medications are administered in low doses, which may be slowly titrated to higher doses, to avoid untoward effects of the drug. Titration is also used to designate incremental release of a client from a locked unit to see whether the client is able to tolerate specified activities on the unlocked unit, or to go to dinner in the dining room off the locked unit, then return (Chapter 20).

Tolerance　The need for greatly increased amounts of a substance used to achieve intoxication or the desired mind-altering effects, or markedly decreased effects with continued use of the same amount of the substance (Chapter 13).

Trait disorders　The diagnoses made on Axis II, which is used exclusively for the description of personality disorders and mental retardation. The symptoms of a personality disorder or mental retardation are not time limited and do not occur only in a time of crisis, but are fixed characteristics (trait versus trait) (Chapter 12).

Transference　The feelings or responses that a client has toward the nurse that are associated with someone significant in the client's life. Although transference may be a natural part of therapy, the nurse needs to be aware of it and manage it to avoid inappropriate behavior of the client toward the nurse (Chapters 7, 19).

Transgenerational violence　When violence within the family is an accepted, everyday occurrence and a natural, normal component of family living, and therefore continues from one generation to the next as if it is normal (Chapter 23).

Transindividual perspective　Looking beyond individuals to the family or community as the unit of care.

Transinstitutionalization　A process in which clients are transferred from one institution to another, such as from a psychiatric hospital to a nursing home.

Transitional objects　Objects that remind one of a significant person. For example, a man keeps a picture of his wife on his desk, which reminds him of her during work hours, or a child keeps pieces of a blanket he/she had as a baby to bring comfort in stressful moments (Chapter 12).

Triggers　In relation to sexual dysfunction, triggers are stimuli that heighten unacceptable sexual cravings (Chapter 17).

Trust　The reliance on the truthfulness or accuracy of the therapeutic relationship developed through the consistency of the nurse's words and actions (Chapter 19).

Trust versus mistrust　Erikson's term for the first developmental crisis that the child tries to resolve. Consistent, predictable, and continuous care results in developing a sense of trust in oneself, others, and the world. Inconsistent, unpredictable, or discontinuous care results in the polar opposite, or mistrust of oneself, others, and the world.

Unconditional positive regard　The stance of the therapist modeling the unconditional acceptance of the client and based on the belief that the client is competent to direct himself or herself in his or her natural tendency to move forward toward integration.

Unconscious suicidal intention　A state outside of awareness during which persons engage in risk-taking behaviors that have a high likelihood of causing their deaths (Chapter 24).

Underselect　The inability of children with psychiatric disorders to select which stimuli are most important; manifested by inappropriate responses to routine events.

Unipolar depression　Disorder characterized by episodes of depression with no mania (Chapter 10).

Vaginal dilators　A graduated series of cylindric dilators introduced into the vagina to decrease involuntary spasm (Chapter 17).

Vaginal plethysmography　A test that uses a vaginal probe to assess blood flow to the female vagina. Blood flow is an indicator of arousal.

Verbal communication   Spoken or written words that compose the symbols of language (Chapter 7).

Vicarious learning   Learning through imagining the experiences of others as if they are one's own.

Victimizer   Another term used to define a sex offender; may be used when discussing familial transmission of the paraphilia (Chapter 17).

Vigilance   The ability to sustain attention over long periods of time.

Violence   A term used to describe behavior that is physically, psychologically, or sexually harmful, injurious, or assaultive (e.g., child abuse, domestic violence, elder abuse, family violence).

Viral load   Viral load or viral burden is a measure of the quantity of HIV in the blood. Viral load tests measure the amount of HIV-1 RNA in a small amount of blood. These tests are used by health care providers to assess the effectiveness of current antiretroviral therapies and to determine when to start therapy and when to change therapies.

Warm-up   A stage of psychodrama and movement/dance therapy that focuses on introducing group members, increasing the comfort level, and determining the theme or issue to be addressed.

White matter   Brain tissue composed of the myelinated axons of neurons (Chapter 3).

Xenophobia   A morbid fear of strangers and those who are not of one's own ethnic group (Chapter 5).

Yohimbine   An alpha-adrenoreceptor blocker that may facilitate blood flow to the genitalia and therefore improve sexual arousal.

Index

Asendin. *see* Amoxapine
Asian Americans, 75, 76t
Asperger's disorder, 354
Aspiration
  in Alzheimer's disease patients, 338
  silent, 338b
Assertiveness, 123-124, 124b
Assertiveness training, for
    schizophrenia, 267
Assessment
  acquired immunodeficiency syndrome,
      595-596
  adjustment disorders, 420-421
  Alzheimer's disease
    attention span, 336
    behavior-based, 337
    cognitive, 335-336
    dementia severity rating scale, 336
    emotional control, 337
    emotional status, 337
    environment for, 334-335
    functional ability, 338
    geriatric depression scale, 336
    judgment, 337
    language, 336
    memory, 336
    Mini-Mental Status Examination, 336
    mood, 336-337
    neurologic deficits, 335-337
    organization, 336
    perception, 336
    reasoning, 337
    state of mind, 336-337
  anxiety, 185
  battered woman, 524-525
  bipolar disorder, 216-217
  child abuse, 531-532
  depression, 216-217
  eating disorders, 382
  elder abuse, 542
  grief, 581-582
  human immunodeficiency virus, 595-
      596
  instrumental activities of daily living,
      159, 159b
  mania, 216-217, 218b
  mood disorders, 216-217, 218b
  multisystem, 93
  nursing process
    case study of, 85
    components of, 94, 95b
    description of, 78, 79, 94
    frameworks for, 95-97, 97t
    functional health pattern framework
        for, 95-96
    human response patterns framework
        for, 96-97
    nurse-client interview, 94, 96f
    purpose of, 94
    racial influences on, 79
    settings for, 94

Assessment *(Continued)*
  paraphilias, 407
  personality disorders, 282-285
  schizophrenia, 260-261, 261b
  sexual abuse, 537-539
  sexual dysfunctions, 397, 397b
  spirituality, 83-85, 84b
  substance abuse, 311-313
  suicidal behaviors, 561-564
  suicide, 561-564
Assimilation, 66, 143
Assisted living
  adult family homes, 610t, 610-611
  adult residential treatment programs,
      609-610, 610t
  congregate care facilities, 610, 610t
Association cortex, 36-37
Attachment theory, 144
Attending, 430
Attention-deficit/hyperactivity disorder,
    355-356, 627
Attention span, 162
Atypical antipsychotics
  anticholinergic effects, 242
  clozapine. *see* Clozapine
  definition of, 264
  description of, 457
  dopamine receptor blocking by, 240
  inappropriate use of, 467
  indications, 457
  mania treated with, 484
  mechanism of action, 240-241, 241f
  olanzapine. *see* Olanzapine
  quetiapine, 459t, 466
  risperidone. *see* Risperidone
  schizophrenia treated with, 240-242,
      241f, 259
  side effects of, 264
  typical antipsychotics vs., 242
  ziprasidone, 242, 459t, 466-467
Atypical depression, 214, 214b
Autistic disorder, 353-354
Autistic thinking, 238b
Autoantibodies, 154
Autodiagnosis, 14
Autonomy
  description of, 61
  shame and doubt vs., 140, 141t
Aventyl. *see* Nortriptyline
Averse conditioning, 321
Avoidant personality disorder
  epidemiology of, 281b
  nursing diagnoses for, 286
Axon, 39, 39f
Ayurveda/Ayurvedic medicine, 501

B

Backward masking, 278
Bandura, Albert, 145, 522-523
Barbiturates, 306, 485t
Basal ganglia, 37

Battered woman
  batterer
    assessment of, 524-525
    characteristics of, 524b, 524-525
  case study of, 527
  cultural considerations, 524
  definition of, 523-524
  epidemiology of, 522b
  feminist theory of, 523
  indicators, 525, 526b
  laws regarding, 528
  nursing interventions for, 528, 529t
  nursing process for
    assessment, 524-527
    DSM-IV-TR diagnoses, 527
    evaluation, 528-529
    implementation, 528
    nursing diagnoses, 527
    outcome identification, 527-528
    planning, 528
  physical examination of, 525
  during pregnancy, 523
  preventive strategies, 528
  statistics regarding, 520, 523
Behavior(s)
  aggressive
    antipsychotics for, 489
    in conduct disorder, 360
    drug treatment for, 489-490
    in personality disorders, 278
    in schizophrenia, 266t, 270
    serotonergic activities and, 278
  anxiety effects, 176t
  of attention-deficit/hyperactivity disor-
      der, 355-356
  of autistic disorder, 353-354
  of conduct disorder, 360-361
  depression effects, 208
  dysthymic disorder effects, 209
  limiting of, 30
  manic episode effects, 210
  of oppositional defiant disorder, 362
  of Tourette's disorder, 359
Behavioral genetics theory of aging, 156
Behavioral model of anxiety, 176
Behavioral theories
  classical conditioning, 144-145
  description of, 144
  operant conditioning, 144-145
  social learning theory
    Bandura's work, 145-146
    description of, 145
    Rotter's work, 145
Behavioral therapy
  anxiety treated with, 192
  eating disorders treated with, 389
  mood disorders treated with, 231
  for substance abuse disorders, 320-321
Behavior modification
  description of, 370
  for schizophrenia, 267